OXFORD MEDICAL PUBLICATIONS

Oxford Desk Reference
Rheumatology

Oxford University Press makes no representation, express or implied, that the drug dosages in this book are correct. Readers must therefore always check the product information and clinical procedures with the most up-to-date published product information and data sheets provided by the manufacturers and the most recent codes of conduct and safety regulations. The authors and the publishers do not accept responsibility or legal liability for any errors in the text or for the misuse or misapplication of material in this work.

▶ Except where otherwise stated, drug doses and recommendations are for the non-pregnant adult who is not breast-feeding.

Oxford Desk Reference
Rheumatology

Richard Watts
Consultant Rheumatologist
Ipswich Hospital NHS Trust
Ipswich and Clinical Senior Lecturer
University of East Anglia
Norwich

Gavin Clunie
Consultant Rheumatologist
Ipswich Hospital NHS Trust
Ipswich

Frances Hall
University Lecturer and Honorary Consultant in Rheumatology
University of Cambridge
Addenbrooke's Hospital
Cambridge

and

Tarnya Marshall
Consultant Rheumatologist
Norfolk and Norwich University Hospital
Norwich

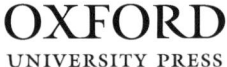

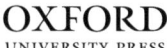

Great Clarendon Street, Oxford OX2 6DP
United Kingdom

Oxford University Press is a department of the University of Oxford.
It furthers the University's objective of excellence in research, scholarship,
and education by publishing worldwide. Oxford is a registered trade mark of
Oxford University Press in the UK and in certain other countries

© Oxford University Press 2009

The moral rights of the authors have been asserted
Database right Oxford University Press (maker)

Reprinted 2013

All rights reserved. No part of this publication may be reproduced,
stored in a retrieval system, or transmitted, in any form or by any means,
without the prior permission in writing of Oxford University Press,
or as expressly permitted by law, or under terms agreed with the appropriate
reprographics rights organization. Enquiries concerning reproduction
outside the scope of the above should be sent to the Rights Department,
Oxford University Press, at the address above

You must not circulate this book in any other form
and you must impose this same condition on any acquirer

British Library Cataloguing in Publication Data
Data available

Library of Congress Cataloging in Publication Data
Data available

ISBN 978-0-19-922999-4

Preface

Rheumatology covers a very broad range of conditions ranging from soft tissue rheumatology, through the inflammatory arthritides to complex multi system disease.

Our aim in writing this volume is to provide easily accessible and practical information in a single desk-sized book. We aim to help the specialist rheumatologist with the diagnosis and management of these problems. We emphasize the clinical presentations of these conditions, approaches to investigation and diagnosis, and up to date management. Treatment protocols, where ever possible, are evidence-based and we provide the evidence base for the use of drug therapy. We hope that the information provided, will help the clinician in managing patients and thus reduce the impact of these diseases.

We are grateful for the long suffering support of our families during the writing of this book.

Brief contents

Detailed contents *ix*
Abbreviations *xiii*
Contributors *xix*

1 **Clinical assessment of rheumatological disease** — 1
2 **Investigation of rheumatic disease** — 23
3 **Organ involvement in rheumatological disease** — 47
4 **Rheumatological procedures: injection therapy** — 105
5 **Regional musculoskeletal anatomy and conditions** — 117
6 **Rheumatoid arthritis** — 197
7 **The spondylarthropathies** — 209
8 **Autoimmune connective tissue diseases** — 239
9 **Vasculitis** — 313
10 **Juvenile idiopathic arthritis** — 351
11 **Pregnancy and the rheumatic diseases** — 365
12 **Osteoarthritis and related disorders** — 371
13 **Crystal arthritis** — 383
14 **Bone diseases** — 395
15 **Hereditary diseases of connective tissue** — 437
16 **Musculoskeletal infection** — 445

17 **Chronic pain** 479

18 **Miscellaneous diseases** 491

19 **DMARDs and immunosuppressive drugs** 531

Index 577

Detailed contents

1 **Clinical assessment of rheumatological disease** 1
   Rheumatology history taking 2
   Rheumatological examination 8
   Patterns of rheumatological disease: oligoarticular pains in adults 14
   Widespread pain (in adults) 18

2 **Investigation of rheumatic disease** 23
   Plain radiography 24
   Ultrasound 26
   Computed tomography 30
   Magnetic resonance imaging 34
   Radionuclide imaging 36
   Autoimmune serology 38
   Synovial fluid analysis 42
   Clinical neurophysiology 44

3 **Organ involvement in rheumatological disease** 47
   The eye 48
   The chest 54
   The heart 66
   The kidney 74
   The gut and hepatobiliary disease 82
   The nervous system 90
   The skin 98

4 **Rheumatological procedures: injection therapy** 105
   Aspiration of joints 106
   Procedure 108

5 **Regional musculoskeletal anatomy and conditions** 117
   The spine 118
   Cervical spine: regional musculoskeletal conditions 124
   Thoracic spine and chest wall: regional musculoskeletal conditions 128
   Lumbar spine: regional musculoskeletal conditions 130
   The shoulder 136
   The shoulder girdle: regional musculoskeletal conditions 140
   The elbow 146
   The elbow: regional musculoskeletal conditions 148
   The hand and wrist 152
   Hand and wrist: regional musculoskeletal conditions 158
   Pelvis, hip, and groin 164
   Pelvis, hip and groin: regional musculoskeletal conditions 168
   The knee 174
   The knee: regional musculoskeletal conditions 178
   Lower leg and foot 184
   Lower leg and foot: regional musculoskeletal conditions 188
   Conditions of the ankle and hindfoot 190
   Conditions of the mid and forefoot 194

6 **Rheumatoid arthritis** 197
   Guidelines for the management of rheumatoid arthritis 208

7 **The spondylarthropathies** 209
   The spondylarthropathies: disease spectrum (including undifferentiated spondylarthropathy) 210
   Ankylosing spondylitis 214
   Psoriatic arthritis 220
   Reactive arthritis 226
   Enteropathic spondylarthropathy 230
   Juvenile spondylarthropathy/enthesitis-related arthritis 232
   SAPHO (Le Syndrome Acné, Pustulose, Hyperostose, Ostéite) 236

8 **Autoimmune connective tissue diseases** 239
   Systemic lupus erythematosus 240
   Sjögren's syndrome 254
   Systemic sclerosis 264
   Antiphospholipid syndrome 274
   Polymyositis 282
   Dermatomyositis 290
   Juvenile dermatomyositis 298
   Inclusion body myositis 302
   Undifferentiated (autoimmune) connective tissue disease 306
   Mixed connective tissue disease 307
   Overlap syndromes 308
   Eosinophilic fasciitis 310

9 Vasculitis 313

Introduction 314
Giant cell arteritis 318
Polymyalgia rheumatica 320
Takayasu arteritis 322
Wegener's granulomatosis 324
Churg–Strauss Syndrome 326
Microscopic polyangiitis 328
Treatment of ANCA-associated vasculitis 330
Polyarteritis nodosa 332
Cryoglobulinaemia 334
Primary central nervous system vasculitis 336
Cogan's syndrome 338
Behçet's disease 340
Henoch–Schönlein purpura 342
Kawasaki disease 344
Relapsing polychondritis 346
Thromboangiitis obliterans 348

10 Juvenile idiopathic arthritis 351

Juvenile idiopathic arthritis: overview 352
Oligoarticular juvenile idiopathic arthritis 358
Rheumatoid factor (RF) negative polyarticular JIA 359
Rheumatoid factor (RF) positive polyarticular JIA 360
Systemic onset JIA 362
Juvenile PsA 364

11 Pregnancy and the rheumatic diseases 365

Pregnancy and the rheumatic diseases 366

12 Osteoarthritis and related disorders 371

Osteoarthritis 372
Osteoarthritis-related disorders 380

13 Crystal arthritis 383

Gout 384
Calcium pyrophosphate dihydrate disease 388
The basic calcium phosphate crystals 392

14 Bone diseases 395

Post-menopausal osteoporosis 396
Therapeutics of post-menopausal osteoporosis 402
Osteoporosis in men 406
Glucocorticoid induced osteoporosis (GIO) 408
Osteoporosis in children 412
Primary hyperparathyroidism 414
Paget's disease of bone (osteodystrophia deformans) 418
Osteomalacia and rickets 422
Renal bone disease 426
Osteogenesis imperfecta 428
Miscellaneous bone diseases 1 432
Miscellaneous bone diseases 2 434

15 Hereditary diseases of connective tissue 437

Marfan syndrome 438
Ehlers–Danlos syndrome 440
Joint hypermobility syndrome 442

16 Musculoskeletal infection 445

Practical approach to a hot swollen joint 446
Septic arthritis 448
Gonococcal arthritis 452
Osteomyelitis 454
Soft tissue infection 458
Rheumatic fever 462
Brucellosis 464
Lyme disease 466
Viral arthritis 468
Mycobacterial infection 472
Fungal infection 476

17 Chronic pain 479

Chronic pain 480
Fibromyalgia syndrome 484
Complex regional pain syndrome type I 488

18 Miscellaneous diseases 491

Acromegaly 492
Diabetes mellitus 494
Adult onset Still's disease 496
Amyloidosis 498
Autoinflammatory syndromes 500
Hyperimmunoglobulinaemia D with periodic fever syndrome 502
TNF-receptor-associated periodic syndrome 503
Cryopyrin-associated periodic syndrome 504
Haemochromatosis 506
Haemoglobinopathies 508
Haemophilia 510
Sarcoidosis 512
Panniculitis 514
Alkaptonuria 516

Gaucher's disease *518*
Eosinophilia-myalgia syndrome and toxic oil syndrome *520*
Metabolic myopathies *522*
Synovial osteochondromatosis *526*
Pigmented villonodular synovitis *527*
Bone tumours *528*

19 **DMARDs and immunosuppressive drugs** *531*
Methotrexate *532*
Sulfasalazine *538*
Leflunomide *540*
Anti-malarials (hydroxychloroquine and chloroquine) *544*
Gold: intramuscular (sodium aurothimalate) and oral (auranofin) *546*
Penicillamine *550*
Azathioprine *552*
Mycophenolate mofetil *556*
Ciclosporin (previously cyclosporin A) *558*
Cyclophosphamide *562*
Biologics: anti-TNF (infliximab, etanercept, adalimumab), anti-CD20 (rituximab), anti-IL-1 (anakinra), CTLA4–Ig (abatacept), and anti-IL-6R (tocilizumab) *568*

Index *577*

Abbreviations

β2GPI	β2 Glycoprotein I	BASDAI	Bath ankylosing spondylitis disease activity index
25OHD	25-hydroxyvitamin D	BASFI	Bath ankylosing spondylitis functional index
99mTc	Technetium-99m	BCP	basic calcium phosphate
AA	amyloid A	bd	twice daily
AAS	ANCA-associated vasculitides	BD	Behçet's disease
AAV	ANCA-associated vasculitis	BHPR	British Health Professionals in Rheumatology
ACA	anti-centromere antibodies	BJH	benign joint hypermobility
ACE	angiotensin converting enzyme	BILAG	British Isles Lupus Assessment Group
ACJ	acromioclavicular joint	BMC	bone mineral content
ACL	anterior cruciate ligament	BMD	bone mineral density
aCL	anticardiolipin	BMI	body mass index
ACLE	acute cutaneous lupus erythematosus	BP	blood pressure
ACR	American College of Rheumatology	BSPAR	British Society for Paediatric and Adolescent Rheumatology
AD	autosomal dominant	BSR	British Sociaty of Rheumatology
ABD	adynamic bone disease	BUA	broadband ultrasound attenuation
ADHR	autosomal dominant hypophosphataemic rickets	BVAS	Birmingham Vasculitis Assessment Score
ADM	amyopathic dermatomyositis	CAD	coronary artery disease
ADO	AD osteopetrosis	CAPS	cryopyrin associated periodic syndrome
AECA	anti-endothelial cell antibodies	CBC	Complete blood count
AF	atrial fibrillation	CCF	Congestive cardiac failure
AICTD	autoimmune connective tissue disease	CCP	cyclic citrullinated peptide
AIDS	Acquired immunodeficiency syndrome	CDC	Centres for Disease Control and Prevention
ALL	acute lymphoblastic leukaemia	CF	cystic fibrosis
ALP	Alkaline phosphatase	CGRP	calcitonin gene-related peptide
ALT	alanine transaminase	CHAQ	Childhood Health Assessment Questionnaire
AMA	anti-mitochondrial antibodies	CHB	congenital heart block
AMPD	adenosine monophosphate deaminase	CHCC	Chapel Hill Consensus Criteria
AN	Anorexia nervosa	CINCA	chronic infantile neurological cutaneous and articular syndrome
ANA	Antinuclear antibody	CK	creatine kinase
ANCA	Anti-neutrophil cytoplasmic antibody	CKD	chronic kidney disease
AOSD	Adult Onset Still's disease	CMAP	compound muscle action potential
AoV	Aortic valve	CMAS	Childhood Myositis Assessment Scale
AP	anteroposterior	CMC	carpometacarpal
APC	Antigen-presenting cell	CMCJ	carpometacarpal' joint
APL	antiphospholipid	CMO	cystoids macular oedema
APLS	Antiphospholipid Syndrome	CMV	cytomegalovirus
APTT	activated partial thromboplastin time	CNS	central nervous system
AR	autosomal recessive	CPN	common peroneal nerve
AS	Ankylosing spondylitis	CPPDD	calcium pyrophosphate dihydrate deposition (disease/arthritis)
ASAS	Assessment of Ankylosing spondylitis (group)	CRP	C-reactive protein
ASIF	Ankylosing Spondylitis International Federation	CRPS	Chronic Regional Pain Syndrome
ASIS	Anterior superior iliac spine	CS	Cogan's syndrome
ASOT	anti-streptolysin O titre	CSS	Churg–Strauss Syndrome
AST	aspartate transaminase	CSVV	cutaneous small vessel vasculitis
AVN	Avascular necrosis		
AZA	azathioprine		
BAFF	B cell activating factor belonging to the TNF family		

ABBREVIATIONS

CT	computerized tomography	EIP	extensor indicis proprius
CTD	connective tissue disease	EMG	electromyography
CTPA	CT pulmonary angiogram	EMS	eosinophilia-myalgia syndrome
CTS	carpal tunnel syndrome	EN	erythema nodosum
CTX	C telopeptide [Collagen] crosslinked	ENA	extractable nuclear antigens
CV	conduction velocity	ENT	ear nose throat
CVA	Cerebrovascular accident	EPB	extensor pollicis brevis
CVD	cardiovascular disease	ER	endoplasmic reticulum
CXR	chest X-Ray	ERA	enthesitis related arthritis
CYC	cyclophosphamide	eRA	endothelin receptor antagonists
DAD	diffuse alveolar damage	ERCP	endoscopic retrograde cholepancreatography
DALY	Disability Adjusted Life Years	ESpA	enteropathic spondylarthropathy
DAS	Disease Activity Score	ESR	erythrocyte sedimentation rate
DBPCS	double-blind, placebo-controlled studies	ESRD	end-stage renal disease
DBPRCT	double-blind, placebo-controlled randomised trial	ESRF	end-stage renal failure
dcSSc	diffuse cutaneous systemic sclerosis	ESSG	European Spondylarthropathy Study Group
DES	diethylstilboestrol	EU	endoscopic ultrasound
DEXA	dual energy X-Ray absorptiometry	EULAR	European League Against Rheumatism
DIC	diffuse intravascular coagulation	EUVAS	European vasculitis Study Group
DILS	diffuse infiltrative lymphocytosis syndrome	FAI	femoroacetabular impingement
DIPJ	distal interphalangeal joint	FBC	full blood count
DISH	diffuse idiopathic skeletal Hyperostosis	FCAS	familial cold inflammatory condition
DLE	discoid lupus erythematous	FCR	flexor carpi radialis
DM	dermatomyositis	FCU	flexor carpi ulnaris
DMARD	disease-modifying ant-rheumatic drug	FD	fibrous dysplasia
DML	distal motor latency	FDS	flexor digitorum superficialis
DMOADS	disease modifying OA drugs	FGF	fibroblast growth factor
DMSA	Dimercapto succinic acid	FHL	flexor hallucis longus
DNA	deoxyribonucleic acid	FIO	fibrogenesis imperfecta ossium
DNIC	diffuse Noxious Inhibitory Control	FM	fibromyalgia
D-PCA	D-penicillamine	FMF	familial Mediterranean fever
DRL	drug-related lupus	FMS	fibromyalgia syndrome
DRUJ	distal radio-ulnar joint	FOP	fibrodysplasia ossificans progressiva
DRVVT	Dilute Russell Viper Venom Test	FVC	forced vital capacity
DTPA	Diethylene triamine penta acetic acid	GAVE	gastric antral vascular ectasia
DVT	deep vein thrombosis	GBM	Glomerular Basement Membrane
DXA	dual X-ray absorptiometry	GC	glucocorticoid
DXR	digital X-ray radiogrammetry	GCA	giant cell arteritis
EBT	ethylidene bis[tryptophan]	GFR	glomerular filtration rate
EBV	Epstein–Barr virus	GH	growth hormone
ECG	electrocardiogram	GHJ	glenohumeral joint
ECHO	echocardiogram	GI	gastrointestinal
ECLAM	European Consensus Lupus Activity Measurement	GIO	glucocorticoid-induced osteoporosis
ECRB	extensor carpi radialis brevis	GN	glomerulonephritis
ECRL	extensor carpi radialis longus	GORD	gastro-oesophageal reflux disease
ECU	extensor carpi ulnaris	GTN	glyceryl trinitrate
EDC	extensor digitorum communis	HADS	Health, Anxiety, Depression Score
EDM	extensor digiti minimi	HAQ	Health Assessment Questionnaire (HAQ)
EDS	Ehlers–Danlos syndrome	HBV	hepatitis B virus
EEG	electroencephalography	HCQ	hydroxychloroquine
EH	endosteal hyperostosis	HCV	hepatitis C virus

HDL	high density lipoprotein	JPsA	juvenile psoriatic arthritis
HELLP	haemolysis, elevated liver enzymes, low platelets	JSpA	juvenile spondylarthropathy
		JVP	jugular venous pressure
Hgo	homogenistic acid oxidase	KCO	Carbon monoxide transfer co-efficient
HIDS	hyperimmunoglobulin D with periodic fever syndrome	KD	Kawasaki disease
		KIR	killer cell immunoglobulin-like receptor
HIV	human immunodeficiency virus	KP	keratic precipitates
HLA	human lymphocyte antigen	LA	lupus anticoagulant
HME	hereditary multiple hyperostosis	LAiP	lupus activity index in pregnancy
HMW	high molecular weight	LCL	lateral collateral ligament
HOA	hypertrophic osteoarthropathy	LCPD	Legg–Calvé–Perthes Disease
HPOA	Hypertrophic pulmonary osteoarthropathy	lcSSc	limited cutaneous systemic sclerosis
HR	high resolution	LDH	lactate dehydrogenase
HRCT	high resolution CT	LDL	low density lipoprotein
HRQOL	health-related quality of life	LE	lupus erythematosus
HRT	hormone replacement therapy	LEF	leflunomide
HSP	Henoch–Schönlein purpura	LETM	longitudinally extensive transverse myelitis
HSV	Herpes Simplex Virus	LFT	liver function test
HTLV	human T cell lymphotropic virus	LIP	lymphocytic interstitial pneumonia
HUS	haemolytic uraemic syndrome	LMWH	low molecular weight heparin
IBD	inflammatory bowel disease	LOS	lower oesophageal
IBM	inclusion body myositis	LP	lumbar puncture
IBP	inflammatory back pain	LRP	lipoprotein receptor-related protein
ICAM	intercellular adhesion molecule	LSp	lumbar spine
ICD	International Classification of Disease	LV	left ventricle
lcSSc	localised cutaneous Systemic Sclerosis	LVEF	left ventricular ejection fraction
ICU	intensive care unit	LVH	left ventricular hypertrophy
IE	infective endocarditis	MAA	myositis-associated autoantibodies
IF	immunofluorescence	MAGIC	mucosal and genital ulceration with inflamed cartilage
IFN	interferon		
IGF	insulin related growth factor	MAHA	microangiopathic haemolytic anaemia
IHD	ischaemic heart disease	MAS	macrophage activation syndrome
IIF	immunofluorescence	MASES	Maastricht Ankylosing Spondylitis Enthesitis Score
IIH	idiopathic intracranial hypertension		
IJO	idiopathic juvenile osteoporosis	MC&S	microscopy, culture and (antibiotic) sensitivities
IL	interleukin		
ILAR	International League of Associations for Rheumatology	MCL	medial collateral ligament
		MCP	macrophage chemotactic protein
ILD	interstitial lung disease	MCPJ	metacarpophalangeal joint
IMACS	International Myositis Assessment and Clinical Studies	MCV	motor conduction velocity
		MD	multidetector
INR	International normalized ratio	MDCT	multidetector CT
IP	interphalangeal	MDAAT	Myositis Disease Activity Assessment Tool
ITB	iliotibial band	MDP	methyl diphosphonate
IUGR	Intrauterine growth retardation	MDRD	modification of diet in renal disease
IV	intravenous	MDT	multi-disciplinary team
IVIG	intravenous Immunoglobulin G	ME	myalgic encephalopathy
JAS	juvenile ankylosing spondylitis	MEPE	matrix extracellular phosphoglycoprotein
JDM	juvenile dermatomyositis	MHC	major histocompatibility complex
JHS	joint hypermobility syndrome	MI	myocardial infarction
JIA	juvenile idiopathic arthritis	MIF	macrophage inhibitory factor
JIIM	juvenile idiopathic inflammatory myopathies	MMF	mycophenylate mofetil
		MMP	matrix metalloproteinase

MMSE	mini mental state examination	PCP	pneumocystis pneumonia
MMT	manual muscle testing	PCR	polymerase chain reaction
MPA	microscopic Polyangiitis	PCS	placebo-controlled studies
MPO	myeloperoxidase	PD	peritoneal dialysis
MR	magnetic resonance	PDB	Paget's disease of bone
MRC	Medical Research Council	PDD	progressive diaphyseal dysplasia
MRA	MR angiography	PDGF	platelet-derived growth factor
MRI	magnetic resonance imaging	PE	Pulmonary embolism
MRS	magnetic resonance spectroscopy	PEFR	peak expiratory flow rate
MRSA	methacillin-resistant Staphylococcus aureus	PET	positron emission tomography
		PF	plantar fasciitis
MRV	MR venography	PFK	phosphofructokinase
MSA	myositis specific autoantibodies	PFTs	pulmonary function tests
MSG	minor salivary gland	PHPT	primary hyperparathyroidism
MSU	mid-stream urine	PIN	posterior interosseus nerve
MTB	*Mycobacterium tuberculosis*	PIPJ	proximal interphalangeal joint
MTPJ	metatarsophalangeal joint	PITF	posteroinferior tibiofibular
MTX	methotrexate	PLM	polarized light microscopy
MWS	Muckle Well syndrome	PM	Polymyositis
NCS	nerve conduction studies	PML	progressive multifocal leukoencephalopathy
NFκB	nuclear factor κB		
NHL	non- Hodgkins lymphoma	PMN	polymorphonuclear
NICE	National Institute for Clinical Excellence	PMO	postmenopausal osteoporosis
NK	natural killer (cells)	PMR	polymyalgia rheumatica
NMDA	N-methyl-D-aspartate receptor	POPP	psoriatic onycho pachydermo periostitis
NNO	number needed to offend	PP	pulsus paradoxus
NNT	number needed to treat	PPI	Proton pump inhibitor
NOMID	neonatal onset multi-system inflammatory disease	PR3	proteinase 3
		PCR	placebo-controlled randomised trial
NSAID	non-steroidal anti-inflammatory drug	Ps	psoriasis
NSIP	non-specific interstitial pneumonia	PSA	prostate-specific antigen
NTX	N-teldopeptide [Collagen] Crosslinks	PsA	psoriatic arthritis
OA	osteoarthritis	PSIS	posterior superior iliac spine
OCT	ocular coherence tomography	PSRA	post-streptococcal reactive arthritis
od	once daily	pSS	primary Sjögren's syndrome
OF	osteitis fibrosa	PT	Prothrombin time
OI	osteogenesis imperfecta	PTH	parathyroid hormone
OLT	osteochondral lesion of the talus	PVNS	pigmented villonuclear synovitis
OMIM	Online Mendelian Inheritance in Man	QCT	quantitative computerised tomography
ONJ	osteonecrosis of the jaw	qds	four times daily
OP	organizing pneumonia	QOF	quality and outcome framework
OPLL	ossification of the posterior longitudinal ligament	QUS	quantitative (Heel) ultrasound
		RA	rheumatoid arthritis
OR	Odds ratio	RANK	receptor activator of nuclear factor kB
OSS	Osgood–Schlatter's syndrome	RCA	regulators of complement activation
OT	occupational therapy	RCP	Royal College of Physicians
PACNS	primary angiitis of the CNS	RCT	randomized controlled trial
PADI	posterior atlantodental interval	RDBPCT	Randomized double-blind, placebo-controlled trial
PAH	pulmonary arterial hypertension		
PAN	polyarteritis nodosa	ReA	reactive arthritis
PBC	primary biliary cirrhosis	REMS	
PCL	posterior cruciate ligament	RF	rheumatoid factor
PCNSV	Primary central nervous systemic vasculitis	RNP	ribonucleoprotein

ROD	renal osteodystrophy	TFCC	triangular fibrocartilage
RP	Raynaud's phenomenon/relapsing polychondritis	TFL	tensor of fascia lata
		TGF-β	transforming growth factor beta
RSD	reflex sympathetic dystrophy	TIMP	tissue inhibitors of MMPs
RTA	renal tubular acidosis	TIN	tubulointerstitial nephritis
RVSP	Right ventricular systolic pressure	TLC	total lung capacity
SAA	serum amyloid A	TLCO	transfer capacity
SACLE	subacute cutaneous lupus	TMJ	temporomandibular joint
SaP	serum amyloid P	TNF	tumour necrosis factor
SAP	sensory action potentials	TOE	transoesophagal echocardiogram
SAPHO	(LC) Syndrome Acné, Pustulose, Hyperostose, Ostéite	TPHA	T. palladium haemagglutination assay
		TPMT	thiopurine methyl transferase
SBE	Subacute bacterial endocarditis	TR	tricuspid regurgitation
SC	subcutaneous	TRAPS	tumour necrosis factor receptor-associated periodic syndrome
SCFE	slipped capital femoral epiphysis		
SCJ	sternoclavicular joint	TSH	thyroid stimulating hormone
SCLE	sub-acute cutaneous lupus erythematosus	TSp	thoracic spine
		TTE	transthoracic echocardiogram
SD	standard deviation	TTP	thrombotic thrombocytopenic purpura
SEA	seronegative enthesopathy arthritis	TTR	transthyretin
SERM	selective estrogen receptor modulators	U&Es	urea and electrolytes
SHPT	secondary hyperparathyroidism	UAICTD	undifferentiated autoimmune connective tissue disease
SIJ	sacroiliac joint		
SLAC	scapho-lunate advanced collapse	UCTD	undifferentiated connective tissue disease
SLAM	SLE Lupus Activity Measure	UIP	usual interstitial pneumonia
SLE	systemic lupus erythematosus	US	ultrasound
SLEDAI	SLE Disease Activity Index	USpA	undifferentiated Spondylarthropathy
SLICC	Systemic Lupus International Collaborating Clinics	USS	Ultra sound scan
SNAC	scaphoid non-union and advanced collapse	UTI	urinary tract infection
		VAS	visual analogue scale
SOS	speed of sound	VATS	video-assisted thoracoscopic surgical
SpA	spondylarthropathy	VDI	Vasculitis Damage Index
SPARCC	Spondyloarthritis Research Consortium (Canada)	VDR	vitamin D Receptor
		VEGF	vascular endothelial growth factor
SPECT	single photon emission computerised tomography	VF	vertical fracture
		VFA	vertebral fracture analysis
SR	strontium ranelate	VGKC	voltage-gated potassium channel
SRP	signal recognition peptide	VLCAD	very long-chain acyl-CoA dehydrogenases
SS	Sjögren's syndrome		
SSA	Sjögren's syndrome A	VT	ventricular tachycardia
SSc	systemic sclerosis	vZV	*Varicella zoster* virus
SSRI	selective serotonin receptor antagonists	vWF	von Willebrand factor
SST	supraspinatus tendon	WBC	white blood cell
sSS	secondary Sjögren's syndrome	WG	Wegener's Granulomatosis
SVC	Superior vena cava	WHI	Womens' Health Initiative
SZP	sulphasalazine	WHO	World Health Organisation
TA	Temporal Artery	XLH	X-linked hypophosphataemia
TAO	thromboangiitis obliterans	YP	yak pox
TCE	trichloroethylene	ZCD	Zebra Fish Disease
tds	three times daily		
TENS	transcutaneous electrical nerve stimulation		

Contributors

Dr Ademola Adejuwon
Registrar in Trauma and Orthopaedic Surgery
University College Hospital
London

Dr Kate Armon
Consultant Paediatrician
Norfolk and Norwich University Hospital
NHS Foundation Trust
Norwich

Dr Fraser Birrell
Senior Lecturer in Rheumatology
University of Newcastle upon Tyne
Newcastle

Dr Julian Blake
Consultant Neurophysiologist
Norfolk and Norwich University
Foundation NHS Trust

Dr Marian L Burr
Academic Clinical Fellow in Rheumatology
ARC Epidemiology Unit
University of Manchester
Manchester

Mr Ben Burton
Consultant Opthalmologist
James Paget University Hospital NHS
Foundation Trust
Norfolk

Dr Gavin Clunie
Consultant Rheumatologist
Ipswich Hospital NHS Trust
Ipswich

Dr Carlos Cobiella
Consultant Orthopaedic Surgeon
The Shoulder Unit
Hospital of St John & St Elizabeth
London

Dr Dave Dutka
University Lecturer and Honorary
Consultant Cardiologist
Addenbrooke's Hospital
Cambridge

Dr Amel Ginawi
Specialist Registrar in Rheumatology
Addenbrooke's Hospital
Cambridge

Dr Mark Goodfield
Consultant Dermatologist
Department of Dermatology
Leeds General Infirmary
Leeds

Dr Richard Goodwin
Consultant Radiologist
Norfolk and Norwich University NHS
Foundation Trust
Norwich

Mr Fares S Haddad
Consultant Orthopaedic Surgeon
University College Hospital
London

Dr Frances Hall
University Lecturer and Honorary
Consultant in Rheumatology
University of Cambridge School of
Clinical Medicine
Cambridge

Mr James Hopkinson-Woolley
Consultant Orthopaedic Surgeon
University of Cambridge
Addenbrooke's Hospital
Cambridge

Mr Maxim Horwitz
Specialist Registrar in
Trauma and Orthopaedics
Royal National Orthopaedic Hospital
Stanmore

Dr Sujith Konan
Clinical and Research Fellow
University College Hospital
London

Dr Mark Lillicrap
Consultant Rheumatologist
Addenbrooke's Hospital
Cambridge

Mr Lennel Lutchman
Consultant Orthopaedic Surgeon
Norfolk and Norwich University Hospital
Norwich

Dr Tarnya Marshall
Consultant Rheumatologist
Norfolk and Norwich University Hospital
Norwich

Dr Maninder Mundae
Research Fellow in Rheumatology
Addenbrooke's Hospital
Cambridge

Dr Andrew J K Östör
Consultant Rheumatologist
School of Clinical Medicine
University of Cambridge
Cambridge

Dr Helen Parfrey
University Lecturer and Honorary
Consultant in Medicine
University of Cambridge School of
Clinical Medicine
Cambridge

Dr Shin-Jae Rhee
Orthopaedic Registrar
University College Hospital
London

Dr Nick Shenker
Consultant Rheumatologist
Addenbrooke's Hospital
Cambridge

Mr Elliot Sorene
Consultant Orthopaedic Surgeon
University College London Hospitals
London

Dr Michael Walsh
Clinical Fellow in Lupus and Vasculitis
Addenbrooke's Hospital
Cambridge

Dr Richard Watts
Consultant Rheumatologist
Ipswich Hospital NHS Trust
Ipswich
and Clinical Senior Lecturer
University of East Anglia

Dr Jeremy Woodward
Consultant Gastroenterologist
Addenbrooke's Hospital
Cambridge

Dr Michael Zandi
Neurology Research Fellow
Addenbrooke's Hospital
Cambridge

Chapter 1

Clinical assessment of rheumatological disease

Rheumatology history taking *2*
Rheumatological examination *8*
Patterns of rheumatological disease: oligoarticular pains in adults *14*
Widespread pain (in adults) *18*

Rheumatology history taking

There is a wide spectrum of musculoskeletal and other disease that can present with musculoskeletal symptoms. Given the nature of those symptoms and the context in which they are presented, however, there are some principles of history taking worth highlighting here. The following issues are discussed.
- The complaint of pain.
- The complaint of stiffness.
- Multiple musculoskeletal symptoms.
- Rheumatology Questionnaire tools.
- Additional (non-musculoskeletal) symptoms.
- Reporting styles.
- History from others: assent and necessity.

Pain

Pain is the most common musculoskeletal symptom. It is defined by its subjective description, which may vary depending on its physical or biological cause, the patient's understanding of it, its impact on function, and the emotional and behavioural response it invokes. Pain is also often 'coloured' by cultural, linguistic, and religious differences and beliefs. Therefore, pain is not merely an unpleasant sensation; it is also an 'emotional change'. The experience is different for every individual. In children and adolescents the evaluation of pain is sometimes complicated further by the interacting influences of the experience of pain within the family, school, and peer group.
- Adults usually accurately localize pain, although there are some situations worth noting in rheumatic disease, where pain can be poorly localized.
- Pain may be localized, but caused directly or indirectly (referred) by a distant lesion, e.g.:
  - interscapular pain caused by postural/mechanical problems in the cervical spine;
  - pain from shoulder lesions referred to the area around deltoid insertion in the humerus;
  - lumbosacral pain referred to the area around the greater trochanters;
  - hip joint pain referred (often without pain in the groin) down the thigh, even to the knee.
- Pain caused by neurological abnormalities, ischaemic pain, and pain referred from viscera are less easy for the patient to visualize or express, and the history may be given with varied interpretations.
- Bone pain is generally constant, despite movement or change in posture. In comparison, muscular, synovial, ligament, or tendon pain tends to alter with movement. Fracture, tumour, and metabolic bone disease are all possible causes. Such constant, local, sleep-disturbing pain should always be considered potentially sinister and investigated.
- It is worth noting that certain descriptors of pain (at least in English-speaking patients) have consistently been associated with the influence of non-organic modifiers of pain, the pain experience, and it's reporting. These descriptors can be found in a number of pain evaluation questionnaire tools (Table 1.1.).

Pain in children

The assessment of pain in young children is often difficult. The presence of pain may have to be surmised from behaviour, since young children may not be able to verbalize their pain.
- Children may be fractious and irritable, or quiet and withdrawn; they may be off their food and have disturbed nights. If they can verbalize they often localize pain poorly.
- On examination, a child may not admit to pain, but will withdraw the limb or appear anxious when the painful area is examined. Observing both the child's and parent's facial expression during an examination is very important.
- Although a description of the quality of pain is beyond young children, often an indication of its severity can be obtained through asking them to indicate on a diagram how they feel about it (e.g. the Faces Rating Scale). Older children are often able to score pain from 0 to 10.

Table 1.1 Descriptors of pain that may be relevant in revealing the influence of non-organic/amplifying 'interpretative' factors on the reporting of pain

Organic	Non-organic or pain amplification
Pounding	Flickering
Jumping	Shooting
Pricking	Lancinating
Sharp	Lacerating
Pinching	Crushing
Hot	Searing
Tender	Splitting
Nagging	Torturing
Spreading	Piercing
Annoying	Unbearable
Tiring	Exhausting
Fearful	Terrifying
Tight	Tearing

Stiffness

Stiffness can be an indication of oedema and/or inflammation.
- Stiffness, however, is not specific for inflammatory musculoskeletal lesions. Musculoskeletal stiffness is assumed to be due to accumulation of fluid in structures thus oedema resulting from traumatic or degenerative lesions may produce stiffness in theory.
- Inflammatory-induced stiffness in any musculoskeletal structure often improves with movement.
- Neurological stiffness (increased tone) can mimic stiffness from musculoskeletal lesions. It typically occurs in insidiously developing myelopathy, early Parkinson's Disease and some other extra-pyramidal disorders, for example.
- Some patients with inflammatory diseases complain about stiffness without pain [e.g. in some patients with ankylosing spondylitis, in early or mild rheumatoid arthritis (RA)].

Multiple musculoskeletal symptoms

Multiple symptoms can occur simultaneously or seemingly linked over time (patterns). Either may be due to a single systemic condition or multiple separate musculoskeletal lesions. The assessment of symptoms can be complicated by how long patients have had symptoms (recall bias). The likelihood that each scenario exists depends on a number of variables including:

- The background prevalence of any condition in the reference population.
- The configuration of the healthcare system particularly the ease or difficulty with which patients can access specialist care.
- Individual factors, which may influence presentation to doctors (e.g. ethnic or socio-economic factors).

Patterns of musculoskeletal symptoms

Patterns of musculoskeletal symptoms are recognized in association with certain rheumatic conditions. Patterns are not usually specific, but help in forming a working diagnosis. Patterns can be interpreted from either the simultaneous presentation of symptoms given their distribution or from a presumed link between symptoms over time (common originsee Case 1.1). The latter, of course, is the most difficult situation to unravel. Some examples of patterns include:

- Simultaneous symmetrical small joint inflammation in the hands and wrists [e.g. RA or calcium pyrophosphate dihydrate disease (CPPDD) polyarthritis or pseudo-RA psoriatic arthritis].
- Simultaneous asymmetric, lower limb pains associated with inflammatory low back pain 4 weeks after *Salmonella* infection (e.g. reactive arthritis).
- A history of acute, but also previously recurrent monoarticular, peripheral joint, symptoms over many years (e.g. gout or the pseudogout form of CPPDD arthritis/disease).
- Recurrent 'tennis elbow' and episodic inflammatory back pain symptoms – both for many years, recalcitrant bilateral plantar fasciitis 5 years previously in a patient known to get recurrent bouts of psoriasis presenting now with a single swollen knee (psoriatic arthritis).

Separate co-prevalent conditions

Musculoskeletal conditions are common, particularly in the elderly. It is common for the elderly to present to specialists infrequently and/or late, and have a considerable amount of symptoms. In the elderly, both over- and under-diagnosis of unifying conditions are quite easy mistakes to make given the problems in assessment (see Case 1.2). Common 'degenerative' and other lesions giving (either chronic variable or persistent) symptoms are:

- Osteoarthritis.
- Crystal-induced inflammation or accelerated degeneration of joints and other structures.
- Rotator cuff degeneration/arthropathy.
- Radicular symptoms (usually nerve root exit foramen stenosis in spinal canal lateral recess).
- Frank lumbar spinal stenosis.
- Mild myopathy (e.g. chronic hypovitaminosis-D).
- Various contributors to back pain [osteoarthritis (OA) facet joints, degenerative disc disease, osteoporotic fracture].

Case 1.1. *A 40-year-old woman presents with 6 months achy pain and stiffness of fingers, both hindfeet and lower legs. No back pain is present. She has had fatigue for 5 years (diagnosed with ME), mild myositis was diagnosed 2 years previously on clinical grounds and she has had some rashes over the past 10 years, dry, gritty eyes, and xerostomia.*

Are the symptoms from past history linked or separate? The differential diagnosis needs to be wide and history taking extensive. Primary care physicians may not have referred her to specialists for some of her previous problems. Previous clinical diagnoses may not have been made cognisant of the possibility that autoimmune disease can cause periodic symptoms in different body systems. Consideration of her having either an autoimmune connective tissue disease (e.g. lupus or primary Sjögren's disease), Lyme disease, or chronic sarcoid must be given. Distinction of current symptoms from chronic pain, evidence for pathology at sites of symptoms, and blood tests will be important in determining diagnosis [e.g. compared with fibromyalgia (FM)].

Case 1.2. *An 80-year-old lady known to have type 2 diabetes (20-year history) complicated by CKD3 (renal impairment) and hypothyroidism presents with bilateral shoulder and wrist pain, pain in 2nd and 3rd fingers, swollen knees, and collapsed (valgus) painful swollen hindfeet. She is used to being ill, does not present to doctors early, and many symptoms are long-standing. The time of onset of each symptom cannot be determined accurately.*

Late-onset RA, gout, or CPPDD arthritis might be single causes of all her symptoms; however, it would be wise to initially consider some combination of separate, but common conditions, which could be contributing to her predicament. Conditions might include: osteoarthritis (e.g. knee), carpal tunnel syndrome, Charcot arthritis or diabetic osteolysis (e.g. subtalar joints), adhesive capsulitis (diabetes-associated), and subacromial impingement (e.g. 2nd to a rotator cuff lesion). The situation may be complicated by any diabetic cheirarthropathy in her hands, peripheral neuropathy or cardiac failure (swollen ankles), and her ability to tolerate symptoms (influencing the reporting of symptoms) perhaps influenced by fatigue from diabetes and (undertreated) hypothyroidism!

Evaluating a history of illness in children and young people

A musculoskeletal disorder will affect a growing, developing child differently to an adult. Children with inflammatory disorders, as in adults, will be affected systemically by their illness. Non-musculoskeletal symptoms associated with musculoskeletal disease can occur in children. In addition, specific aspects of a child's life should be addressed.

- **Development**. Is the young child meeting normal developmental milestones? Is walking delayed or has it regressed in any way? Are they keeping up with their peers in toddler groups or nursery?
- **Appetite and growth**. Is the child eating normally and gaining weight? Do they have a record of weight and height with them (red book in the UK)? Does it show good growth or a falling through the centiles? Older children are not often weighed, but you can ask if the clothes

have become loose. Also, is there any change in bowel or bladder function?
- **Energy levels.** Young children who are normally described as '... into everything ...', or '... you can't take your eyes off her for a minute ...' may become '... well behaved ...', and '... now plays quietly in one place...' Establish, therefore, if the child is abnormally fatigued?
- **Is there weakness?** The things the child used to do independently like brushing hair, cutting up their own food, may be lost.
- **Hobbies.** What do they enjoy doing? Have they had to stop doing any activities? Is there anything they want to do, but can't?
- **School.** How much school has been missed? Are they keeping up with their peers at school, both in terms of physical activity and academically? Is there any deterioration in handwriting?
- **Vision.** Has there been any deterioration in vision? Those <10–11 years old often do not notice if the sight in one eye has deteriorated.

Rheumatology Questionnaire tools

Most rheumatologists use some questionnaire tools to assess different aspects of disease in certain (validated) situations. Tools can be used in clinical practice or, in certain examples, to grade outcome in research.

Some questionnaire tools used in assessing rheumatological disease
- Health Activity Questionnaire.
- Short form 36 (SF36).
- Bath Index Questionnaires (AS).
- Quality of Life Questionnaires (RAQoL, ASQoL etc.).
- Hospital Anxiety and Depression Scale (HADS).
- Child Health Assessment Questionnaire (CHAQ).

For more detail on disease-specific assessment tools, see relevant chapter on that disease.

Measuring disability: questionnaire tools
Many questionnaire tools exist that are used to score disability in specific diseases. Usually, a tool has been developed to measure disability in a specific population for a specific reason. Some tools have been well validated for that purpose. It is also true that disability tools get adopted to use in other scenarios in the same disease (e.g. early as opposed to late arthritis or in different countries or cultures), but also adopted/applied in other diseases. The degree to which a tool is validated in situations other than which it was devised for (and by implication applicable to), is variable (examples listed below).

Health Assessment Questionnaire (HAQ)
Self-assessment questionnaire originally developed and validated in hospital populations of RA patients to measure functional disability.
- Easy and quick to complete for patients, the scoring is weighted and a little complicated to summarize for assessors.
- Has been extensively validated in different scenarios in RA populations over the last 25 years.
- Although responsive to change (usually deterioration) in RA when used extensively some years ago, the tool's ability to respond to less overt changes in functional ability, either in disease deterioration or improvement with treatment has been questioned.
- Other tools for RA. Some generic measures do include assessment of features of disability in RA and have been applied as such (Stanford Health Assessment Questionnaire, Nottingham Health Profile, Short Form-36).

WOMAC
The Western Ontario and McMaster Universities Osteoarthritis Index (WOMAC) has been used to assess disability in OA since 1982.
- WOMAC utilizes a 24-question proforma including domains on pain, disability, and stiffness in regard of knee and hip OA.
- For its purpose WOMAC has been extensively validated in clinical practice and research settings, is quickly completed, is reliable and responsive to change. It has been translated into >60 language forms.
- The most recent version of WOMAC (WOMAC™ 3.1 Index) is a joint-targeted version of the index.

Bath Ankylosing Spondylitis Functional Index (BASFI)
Devised over 15 years ago, this self-assessed questionnaire has been validated in measuring Ankylosing spondylitis (AS) disability in different populations and in early and late disease. Its strength is its simplicity.
- BASFI is done by the patient. There are 10 questions and responses are on a visual analogue scale.
- Eight questions cover AS-relevant functional issues and 2 questions refer to overall effects of disability.
- BASFI has not been extensively validated over the long-term in the context of immunotherapy for AS. There is some concern that, with the short-term variation of effects from anti-TNFα therapies, BASFI may be over-responsive on a single assessment.
- Alternative functional indices for AS include The Dougados Functional Index; HAQ-S (HAQ adapted for spondylarthropathies).

The Child Health Assessment Questionnaire (CHAQ)
The CHAQ is a disease-specific measure of functional status that comprises two indices, disability, and discomfort. Both indices focus on physical function. Disability is assessed in eight areas with a total of 30 items with difficulty rated 0–3. Pain is measured on a 100 mm visual analogue scale.
- The reliability and validity of the tool are excellent.
- It takes an average 10 min to complete, and can be completed either by a parent or the older child, since the two raters correlate well.
- The CHAQ is now commonly used in juvenile idiopathic arthritis (JIA) randomized control trials (RCTs) and is helpful in clinic to monitor response to treatments.

Additional (non-musculoskeletal) symptoms

When are non-musculoskeletal symptoms relevant to making (or not making) a diagnosis of a musculoskeletal condition (see Table 1.2)? The diagnostician will need to:
- Have a broad knowledge base of general medical and musculoskeletal conditions.
- Have an in-depth understanding of systemic conditions with musculoskeletal features (see p 47–104).
- Be aware of the potential of some chronic conditions to have relapsing features.

- Be suspicious of previous diagnoses if based on incomplete or erroneous evidence. This works both ways in that previous symptoms can be ascribed to the chronic rheumatological condition or may have been inappropriately ascribed to another diagnosis.

Reporting styles

No two patients ever seem to give the same account, even for the same conditions! Experienced rheumatologists will recognize a number of characteristic patterns of history accounts for some conditions, however. How a history is given can be influenced by a number of factors.
- Whether the patient is verbose or reticent.
- Anticipated gain from the consultation.
- Interpretative styles.

These aspects are discussed below. We do not aim to provide solutions. A detailed discussion is beyond the scope of this text. We aim to provide a framework for further thought and discussion about the issues.

Verbosity or reticence

The skill in history taking with verbose patients is in steering the conversation back to the relevant points. It is important to accept, however, that the verbose historian often requires time initially to explain things in their own way. They may otherwise feel cheated and uncomfortable with a (perceived) shortened consultation. Thus, 'free rein before reining in' should be your maxim.

Reticence on the part of the patient may have a reason or be an intrinsic characteristic. Such consultations often require more closed questioning. Reticence is often associated with stoicism. It's not always right to believe or conclude little is wrong if little is complained about.

Secondary gain

Patients may knowingly or unknowingly look for 'gain' from a consultation, in addition to the process of getting a diagnosis or advice about treatment. Gain, anticipated or not, can imply different things for different people and can affect the way in which a history is provided.
- The simplest form of gain is reassurance. Some aspects of the history can be overlooked if not perceived by the patient as currency in obtaining reassurance.
- Symptom emphasis. The patient's (usually conscious, but not always) objective is that specific symptom recognition and acknowledgement of its' severity by the doctor is important to condone a predicament (such as absence from work, social support application, etc.). Thus, parts of the history are emphasized. Often florid adjectives are used.

Interpretative styles

Many patients have thought about why they have symptoms and will readily tell you their beliefs. This can be helpful or distracting, and sometimes amusing.
- Most people will have little concept of autoimmune or inflammatory disease – illness with no basis in trauma. Patients often try to be 'helpful' by linking the onset of their symptoms to events – often physical trauma or activities – which they regard as important. This can be distracting.
- A previous diagnosis can lead to any new symptoms being interpreted by a patient as secondary to that diagnosis. For example prolonged fatigue put down to 'ME' (± fibromyalgia), but potentially due to primary Sjögren's syndrome or chronic sarcoid, for example. Where there has been 'investment' in a previous diagnosis, even if it is

Table 1.2 Non-musculoskeletal symptoms associated with musculoskeletal diseases

Non-musculoskeletal symptom	For example: possible causes/associations
Fever	Infection, SLE[†] or other AICTD*, Adult Stills Diseasedisease, periodic fevers, post-streptococcal conditions, reactive arthritis
Dry eyes	Sjögren's, sarcoid
Xerostomia	Sjögren's, sarcoid
Headache	Giant cell arteritis, neck disorders, migraine (SLE[†] or APLS**).
Mucocutaneous ulcers	AICTDs, Behçet's, Reactive arthritis
Dysphagia	Scleroderma
Sharp chest pains	Serositis (SLE[†]), pericarditis (AICTDs*)
Cough	Sarcoid, AICTDs*
Dyspnoea	Interstitial lung disease, pulmonary hypertension, pericarditis (AICTDs*)
Abdominal pain	Crohn's disease [enteropathic spondylarthropathy (ESpA)];
Diarrhoea	Crohn's disease (ESpA); Reactive arthritis
Skin burning	Peripheral neuropathy or mononeuritis (AICTDs)*
UV skin sensitivity	SLE[†]
Parasthesias	Radiculopathy, entrapment neuropathies, neuropathy secondary to AICTD*
Fatigue	Can be associated with many severe/chronic musculoskeletal or autoimmune diseases
Dyspareunia or genital discharge	Reactive arthritis
Polyuria/nocturia	Hypercalciuria (Primary hyperparathyroidism)

*AICTD: autoimmune connective tissue diseases. [†]SLE: systemic lupus erythematosus. **APLS: antiphospholipid syndrome.

erroneous, attempts by you to develop the notion of a different diagnosis, through your questions, can be perceived as a threat. Questioning needs to be circumspect.

History from others: assent and necessity

There are four main scenarios whereby people other than the patient may be involved in providing all or part of the history.
- The elderly with communication impairment.
- Linguistic barriers.
- Those who are too ill to give a history.
- Paediatric history taking.

The elderly
History taking from an elderly patient can be challenging. Consultations can, and often should, take time. The most appropriate approach to take is important to determine early on. For example, knowing whether there are intransigent fears about being admitted to hospital or undergoing surgery can be important in determining where a consultation goes.
- It may be appropriate to aim for pragmatic solutions without necessarily basing therapeutic choices on invasive investigations. History taking should be tailored accordingly (and, thus, often needs to be more comprehensive and carefully taken compared with normal).
- Symptom reporting and its location is not always exact or in an expected distribution in the elderly. For example, co-prevalent pathology can complicate the report of specific symptoms (e.g. the report of pain in feet where dependent oedema and small fibre peripheral neuropathy have been present for a long time).
- Be aware of multiple, often age-related, pathologies.

Linguistic barriers
There are two aspects to communication. The first is general comprehension and communication given the language barrier. The second aspect is an ability of a language to adequately explain medical symptomology (for your purposes) – blunted either because of the intrinsic properties of their language and/or socio-ethnic influences.
- Linguistic barriers to obtaining a history can be lowered by predicting and addressing certain situations. Alerting patients or clinic staff of the need to arrange an interpreter to attend the consultation (and also the need to establish whether it should be male or female); providing written material about how your clinic works in (the appropriate) language, etc.
- Consider provision of access to a female doctor for women from certain ethnic backgrounds.
- Know the likely regard that certain ethnic groups have for 'a doctor'. The success of a consultation may stem from following a patient's certain perceived ideals about the role you, as a man or woman, follow in conducting the consultation.
- Be aware of likely family/social interactions in relevant situations. History giving from a relative may be influenced by established communication patterns within a family or group (even if another is not present), and there may even be barriers to the patient advocating a role for their relative in such situations.

The ill patient
There will be a need occasionally to assess either a patient who cannot communicate because of previous serious illness (e.g. severe stroke) or because they are critically ill (e.g. ventilated in an intensive care facility).
- Predicting the situation in your clinic can reduce the problems associated with communicating with severely ill patients. The main barrier to achieving a valuable assessment is often lack of time.
- Usually the main carer will attend the clinic. The patient's comprehension may be fine, but their language compromised; however, directing all questions to the carer is impolite. Don't exclude the patient!
- Obtaining previous medical records will be helpful in many cases. This can be a key issue if you're being asked the diagnosis of a critically patient on the intensive (critical) care unit (ICU).
- In the situation of a ventilated or sedated ICU patient it may be important to actively seek relatives and contacts of the patient to establish the history of the current, and if necessary previous, illness. The most important account may not come from relatives, but the person who has seen the patient most, recently.

Paediatric history taking
Talking with children and adolescents
Children are not small adults and their assessment should be different to that in adults. Concepts of pain may be well developed, but of stiffness and swelling not. You will need to obtain a history both from the child and a carer.
- Talking with the carer who spends most time with the young child is ideal. If the child is in full-time childcare, reports from nursery and childminder can be useful.
- Picture clues are often helpful in obtaining information from young children. For example, showing a range of facial expressions (happy to very sad) and asking which picture reflects their experience regarding pain (of a specific joint, for example) has been shown to help ('Faces' rating scale). The parent can clarify.
- Obtaining a history from adolescents can be challenging. Have a well thought-out strategy, but note the presence of a parent doesn't always help:
  - some teenagers' communication habits with their parents can impair a consultation;
  - it is often best, once trust has been established (may be several consultations), to see the young person alone first, then with the parent – talk to the teenager first or you risk alienating them, even if they are reticent;
  - try not to allow the parent to 'jump in' too quickly; clarification of history with the parent is important, but probably later in the consultation and with the teenager present;
  - in the rare circumstance when you think its necessary to speak with the parent alone, obtain consent from the young person first; they, like all of us, wish to be treated with dignity and respect.

Pattern recognition
Localized or diffuse pain
There is merit and utility in considering initially whether the child is well or unwell, and then discriminating whether any condition is local or widespread.
- Localized pain in a well child might be due to soft-tissue injuries, oligoarticular JIA, growing pains, and perhaps bone tumours.
- If unwell, but pain and other symptoms localized, consider septic arthritis or osteomyelitis.

- Widespread pain in a well child might be secondary to hypermobility or pain syndromes.
- Unwell children with widespread symptoms are the group most likely to have serious pathology, including leukaemia, systemic JIA and AICTDs.
- Children with hypermobility can have recurrent quite widespread symptoms, but there is no accepted definition of hypermobility in children.
- Growing pains are common and are a frequent reason for parents to consult, as symptoms, although short-lived, can appear severe and can cause children some distress.

Typical features of growing pains
- Occur age 3-11 years old.
- The child is systemically well.
- Growth and motor milestones are normal.
- Activities not limited by symptoms.
- Pains are usually symmetrical in the legs.
- Pains never occur in the morning after waking.
- The child does not limp.
- The examination is normal.

Rheumatological examination

Setting and resources
An ideal examination environment requires certain basic facilities and some relevant equipment.

Place
In addition to the general requirements of privacy and comfort then rheumatological examination can be completed almost anywhere.
- It is essential to have sufficient space to examine gait and lower limb/foot biomechanics when the patient is walking. Patients will need to be barefoot so a hard but clean floor is required.
- Space is also important. Shoulder and spine examination is best done with the patient standing.
- A couch that is height-adjustable with an additional adjustable back-rest is essential.
- An area for joint and other connective tissue injections, which is kept clean (although strict sterile conditions are not generally needed).
- There should be a controlled facility to dispose of human waste material (e.g. synovial fluid after joint aspirate), and a wash-basin with antibacterial gel and soap.

Kit
There are only a few necessary pieces of equipment. Ideally, the following should be provided:
- **Tape measure for measuring:** limb circumference and leg-length; chest expansion at nipple height [for chest restriction in ankylosing spondylitis (AS)]; Schöber's test (lumbar spine forward flexion range in AS); span (3rd finger tip to opposite 3rd finger with patient's arms outstretc.hed) in assessing for Marfan syndrome.
- **Neurology kit:** tendon hammer, 128 Hz frequency tuning fork, sensory skin testing pins, and cotton wool.
- **Ophthalmoscope** (signs of vasculitis).
- **Goniometer** for joint angle measurement.
- **Diagnostic injection kit (1):** 1% lidocaine 5- or 10-ml vials, 5-ml syringes, and a range of hypodermic needles [21, 23, and 25 gauge, ideally long (40 mm/1.5')] for injections.
- **Injection therapy kit (2):** long-acting glucocorticoid for joint and intramuscular injection (e.g. triamcinolone acetonide 40 mg/ml vials); hydrocortisone vials for superficial connective tissue, tendon, enthesis and small joint injections (25–50 mg); alcohol swabs; plasters; a variety of syringe sizes and needles.
- **General medical examination:** for assessing cardiac and lung function in patients with autoimmune joint or connective tissue disease, a stethoscope, peak flow meter and blood pressure sphygmomanometer are important.
- **Shirmer's tear test strips** (Sjögren's, see p. 256).
- **Multistix for urinalysis** is important. Screening for renal disease in SLE, vasculitis and RA starts with testing for blood and protein on a simple urine dipstick analysis.
- **Diagnostic ultrasound** (US) in the clinic is commonplace in many centres and is a highly desirable facility used in conjunction with musculoskeletal examination. Ideally, there should be facility to use Doppler with it to gauge the vascularity of thickened soft-tissue/synovium.
- For children it is necessary to have a selection of different age-appropriate toys to keep them (or their siblings) occupied and content during the consultation.

Principles of musculoskeletal examination

What is normal?
With some experience it is possible to develop a good appreciation of what is within the boundaries of a normal examination. Age, gender, and ethnicity can all influence the range of normal findings both in appearance and movement of musculoskeletal structure.
- There is wide variation in musculoskeletal features, many of which cannot be classed as 'abnormal' and never cause problems. Other features, however, might be within the range of 'normality', but do increase the risk of subsequent abnormality. Both types of features are often inherited.
- Some common examples of the normal variation in musculoskeletal features that dictate differences in skeletal appearance:
  - limb length;
  - protracted (sloping) shoulders;
  - lumbosacral lordosis/pelvic tilt;
  - femoral neck ante or retroversion;
  - flat feet (but with ability to re-form longitudinal plantar arch when non-weight bearing).
- Children are far more flexible than adults and usually girls more flexible than boys. This underscores the difficulty in coming to a consensus as to what constitutes (mild or moderate) hypermobility in children.
- Generally, women retain greater flexibility than men as they age. Greater muscle bulk and tension may determine more resistance of 'end-feel' at the extreme of range of passive joint movement.
- People of South Asian descent often show greater flexibility in joint movement, and connective tissue flexibility than Caucasians and Afro-Caribbeans.

Symmetry
The vast majority of people start off life broadly symmetrical (left to right)! Development of dominant right- or left-sided function can change symmetry slightly, and certainly previous disease or injury can lead to obvious asymmetry. Examining both sides when presented with unilateral locomotor symptoms is important to orientate the examiner as to what is 'normal' for the person being examined. Important examples include:
- **Shoulder movement range.** Subtle degrees of shoulder restriction can accompany rotator cuff lesions. There is, however, a variation in normal shoulder movements in the population. It is always important to examine a patient's good shoulder first.
- **Subtle degrees of loss of knee joint movement can be missed**. It within the accepted 'normal' range to have a little extension at the knee. The conclusion that a 'fully straight' knee on the couch is normal would therefore be erroneous, without testing for extension in the symptomatic and unaffected knee.
- Similarly, given that early loss of hip movement is often only appreciated from restriction of hip extension, it is important to examine patients with hip symptoms while

they are lying prone. Extension range of the hip, however, is sometimes hard to interpret given the tendency for additional pelvis tilt and back arching when the leg is lifted. Compare sides.

Examining the proximal moving part
There is a tendency for musculoskeletal lesions around certain joints to present with relatively few symptoms at that joint but present with referred pain to more distal structures. Examples:
- Neck lesions causing referred pain into the arm (separate to radicular distribution sensory symptoms and pain from any nerve root lesion).
- Rotator cuff lesions causing referred pain to the area around the deltoid insertion.
- Hip lesions causing pain and stiffness in the anterior thigh and knee. Occasionally, you might come across patients deny having groin or hip area pain at all.

Passive vs active examination
When patients move their own joints (active movement) structures can move differently compared with when an examiner moves them (passive). This is a key issue appreciated well by physical therapists and musculoskeletal physicians, and developed initially by Cyriax.
- Pain elicited by passive examination (which usually is, although may not be, present during active movement of the same structure) suggests an intra-articular lesion. The proviso here is that your patient's peri-articular tissues are completely relaxed for your examination.
- Patient-initiated painful movement of the joint (active movement), which lessens or disappears on passive joint examination, suggests involvement of extra-articular tissues that have a moment of force around that joint (e.g. ligament or tendon).
- The integrity of systems of joint prime movers and secondary stabilizers can only be examined actively (although isolated specific lesions can be complex and signs are often not specific). Physiotherapists refer to weight bearing leg examination as 'closed chain'.
- Knowledge of the stabilizers (e.g. isometrically operating muscles) around certain joints is essential for Rheumatologists (e.g. the role of short hip abductors in stabilizing the pelvis and avoiding a Trendelenberg gait).

Functional assessment
An assessment of the musculoskeletal (locomotor) system requires an examination of moving parts. Functional anatomy and regional functional assessments are included in Chapter 5. General function is dealt with here.

General observation
Observing patients even before they enter the consultation room can be helpful in the functional examination.
- **Body habitus/posture**. Check for patient walking stooped with kyphosis (intervertebral disc disease or osteoporosis). Does the patient walk bow-legged or with difficulty, what walking aids are used, what shoes are being worn, who is accompanying them and what is their role in helping the patient?
- Is the patient accommodating or protecting painful areas? For example, how does the patient rise from the waiting room chair or do they depend on others to help movement? How is the coat taken off (?shoulder pain)?

How (whether) is your hand is shaken. Does the patient sit skew (?unilateral back/hip pain)?

Gait

Antalgic
A limp can be obvious and accentuates the indication of pain a patient may be getting from a weight-bearing joint. The period of stance phase of the gait is reduced on the affected side. Look to see if any walking aid is being used correctly. For a right-sided knee or foot problem a stick will be most helpful used in the left hand, for example.

Trendelenberg
Leaning over on a painful or weakened hip might indicate a Trendelenberg effect. Normally, gluteus medius and minimus, which arise from the ileum and insert on the greater trochanter, isometrically contract when weight is put on their side to stabilize (abduct) the femur against the pelvis. This prevents the pelvis sagging on the other side when the leg is lifted on that other side for the swing phase of the gait. If gluteus medius is weak or denervated, or there is reduced lever-arm capacity of abduction (shortened femoral neck, hip instability, pain, etc.) the pelvis can sag on the other side and there is difficulty swinging the leg through on walking. The patient can compensate by leaning over the affected side to reduce the (lever arm effect or ground reaction force) needed to stabilize the pelvis – a compensated Trendelenberg gait.

Myopathic
A myopathic gait is most obvious when there is significant quadriceps weakness. The difficulty in lifting the legs is compensated for by leaning back slightly and tilting the pelvis forward. Gait can be high stepping if associated with significant weakness of tibialis anterior or peroneal muscles, and can be associated with a Trendelenberg lurch if associated with hip abductor muscle weakness.

High-stepping or foot slap gait
The leg is lifted high on swing phase of gait because the ability to actively dorsiflex and evert the foot to prevent the toe dragging on the ground is compromised by muscular weakness. Most often due to peroneal nerve damage or compromise (e.g. L5/S1 radiculopathy). The poor dorsiflexor control can results in the foot slapping down.

The adult 'GALS' screening examination
The locomotor system is complex and difficult to examine. The gait, arms, leg, and spine (GALS) examination is a selective clinical process to detect important locomotor abnormalities and functional disability. It is based on a tested 'minimal' history and examination system with a simple method of recording. The screen is fast and easy to perform, and includes objective observation of functional movements relevant to activities of daily living. The GALS screen has been well validated and accepted into the core undergraduate curriculum in UK Medical Schools, and has been taught as a quick and pragmatic screening assessment for use in general practice.

Screening history
If patients answer 'no' to the following three questions then there is unlikely to be any significant musculoskeletal abnormality or disability.
- Have you any pain or stiffness in your muscles, joints or back?
- Can you dress yourself completely without difficulty?
- Can you walk up and down stairs without difficulty?

Examination
The patient is examined with him/her wearing only underwear. The sequence is unimportant. Logically, it is most appropriate to examine gait, spine, arms then legs.

Gait: inspect the patient walking, turning, and walking back. Look for:
- Symmetry and smoothness of movement.
- Normal stride length and ability to turn quickly.
- Normal heel strike, stance, toe-off, and swing through.

Spine: inspect from three views. From the back inspect for:
- A straight spine (no scoliosis).
- Normal symmetrical para-spinal, shoulder and gluteal muscles.
- Level iliac crests.
- No popliteal swelling and no hind-foot swelling or deformity.

From the side ensure there is a normal cervical and lumbar lordosis and very slight thoracic kyphosis. The patient is then asked to touch his/her toes keeping the knees straight. Lumbar forward flexion should be smooth and the lumber spine should adopt a smooth curved shape.

Arms: from the front first ask the patient '… to try to place his/her ear on first the right then the left shoulder…' This tests for cervical flexion. From the front ask the patient to complete the following:
- 'Place both hands behind your head, elbows back'. This tests shoulder abduction and external rotation. A major glenohumeral or rotator cuff lesion will impair this movement.
- 'Place both hands down by your side, elbows straight'. This tests for full elbow extension.
- 'Place both hands, out in front, palms down, fingers straight, then turn both hands over'. You can identify major wrist or finger swelling, or deformity, palmar muscle wasting or erythema, the ability to supinate the forearms from the elbow, and fully extend fingers.
- 'Make a tight fist with each hand then, with both hands, place the tip of each finger in turn onto the tip of your thumbs'. You can identify any major deficit in the power grip and evaluate the fine precision pinch movement (thumb opposition).
- The examiner squeezes across the 2nd to 5th metacarpal. From this tenderness might be elicited, which might signify synovitis of metacarpophalangeal joints (which might not be detectable by inspection alone).

Legs: with the patient standing inspect the legs from the front checking for symmetry, obvious knee swelling, knee or hind-foot valgus or varus, and changes to muscle bulk and skin rashes. Then ask the patient to lie flat, supine on the couch. The remainder of the assessment involves the examiner moving joints (passive joint examination).
- Flex the hip to 90° with the leg bent holding the knee also at 90°. Repeat for other side.
- Rotate each hip in flexion (swing the foot out). Hips should flex and rotate symmetrically if normal without restriction or pain.
- During the above manoeuvre depress the patella, feeling for crepitus (often present with knee effusion).
- Squeeze across metatarsals for tenderness at toe bases (typically present if there is metatarsophalangeal joint synovitis) and inspect soles of feet for callosities. An abnormal distribution of callosities can reflect abnormal weight bearing owing to deformities, etc.

Rheumatological examination in children

The examination of a child with a musculoskeletal problem is often opportunistic as they may be in pain. You will gain the best information from close observation that starts when the child and family walk in to your consulting room.
- The child should have their weight and height measured accurately, and plotted onto centile charts. The biological aim of childhood is growth and development, and if either are failing, there are major concerns.
- The essence of the examination is keeping the child engaged and not losing their trust by hurting them.
- Gait (in the mobile child) should be observed with the child undressed (but preserving dignity). Pre-school age children are usually happy to walk about in their underpants; those less confident need to hold a parent's hand. Older children will want more clothes on and it is wise to ask children to bring shorts to change into.
- It is normal for toddlers to be 'bow legged' and 'flat footed'. In-toeing, out toeing, 'curly toes', and 'knock knees' are all common normal variants. The toddler should, however, be symmetrical and, where there is asymmetry, look carefully for pathology.
- Intoeing has many causes, but almost all are simple often age-related biomechanical reasons:
  - femoral anteversion (age 3–8 years);
  - internal tibial torsion (up to age 3–4 years);
  - bow legs – most resolve by age 3 years;
  - knock knees – most resolve by age 7 years;
  - flat feet – most resolve by age 6 years and normal arches are seen on standing on tiptoe.
- Unilateral 'out toeing' can be because of ankle arthritis; severe or asymmetrical leg bowing may indicate rickets (more common in the UK in dark skinned children). Asymmetrical skin creases at the groin with leg length discrepancy suggests a late diagnosis of developmental dysplasia of the hip.
- In juvenile idiopathic arthritis (JIA) an antalgic gait and asymmetry due to leg length discrepancy are common.
- Ask the child to sit on the floor then get up unaided. If the child has to turn onto 'all fours' and then 'walk up' their legs using their hands there is proximal muscle weakness (Gower's sign).
- Perform a general examination, particularly noting any skin rashes, nail changes, oral ulceration, heart murmurs, lymphadenopathy, and organomegaly.
- Examine peripheral neurology, muscle bulk, and strength. An unassisted sit-up or flexing the head against resistance are valuable in assessing truncal weakness as found in dermatomyositis (DM).
- In the musculoskeletal examination, check every joint. Because of poor localization of pain, there may be unexpected findings.
- Check for tenderness over entheses.
- Subtle swelling of the ankle joint is best detected from behind the child with the child standing.
- If a joint looks, feels, and moves normally then it probably is normal!

CHAPTER 1 Clinical assessment of rheumatological disease

The paediatric GALS examination
The pGALS examination provides an easy screening examination, validated to detect significant abnormality with high sensitivity. Following detection of an abnormality there may be a detailed focus on it.
- It is best done by getting the child to copy the examiner.
- It is important to register both non-verbal and verbal indicators of discomfort.
- A key finding is asymmetry.

Neurological examination (adults)
A detailed view of neurological examination technique is beyond the scope of this text. However, knowledge of patterns of presentation of neurological disease – particularly spinal cord and peripheral nerve lesions – is essential.

Stiffness
Stiffness is a common musculoskeletal symptom. It can also be reported in early neurological disease.
- Back and general, mainly proximal, limb stiffness is a well-recognized features of early Parkinson's Disease. Think of assessing:
  - facial expressivity (?lacking);
  - gait (?lack of arm swinging, shuffling);
  - limb rigidity;
  - resting tremor (e.g. thumb and forefinger);
  - passive elbow movement for 'cogwheeling'.

Stiffness is also a feature of slowing evolving myelopathy. Patients with lesions causing myelopathy present occasionally to rheumatologists. Lesions include axial and subaxial cervical spine stenosis owing to disc and degenerative spine disease or instability in the spine associated with rheumatoid arthritis. Key points in the history worth exploring might be:
- Any previous spinal trauma.
- Radicular peripheral limb parasthesias, numbness, or burning pain.
- Any long-standing neck or thoracic spine symptoms.
- Progressive abnormalities in bladder control.

The examination of patients with potential myelopathy is necessary detailed. However, often with a slowly evolving lesion, signs can be atypical and in some patients, difficult to elicit.
- Tone and reflexes in limbs can be difficult to assess owing to co-existent joint disease.

Table 1.3 The pGALS musculoskeletal screening examination

Screening questions
Do you (or does your child) have any pain or stiffness in your (their) joints, muscles or back?
Do you (or does your child) have any difficulty getting yourself (him/herself) dressed without any help?
Do you (or does your child) have any problem going up and down stairs?

Screening manoeuvres	Features assessed	Examples of abnormalities
Observe the child standing (from front, back and sides)	Posture	Knock knees, bow legs.
	Habitus	Leg length discrepancy, Scoliosis, kyphosis
Observe the child walking and 'Walk on your tip-toes/walk on your heels'	Feet and ankles	Flat feet, antalgic gait, Inflammatory arthritis, enthesitis-related arthritis (ERA), sever disease, tarsal coalition
'Hold your hands out straight in front of you'	Shoulders, elbows, wrists, hands	Inflammatory arthritis
'Turn your hands over and make a fist'	Wrists, elbows, small joints of hands	
'Pinch your 1st finger and thumb together'	Small joints index finger and thumb	
'Touch the tips of your fingers'	Small joints of fingers	
Squeeze the metacarpophalangeal joints (MCP) joints	MCP joints	
'Put your hands together palm to palm and then back to back'	Small joints of fingers, wrists	
'Reach up, "touch the sky", and look at the ceiling'	Neck, shoulders, elbows, wrists	Hypermobility, inflammatory arthritis
'Put your hands behind your neck'	Shoulders, elbows	Hypermobility, inflammatory arthritis
Feel for effusion at the knee	Knee	Inflammatory arthritis
Active movement of knees and feel for crepitus	Knee	Anterior knee pain
Passive movement (full flexion and internal rotation of hip)	Hip	Perthes, slipped femoral epiphysis, hip dysplasia, inflammatory arthritis (ERA)
'Open wide and put three (child's own) fingers in your mouth'	Temporomandibular joints	Inflammatory arthritis
'Try and touch your shoulder with your ear'	Neck	Inflammatory arthritis, torticollis
'Bend forwards and touch your toes'	Thoracolumbar spine	Spondylolysis, spondylolisthesis, mechanical back pain, Inflammatory arthritis (ERA)

Table reproduced, with permission, from: Foster HE, Jandial S. pGALS – a screening examination of the musculoskeletal system in school-aged children. *Reports on the Rheumatic Diseases (Series 5), Hands On 15*. Arthritis Research Campaign; 2008 June.

RHEUMATOLOGICAL EXAMINATION

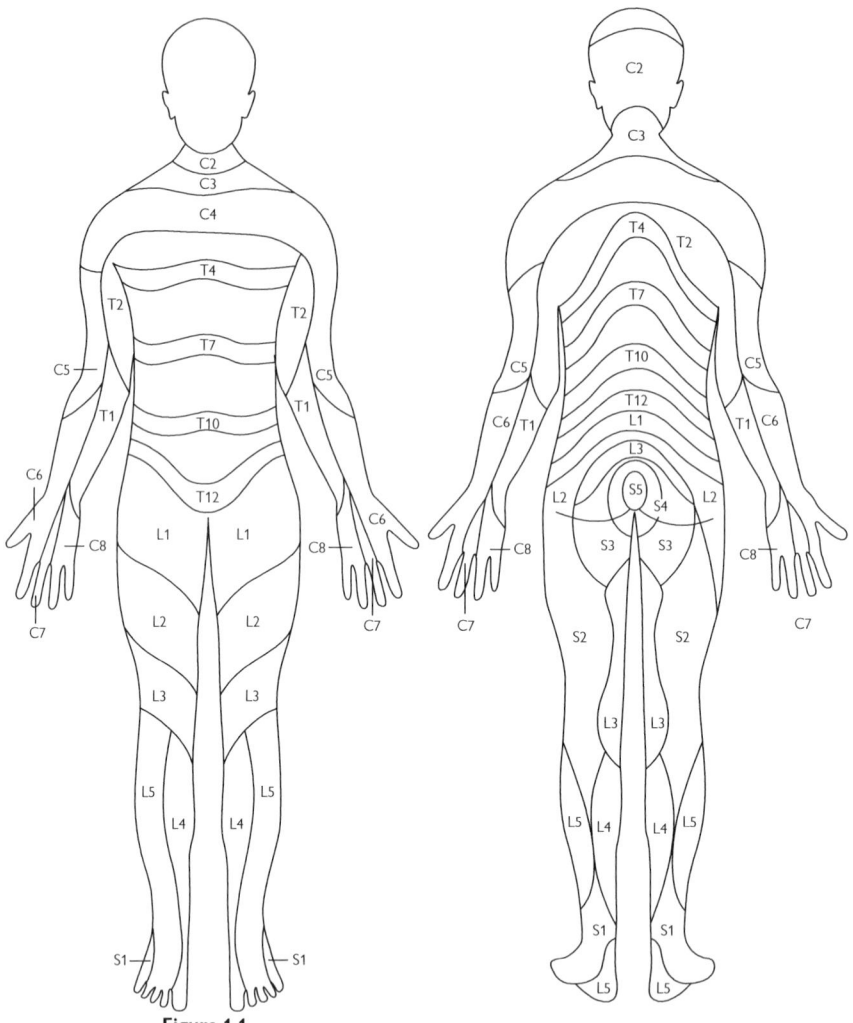

Figure 1.1

- Testing clonus is often inappropriate in patients with joint disease.
- Plantar responses are not necessarily extensor.
- Sensory skin testing requires time and a fairly detailed approach. Patients with RA and other arthritides and AICTDs may have additional (or longstanding) radicular signs or changes in sensory changes from other causes of neuropathy.

Peripheral limb pain

Discriminating pain from musculoskeletal causes, and neurological radicular or other peripheral nerve lesions can be difficult. Often multiple lesions exist.

- Common scenarios include
  - diagnosing carpal tunnel syndrome;
  - establishing whether neurogenic pains in the hand are from median or ulna nerve lesions or nerve root lesions in the neck;
  - discriminating the cause of leg pain (joint or muscle pain or lumbar nerve root).
- Neurogenic pain is often described as 'burning', and is associated with parasthesias ('tingling') or 'numbness'.
- A positive Tinnel's test (parasthesias from percussion over peripheral nerve course at possible sites of entrapment) is an important sign in peripheral nerve entrapment lesions.
- Knowledge of radicular and peripheral nerve distribution and function is important (see Appendix).

Resources

ARC pGALS DVD. Available at: www.arc.org.uk/arthinfo/emedia.asp#pGALS

ARC. Available at: http://www.arc.org.uk/arthinfo/medpubs/6535/6535.asp

Examining the central nervous system. Available at: http://www.scribd.com/doc/19826/Examination-of-the-Central-Nervous-System;

Further reading

Bellamy N. WOMAC *Osteoarthritis Index*. Available at: www.womac.org.

Calin A, Garrett S, Whitelock H, et al. A new approach to defining functional ability in ankylosing spondylitis: the development of the Bath Ankylosing Spondylitis Functional Index. *J Rheumatol* 1994; **21**: 2281–5.

Doherty M, Dacre J, Dieppe P, Snaith M. The 'GALS' locomotor screen. *Ann Rheum Dis* 1992; **51**: 1165–9.

Foster HE, Kay LJ et al. Musculoskeletal screening examination (pGALS) for school-age children based on the adult GALS screen. *Arthritis Care Res* 2006; **55**: 709–16.

Jandial S, Foster H. Examination of the musculoskeletal system in children – a simple approach. *Paed Child Health* 2007; **18**(2): 47–55.

Observational gait analysis. Available at: http://www.iol.ie/~rcsiorth/journal/volume2/june/gait.htm;

Scott DL, Garrood T. Quality of life measures: use and abuse. *Baillieres Best Pract Res Clin Rheumatol* 2000; **14**: 663–87.

Patterns of rheumatological disease: oligoarticular pains in adults

Background
Inflammation may be a consequence of a range of cellular processes but there are no clinical features that are both frequent and specific enough to allow a diagnosis to be made of its cause in any single joint.
- In any given joint synovitis may not be the only inflamed tissue. Enthesitis of insertions of joint capsules, intra-articular and peri-articular ligaments/tendons may be the primary site of inflammation in some disorders.
- The differential diagnosis of synovitis includes haemarthrosis and other synovial processes, e.g. pigmented villonodular synovitis (PVNS).

History: general points
- Pain and stiffness are typical, although not invariable features of synovitis and enthesitis. Pain and stiffness are often worse during or after a period of immobility. The presence or absence of stiffness does not discriminate between diagnoses. Pain is often severe in acute joint inflammation.
- There are no descriptors that discriminate pain from synovitis or enthesitis.
- Swelling, either due to synovial thickening or effusion, often accompanies synovitis. Enthesitis may be associated with peri-articular soft tissue swelling. A patient's report of swelling is not always reliable.

Examination: general points
- Skin erythema and heat are common with crystal and septic arthritis.
- Severely tender swelling suggests joint infection, haemarthrosis or an acute inflammatory reaction to crystals. Inflammation of entheses results in 'bony' tenderness at joint margins and sites of tendon or ligament insertion.
- The degree to which passive and active joint mobility is reduced depends on a number of interdependent factors (e.g. pain, size of effusion, peri-articular muscle weakness or pain).
- Symptoms elicited by movement of a joint affected by synovitis or enthesitis include pain and stiffness, although neither may be specific.
- Reaching the end of (reduced) joint range, whether elicited passively or actively, invariably causes pain (although it should be noted that if any normal joint is forced through the end of range, pain can result).

History
Age and gender
- Oligoarthritis is uncommon in young adults. Spondylarthropathy (SpA), especially reactive arthritis, is likely to be the main cause (e.g. 75% of patients who develop reactive arthritis are <40 years).
- Gout typically occurs in those over 40 years and is the commonest cause of inflammatory arthritis in men (self-reported in 1 in 74 men and 1 in 156 women).
- The mean age of patients with (CPPDD) arthritis is about 70 years (range 63–93 years).

Table 1.4 The causes of oligoarticular (including monoarticular) joint pain and typical patterns of presentation

Disease	Typical pattern
Gout (p. 383)	Age >40 years. Initially acute monoarthritis. Association with hyperuricaemia, renal impairment, diuretics. General symptoms can mimic sepsis. Possible family history. High acute phase response. Neutrophilia. Joint fluid urate crystals seen by polarized light microscopy (PLM). Joint erosions (typical) and tophi occur in chronic disease.
SpA (p. 209)	Age <40 years, men > women. Mostly oligoarticular lower limb joint enthesitis/synovitis. May occur with sacroiliitis, urethritis or cervicitis, uveitis, gut inflammation, psoriasis. Possible family history. ESR/CRP can be normal. More severe in HLAB27 positive people.
CPPDD arthritis (p. 383)	Mean age 72 years. Oligoarticular, acute monoarticular (25%) and occasionally polyarticular patterns. Haemarthrosis. Obvious trauma does not always occur. Swelling usually considerable. Causes include trauma (e.g. cruciate rupture or fracture), PVNS, bleeding diatheses and chondrocalcinosis.
Osteoarthritis (p. 371)	Soft tissue swelling is usually not as obvious as bony swelling (osteophytes). Typical distribution (e.g. first carpometacarpal and knee joints).
Rheumatoid arthritis (p. 197)	Unusual presentation in a single joint. Can present with just a few (usually symmetrical) joints.
Septic arthritis (excluding N. gonorrhae)	Commonest cause *Staphylococcus aureus*. Associated with chronic arthritis, joint prostheses and reduced host immunity. Peak incidence in elderly. Systemic symptoms common and sometimes overt, thoughalthough may not occur. Synovial fluid is Gram stain positive in 50% of cases and culture positive in 90% of cases.
Gonococcal arthritis	Age 15–30 years in urban populations and with inherited deficiency of complement C5 to C9. One form presents as an acute septic monoarthritis. Organism detected by Gram stain of joint fluid (25%) or culture (50%).

Different joints?
- Shoulder synovitis is typical in hydroxyapatite arthritis and AL amyloidosis.
- Involvement of a shoulder or hip is unusual in gout.
- CPPDD arthritis (as pseudogout) occurs rarely in the small finger joints.
- The knee is the commonest site of acute CPPDD arthritis, and is the site of about 50% of septic and the majority of gonococcal arthritis cases.
- Acute massive swelling of the knee is typical in Lyme arthritis and can occur with septic arthritis. Massive swelling of the knee can also occur in psoriatic arthritis but the history is usually chronic.
- There are many theoretical causes of synovitis in a single first metatarsophalangeal joint (MTPJ), but the majority

of cases are due to gout (50–70% of first attacks occur in this joint).

Preceding factors
Factors preceding oligoarthritis may be relevant. These include infection and trauma.
- Acute non-traumatic monoarticular synovitis is most commonly due to crystal-induced synovitis or associated with SpA.
- A preceding history of trauma might suggest intra-articular fracture, meniscus tear (knee) or an intra-articular loose body (e.g. osteochondral fragment).
- Twinges of joint pain often precede an acute attack of gout. Acute arthritis occurs in 25% of patients with CPPDD arthritis.
- An acute monoarthritis with fever in familial Mediterranean fever (FMF) is a mimic of septic arthritis. Such joint manifestations are a common (75% of cases), but not invariable feature.

Crystal arthritis?
Crystal arthritis is associated with other conditions.
- Hyperuricaemia, causes of which include obesity, renal insufficiency, tumour lysis syndrome, myeloproliferative diseases are associated with gout.
- Hypertension, hypertriglyceridaemia, and a history of urate renal stones are associated with gout.
- Attacks of gout and CPPDD arthritis can be precipitated by any non-specific illness, trauma, and surgery. The commonest associated disorder of CPPDD is primary hyperparathyroidism (10% of cases).
- Though uncommon, hypomagnesaemia, hypophosphatasia [low alkaline phosphatase (ALP) activity], haemochromatosis, Wilson's disease, and ochronosis are all associated with CPPDD arthritis.

Link with infection
Many types of infection are linked to oligoarticular arthritis.
- Viruses, bacteria, protozoa, helminthes, and fungi can all directly invade joints. The range of systemic features is wide and pathogens can cause both polyarticular and oligoarticular joint conditions.
- The infections recognized to trigger reactive arthritis are *Salmonella, Yersinia, Shigella, Campylobacter*, and *Chlamydia*. Reactive arthritis in those who acquire chlamydial (non-gonococcal) urethritis is relatively uncommon (about 1 in 30).
- Acute HIV infection is associated with a subacute oligoarticular arthritis (usually knees and ankles).
- Chronic arthritis of any type, diabetes, immunodeficiency, regular dialysis, chronic renal failure, and joint prostheses are risks for septic arthritis.
- Lyme disease should be considered a cause of oligoarthritis in patients with a history (weeks to years ago) of erythema chronicum migrans [macule/papule initially, expanding 0.5–1 cm/day to a mean diameter of 15 cm (range 3–68 cm) fading often without treatment in 3–4 weeks].
- A history of circumcorneal eye redness with pain, photophobia, and blurred vision may be due to anterior uveitis – associated with SpA, but also sarcoid, Behçet's, and Whipple's disease.

Family and social history
There may be important clues from the family and social history.

- Both gout and SpA may be familial. About 10% of patients with gout have a family history.
- Gout in young adults suggests an inherited defect (usually increased urate from increased 5-phosphoribosyl-1-pyrophosphate synthetase, because other deficiencies present in childhood).
- Excessive alcohol consumption is associated with gout. Alcohol can also contribute to lactic acidosis that inhibits urate breakdown.
- Consider Lyme disease if patients live, work or visit endemic areas for infected ticks (within the northeast rural United States, Europe, Russia, China, and Japan). Peak incidence of infection is June/July.
- Brucellar arthritis is generally monoarticular and occurs in areas where domesticated animals are infected and poor methods of animal husbandry, feeding habits and hygiene standards co-exist.

Other associated features
Associated features include previous eye, gastrointestinal, cardiac, and genitourinary symptoms.
- Low-grade fever, malaise, and anorexia occur in septic arthritis and gout. Marked fever occurs in only about a third of patients with septic arthritis.
- Marked fever, hypotension, and delirium can occur (rarely) in acute flares of CPPDD arthritis.
- Try eliciting a history of SpA:
  - back or buttock pain (enthesitis or sacroiliitis);
  - swelling of a digit (dactylitis);
  - plantar heel pain (plantar fasciitis);
  - red eye with irritation (anterior uveitis);
  - urethritis, balanitis, cervicitis, or acute diarrhoea (reactive arthritis);
  - psoriasis;
  - symptoms of inflammatory bowel disease.
- Behçet's disease is a cause of oligoarticular synovitis. Other features include painful oral and genital ulcers, and uveitis.
- The involvement of more than one joint does not rule out septic arthritis. In up to 20% of cases, multiple joints can become infected.

Examination

General
Always compare sides. Establish whether there is true synovial swelling. A history of swelling is not always reliable. Enthesial inflammation in SpA does not usually cause swelling.

Affected joints
Examine for tenderness. Check the range of (passive) movement, for locking and instability.
- Acute processes, such as crystal arthritis and infection often lead to a painful swelling, marked tenderness of swollen soft-tissues, and painfully restricted active and passive movement of the joint. Features are usually less overt with chronic arthritis.
- Instability of an acutely inflamed joint or tests for cartilage damage in the knee may be difficult to demonstrate. Further examination will be necessary after drainage of joint fluid/haemarthrosis.
- Detection of enthesis tenderness around the affected joints or at other sites is a useful clue to the underlying diagnosis of SpA.

Examination of other musculoskeletal structures
- Examine the back and for sites of bony tenderness. Sacroiliitis and enthesitis are common in SpA.
- Tendonitis is not specific and can often occur in gout, CPPDD arthritis, SpA, and gonococcal infection.

Skin rashes and other features of inflammation
Oligoarthritis may be part of a systemic inflammatory/infective condition.
- Temperature and tachycardia can occur with non-infective causes of acute arthritis (e.g. crystal arthritis), although their presence with oligoarticular joint swelling requires exclusion of joint infection.
- Gouty tophi may be seen in the pinnae, but also anywhere peripherally. They can be difficult to discriminate clinically from rheumatoid nodules. Polarized light microscopy (PLM) of material obtained by needle aspiration will be diagnostic for tophi.
- The hallmark of relapsing polychondritis is lobe-sparing, full thickness inflammation of the pinna.
- Mouth ulcers can occur with any illness; however, crops of large painful lesions associated with oligo-articular arthritis suggests Behçet's disease.
- A typical site for osteitis associated with axial sarcoid or SAPHO (Le Syndrome, Acné, Pustulose, Hyperostose et Ostéité) is manubriosternal.
- Erythema over a joint suggests crystal or infection.
- Associated skin rashes may include erythema nodosum (associated with ankle pains in sarcoid), the purpuric pustular rashes of Behçet's, gonococcal infection (single pustules) and Le SAPHO, erythema marginatum (rheumatic fever), or keratoderma blenhorragica (aggressive-looking psoriasis-like rash of the sole of the foot in reactive arthritis disease).
- Psoriasis may be associated with synovitis, enthesitis or periostitis.

Investigations
Doubt about the presence of synovitis can be addressed by obtaining US or magnetic resonance (MR) imaging of the joint(s) in question.

Joint aspiration (see Table 1.5)
Fluid should be sent in sterile bottles for microscopy and culture.
- Synovial fluid appearances are not specific. Blood or blood-staining suggests haemarthrosis from trauma (including the aspiration attempt), haemangioma, PVNS, synovioma, or occasionally CPPDD arthritis.
- Turbidity of fluid relates to cellular, crystal, lipid, and fibrinous content, and is typical in septic arthritis and acute crystal arthritis owing to the number of polymorphonuclear (PMN) leucocytes.
- Cell counts give some diagnostic guidance, but are non-specific. There is a high probability of infection or gout if the PMN differential is >90%.
- Joint fluid eosinophilia is not specific.
- Compensated PLM of fluid can discriminate urate (3–20 µm, needle-shaped, negatively birefringent – blue and then yellow as the red plate compensator is rotated 90°) and calcium-containing crystals, e.g. CPPDD (positively birefringent, typically small, and rectangular or rhomboid in shape).

- Lipid and cholesterol crystals are not uncommon in joint fluid samples, but their significance is unknown.
- Crystals seen less commonly, but in typical settings include hydroxyapatite associated with Milwaukee shoulder (or knee) syndrome (alizarin red-S stain positive), calcium oxalate in dialysis patients (may need scanning electron microscopy), cystine in cystinosis, and xanthine in xanthinosis.
- The presence of crystals in joint fluid does not exclude infection.
- The commonest causes of non-gonococcal septic arthritis in Europe and North America are *Staph aureus* (40–50%), *Staph epidermidis* (10–15%), *Strep* species (20%), and Gram-negative bacteria (15%).

Table 1.5 Features of joint fluid

Feature	Normal	Non-inflammatory	Inflammatory	Septic
Viscosity	V high	High	Low	Varies
Colour	None	Straw	Straw	Varies + orgs
Clarity	Clear	Clear	Opaque	Opaque
Leucocytes (cells/mm^3)	200	200–2000	2000–50 000	>50 000
PMNs (%)	<25	25	Often >50	>75

Radiographs
Radiographs can confirm an effusion, show characteristic patterns of chondral and bone destruction (e.g. in infection or erosive gout), and show intra-articular calcification from CPPDD or hydroxyapatite.
- If septic arthritis is suspected radiographs are essential. Patchy osteopaenia and loss of bone cortex are cardinal signs.
- Punched-out (Lulworth Cove) erosions, soft tissue swellings (tophi) and patchy calcification are hallmarks of chronic gout.
- Intra-articular calcification may be either chondrocalcinosis (fine linear or punctate fibrocartilage calcification) or larger loose bodies (often with osteophytes). Both associate with CPPDD arthritis.
- Numerous round-shaped calcific masses in a joint can be due to synovial chondromatosis (commonest in middle-aged men, 50% of cases – knee).
- The presence of erosions per se does not imply RA. Erosions can be due to erosive enthesitis associated with SpA, CPPDD arthritis, and gout.

MR
Further MR imaging should be discussed with your radiologists.
- Confirmation of traumatized structures, such as meniscus damage in the knee and labral damage in the shoulder should be sought if suspected.
- MR can confirm synovitis, although appearances are usually non-specific. Focal high signal in bone on T2 and fat suppressed images ('bone bruising') if in sub-enthesial sites can indicate osteitis in SpA.

CHAPTER 1 Clinical assessment of rheumatological disease

Ultrasound

Many rheumatologists use US to aid diagnosis and characterize inflammatory arthritis in the clinic.
- Joint and tendon thickening, and changes in appearance of soft-tissues are all identifiable with US.
- US is more sensitive than clinical examination and radiographs at detecting small joint synovitis in RA.
- The addition of patterns of abnormality with Doppler is useful in assessing the activity of synovitis in joints in RA and inflammatory arthritis.
- Erosions at small joints are detectable in patients with inflammatory arthritis at an earlier stage compared with radiographs.
- At the wrist US can also show features suggestive of median nerve entrapment.
- In experienced hands US can be used to show clinical and asymptomatic entheseal changes around the hindfoot in SpA patients.
- Ultrasound-guided glucocorticoid injections into different structures (including sub-acromial space) has been shown to be more accurate than bedside injection without imaging.

Laboratory investigations to consider
- Full blood count (FBC), erythrocyte sedimentation rate (ESR), C-reactive protein (CRP). Neutrophilia is not specific for infection and can occur in crystal arthritis.
- Blood urea, electrolytes, creatinine and urate (e.g. hyperuricaemia and renal impairment with gout).
- Blood calcium, phosphate, albumin, ALP [± parathyroid hormone (PTH)], thyroid function tests, and ferritin to screen for hyperparathyroid or thyroid disease or haemochromatosis associated with CPPDD arthritis.
- Autoantibodies: rheumatoid factor (RF) is not specific for RA. Cyclic citrullinated peptide (CCP) antibodies are probably more sensitive for a diagnosis of RA in early inflammatory arthritis patients. However, acuity of findings is still likely to be blunted by suboptimal case ascertainment. Low titre CCP antibodies do occur in non-RA inflammatory arthritides.
- Serum angiotensin converting enzyme (sACE) (occurs in, although is not specific for, sarcoid), IgM *Borellia burgdorferi* serology (acute arthritis or history of migratory arthritis in Lyme disease).
- Antibodies to the streptococcal antigens streptolysin O (ASOT) DNAase B, hyaluronidase, and streptozyme in patients who have had sore throat, migratory arthritis or features of rheumatic fever.

Synovial biopsy
- If there is a haemarthrosis or suspicion of PVNS, MR of the joint is necessary before undertaking a biopsy to characterize the vascularity of a lesion.
- Consider a biopsy in the following situations: undiagnosed monoarthritis, suspicion of: sarcoid arthropathy, infection despite negative synovial fluid microscopy and cultures, gout despite failure to detect crystals in synovial fluid and amyloid.
- Formalin fixation of samples is sufficient in most cases. Samples for PLM are fixed in alcohol (urate is dissolved out by formalin). Snap freezing in nitrogen is essential if immunohistochemistry is required.
- Arthroscopic biopsy will yield more tissue than needle biopsy; it may add diagnostic information and joint irrigation can be undertaken.
- Congo red staining of synovium, ideally with PLM, should be requested if AA, AL or β_2-microglobulin amyloid is a possibility. Typical situations are in myeloma (AL) and long-term dialysis patients (β_2-microglobulin). AA amyloid (in long-standing RA, AS, FMF and Crohn's disease) is a rare, although recognized complication of each condition.

Widespread pain (in adults)

Many conditions are characterized by musculoskeletal symptoms, some of which may be diffuse or multicentric. Also, the interpretation and reporting of symptoms varies and can be a source of confusion.

Background

History: general points

Widespread symptoms can be due a variety of conditions, not all affecting joints. Assessment requires consideration of disease characterized by:
- Polyarticular disorders such as RA, prostate specific antigens (PSA), and CPPDD polyarthritis.
- Conditions of muscle [e.g. polymyositis, polymyalgia (PMR), sarcoid, statin-induced myalgia].
- Polyenthesopathies primarily psoriasis-associated but also enteropathic SpA, SAPHO, and sarcoid.
- Pain from a combination of muscle, joint, and tendon complicated by fatigue (e.g. SLE, Sjogren's).
- Neurological disease, such as cervical myelopathy (mimicking musculoskeletal – 'stiffness') and inflammatory dural disease (e.g. 'burning pain' dysaesthesia in neurosarcoid).
- Chronic pain amplification and fatigue.

Examination: general points

Assessment needs to be comprehensive if joint disease is not evident on examination. Full neurological examination is often necessary.
- An appreciation of the distribution of lesions likely with polyenthesopathy, the neurological signs of neuromeningeal sarcoid and distribution of fibromyalgia tender points is important.
- Slowly evolving myelopathy can result in few hard signs. The 'flavour' of increased tone in limbs, generalized increase in reflexes and blunted skin sensation to fine pinprick or light touch in the legs is often all that is detected.

History

Age, gender, and racial background

The degree to which these factors influence the likelihood of disease varies according to the background disease occurrence in the (local) population.
- There is a low incidence of ankylosing spondylitis (AS) in patients aged >65 years with back and joint pains.
- Generalized OA is rare in young men and unusual in women <40 years.
- With an incidence of less than $1:10^6$ autoimmune polymyositis (PM) is rare compared with PMR which has an incidence of about 1:10 000 (age >50 years).
- SLE is up to 5 times more common in black than in white races.
- Osteomalacia occurring in temperate zone 'western' populations is more likely in economically deprived than in affluent areas, in the institutionalized elderly than in young adults, and in some Asian ethnic groups, rather than Caucasians.

The history of the pain at different sites

- A good history should give you the anatomical site of pains and should be able to reveal the tissue of origin in the majority of cases.
- Widespread pain due to bone pathology alone should be considered. Bony pain is often unremitting, day and night. It changes little with changes in posture and movement.
- Discriminating whether there is a single process causing the widespread pain may depend on whether the same types of lesions are consistently present. Are all symptoms only from joints? Is there a combination of enthesial and joint pains?
- Problems may arise if it is assumed that all pains arise from a single pathological process. In children and young adults this would be likely, but in the elderly, particularly where there is late presentation, multiple pathologies are often present.

Establish which joints are affected

- A symmetrical pattern of small joint synovitis is typical of, but not specific for, RA. Chronic arthritis from parvovirus B19 infection, pseudo-rheumatoid PSA, polyarticular gout (particularly in postmenopausal women) and CPPDD polyarthritis in the elderly may mimic RA in this respect.
- Small hand joint pain occurs in nodal generalized OA and PSA. PIPJ and thumb CMC joints can be affected in both. PSA patients often have additional enthesitis and inflammatory lesions in feet. The latter would be more unusual in OA.
- The combination of sacroiliac pelvic and lower limb joint/enthesis pain, typically in an asymmetrical oligoarticular pattern, is suggestive of SpA.
- Large and medium-sized joints are typically affected in CPPDD disease, but a picture of multiple joint involvement similar to that in RA is possible (including tenosynovitis).
- CPPDD disease can affect spinal structures.
- Widespread arthralgia/arthritis occurs in patients with leukaemias, lymphoma, and myeloma, and with certain infections (see Table 1.6). Lesions may be a complex combination of involving joint, muscle, and bone.

Ask about the pattern of joint symptoms over time

- A short, striking history of marked, acute polyarticular symptoms often occurs with systemic infection. Malaise and fever should raise suspicion of infection.
- Migratory arthralgia occurs in 10% of RA patients initially: a single joint becomes inflamed for a few days then improves and a different joint becomes affected for a few days and so on. A similar pattern can occur in poststreptococcal arthritis, occasionally in acute sarcoid, is not unusual before frank oligoarthritis develops in Lyme disease.
- A history suggestive of recurrent enthesial lesions (e.g. previous tennis elbow or plantar fasciitis) or 'injuries', which have been 'slow to heal' and episodic or persistent inflammatory back or neck pains is typical in patients with PSA.
- Recurrent pains from various musculoskeletal lesions, which have occurred either from injury or developed insidiously, are typical in patients with underlying hypermobility. Lesions are often mild and signs slight. Chronic pain is well recognized.

Table 1.6 Common infections associated with arthralgias and an acute phase response

Infection	Features
Rheumatic fever (group A β haemolytic Strep)	Acute infection 1-2/52 earlier; fever, rash, carditis. High ASOT (80%), +ve anti-DNAaseB IgM, throat swab culture +ve.
Post-streptococcal	Acute infection 3–4/52 earlier, tenosynovitis.
Parvovirus B19*	Severe flu-like illness at outset, rashes. Anti-B19 IgM.
Rubella (also post-vaccine)	Fever, coryza, malaise, rash. Culture and anti-Rubella IgM.
Hepatitis B	Fever, myalgia, malaise, urticaria, abnormal LFTs. Bilirubin and ALT elevated; anti-HbsAg/HbcAg +ve.
B burgdorferi (Lyme)	Tick bites, fever, headache, myalgia, fatigue, nerve palsies. Anti-Borrelia IgM.
Toxoplasma gondii	Myositis, parasthesias, anti-toxo IgM.

*The features of parvovirus infection can be quite different in children

Widespread 'muscle' pain (see Table 1.7)
Patients who report muscle pains may have muscle pains, but also radicular, referred, and enthesial pains can be mistaken as arising from muscle.
- The myalgia may be fibromyalgia or enthesitis.
- Neuromeningeal inflammation in neurosarcoid might result in perceived muscle pains.
- Pain locating to muscle group areas may be ischaemic in origin (particularly neural claudication type pains in legs).
- The differential of polymyositis and dermatomyositis is wide, although many conditions are rare.

Features of a history of myalgia
- PMR (rare <55 years), myositis, and endocrine/meta-bolic myopathies typically affect proximal limb and truncal musculature, but PMR is also associated with giant cell arteritis (GCA), and therefore may present with headache, fatigue, and lassitude.
- Though rare, truncal muscle pain and stiffness can be a presenting feature of Parkinson's disease.
- Cramp-like pains may be a presenting feature of any myopathy. Some patients can interpret radicular (nerve root) pains as 'cramp-like' and, therefore, explain their presence in a muscular distribution.
- Inflammatory and endocrine/metabolic myopathies are not always painful.
- Some genetic muscle diseases (e.g. myophosphorylase, acid maltase deficiency), can present atypically late (in adults) with progressive muscle weakness.
- Severe acute muscle pain is commonest in viral, neoplastic and drug-induced myopathies. Some toxic causes may result in rhabdomyolysis, myoglobinaemia, and renal failure.
- In severe, acute myopathy consider also the rare eosinophilic fasciitis or eosinophilic-myalgia syndrome (toxic reaction to L-tryptophan).
- Low-grade episodic muscle pain might denote an undisclosed hereditary metabolic myopathy.

Table 1.7 The major myopathies

Process	Conditions
Infectious	Viruses (e.g. influenza, Hep B/C, Cocksackie, HIV)
	Bacteria (e.g. B burgdorferi)
	Other (e.g. malaria, toxoplasmosis)
Endocrine or metabolic	Hypo/hyperthyroidism, hypercortisolism, hyperparathyroidism
	Hypokalaemic, hypocalcaemic
Autoimmune	Polymyositis, dermatomyositis, SLE, scleroderma, Sjogren's
	Vasculitides, myasthenia gravis, eosinophilic fasciitis
Neoplastic	Carcinomatous paraneoplastic
Drug-induced	Anti-lipid (statins, clofibrate, etc.), colchicines, *D-penicillamine, AZT, *chloroquine, ciclosporin, alcohol and opiates (rhabdomyolysis)
Muscular dystrophies	Limb-girdle, fascioscapulohumeral
Congenital	Mitochondrial myopathy, myophosphorylase deficiency, lipid storage

*Drugs most likely to cause a painful myopathy

Ischaemic pains
- Patients may have little concept of ischaemia and might describe their symptoms in the context of muscles, and in a muscular distribution.
- Ischaemic muscle pain often occurs predictably in association with repeated activity, and eases or resolves on rest.
- The distribution of pains may give clues as to sites of underlying pathology, e.g. upper limbs in subclavian artery stenosis or thoracic outlet syndrome or, typically, thighs, and calves in atherosclerotic vascular disease or lumbosacral spine/lumbar nerve root stenosis. Sitting forward may relieve the latter.
- Ischaemic pains in the context of a rash may suggest systemic vasculitis.

Widespread pain due to bone pathology
- Bone pains are unremitting and disturb sleep. They could denote malignancy.
- Major diagnoses to consider include disseminated malignancy, multiple myeloma, metabolic bone disease (e.g. renal osteodystrophy, hyperparathyroidism, osteomalacia), and polyostotic Paget's disease.

Past medical history
Direct questioning is often required, as previous problems may not be regarded as relevant by the patient.
- Previous lesions that *could* have been due to enthesitis, previous psoriasis even if mild and a family history of psoriasis are all relevant to making a diagnosis of PSA.
- Previous inflammatory bowel disease, diarrhoeal or dysenteric illness, uveitis, or urogenital infection symptoms might be relevant to a diagnosis of SpA.
- For those in whom myalgia/myositis seems likely: preceding viral illness, foreign travel, previous erythema nodosum, i.e. previous sarcoid, drug, and substance use or abuse – all might be relevant.

- For all patients: weight loss or anorexia (?malignancy); temperatures or night sweats (?vasculitis or infection); sore throat (?post-streptococcal condition); rashes (?Lyme disease, SLE, DM, PSA, vasculitis, sarcoid, SAPHO, Behçet's Disease).
- For those with widespread bony pain: history of rickets (?privational osteomalacia); chronic renal disease (will precede renal osteodystrophy and may predispose to osteoarticular deposition of β_2-microglobulin and crystal arthritides.

Psychosocial and sexual history
- Preceding sexual contact and genital infection is important primarily because of an association of *Chlamydia trachomatis* infection with reactive arthritis and enthesitis/SpA.
- Reactive arthritis has an association with HIV. HIV can cause acute myositis and is a risk factor for pyomyositis and severe PSA.
- There is an association of anxiety and depression with FM (p. 479).
- Asking specifically about genital lesions can disclose a history of recurrent ulcers in Behçet's Disease.

Family history
- There is an hereditary component to large joint, and generalized nodal OA, PSA, and the SpAs and gout.
- The risk of developing any autoimmune condition is higher in families of patients with autoimmune diseases than generally.

Drug history
- The following have been reported, to cause a myopathy: lithium, chloroquine*, clofibrate, statins, salbutamol, penicillin, colchicine, D-penicillamine*, sulphonamides, hydralazine, ciclosporin, phenytoin, cimetidine* (muscle cramps), zidovudine, carbimazole, and tamoxifen (*painful).
- Myositis from D-penicillamine is not dose- or cumulative dose-dependent. It can be life threatening.
- Drug-induced SLE, which is characterized commonly by arthralgia, aching and malaise, and polyarthritis, occurs with a number of drugs, including hydralazine, procainamide, isoniazid, and minocycline. Quinidine, labetalol, captopril, phenytoin, methyldopa, and sulphasalazine are among others that probably cause the condition.
- Alcohol in excess can cause severe toxic myopathy occasionally resulting in rhabdomyolysis.

The relevance of cardiovascular and respiratory symptoms and diseases
- Cardiac abnormalities are features of autoimmune rheumatic and connective tissue diseases, although infrequent at initial presentation. Cardiac infection is associated with widespread aches and pains (e.g. rheumatic fever/post-streptococcal myoarthralgia, infective endocarditis).
- Exertional dyspnoea owing to interstitial lung disease occurs in many patients with autoimmune connective tissue and rheumatic diseases. Up to 40% of RA patients may have CT evidence of lung fibrosis. In the majority of (usually sedentary) RA patients, symptoms are often mild.
- Ventilatory failure and aspiration pneumonia (?postural/nocturnal cough) can occur as a result of a combination of truncal striated, diaphragmatic and smooth muscle weakness in PM.

- RA is associated with bronchiectasis.
- Pericardial pains and pericarditis is not unusual in SLE patients prone to get serositis.
- The commonest neoplasm in patients diagnosed with carcinomatous myositis, is of the lung.
- Chronic dry cough can be associated with interstitial lung disease and dryness of airways (Sjögren's).

The relevance of gastrointestinal symptoms and diseases
- Patients may have overlooked volunteering abdominal and gut symptoms especially if symptoms have resolved. There are many links between bowel disease and polyarthralgia/polyarthritis (e.g. Crohn's Disease, UC, Sjögren's, Whipple's).
- Ask specifically about previous severe diarrhoeal or dysenteric illnesses, which, if due to *Campylobacter, Yersinia, Shigella,* or *Salmonella,* may be relevant to diagnosing reactive arthritis/SpA.
- Gut smooth muscle may be affected in PM and scleroderma (dysmotility), and give rise to dysphagia and abdominal pain.
- Non-specific bowel symptoms are relatively common in Sjögren's (?pancreatic exocrine dysfunction), unusual in SLE, but occur (?serosal lesions or thromboembolic lesions)

The relevance of neurological symptoms and diseases
- Widespread pain accompanying neurological disease is unusual, but occurs in a few scenarios.
- Slowly evolving cervical myelopathy often presents with widespread stiffness and discomfort with pain ensuing relatively late in the progression of disease. Sometimes sensory symptoms are not volunteered.
- Patients with a lesion in the cord (e.g. post-traumatic syrinx) can also complain about a discomfort in all four limbs, which can mimic musculoskeletal stiffness. Pain can be prominent but is not necessarily the main complaint.
- Sarcoidosis can affect the meninges and produce fluctuating sensory symptoms often characterized by diffuse dysaesthesia. Symptoms are not necessarily radicular or dermatomal.

Examination
In patients with widespread pain a full medical examination is always necessary.

Skin and nails
- Nails may show prominent ridges or pits in psoriatic arthropathy, splinter haemorrhages in infective endocardtis, rheumatoid vasculitis, or antiphopholipidsyndrome (APLS), or periungual erythema.
- Skin rashes that occur in conditions characterized by widespread pain, e.g. erythema migrans in Lyme disease, erythema marginatum in rheumatic fever, UV sensitive rash on face/arms in SLE, violacious rash on knuckles/around eyes/base of neck in dermatomyositis (DM), livedo reticularis in SLE/APLS, purpuric rash in vasculitis.
- Psoriasis is often mild and in discrete places such as the hairline, around the waist or natal cleft.
- Signs of anaemia are a non-specific finding in many chronic systemic autoimmune diseases.
- Clubbing of the digits may be present in Crohn's disease and ulcerative colitis (associated with SpA), hypertrophic

osteoarthropathy and bronchiectasis (associated with RA).
- Oedema can occur in both upper and lower limb peripheries in a subset of patients presenting with inflammatory polyarthritis/tenosynovitis. The condition has been termed RS3PE (remitting seronegative symmetrical synovitis with pitting oedema) syndrome. This condition occurs suddenly, often in patients between 60 and 80 years old, and is very disabling. It can be associated with haematological or neoplastic disease.
- Acneiform rashes occur in Behçet's disease, SAPHO and in sarcoid.

Musculoskeletal examination
Note the *specific cause* of joint swelling, site of tenderness, distribution of affected sites, and any intrinsic hypermobility.
- Bony swelling at DIPJs (Heberden's nodes) and PIPJs (Bouchard's nodes) is a feature of OA, but signs can mimic PSA. Look for any dactylitis (can be acute or indolent) and tenderness of phalanges distant from joint (enthesitis/dactylitis) in PSA. Periosteal new bone at sites of chronic enthesitis may be palpable and tender in PSA, but not OA.
- Non-bony nodules may occur in RA, polyarticular gout, multicentric reticulohistiocytosis, or hyperlipidaemia (xanthomata).
- The 'painful joints' may be inflamed tendons or entheses. Tender tendon insertions and peri-articular bone tenderness, without any joint swelling, may denote enthesis inflammation associated with SpA.
- Tendonitis may be part of many autoimmune rheumatic or connective tissue diseases (e.g. thickening of the digital flexors and swelling of the dorsal extensor tendon sheath in the hand and tenderness/swelling of both peroneal and posterior tibial tendons in the foot.
- Gross swelling with painful restriction of small joints is unusual in SLE. Often there is little to find on examination of joints.
- General joint hypermobility may account for, or contribute to, joint and other soft tissue lesions. An examination screen for hypermobility (p. 442) may be helpful.

If widespread myalgia is more likely than joint pain
- Establish there is muscle pathology rather than symptoms perceived in muscles and occurring in other structures (e.g. entheses) or referred from elsewhere (e.g. neurological or vascular disease).
- The characteristic sites of tenderness in FM (p. 442) should be recognized. However, in FM despite discomfort muscles should be strong.
- Be careful about diagnosing FM if there are tender points at entheses, which can occur in SpA or sarcoidosis. Tenderness of plantar fascia origin and around hind feet would be relevant in this respect.
- The strength testing of truncal and some limb muscles may be difficult in the presence of pain.
- Patterns of muscle weakness are not disease specific. Characteristic patterns: symmetrical proximal limb and truncal in PM/DM (p. 282 and p. 290); quadriceps and forearm/finger flexors in inclusion body myositis; limb muscles in mitochondrial myopathy.
- Muscles in PMR are not intrinsically weak.
- Muscle wasting is not specific, but if profound and associated with a short history consider neoplasia.

- Increased limb tone and rigidity, most evident by stiff passive movement at a joint, is consistent with extrapyramidal disease. There may be resting tremor in the hand, facial impassivity and 'stiff' gait.
- Diagnostic testing for fatiguability in myasthenia (strictly) requires examination before and after a placebo-controlled, double blind injection of an anticholinesterase.
- In suspected cases of PM/DM examine carefully for cardiorespiratory abnormalities. Other associated features in DM include periungual erythema/telangiectasias, (see Plate 11) erythematous violacious rash and skin calcinosis, dysphagia and dysphonia.
- Because of its associations, patients with myositis should be carefully examined for the following signs: dry eyes/mouth (Sjögren's, p. 254), skin thickening/tenderness or discolouration (scleroderma), skin rashes (SLE), thyroid tenderness/enlargement (endocrine myopathy).

Investigations
General points
- ESR and CRP may be raised in either infection or autoimmune connective tissue or rheumatic diseases. A slightly increased ESR is a common finding in healthy elderly people.
- Antinuclear antibody (ANA) may occur in association with many autoimmune conditions, in other diseases and in some healthy people. It is, therefore, not diagnostic for SLE or any single condition; however, high-titre ANA is often significant and, from a converse perspective, SLE without ANA is rare (IF on Hep2).
- Rheumatoid factor (RF) is not specific for RA. For example 1:6 people with infection or an inflammatory condition produce detectable RFs. Low titre RF occurs increasingly with age in healthy people. RFs occur in smokers. High titre RF occurs in Sjögren's syndrome, cryoglobulinaemia, and other systemic vasculitides notably.
- Controversy exists about the existence and diagnosis of FM. It is prudent only to make a diagnosis of FM in the presence of normal ESR, CRP, FBC (CBC), urea, electrolytes, liver function, and thyroid function tests, and if enthesitis-related disorders (e.g. SpAs and sarcoid) can be confidently excluded. Blood calcium, phosphate, serum immunoglobulins, ACE, and protein electrophoresis may reasonably be added to this list.
- Persistently elevated complement C3 and/or serum amyloid A (SAA) would call into question the existence of FM alone without an underlying chronic inflammatory condition.

Basic tests in patients with polyarthropathy
- Urinalysis (dipstick) can show proteinuria or haematuria – glomerular or tubular damage are possible.
- ESR and CRP are often raised in autoimmune rheumatic/connective tissue diseases, although they are non-specific and may be normal in the early stages of these conditions. If very high (e.g. ESR > 100 mm/h) be suspicious of infection or malignancy. ESR >50 mm/h is one diagnostic criterion of giant cell arteritis. There is often no acute phase response in patients with enthesitis (even although pain and bony tenderness may be widespread).
- A mild normochromic normocytic anaemia often accompanies autoimmune connective tissue or rheumatic diseases, infections, and malignancy.
- Throat swab, ASOT, anti-DNAaseB antibodies (post-streptococcal condition).

- Other simple blood tests, which should be considered given appropriate clinical evidence for the relevant disease: random blood sugar, thyroid function tests/thyroid antibodies, liver function tests, and prostatic specific antigen.
- Joint fluid aspiration and culture is mandatory for patients in whom sepsis is a possibility. Fluid should be examined by polarized light microscopy in suspected cases of crystal-induced synovitis.
- Testing serum for extractable nuclear antigens (ENAs) may be useful for characterizing the type of autoimmune process. None should be considered alone to be diagnostic or specific for any disease, although diagnostic information is available from certain positive or negative associations.
- In most patients presenting with a short history of widespread joint pains, radiographs will be normal.
- Referral to a sexual health clinic for detailed investigations if there's a suggestion of recent or recurrent genital infection/symptoms may help to strengthen the evidence for a diagnosis of reactive arthritis.

Basic laboratory tests in patients with widespread muscle pain/weakness

- Dipstick urinalysis: to screen for haematuria or myoglobinuria.
- FBC (CBC) and measures of acute-phase response.
- An endocrine and metabolic screen: urea, electrolytes, creatinine, thyroxine and thyroid-stimulating hormone (TSH), blood calcium, phosphate, and 25-hydroxyvitamin D, LFTs.
- Elevated CK occurs in most cases of PM. Creatine kinase (CK), ALT, AST, LDH are non-specific markers of muscle damage. Specific muscle iso-enzymes of CK and LDH exist and normal range of all enzymes may vary in different populations probably mainly as a function of muscle bulk (e.g. Afro-Caribbean > Caucasian).
- Muscle enzymes can be elevated after non-inflammatory muscle damage, e.g. exercise/trauma.
- Check for ANA and, if positive, screen for ENAs. Antibodies to certain (cytoplasmic) tRNA synthetases (e.g. Jo-1) are myositis-specific.
- All of the above tests may reasonably be done in cases where muscle pains might be due to fibromyalgia, but other pathology needs excluding.
- Check for urinary myoglobin in cases where acute widespread muscle pain may be associated with excessive alcohol or ingestion of certain drugs (cocaine, amphetamines, ecstacy, heroin), exercise or trauma. Patients will be at risk of renal failure.
- PM can be the presenting feature of HIV disease. Consider testing HIV serology. In HIV-positive patients, infections causing muscle disease include TB and microsporidia.
- Viral myositis is often clinically indistinguishable from PM. Serology, and PCR of muscle tissue or inflammatory cells may reveal diagnostic clues.

Electrophysiology and imaging in patients with muscle conditions

- Electromyographic abnormalities occur in 60–70% of patients with muscle inflammation. More information is likely if studied in the acute rather than the chronic phase of the illness. In the acute condition denervation and muscle degeneration give rise to fibrillation potentials in 74% of PM and 33% of DM patients. Other features include low-amplitude short-duration motor unit and polyphasic potentials.
- Electromyography is poor at discriminating on-going muscle inflammation in myositis from steroid-induced myopathy.
- There are characteristic MR patterns of abnormality in PM/DM. Images can be used to identify potential muscle biopsy sites to avoid false-negative results associated with patchy muscle inflammation.

Muscle biopsy

- With sizeable tissue samples from affected muscle and judicious use of a range of laboratory techniques, diagnostic information can be provided. Differential diagnosis needs to be discussed with the pathologist whilst planning the biopsy.
- Myositis may be patchy and biopsy may miss affected muscle. MR is sensitive in identifying areas of muscle inflammation.
- In PM, inflammatory infiltrates predominate in the endomysial area around muscle fibres without perifascicular atrophy. In DM inflammation is prominent in the perimysial area and around small blood vessels and there is typically perifascicular atrophy.
- Routine tests do not reliably distinguish PM from cases of viral myositis. Some of the glycogenoses will become obviously apparent from light microscopy of biopsy material.

Investigations for malignancy

Investigations in adults with widespread muscle or bony pain should aim to rule out malignancy, particularly myeloma and 2° malignancies from breast, renal, and prostate cancers.

- Investigations may include breast US, mammography and MR, urine cytology, PSA, renal US, serum, and urinary protein electrophoresis.
- Hypercalcaemia may accompany these conditions, thus check blood calcium, phosphate, and albumin.
- PTH should be checked in suspected cases of osteomalacia (raised 2° to calcium/vitamin D deficiency) together with 25-hydroxyvitamin D levels (low or low/normal), and ALP (high/normal).
- Bone scintigraphy can identify sites of neoplasia, Paget's disease, severe osteomalacia.
- Bone biopsy (maintained undecalcified by placing sample in 70% alcohol) of affected sites will be diagnostic in some, but not all, cases of osteomalacia, osteoporosis, renal osteodystrophy, malignancy, and Paget's disease. Good samples are hard to obtain. The best samples are obtained from a transiliac biopsy. Bone marrow can be aspirated for examination at the same time.

Chapter 2

Investigation of rheumatic disease

Plain radiography 24
Ultrasound 26
Computed tomography 30
Magnetic resonance imaging 34
Radionuclide imaging 36
Autoimmune serology 38
Synovial fluid analysis 42
Clinical neurophysiology 44

Plain radiography

Plain films remain the most commonly used imaging modality for the investigation of rheumatic disease despite the advent of more complex techniques. There are a number of reasons for this:

- Plain films are convenient for patients, cheap and reproducible. This allows direct comparison between films taken at different times and at different sites in the follow-up of patients.
- The resolution of X-ray film exceeds that of MRI, CT, ultrasound or nuclear medicine, providing exquisite detail of fine bony architecture.
- The body of knowledge of the radiology of rheumatic disease is based on plain film appearances, and it remains the most useful imaging technique for discriminating between the various arthropathies.

Disadvantages

- Plain films involve ionizing radiation and this needs to be taken into consideration in their use. For instance a lumbar spine film has the equivalent radiation dose of 50 chest X-rays.
- They are insensitive in the early stages of many diseases.
- They provide at best limited evidence of soft tissue pathology, such as tendon rupture.

Indications

Plain films are the usual imaging technique for the initial investigation of a symptomatic joint or joints, and serial imaging allows assessment of disease progression or response to therapy.

Whilst plain films are commonly used in the investigation of any symptomatic joint, the hands are most often imaged for initial assessment and follow-up of localized and more generalized arthralgia. The standard view is the antero-posterior (AP) projection of both hands. This allows assessment of both the nature of any radiographic change and its distribution.

Plain films can also be useful in the evaluation of joint stability. For example, lateral views of the cervical spine in flexion and extension allow assessment of instability at the craniocervical junction in patients with rheumatoid arthritis.

Plain film findings

The following are the major findings seen on plain films in rheumatological disease. They are described in relation to the hands in line with clinical practice and for ease of comparison, except where otherwise specified.

Soft tissue swelling (Figure 2.1)
Peri-articular soft tissue swelling often reflects synovitis, and until the advent of ultrasound and MRI was often the earliest radiological finding in arthritis. It also occurs in:

- Joint effusions or bursal distention (e.g. pre-patellar bursitis).
- Dactylitis.
- Soft tissue injuries.
- Crystal arthropathy, when calcific deposits may be seen in the soft tissues or cartilage (CPPDD).

Osteopaenia (Figure 2.2)
Osteopaenia is defined as reduction of bone quantity whilst maintaining quality, whereas osteoporosis specifically reflects reduced osteoid production.

Localized osteopaenia occurs in:
- Rheumatoid arthritis, when it occurs in a peri-articular distribution and reflects increased bone turnover and resorption.
- Regional migratory osteoporosis.
- Complex regional pain syndrome and disuse atrophy.
- The initial stages of osteomyelitis.
- Early lytic Paget's disease (osteoporosis circumscripta).
- Focal lesions of bone, such as metastases and myeloma.

Generalized osteopaenia occurs in:
- Senile osteoporosis with subsequent fracturing.
- Osteomalacia as a result of poor quality osteoid.
- Hyperparathyroidism.
- Haemochromatosis.
- Diffuse metastatic disease or myeloma.
- Drug therapy, particularly long-term high dose steroids.
- Osteogenesis imperfecta.

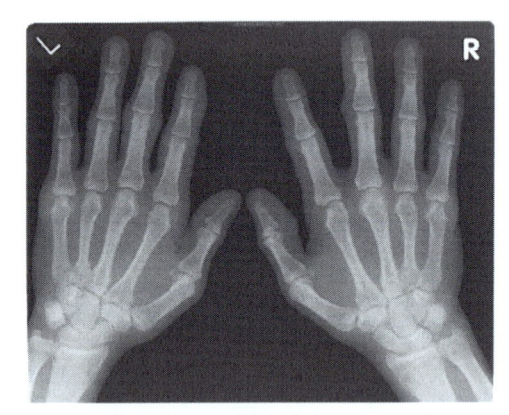

Figure 2.1 Early gout arthropathy with peri-articular soft tissue swelling and calcification.

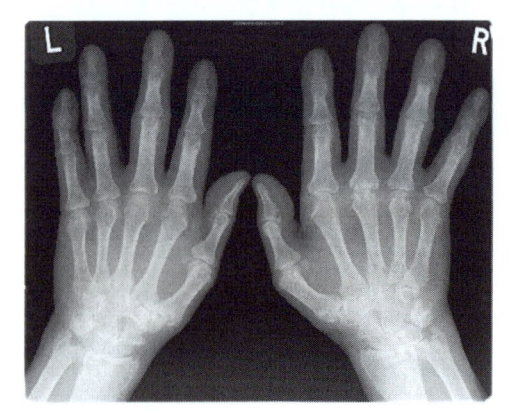

Figure 2.2 Rheumatoid arthritis with subtle ulnar deviation of MCP joints and peri-articular osteopaenia and erosions.

CHAPTER 2 **Investigation of rheumatic disease**

Sclerosis (Figure 2.3)
Subchondral sclerosis is seen in osteoarthritis accompanied by reduced joint space and subchondral cyst formation, but localized sclerosis may also occur in:
- Avascular necrosis and bone infarcts.
- Osteomyelitis.
- Paget's disease.
- Fibrous dysplasia.
- Benign focal lesions, such as bone island, osteoid osteoma and healing fractures.
- Primary and secondary bone tumours.
Generalized sclerosis is seen in:
- Myelofibrosis.
- Diffuse metastatic disease.
- Sickle cell disease.
- Advanced Paget's disease.
- Polyostotic fibrous dysplasia.
- Renal osteodystrophy.
- Hypoparathyroidism and pseudohypoparathyroidism.

Erosions (Figure 2.2)
Erosions represent focal cortical lucencies and occur as a result of local inflammation. They are seen in:
- Rheumatoid arthritis.
- Psoriatic arthritis, unlike rheumatoid arthritis (RA) tending to affect the DIP joints.
- Reiter's syndrome, which primarily affects in the feet.
- Erosive (inflammatory) osteoarthritis.
- Ankylosing spondylitis, especially at the margins of vertebrae (preceding the sclerotic 'shining corner' or Romanus lesion).
- Gout, in which the erosions are adjacent to the articular surface and have the typical appearance of an overhanging edge and sclerotic margin ('rat bite' erosion).
- Haemophilia.
- Acro-osteolysis (erosion of the terminal tufts) occurs in psoriatic arthritis, scleroderma, hyperparathyroidism and Sjögren's syndrome (Figure 2.4).

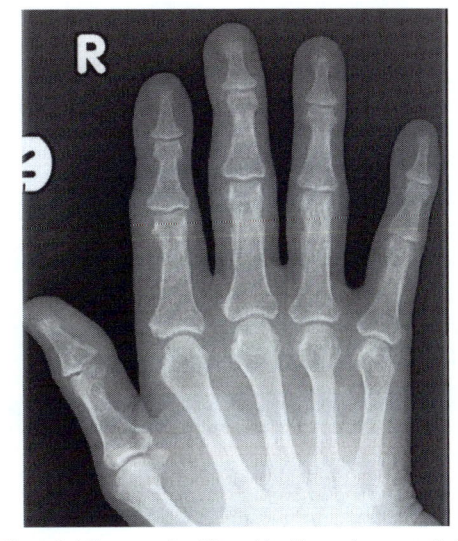

Figure 2.4 Hyperparathyroidism with widespread acro-osteolysis, and sub-periosteal resorption of bone affecting the index finger middle phalanx.

Bone proliferation (Figure 2.3)
The osteophyte is the hallmark of osteoarthritis, but bony proliferation may also be seen in:
- Inflammatory spondyloarthropathy, in which there is new bone formation at the enthesis (e.g. syndesmophyte).
- Diffuse idiopathic skeletal hyperostosis (DISH).
- Healing fractures.
- Bone-forming tumours.

Other findings

Joint Space (Figure 2.3)
The joint space may be increased in the presence of active synovitis which distends the joint. Joint space reduction is a hallmark of osteoarthritis, and is also a feature of psoriatic arthritis, CPPDD, and haemochromatosis. It is less common in gout, sarcoidosis, scleroderma, and is seen only late in rheumatoid arthritis.

Malalignment (Figure 2.3)
Joints may become malaligned sue to asymmetric loss of joint space, such as in the *genu vara* deformity seen in osteoarthritis. Subluxation and dislocation may occur in advanced rheumatoid arthritis as a result of ligamentous instability (Figure 2.2).

Periosteal reaction
In rheumatological practice this is seen in Reiter's syndrome, juvenile idiopathic arthritis (JIA) and psoriatic arthritis. It is also seen in bone tumours, osteomyelitis, healing fractures, hypertrophic osteoarthropathy, thyroid acropachy, and venous stasis. Subperiosteal resorption of bone is a characteristic feature of hyperparathyroidism (Figure 2.4).

Lucencies
Subchondral cysts are a hallmark of osteoarthrosis, and are also seen in haemophilia, amyloidosis, and haemochromatosis.

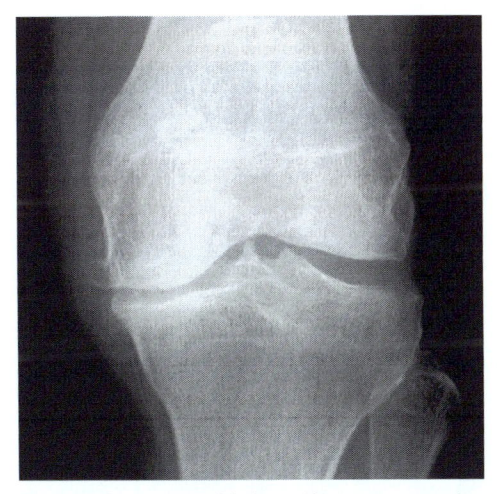

Figure 2.3 Osteoarthritis of the knee with joint space narrowing, subchondral sclerosis, peripheral osteophyte formation, and varus deformity.

Ultrasound

Ultrasound has only fairly recently been introduced in musculoskeletal cases and its use is expanding rapidly. Unlike other modalities ultrasound enables clinical correlation as the radiologist is with the patient while performing the scan.

Advantages
- Unlike plain films, computerized tomography (CT) and nuclear medicine, it does not involve ionizing radiation.
- It is quick to perform and well tolerated by patients.
- It is cheaper to perform than CT and magnetic resonance imaging (MRI).
- The apparatus is portable and so can be used in clinic or at the bedside.
- It provides excellent resolution of soft tissues, including assessment of neovascularity with Doppler imaging.
- It allows precise real-time targeting of needles for diagnostic and therapeutic intervention.

Disadvantages
- It is operator dependant to a greater extent than other modalities, which may make follow-up assessment less accurate.
- It is only able to assess the bone surface so cannot identify marrow oedema or pure bony abnormalities.

Indications
Clinical indications for ultrasound in rheumatological practice include, but are not limited to:
- Assessment for synovitis and/or taenosynovitis in early arthralgia, thereby allowing prompt initiation of disease-modifying antirheumatic drugs. Erosions are also well demonstrated.
- Assessment of rotator cuff pathology. Unlike MRI, ultrasound allows dynamic scanning to investigate impingement, and is the initial investigation of choice for rotator cuff pathology in many institutions in the UK.
- Investigation of masses such as ganglia.
- Investigation of functional problems such as trigger finger.
- Guiding diagnostic and/or therapeutic injections, including bursal injections and joint aspirations.

Joints (Figure 2.5)
Synovitis
Ultrasound is becoming increasingly utilized in the investigation and management of early arthralgia as it can detect synovitis at an earlier stage than plain films, and is of comparable sensitivity to MRI, but significantly more convenient and cheaper.

Synovitis is seen as soft tissue proliferation arising from a joint with or without an effusion (see Figure 2.6). As expected it is hyperaemic on power Doppler scanning.

Other findings
In addition to synovitis, ultrasound is accurate in assessment for the presence of joint effusions and the constellation of abnormalities seen in osteoarthrosis including osteophytes, loose bodies, capsular proliferation and joint space narrowing.

Tendon abnormalities
Tendon degeneration spans a continuum from mild tendinosis through partial tears to complete rupture.

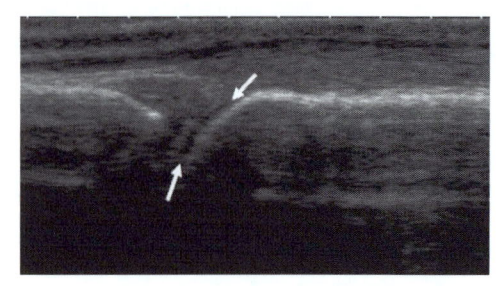

Figure 2.5 Normal MCP joint with the articular cartilage clearly seen as a thin black stripe on the metacarpal head (arrows).

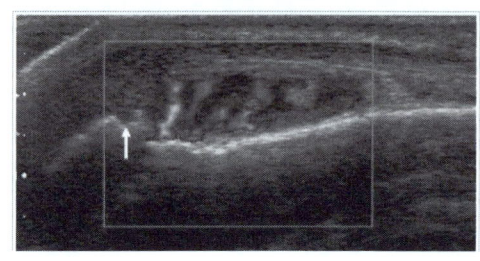

Figure 2.6 Synovitis of the thumb macrophage chemotactic protein (MCP) joint with an effusion and hyperaemia. An erosion is present (arrow).

Each of these stages can be accurately identified on ultrasound. The earliest signs are thickening, hypo-echogenicity and loss of the normal fibrillar pattern. Tears are seen as focal hypo-echoic clefts or defects, and the frayed ends of ruptured tendons can be localized prior to repair or reconstruction (Figure 2.7). Normal tendons contain no identifiable blood vessels, and their presence is a further indicator of tendon pathology.

Taenosynovitis usually appears as hypo-echoic fluid distending the sheath surrounding the tendon. It can contain echogenic hypertrophied synovium (Figure 2.8) and may or

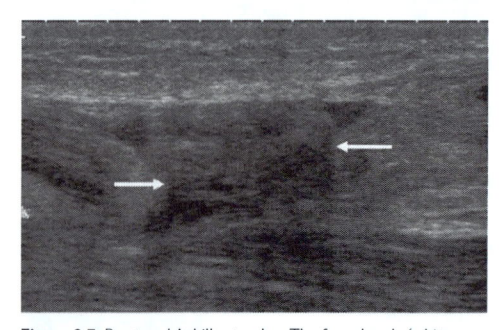

Figure 2.7 Ruptured Achilles tendon. The frayed ends (white arrows) are clearly seen and can be marked prior to reconstruction. The defect is filled with echogenic haematoma.

CHAPTER 2 Investigation of rheumatic disease

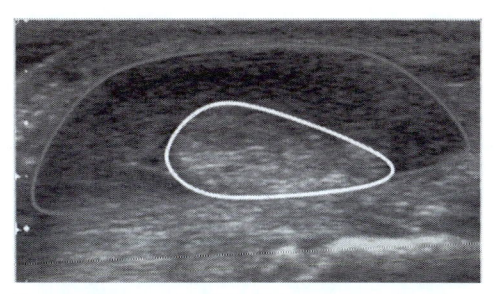

Figure 2.8 Taenosynovitis of the tibialis posterior tendon (white outline). The tendon sheath (red outline) is distended and contains echogenic synovium.

may not be associated with tendon abnormalities. The exception is De Quervain's taenosynovitis, which affects the extensor group one tendons at the wrist (abductor pollicis longus and extensor pollicis brevis). This is a stenosing taenosynovitis, which appears as a thickening of the tendon sheath with little or no associated fluid. Type 1 tendons, such as the Achilles are not surrounded by a tendon sheath, instead there is a layer of loose areolar tissue called paratenon. This too can become distended with fluid (paratendonitis).

Functional tendon abnormalities such as triggering and subluxation are well demonstrated using dynamic scanning, when tendon excursion can be observed during active and passive movement.

Bursae

Bursae usually occur in recognized locations and are easily assessed with ultrasound. When inflamed they are usually seen as hypoechoic foci with a hyperechoic margin. The subacromial-subdeltoid bursa (Figure 2.9) is often distended in patients with rotator cuff symptoms, and can be seen overlying the supraspinatus tendon. Dynamic scanning during shoulder abduction may show filling of the bursa and/or bunching up of the tendon fibres under the acromion and/or coraco-acromial ligament and confirms impingement.

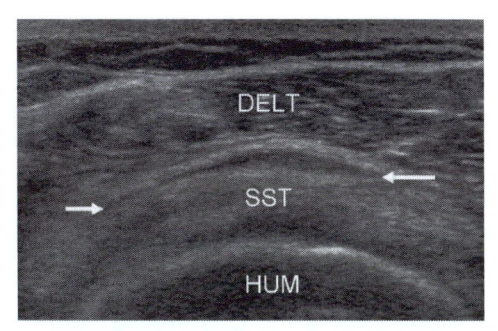

Figure 2.9 Distended and inflamed subacromial-subdeltoid bursa (white arrows). The humeral head (HUM), supraspinatus tendon (SST) and overlying deltoid (DELT) are shown.

The pre-Achilles, pre-patellar, intermetatarsal, iliopsoas, trochanteric, olecranon, and semimembranosus-medial head of gastrocnemius (Baker's cyst) bursae are amongst those also frequently visualized. They may contain hypertrophied synovium or loose bodies.

Soft tissue masses

Ultrasound is a valuable tool in the investigation of superficial soft tissue masses due to its excellent spatial resolution and Doppler assessment. Ganglia are seen as lobulated, septated fluid collections in characteristic locations such as the dorsum of the wrist (Figure 2.10). The neck of the ganglion can usually be followed to an underlying joint or ligament. Lipomas are also well seen, except benign unencapsulated superficial lipomas, which are indistinguishable from the normal subcutaneous fat. Vascular malformations are usually soft masses with varying amounts of fat but are strikingly hypervascular (Figure 2.11). Their feeding vessels can often be traced. Malignant soft tissue masses are also well seen, but ultrasound has limited specificity and MRI scanning is usually required.

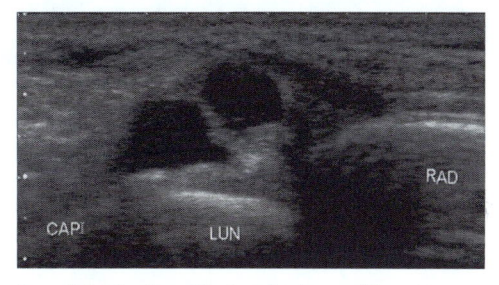

Figure 2.10 Ganglion arising from the dorsum of the wrist, seen as a lobulated and septated fluid collection. The distal radius (RAD), lunate (LUN) and capitate (CAP) have been marked.

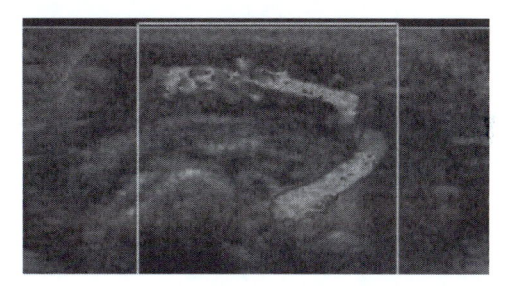

Figure 2.11 Vascular malformation over the thenar eminence with a prominent feeding vessel.

Intervention

The use of ultrasound to guide interventional procedures in the musculoskeletal system is increasing rapidly. It enables real-time visualization of needle position and so is likely to reduce the risk of injections or biopsies being inaccurate.

Interventional procedures performed with ultrasound include:

- Therapeutic injection of corticosteroid into tendon sheaths, joints or bursae (Figure 2.12).
- Diagnostic injection of local anaesthetic into joints, for example, into the hip to distinguish between lumbar and hip origins of leg pain.
- Aspiration of joints, tendon sheaths, or soft tissue collections when infection is being considered.

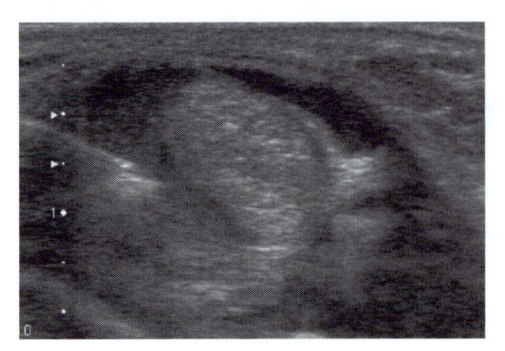

Figure 2.12 Ultrasound-guided injection of corticosteroid into the tendon sheath of tibialis posterior. The needle is seen entering from the left with echogenic steroid filling the distended sheath.

- Dry needling of tendonitis and enthesitis, e.g. tennis elbow, plantar fasciitis, and Achilles tendonitis. This is usually accompanied by steroid infiltration into the adjacent soft tissues. The injection of autologous blood into damaged tendon may be used in refractive cases.
- Barbotage and aspiration of calcific tendonitis.
- Aspiration and barbotage of ganglia.
- Biopsy of soft tissue masses. This is often done to confirm or exclude a sarcoma, in which case it should only be performed under the clear direction of the surgeon who would perform any subsequent resection. This is important because the biopsy tract needs to be excised at operation, and the procedure needs to be planned to avoid contamination of adjacent compartments.

Computed tomography

CT is a well established modality for imaging across the clinical spectrum. The recent introduction of multislice scanners allows detailed imaging of the musculoskeletal system.

Advantages
- Excellent detail of bone.
- Greater spatial resolution than MRI.
- Quick and generally well tolerated by patients.
- Widely accessible modality.
- Multidetector CT (MDCT) scans with multiplanar reconstructions allow joints to be viewed from many angles (Figure 2.13). 3D reconstructions can also be made and are particularly useful in trauma.
- High resolution CT (HRCT) of the chest is more sensitive than chest X-ray in assessing for the presence of pulmonary fibrosis or other interstitial processes.
- May be helpful if MRI is contraindicated (e.g. CT arthrogram in lien of MRI Knee).
- Can be used to guide interventional procedures, particularly in the spine.

Disadvantages
- CT involves ionizing radiation in significant dose. For example a CT of the lumbar spine is equivalent to 500 chest X-rays.
- Limited soft tissue detail, and early changes such as marrow oedema cannot be identified.
- Image quality is degraded in the presence of metallic prostheses or fixation devices.

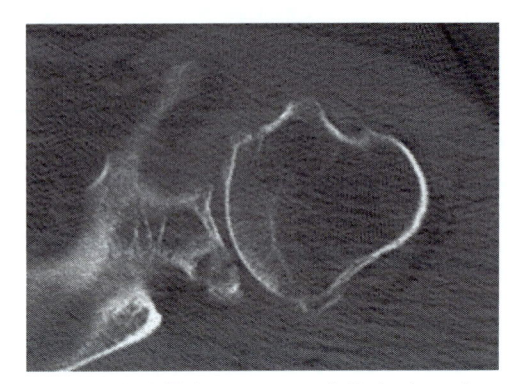

Figure 2.14 Axial CT showing an osteoarthritic glenohumeral joint prior to replacement. Note the reduced joint space, marginal osteophytes and subchondral sclerosis of the humeral head, and subchondral cysts in the glenoid.

- In assessing advanced inflammatory spondyloarthritis, in particular the extent of any ankylosis in the spine. It provides excellent detail of the sacroiliac joints, but MRI is often preferred in the early stages when marrow oedema precedes structural bone alteration.
- To accurately localize a lesion within bone, such as a cortically-based osteoid osteoma.

Trauma
CT imaging of the body is widely used in the context of acute trauma to exclude visceral or head injury. While plain films are usually the initial modality for skeletal trauma, CT is used to assess complex fractures, to exclude fractures where plain films are inconclusive, and for follow-up of fractures and their fixation. Examples include:
- Assessment of bony detail in spinal injuries. Sagittal and coronal reconstructions are especially useful (Figure 2.15) particularly if there is pre-existing spinal disease, such as ankylosing spondylitis.
- Assessment of pelvic fractures, when 3D reconstructions are often performed (Figure 2.16).

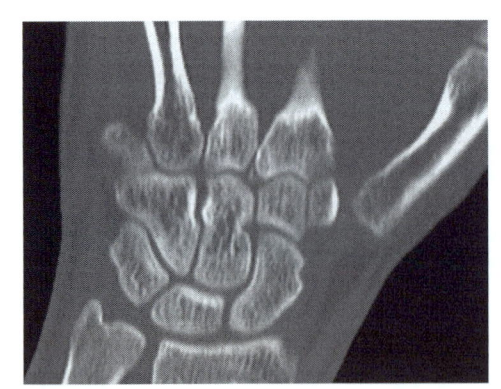

Figure 2.13 Single image from a CT of a normal wrist reconstructed in the coronal plane. Note the excellent bone but limited soft tissue detail.

Clinical applications
CT is useful in a number of clinical scenarios.

Arthropathy
- CT is particularly useful prior to joint replacement in order to assess the state of the articular surfaces, e.g. the glenoid prior to shoulder replacement (Figure 2.14).
- To quantify the extent of bone destruction in processes such as septic arthritis.

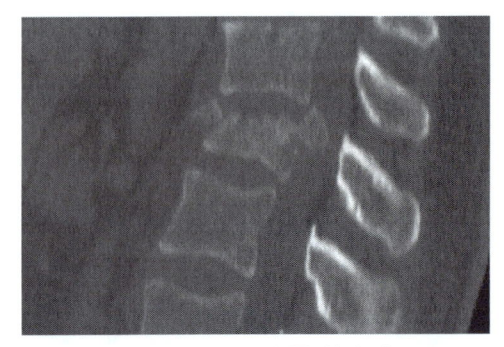

Figure 2.15 Sagittally reconstructed CT of the lumbar spine showing a burst fracture of L1, with a large retropulsed fragment lying in the spinal canal.

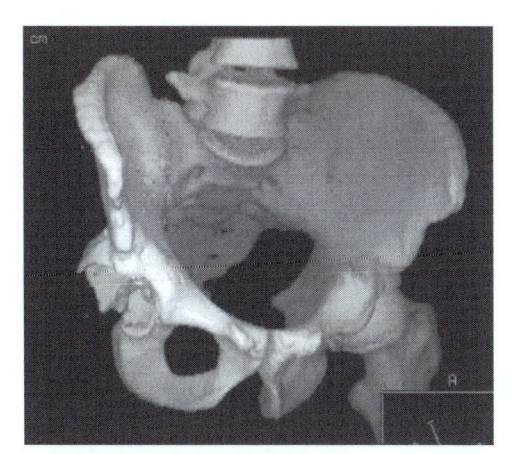

CHAPTER 2 **Investigation of rheumatic disease** 31

Figure 2.16 3D reconstruction of the bony pelvis showing a fractured posterior right acetabular wall.

- To confirm or exclude non-union of fractures.
- In the investigation of pars defects, particularly if surgery is being considered (Figure 2.17).
- CT arthrography or myelography is occasionally used in patients in whom MRI is contraindicated (Figure 2.18).

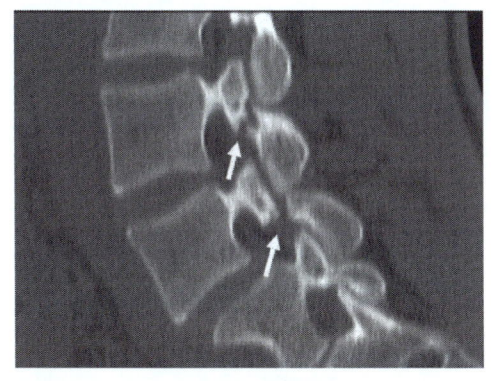

Figure 2.17 Sagittally reconstructed CT of the lumbar spine showing pars defects at L4 and L5 (white arrows).

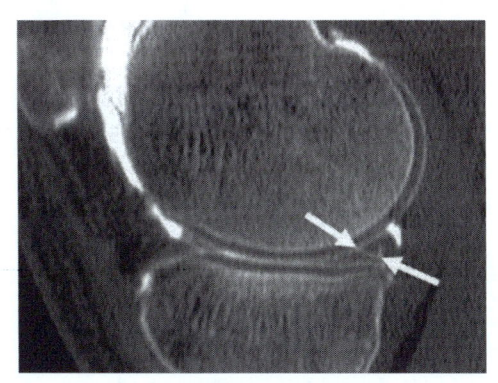

Figure 2.18 CT arthrogram of the knee showing a tear of the medial meniscus (white arrows).

Intervention
CT is used to guide interventional procedures in the musculoskeletal system and elsewhere, for example:
- Spinal nerve root blocks and facet joint injections.
- Bone biopsy.
- Lung and other visceral biopsy, particularly in the pelvis and retroperitoneum.

Chest imaging
CT of the chest is used to further assess masses or other abnormalities seen on chest X-ray. In rheumatological practice these may include:
- Granulomas in Wegener's disease.
- Nodules or pleural effusions in rheumatoid arthritis.
- Parenchymal masses, and/or mediastinal or hilar lymph nodes in sarcoid.
- Primary or secondary malignancy.

High resolution CT (HRCT) is the optimum modality for imaging the pulmonary parenchyma in the context of suspected interstitial lung disease. It achieves resolution of up to 300 μm and visualizes the secondary pulmonary lobule. Typical findings include:
- Basal fibrosis and 'honeycombing' in usual interstitial pneumonia (UIP, Figure 2.19), which is associated with rheumatoid arthritis and some drugs.
- Basal fibrosis and a dilated oesophagus in scleroderma.
- Upper lobe fibrosis in ankylosing spondylitis or sarcoidosis.
- Perilymphatic nodules, irregular septal thickening and traction bronchiectasis amongst other findings in sarcoidosis.

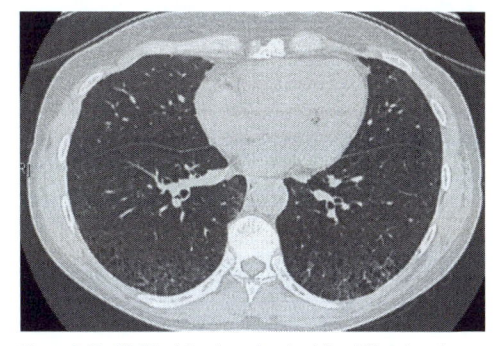

Figure 2.19 HRCT of the chest showing bibasal fibrosis and honeycombing. These appearances may be seen in rheumatoid arthritis and other collagen vascular diseases.

Other applications
Further applications of CT in rheumatological practice include:
- To investigate the sinuses and orbits in, for instance, Wegener's granulomatosis or lymphoma (Figure 2.20).
- CT angiography may be helpful in imaging the vascular system in polyarteritis nodosum or other vasculitides.
- To investigate abdominal masses, such as splenomegaly in SLE, rheumatoid arthritis, or sarcoidosis.
- To accurately assess the craniocervical junction in rheumatoid arthritis, particularly in the pre-operative situation.

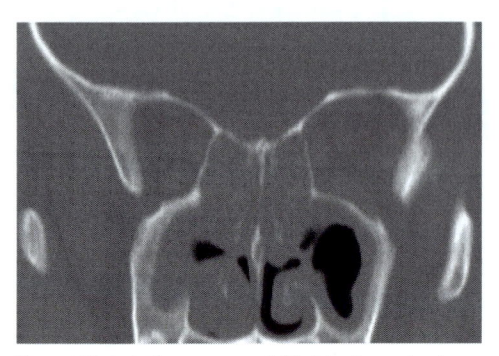

Figure 2.20 Sagittally reconstructed CT of the sinuses showing gross mucosal thickening and destruction of the inferior turbinate on the right in Wegener's.

Magnetic resonance imaging

MRI has only become widely available in the NHS within the last 10 years. It has a wide range of applications, with musculoskeletal imaging (including spine) forming a significant proportion of cases scanned.

Advantages

- It does not involve ionizing radiation, but instead forms images from electromagnetic radiation. This makes it a generally safe technique;
- Excellent soft tissue detail and contrast (Figure 2.21).
- It is the best modality for assessing bone marrow, and so is sensitive in the early stages of many diseases.
- Its ability to assess soft tissue and bone together, and in detail sets it apart from other modalities.
- MR arthrography has largely replaced conventional diagnostic arthroscopy, e.g. in imaging the glenoid labrum.

sensitive in the early stages of the process. However it remains unclear whether all those with an abnormal MRI will go on to develop a full-blown inflammatory spondyloarthopathy. Other advantages include:

- The ability to assess adjacent structures in the same examination, e.g. hips, pelvis and prevertebral structures.
- Repeat imaging can be used to assess disease response or progression.
- Reliable distinction between degenerative and inflammatory processes.
- Infective discitis and osteomyelitis are well seen (Figure 2.23).

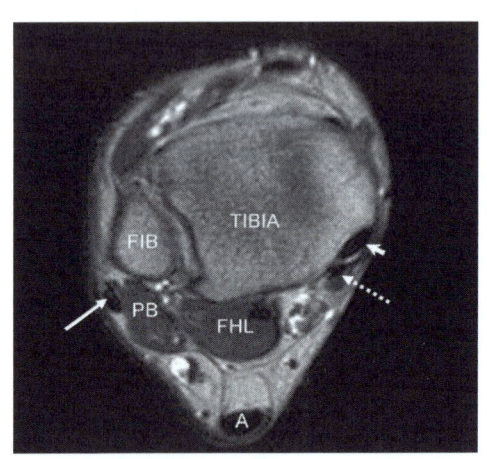

Figure 2.21 Axial T2-weighted MRI of a normal ankle showing the tendons of peroneus longus (solid arrow), peroneus brevis (PB), flexor hallucis longus (FHL), Achilles (A), flexor digitorum longus (broken arrow), and tibialis posterior (short arrow). The posterior tibial neurovascular bundle lies between FHL and FDL. The extensor tendons are seen anteriorly.

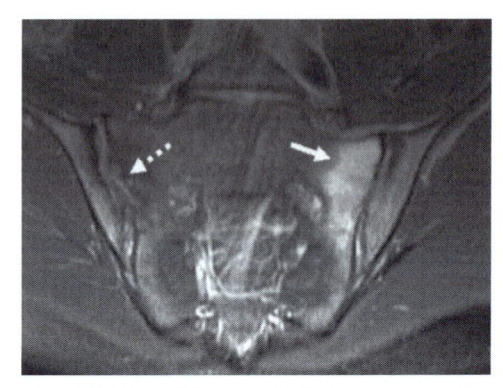

Figure 2.22 Coronal T2 fat saturated MRI of asymmetric sacroilitis, with marrow oedema (solid arrows) and erosions (broken arrows).

Disdvantages

- It is more expensive than other modalities.
- It is time consuming, with scans lasting from 20 min to 1 hour. It is also very sensitive to movement artefact.
- Many patients suffer from claustrophobia and cannot complete the examination.
- It is absolutely contraindicated in patients with devices such as cardiac pacemakers and neural stimulators.
- Whilst very sensitive to early disease processes, specificity can be limited. For example a joint effusion and synovial proliferation require contrast to be distinguished as both are of similar signal on unenhanced imaging.

MRI in inflammatory disease

Spine

MRI plays an important role in the investigation of inflammatory spondyloarthropathy (Figure 2.22). Whilst plain films and CT can only detect established bony changes, the ability of MRI to detect marrow oedema makes it very

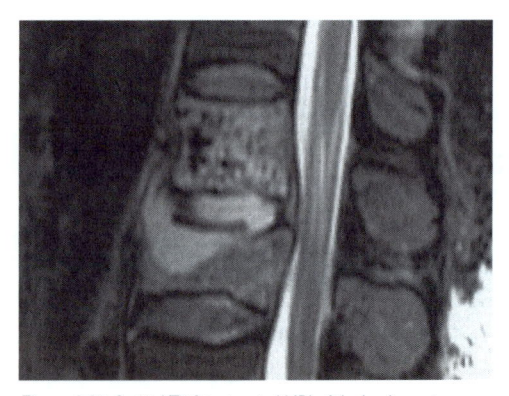

Figure 2.23 Sagittal T2 fat saturated MRI of the lumbar spine showing endplate destruction and a fluid collection in acute infective discitis.

Appendicular skeleton

Inflammatory disease of bone, joints and soft tissues in the peripheral skeleton is well demonstrated on MRI. Examples include:

- Hip pathologies such as avascular necrosis, synovitis and trochanteric bursitis (Figure 2.24);
- Tendinopathy and taenosynovitis, e.g. at the ankle;
- Subacromial bursitis and rotator cuff pathology;
- Inflammatory arthropathy with synovitis (Figure 2.25);

CHAPTER 2 **Investigation of rheumatic disease**

- Entheseal changes, e.g. tennis elbow
- Muscle abnormalities such as myositis or wasting with fatty infiltration.

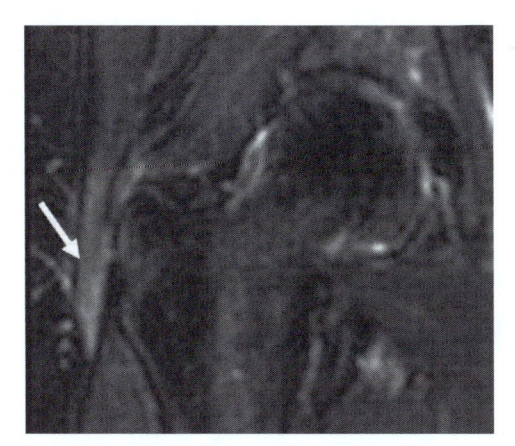

Figure 2.24 Coronal T2 fat saturated image of the left hip showing high signal adjacent to the greater trochanter indicating trochanteric bursitis and/or gluteal tendinopathy (arrow).

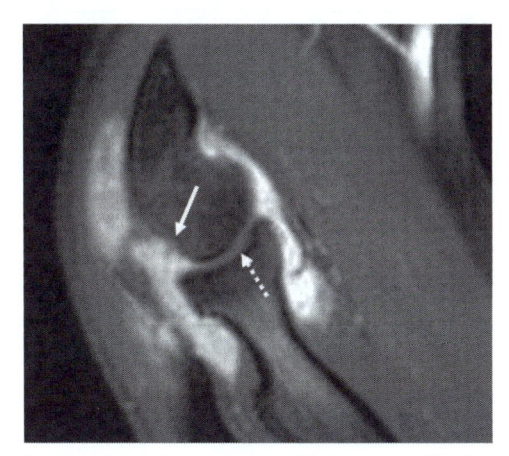

Figure 2.25 Sagittal contrast-enhanced T1 fat saturated MRI of the elbow in rheumatoid arthritis, showing prominent enhancing synovitis (high signal) with erosions of the capitellum (solid arrow) and cartilage thinning on the radius (broken arrow).

Degenerative disease

Spine

MRI is a fundamental part of the assessment of back pain, the majority of which is due to degenerative change affecting the intervertebral discs and/or the facet joints, with or without subsequent neural compression. MRI findings include:
- Loss of signal in and height of the intervertebral discs.
- Herniation of disc material causing compression of nerve roots in the lateral recess or exiting nerves in the intervertebral foramen (Figure 2.26).
- Spinal stenosis, which may cause cord compression, cauda equina syndrome or myelopathy.
- Spondylolisthesis, which may be due to facet joint degeneration or pars interarticularis defects.
- Vertebral end plate reactive changes.

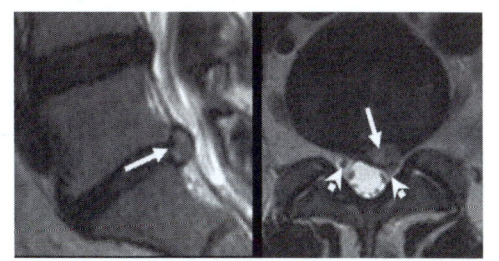

Figure 2.26 Coronal and sagittal T2 weighted images of a left paracentral disc herniation at L5/S1 compressing the traversing left S1 root in the lateral recess (arrowheads comparing both). Less severe degenerative changes affect the L4/5 disc.

Appendicular skeleton

MRI is also very sensitive in the early stages of the degenerative process in the remainder of the skeleton. Areas commonly imaged include:
- Hips
- Knees
- Ankles
- Shoulders
- Wrist

MR arthrograms are sometimes performed to assess cartilaginous structures, such as the labrum in the shoulder and hip, and articular cartilage surfaces in other joints, triangular fibrocartilagenous complex in the wrist.

MRI is also commonly used in trauma, both acute and chronic. A good example is in the investigation of osteochondral lesions which are most commonly seen in the knee and ankle (Figure 2.27).

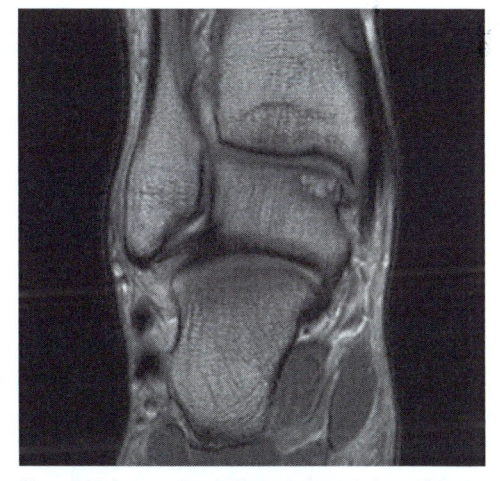

Figure 2.27 An osteochondral lesion is shown in the medial aspect of the talar dome. There is chondromalacia of the overlying articular cartilage.

Radionuclide imaging

Gamma camera imaging using radionuclides in the investigation of musculoskeletal cases is long established. Positron emission tomography (PET) imaging is a recent development whose role is expanding rapidly. All methods involve ionising radiation with a dose to each patient. For example the effective dose from a bone scan equates to 200 chest X-rays. The images generated are physiological, rather than anatomical as provided by other modalities (i.e. a bone scan is an image of the distribution of osteoblastic activity, rather than of the bones themselves).

Nuclear medicine

Bone scan (Figure 2.28)
Technetium-99m-labelled methylene diphosphonate (^{99m}Tc-MDP) is incorporated into bone at a rate dependant on blood flow and osteoblastic activity.

Advantages

- Cheap compared to MRI.
- Readily available with most radiology departments having gamma cameras on site.
- Excellent sensitivity to bone turnover. Increased uptake often precedes plain film changes.
- Whole body imaging allows investigation of non-specific abnormalities such as raised serum alkaline phosphatase.
- Early synovitis is seen as increased activity in the affected joint(s) and can be useful as a 'one shot' view, although it has largely been superseded by ultrasound or MRI.
- Early images visualize perfusion and blood pool phases, and so identify hyperaemia in infection/inflammation.
- Serial imaging enables follow-up.
- Improved anatomical detail with single photon emission computed tomography (SPECT) imaging, in which the gamma camera rotates 360° around the patient provides improved lesion conspicuity and spatial resolution at the expense of increased time for image acquisition.

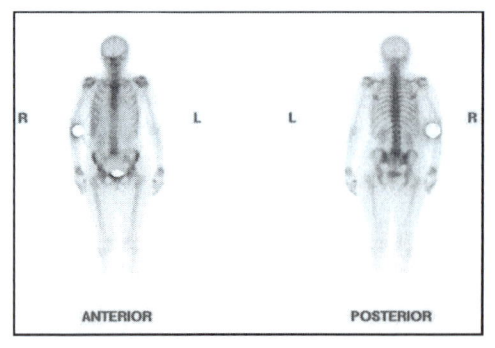

Figure 2.28 Bone scan showing mildly increased uptake of tracer at the CMC joints of both thumbs in keeping with osteoarthritis, but otherwise normal distribution of tracer.

Disadvantages

- Although sensitive to osteoblastic activity, it is not specific, with increased uptake seen in any area of increased bone turnover, including healing fractures, OA and other arthropathies, neoplastic lesions (both primary and secondary), infection, and avascular necrosis. Correlation with plain films or other modalities is often required. Improved specificity has been reported using ^{99m}Tc-labelled IgG.
- The radiation dose is higher than plain films.
- Limited anatomical detail.
- Lesions where there is not increased osteoblastic activity will not demonstrate increased activity may be missed, e.g. plasmacytoma.
- 'Cold spots' are areas of photopenia and occur where there is reduced osteoblastic activity compared with the surrounding bone and may be difficult to detect. Examples include fibrous dysplasia and prostheses.
- Interpretation in the immature skeleton is hampered by normal increased activity at the growth plates.

Rheumatological indications
Indications for bone scan in rheumatological practice include:

- Elevated serum markers but no localizing information (e.g. in Paget's disease).
- Investigation of painful prostheses.
- In complex regional pain syndrome (CRPS).
- Investigation of metastatic disease (Figure 2.29).

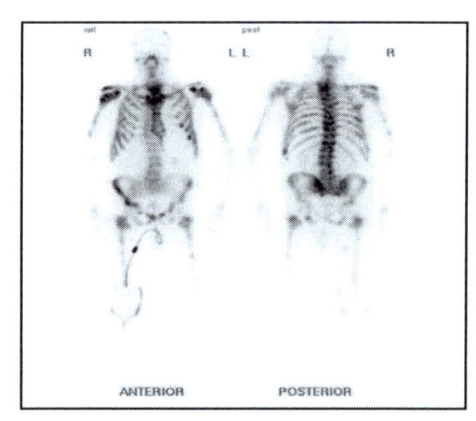

Figure 2.29 Bone scan showing multiple areas of increased uptake of ^{99m}Tc-MDP in a patient with extensive skeletal metastases. A urinary catheter is in place.

Other nuclear medicine applications

Other applications of nuclear medicine include:

- Ventilation-perfusion (V/Q) scans using ^{99m}Tc-labelled MAA for perfusion and aerosolized ^{99m}Tc-DTPA for ventilation in the investigation of pulmonary emboli. A normal chest X-ray is required to obtain adequate information, otherwise a CT pulmonary angiogram is performed.
- Indium-111 or ^{99m}Tc can be used to label white blood cells in imaging for infection or inflammation, e.g. in pyrexia of unknown origin, inflammatory bowel disease, infected grafts (Figure 2.30) or osteomyelitis.
- ^{99m}Tc-pertechnetate and occasionally Iodine-123 are used to image the thyroid in the investigation of a palpable mass, hyperthyroidism or thyroid malignancies. Iodine-131 is much higher energy and is used to treat active nodules, diffuse toxic goitre and thyroid cancer.

CHAPTER 2 **Investigation of rheumatic disease**

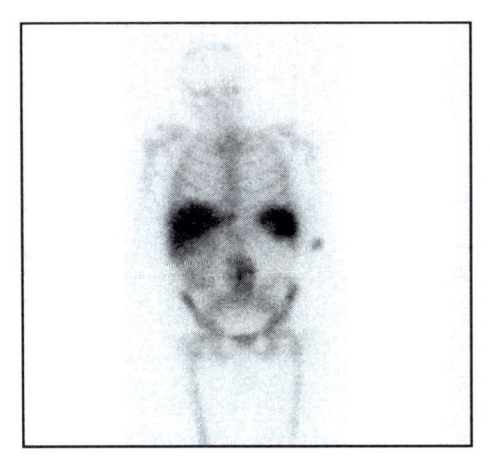

Figure 2.30 Indium-111 labelled WBC scan showing increased uptake around an infected aortic graft. Normal hepatic and splenic reticuloendothelial uptake.

- ^{99m}Tc-sestamibi imaging is used in parathyroid imaging.
- ^{99m}Tc-sestamibi is used in cardiac imaging to assess myocardial perfusion.
- ^{99m}Tc-labelled red blood cells, ^{99m}Tc sulphur colloid or ^{99m}Tc pertechnetate are used in the investigation of gastrointestinal bleeding.
- ^{99m}Tc-labelled DMSA or MAG-3 are used to investigate the renal tract in obstructive uropathy, renal failure, renal masses, or vesico-ureteric reflux.
- ^{99m}Tc-labelled albumin is injected intradermally and the activity traced proximally in the investigation of lymphoedema (Figure 2.31).

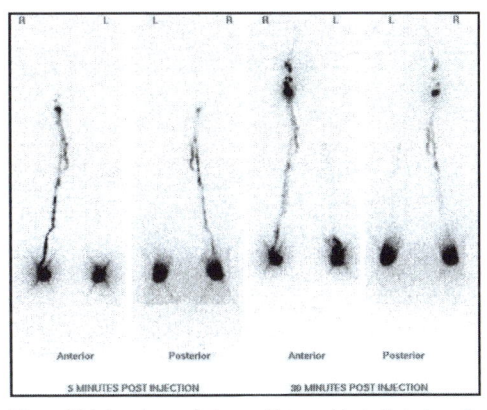

Figure 2.31 Lymphangoscintigram with tracer injected intradermally in both feet, showing hypoplasia of the lymphatics on the left.

Positron emission tomography (PET)
PET scanning is a recent development and is a functional modality that most commonly uses ^{18}F-FDG, a glucose analogue tracer with a short half-life whose distribution corresponds to glucose metabolism. The images obtained therefore identify areas of increased glycolysis, such as many malignancies. It is now usually combined with CT scanning (PET-CT) with co-registration of images to better localize the areas of increased activity improving accuracy of the technique.

Advantages
- The ability to assess function, rather than simple morphology as with other modalities.
- This enables more accurate staging of tumours with uptake seen in the primary tumour, and involved lymph nodes or metastatic deposits. Whole body scans are currently most commonly used in non-small cell lung cancer, lymphoma, recurrent colorectal cancer, and melanoma. It is not effective in tumours with low metabolic activity, such as many bronchoalveolar cell and renal cell carcinomas.
- Early serial imaging is increasingly used to assess response to treatment and allow an early switch to second line chemotherapy in non-responders.

Disadvantages
- Expensive modality with cyclotrons needed to produce the radionuclide.
- Short half-life of most of the radionuclides means these need to be sited close to the hospital. This has meant that scanners have tended to be located at specialist centres. FDG has a relatively long half-life allowing remote imaging, e.g. with the increasing utilization of mobile PET/CT services in many areas.
- High radiation dose to patients, with a PET scan of the head equivalent to 250 chest X-rays.
- Major radiation protection issues in relation to staff manning the facility.

Applications in rheumatology
The role of PET is expanding and includes both oncological and other patient groups in whom the accurate detection of inflammatory processes is important. Examples that may be encountered in rheumatological practice include:
- Investigation of unexplained lymphadenopathy, e.g. in sarcoidosis, TB or lymphoma.
- In large vessel vasculitis, where the inflammatory process is detected before the structural changes that are required for detection using conventional modalities.
- Assessment of bone and soft tissue tumours.

Acknowledgements
My thanks to Dr Duncan MacIver for his help in preparing this chapter.

Autoimmune serology

Antinuclear antibodies
The identification of antinuclear antibodies (ANA) is an important part of clinical rheumatology. ANA testing is one of the most frequently performed antibody tests.

The traditional substrate was rodent tissue, but over the past 20 years their use has been superseded by HEp-2 cells. These are immortalized cells, which originate from a human laryngeal carcinoma (human epithelioma type 2 cells) and are grown as monolayers.

HEp-2 cells advantages
- More sensitive enabling identification of more patterns.
- Human origin ensures better specificity than animal tissues.
- Nuclei are larger.
- Cell monolayer ensures all nuclei are visible.
- Cell division rates are higher so that antigens produced only in cell division are easily located.
- No obscuring intracellular matrix.
- Antigen distribution is uniform.

Methods of detection
ANA in serum are detected using an indirect immunofluorescence (IIF) assay. The intensity and patterns of fluorescence are reported. Many centres only report the presence or absence of ANA with a 3- point scale – negative, weak positive, strong positive. Semi-quantitative evaluation can be obtained using serial dilutions to endpoint fluorescence (the titre = reciprocal of dilution. A titre >1:80 is suggestive of an autoimmune connective tissue disease.

Standard reference sera are available for laboratory standardization.

Disease and autoantibodies are associated with HEp-2 patterns.

Specific ANA patterns
Homogeneous nuclear
Uniform diffuse fluorescence of the entire nucleus of interphase cells. Surrounding cytoplasm is negative.

Clinical association
Common in systemic lupus erythematosus (SLE), drug induced rheumatoid arthritis (RA), juvenile idiopathic arthritis (JIA), and systemic sclerosis.

Antigen
Antibodies to dsDNA (confirm by ELISA or *Crithidia luciliae* IIF), histones mainly [H2A-H2B]-DNA complex, Ku.

Homogeneous nuclear with rim
Similar to homogeneous with uniform diffuse fluorescence of the entire nucleus of interphase cells, but with greater intensity at the nuclear rim. Surrounding cytoplasm is negative.

Clinical association
Common in SLE especially if active.

Antigen
Antibodies to dsDNA and other antigens producing nuclear staining.

Coarse speckled
Dense, intermediate-sized particles, together with large speckles. Metaphase cells show no staining of the condensed chromatin region.

Table 2.1 Principal associations of HEp-2 positive sera

Disease	% Incidence
Chronic discoid lupus	5–50
Chronic infections	10–50
Dermatomyositis/polymyositis	30–40
Drug induced SLE	<50
Felty's syndrome	95–100
Healthy population	<5
Healthy relatives SLE patients	25
Juvenile idiopathic arthritis	15–30
Lupoid hepatitis	95–100
Neonatal lupus syndrome	<90
Neoplastic diseases	10–30
Normal elderly	<30
Polyarteritis nodosa	15–25
Pregnancy	5–10
Primary biliary cirrhosis	95–100
Rheumatoid arthritis	>95
Rheumatic fever	<5
Sjögren's syndrome	>95
SLE	95–100
Scleroderma (SSc)	>90

From Bradwell et al. (1995).

Clinical association
Common in SLE and SLE overlap syndromes.

Antigen
Particularly U1-snRNP or Sm proteins, but also produced by other antinuclear antibodies. Antigens are located in the small ribonuclear proteins (snRNPs).

Fine speckled
Fine to discrete speckled staining of interphase cells in a uniform distribution.

Clinical association
Common pattern found in SLE, Sjögren's syndrome, subacute LE, and scleroderma.

Antigen
Common to many nuclear proteins including SS-A (Ro) and SS-B (La) and RNA polymerases II and III.

Centromere
40–60 discrete speckles distributed throughout the interphase nuclei and characteristically found in the condensed nuclear chromatin during mitosis.

Clinical association
Found almost exclusively in limited cutaneous systemic sclerosis.

Antigen
Centromere proteins are located at the inner and outer kinetochore plates, which interact with mitotic spindle apparatus during cell division. Antibodies recognize three proteins CENT-B, CENT-A, and CENT-C. Kinetochore antigens

duplicate during G2 of interphase leading to the typical pattern seen in mitosis.

Nucleolar homogeneous
IIF staining of the entire nucleolus.

Clinical association
Found in 50% of patients with polymyositis-scleroderma overlap syndrome.

Antigen
The target antigen is PM-SCl.

Fine speckled
Fine granules condensed around the nucleus which reduces towards the periphery is typical of the tRNA synthetases.

Clinical association
Seen in around 20–40% of patients with polymyositis, especially associated with polyarthralgia and interstitial lung disease (tRNA synthetase syndrome).

Antigen
Jo-1 antibodies are targeted against the reactive site of histydyl tRNA synthetase, the cytoplasmic enzyme responsible for complexing histidine to its cognate transfer RNA. Other tRNA synthetase antibodies are PL7 (threonyl-tRNA), PL12 (alanyl-tRNA synthetase), EJ (glycyl-tRNA synthetase, OJ (isoeucyl-tRNA synthetase). Signal recognition particle antibodies give a similar pattern.

Mitochodrial
Numerous course granular filamentous cytoplasmic speckles extending around the nucleus and throughout the cytoplasm. Rodent kidney sections are more sensitive and should be used to confirm the pattern.

Clinical association
Commonly found in primary biliary cirrhosis, scleroderma (40%) and rarely in overlap syndromes.

Antigen
M2 is the commonest target antigen. M2 comprises a cluster of mitochondrial inner membrane proteins of which pyruvate dehydrogenase is the antigen in primary biliary cirrhosis.

DNA antibodies

The detection of antibodies to double stranded (ds) DNA is central to the diagnosis of SLE. Their presence in the serum of patients with SLE was first described 50 years ago. Very early it was recognized that they might be pathogenic as they could be eluted from the kidneys of patients with lupus nephritis. Antibodies to single stranded DNA are found in wide variety of autoimmune and infectious conditions.

Methods of detection
A number of different assays have been described for detection of DNA antibodies (reviewed in Isenberg & Smeenk, 2002). Described assays include IIF using HEp2 cells, *Crithidia luciliae* IIF, radioimmunoassay and ELISA. The technique used in most routine laboratories is ELISA, but the crithidia assay has a role in confirming the presence of dsDNA antibodies.

Crithidia luciliae assay
Crithidia luciliae is a haemoflagellate protozoan with a kinetoplast, which contains pure circular dsDNA, and no histone or other common autoantigens. This is considered the 'gold standard' immunofluorescence shows bright staining of the kintoplast. The assay is less sensitive than ELISA but is more specific.

ELISA
Solid phase ELISA is the most widely used test to detect dsDNA antibodies. It is cheap, easily automated and is quantifiable.

Clinical association
Antibodies against dsDNA are the characteristic autoantibodies in SLE, with a specificity of 95%, occurring in 70% of patients at some stage of their disease. They are associated with renal involvement. dsDNA antibody levels measured by ELISA fluctuate with disease activity and can be used to guide treatment decisions, but changes in treatment should not be made solely on the basis of changes in dsDNA levels. It is unclear whether a rise in anti-dsDNA antibody levels predicts a flare. Immunosuppressant treatment aimed solely at normalising anti-dsDNA antibody levels is associated with high drug toxicity.

Extractable nuclear antigens
Detection of antibodies against the extractable nuclear antigens (ENA) is useful in the diagnosis of several autoimmune rheumatic diseases. These antibodies were traditionally detected using immunodiffusion techniques, although ELISAs are now very widely used. Enzyme digestion studies showed that these antigens were sensitive to RNase and trypsin and are composed of ribonucleoprotein (RNP). The Sm (or Smith antigen; Sm, Ro, and La antigens were each named after the first two letters of the surname of the patients in whom antibodies to them were first found) is resistant to RNase and trypsin. The RNP antigenic determinants are found in association with U1 RNA, whereas Sm determinants are present on U1, U2, and U4–6 RNA. The other two important nuclear antigens are Ro and La, these are identical to the independently identified antigens Sjögren's syndrome A (SS-A) and Sjögren's syndrome B (SS-B).

Clinical association
The clinical associations of the ENA are given in Table 2.2.

Antiphospholipid (anticardiolipin) antibodies

Antibodies to phospholipids particularly cardiolipin (ACA) are responsible for the false positive Wasserman reaction and lupus anticoagulant seen in patients with the primary antiphospholipid antibody syndrome (APS) and in some patients with SLE. The interaction of phospholipid and a co-factor beta 2-glycoprotein is necessary for the antienic site to be available for binding of antibody.

Methods of detection
ACA are typically detected by an ELISA method. A positive IgG anticardiolipin test present on more than one occasion at least 6 weeks apart is most specific for APS, but some patients are only IgM antibody positive.

Clinical association
Antiphospholipid antibodies are associated with an increased risk of vascular thrombosis, recurrent foetal loss, livedo reticularis, and thrombocytopaenia.

Anti-C1q antibodies

C1q is the first component of the classical pathway of complement activation, hereditary deficiency is a risk factor for SLE.

Table 2.2

Antibody	Disease	Prevalence	Specificity	Clinical associations
dsDNA	SLE	70%	High	Lupus nephritis
Sm	SLE	5% (Caucasian)	High	Lupus vasculitis
		30–50% Afro-Caribbean		CNS lupus
Ro (SS-A)	SLE	40%	Low	Photosensitivity, subacute cutaneous. LE, congenital heart block, neonatal LE.
	Sjögren's	80%	High	Extraglandular disease
La (SS-B)	SLE	15%	Low	as for Ro
	Sjögren's	50%	High	as for Ro
U1RNP	SLE	30%	Low	Raynaud's phenomenom, swollen fingers
rRNP	SLE	15%	High	CNS lupus (psychosis, depression)
PCNA (cyclin)	SLE	5%	High	Proliferative glomerulonephritis
Phospholipid	SLE		High	Thrombosis, foetal loss, thrombocytopaenia
C1q	SLE	40%	Moderate	Lupus nephritis
Centromere	SSc	30%	Moderate	Limited cutaneous variant
Topoisomerase 1	SSc	30%	Moderate	Limited cutaneous variant. Absence of lung disease
RNA-polymerases	SSc	20%	High	Diffuse variant, visceral involvement
PM-SCL	SSc	5%	High	Scleroderma/polymyositis overlap
Jo-1	Polymyositis	30%	High	Polymyositis with interstitial lung disease
SRP	Polymyositis	4%	High	Severe myositis
Mi-2	Polymyositis	10%	High	Dermatomyositis
CCP	RA	80%	High	Erosive RA
PR3	Vasculitis	90%	High	Wegener's granulomatosis
MPO	Vasculitis	50%	Moderate	Microscopic polyangiitis
M2	Liver	80%	High	Primary biliary cirrhosis

SS = systemic sclerosis; SLE = systemic lupus erythematosus; SRP = signal recognition particle; PR3 = proteinase 3; MPO = myeloperoxidase; ccp = cyclic citrullinated peptide.

Clinical association
Antibodies against C1q are present in the serum of patients with SLE (up to 47%) and are associated with renal involvement. Monitoring anti-C1q may be useful to detect renal flares.

Rheumatoid factor
The detection of rheumatoid factor (RF) has been a key diagnostic tool in the diagnosis of RA. It pre-eminence has recently been challenged by the development of anti-CCP antibodies (vide infra). RFs are directed against the Fc part of IgG. Conventional assays detect IgM RF but IgG and IgA RF can be detected using specialized assays (see Plate 25).

Methods of detection
The presence of RF can be detected by agglutination of IgG-sensitized sheep red cells or latex coated with human IgG. Other assays are radioimmunoassays, ELISA or nephelometry.
Increasingly ELISAs are being used because they are cheap, reliable and easily automated.

Clinical association
RF has relatively low specificity for RA, however it is a good predictor of persistence of disease. RF is often detected in other chronic inflammatory conditions such as SLE, Sjögren's syndrome (60%), chronic osteomyelitis, and up to 10% of the general population especially the elderly. RF activity is often detected in patients with hepatitis C virus (HCV) associated cryoglobulinaemia. Cryoglobulins are formed of HCV core protein plus IgG antibody, which are then precipitated by IgM RF.

Anti-cyclic citrullinated peptide (CCP) antibodies
The relatively poor specificity of traditional RF assays for RA has led to the development of new serological markers. The most promising of these are antibodies directed against citrullinated antigens. The citrulline moiety the key component of the antigenic determinant is post-translationally generated by peptidylarginine deaminases from arginine. Proteins that normally include citrulline residues include myelin basic protein, filaggrin and some histones. Proteins such as fibrin and vimentin may citrullinated following inflammation, cell death or injury.

Methods of detection
Several ELISA assays have been developed and the second generation assays are being increasingly used.

Clinical association
Anti-CCP antibodies are present in 80% of patients with established RA. The specificity is around 95–98% with a sensitivity of 70–80% (Avouac et al, 2006). The prevalence in other diseases, which may be confused with RA is low and they are present in 0.4% of the general population. Anti-CCP antibody positivity is strongly associated with the shared epitiope.

A positive anti-CCP test appears to predict the development of erosive RA and this predictive value is independent of RF.

Anti-neutrophil cytoplasmic antibodies

Antineutrophil cytoplasmic antibodies (ANCA) were first detected in the sera of patients with systemic vasculitis in the early 1980s and have become an important tool in the diagnosis of patients with systemic vasculitis.

Methods of detection

ANCA in serum are detected using an IIF assay on ethanol fixed human neutrophils. The intensity and patterns of fluorescence are reported. Many centres only report the presence or absence of ANCA with a three point scale – negative, weak positive, strong positive. Semi-quantitative evaluation can be obtained using serial dilutions to end-point fluorescence (the titre = reciprocal of dilution. A titre >1:80 is suggestive of a systemic vasculitis.

Standard reference sera are available for laboratory standardization.

Specific ANCA patterns

Cytoplasmic

There is uniform staining of the cellular cytoplasm.

Antigen

The cytoplasmic pattern of staining on IIF (cANCA) is associated with the antigen proteinase 3 (PR3).

Perinuclear

The staining is located around the rim of the nucleus-perinuclear pattern (pANCA).

Antigen

The major target of pANCA is myeloperoxidase (MPO). There are a number of other antigens associated with pANCA (e.g. lactoferrin), but with less clinical significance.

Antigen specific ELISAs have been developed for the detection of the two main antigenic targets of ANCA. It is recommended that a positive result for ANCA by IIF is confirmed by antigen specific ELISA. This is especially important in pANCA positive sera where there may be confusion with a rim pattern ANA (Savige et al., 1999).

Clinical associations

The combination of cANCA and PR3 is highly specific (>90%) for Wegener's granulomatosis, whilst pANCA-MPO occurs in microscopic polyangiitis and Churg–Strauss syndrome, but is less specific (Hagan et al., 1998).

Levels of PR3-ANCA and MPO-ANCA fluctuate with disease activity, but an increase in level should not alone be used as indication to change treatment.

Further reading

Avouac J, Gossec L, Dougados M. Diagnostic and predicitive value of anti-cyclic citrullinated protein antibodies in rheumatoid arthritis: a systematic review of the literature. *Ann Rheum Dis* 2006; **65**: 845–51.

Bradwell AR, Stokes RP, Johnson Gd. *Atlas of HEp-2 cell patterns.* Binding Site, Birmingham, 1995.

Hagen EC, Daha MR, Hermans J, Andrassy K, Csernok E, Gaskin G, et al. Diagnostic value of standardized assays for anti-neutrophil cytoplasmic antibodies in idiopathic systemic vasculitis. EC/BCR Project for ANCA Assay Standardization. *Kidney Int* 1998; **53**: 743–53.

Isenberg DA, Manson JJ, Ehrenstein MR, Rahman A. Fifty years of anti-ds DNA antibodies: are we approaching journey's end? *Rheumatology* 2007; **46**: 1052–6.

Isenberg DA, Smeenk R. Clinical laboratory assays for measuring anti-ds DNA antibodies. Where are we now? *Lupus* 2002; **11**: 797–800.

Savige J, Gillis D, Benson E, Davies D, Esnault V, Falk RJ, et al. International consensus statement on testing and reporting of antineutrophil cytoplasmic antibodies (ANCA). *Am J Clin Pathol* 1999; **111**: 507–13.

Symmons DPM. Classification criteria for rheumatoid arthritis – time to abandon rheumatoid factor? *Rheumatology* 2007; **46**: 755–6.

Westwood OMR, Nelson PN, Hay FC. Rheumatoid factors: what's new? *Rheumatology* 2006; **45**: 379–85.

Synovial fluid analysis

Definition
Normal synovial fluid is a transudate of plasma that additionally contains high molecular weight sugar-rich molecules mainly hyaluronans.

Normal synovial fluid
In the normal joint synovial fluid production is balanced by drainage via synovial lymphatics. Macrophage derived type A synoviocytes keep the fluid clear of debris. Fibroblast derived type B synoviocytes produce hyaluronans.

Synovial fluid in the diseased joint
In the diseased joint there is a change in the volume and composition of the synovial fluid.

Synovial fluid examination
Simple examination of the fluid may be performed in the consulting room or at the bedside; more detailed analysis requires access to the laboratory. Examination of synovial fluid comprises four parts. visual analysis, nucleated cell count, 'wet' preparation, cytocentrifuge preparation,

Visual analysis
Volume
Volume is usually increased in active disease. A low volume does not exclude significant disease. Effusions may be difficult to aspirate because fibrin clots rice bodies or other debris are present and clog the needle. Long-standing effusions may be become loculated and inaccessible through the chosen route of access.

Colour
Normal synovial fluid is a pale yellow colour. A diffusely red or orange effusion suggests a haemarthrosis. Damage to cartilage or a vessel during aspiration will result in an initially clear effusion, which becomes blood stained. A inflammatory effusion will appear white or creamy in colour. A septic effusion may be pigmented by bacterial products.

Clarity
Normal synovial fluid is clear and print can be read through it. As the cell count increases the fluid becomes progressively more opaque.

Viscosity
Normal synovial fluid is viscous because it contains complex sugars. In inflammatory disease there is enzymatic breakdown of these sugars and consequent fall in viscosity.

Highly viscous fluid can be obtained from ganglia and mucous cysts.

Nucleated cell count
A nucleated cell count can be performed simply using a haemocytometer chamber. The number of cells can be used to classify an effusion.
- Normal synovial fluid contains <200 cell/mm^3 (<0.2 × 10^9/l).
- Non-inflammatory effusions contain 200–1000 cells/mm^3 (0.2–1.0 × 10^9/l).
- Inflammatory effusions contain >1000 cells/mm^3 (>1.0 × 10^9/l).
- Cell counts > 50 000 cells/mm^3 (50 × 10^9/l) raise the suspicion of infection but can occur in RA, crystal arthritis and reactive arthritis.

Wet preparation
Direct microscopy of an unstained fresh specimen enables cells and crystals to be detected.

Routine light microscopy
Erythrocytes and white cells may be observed and counted. Ragocytes containing intracytoplasmic granules are seen in RA and other inflammatory arthritides. Crystals of monosodium urate, and oxalate can also be seen.

Polarizng light microscopy
Polarizing light microscopy is required to distinguish various types of crystal. Monosodium urate crystals are needle shaped and highly birefringent. The crystals when viewed through crossed polarizers with an interposed quarter wave plate appear yellow or blue against a red background. Urate crystals when intracytoplasmic are diagnostic of gout.
Calcium pyrophosphate dihydrate crystals are also birefringent, but are rhomboid in shape
Hydroxyapatite crystals are too small to be with plain light microscopy, but if stained with alizarin red can be seen as red birefringent clumps.
Lipid crystals may be seen as Maltese cross-shaped deposits.

Cytocentrifuge preparation
Detailed cell analysis must be performed on a cytocentrifuge preparation. Neutrophils account for 60–80% of cells in inflammatory arthritides. In septic arthritis neutrophil counts may be 95% of nucleated cells present. Macrophages are predominant in viral arthritis.

Table 2.3 Feature of synovial fluid crystals

Crystals	Size (μm)	Shape	Birefringence	Disease associations
MSU	2–10	Needle, rod	Strongly negative	Acute and chronic gout
CPPDD	2–10	Rhomboids, rods	Weakly positive	CPPDD crystal deposition disease, OA
Apatite-like clumps	5–20	Round, irregular	None	Periarthritis, OA, clumps
Calcium oxalate	2–10	Polymorphic,	Positive	Renal failure dipyramidal
Cholesterol	10–80	Rectangles, needles	Negative or positive	Chronic RA or OA
Depot glucocorticoids	4–15	Irregular rods, rhomboids	Strongly positive or negative	Iatrogenic post-injection flare
Lipid liquid crystals	2–8	Maltese crosses	Strongly positive	Acute inflammation, bursitis

MSU = monosodium urate; CPPDD = calcium pyrophosphate dehydrate.

Micro-organisms can be identified in 85% of clinically infected aspirates. Gram staining should be performed on aspirates to exclude infection by Gram-positive organisms, which account the majority of joint infections. Gram negative organisms and organisms in previously or partially treated effusion may be difficult to detect.

Use of synovial fluid examination

Examination of synovial fluid is most useful.
- To distinguish non-inflammatory joint disease from inflammatory causes.
- Identification of crystal arthropathy.
- Identification of septic arthritis.

Further reading

Dieppe P, Swan A. the identification of synovial crystals in synovial fluid. *Ann Rheum Dis* 1999; **58**: 261–3.

Clinical neurophysiology

Definition
Clinical neurophysiology is the diagnostic study of evoked and spontaneous bioelectrical signals from the central and peripheral nervous systems and from skeletal muscle. It encompasses nerve conduction studies (NCS), needle electromyography (EMG), electroencephalography (EEG) and evoked central, and cortical responses (SSEPs, VEPs and BAEP). In the context of rheumatology only those aspects related to the study of the peripheral nervous system and neuromuscular function are most often required.

Nerve conduction study
Action potentials and conduction velocity
Action potentials are evoked by stimulating a peripheral nerve with a supra-maximal electrical square wave current of 0–100 mA usually of 0.1 ms duration (in some circumstances the duration may be increased up to 1 ms). The resultant evoked action potential is recorded with surface electrodes at a measured distance from the stimulating surface electrode. The amplitude of the evoked response is recorded and the conduction velocity calculated. The action potential recorded is a compound action potential generated by the summation of all the individual axon action potentials in a particular nerve or muscle.

Both sensory nerves and motor nerves can be studied. The amplitude of the compound action potential gives an estimate of the number of axons stimulated. Each nerve and muscle has its own normal reference range for amplitude. Sensory amplitudes are measured in microvolts (µV) and motor amplitudes in millivolts (mV). The sensory reference ranges are very wide and dependent on body weight, occupation, age and race. Conduction velocities are measured to the onset of the action potential and are those of the fastest axons stimulated, giving information about the integrity of the myelin. Conduction velocities are much less variable between patients and nerves. In the upper limb velocities are in the range of 50–60 m/s, whereas in the lower limb the velocities are generally slower, around 40–50 m/s. Only the largest myelinated fibres can be studied by routine nerve conduction.

Sensory action potentials (SAP) are measured with surface electrodes over the sensory nerve at a measured distance from the stimulating electrode allowing calculation of the conduction velocity (CV). Motor function is studied by stimulating a nerve and measuring the elicited compound muscle action potential (CMAP) amplitude recorded with surface electrodes over a muscle. The time taken between stimulus and response is the distal motor latency (DML). Motor conduction velocity (MCV) is determined between any two accessible points along a nerve, which can be divided into multiple segments along the limb from the most distal stimulus point up to the nerve root. This allows the demonstration of any focal slowing, motor conduction block or patchiness of abnormality.

F wave
Although in principle very proximal conduction velocities can be measured, the latency of the F wave is most often used as an indirect measure of proximal conduction. The F wave is a non physiological reflex dependent on the retrograde stimulation of the motor nerve. A motor action potential can travel the wrong way along the axon to the anterior horn cell where it can generate a reflex action potential which then travels back down the motor axon in the normal physiological direction evoking a recordable motor response distally. Any delay in the time taken for this reflex (F latency) with normal distal conduction implies proximal slowing and demyelination.

H reflex
The Hoffman reflex (H reflex) is used in a similar way, but is a physiological response dependent on the stretch reflex arc. It is the neurophysiological counterpart of the tendon reflex.

Other techniques
Repetitive motor nerve stimulation is used to study the function of the neuromuscular junction. Stimulation at a rate of 3 Hz normally elicits a compound muscle action potential of near identical amplitude with each successive stimulus. If there is failure of transmission at the neuromuscular junction, as occurs in myasthenia gravis, the amplitude of the compound action potential progressively falls with each stimulus, producing an amplitude 'decrement'.

Needle electromyography
With a needle electrode placed in a muscle the individual muscle fibre or motor unit action potentials can be recorded in response to a voluntary contraction (a motor unit is the group of muscle fibres supplied by one axon). The shape, duration, firing rate, and amplitude of the individual action potentials are assessed. At maximal voluntary contraction the number of motor units is assessed by measuring the amplitude of the overall envelope of electrical activity referred to as the interference pattern. Although there are objective quantitative techniques for this, in routine clinical practice this assessment is most often performed subjectively by observation of the action potential representation on a display and through a loudspeaker. EMG is used to determine if a deficit of motor function is secondary to nerve dysfunction (neurogenic) or due to primary muscle disease (myopathic). It also allows one to work out the anatomy of a nerve lesion.

Spontaneous activity is initially recorded. The muscle being studied must be completely relaxed. Normally, a muscle should be near silent on insertion of the needle. If one is near the neuromuscular junction, a characteristic 'end plate noise' is heard. In acutely denervated muscle, myositis and many myopathies, muscle fibres generate spontaneous low amplitude very brief potentials called fibrillations, which are a relatively non-specific feature of disturbed muscle physiology. Fibrillations may occur from months to years if a denervated muscle does not reinnervate.

Other spontaneous activity is also seen which may imply more specific diagnoses. Spontaneously firing motor units (fasciculations) when seen infrequently are normal, but if plentiful they suggest chronic, but ongoing denervation as seen in motor neurone disease. Some types of spontaneous and rapidly firing motor units, complex repetitive discharges, and myokimic or neuromyotonic discharges may be seen in proximal compressive lesions, denervation and peripheral demyelination. Myotonic discharges are seen with clinical myotonia.

Acute denervation
Acute denervation from any cause results in the reduction of the number of motor units that can be activated and thereby also a reduction of the interference pattern. Any remaining motor units will fire more rapidly than normal to compensate. The morphology of these units will

nevertheless remain normal for several weeks until the muscle becomes chronically denervated. Chronic denervation results in the reinnervation of previously denervated motor units by axonal regeneration and intra-muscle collateral axonal sprouting, with consequent increase in their amplitude and complexity resulting in polyphasia.

Muscle disease
Primary muscle disease is characterized by the presence of many low amplitude and highly polyphasic motor units that fire very easily and rapidly in response to voluntary activation, but with the generation of low levels of force as assessed by the neurophysiologist. This results in a very full interference pattern of low amplitude.

Specific conditions

Carpal tunnel syndrome and other entrapments
The neurophysiological examination of patients with carpal tunnel syndrome (CTS) represents a paradigm of neurophysiology and of other entrapment neuropathies. The aim is to confirm the focal nature of the neuropathy at the wrist and grade its severity. The median nerve SAP is normally recorded by stimulating digit 2 or 3, and recording over the median nerve proximal to the carpal tunnel. In a mild or early neuropathy only slowing of conduction may be seen due to a degree of demyelination, but as the condition progresses axonal degeneration occurs with a fall in SAP amplitude. The median nerve SAP is compared with either the ulnar or radial SAP. The DML to abductor policis brevis is measured to determine the degree of distal motor slowing. As with sensory conduction evidence of motor slowing and demyelination normally occurs before loss of axons and CMAP amplitude reduction. A variety of short segment nerve studies are used to demonstrate focal carpal tunnel slowing such as a median palm to wrist sensory conduction velocity and a comparison of the DML from the second lumbrical (median innervated) to that of the second interosseous (ulnar innervated) muscles. End stage carpal tunnel syndrome results in the loss of any recordable motor or sensory response distally preventing confirmation of the focal nature of the original lesion. Neurophysiology for carpal tunnel syndrome is not usually required for diagnosis but is needed for planning treatment and predicting outcome.

With some entrapment nerve lesions conduction block may be seen. With an acute lesion of the ulnar nerve at the elbow or common peroneal nerve at the fibular head, it may be possible to demonstrate a normal functioning nerve segment distal to the lesion by virtue of normal SAP and CMAP amplitudes and CV, but with slowing of CV through the compressed region. With stimulation proximal to the lesion there is attenuation of motor and sensory amplitudes indicating a segment of significant demyelination. If left untreated such lesions may progress to axonal degeneration and loss of focal slowing making it difficult to localize the site of entrapment as with late carpal tunnel syndrome.

Radiculopathy
Study of patients with possible radiculopathies is often requested. This is usually to exclude an alternative diagnosis as MRI scanning is a more appropriate investigation to show a root lesion. Nevertheless, neurophysiology may confirm a radiculopathy by demonstrating a normal dermatomal sensory response accompanied by denervation changes confined to muscles supplied by the corresponding myotome. Root lesions are usually proximal to the dorsal root ganglion (preganglionic) resulting in a normal functioning distal sensory axon despite sensory disturbance or numbness. Any lesion distal to the dorsal root ganglion is referred to as post-ganglionic.

Myopathy
Needle EMG is frequently requested for the assessment of possible myopathic conditions, such as polymyositis and Statin, induce muscle disease. It is a very sensitive method and should be performed prior to muscle biopsy as it may direct which muscle to sample. Myopathic needle EMG abnormalities are, however, seldom found in the absence of weakness. Mild or even modest rises in creatinine kinase may not be accompanied by clear EMG changes if there are no other clinical abnormalities.

What to tell patients
Clinical neurophysiology examination involves the use of small electrical currents to stimulate nerves in order to assess the cause of symptoms. The electrical currents used are safe and feel a bit like a TENS machine or a muscle toner. Special care is needed with pacemakers and patients may need cardiac monitoring during the examination and a pacemaker check afterwards. The presence of implantable defibrillators is a significant contraindication. Pregnancy is not a contraindication to electrical stimulation. Needle EMG is often likened to acupuncture and is of similar discomfort to a venepuncture. Warfarin is a relative contraindication to needle examination and a recent INR (less than 2.5) is desirable. Some patients find the examination uncomfortable and they should be warned about this, but it should not be over emphasized as anxiety prior to the examination undoubtedly increases the discomfort.

Acknowledgements
My thanks to Dr Julian Blake for his help in preparing this chapter.

Further reading
Neuromuscular Home Page, Neuromuscular Diseases Center, Washington University, St Louis, MO USA. Available at: http://neuromuscular.wustl.edu

British Society for Clinical Neurophysiology. Available at: http://www.bscn.org.uk

American Association of Neuromuscular and Electrodiagnostic Medicine. Available at: http://www.aanem.org

Preston DC, Shapiro BE. *Electromyography and Neuromuscular Disorders*, 2nd edn. Philadelphia: Elsevier, Butterworth Heinemann, 2005.

Making the best use of Clinical radiology service. (Sixth Ed.). Royal College of Radiologists 2007.

Chapter 3

Organ involvement in rheumatological disease

The eye *48*
The chest *54*
The heart *66*
The kidney *74*
The gut and hepatobiliary disease *82*
The nervous system *90*
The skin *98*

The eye

Although serious eye problems are rare in rheumatology clinics, failure to spot warning signs and symptoms can have catastrophic consequences for the patient. This chapter will consider rheumatological conditions affecting the eye and highlight those, which require urgent referral and treatment. High dose immunosuppression is often required to prevent ocular pathology due to the very limited ability of the eye to recover function following damage.

Classification

Table 3.1 Anatomical classification of eye involvement in rheumatological disease

	Uveitis	Scleritis	Ocular surface	Optic neuropathy	Retinal changes	Other
Rheumatoid arthritis	No	Painful or painless	PUK, dry eye	Very rare	Very rare retinal vasculitis	
Ankylosing spondylitis	Anterior uveitis, bilateral in 80% hypopyon is common	Anterior scleritis	Conjunctivitis			
Systemic lupus erythematosus		Yes	Dry eye	Very rare	CWS, haemorrhages, oedema, vascular occlusion	
Systemic sclerosis			Dry eye			
Sjögrens syndrome			Dry eye			
Dermato- and polymyositis		Yes			CWS, haemorrhages, oedema	Orbital myositis
Behçet's disease	Panuveitis, hypopyon is common	Rarely		Rare	Retinal vein occlusions, white ischaemic retinal patches	Cerebral sinus thrombosis (bilateral papilloedema)
Relapsing polychondritis		Yes 43% of RP	PUK	Rare	Rare CWS, haemorrhages	
Polyarteritis nodosa	Rarely	Yes	PUK	Rarely AION	CWS, exudates	Rarely orbital inflammation
Sarcoidosis	Acute or chronic pan-uveitis	Rarely	Dry eye	Yes	Choroidal granulomas, periphlebitis, optic neuropathy	Facial nerve palsy
Reactive arthritis	Mainly anterior uveitis (in 30%) often unilateral	Rarely	Conjunctivitis (rarely keratitis)			
Giant cell arteritis		Rarely		Yes	CWS occasionally	Transient obscurations 10%
Wegener's granulomatosis	Rarely causes uveitis	Yes	PUK	Yes	Retinal vasculitis	Orbital involvement common
Juvenile idiopathic arthritis	Chronic anterior uveitis					Glaucoma, band keratopathy
Anti-phospholipid syndrome (APS)				Rarely AION	Retinal vascular occlusions	Amaurosis fugax, TIA
Psoriatic arthritis	Anterior uveitis	Rarely				
Inflammatory bowel disease	Anterior or posterior uveitis	Rarely				

Abbreviations: PUK; Peripheral ulcerative keratitis; CWS = Cotton wool spots; AION = anterior ischaemic optic neuropathy.

CHAPTER 3 Organ involvement in rheumatological disease

Definitions and disease associations
Nomenclature describing anatomy of the eye is shown in Figure 3.1.

Conjunctivitis
Infection or inflammation of the conjunctiva (usually viral, bacterial or allergic).

Blepharitis
Inflammation of eyelid margins often with colonization of 'harmful bacteria', such as staphylococcus. Exacerbates dry eye problems.

Episcleritis
Inflammation of episclera. Is usually idiopathic, but can be seen in rheumatoid arthritis (RA), spondylarthropathies (SpAs), and gout.

Scleritis
Inflammation of sclera, may be anterior (red eye) or posterior (eye may be white), nodular, diffuse, necrotizing or non-necrotizing.

30–50% cases are idiopathic but scleritis can be associated with RA, Wegner's granulomatosis (ANCA-associated vasculitis, AAV), SpAs, relapsing polychondritis (RP), polyarteritis nodosa (PAN), systemic lupus erythematosus (SLE), Behçet's, sarcoidosis, and very rarely ulcerative colitis, gout, Mycobacterium tuberculosis (MTB), Lyme disease and syphilis.

Peripheral ulcerative keratitis
Inflammation, thinning, and ulceration of sclera and cornea (corneal inflammation = keratitis). Is similar to scleritis.

Anterior uveitis (iritis, iridocyclitis)
Inflammation centred on the anterior chamber of the eye/iris (may be granulomatous or non granulomatous). Intermediate uveitis is inflammation centred on the vitreous. Occurs in SpAs, sarcoidosis, Lyme disease, MTB, multiple sclerosis, pars planitis and in association with juvenile idiopathic arthritis (JIA). Many cases are idiopathic however.

Posterior uveitis
Inflammation centred on the posterior chamber of the eye/retina/choroid. Panuveitis – posterior uveitis with vitreous cells and anterior uveitis. Posterior uveitis occurs in sarcoid, Behçet's (esp. Turkish). It occurs, too, in SLE, PAN, and dermatomyositis, but is very rare.

Cataract
Opacification of the lens. Common in elderly patients, secondary to glucocorticoids (GCs) or uveitis.

Glaucoma
Raised intraocular pressure with associated visual field loss and optic disc cupping. Glaucoma is often secondary to GC use and uveitis, particularly in JIA and sarcoidosis. It is more common if there is a family history of glaucoma or in short-sighted patients.

Retinovascular disease
Causes. Inflammation and/or occlusion of retinal blood vessels, branch, or central retinal artery occlusion or vein occlusion.
- Retinal vessel inflammation is usually referred to as retinal vasculitis, whilst 'retinitis' refers to mainly viral retinal infections (cytomegalovirus, CMV) or as a misnomer in retinitis pigmentosa.
- Maculopathy is a non-specific term denoting any pathology affecting the central retina (e.g. diabetes, genetic conditions, ageing change).
- Commonly due to diabetes or hypertension, but also seen in association with rheumatological conditions, such as Behçet's, SLE, antiphospholipid syndrome (APLS), Sarcoidosis, etc.

Sarcoidosis
Sarcoid can cause granulomas to form anywhere in the eye including the optic nerve, lacrimal gland or eyelids. Granulomatous uveitis is typical. Sarcoid is arguably the commonest cause of posterior uveitis in rheumatology patients and is a cause of retinovascular disease.

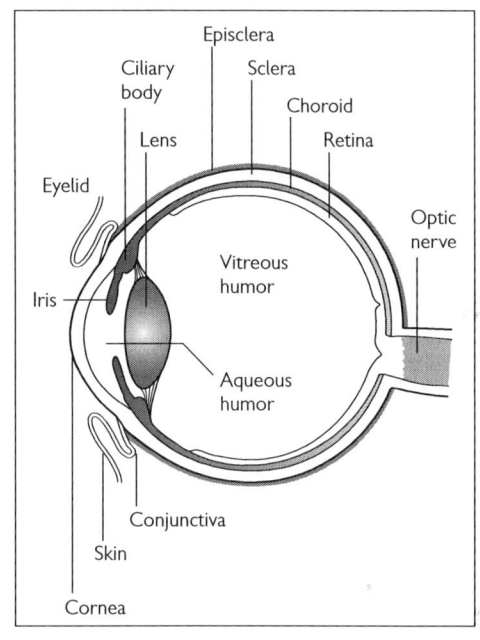

Figure 3.1 Diagrammatic representation of the eye shown in cross-section.

SLE
May cause cotton wool spots in retina. Vascular occlusion, such as blockage of the central retinal artery may occur presenting with sudden onset severe loss of vision in one eye. Retinal neovascularization with subsequent vitreous haemorrhage may also occur.

Rheumatology drug associated effects on the eye
- GCs cause cataract, glaucoma, and rarely central serous retinopathy.
- Hydroxychloroquine rarely causes a bullseye appearance maculopathy with retinal cell death.
- Bisphosphonates (especially pamidronate) have been reported to cause uveitis or unilateral scleritis.
- Etanercept may rarely be associated with uveitis.
- Potent immunosuppression (e.g. cyclophosphamide) increases risk of viral retinitis (HSV, CMV), which may present with blurred vision, field loss, flashing lights, or floaters. Although rare, this is potentially very serious and merits immediate referral for ophthalmological examination.
- Penicillamine can cause myasthenic diplopia.

Risk factors
- Human lymphocyte antigen (HLA) B27 is strongly associated with anterior uveitis.
- All JIA patients should be screened for uveitis.
- In giant cell arteritis (GCA), in 70% of untreated cases, visual loss in one eye is followed within 1 week by visual loss in the second eye.
- In RA, rheumatoid factor (RF) seropositivity is a risk factor for scleritis.

Clinical features
Key features in the history
- Presence/severity of pain:
  - photophobia is common in uveitis;
  - if woken from sleep by severe pain 'like someone drilling into my eye socket' then consider symptom very typical for scleritis;
  - mild tenderness to touch can mean episcleritis, though scleritis is more severe and serious;
  - grittiness and stinging suggest dry eye or other ocular surface problems; blepharitis is the commonest cause of dry eye symptoms with grittiness, watering, crusting of eyelid margins, mild redness with normal vision. [Warning: blepharitis is so common that many patients with serious eye problems also have blepharitis – it is a diagnosis of exclusion.]
- Visual disturbance: with loss of vision for a few seconds only consider GCA.
- Blurred vision can be due to uveitis, cataract, retinovascular disease, and rarely scleritis.
- Never diagnose episcleritis, blepharitis, or conjunctivitis if vision is blurred and does not clear on blinking.
- A sticky discharge occurs with conjunctivitis, is copious, foul smelling, and purulent in gonorrhoeal conjunctivitis, and manifests as stringy threads in allergic conjunctivitis.
- History of use of eye drops/other ophthalmic preparations might suggest allergic conjunctivitis. It causes red itchy eye and skin around lids (develops if patients are allergic the preservative in artificial tear drops). A preservative-free preparation such as celluvisc 0.5% should be tried.
- New headache, scalp tenderness, jaw claudication, tongue claudication, shoulder/hip girdle stiffness may indicate GCA [with or without polymyalgia rheumatica (PMR)). More often, patients have had sudden loss of vision in one eye to 'count fingers' vision or worsens with a recent onset new headache.

Key features on examination
All patients complaining of any eye symptoms at all must have some record of their visual acuity in each eye (Snellen chart ideally ± pinhole or if not available ability to read small print with glasses on).
- Red eye is caused by conjunctivitis, blepharitis, episcleritis, anterior scleritis, or uveitis (not always).
- White eye is from posterior scleritis and some chronic uveitides (e.g. sarcoid, JIA, intermediate uveitis).
- Check for distribution of 'redness'. Diffuse is unhelpful in differentiating cause. Quadrantic is typical for episcleritis, scleritis or trichiasis, whilst circumlimbal flush occurs in anterior uveitis, but is not a reliable sign.
- The redness of scleritis will persist after one drop of 10% phenylephrine is administered, whereas the redness of episcleritis will disappear after 10 min as the more superficial episcleral vessels are constricted by the phenylephrine. The scleral vessels are too deep to be affected (phenylephrine causes blurred vision and pupil dilation for 8 h).
- With a direct ophthalmoscope, detect the presence or absence of optic disc swelling, atrophy, disc cupping (in glaucoma), retinal haemorrhages, and cotton wool spots. Large keratic precipitates (KPs) will be visible with an ophthalmoscope. Pull lower lid down to look for a hypopyon.
- Pus in the anterior chamber (hypopyon) is typically seen in HLA B27 positive anterior uveitis, particularly with AS. Also seen with Behçet's and endophthalmitis.
- To detect mild anterior or posterior uveitis requires examination with a slit lamp, as cells in the anterior chamber are not visible with a direct ophthalmoscope.
- Confrontation visual field testing will only pick up gross pathology like a homonymous hemianopia from a CVA. It will not detect early glaucoma.
- A relative afferent papillary defect denotes serious pathology affecting the visual pathway between the optic chiasm and the retina (GCA, sarcoid optic neuropathy, retinal detachment).
- A cloudy cornea can occur with very high intraocular pressure (acute glaucoma), confluent KPs (uveitis), infection, trauma, band keratopathy, and corneal decompensation (post-surgery).
- Irregular pupil shape from posterior synechiae or KPs imply that the patient has had anterior uveitis. They do not always disappear following treatment sometimes becoming pigmented and permanent. Only treat if active uveitis is confirmed with slit lamp examination.

Fundoscopy
Macula
Cystoid macular oedema (CMO; fluid cysts at fovea with a petalloid appearance) occurs with uveitis but is difficult to see with an ophthalmoscope and is best demonstrated using ocular coherence tomography or fluorescein angiography. Flame haemorrhages and cotton wool spots require investigation to check blood pressure (BP) and for hyperglycaemia before looking for a vasculitic or autoimmune process.

Disc
GCA may present with severe unilateral loss of vision, an afferent pupillary defect and a pale swollen optic disc caused by arteritic anterior ischaemic optic neuropathy (occlusion of the small blood vessels supplying the optic nerve anteriorly in the orbit).

Retinovascular disease
- Asymptomatic vascular sheathing is most commonly caused by sarcoidosis (venous 'candle wax dripping').
- Arterial sheathing is rare, but may be seen with SLE, PAN, AAV, Behçet's, syphilis, and acute retinal necrosis.
- Vascular occlusions are usually painless and may not be noticed by the patient (branch retinal vein occlusions affecting peripheral veins) or may cause profound visual loss as in central retinal artery occlusion.
- Vein occlusions with uveitis suggest Behçet's, sarcoidosis or syphilis. Vein occlusions without uveitis are usually secondary to atherosclerosis in the retinal artery, which compresses the vein as it crosses it on the retina.
- Retinal arterial occlusion is commonly secondary to emboli from the carotid arteries, but can occur in GCA, SLE and some forms of vasculitis.

CHAPTER 3 Organ involvement in rheumatological disease

- Central retinal artery occlusion results in 'count fingers' vision or worse, and a pale retina with a cherry red spot at the fovea. The retinal appearance returns to normal within 2 weeks.
- Vein occlusions do not allow blood to leave the eye, hence there are multiple retinal haemorrhages, often flame-shaped.

Conjugate gaze/double vision
Unless long-standing double vision requires that the patient is referred to an ophthalmologist.
- Usually caused by thyroid eye disease, cranial nerve palsies, decompensating squint, decompensating congenital fourth nerve palsy, or trauma.
- Rare causes of diplopia that could present in the rheumatology clinic include rheumatoid nodule on superior oblique tendon causing vertical diplopia, penicillamine-induced myasthenia, orbital mass from AAV, central nervous system (CNS) lesions, or a nerve palsy from vasculitis, Whipple's, sarcoidosis, Lyme disease, Behçet's, or MTB.

General examination
The approach to a general examination will depend on the history and ocular findings, but should include looking for joint pathology (e.g. RA), skin (Psoriasis, erythema nodosum, vasculitis, scalp tenderness), lungs (sarcoidosis, AAV). All patients with scleritis should have BP and urinalysis to exclude renal involvement, which may be life threatening.

Investigations

Slit lamp examination
Dry eye can be detected using 2% fluorescein drops. These reveal inferior punctuate staining and sometimes corneal droplet like threads called filamentary keratitis. Rose–Bengal drops cause eye pain and are best avoided.

Schirmer's test (Figure 8.4)
A Schirmer strip (filter paper) is tucked under the lower eyelid and soaks up the tears. The length of staining in mm gives a measure of tear production. Less than 5 mm wetting in 5 min denotes aqueous tear deficiency (as seen in Sjögren's), 5–10 mm is equivocal, greater than 10 mm is normal (without anaesthetic eye drop use).

Tonometry
All uveitis patients need their intraocular pressures checked by Goldman tonometry. Digital tonometry (using 2 fingers to press on the eyeball) is only reliable to distinguish between normal pressure (<21 mmHg) and extremely high pressures (>45 mmHg).

Fluorescein angiography
Is used to investigate uveitis (CMO and vasculitis) and visual loss in scleritis. May also show delayed choroidal perfusion in cases of visual loss in suspected GCA.

Ocular coherence tomography (OCT)
Allows 3D imaging of the retina down to the level of the choroid. Very useful for showing retinal fluid (CMO).

Microbiology
- Borrelia serology is rarely positive, but worth doing in endemic Lyme Disease areas.
- TPHA is always worth checking as it alters treatment.
- If viral retinitis is suspected, then a vitreous tap should be taken and sent for PCR for varicella-zoster, CMV, Epstein Barr virus (EBV), syphilis, and toxoplasmosis.
- If taking a swab for conjunctivitis then culture for *Chlamydia*, as well as the usual organisms.

Histology
- Orbital biopsy may be required to diagnose AAV.
- Sarcoid granulomas can be seen on conjunctival biopsy or lacrimal gland biopsy in dry eye patients.
- Temporal artery biopsy may be useful in GCA, although a negative biopsy does not exclude the diagnosis.

Other laboratory tests
Tests requested should be determined once the ophthalmological differential diagnosis has been formed. All systemic rheumatological diseases associated with eye lesions are appropriately evaluated with full blood count (FBC), ESR, CRP, LFTs, U&Es, and creatinine.
- ESR, FBC, LFTs, and CRP should be tested if GCA suspected. A normal ESR and/or CRP does not rule out the diagnosis. A raised platelet count is suggestive in younger patients.
- A raised ACE is associated with, but not specific for sarcoid. Some people with sarcoid have an ACE in the reference range.
- If AICTD suspected then consider checking ANA, ENAs, C3, and C4, RF, a functional assay for lupus anticoagulant (e.g. Dilute Russell Viper Venom Test, DRVVT) and aCL antibodies.
- If RA suspected check RF and CCP antibodies.

Treatment

Uveitis
- Anterior uveitis can usually be managed by topical glucocorticoid (GC) eye drops and dilating drops (cyclopentolate) to prevent posterior synechiae forming. A reducing course of GCs over 5–6 weeks is typical, although some patients require GC eye drops for many years to prevent flare-ups. Occasionally subconjunctival GC injections are required.
- Children with JIA can get anterior uveitis which causes damage to the eye without the patient having symptoms or causing red eye (see below).
- Posterior uveitis may also require orbital floor depot steroid injections (triamcinolone), systemic steroids, steroid sparing agents (ciclosporin, mycophenolate mofetil, tacrolimus, and azathioprine) and biologics (infliximab preferred to etanercept in eye patients). Intravitreal GC injections are also used.
- A rare complication of posterior uveitis is the development of a choroidal neovascular membrane – this presents with unilateral blurred vision and distortion (assessed with Amsler grid). Urgent ophthalmology opinion is needed to consider increased immunosuppression, photodynamic therapy or the use of intra-vitreal anti-VEGF agents.
- Sarcoid usually responds well to topical and systemic steroids, methotrexate may have some advantages as a steroid sparing agent in this condition.
- Sarcoid uveitis often is chronic. HLA B27 associated anterior uveitis has a relapsing remitting course.
- Behçet's patients often require high dose systemic GCs and ciclosporin. Azathioprine reduces the incidence of ocular attacks. Chlorambucil may cause long-term remission, but causes infertility. Infliximab or interferon-α2a may prove useful for ocular disease in the future.
- About 90% of patients with ocular Behçet's go blind in 4 years if not treated.

Scleritis and episcleritis

- Episcleritis is usually self-limiting or resolves with flurometholone eye drops (mild GC) or oral non-steroidal anti-inflammatory drugs (NSAIDs). It is sensible to refer to an ophthalmologist to check diagnosis unless there is a convincing and documented history of previous episcleritis.
- Scleritis may resolve with an NSAID or systemic GCs (reducing course over many months).
- Severe cases of scleritis may need IV methylprednisolone 1 g daily for 3 days followed by oral GCs and GC-sparing agents. Cyclophosphamide may be needed in very aggressive cases.
- Urgent ophthalmology referral is required as severe scleritis cases can rapidly result in scleral melting, globe perforation, and loss of vision. PUK is treated along similar lines to scleritis.
- There is no ocular treatment for scleromalacia perforans (painless necrotizing scleritis in late stage RA).
- RA scleritis patients have an increased risk of mortality.

Giant cell arteritis

In suspected cases with ocular symptoms immediate ophthalmology referral is mandatory. Also do not delay starting glucocorticoids (GCs), while waiting for an ophthalmologist to review the patient or a biopsy. In GCA it is very unusual for any significant visual recovery to take place once vision is lost.

- Observational studies support the use of high dose GCs in GCA. Recently, guidelines on the management of large vessel vasculitis have been produced by EULAR (Mukter et al., 2008).
- In patients without ocular symptoms, oral GCs starting at 0.7–1 mg/kg (maximum dose 60–80 mg) should be prescribed. In patients with ocular symptoms IV methylprednisolone 1 g daily for 3 days should be used in addition to oral GCs.
- The headache should resolve rapidly (<48 h).
- A recent randomized study suggested that use of IV methylprednisolone (15 mg/kg) for 3 days in addition to oral prednisolone 40 mg/day permitted more rapid GC taper.
- Oral GCs should be tapered quickly aiming for 10 mg/day at 6 months.
- In patients with fluctuating visual loss, plasma expanders, fragmin, aspirin, lying the patient down with foot of bed raised, and oral acetazolamide to reduce intraocular pressure, have been tried. Data from robust studies is lacking however.

Keratoconjunctivitis sicca

Most patients benefit from eye drops. There are many different preparations from which to choose.

- Short-acting preparations contain polyvinyl alcohol (SnoTears, Liquifilm) or carboxycellulose (hypromellose, Tears Naturale). Longer-acting preparations contain carbomer gels (e.g. Viscotears, Geltears) or paraffin (e.g. Lacrilube, Lubri-Tears); these are stickier and patients may prefer to use them at night. Some patients are intolerant of preservatives in aqueous drops and preservative-free Liquifilm may be tolerated.
- Blepharitis is common and frequently exacerbates the symptoms of dry eyes. Treat with daily lid hygiene cleaning eyelid margins with a cotton bud dipped in dilute baby shampoo. Ocular chloramphenicol bd for 2 weeks ± GC eye drops when necessary. Oral doxycline can be used in more severe cases with rosacea.

Surgery

- Cataract surgery in patients with uveitis requires adequate GC cover and management by an ophthalmologist with some experience of managing uveitis.
- Lacrimal duct plugging/ablation is useful in more severe cases of dry eye.
- Intraocular GC slow-release devices are being developed but have a high rate of secondary glaucoma.

Retinovascular disease in AICTDs/vasculitis

Active retinopathy in the context of an AICTD or vasculitis should prompt a review of disease activity by both medical ophthalmologist and rheumatologist. The retina is the only part of the body, apart from the nailfolds, where capillaries vessels can be viewed directly.

- Care should be taken to distinguish hypertensive retinopathy from that caused by systemic vasculitis.
- SLE retinopathy usually has a good prognosis for vision, although a small group has an occlusive vasculopathy and cerebral vasculitis with a poor prognosis.

Juvenile idiopathic arthritis

- Anterior uveitis can be asymptomatic.
- JIA-associated uveitis can start soon after the onset of the arthritis or may already be present at the time of diagnosis of JIA. It can be severe with few symptoms.
- Referral for ophthalmological screening by a specialist experienced in seeing children with the condition is therefore urgent.
- Children should be screened by an ophthalmologist according to the BSPAR protocol (see Assessment tools, below).
- Treatment is challenging and children can go blind with this condition. Systemic GCs, eye drops, and methotrexate have been used extensively.
- If methotrexate is discontinued for any reason then the ophthalmologist should be informed as more frequent ocular screening is required at this point
- In addition to chronic anterior uveitis, ocular damage and even blindness can be caused by cataract, secondary glaucoma, band keratopathy and ultimately phthisis bulbi.

Resources

Assessment tools

A reading chart (test with reading glasses on and record distance, e.g. 20 cm) or Snellen chart should be available to check visual acuities.

Hydroxychloroquine screening

- Check patient's vision is normal in each eye before starting treatment and document this. If not normal then ask them to see their high street optician (optometrist) who can provide a report on their vision and eyes.
- Check visual acuity annually. If vision deteriorates then stop treatment, send patient to their optometrist who can refer on to an ophthalmologist if new glasses are not the answer.

CHAPTER 3 Organ involvement in rheumatological disease

- If exceeding the maximal daily dosage of 6.5mg/kg of lean body weight or in patients who have taken the drug, even in recommended doses, for >6 years then annual screening by an ophthalmologist is prudent. The Royal College of Ophthalmology guidelines are available free of charge at: http://www.rcophth.ac.uk/docs/publications/published-guidelines/Oculartoxicity2004.pdf;
- Children with JIA should be screened for uveitis by an ophthalmologist according to the BSPAR protocol (available at: http://www.bspar.org.uk/downloads/clinical_guidelines/BSPAR_guidelines_eye_screening_2006.pdf).

Guidelines/NICE
Hydroxychloroquine Monitoring Guidelines: Royal College of Ophthalmology. Available at: http://www.rcophth.ac.uk/docs/publications/published-guidelines/Oculartoxicity2004.pdf

BSPAR protocol for screening children with JIA: Available at: http://www.bspar.org.uk/downloads/clinical_guidelines/BSPAR_guidelines_eye_screening_2006.pdf.

ICD-10 codes
H04.1 Dry eye.
H15.0 Scleritis.
H15.1 Episcleritis.
H20.0 Acute anterior uveitis.
H20.1 Chronic anterior uveitis.
H30.1 Posterior uveitis.
H35.0 Retinal vasculitis.

See also
- Rheumatoid arthritis.
- Ankylosing spondylitis/SpA.
- Reactive arthritis (spondylarthropathy).
- Systemic lupus erythematosus.
- Sjögren's syndrome.
- Wegener's granulomatosis (ANCA-associated vasculitis).
- Behçet's disease.
- Sarcoidosis.
- Juvenile idiopathic arthritis.
- Anti-phospholipid antibody syndrome (APLS).
- Polyarteritis nodosa.

Further reading
Jabs DA, Nussenblatt RB, Rosenbaum JT. Standardization of Uveitis Nomenclature (SUN) Working Group. Standardization of uveitis nomenclature for reporting clinical data. Results of the First International Workshop. *Am J Ophthalmol.* 2005; 140: 509–16.

Krause L, Altenburg A, et al. Long-term visual prognosis of patients with ocular adamantiades-Behçet's disease treated with interferon-alpha-2a. *J Rheumatol* 2008; 35: 896–903.

Mavrikakis I, Sfikakis PP, et al. The incidence of irreversible retinal toxicity in patients treated with hydroxychloroquine: a reappraisal. *Ophthalmology.* 2003; 110: 1321–6.

Mukhtyar C, Guillevin L, Cid MC, et al. EULAR recommendations for the management of large vessel vasculitis. *Ann Rheum Dis* 2008. Epub ahead of print: doi:10.1136/ard.2008.088351.

Niccoli L, Nannini C, et al. Long-term efficacy of infliximab in refractory posterior uveitis of Behçet's disease: a 24-month follow-up study. *Rheumatol (Ox)* 2007; 46: 1161–4.

The chest

Chest disease is a significant cause of morbidity and mortality in rheumatological conditions, and the disease may sometimes present with respiratory symptoms. Chest involvement may occur in patients with congenital, or acquired deformity of the spine or rib cage, in RA, autoimmune connective tissue connective tissue diseases, ankylosing spondylitis (AS), ANCA-associated vasculitides (AASV), RP, and other systemic inflammatory conditions, such as sarcoidosis. The management reflects the location of pathology and its pathophysiology. This section will consider those rheumatological conditions affecting the chest wall, pleura, airways, lung parenchyma, lung vasculature, and lymphatics.

Classification

Conditions may be classified arbitrarily according to their disease associations or on their anatomical basis (Table 3.2).

Table 3.2 Anatomical Classification of Lung Involvement in Rheumatological Disease

	Chest Wall	Pleura	Airways	Parenchyma	Pulmonary Vasculature & Lymphatics
Rheumatoid Arthritis (RA)	Respiratory muscle weakness	Pleurisy ± effusion; Empyema; Nodules	Follicular and/or obliterative bronchiolitis; Bronchiectasis; Cricoarytenoid arthritis; Vocal fold nodules	ILD (UIP > NSIP > OP, LIP); Drug-induced pneumonitis; Nodules; Infections – pneumonia and tuberculosis	PAH
Ankylosing Spondylitis (AS)	Costovertebral arthritis	Pleural thickening; effusion	Obliterative bronchiolitis	Upper lobe fibrosis	
Systemic Lupus Erythematosus (SLE)	Shrinking Lung; Costochondritis	Pleurisy ± effusion	Upper airways dysfunction; Obliterative Bronchiolitis; Bronchiectasis	ILD (NSIP or DAD > OP, UIP or LIP); Diffuse alveolar haemorrhage/ acute lupus pneumonitis.	PAH; Pulmonary embolus (APLS)
Systemic Sclerosis (SSc)	Hidebound chest (diffuse cutaneous SSc)			ILD (NSIP >> UIP > DAD); Aspiration pneumonia	PAH
Sjögren's Syndrome		Pleurisy ± effusion	Bronchiectasis	ILD (NSIP > LIP > OP, UIP or DAD)	Lymphadenopathy; Lymphoma
Dermato- and Polymyositis (DM, PM)	Respiratory muscle and diaphragm weakness			ILD (NSIP >OP > DAD or UIP); Aspiration pneumonia	PAH
Behçet's Disease		Pleurisy		OP	Pulmonary artery aneurysm; Arterial and venous thrombosis
Relapsing Polychondritis	Costochondritis		Laryngeal destruction; Tracheomalacia	Pneumonia	
Systemic Vasculitides		Effusion (CSS)	Large airway stenoses (AASV)	Haemorrhage; Cavitating lesions (AASV)	Mediastinal lymphadenopathy
Sarcoidosis	Respiratory muscle and diaphragm weakness	Effusion	Airflow obstruction due to endobronchial sarcoidosis	Pulmonary fibrosis	Bilateral hilar lymphadenopathy (Löfgren's syndrome); PAH
Periodic Fevers		Pleurisy ± effusion			
Chest wall deformity	Congenital or acquired kyphosis; scoliosis; pectus excavatum			Pneumonia	Secondary PAH

Abbreviations: ILD: interstitial lung disease; UIP: usual interstitial pneumonia; NSIP: non-specific interstitial pneumonia; OP: organising pneumonia; LIP: lymphocytic interstitial pneumonia; DAD: diffuse alveolar damage, APLS: antiphospholipid antibody syndrome; PAH: pulmonary arterial hypertension; SSc: Systemic sclerosis; CSS: Churg Strauss Syndrome.

Epidemiology

Chest wall and pleura
- Costochondritis occurs in patients with SpAs, sarcoid, and SAPHO.
- The hidebound chest is a complication of truncal scleroderma in diffuse cutaneous systemic sclerosis.
- Myopathy/myositis.
- Involvement of respiratory muscles occurs in about 25% of patients with inflammatory muscle diseases; this predisposes the patient to pneumonia, but is a rare cause of ventilatory failure.
- >50% of patients with sarcoidosis have granulomas in their muscles, but <1% are symptomatic.
- The 'shrinking lung' syndrome has been reported as a rare (<0.3%) complication of SLE.
- Pleurisy, pleuritis, and effusions are the commonest pulmonary manifestations of SLE, affecting up to 35%. RA pleural effusions are usually small and asymmetric, occurring in 5% of patients, in particular males with long-standing articular disease and those with subcutaneous nodules.
- Apical pleural thickening is an early feature of AS; effusions are rare. Up to 10% of cases of Wegener's granulomatosis (WG) will develop an effusion.
- Pectus excavatum is the commonest congenital chest wall deformity, affecting 1 in 300 live births.
- Scoliosis is usually idiopathic, but can be associated with neuromuscular diseases, e.g. poliomyelitis.

Airways
- Cricoarytenoiditis occurs commonly (>25%) in RA and has been reported in SLE and in SpAs.
- Vocal fold lesions, including nodules and bamboo nodes, occur in RA.
- Recurrent laryngeal neuropathy may occur in any condition associated with mononeuritis (including SLE and small vessel vasculitides).
- Tracheomalacia and bronchomalacia are features of RP. A retrospective review of dynamic chest CT scans in patients with RP indicates intra-thoracic airway abnormalities in 94% (17/18) and extra-thoracic (tracheal and proximal bronchial) involvement in 44% (8/18).
- Large airway stenosis. Tracheal stenosis occurs commonly in patients with WG.
- Follicular and/or obliterative bronchiolitis: Small airways obstructive lung disease is most commonly seen in RA compared with other rheumatological conditions.
- Bronchiectasis is found in RA patients with severe, chronic nodular disease. HRCT studies indicate a prevalence of 30% in RA and 20% in SLE patients.

Lung parenchyma
Interstitial lung disease (ILD)
The prevalence and clinical significance of ILD varies in the autoimmune connective tissues diseases. With the advent of HRCT, ILD is becoming increasingly recognized.
- In post-mortem studies of SSc, ILD is present in up to 80%, although clinically significant fibrosis occurs in approximately 40% of patients.
- In SSc, anti-topoisomerase antibody (Scl-70) is associated with ILD, whereas anti-centromere antibody is protective.
- ILD is less common (30%) in dermato- (DM) and poly-myositis (PM), SLE (30%), RA (20%), and Sjögren's syndrome (10%).
- In RA, ILD is more common in men, in late-onset disease and in those with high titre RF.
- In sarcoidosis, 25% will develop pulmonary fibrosis.

Other parenchymal lesions
- Rheumatoid nodules are reported in up to 20% of patients.
- Diffuse alveolar haemorrhage is rare, occurring in 1-5% of SLE patients.
- Nodular lesions are found in 55–70% of those diagnosed with ANCA-associated systemic vasculitis (AASV) and cavitating lesions occur in 35–50% of patients with WG.
- Pneumonia is a primary concern in patients treated with immunosuppression. In addition, some patients with SLE have an increased risk of infection with encapsulated bacteria.
- Aspiration pneumonia may be a complication both of oesophageal dysmotility in SSc and weak upper pharyngeal muscles in DM and PM.

Pulmonary vasculature and lymphatics
- Pulmonary arterial hypertension (PAH) due to a vasculopathy is most frequently occurs in limited cutaneous SSc (~12%) and mixed connective tissue disease (MCTD), less commonly in SLE (~4%) and APLS (~2%), and rarely in RA and PM.
- Pulmonary capillaritis (small vessel vasculitis) is associated with RA, PM, and SLE.
- Thromboembolism occurs in 25% of SLE (most with APLS) patients and is a major cause of death.
- In Behçet's disease, the reported prevalence of pulmonary complications ranges from 1 to 8%. The pulmonary arteries are the second commonest site for aneurysms particularly in young men. Superior vena cava obstruction can result from thrombosis of innominate and sub-clavian veins.
- Although it can occur at any age, sarcoidosis has a peak incidence between 20 and 39 years. All racial and ethnic groups are affected, in particular northern Europeans (5–40/100 000) and African Americans (35.5/100 000). PAH has been identified in up to 23% of patients at rest and 43% with exertion.

Aetiology/pathophysiology

Chest wall and pleura
- Costochondritis in RP is characterized by recurrent, destructive inflammation of cartilaginous structures.
- 'Shrinking lung' syndrome is attributed to diaphragmatic weakness, however a myopathy is present only in a third of SLE patients and muscle enzymes are normal. Phrenic nerve neuropathy, involving immune complex deposition and ischaemic lesions, has also been reported.
- The aetiology of congenital and acquired chest wall deformities is largely obscure. Polymorphisms in the oestrogen receptor gene have been implicated in adolescent idiopathic scoliosis.

Pleuritis and pleural effusions
The presence of immune complexes, complement activation products, and immune deposits within the parietal pleura suggest an immune-mediated mechanism is a common pathway in the development of pleural disease.

- In RA, immune complexes are probably generated locally in the pleura, whereas they are derived from the circulation in SLE.
- RA-associated effusions have a high concentration of IL-2, which suggests that a local T cell mediated immune reaction maybe a more important mechanism than in SLE.
- Both sterile and septic empyemas have been reported in RA.

Airways
- Dysphonia may result from synovitis/subluxation of the cricoarytenoid joint, rheumatoid nodules of the larynx, or arteritis of the vasa nervorum of the recurrent laryngeal and vagus nerves.
- Laryngeal paralysis and destruction, and tracheomalacia are consequences of recurrent inflammation of the airway wall cartilage.
- Upper and large airways inflammation can occur with AASV. Tracheobronchial ulceration, intra-luminal pseudotumour and bronchiomalacia due to necrotizing granulomas of the cartilage result. The subglottic region of the trachea is most frequently involved, usually in younger patients. Scarring here leads to airway stenosis and obstruction.
- Follicular bronchiolitis is characterized by peribronchiolar inflammation with lymphoid follicles situated between bronchioles and pulmonary arteries. External compression of the airway lumen results, leading to small airways obstruction.
- Obliterative bronchiolitis occurs as a result of direct occlusion of the airway lumen by fibrotic tissue. The small airways proximal to the terminal bronchiole are involved. The aetiology is unknown.
- Bronchiectasis: dilatation and thickening of the airways proximal to the terminal bronchioles occurs as a result of chronic inflammation.

Lung parenchyma
ILD associated with autoimmune connective tissue disease is classified histologically in accordance with the ATS/ERS consensus statement. The aetiology, the role of autoantibodies and underlying disease pathogenesis, remains to be determined.
- Epithelial injury is a common feature that triggers a number of inflammatory cytokine, coagulation, and mechano-sensing cascades.
- This activates stem cells, epithelial to mesenchymal transition, fibrocyte recruitment from the bone marrow, and differentiation of fibroblasts to myofibroblasts.
- Excessive collagen and extra-cellular matrix is produced ultimately leading to fibrosis.

NSIP (non-specific interstitial pneumonia)
This is the commonest ILD associated with autoimmune connective tissue diseases, particularly SSc. Both cellular (interstitial inflammation with lymphoid aggregates and minimal fibrosis) and fibrotic (dense interstitial collagen deposition leading to distortion of the lung architecture) forms occur. NSIP can be distinguished from UIP by its temporal uniformity.

UIP (usual interstitial pneumonia)
The characteristic histological features are architectural destruction, fibrosis with honeycomb formation, fibroblastic foci, and a peripheral, patchy distribution. These areas of fibrosis are interspersed with normal lung and connect to form a reticulum.

LIP (lymphocytic interstitial pneumonia)
Diffuse infiltration of the alveolar septa by a dense polyclonal lymphocytic infiltrate. Both B and T cells are present. T cells predominate in the alveolar septum; B cells are found in the lymphoid follicles. Viral infections, including EBV, may have a role in disease pathogenesis. It is important to exclude lymphoma.

Organizing pneumonia (OP)
This is most frequently reported with DM or PM. Organizing granulation tissue fills the alveolar ducts and alveoli. It is a patchy process and overall the lung architecture is preserved. Although OP usually resolves, it can progress to fibrosis.

Diffuse alveolar damage (DAD)
This is a rapidly progressive form of ILD with a high mortality. It has a diffuse distribution with hyaline membrane formation, septal thickening, and organization of the air spaces. Granulomas, viral inclusions, and neutrophilic abscesses suggest an infective aetiology.

Other parenchymal pathology
- Drug-induced pneumonitis is a diagnosis made after exclusion of infection, haemorrhage, or other pulmonary disease, in the setting of an appropriate drug exposure history. Risk factors include age, diabetes mellitus, pre-existing lung disease, hypo-albuminaemia, renal impairment, and use of disease-modifying anti-rheumatic drugs (DMARDs). The mechanism is unknown. Histological patterns of NSIP, OP, granulomas, and eosinophilic infiltrates have been reported.
- Rheumatoid nodules occur in the interlobular septa, subpleural regions and lung parenchyma. They can be single or multiple, can cavitate and must be differentiated from a pulmonary neoplasm. Caplan described multiple nodules that rapidly cavitated in 25% of Welsh coal miners with RA. Other occupational dust exposures have been associated with this syndrome.
- Pulmonary haemorrhage occurs is due to involvement of small vessels in AASVs (WG, microscopic polyangiitis [MPA] and Churg–Strauss syndrome [CSS]). Fibrinoid necrosis, necrotizing granulomas and neutrophilic infiltrates occur within the vessel walls. The resulting nodular lesions may cavitate and either resolve or repair with fibrosis. ANCAs have been implicated in the disease pathogenesis.
- Infection: hyposplenic SLE patients are susceptible to encapsulated organisms. Those patients receiving anti-TNFα regimens are at an increased risk of severe common infections, atypical mycobacterial and MTB infections. Fungal colonization and aspergillomas can occur in pulmonary cavities (e.g. AS, WG).
- The susceptibility for, and phenotype of, sarcoid depends on both genetic and environmental factors.

Aetiology and pathophysiology of lung sarcoid

Genetic factors
Macrophage HLA class II antigens encoded by HLA-DRB1 and DQB1, butyrophilin-like 2 (*BTNL2*) gene on chromosome 6p and chromosomes 3p, 5p, 5q

Environmental factors
Inorganic particles, metalworking, moulds, mycobacterial, and propionibacterial infections.

CHAPTER 3 Organ involvement in rheumatological disease

Granulomas
CD4+ T cells interact with antigen presenting cells to form and maintain epitheloid, non-caseating granulomas. These activated CD4+ cells can differentiate into Th-1 like cells secreting IL-2 and IFNγ, to propagate the local cellular immune response. Sarcoid granulomas may resolve, persist or lead to fibrosis, and can, depending on their site, lead to lymphadenopathy and pulmonary hypertension.

Matrix changes
Activated alveolar macrophages stimulate fibroblast proliferation and collagen production via secretion of fibronectin and CCL18. Matrix metalloproteinases 8 and 9 are increased in bronchoalveolar lavage specimens. Sputa from these patients can contribute to extra-cellular matrix degradation and remodelling that ultimately results in fibrosis.

Pulmonary vasculature and lymphatics
Pulmonary arterial hypertension (PAH)
Of greatest relevance in SSc, PAH evolves following fibrocollagenous intimal and medial arterial thickening, alterations in the elastic lamina and luminal narrowing.
- In SSc, endothelial injury appears to be an early event and aberrant 'cross-talk' between endothelia, underlying vascular smooth muscle cells and other stromal cells orchestrates the proliferative vasculopathy and fibrosis.
- Vasoconstrictive, pro-inflammatory and prothrombotic endothelial products, including endothelin-1 (ET-1) and von Willebrand factor are elevated.
- Anti-inflammatory, anti-thrombotic, vasodilators, such as nitric oxide are reduced.
- The proliferative vasculopathy serves to increase pulmonary vascular resistance and to cause PAH. Anti-endothelial cell antibodies (AECA), including antibodies specific for the platelet-derived growth factor (PDGF) receptor have also been implicated in the initiation of endothelial cell injury in SSc.
- The development of PAH in SSc is also associated with the presence of anti-cardiolipin antibodies.
- In SLE-related PAH, granular deposits of IgG and the complement protein C1q have been identified in vessel walls, suggesting that immune deposits may be involved in the pathogenesis.
- In sarcoidosis, granulomatous infiltration of the pulmonary arterioles has been observed.
- Secondary PAH can result from long-term sequelae of chronic hypoxia, secondary to severe airway, parenchymal or chest wall disease.
- Pulmonary artery aneurysm: Histopathological features of Behçet's disease include a systemic vasculitis of all vessels of both the arterial and venous circulations, and perivascular inflammatory infiltrates. Inflammatory thrombotic occlusion, recanalization and fresh thrombi can be found within arterial aneurysms.

Thromboembolic disease
- In SLE/APLS, anti-phospholipid antibodies promote thrombo-embolic disease by up-regulating endothelial cell adhesion molecules, increasing expression of pro-coagulant endothelial cell products (tissue factor, von Willebrand factor, thromboxane A_2) and decreasing anti-coagulant products (thrombomodulin, protein C).
- In Behçet's disease, a number of mechanisms have been implicated in thrombosis, including increased platelet reactivity and homocysteine levels, and reduced activated protein C and tissue plasminogen activator levels.

Lymphadenopathy
- Lymphadenopathy results from recruitment and proliferation of lymphocytes in an adaptive immune response, as in autoimmune connective tissue diseases or due to development of epitheloid granulomas (e.g. hilar lymphadenopathy in sarcoidosis).
- Lymphoma represents malignant transformation of lymphoid elements. This may manifest as hilar lymphadenopathy. Approximately 5% of patients with Sjögren's syndrome develop lymphoma.

Risk factors
- Smoking, in particular patients with RA.
- Pets.
- **Occupational exposures**: asbestos, coal dust and hard metal pneumoconiosis.
- Pneumotoxins: azathioprine, methotrexate, cyclophosphamide, celecoxib, sulphasalazine, leflunomide, D-penicillamine, gold, and anti-TNFα therapies – infliximab, etanercept.
- Susceptibility to encapsulated bacterial infection (hyposplenism or mannose binding protein deficiency in SLE).
- Left ventricular failure is more likely to occur in patients with accelerated atherosclerosis (SLE, RA) or with cardiomyopathies, or in those patients treated with glucocorticoids (GCs).
- Anticardiolipin antibodies and/or lupus anticoagulant are risk factors for thromboembolic disease and the development of PAH.
- Anti-Jo-1 antibodies are associated with the development of ILD in DM and PM.

Clinical features

The exercise capacity of patients with rheumatological diseases is often limited by musculoskeletal disease. Hence, exertional dyspnoea may be masked. For all patients, assess the respiratory rate, the presence of central cyanosis and oxygen saturations (either on air or inspired FiO_2).

Chest wall and pleura
- Dyspnoea from chest wall restriction.
- Orthopnoea and dyspnoea exacerbated by being in a bath of water suggest diaphragmatic weakness.
- Chest pain needs clarifying whether it is parasternal/paravertebral (costochondral/costovertebral) or whether it is more diffuse and worse on deep inspiration (pleuritic).
- Chest pain referred from general lower neck and upper spinal pathology is common (e.g. degenerative disease or vertebral fracture).
- History of chest wall deformity and trauma.

Examination features
- Costovertebral tenderness (costochondritis in SpAs or SAPHO).
- Manubriosternal and sternoclavicular joint (SCJ) tenderness and swelling is a feature of SpAs, SAPHO, and axial sarcoid.
- Reduction of chest expansion in AS, SSc, DM, PM, or SLE shrinking lung. Serial measurements of chest expansion are useful for monitoring thoracic restriction involvement in AS.

- Paradoxical abdominal movement occurs with diaphragmatic weakness.
- Stony dull percussion note, reduced breath sounds and vocal resonance indicates pleural effusion.
- A pleural rub is characteristic of inflammation of pleura (pleurisy alone, or in association with pneumonia or pulmonary embolus).

Airways
- Shortness of breath, particularly on exertion.
- Persistent productive cough or recurrent lower respiratory tract infections suggests bronchiectasis.
- Wheeze: establish diurnal variation and relationship to exercise.
- Hoarseness may indicate arthritis of cricoarytenoid joints or vocal fold nodules (e.g. RA).
- Cough is a non-specific symptom associated with different airways diseases.

Examination features
- Inspiratory stridor with large airway obstruction.
- Monophonic (tracheal) inspiratory wheeze, associated with a bovine cough may indicate tracheomalacia in relapsing polychondritis (rare).
- Expiratory polyphonic wheezing indicates bronchospasm.
- High-pitched, end-inspiratory basal squeaks, in the absence of wheezing, are characteristic of obliterative bronchiolitis (usually with RA).

Lung parenchyma
- Cough: usually persistent and non-productive.
- Exertional dyspnoea.

Examination features
- Finger clubbing occurs in ~70% of patients with pulmonary fibrosis.
- Reduction in chest expansion in severe disease.
- Inspiratory crepitations: basal in pulmonary fibrosis associated with RA, SLE, systemic sclerosis (SSc), Sjögren's syndrome, DM, and PM.

Pulmonary vasculature and lymphatics
- Shortness of breath, particularly on exertion.
- Haemoptysis.

Examination features
- Signs of right heart strain may be evident in PAH (large 'a' and 'v' waves in JVP, parasternal heave, right ventricular gallop rhythm, loud P2, pansystolic murmur loudest over left sternal edge).
- Right heart failure (elevated JVP, peripheral pitting oedema) occurs in decompensated PAH. Systolic waves in the JVP and a pulsatile liver indicate tricuspid regurgitation.
- Parotid enlargement and palpable lymphadenopathy (cervical, axillary, and/or inguinal) may be present in cases of Sjögren's syndrome or sarcoidosis, in which hilar lymphadenopathy can be demonstrated by radiological imaging.

Investigations

Chest wall and pleura

Lung function tests: spirometry
Measures such as the forced vital capacity (FVC) and total lung capacity (TLC) are used to detect a restrictive defect, which may be attributable to chest wall, pleural or fibrotic lung disease. In restrictive disease, the FEV_1/FVC ratio is preserved or elevated (although absolute values of FEV_1 decrease). FVC is used to monitor respiratory function in patients with DM or PM. Ventilatory support should be considered when FVC <50% and/or hypercapnic respiratory failure.

Respiratory muscle function testing
Sniff test. Maximal inspiratory and expiratory pressures measure respiratory muscle, including diaphragmatic, function. Fluoroscopy can be used to assess for the presence of diaphragmatic weakness or paralysis.

CXR
500 ml pleural effusion will be detectable as blunting of the costophrenic angle. Larger effusions are obvious. Raised hemidiaphragm suggests diaphragmatic weakness.

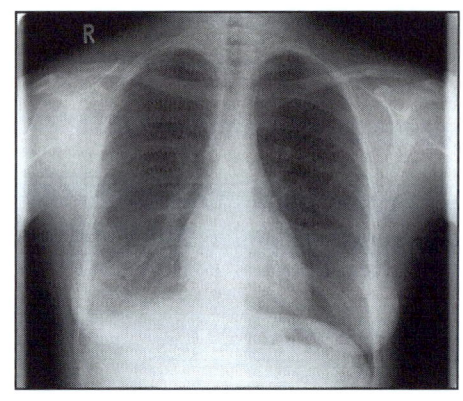

Figure 3.2 Right sided pleural effusion in SLE.

HRCT chest
Ankylosis of costochondral and costovertebral joints is visible (AS). Pleural thickening alone or in the presence of a pleural effusion can be detected.

Pleural aspirate and Abrams pleural biopsy.
- In RA and SLE, the pleural fluid is usually an exudate (protein >30 g/l).
- RA associated pleural effusions can become a sterile empyema, characterized by a reduced glucose concentration (<30 mg/dl), elevated lactate dehydrogenase (LDH), and cholesterol levels, high titre RF and low pH.
- SLE effusions have a raised glucose level (>60 mg/dl) and the pleural fluid/serum glucose ratio is >0.5. Note that in right heart failure, secondary to pulmonary hypertension, the pleural fluid may be a transudate.
- For all pleural aspirates request microscopy, culture and sensitivity and in patients who are immunosuppressed, especially with anti-TNFα, request a Ziehl–Nielsen stain for acid-fast bacilli, mycobacterial cultures, and consider other assays, including PCR.
- The pleural biopsy should be cultured in addition to histological assessment. Request cytology where malignancy, including lymphoma, is suspected.

T-spot assay if M. tuberculosis (MTB) is suspected.
This assay of the patient's T cell responses to mycobacterial antigen, ESAT-6, is particularly useful for discriminating

CHAPTER 3 Organ involvement in rheumatological disease

Table 3.3 Lung function test: spirometry, characteristics in disease associated with rheumatological conditions

Lung involvement	FEV₁	FVC	FEV₁/FVC	TLC	RV	TLCO	KCO
Chest wall/pleura	N or ↓	↓	N or ↑	↓	N or ↓	N or ↓	N or ↑
Bronchiectasis	↓	N or ↓	↓	N or ↑	N or ↑	N or ↓	N
OB	N or ↓	N or ↓	↓ or ↑	N or ↑	↑	↓	N
ILD	N or ↓	↓	↑	↓	N or ↓	↓	↓
Alveolar haemorrhage	N	N	N	N	N	N or ↑	↑
Pulmonary vascular	N	N	N	N	N	↓	↓

FEV₁: Forced expiratory volume in 1 second; FVC: Forced vital capacity; TLC: Total Lung Capacity; RV: Residual Volume; TLCO: Gas Transfer Factor; KCO: Gas transfer factor adjusted for lung volume (KCOc is also corrected for Hb)

between exposure to MTB and BCG (the latter lacks expression of the ESAT-6 antigen).

Arterial blood gases
For assessment of oxygenation and the presence of hypercapnic respiratory failure.

Airways
Lung function tests: spirometry
In healthy individuals, the FEV₁/FVC ratio is usually 75%, falling to ~65% in those aged over 70 years. In obstructive ventilatory defect, the FEV₁/FVC ratio is <70%, whereas a ratio >80% indicates restrictive lung disease. Upper airway obstruction is suggested by FEV₁(L)/PEFR(l/min) ratio >10 (e.g. in RP).

Serial peak expiratory flow rate (PEFR) measures.
PEFR should be measured on at least three occasions throughout the day, including an early morning reading to assess for diurnal variation and are used to diagnose reversible obstructive airways disease.

Flow-volume loop (Figure 3.3)
Used to investigate upper (fixed or variable) or lower airway obstruction, or restrictive disease.

HRCT
Lung windows can be used to examine abnormal airway architecture, e.g. bronchiectasis, tracheomalacia. Expiratory images are helpful in the detection of air trapping, as occurs with small airways disease. Obliterative bronchiolitis is characterized by a 'mosaic attenuation pattern' on HRCT, whereas 'tree in bud' typifies follicular bronchiolitis. HRCT may also be used to examine the larynx for signs of cricoarytenoiditis, subluxation, or deformity.

Sputum analysis
Microscopy, culture, and sensitivities, including Ziehl–Nielsen stain for acid-fast bacilli, mycobacterial cultures and, possibly, PCR analysis should be requested in patients at risk of MTB.

Fibre optic bronchoscopy
Used to determine the presence of tracheal stenosis. Endobronchial sarcoid granulomas have a characteristic cobblestone appearance. Airway abnormalities should be biopsied for histological assessment.

Lung parenchyma
Lung function tests: spirometry
The transfer factors (TLCO and KCO) measure the efficiency of gas exchange. The KCO is corrected for lung volume and KCOc corrected for both lung volume and haemoglobin concentration.

HRCT (Figures 3.4–3.6)
Lung windows enable the detection of parenchymal disease. Ground glass change represents alveolitis (NSIP, LIP, DAD), pulmonary haemorrhage, or infection (PCP, viral). Reticulations, traction bronchiectasis, honeycombing, and architectural distortion are found in the presence of fibrosis. Septal thickening, centrilobular nodules, and cysts are features of LIP, whereas consolidation occurs with organizing pneumonia.

Other imaging modalities
- ¹⁸FDG-PET and MR with gadolinium may be used to determine neurological and cardiac involvement in sarcoidosis.

Upper panel: Airflow obctructions as occurs with airways disease, e.g. obliterative bronchiolitis.

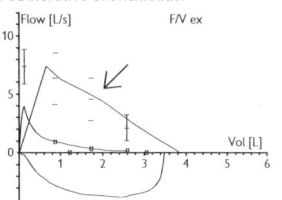

Middle panel: Restrictive ventilatory defect as seen with fibrosing ILD, pleural, or chest wall involvement.

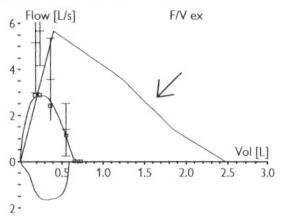

Lower panel: Fixed extrathoracic upper airway obstruction.

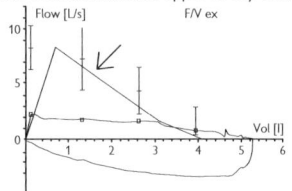

Figure 3.3 Patterns of Flow-volume loops (In each panel, the arrow indicates normal flow volume loop).

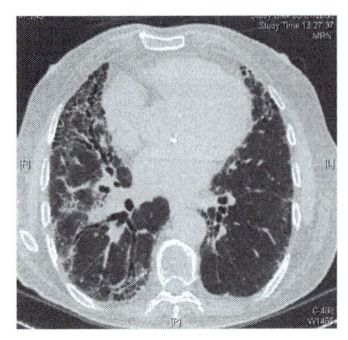

Figure 3.4 HRCT showing pulmonary fibrosis (UIP) in a patient with SLE.

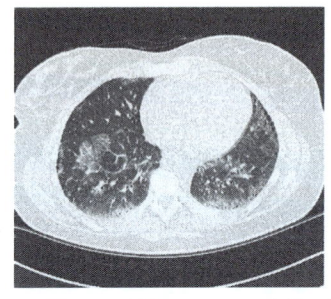

Figure 3.5 HRCT showing NSIP in a patient with SSc-related ILD.

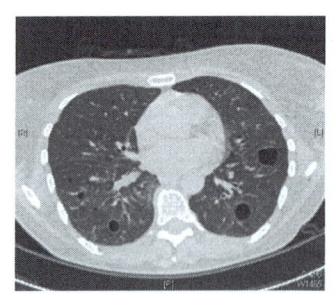

Figure 3.6 HRCT showing LIP in Sjögren's Syndrome.

- Oesophageal manometry, barium swallow and gastroscopy to assess for aspiration and upper GI tract involvement.

Fibre optic bronchoscopy with bronchoalveolar lavage (BAL) and transbronchial biopsy
- Differential cell count of BAL provides diagnostic and prognostic information. BAL neutrophilia in the presence of fibrosis is associated with a poor prognosis. Lymphocytic lavages are found with cellular NSIP, OP, LIP, and sarcoidosis. The presence of eosinophils (>5%) may be associated with drug-induced pneumonitis. A blood-stained lavage signifies pulmonary haemorrhage.
- Transbronchial biopsies have a diagnostic yield >85% for sarcoidosis when multiple lung segments are sampled.

A video-assisted thoracoscopic surgical (VATS) lung biopsy may be required for diagnosis (if atypical features on HRCT) for other ILDs and pulmonary vasculitis.

Other useful investigations
- Serum ACE, serum, and 24-h urinary calcium may be elevated in sarcoidosis. ACE levels are increased in 60% of patients and are influenced by ACE gene polymorphisms. Its role in diagnosis and management of sarcoidosis remains controversial.
- Avian and aspergillus precipitins in those with appropriate clinical history or suggestive radiological features.

Pulmonary vasculature and lymphatics
Lung function tests: spirometry.
If the KCO is decreased disproportionately compared to lung volume (e.g. TLC or FVC), this may reflect a pulmonary vascular defect.

CXR (Figure 3.7)
Hilar and paratracheal lymphadenopathy can be detected. CXR is used to stage sarcoidosis.
- **Stage 1:** bilateral hilar lymphadenopathy.
- **Stage 2:** lymphadenopathy and parenchymal disease.
- **Stage 3:** parenchymal disease alone
- **Stage 4:** fibrosis.

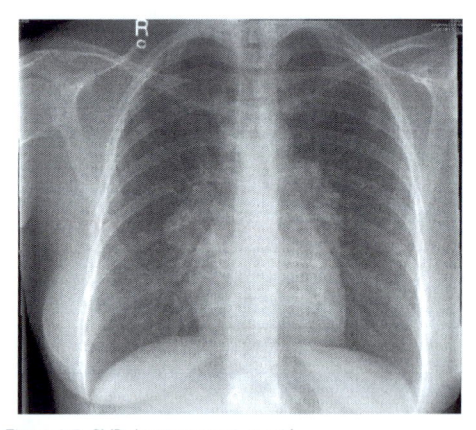

Figure 3.7 CXR showing stage 1 sarcoid.

Ventilation-perfusion scan (Figure 3.8)
This is the investigation for a suspected pulmonary embolus in a patient with a normal plain CXR.

Other CT examinations
CT pulmonary angiogram (CTPA) is used for a suspected pulmonary embolus in patients with pre-existing pulmonary disease and/or an abnormal plain CXR and to identify pulmonary artery aneurysms. Mediastinal windows can assess for hilar and mediastinal lymphadenopathy.

Echo and right heart catheterization studies
Used to evaluate pulmonary hypertension both at rest and with exercise.

CHAPTER 3 Organ involvement in rheumatological disease

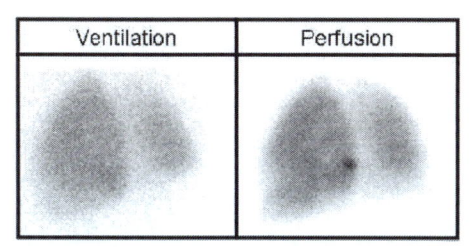

Figure 3.8 Ventilation/perfusion (V/Q) scan from patient with APLS showing multiple areas of impaired perfusion.

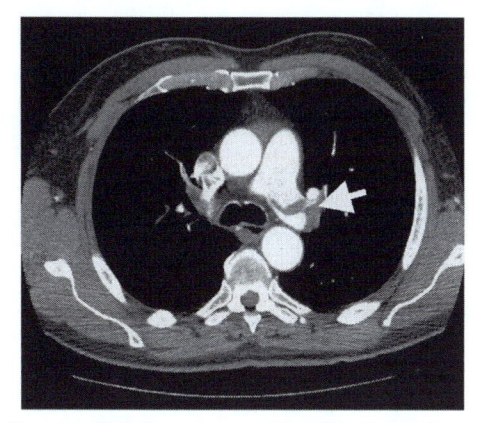

Figure 3.9 CTPA demonstrates a saddle embolus (arrowed).

Other pulmonary or related assessments
- **Pulse oximetry:** non-invasive assessment of oxygen saturation of haemoglobin.
- **Blood gases:**

	Normal	Type I respiratory failure	Type II respiratory failure
H⁺ (nmol/l)	35–45	35–45	≥45
PO$_2$ (kPa)	10–13.3	<8.0	<8.0
PCO$_2$ (kPa)	4.8–6.1	<6.6	>6.6
Plasma HCO$_3^-$ (mmol/l	22–26	22–26	>26
O$_2$ saturation (%)	92–100	<92	<92

- **FBC:** investigation for anaemia is important in the breathless patient.
- **Exercise tests:** the 6-min walk test is often used as a serial assessment of function in patients with known ILD and/or PAH. Note that patients with rheumatological conditions may be limited by musculoskeletal pathology.
- **Sleep studies:** overnight oximetry to assess for evidence of oxygen desaturation. Detailed polysonography is required for obstructive sleep apnoea and sleep disorders.
- **Fitness to fly assessments:** hypoxic challenge should be performed in patients with resting sea level SpO$_2$ 92–95% who have an additional risk factor (hypercapnia, FEV$_1$<50%, restrictive lung disease, cerebrovascular or cardiac disease, or discharged within 6 weeks for an exacerbation of chronic lung or cardiac disease). SpO$_2$<92% at rest or use of supplemental oxygen at sea level indicates the need for in-flight oxygen. Patients with infectious mycobacterial disease must not travel by public air transportation until rendered non-infectious.
- ECG is used to detect signs of right heart strain (right axis deviation, dominant secondary R wave in V1); P pulmonale, right bundle branch block and atrial conduction abnormalities, such as atrial fibrillation, may also occur.
- Echocardiography is used as a screening test for PAH, signs of which include right ventricular dilatation or hypertrophy and tricuspid regurgitation (TR). If TR is present, it is possible to measure the peak pulmonary artery systolic pressure indirectly with Doppler echocardiography.
- Right heart catheterization is used to measure pulmonary artery pressure to enable diagnosis, assess patient response to vasodilators and facilitate monitoring of pulmonary arterial hypertension.

Treatment
In all cases exposure to exacerbating factors should be reduced or stopped.
- Stop smoking.
- Minimize/remove occupational or recreational exposures.
- Stop pneumotoxic drugs.
- Review other drugs that may be exacerbating respiratory disease (e.g. GCs and NSAIDs in left ventricular failure; immunosuppressants in bronchiectasis, pneumonia and empyema).
- Assess need for supportive measures including O$_2$, analgesia and the need for ventilatory support.
- Influenza and pneumococcal vaccinations should be considered for patients who are either immunosuppressed or have pulmonary disease.

Chest wall and pleura
Costochondritis/enthesitis
Topical administration of NSAID gel may provide local relief. Oral NSAIDs. Judicious use of manubriosternal and SCJ GC injection in SAPHO.

SSc hidebound chest
The patient may be advised to perform daily deep breathing exercises, but there is no evidence base that this or pharmacological intervention affects the SSc progression.

SLE shrinking lung
There are no specific treatments, although GCs, high-dose inhaled β-agonists, and theophylline have been tried. Generally, the prognosis is good

Myositis-related chest wall/diaphragmatic weakness.
Treatment is of the underlying condition, plus the provision of chest physiotherapy to aid clearance of retained secretions. Non-invasive ventilation may be required if there is evidence of hypercapnic respiratory failure, as may occur following an acute presentation of myositis.

Pleural effusions
Review other evidence of RA disease activity (e.g. DAS28, CRP, ESR) or SLE disease activity (e.g. BILAG, SLEDAI, ESR, C3 and C4, CRP (CRP often rises in SLE serositis, in the absence of infection). In the presence of active disease, adjust or change immunosuppressive regimen to control systemic symptoms. Thoracocentesis with a chest drain is

required for large effusions or those refractory to medical treatment. Consider pleurodesis and/or pleurectomy for recurrent, non-infective effusions.

Empyema
Thoracocentesis with a chest drain together with appropriate antibiotic treatment of the underlying infection. The presence of pleural thickening (>1 mm on CT images) or an extensively loculated effusion may indicate the need for surgical intervention. Review underlying rheumatological disease activity and assess the nature of and reasons for immunosuppression (e.g. neutropaenia, lymphopenia, hypogammaglobulinaemia). Review the use of conventional and biologic immunosuppressants.

Congenital/acquired scoliosis, kyphosis and pectus excavatum
Physiotherapy to aid draining of secretions from hypoventilated regions and to retard progression of deformity. If spinal deformity is progressive, refer to spinal surgeon for assessment.

Airways

Cricoarytenoid arthritis, laryngeal destruction, tracheomalacia
Maintaining adequate ventilation is the mainstay of treatment. Tracheostomy is required if there is significant laryngeal involvement. Surgery or the insertion of airway stents has been described to relieve severe airflow obstruction. Chest physiotherapy is important to aid with clearance of secretions. Steroids and immunosuppression have been used in the management of acute inflammatory episodes.

Proximal airway stenosis
Control the systemic disease with immunosuppressive treatments. Additional measures include dilatation and local injections of long-acting GCs to the involved sites of the trachea, performed via rigid or flexible bronchoscopy. If there is severe airflow obstruction, airway stents or tracheostomy may be necessary.

Bronchiectasis
Physiotherapy with postural drainage and appropriate antibiotic regimes form the basis of treatment. Inhaled corticosteroids and long-acting β-agonists are helpful for obstructive airways disease.

Follicular bronchiolitis
Antibiotics and inhaled GCs are of no proven benefit. Oral GCs have varying results (see obliterative bronchiolitis).

Obliterative bronchiolitis
This responds poorly to oral or inhaled GCs. Macrolides (clarithromycin) and immunosuppressants including cyclophosphamide, sirolimus and mycophenolate mofetil (MMF) have been used with limited success. Overall prognosis is poor.

Lung parenchyma (ILD)
The decision to treat is often challenging and should be based on the evaluation of disease severity (as determined by extent of disease on HRCT and TLCO), longitudinal disease behaviour (change in FVC) and the histological type of ILD. There are few data from few therapeutic trials in these patients.

SSc
One open-label prospective and two retrospective analyses suggest that MMF is associated with reduced progression of ILD in SSc. A pilot study of MMF given with methylprednisolone pulses followed by low-dose prednisolone supports this. Although a small study (45 patients), cyclophosphamide followed by azathioprine compared to GCs alone failed to reveal any different between the two randomized arms.

SLE and RA associated ILD
There are no placebo-controlled trials of therapy. One small, open-labelled study of prednisolone treatment (60 mg/day for 4 weeks) showed resolution or improvement of symptoms in >60% of patients. Based on a series of case reports, treatment regimes involve a trial of GCs with an immunomodulatory agent, including cyclophosphamide, methotrexate, azathioprine, MMF, and rituximab (used for GC-resistant LIP). The role of anti-oxidant therapy in rheumatological disease associated UIP is unknown.

Lung parenchyma: other diseases

Sarcoidosis
Treatment is usually determined by stage of pulmonary disease and organ involvement.
- Löfgren's syndrome (stage 1 disease) symptoms are treated with NSAIDs. In these patients, >90% will undergo spontaneous resolution.
- Inhaled GCs are used for airways involvement (cough, wheeze, endobronchial sarcoidosis).
- A 3-month trial of oral GCs is required when there is ILD (stage 2, 3 or 4 disease). If lung function improves, taper the GC dose to 5–15 mg/day and treat for at least 12 months.
- GC-sparing agents including methotrexate, azathioprine and MMF have all been used in refractory disease. One RCT of anti-TNFα treatment showed modest improvement in FVC at 6 months.

Drug-induced pneumonitis
The most important treatment is stopping the offending drug and supportive measures (oxygen). GCs may have a role in methotrexate induced pneumonitis and eosinophilic diseases. Folinic rescue is often used when there is suspicion of underlying folate deficiency.

Rheumatoid nodules
Treatment is aimed at controlling the underlying systemic disease.

Pulmonary haemorrhage
Respiratory supportive therapy including mechanical ventilation may be required if there is evidence of respiratory failure.
- Treatments are directed for either the remission-induction or maintenance phase according to disease severity as determined by the European Vasculitis Study Group (EUVAS).
- Remission-induction phase:
  - limited disease: use a single agent, e.g. GCs, azathioprine or methotrexate;
  - early generalized disease – use oral GCs and cyclophosphamide or methotrexate;
  - active generalized disease – pulses of IV GCs and cyclophosphamide;
  - severe disease – as for active generalized disease plus plasma exchange therapy;
  - refractory disease – if the above treatments fail, consider infliximab, rituximab, antithymocyte globulin or IVIG. In one study, infliximab induced remission in 88% of patients but it was associated with a high rate of infection (21%) and disease relapse (20%). In a small

study with rituximab, remission was induced in all 11 patients and 8 of them had undetectable ANCA titres. Larger, randomized controlled studies are required to assess these treatments further.
- Maintenance phase once clinical remission has been established for 3–6 months. Usual maintenance therapy consists of low dose GCs with azathioprine or methotrexate. If intolerant, consider second line agents MMF, cyclophosphamide or leflunomide.
- Septrin (to treat *Staph. aureus* infection) has been shown to reduce the rate of relapses.

AASV cavitating lung lesions
Exclude infection and treat as above. Anti-TNFα therapies and rituximab have shown promising results.

Infections
- Treat pneumonia with appropriate antibiotics.
- Supportive measures including oxygen, analgesia, and chest physiotherapy may be required.
- Treat atypical mycobacterial disease or MTB in accordance with British Thoracic Society or American Thoracic Society guidelines. Referral to respiratory physician is recommended.
- For aspiration pneumonia, lifestyle measures (avoid large meals, and elevate the head of the bed) in addition to reflux treatment (PPI or ranitidine) and gastric motility stimulants are used.

Pulmonary vasculature and lymphatics
PAH Secondary to AICTDs
Supportive treatments include warfarin, diuretics, digoxin, oxygen, and lifestyle advice.
- For SSc-related PAH, bosentan, sildenafil, prostanoids and sitaxsentan are used (see p. 269–270).
- For other AICTDs, immunosuppress if evidence of active disease. Small, randomized studies of cyclophosphamide alone or in combination with GCs have shown a fall in pulmonary artery pressure.
- Patients with positive vasodilator challenge during right heart catheterization studies might benefit from a calcium channel blocker. Otherwise treatment pathways are as for SSc-related PAH.

Secondary PAH
Optimize treatment for the underlying lung disease. Supportive treatments as above.

Pulmonary embolism
Anticoagulate with warfarin; however, the duration of treatment and intensity of anticoagulation remains controversial. Beware of the development of aneurysms in patients with Behçet's syndrome (see below). Aspirin is a useful alternative in this group. Hydroxychloroquine may be added to the anticoagulant regime of patients with inflammatory rheumatological disease and thromboembolic disease, since there is some evidence that it has anticoagulant effects.

Pulmonary arterial aneurysm
A combination of prednisolone and cyclophosphamide therapy is used, although there are no RCT data on which to base management. Anticoagulation carries a significant risk and should be used only after systemic immunosuppressives have been started. Embolization is limited by the size and number of aneurysms.

Lymphoma
Refer to haematologist for appropriate management.

Prognosis/natural history
Pulmonary involvement in Rheumatological Disease is invariably associated with significant mortality.
- The histological type of ILD is the most important predictor of early mortality, with patterns characterized by fibrosis (UIP, fibrosing NSIP) having a worse prognosis than those demonstrating cellular disease (cellular NSIP, LIP, OP).
- RA patients with UIP type ILD have a survival similar to those with idiopathic pulmonary fibrosis (50% 3-year mortality).
- Diffuse alveolar haemorrhage that is associated with SLE has a 50% in hospital mortality.
- The development of PAH is associated with significant mortality, particularly in SSc.
- In Behçet's disease, pulmonary artery aneurysm formation has a poor prognosis, with a 2-year mortality of 30%.

Monitoring disease activity
In addition to clinical assessment, the monitoring of lung disease activity involves serial CXRs, lung function tests (the rate of decline of FVC is of prognostic importance in ILD), 6-minute walk tests and echocardiogram.

Transplantation should be considered for those with progressive ILD or PAH (TLCO <35%) in whom the systemic disease is well controlled.

Resources
Respiratory physiotherapy resources are available from the British Thoracic Society website. Available at: http://www.brit-thoracic.org.uk

Information related to drug induced lung diseases. Available at: www.pneumotox.com/base.php?fich=new&lg=en

Assessment tools
New York Heart Association (NYHA) Functional Classification system.

Class	Patient symptoms
I	No limitation of activity. Ordinary physical activity does not cause undue fatigue, palpitation, or dyspnoea.
II	Slight limitation of activity. Comfortable at rest, but ordinary physical activity results in fatigue, palpitation or dyspnoea.
III	Marked limitation of physical activity. Comfortable at rest, but less than ordinary activity causes fatigue, palpitation or dyspnoea.
IV	Symptomatic at rest. Any physical activity increases fatigue, palpitation, or dyspnoea.

Guidelines
British Thoracic Society (BTS) Guidelines for management of the Interstitial Lung Diseases (new version available 2008), Pulmonary hypertension, TB and Fitness to fly. Available at: http://www.brit-thoracic.org.uk/guideline-download.html
American Thoracic Society (ATS) guidelines for the management of mycobacterial disease. Available at: http://www.thoracic.org

ICD-10 codes
- J99.1 Respiratory disorder in diffuse CTD (DM, PM, SS, SLE, WG).
- J99.0* Rheumatoid lung disease.

- J99.8* Respiratory disorders in ankylosing spondylitis or cryoglobulinaemia.
- M95.5 Acquired deformity of chest and rib.

See also:

Rheumatoid arthritis	p. 197
Systemic lupus erythematosus	p. 240
Systemic sclerosis	p. 264
Dermatomyositis	p. 290
Polymyositis	p. 282
Sjögren's syndrome	p. 254
ANCA-associated vasculitis	p. 330
Behçet's disease	p. 340
Relapsing polychondritis	p. 346
Sarcoidosis	p. 512
The heart in rheumatological disease	p. 66

Further reading

Abraham D, Distler O. How does endothelial cell injury start? The role of endothelin in systemic sclerosis. *Arthr Res Ther* 2007; **9**(Suppl 2): S2.

American Thoracic Society/European Respiratory Society International Multidisciplinary Consensus Classification of the Idiopathic Interstitial Pneumonias. *Am J Respir Crit Care Med* 2002; **165**: 277–304.

Ansari A, Larson PH, Bates HD. Vascular manifestations of systemic lupus erythematosus: current perspective. *Angiology* 1986; **37**: 423–32.

Bayar N, Kara SA, et al. Cricoarytenoiditis in rheumatoid arthritis: radiologic and clinical study. *J Otolaryngol* 2003; **32**: 373–8

Gerbino AJ, Goss CH, Molitor JA. Effect of mycophenolate mofetil on pulmonary function in scleroderma-associated interstitial lung disease. *Chest* 2008; **133**: 455–60

Hoyles RK, Ellis RW, et al. A multicenter, prospective, randomised, double-blind, placebo-controlled trial of corticosteroids and intravenous cyclophosphamide followed by oral azathioprine for the treatment of pulmonary fibrosis in scleroderma. *Arthr Rheum* 2006; **54**: 3962–70.

Karim MY, Miranda LC, et al. Presentation and prognosis of the shrinking lung syndrome in systemic lupus erythematosus. *Semin Arthritis Rheum* 2002; **31**: 289–98.

Lee KS, Ernst A, et al. Relapsing polychondritis: prevalence of expiratory CT airway abnormalities. *Radiol* 2006; **240**: 565–73.

Liossis SN, Bounas A, Andronopoulous AP. Mycophenolate mofetil as first-line treatment improves clinically evident early scleroderma lung disease. *Rheumatol* 2006; **45**: 1005–8.

Nihtyanova SI, Brough GM, et al. Mycophenolate mofetil in diffuse cutaneous systemic sclerosis – a retrospective analysis. *Rheumatol* 2007; **46**: 442–5.

Quismorio FP Jr, Sharma O, et al. Immunologic and clinical studies in pulmonary hypertension associated with systemic lupus erythematosus. *Semin Arthritis Rheum* 1984; **13**: 349–59.

Utzig MJ, Warzelhan J, et al. Role of thoracic surgery and interventional bronchoscopy in Wegener's granulomatosis. *Ann Thorac Surg* 2002 **74**: 1948–52.

Vanthuyne M, Blockmans D, et al, A pilot study of myophenolate mofetil combined to intravenous methylprednisolone pulses and oral low-dose glucocorticoids in severe early systemic sclerosis. *Clin Exp Rheumatol* 2007; **25**: 287–92.

The heart

Cardiovascular disease accounts for the majority of premature mortality in several inflammatory Rheumatological conditions. Pericardial, myocardial and endocardial tissues are affected by the processes, which cause the underlying multisystem inflammatory diseases; Cardiac disease may also arise as a result of coronary or systemic/pulmonary arterial diseases.

Classification

Table 3.4 Anatomical classification of cardiac involvement in rheumatological disease

	Pericardial disease	Myocardial and conduction system disease	Endocardial (valvular) disease	Coronary artery disease	Pulmonary arterial hypertension	Aortitis
Rheumatoid arthritis (RA)	+++	+?	+	++	rare	+
Ankylosing spondylitis (AS)	±	+	++	+	rare	++
Reactive arthritis	±	±	±	±		+
Systemic lupus erythematosus (SLE)	+++	++	++	++		
Neonatal lupus		++				
APLS			+++			
Systemic sclerosis (SSc)	++	++	+	+	++	
Sjögren's syndrome (SS)	+	+	±			
Dermato- (DM) and polymyositis (PM)	±	+	±	±		
Behçet's disease	+		+	+		+
Kawasaki disease				+++		
Wegener's granulomatosis (WG)				+		
Churg–Strauss syndrome (CSS)		+		+		
Takayasu's disease		+	++	+		+++
Polyarteritis nodosum (PAN)	±	+++	±	+++		
Relapsing polychondritis			+			
Giant cell arteritis (GCA)		+++	+	+		+
Adult Still's disease	++	±	±			
Rheumatic fever	++	+++	+++	++		
JIA	++					
Haemachromatosis		++				
Sarcoidosis	+	+	?			
Hereditary connective tissue disease*			++			
Gout		?	?			

Abbreviations: APLS, antiphospholipid syndrome; JIA, Juvenile idiopathic arthritis; * e.g. Marfan syndrome, Ehlers–Danlos

Epidemiology

Pericardial involvement
Pericardial effusions occur commonly in RA, SLE, SSc, and Adult Still's disease, but most are asymptomatic.

Myocardial and conduction system disease
- Cardiomyopathy is rare in RA. Amyloid can occur in patients with persistent elevation of inflammatory markers.
- Haemochromatosis may present with arthritis and cardiomyopathy.
- Myocarditis occurs in ~10% of patients with SLE.
- In sarcoidosis, cardiac involvement has been reported in >25%, but this is rarely clinically significant.
- Giant cell myocardiits is rarely associated with RA, SLE, Sjögren's syndrome, GCA, and Takayasu's arteritis.
- In RA, ventricular arrhythmias or sudden cardiac death may be secondary to ischaemia, nodules, amyloidosis, increased sympathetic drive, and drugs.

- In SLE, sinus tachycardia, atrial fibrillation, and atrial ectopics are the most common dysrhythmias.
- In SSc, ventricular arrhythmias occur in about a half of patients and sudden cardiac death has been estimated to occur in ~5%.
- Atrial arrhythmias [atrial fibrillation (AF), atrial flutter or paroxysmal supraventricular tachycardia (SVT)] are present in about a quarter of SSc patients.
- Conduction disturbances occur in about a third of RA, SSc (bundle branch block) and SLE [first degree atrioventricular (AV) block] patients.
- Congenital heart block (CHB) is the most serious manifestation of neonatal lupus and occurs in ~2% of mothers with anti-Ro antibodies (~20% in a mother with a previous, affected child). CHB is reported to be associated with ~20% mortality and about two-thirds of live-born children require a pacemaker. Incomplete blocks may progress postnatally. Complete CHB, once established, is irreversible.
- Drug-induced cardiomyopathy may occur with corticosteroids or antimalarials.

Valvular disease
- In RA mitral and aortic valve regurgitation are common echocardiogram findings, but significant in a minority.
- In SLE, Libman-Sacks endocarditis is a verrucous endocarditis of valve leaflets, papillary muscle, and/or endocardium.
- Valvular disease occurs in about 50% of SLE patients with antiphospholipid antibodies. Exclude infective endocarditis (IE).
- In APLS valvular disease is estimated to occur in about a third by transthoracic (TTE) and ~80% by transoesophageal echocardiogram (TOE). Only ~5% patients require surgery. Exclude IE.
- Cardiac conduction defects, aortic valve incompetence and cardiomegaly occur in AS. Anatomic evidence of aortic valve involvement can be seen in up to 20% AS patients, but few have valvular dysfunction. About 50% patients with isolated aortic valve incompetence are HLA B27 positive.
- In rheumatic fever 70% of patients have valvulitis and mitral stenosis is the commonest sequelae. This is rare in the developed world.

Coronary artery disease (CAD)
- In RA, the risk of myocardial infarction (MI) is increased ~2-fold. Silent MI is more common and recurrence of cardiac events is higher in RA compared with controls. Treatment with methotrexate (MTX) appears to be associated with a decreased cardiovascular mortality and morbidity. This probably reflects the association of plaque instability and vasculitis with active RA.
- CAD occurs in ~10% SLE patients (risk 4–8-fold of controls).
- In APLS CAD occurs in ~5%.

Pulmonary arterial hypertension (PAH)
Refer to 'The Chest' in the chapter on Organ involvement in rheumatological disease. (Refer to 'The chest and also see SSc, p. 264–272.)

Aortitis
Takayasu's arteritis, AS, GCA, and relapsing polychondritis are all associated with aortic root/arch involvement.

Aetiology/pathophysiology
Pericardial disease
In SLE, deposition of immunoglobulin and complement C3 on pericardial tissue has been demonstrated.

Myocardial and conduction system disease
- In SLE myocarditis, immunofluorescence demonstrates granular deposition of immunoglobulin and complement component, suggesting immune complex disease. Deposits are predominantly in the wall of myocardial blood vessels. In giant cell myocarditis, multicellular giant cells are prominent in the infiltrate.
- Abnormalities of depolarization and repolarization of pacemaker tissue and myocytes together with abnormal autonomic tone may result from the effects of autoantibodies (e.g. anti-Ro) binding to the tissues, or of other circulating inflammatory mediators, which may have excitatory and/or cytotoxic effects on excitable tissues.
- In SSc, patchy myocardial fibrosis promotes the development of re-entrant tachycardias.
- Drugs may also contribute to arrhythmias, e.g. hydroxychloroquine is associated with QT prolongation and refractory ventricular arrhythmias. Rarely sulphasalazine is associated with causing a cardiomyopathy.
- Conduction tissue may be infiltrated by mononuclear cells or disrupted by vasculitis of arterial supply in RA.
- Antibodies (e.g. anti-Ro antibodies) specific for cardiac conducting tissue may also bind to cardiac myocytes and disrupt the function of calcium channels.
- In SSc, fibrosis of the sino-atrial node and other conducting tissue underlies the high incidence of conduction disturbance.

Valvular disease
- In SLE and APLS, deposition of autoantibodies, including anti-endothelial antibodies, anti-phospholipid antibodies, and immune complexes is believed to be responsible for contributing to endocardial inflammation and valvular disease.
- In APLS, intravalvular capillary thrombosis or superficial thrombosis on luminal surface of valve leaflets have been reported. Fibrosis and calcification are thought to be sequelae of chronic damage/inflammation.
- In AS, aortic incompetence results from inflammation and dilatation of the aortic root.

Coronary artery disease (CAD)
- In RA, traditional risk factors are increased and contribute to risk of CAD, e.g. systemic inflammation contributes to atherogenic lipid profiles and insulin resistance, reduced mobility in patients with arthritis increases the incidence of obesity; decreased exercise increased weight and some drugs (NSAIDs, glucocorticoids [GCs], leflunomide) promote development of hypertension.
- Also in RA, circulating inflammatory mediators, e.g. CRP and TNFα may cause direct endothelial damage. CD4+CD28-T cells are increased in RA and some other patients with unstable angina; they have been implicated in plaque destabilization.
- In SLE, circulating inflammatory mediators may be directly involved in endothelial damage.
- Anti-phospholipid or anti-β2GPI antibodies have been reported to bind to endothelial cells.

Pulmonary arterial hypertension
Refer to 'The Chest' in the chapter on Organ involvement in rheumatological disease (Refer to 'The Chest' and also see SSc, p. 264–272.)

Aortitis

Aortitis may result from vasculitis in the vasa vasorum of the adventitia or, in GCA, as a result of a local immune response generated by over-reactivity of dendritic cells resident in the adventitia. Inflammation may give rise to disintegration of the aortic media, with aneurysm formation, or fibrosis with resultant stenosis of the aorta or arteries originating from it.

Risk factors

- Traditional risk factors for ischaemic heart disease (smoking, hypertension, hyperlipidaemia, family history, obesity) also apply to RA and SLE patients, and are likely to contribute to ischaemic heart disease (IHD) in all patients with rheumatological disease.
- Lupus anticoagulant and anti-β2GPI are risk factors for MI in SLE patients.
- Left heart valvular disease is a risk factor for stroke, and possibly epilepsy, in patients with APLS.
- Anti-Ro antibodies in pregnancy confer about a 2% risk of CHB (15–20% if the mother already has an affected child).
- HLA-B27 is a risk factor for aortitis.

Clinical features

Pericardial disease

- Pericarditic pain is classically positional, precordial, and relieved by sitting forward.
- Dyspnoea with pericardial effusion raises the possibility of tamponade.
- Fever and tachycardia are common.
- Pericardial rub occurs in the early stages but is lost as fluid accumulates – a stage that is associated with reduced heart sounds.
- Development of tamponade is indicated by raised jugular venous pressure (JVP) with a sharp rise and y descent. Kussmaul's sign, pulsus paradoxus, and reduced pulse volume are also detectable.

Myocardial and conduction system disease

Cardiomyopathies of all causes may present with dyspnoea, orthopnoea, and palpitations.

- Heart failure is associated with tachycardia, reduced pulse volume, elevation of the JVP, gallop rhythm, hyperdynamic, and/or displaced apical impulse.
- Left ventricular failure is usually associated with signs of pulmonary oedema or pleural effusion.
- Right heart failure is associated with raised JVP, pitting oedema of the ankles/legs; a pulsatile liver.
- The pulse rate and rhythm should be carefully assessed in patients with a history of palpitations.
- Manual (rather than automated) blood pressure measurement may reveal hypertension, hypotension, or a pulsus alternans.
- CHB *in utero* may manifest with a fetal bradycardia.

Valvular disease

Valve problems can present with palpitations, clinical features of cardiac failure or syncopal episodes (e.g. with aortic stenosis).

- Fevers and sweats and 'new' murmurs may indicate IE.
- Pulse character and volume should be carefully assessed.
- Blood pressure assessment may reveal wide pulse pressure in aortic regurgitation.

- Cardiac auscultation for murmurs.
- Check for signs of IE – fever, splinter haemorrhages, splenomegaly.

Coronary artery disease (CAD)

CAD can present as central tight chest pain and/or dyspnoea on exertion.

- The incidence of silent MI is increased in RA and SLE patients relative to controls.
- Left ventricular dysfunction must be considered and the cause identified, i.e. ischaemia, myocarditis, or valvular dysfunction.
- On examination look for signs of arrhythmias, cardiac failure, hypertension, and hypercholesterolaemia.

Pulmonary arterial hypertension (PAH)

Refer to 'The Chest' in the chapter on Organ involvement in rheumatological disease. (Refer to 'The Chest' and also see SSc, p. 264–272).

Aortitis

Aortitis might be 'silent' or present with chest pain, radiating to the back.

In the examination assess radial and carotid pulses; listen for subclavian bruit and aortic incompetence. Measure BP in both arms (may be discrepant), and there may be pulse delay between radial pulses or radio-femoral delay.

Cardiac signs

Kussmaul's sign (Adolf Kussmaul 1822–1902)

Normally, the JVP falls with inspiration (reduced pressure in the expanding thoracic cavity). Where there is impaired right ventricle filling (e.g. restrictive pericarditis, pericardial effusion, tamponade), JVP can rise with inspiration (Kussmaul's sign).

Pulsus paradoxus (PP)

PP is an exaggeration of the normal variation in the pulse during the inspiratory phase of respiration, in which the pulse becomes weaker as one inhales and stronger as one exhales. It is a sign that is indicative of several conditions including cardiac tamponade, pericarditis, chronic sleep apnoea, and obstructive lung disease (e.g. asthma, COPD). The paradox in PP is that one can detect extra beats on auscultation during inspiration, when compared with the radial pulse. It results from an accentuated decrease of the blood pressure. PP has been shown to be predictive of the severity of cardiac tamponade.

PP is quantified using a blood pressure cuff and stethoscope, by measuring the variation of the pressure in systole with respiration. PP is an inspiratory reduction in systolic pressure >10 mmHg.

Causes include tamponade, pericardial effusion, asthma, tension pneumothorax, PE, SVC obstruction.

Pulsus alternans

The arterial pulse waveform has alternating strong and weak beats. It is almost always indicative of left ventricular systolic impairment and carries a poor prognosis.

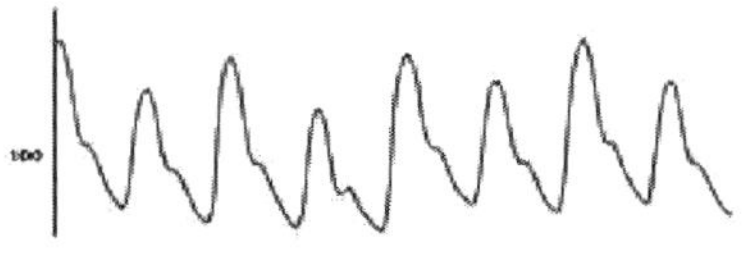

Figure 3.10 Key findings in valve disease in rheumatology patients

CHAPTER 3 Organ involvement in rheumatological disease

> *Chronic aortic insufficiency/regurgitation* causes an early diastolic and decresendo murmur, which is best heard at aortic area when the patient is seated and leans forward with breath held in expiration. The murmur is usually soft and seldom causes thrill.
>
> *Chronic mitral regurgitation* typically causes a pansystolic murmur (usually high-pitched) heard at the apex radiating to the axilla and is associated with an apical thrill and 3rd heart sound. Patients with mitral valve prolapse (e.g. Marfan syndrome) often have a mid-to-late systolic click and a late systolic murmur
>
> *Signs in PAH (e.g. in SSc)*
> Altered heart sounds, such as a widely split S_2 or 2nd heart sound, loud P_2, (para)sternal heave, possible S_3 or 3rd heart sound, and pulmonary regurgitation. Other signs include an elevated JVP, peripheral oedema, ascites, hepatojugular reflux, and clubbing.

Investigations

Pericardial disease

- ECG: in acute pericarditis - saddle-shaped ST elevation. Subsequently, the ST segments normalize but T waves flatten and the amplitude of the QRS complex alternates (QRS alternans).
- Echocardiography shows pericardial fluid, thickening and calcification. Tamponade is suggested by diastolic compression of right heart chambers, lack of inspiratory collapse of inferior vena cava and swinging of the whole heart. Doppler assessment of diastolic flow patterns may suggest constrictive pericarditis.

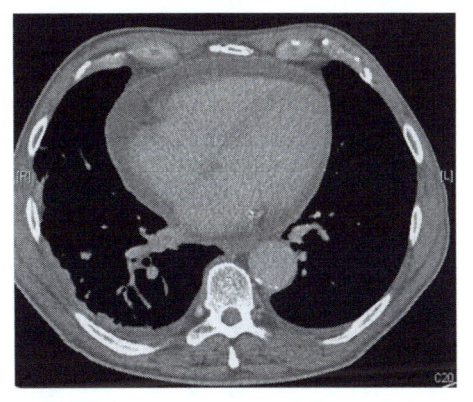

Figure 3.11 CT chest showing pericardial effusion in RA

- CXR reveals increased cardiothoracic ratio in cardiac failure and prominent upper lobe pulmonary veins in pulmonary venous hypertension.
- Cardiac enzymes should be measured to assess for a myocardial infarction or myocarditis.
- Pericardiocentesis should be considered when purulent, tuberculous, or malignant effusion is suspected.
- MR is useful for loculated effusion, haemopericardium, or constrictive pericarditis. MR also evaluates severity of valvular regurgitation.
- CT can also be used to assess pericardial anatomy and may be used to guide aspiration of small effusions.
- Pericardial biopsy is indicated if MTB is still suspected, but not confirmed after pericardiocentesis (particularly relevant in patients treated with anti-TNFα agents).
- Endomyocardial biopsy may rarely be required to distinguish constrictive pericarditis from restrictive cardiomyopathy. Patchy disease can be missed. Biopsy should only be done if supported by appropriate pathology expertise.
- Cardiac catheterization is used to assess end-diastolic pressures in the RV and LV in the investigation of constrictive pericarditis.
- Screen for autoimmune, infective, and malignant diseases. Include: FBC, renal function, liver function tests, serum ACE and calcium (sarcoidosis), ferritin (very high in Adult Still's), lactate deyhydrogenase (leukaemia, lymphoma) blood/urine/sputum cultures, ANA & ENAs, RF, anti-CCP antibodies (RA), Igs, ANCA, and complement components C3 and C4.

Myocardial and conduction system disease

- Troponin-I is a specific indicator of myocardial damage.
- Ferritin – if adult Still's suspected.
- Serum ACE, PTH and plasma and 24 h urinary calcium if sarcoidosis suspected (and 1,25-dihydroxyvitamin D).
- Thyroid function tests in AF or sinus tachycardia.

ECG

- Annual ECGs are recommended in all rheumatological patients at risk of myocardial and conduction tissue disease; this includes apparently unaffected offspring of mothers with anti-Ro antibodies.
- 24-h Holter monitoring is used to evaluate patients with intermittent palpitations.

Echocardiography

- Shows nodules, dilation of chambers, and hypertrophy of chamber walls and estimates function (e.g. LVEF).
- A 'sparkling' pattern can indicate amyloid.
- Global hypokinesis suggests myocarditis in associated disease.

Cardiovascular MR

- Can be used to evaluate LV function, myocardial perfusion, and distinguish causes of cardiomyopathy.
- T2 values indicate abnormal myocardial relaxation.

Other investigations

- Anti-microbial antibody titres (e.g. CMV, EBV, influenza, hepatitis C, Coxsackie B, *Borrelia burgdorferia*, *Chlamydia pneumonia*); elevated IgM indicates acute infection; elevated IgG is evidence for previous exposure.
- Exercise stress testing for suspected ischaemia often not possible due to locomotor issues – use other non-invasive test such as MIBI, stress echo or MR perfusion.
- Serial fetal echocardiography should be performed in mothers with anti-Ro antibodies; a recommendation is for weekly scans between 16–26 weeks of gestation and alternate week scans from 28–34 weeks).
- SAP (serum amyloid P) *scan* should be performed if the diagnosis of amyloid is considered.
- Endomyocardial biopsy if myocarditis is suspected. Samples should be sent for PCR for microbial DNA or RNA (enterovirus, adenovirus, echovirus, HSV, CMV, EBV, HIV, *Borelia*, MTB, *Chlamydia* pneumonia).

Dallas criteria for classification of (PCR -ve) myocarditis

Initial biopsy
- *Myocarditis* myocyte necrosis, degeneration, or both in the absence of significant coronary artery disease, with adjacent inflammatory infiltrate ± fibrosis.
- *Borderline myocarditis* inflammatory infiltrate too sparse or myocyte damage not apparent.
- *No myocarditis*.

Subsequent biopsy
- On-going myocarditis ± fibrosis.
- Resolving myocarditis ± fibrosis.
- Resolved myocarditis ± fibrosis.

The inflammatory infiltrate is sub-classified by dominant cell type (lymphocytic, neutrophilic, giant cell, granulomatous or mixed), severity (mild, moderate, severe) and distribution (focal, confluent or diffuse).

Valvular disease
- Echocardiography (both TTE and TOE) is used to screen for valve lesions in predisposing conditions (e.g. aortic regurgitation in AS) or on the finding of a new murmur (e.g. suspected rheumatic fever).
- Also use TTE/TOE to seek vegetations in suspected IE and in APLS (Libman-Sacks endocarditis; TOE is more sensitive than TTE).
- Blood cultures – multiple sets to exclude IE.

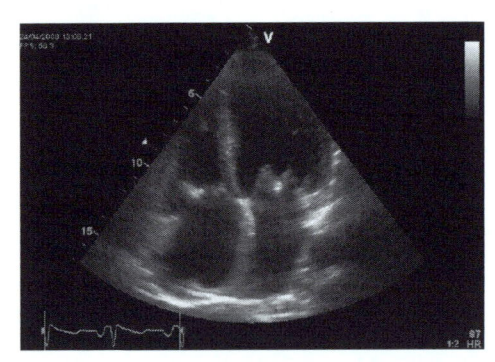

Figure 3.12 TTE: apical four-chamber view demonstrating vegetations in Libman-Sacks endocarditis.

Coronary artery disease
- ECG for typical signs of ischaemia.
- Troponin I.
- In patients who are unable to exercise, stress TTE can be performed using sympathomimetic agents. For example, a dobutamine stress test has a sensitivity of 74% and specificity of 70% for ischemia-induced wall motion abnormalities). Vasodilators (dipyridamole or adenosine) can also be used.
- Non-invasive assessment includes stress nuclear echo or MR, or multi-detector (MD) CT.
- Coronary angiography remains the gold standard for the visualization of the coronary arterial tree.
- Dobutamine MR has a greater sensitivity (86%) and specificity (86%) for ischaemic-related wall motion defects than dobutamine transthoracic echocardiography.

Pulmonary arterial hypertension
Refer to 'The Chest' in the chapter on Organ involvement in Rheumatological Disease (Refer to 'The Chest' and also see SSc, p. 264–272).

Aortitis
- Echocardiography.
- MR appearances of aortitis in Takayasu's arteritis have been described. It may be possible to discriminate appearances of Takayasu's from aortitis in other conditions though clarifying studies are required.
- ^{18}Fluorodeoxyglucose positron emission tomography (^{18}FDG-PET) is used in some specialist centres to characterise GCA and Takayasu's arteritis, but its precise role in diagnosis and monitoring, particularly in GCA, remains to be clarified.
- Mild to moderate uptake of ^{18}FDG tracer in vessel walls in atherosclerotic disease can occur and, especially in the elderly, this can confuse the picture further – leading to false positive results. Care in reporting is essential and interpretation should be made in light of other clinical information.

Treatment

Pericardial disease
Refer to cardiologist if pericarditis is associated with compromised cardiac performance.
- Analgesia: either NSAIDs (beware increased risk of peptic ulcer disease in RA, and of oesophageal dysmotility in SSc) or course of GCs.
- Treat underlying condition, usually with high-dose oral or pulsed intravenous GCs, initially, followed by introduction of GC-sparing immunosuppression.
- Therapeutic pericardiocentesis ± temporary drain in tamponade.
- Pericardial fenestration in recurrent tamponade.
- Intra-pericardial triamcinolone and oral colchicine have been used in large, recurrent effusions.
- Resection of the pericardium is required in rare cases of constrictive pericarditis.

Myocardial and conduction system disease
Common themes in the management of myocardial disease are:
- Management of cardiac failure with diuretics, ACE inhibitors, nitrates, and, if required, inotropic support.
- Monitor potassium especially carefully in patients with renal disease, and those on GCs or mycophenolate mofetil.
- Management of arrhythmias by conventional means, since no RCTs have been performed on patients with arrhythmias in inflammatory Rheumatological disease:
  - SVT – use verapamil-type calcium channel blockers or β-blockers;
  - for AF digoxin and other rate-controlling agents as per NICE guidance; AV nodal ablation may used to control ventricular response rate in patients with AF or atrial flutter, and is successful in >80%;
  - in sinus tachycardia treat underlying cause (e.g. hyperthyroidism or active inflammatory disease); otherwise use β-blockers;
  - for recurrent ventricular fibrillation (outside the context of acute MI), consider an implantable cardioverter defibrillator;

CHAPTER 3 Organ involvement in rheumatological disease

- ventricular tachycardia (VT) – **involve cardiology team urgently!** Sustained, symptomatic, drug-resistant, monomorphic VT, re-entrant VT, and occasionally severely symptomatic premature ventricular contractions, can be treated with radiofrequency ablation.
- Prevention of mural thrombus with anticoagulants.
- Control of underlying condition. For chronic inflammatory conditions, this includes high-dose GCs (usually pulsed intravenous methylprednisolone) in the early stages, followed by introduction of immunosuppressants such as azathioprine, mycophenolate mofetil, cyclophosphamide, ciclosporin, tacrolimus, or sirolimus.
- Intravenous immunoglobulins are sometimes used (beware of volume overload in cardiac failure), although evidence for their efficacy is anecdotal only.

Management of specific conditions
- **Viral myocarditis.** Supportive treatment, but if there are concerns, involve cardiologist.
- **Cardiac amyloid.** Increase immunosuppression to reduce progression. Poor prognosis once confirmed.
- **Cardiac nodules.** There is no evidence that immunosuppression alters nodules. Surgery may occasionally be indicated.
- **Sinus tachycardia** in SLE may respond to GCs.
- **Incomplete CHB** in utero may respond to fluorinated GCs (dexamethasone or betamethasone), which cross the placenta. Some studies suggest that betamethasone is preferable since high-dose dexamethasone may be neurotoxic.
- **Complete CHB** may require pacing (~33% within the first week post-partum). **Refer to cardiologist**.
- **Prophylactic treatment of pregnant women** with anti-Ro antibodies (even those with previous children with CHB) is not currently recommended because of the risk of spontaneous abortion, growth retardation, stillbirth and, possibly, neurotoxicity with dexamethasone.
- **Defibrillator and/or pacemaker implantation** may be required for a range of conduction disturbances, e.g. recurrent VT, bradyarrhythmias.
- **Maintain a low threshold for referral of patients with myocardial and conduction system disease to cardiologists; remember ischaemia is often silent in RA and SLE.**

Valvular disease
- Aspirin has been suggested for APLS patients with asymptomatic valvular disease, but the evidence base is lacking. Consider the risk-benefit ratio.
- Prophylactic antibiotics are not recommended by current guidelines.
- Valve replacement surgery is occasionally indicated. Refer to cardiology for assessment.

Coronary artery disease (CAD)
General measures in CAD include nitrates, aspirin, statins, and anti-hypertensives, to maintain blood pressure <140/85.
- The UK Primary Care Quality and Outcomes Framework (QOF) for cardiovascular risk reduction, sets targets for blood pressure and lipids, which are less stringent than other recognised national guidelines.
- Furthermore more stringent guidance (e.g. Joint British Society guidelines) takes no account of the increased risk associated with inflammatory rheumatological disease, e.g. RA and SLE. An algorithm for cardiovascular risk reduction in RA and SLE has been proposed.

Rheumatoid arthritis (RA)
- Optimize control of disease activity, with minimal use of GCs.
- MTX treatment appears to reduce cardiovascular risk.
- Use of anti-TNFα agents may also reduce risk of cardiovascular events, but may exacerbate severe CCF.
- Antimalarials may have anti-atherogenic activity and can be used in combination with other DMARDs.
- Use NSAIDs only when necessary and discuss potential cardiovascular risks with patient. COX2 selective NSAIDs increase cardiovascular disease risk and use should be discussed on an individual basis.
- Aspirin should also be used carefully, since RA is associated with ~5-fold increase in the risk of gastrointestinal haemorrhage.
- Monitor and modify traditional risk factors, including smoking, hypertension, hyperlipidaemia, obesity, diabetes mellitus, and hypothyroidism.
- A cardiovascular risk reduction algorithm has been proposed (see resources).

Systemic Lupus erythematosus (SLE)
- Optimize control of disease with minimal use of GCs.
- Antimalarials may have anti-atherogenic and anticoagulant activity, and can be used alone or in combination with other immunosuppressants.
- Aspirin prophylaxis may be beneficial. A cohort study suggested that aspirin was associated with a 70% reducton in cardiovascular mortality. Monitor and modify traditional risk factors, as for RA.

Antiphospholipid syndrome (APLS)
As for SLE but aspirin ± antimalarials are used in patients who have not had frank thromboembolic disease. Warfarin ± antimalarials are used in patients who have.

Table 3.5 Recommendations for anti-TNFα use in RA patients with congestive cardiac failure

Scenario	Recommendation
RA with no history of CCF	No echocardiographic screening required.
RA with mild CCF (NYHA class I and II)	Doppler echocardiography prior to anti-TNFα.
If LVEF >50% then treat following informed discussion and monitor with TTE.	
RA with severe CCF (NYHA class III and IV)	Avoid anti-TNFα. Consider using Rituximab.
Investigate and treat CCF.	
Development of CCF while receiving anti-TNFα treatment.	Stop anti-TNFα and investigate and treat CCF.

Other conditions
- For Kawasaki Disease – refer to Chapter 9, Vasculitis.
- Sarcoidosis – refer to section on Chapter 18, p. 512, Sarcoidosis in miscellaneous rheumatological disease.
- The frequency of CAD and other cardiovascular disease is increased in a number of inflammatory rheumatological conditions. Careful management of conventional

cardiovascular risk factors is recommended (BP, lipids, smoking), as well as screening for hyperglycaemia and hypothyroidism.

Pulmonary arterial hypertension
Refer to both section on SSc (p. 264–272), and the section on 'The Chest' in Chapter 3, p. 54

Aortitis
Treat underlying inflammatory disease since dilatation of aorta increases the risk of vessel rupture.

Resources
British Heart Foundation information online. Available at: www.bhf.org.uk/default.aspx

Cardiovascular risk reduction algorithm for patients with RA and SLE. Available at: www.medschl.cam.ac.uk/medtools/chd1.php

Panoulas *et al*. Algorithm for management of hypertension in RA. 2008; see references.

Assessment tools
New York Heart Association (NYHA) Functional Classification system

Class	Patient symptoms
I	No limitation of activity. Ordinary physical activity does not cause undue fatigue, palpitation, or dyspnoea.
II	Slight limitation of activity. Comfortable at rest, but ordinary physical activity results in fatigue, palpitation, or dyspnoea.
III	Marked limitation of physical activity. Comfortable at rest, but less than ordinary activity causes fatigue, palpitation, or dyspnoea.
IV	Symptomatic at rest. Any physical activity increases fatigue, palpitation, or dyspnoea.

Guidelines
Joint British Societies' guidelines on prevention of cardiovascular disease in clinical practice (see refs).

NICE Clinical Guideline CG64: Prophylaxis against infective endocarditis (www.nice.org).

Further reading
Bidani AK, Roberts JL. Immunopathology of cardiac lesions in fatal systemic lupus erythematosus. *Am J Med* 1980; **69**: 849–58.

Hall FC, Dalbeth N. Disease modification and cardiovascular risk reduction: two sides of the same coin? *Rheumatol* 2005; **52**: 3678–9.

JBS2. Joint British Societies' guidelines on prevention of cardiovascular disease on clinical practice. *Heart* 2005; **91**: 1–52.

Khanna D, McMahon M. Anti-tumour necrosis factor alpha therapy and heart failure. *Arthritis Rheum* 2004; **50**: 1040–50

Maisch B, Pankuweit S, *et al*. Invasive techniques – from diagnosis to treatment. *Rheumatology* 2006; **45**: iv32–38.

Maksimovic R, Seferovic PM, et al. Cardiac imaging in rheumatic diseases. *Rheumatology* 2006; 45 iv26–31.

Panoulas VF, Metsios GS, *et al*. Hypertension in rheumatoid arthritis. *Rheumatol* 2008; in press.

Rosenstein ED, Zucker MJ, Kramer N. Giant cell myocarditis: most fatal of autoimmune diseases. *Semin Arthritis Rheum* 2000: **30**: 1–16.

Seferovic PM, Ristic AD, *et al*. Cardiac arrhythmias and conduction disturbances in autoimmune rheumatic diseases. *Rheumatol* 2006; **45**: iv39–42.

Slobodin G, Naschitz JE, *et al*. Aortic involvement in rheumatic diseases. *Clin Exp Rheumatol* 2006; **24**: S41–7

Soltesz P, Szekanecz Z., *et al*. Cardiac manifestations in antiphospholipid syndrome. *Autoimmun Rev* 2007; **6**: 379–86.

Tincani A, Rebaioli CB, *et al*. Heart involvment in systemic lupus erythematosus, anti-phospholipid syndrome and neonatal lupus. *Rheumatology* 2006; **45**: iv8–13

Van Doornum S, McColl G, Wicks IP. Accelerated atherosclerosis. An extraarticular feature of rheumatoid arthritis? *Arthritis Rheum* 2002; **46**: 862–73.

Voskuyl AE. The heart and cardiovascular manifestations in rheumatoid arthritis. *Rheumatology* 2006; **45**: iv4–7

Weyand CM, Gornzy JJ. Medium and large-vessel vasculitis. *N Engl J Med* 2003; **349**: 160–9.

Organ involvement in rheumatological disease

The kidney

Renal involvement in rheumatological disease is a significant cause of morbidity and predictor of mortality. These complications can arise as a result of the direct effects of the disease or as a result of the treatment. Diseases with particularly strong associations with kidney involvement include: systemic lupus erythematosus (SLE), systemic vasculitides, rheumatoid arthritis (RA), systemic sclerosis, Behçet's disease, anti-phospholipid antibody syndrome (APLS), Sjögren's syndrome (SS) and sarcoidosis. Medications commonly used in rheumatological diseases and commonly associated with renal complications include: non-steroidal anti-inflammatory drugs (NSAIDs), D-penicillamine, and gold.

Rheumatological diseases that affect the kidney can present as any one of several syndromes. Major renal syndromes include the nephritic syndrome, the nephrotic syndrome, tubulointerstitial nephritis, and acute or chronic renal failure.

Nephritic syndromes (glomerulonephritis)

Definition

The nephritic syndrome is characterized by new onset or worsening hypertension, acute renal failure and abnormalities of urine sediment, primarily glomerular haematuria, cellular casts and non-nephrotic range proteinuria (<3.5 g/day). Renal dysfunction is an insensitive marker of renal involvement due to the inherent large reserve of renal function in most people. Also, nephrotic range proteinuria does not exclude a nephritic syndrome.

Rheumatological diseases associated with the nephritic syndrome include proliferative lupus nephritis, anti-neutrophil cytoplasm antibody associated vasculitis [(AAV), which include Wegener's granulomatosis (WG), microscopic polyangiitis (MPA) and Churg–Strauss syndrome [CSS]), Henoch–Schönlein purpura (HSP), cryoglobulinemic vasculitis and, rarely, RA or Behçet's disease. The nephritic syndrome results from immunological lesions of the glomerulus in these diseases.

Epidemiology

- 75% of patients with SLE will have abnormalities of urinalysis at some point.
- 16% of patients in large European cohorts have significant proteinuria at diagnosis of SLE and 35% will develop proteinuria within 10 years of diagnosis.
- Renal involvement in drug-induced lupus is rare.
- ANCA associated vasculitis (AAV) has a an overall incidence of 10–14 per million in Europe and 80% will have some form of renal involvement but this may vary from isolated urinary abnormalities to rapidly progressive glomerulonephritis and end-stage renal disease
- The incidence of AAV peaks in the 6–7th decade of life.
- ANCA determined by immunofluorescence is manifest by either a cytoplasmic pattern (C-ANCA), associated with reactivity to proteinase 3 (PR3-ANCA) by ELISA, or a peri-nuclear pattern (P-ANCA) associated with reactivity to myeloperoxidase (MPO-ANCA).
- Approximately 90% of patients with WG will have a detectable ANCA (the majority are PR3-ANCA positive), while approximately 70–80% of patients with MPA will have a detectable ANCA (usually MPO-ANCA positive). Less than 50% of patients with CSS are ANCA positive (usually MPO-ANCA).
- HSP is seen primarily in children aged 3–15 years with an annual incidence of approximately 20/100 000 children. HSP is uncommon in adults. HSP is slightly more common in males.
- Renal disease complicates approximately 20% of cases of cryoglobulinemia (50% have a nephritic syndrome).
- Nephritis is a very rare complication of RA and may result from a focal mesangial lesion, a rheumatoid vasculitis or from D-penicillamine treatment.

Aetiology/pathophysiology

The nephritic syndromes result from perturbation of the glomerular endothelium resulting in red blood cells leaking into the urinary space (causing haematuria and cellular casts), and obstruction of the capillaries from either endocapillary proliferation or the proliferation of extracapillary components of the glomerulus (see Plate 35). Obstruction of the capillary lumens leads to renal dysfunction and hypertension.

SLE

- Renal involvement in SLE is characterized by immune complex deposition.
- Immune complexes are composed of DNA-anti-DNA and may include composites of nucleosomes, C1q, chromatin, and other nuclear antigens.
- The pattern of deposition of immune complexes largely determines the phenotype of the renal disease.
- Large and anionic immune complexes deposit in the subendothelial and mesangial compartments of the glomerulus, and subsequent activation of the immune systems provokes a proliferative glomerular lesion the severity of which is determined by the amount deposited. Severe proliferative lesions are characterized by dysmorphic haematuria, red blood cell casts, proteinuria, hypertensions, and eventually renal dysfunction.
- Kidney involvement in SLE may be due to specific subclasses of IgG in specific patients. IgG1 and IgG3 autoantibodies more avidly fix complement, and are more commonly associated with severe renal lesions.

AAV

- The pathogenicity of ANCA is debated.
- Murine models of MPO-induced glomerulonephritis provide the strongest evidence that ANCA are pathogenic. This evidence is supported in humans by a case report of in utero transfer of ANCA causing a pulmonary-renal syndrome. However, ANCA alone may be insufficient in humans to cause disease and other abnormalities, such as a neutrophil priming event (an infection or environmental exposure), endothelial dysfunction, B cell dysfunction, and Fc-RIIIB polymorphisms are implicated in the pathogenesis. Whether these abnormalities are required to initiate vasculitis or are a consequence of the vasculitic damage are unclear.

HSP

- Renal damage is mediated by the deposition of immune complexes, primarily immunoglobulin A1.
- IgA deposition may result from increased IgA secretion following a mucosal infection and/or abnormal glycosylation of IgA.

CHAPTER 3 Organ involvement in rheumatological disease

Cryoglobulinaemia
- Antigen-antibody complexes are deposited in small and medium arteries including glomerular capillaries.
- Hepatitis C virus (HCV) is a common cause.

Risk factors
- Patients of black African or Hispanic descent are more likely to have lupus nephritis, and it is more likely to follow a severe course.
- AAV patients with nasal *Staphylococcus aureus* carriage are at higher risk of relapse. α1-antitrypsin deficiency is associated with a more severe course. The NA1 polymorphism of the Fcγ-RIIIB allele also appears over-represented in patients with severe AAV.
- AAV may result as a complication of medications used in hyperthyroidism, such as propylthiouracil or more rarely with the use of hydralazine or minocycline. Exposure to silica has also been associated with the development of AAV.
- HSP occurs rarely in the summer and is commonly preceded by an upper respiratory tract infection.

Key features in the history
Features associated with the nephritic syndrome.
- New onset hypertension or hypertension that has become increasingly difficult to control.
- Hypertension may be severe and present as an emergency (headache, visual changes, chest pain, dyspnoea).
- Advanced and chronic renal failure is associated with fatigue, anorexia, and pruritis.
- Abnormalities of the urinalysis: haematuria and cellular casts and sub-nephrotic levels of proteinuria.
- Cellular casts are often missed in routine urine samples, but are quite specific for a nephritic process.
- The protean manifestations of renal dysfunction or a systemic immunological process are often mistaken for an infection. Patients commonly report being treated with antibiotics for upper respiratory or urinary tract infections repeatedly with no improvement in their symptoms. This is particularly true of patients with abnormalities of the urinalysis, but without a documented microbiologic diagnosis.
- Extra-renal manifestations of systemic diseases are often more pronounced during periods when the kidneys are also involved.

Table 3.6 International Society of Nephrologists/Renal Pathology Society classification of glomerulonephritis due to SLE. Classes III and IV are proliferative

Class	Major pathological findings
I	Glomeruli normal by light microscopy (LM), but immune complex deposits seen by immunofluorescence (IF)
II	Light microscopy reveals expansion of mesangial cell or the mesangial matrix
III	<50% of glomeruli demonstrate endocapillary or extracapillary glomerulonephritis in addition to mesangial expansion
IV	≥50% of glomeruli demonstrate endocapillary or extracapillary glomerulonephritis in addition to mesangial expansion
V	Subepithelial immune complex deposits are seen on LM, electron microscopy or IF. Class V can occur with other classes.
VI	At least 90% of glomeruli are sclerosed

Special investigations
- Serum creatinine should be performed in all patients suspected of having nephritis, but are not sensitive even in cases of severe disease, as abnormalities of renal function tend to occur late in the disease course.
- Urinalysis demonstrating dysmorphic haematuria with proteinuria and/or cellular casts support the presence of glomerulonephritis.
- Quantification of proteinuria – either a 24-h urine collection or a spot morning urine protein to creatinine ratio should be performed in patients with suspected nephritis and dipstick positive proteinuria.
- Blood tests aim to determine the cause of nephritis and should include hepatitis B, hepatitis C, HIV, ANCA, anti-glomerular basement membrane antibodies, ANA, anti-DNA antibodies, extractable nuclear antigens, APL antibodies, RF, complement levels, protein electrophoresis, and cryoglobulins.
- Anti-double stranded DNA antibodies and hypocomplementemia occur frequently in patients with SLE.
- ANCA indirect immunofluorescence, and an ELISA for PR3 and MPO antibodies should be done in all cases. A negative test does not exclude a diagnosis of vasculitis.
- A renal biopsy should be used to confirm the diagnosis whenever possible, since no serological or urine laboratory work are sufficiently sensitive and specific. A renal biopsy will also provide prognostic information and is used to stratify treatment (see colour plates).

Treatment
Supportive treatment for all patients with nephritis includes the management of volume status, electrolyte abnormalities, and hypertension. Renal replacement therapy in the form of dialysis or renal transplantation may be required for patients with advanced renal failure. The treatment of lupus nephritis is usually predicated by renal biopsy findings.
- Class I and II lesions typically have an excellent renal prognosis even without treatment and are not specifically treated.
- Proliferative lupus nephritis (Class III and IV) is treated with a combination of an immunosuppressive and a tapering course of glucocorticoids (GCs).
- The immunosuppressive of choice has been intravenous cyclophosphamide for 3–6 months on the basis of data demonstrating a longer time to the doubling of creatinine in landmark NIH studies. More recently, there is accumulating data for the use of mycophenolate mofetil. Mycophenolate mofetil or azathioprine (AZA) are most frequently used to maintain remission.
- Consideration of prophylaxis against osteoporosis should be given to patients on GCs and to *Pneumocystis jirovecii* for patients on immunosuppressants.
- The treatment of AAV with renal involvement includes the use of an immunosuppressive agent and a tapering course of GCs. As with proliferative lupus nephritis, immunosuppressive medications are administered sequentially with cyclophosphamide used to induce a remission followed by AZA to maintain remission.
- Cyclophosphamide has been administered orally with frequent monitoring for the induction of leukopenias, but there is mounting evidence that intravenous pulse cyclophosphamide may be equally efficacious with fewer toxicities due to its lower cumulative dose.

- AZA is used after 3–6 months of treatment with cyclophosphamide once a clinical remission has been induced. The optimal duration of AZA is unknown.
- Plasma exchange should be considered for those patients who present with severe renal dysfunction due to AAV or who have a lung haemorrhage.
- The optimal duration of GC therapy is unknown, but longer durations of low-dose therapy has been associated with fewer relapses of disease.
- The treatment of HSP is supportive and includes adequate hydration, rest, and symptomatic relief of pain. Hospitalization may be required for renal insufficiency.
- The role of GCs in HSP in children is controversial, but may decrease the likelihood of renal involvement.
- Children with HSP who present with renal involvement have a poorer renal prognosis, but no therapy has been shown efficacious in randomized controlled trials. Consideration of GCs, immunosuppression, IVIG, or plasma exchange should be given to these patients.
- Treatment of cryoglobulinaemia with renal involvement includes plasma exchange, GCs and immunosuppressants. Treatment of the underlying disease (e.g. HCV or non-Hodgkin's lymphoma) can result in remission. There's some evidence that B cell depletion can be effective in the treatment of cryoglobulinaemic vasculitis.

Prognosis
- The prognosis of proliferative lupus nephritis before the use of immunosuppressants/GCs was poor – the majority of patients developing end-stage renal failure in <5 years. Those treated have 5-year renal survival rate of 90%. Despite advancements in preventing end-stage renal disease, patients who develop proliferative lupus nephritis are at a 5-fold higher risk of death over 10 years compared with patients without nephritis.
- Untreated, AAV has a dismal prognosis (1-year mortality >90%). End-stage renal disease is a common complication of late diagnosis – also a poor prognosis.
- With treatment, the prognosis of AAV has improved dramatically. Patients with very poor renal function at diagnosis (serum creatinine >500 μmol/l) still have a 1-year mortality of 25% with an additional 25% developing end-stage renal disease in randomized clinical trials. Patients with AAV, but a serum creatinine <500 μmol/l have a 1-year mortality of 10% or less. Some cohorts of unselected patients with AAV report 5-year mortality rates of <20%, but many of the patients in these cohorts do not have renal involvement.
- The short-term prognosis of HSP in most patients is favourable with 94% of children and 89% of adults completely recovered by 18 months. One-third of patients will, however, have a relapse of HSP, and this is more common in adolescent or adult patients.
- Persistent and progressive HSP can be poorly responsive to treatment and up to 18% of adults will require dialysis, while only 7% of children will become dialysis dependent. Prognosis is worse among patients presenting with nephrotic syndrome, renal insufficiency, hypertension, tubulointerstitial nephritis, or crescentic glomerulonephritis on biopsy.
- The prognosis of patients with cryoglobulinemic vasculitis is not yet well documented due to relatively recent changes in the standard of care of HCV.

Monitoring
- Monitor for neutropaenia (the nadir after cyclophosphamide is between 10 and 14 days) and infections.
- In the longer term, particularly in patients who receive multiple or extended courses of immunosuppression, the development of pre-malignant or malignant skin lesions, and solid organ malignancies, in particular, bladder cancer, should be excluded.
- Patients with nephritis should have their renal function, urinalysis and proteinuria monitored regularly. Additional monitoring should be disease specific.
- In lupus nephritis, monitoring of complement levels is warranted as persistent hypocomplementemia portends a poor prognosis.
- In lupus nephritis repeating the renal biopsy should be considered for patients with persistent serological or urinary abnormalities after a year of treatment. Persistent immunological activity in repeat renal biopsies may require escalating or prolonged immunosuppression.
- In AAV, monitoring of ANCA is of uncertain significance. Patients may relapse, while ANCA negative or fail to relapse after significant rises in ANCA.

Nephrotic syndromes
Definition
The nephrotic syndrome is characterized by peripheral edema, hypoalbuminemia, hyperlipidemia, lipiduria, and nephrotic range proteinuria (≥3.5 g/day). Lower levels of proteinuria do not exclude the nephrotic syndrome, but the urinalysis is generally dominated by proteinuria.
- Rheumatological diseases associated with the nephrotic syndrome include membranous lupus nephritis, RA (either due to its treatment or AA amyloidosis) and AL amyloidosis. The nephrotic syndrome can also result as a rare complication of non-steroidal anti-inflammatory drug (NSAID) or pamidronate use.
- Other very rare causes of the nephrotic syndrome include dermatomyositis, mixed connective tissue disease, mixed cryoglobulinemia, Sjögren's syndrome, Takayasu arteritis, sarcoidosis, Fabry's disease, and AAV
- The nephrotic syndrome is thought to result from a loss of plasma proteins and a subsequent derangement of renal sodium handling. Several specific pathologic lesions arising from rheumatological diseases result in the nephrotic syndrome and include membranous nephropathy, minimal change disease, and focal and segmental glomerulosclerosis.

Epidemiology
- Membranous lupus nephritis affects 10–20% of patients with SLE and renal involvement.
- Membranous lupus nephritis often occurs in conjunction with a proliferative lesion (e.g. Class III + V).
- Gold and D-penicillamine are known to induce membranous lesions. Incidence, respectively, 3% and 7%.
- Secondary AA amyloidosis is a rare complication of RA or Behçet's disease and may affect the kidneys. Although this complication is usually thought of as a result of long-standing disease, there are few data to support this. Secondary amyloidosis may occur in up to 10% of RA patients, but is only rarely clinically evident.
- Primary AL amyloidosis commonly affects the kidneys and up to 75% of patients will present with proteinuria.
- NSAIDs can induce a minimal change lesion or membranous lesion that causes nephrotic syndrome rarely.

- Case series' of patients with a severe form of focal and segmental glomerulosclerosis due to the use of IV bisphosphonates exist, but the incidence is unknown

Aetiology
The pathogenic mechanisms responsible for the nephrotic syndrome vary according the specific pathologic lesion. In all cases, there appears to be excess filtration of plasma proteins (notably albumin) and reduced tubular reabsorption. The excess filtration of albumin increases tubular sodium reabsorption. This excess sodium reabsorption and concomitant excess water reabsorption combined with the reduced intravascular oncotic pressure is thought to cause peripheral oedema.
- Central to the excess filtration of plasma proteins has been the identification of widespread podocyte effacement. Podocytes form an important component of the filtration barrier to the urinary space and effacement may result in loss of both the mechanical barrier and/or the electrostatic barrier to protein filtration.
- In SLE, small or cationic immune complexes deposit in the subepithelial space or may be directed against subepithelial antigens and provoke a membranous lesion. A similar process is thought to happen in medication related membranous lesions.
- In amyloidosis, abnormal proteins are generated either at an increased rate, or a decreased rate of clearance. These abnormal proteins are deposited in the glomerular basement membrane disrupting the filtration barrier and in the tubules and interstitium disrupting normal plasma protein reabsorption.

Key features in the history and on examination
In nephrotic syndromes, renal failure may also occur as a result of the underlying immunologic insult, but nephrotic syndromes tend to have a slower course than nephritic syndromes except in the case of NSAID induced injuries.
- Peripheral oedema including oedema of the hands and periorbital – can be reported as 'tightness' or 'swelling'.
- Excessive frothing of the urine may indicate proteinuria, but is not always noticed by the patient.
- Patients may report fatigue (non-specific), weight gain, repeated bacterial infections, and reduced appetite.
- The development of hypothyroidism or marked hyperlipidemia by the patient's Primary Care doctor, that is difficult to treat with standard antihyperlipidemic agents, is a pointer toward the diagnosis.
- A recent history of venous thromboembolic disease may be relevant.
- Lipemic blood samples may be noticed.

Special investigations
- Serum creatinine should be checked in all patients with the nephrotic syndrome, but the measure is not a sensitive measure, even of severe disease, as abnormalities of renal function can occur late in the disease course.
- Urinalysis demonstrating fatty casts or fat droplets supports the diagnosis of a nephrotic syndrome.
- Renal ultrasound (US) and Doppler US studies to exclude renal vein thrombosis, a complication of severe nephrotic syndromes, especially membranous lesions, and in preparation for kidney biopsy.
- Quantification of proteinuria by either a 24-h urine collection or a spot morning urine protein:creatinine ratio should be checked.
- Blood tests to exclude other causes of the nephrotic syndrome should include tests for hepatitis B, HCV, HIV, ANA, anti-DNA antibodies, extractable nuclear antigens, RF, complement levels, protein electrophoresis, and cryoglobulins.
- Anti-double stranded DNA antibodies and hypocomplementemia are frequently in lupus nephritis.
- A renal biopsy can confirm the diagnosis possible since no serologic or urine laboratory work are sufficiently sensitive or specific. A renal biopsy will provide prognostic information and is used to stratify treatment.

Treatment
Treatment of nephrotic syndrome can be divided into treatment of symptoms due to the syndrome and treatment of the underlying cause. In some cases, treating the underlying cause results in relatively rapid resolution of the syndrome and, therefore, treatment of the symptoms may be less important as they are short lived.

General management
- **Symptomatic control of peripheral oedema using diuretics.** Loop diuretics are likely the most effective. The efficacy of loop diuretics will be reduced by intratubular binding with albumin. Large doses of diuretic may be needed. Combining a loop diuretic with a non-loop diuretic may improve the diuresis.
- **Treatment of hypertension.** Hypertension usually occurs only after some reduction in renal function. Hypertension in these cases may be volume dependent and resolve with effective dieresis. Angiotensin blockade may effectively reduce proteinuria, as well as control blood pressure and is an important therapy.
- **Lipid lowering medication** can be used to control cholesterol in high-risk patients, but cholesterol levels usually respond rapidly to reductions in proteinuria. If a lipid lowering medication is used, its necessity needs reviewing after a significant reduction in proteinuria.
- **Prophylactic anticoagulation is highly debated.** Data on the relative risk of thrombosis is lacking. Most experts agree that the risk of thrombosis is minimal when serum albumin levels are >20 g/l. The decision to use anti-platelet or anti-coagulant therapy must be weighed for each individual patient.
- There are no data to suggest prophylactic antibiotics are necessary.
- If patients progress to end-stage renal disease, renal replacement therapy may be necessary. This is particularly relevant for patients with amyloidosis.

Treatment of specific causes of the nephrotic syndrome
- The treatment membranous lupus is controversial owing to its frequent overlap with proliferative lesions in epidemiological cohorts. The treatment approach to this variant is disputed because the prognosis of pure Class V disease is not well understood. A common approach for membranous lupus is to use GCs in severe cases and to add immunosuppression if the nephrotic syndrome persists despite 3–6 months of treatment.
- Non-lupus-related membranous nephropathy is frequently treated with 6 months of alternating GCs and cyclophosphamide, an approach shown to reduce end-stage renal disease, but has not been validated in a lupus population.
- Ciclosporin has been advocated by some for primary or secondary membranous nephropathy, but lacks randomized control trial evidence as a first line agent.

- Discontinuation of the causative drug in drug-induced nephrotic syndromes is essential. Treatment with GCs may still be used to reduce the duration of the nephrotic syndrome in severe or prolonged cases, particularly in those with associated renal dysfunction.
- Primary amyloidosis is a plasma cell dyscrasia and as such, therapies are similar to those for multiple myeloma. Treatment options include melphalan with or without GCs, thalidomide and dexamethasone with or without cyclophosphamide, lenalidomide with dexamethasone, and haematopoietic stem cell transfer.
- The treatment of secondary amyloidosis is to control the underlying disease with or without adjunctive therapy. Adjunctive therapies have included colchicine and cyclophosphamide, but the data supporting these approaches is limited. New products such as eprodisate have shown promise in reducing poor renal outcomes in patients with secondary amyloidosis

Prognosis
- The prognosis of Class V lupus is variable in the reported literature, but this may be due to classification systems that overlap membranous variants with proliferative variants. Pure Class V cases appear to have a good prognosis for renal function, but may have difficult to control nephrotic syndrome.
- Nephrotic syndrome resolves after stopping causative gold, D-penicillamine or NSAIDs in virtually all cases.
- The prognosis of patients with secondary amyloidosis is poor with a median survival of about 5 years and a mean time to developing end-stage renal disease of 18 months. More recent epidemiological data suggests that the median survival in the UK is closer to 10 years.
- The prognosis of patients with primary amyloidosis appears worse in patients with higher peripheral blood plasma cell counts (>0.5/µl or >1%), higher serum β2-microglobulin (>2.7 µg/ml), higher bone marrow plasma cell percentage (>10%) and/or dominant cardiac involvement. Survival on haemodialysis is 68% at 1 year and 30% at 5 years.

Monitoring
Patients with nephrotic syndrome should have their renal function, urinalysis, and proteinuria monitored regularly. Additional monitoring should be disease-specific.
- In SLE, monitoring complement levels is prudent as persistent hypocomplementemia suggests a poor prognosis. Consideration to a repeat renal biopsy should be given to patients with persistent serologic or urinary abnormalities after a year of treatment.
- Persistent immunological activity or class switching (the addition of a proliferative lesion) in repeat renal biopsies may require escalating or prolonged immunosuppression in SLE.
- Monitoring of serum amyloid protein in secondary amyloid may be a useful way of tracking disease progression and response to therapy.

Tubulointerstitial nephritis

Tubulointerstitial nephritis (TIN) refers to inflammation of the interstitial compartment of the kidney. It may present very subtly with few abnormalities of the urinalysis and slowly progressive renal failure. It is classically characterized by white blood cell casts in the urine sediment with or without non-nephrotic range proteinuria and renal dysfunction. Several rheumatological diseases are associated with the development of TIN, including Sjögren's syndrome, NSAID or allopurinol use, sarcoidosis, uveitis (TINU), or rarely Behçet's disease.

Epidemiology
- Sjögren's syndrome can involve the kidneys rarely but there are no precise estimates of frequency. The most common lesion is TIN, but there can also be isolated metabolic abnormalities (type 1 renal tubular acidosis or isolated hypokalemia), nephrogenic diabetes insipidus, or very rarely a glomerular lesion.
- Granulomatous interstitial nephritis is common in sarcoidosis, but it rarely results in clinically apparent disease. Additionally, sarcoidosis can result in nephrolithiasis due to related hypercalciuria, nephrotic syndrome due to membranous lesions or urinary obstruction due to retroperitoneal fibrosis. Sarcoidosis may also be related to the tubulointerstitial nephritis and uveitis syndrome (TINU).
- NSAID-related TIN was seen most commonly with fenoprofen, but is probably equally likely with all non-selective NSAIDs. There are reports of COX-2 selective NSAIDs also causing TIN.

Aetiology
- TIN in Sjögren's syndrome is characterized by a lymphocytic infiltrate invading and damaging the tubules. In some cases, granuloma formation is seen.
- Granulomatous inflammation is common in sarcoidosis. The aetiology is unclear.
- The interstitial infiltrate in NSAID-induced TIN is primarily composed of T cells. It is postulated that cyclooxygenase inhibition results in the conversion of arachidonic acid to leukotrienes, which activate Th cells. TIN is complicated in NSAID use by a concomitant haemodynamic injury.

Key clinical features
- Isolated renal manifestations of Sjögren's syndrome or sarcoidosis are rare. A history should include a detailed search for extra-renal disease activity.
- Patients with Sjögren's syndrome may have hypokalemia causing general muscle weakness or nephrogenic diabetes insipidus causing hypotension, low volume status and fatigue.
- Patients with sarcoidosis may have a history of nephrolithiasis due to persistent hypercalciuria.
- Patients with drug-related TIN may develop a rash (15%), fever (27%), eosinophilia (23%), or all 3 (10%).
- Other causes of TIN should be excluded (e.g. antibiotic or infection-related (legionella, cytomegalovirus).
- Owing to the often-insidious nature of the renal injury, advanced renal failure may be present at the time of diagnosis. Advanced renal failure may present as fatigue, anorexia, pruritis, or peripheral oedema.

Investigations
TIN is classically characterized by the presence of white blood cell casts in the urinalysis. Haematuria and proteinuria are also commonly found, although red blood cell casts would be very uncommon.
- Blood biochemistry may reveal an acidosis or hypokalemia in Sjögren's syndrome. Urine biochemistry is helpful in confirming a type 4 renal tubular acidosis.
- Urine eosinophils are commonly associated with drug induced TIN, but are not usually found in NSAID related TIN.

- Gallium scanning has been advocated in drug-induced interstitial nephritis, but its role is incompletely defined.
- A renal biopsy should be used to confirm the diagnosis if the cause of the renal dysfunction is unclear. A renal biopsy will also provide prognostic information and is used to stratify treatment.

Treatment
- There is little evidence for the treatment of renal Sjögren's syndrome or sarcoidosis. In general, patients with clinically apparent renal manifestations of these diseases are treated with GCs, often for a prolonged period.
- Hydroxychloroquine is often an effective treatment for patients with isolated hypercalciuria due to sarcoidosis.
- The primary treatment for drug-induced TIN is withdrawal of the offending agent. The value of a course of GCs is debated, but several weeks of therapy may decrease the time to renal recovery in patients not recovering quickly.

Prognosis
- The prognosis of TIN in Sjögren's syndrome is good with few cases progressing to end-stage renal disease.
- GCs often arrest the progression of TIN in sarcoidosis, but there is often incomplete renal recovery due to chronic scarring. Relapses appear more likely in patients who receive less than 20 mg/day of prednisolone for the first 3 months of treatment.
- End-stage renal disease from acute TIN secondary to medications is uncommon, but chronic TIN from NSAID use or from chronic analgesic nephropathy is common and there is only limited recovery of renal function after discontinuing the offending agent.

Monitoring
- Patients with any form of TIN should have their renal function monitored closely.
- Urine calcium is thought to be a sensitive measure of sarcoidosis activity due to increased vitamin D activity in active granulomata.
- Patients on prolonged courses of GCs require monitoring for the development of diabetes mellitus and glaucoma. Adequate calcium and vitamin D3 supplements and, if necessary specific osteoporosis therapy needs to be given as per guidelines [e.g. American College of Rheumatology Guidelines or Royal College of Physicians (RCP) (UK)].

Acute renal failure

Acute renal failure, renal dysfunction developing and/or worsening over a period of days, can complicate several rheumatological disorders in the absence of abnormalities of the urinalysis. This presentation occurs in systemic sclerosis (SSc; see also p. 264–272, the antiphospholipid syndrome (APLS; see also p. 274–280 and vascular disease, and also, following diagnoses, commonly considered to have a nephritic, nephrotic or TIN presentation when they have a benign or non-diagnostic urine sediment.

Epidemiology
- Autopsy studies indicate up to 80% of patients with diffuse cutaneous SSc have renal damage, although only 50% will have a clinical manifestation.
- Severe renal crisis can develop in a substantial minority of patients with SSc (mainly diffuse cutaneous disease).
- Renal involvement from APLS can occur in up to 25% of patients – affecting blood vessels of all sizes.
- Renal disease in APLS associated with SLE is found in only 10% of renal biopsies from patients with SLE.
- Accelerated vasculopathy influences the long-term prognosis of many patients with rheumatological diseases and can result in chronic kidney disease.

Aetiology
- SSc results in intimal proliferation and thickening of the small arcuate and interlobular arteries. This finding is commonly referred to as 'onion-skin' hypertrophy.
- SSc renal crises result from a thrombotic microangiopathy. Endothelial damage in small vessels causes fibrin clots and renal hypoxia/ischemia. This results in rapidly increasing blood pressure through activation of the renin-angiotensin that worsens the endothelial damage.
- APLS with renal damage is also a thrombotic microangiopathy and may be clinically indistinguishable from a SSc renal crisis (aside from the presence of SSc) or other causes of thrombotic microangiopathy.
- In APLS affected arteries demonstrate thrombotic lesions with intimal mucoid thickening, subendothelial fibrosis and medial hyperplasia.
- Delayed diagnosis/treatment in either SSc renal crisis or APLS may result in sclerotic lesions forming and a biopsy would thus show focal and segmental glomerulosclerosis, rather than the primary findings of a thrombotic microangiopathy.
- Accelerated vascular disease in any rheumatological disease can be caused by prolonged periods of inflammation causing endothelial dysfunction, exposure to GCs (direct effects, and effects on blood pressure and serum lipids), and exposure to immunosuppressants that adversely affect vascular function.

Risk factors
- Diffuse skin involvement, GC use, ciclosporin, and joint contractures are associated with an increased risk of SSc renal crisis.
- SSc renal crisis is associated with autoantibodies to RNA polymerase III and is less frequent in the presence of anti-centromere antibodies.
- In APLS, presence of coagulation factor mutations such as factor V Leiden, are associated with an increased risk of clinical activity including renal disease.
- There is an association between APLS and HLA-DR7 in several ethnic groups and HLA-DQ7 in some groups.

Key clinical features
- Thrombotic microangiopathies are characterized by haemolytic anaemia and thrombocytopaenia.
- Both SSc renal crisis and APLS may result in dramatic elevations in blood pressure and acute retinal changes, proteinuria and haematuria and pulmonary oedema.
- Not all patients with SSc renal crisis will have typical skin manifestations of SSc.
- Other causes of microangiopathy must be excluded: haemolytic-uraemic syndrome/thrombotic thrombocytopaenic purpura and malignant hypertension.
- Use of medications known to increase the risk of SSc renal crisis, such as GCs or ciclosporin. Ciclosporin and other calcineurin inhibitors may induce thrombotic thrombocytopaenic purpura independent of SSc.

Investigations
- Clinical details are of primary importance in the rapid and accurate diagnosis of these conditions. The underlying medical condition must be established.
- Renal biopsy confirms a microscopic angiopathy, but will not distinguish between causes.

Treatment
- Angiotensin converting enzyme inhibitor-based anti-hypertensive treatments are the mainstay of treating SSc renal crisis. Serum creatinine may rise initially, but the relaxation of the efferent arteriole will reduce intraglomerular pressure and reduce scarring, as well as increase interstitial blood flow.
- Control of blood pressure with other agents may also be required.
- Intravenous prostacyclin can help improve microvascular lesions in SSc renal crisis, but experience remains largely anecdotal.
- Rapidly progressive renal failure in APLS may respond to plasma exchange.
- Chronic anticoagulation in patients with APLS with a significant thrombotic complication, such as renal involvement, should be considered.

Prognosis
Left untreated, SSc renal crisis may result in rapid loss of renal function and end-stage renal disease in <8 weeks.

Monitoring
- Regular blood pressure monitoring is essential.
- Full blood count, fibrin degradation products, and blood smear are useful in monitoring microangiopathy.
- Antiphospholipid antibody binding levels are of uncertain significance.

Chronic kidney disease (CKD)

Some patients will present with a chronic elevation in serum creatinine reflecting a reduced glomerular filtration rate (GFR). This reduction in kidney function may be stable or slowly progressive, and is usually associated with a bland urine sediment. In patients with rheumatological diseases, the chronic glomerulopathy of RA, SSc, amyloidosis, chronic urate nephropathy/saturine gout results from chronic inflammation, and is associated with micro-vascular arteriopathy and interstitial fibrosis in the kidney. Chronic NSAID use may exacerbate this chronic injury by promoting hypertension and hyperglycaemia. The severity of chronic kidney disease is classified on the basis of the patient's GFR (or estimate of glomerular filtration rate on the basis of a stable serum creatinine).

Table 3.7 Chronic kidney disease (CKD) staging.

Stage	Glomerular filtration rate (ml/min)
I	>90, but some sign of kidney damage on another test (e.g. proteinuria)
II	60–90
III	30–59
IV	15–29
V	<15 or requires dialysis

Advanced chronic kidney disease (CKD) can be a cause of rheumatologic diseases. For example, severe chronic renal dysfunction is associated with hyperparathyroidism that can cause bone pain and arthralgia or haemodialysis may be associated with the accumulation of β2 microglobulin leading to a secondary amyloidosis.

The vast majority of patients with CKD do not progress to end stage renal failure but die of cardiovascular disease. The management of cardiovascular risk is a important in managing these patients.

Epidemiology and aetiology
- Chronic glomerulopathy is an uncommon complication of RA. The most common pathologic lesion in this disorder is a mesangial proliferative lesion.
- Chronic urate nephropathy is now uncommon. The decrease in urate nephropathy may be partially attributed to the decline in chronic lead exposure, an important aetiological agent in saturnine gout in which lead was a major contributor to renal dysfunction.
- Urate nephropathy is characterized by an elevation in serum urate out of keeping with the degree of renal dysfunction (urate >535 µmol/l in patients with mild renal disease and >700 µmol/l in patients with a creatinine >176 µmol/l).
- Up to 80% of patients with diffuse cutaneous SSc will have renal damage and up to 50% will have chronic hypertension, mild proteinuria, or CKD.
- Although hyperparathyroidism is common in advanced CKD, clinically apparent bone disease is rare outside the dialysis population. Within the dialysis population, disorders of parathyroid hormone (PTH) that can result in fractures and bone pain include osteitis fibrosa (due to excess PTH), osteomalacia (due to inadequate mineralization), and adynamic bone disease (due to over suppression of PTH). See Chapter 14, p. 426.
- Haemodialysis related amyloidosis is a rare complication that is more common with increasing years on dialysis. This disorder is related to the increased generation of β2 microglobulin due to increased levels of inflammation (perhaps due to contact of blood with the dialysis apparatus) and decreased clearance due to poor transport across the dialysis membrane.
- Atherosclerotic renal disease may affect any size blood vessels, but is most common in small vessels. The excess of atherosclerotic disease may be due to chronic inflammation causing endothelial dysfunction and/or the effects of commonly used medications, such as non-NSAIDs, which cause hypertension, or GCs, which cause hypertension and hyperglycaemia.

Key clinical features
The duration and evolution of renal dysfunction is the most important component of the evaluation of renal disease. Patients with CKD that is not progressive can be investigated less aggressively than patients with new onset dysfunction or rapidly deteriorating renal function. In patients with advanced CKD (stage V) enquiry about uraemic symptoms is mandatory, as they will determine the need for initiating renal replacement therapy. Such symptoms include worsening fatigue, anorexia, generalized pruritus, a metallic taste to food, and worsening oedema. Monitoring of fluid, electrolyte, particularly serum potassium, and acid-base balance is important.

Investigations
- Renal biopsies are infrequently required in CKD, but patients with chronic inflammatory diseases, are more likely to require a biopsy.

- Urinalysis and the quantification of proteinuria should be checked in all patients.
- Blood pressure should be monitored closely.
- Patients with stage V disease should have periodic monitoring of serum electrolytes and bicarbonate.
- Patients with stage III-V disease should have periodic monitoring of serum PTH (see p. 426).
- Dialysis related amyloidosis has a predilection for the cervical spine, scapulohumeral region and the carpal tunnels. Cystic bone disease is also common.
- Urinary lead levels in patients with lead exposure.
- Serum urate to guide allopurinol or other anti-hyperuricaemic therapy.

Treatment
- Early referral to a nephrologist is indicated in patients with renal disease and a concomitant rheumatological disease. In CKD referral may expedite a diagnostic biopsy or, when necessary, preparation for renal replacement therapy or renal transplantation.
- The cornerstones of management are adequately managing any underlying chronic disease, renal protection and the management of cardiovascular risk. This includes careful management of blood pressure, hyperlipidemia, diabetes mellitus, and smoking cessation. Aspirin use is warranted on the basis of trials in patients without CKD.
- There is some evidence for the preferential use of angiotensin blockading drugs in patients with hypertension and proteinuria, but this continues to be debated, particularly in the non-diabetic patient.

See also: CKD metabolic bone disease (p. 426).

Resources
Information and internet sites
European Vasculitis Study Group. Available at: http://www.vasculitis.org
Vasculitis Foundation. Available at: http://www.vasculitisfoundation.org
UK Renal association. Available at: http://www.renal.org
NICE (UK) chronic kidney disease guidance. Available at: http://www.nice.org.uk/guidance/

ICD10 codes
N00-08   Glomerular diseases
M32.1+   SLE with organ involvement
N08*5   Glomerular disorders in systemic AICTDs
M31.3   Wegener's Granulomatosis
N04   Nephrotic syndrome

Further reading
Austin HA, III, Klippel JH, et al. Therapy of lupus nephritis. Controlled trial of prednisone and cytotoxic drugs. *N Engl J Med* 1986; **314**: 614–19.

Balow JE, Austin HA, III. Therapy of membranous nephropathy in systemic lupus erythematosus. *Semin Nephrol* 2003; **23**: 386–91.

Boumpas DT, Austin HA III, et al. Controlled trial of pulse methyl-prednisolone versus two regimens of pulse cyclophosphamide in severe lupus nephritis. *Lancet* 1992; **340**: 741–5.

Contreras G, Pardo V, et al. Sequential therapies for proliferative lupus nephritis. *N Engl J Med* 2004; **350**: 971–80.

Fauci AS, Haynes BF, Katz P, Wolff SM. Wegener's granulomatosis: prospective clinical and therapeutic experience with 85 patients for 21 years. *Ann Intern Med* 1983; **98**: 76–85.

Helin HJ, Korpela MM, Mustonen JT, Pasternack AI. Renal biopsy findings and clinicopathologic correlations in rheumatoid arthritis. *Arthritis Rheum* 1995; **38**: 242–7.

Houssiau FA, Vasconcelos C, et al. Immunosuppressive therapy in lupus nephritis: the Euro-Lupus Nephritis Trial, a randomized trial of low-dose versus high-dose intravenous cyclophosphamide. *Arthritis Rheum* 2002; **46**: 2121–31.

Jayne D, Rasmussen N, et al. A randomized trial of maintenance therapy for vasculitis associated with ANCA autoantibodies. *N Engl J Med* 2003; **349**: 36–44.

Lachmann HJ, Goodman HJ, et al. Natural history and outcome in systemic AA amyloidosis. *N Engl J Med* 2007; **356**: 2361–71.

Walsh M, James M, et al. Mycophenolate mofetil for induction therapy of lupus nephritis: a systematic review and meta-analysis. *Clin J Am Soc Nephrol* 2007; **2**: 968–75.

Weening JJ, D'Agati VD, et al. The classification of glomerulonephritis in systemic lupus erythematosus revisited. *J Am Soc Nephrol* 2004; **15**: 241–50.

The gut and hepatobiliary disease

The gut is frequently involved in autoimmune and hereditary connective tissue diseases (CTDs), and in both large and small vessel vasculitides. Clinical features reflect the defective connective tissue components in hereditary CTD, or the processes of chronic inflammation, aberrant repair, vascular damage, and adverse drug reactions in the autoimmune CTDs (AICTDs)/vasculitic syndromes. In addition, rheumatological disease often complicates infective or inflammatory disorders, which are predominantly gastroenterological.

Table 3.8 Anatomical classification of gastrointestinal involvement in rheumatological disease

	Mouth/pharynx	Oesophagus	Stomach	Small Intestine	Large intestine	Liver/pancreas/gallbladder
Rheumatoid arthritis (RA)	+	+	++	+	+	+
SLE	+++	+	+	+	+	+
Systemic sclerosis (SSc)	++	+++	+	++	++	+/−
Dermato- & polymyositis	++	++	+	+	+	
Sjögren's syndrome (SS)	+++	++		+		++
Wegener's granulomatosis (WG)			+	+	+	
Churg–Strauss syndrome (CSS)			+	+	+	
Polyarteritis nodosa (PAN)	+		+	++	+	+
Henoch–Schönlein purpura (HSP)			+	++	+	+
Behçet's disease	+++			+	++	
Kawasaki disease				+	+	
Giant Cell Arteritis (GCA)				+	+	
Cryoglobulinaemia				+	+	+
Reiter's Syndrome				+	++	
Marfan's/Ehlers–Danlos		+		++	++	
Whipple's disease				++	++	

Classification

Epidemiology

Mouth
- Ulcers occur in SLE, Behçet's disease, RA, DM, and PM, PAN, and occasionally other vasculitides.
- Oral fissures occur in Sjögren's syndrome (SS) and in cases of iron deficiency (angular cheilosis).
- Xerostomia is common in SS and sarcoidosis.
- Temporomandibular arthritis may cause pain and limitation of mastication in RA and JIA.
- Drugs used in inflammatory rheumatological disorders may be associated with oral ulceration, candidiasis or (rarely) taste disturbance (dysgeusia).

Oesophagus
- Oesophageal dysmotility occurs in ~90% of SSc and is symptomatic in ~80%. It is also frequently problematic in SS (associated with impaired lubrication of bolus) and in DM and PM. Oesophageal dysmotility also occurs in RA and SLE, but may not correlate with manometric abnormalities. Swallowing may be impaired by cervical spine and laryngeal involvement in RA.
- Megaesophagus occurs in Marfan Syndrome and some forms of Ehlers–Danlos syndrome (EDS).
- Oesophageal perforation can occur in Behçets.
- Aspiration can result from oesophageal dysmotility in SSc, DM or PM. Mega-oesophagus occurs in Marfan Syndrome and EDS.
- Barrett's metaplasia occurs in >33% of SSc patients.
- Oesophageal candidiasis may occur in immunosuppressed patients, especially if neutropaenic; glucocorticoids increase the risk.
- Oesophageal varices (and upper GI haemorrhage) occur as a result of portal hypertension in primary biliary cirrhosis (PBC), which is particularly associated with SSc and SS.
- Hepatic fibrosis and portal hypertension may also follow autoimmune hepatitis (see below) and drug-related hepatitis and fibrosis.
- Portal vein thrombosis occurs in Behçets and SLE. It results in portal hypertension. Nodular regenerative hyperplasia (RA, SLE) can cause portal hypertension.

CHAPTER 3 Organ involvement in rheumatological disease

Stomach
- *Gastritis* is common across the range of autoinflammatory conditions and in response to many disease-modifying or anti-inflammatory drugs
- *Gastric ulcers* are particularly associated with RA, PAN, Behçet's disease, CSS, HSP.
- *Gastric antral vascular ectasia (GAVE)* can occur in portal hypertension, or primarily in SS or SSc.
- *Delayed gastric emptying* is common in SSc (~75%) and occurs in DM/PM, or from secondary amyloidosis.
- Eosinophilic infiltration of the stomach can result in discrete masses in Churg–Strauss syndrome (CSS).

Small intestine
- **Malabsorption** is characteristic of Whipple's disease, and complicates RA, SLE, SS, Marfan syndrome, and EDS.
- **Coeliac disease** (CD) frequency is increased in SS. CD may be association with Spondylarthropathies (SpAs).
- **Whipple's disease** classically presents with weight loss, diarrhoea, abdominal pain, and arthralgia or arthritis; neurological and constitutional features may also occur. Whipple's disease may manifest as arthritis without GI symptoms.
- **Obstruction** may rarely occur as a result of strictures following mucosal ulceration (RA, SLE, PM, DM, SS, PAN, CSS, Behçet's disease).
- **Pseudo-obstruction** may arise in dysmotility syndromes (SSc, Marfan syndrome, EDS, and also RA.
- **Intussusception** may occur in SSc, SLE, and HSP.
- **Mucosal ulceration** may complicate RA, SLE, PM, DM, CSS, HSP, Behçet's disease.
- **Small bowel ischaemia or infarction** may complicate PAN, CSS, WG, cryoglobulinaemia, Behçet's disease, and Giant Cell Arteritis (GCA).
- **Vasculitis of the small intestine** may manifest as fever, abdominal pain, acute malabsorption, and nephrotic syndrome (with hypogammaglobulinaemia and hypocomplementaemia) owing to protein-losing enteropathy or peritonitis.
- **Mesenteric arterial rupture** (leading to an acute abdomen and shock) may occur in Marfan Syndrome, EDS.
- **Perforation** has been associated with RA, SLE, SSc, DM, PM, PAN, CSS, HSP, WG, Behçet's disease, Marfan syndrome, and EDS, and this rarely may be accompanied by *pneumatosis intestinalis*.
- **Amyloid**, with resultant protein-losing enteropathy is a rare complication of RA and SpAs.

Large intestine
- **Colitis** is associated particularly with Behçet's disease and SpA (often clinically silent), but may also complicate RA, SLE, WG, and other vasculitides. Colitis may be complicated by perforation.
- **Appendicitis** is common in the general population, but may present more frequently in PAN and HSP.
- **Constipation and diarrhoea** are prominent problems in dysmotility syndromes (SSc, Marfan Syndrome, EDS), but also complicate SLE, PM, DM, and vasculitides.
- **Faecal incontinence** is a common, but under-reported symptom in SSc.
- **Megacolon and giant diverticulae** may occur in Marfan Syndrome EDS and joint hypermobility syndrome (JHS); these carry an increased risk of perforation.

- **Mucosal telangectasiae** in SSc may be a cause of chronic blood loss and iron-deficiency anaemia.

Liver/pancreas/gallbladder
- **Hepatitis** and transaminitis occurs in RA, Adult Still's disease, SLE, and SS. Hepatitis is generally mild in these conditions, although in Adult Still's disease can follow a fulminant course. Hepatotoxicity is a common adverse effect of drugs used in Rheumatological patients.
- **Secondary amyloidosis** can result in hepatosplenomegaly in RA.
- **Non-specific hepatosplenomegaly** occurs in RA (Felty's syndrome), SLE, and SS.
- **Primary biliary cirrhosis** is associated with SS and SSc.
- **Acalculous cholecystitis** occurs in RA, PAN, WG, and HSP.
- **Exocrine pancreatic insufficiency** occurs in ~25% patients with SS.
- **Pancreatitis** may complicate SS, SLE, PAN, and pancreatic necrosis has been reported in SSc. Drugs may also cause pancreatitis.

Table 3.9 Rheumatological manifestations of gastroenterological and hepatic diseases

GI disease	Rheumatological manifestation
Crohn's disease	SI ~25%; AS ~10%. Peripheral arthritis ~20%
Ulcerative colitis	SI ~15%; AS ~7%. Peripheral arthritis ~20%
Whipple's disease	Migratory arthritis >60%
Enteric infection	Reactive arthritis, septic arthritis, osteomyelitis
Intestinal bypass surgery	Symmetrical polyarthralgia or polyarthritis >50%
Pancreatic arthritis syndrome	Lipid crystal polyarthritis. Bone infarction by fat embolism.
Haemochromatosis	Chrondrocalcinosis and CPPDD disease
Wilson's disease	Chrondrocalcinosis and CPPDD disease
Primary biliary cirrhosis	Polyarthritis ~ 20%; SSc ~20%. Sjögren's syndrome ~ 50%
Hepatitis A	Prodromal polyarthralgia. Arthritis/vasculits rarely
Hepatitis B	Prodromal polyarthralgia. Arthritis ~ 10%; PAN (rare)
Hepatitis C	Polyarthralgia ~10%. Polyarthritis ~ 5%. Mixed cryoglobulinaemia 10–50%; SLE-like syndrome

Aetiology/pathophysiology
Mouth/pharynx
Oral ulcers may reflect the generalized aberrant interaction of leucocytes and endothelium, and an over-reactive local inflammatory response to minor mucosal trauma.
- In RA, mouth ulcers are often associated with antiproliferative DMARDs, which are toxic to rapidly-dividing cells, including mucosal epithelium.
- Oral ulcers in SLE may reflect deposition of local immune complexes and ensuing inflammatory response with mucosal breakdown.
- Deficiency of vitamin B12, folic acid, and iron can also result in oral ulceration.

Oesophagus
- Manometric abnormalities include low amplitude peristaltic waves and reduced lower oesophageal (LOS) pressure in RA.
- Atrophy and fibrosis of the oesophageal wall and damage to intrinsic nerves result in dysmotility ranging from incoordination to complete paralysis in SSc.
- Loss of LOS pressure results in gastro-oesophageal reflux disease (GORD) and peptic stricture in ~8% of RA and SLE patients..
- Inflammatory myopathy predominantly results in impaired deglutition in PM and DM, but also affects smooth muscle of the oesophagus.

Stomach
- Delayed gastric emptying can occur due to infiltration with secondary amyloid (RA), eosinophilia, and fibrosis (CSS), atrophy, and scarring of the muscle layers (SSc), or inflammatory myopathy in PM or DM.
- Ulceration in RA is secondary to medication use (without, which it is no more common than in OA). Local mass-like lesions can occur in CSS.

Small intestine
Inflammatory bowel disease (IBD)
IBD and spondylarthritis (SpA) probably arise as a result of aberrant responses to gut bacteria and the development of an excessive pro-inflammatory T cell response, in particular mediated by the Th17 subset.
- This model can be integrated with known genetic associations with IBD/SpA since variants of pattern recognition receptors (NOD2/CARD15 polymorphism associated with Crohn's disease) and/or cytokine receptors (e.g. IL-23R polymorphism associate with Crohn's disease and AS) could alter the dendritic cell response to micro-organisms and to the inflammatory mileu itself.
- The well-recognized association of these diseases with HLA-B27 could reflect the ability of this HLA molecule to influence the innate response of dendritic cells to micro-organisms.

Bacterial over-growth
Occurs as a result of impaired motility of the intestine in amyloidosis, SSc, DM, and PM; and can be due to diverticular disease in SSc, Marfan syndrome, and EDS.
- It may be exacerbated by the use of PPI in RA and SSc for gastro-protection from NSAIDs or GORD.
- Focal bowel wall thickening or intramucosal haemorrhage can lead to intussusception in HSP, CSS, and SLE.

Whipple's disease
Caused by a bacterium *Tropheryma whipplei*. Affected tissues are infiltrated with foamy macrophages. It appears that aberrant activation of dendritic cells and macrophages, following ingestion of *T. whipplei* may result in a defective Th1 response with persistence of both the bacterium and the aberrant inflammatory response.

Large intestine
- Colitis resembling Crohn's disease can occur in Behçet's with mucosal aphthae.
- Vasculitis resulting in mucosal or full-thickness ischaemia can occur in RA, SLE, WG, PAN, HSP, and other vasculitides.
- Scarring and atrophy of the ano-rectal musculature can result in faecal incontinence in SSc.

Liver/pancreas/gallbladder
Small vessel vasculitis resulting in patchy hypoperfusion leads to nodular regenerative hyperplasia of the liver in RA and SLE, and can cause portal hypertension.

Table 3.10 Gastrointestinal effects associated with drugs used in rheumatological patients

Drug	Effect
NSAIDs	Dyspepsia, nausea, peptic ulcer, abnormal liver function tests, protein-losing enteropathy. NSAIDs **reduce** the risk of colonic carcinoma.
Glucocorticoids	Peptic ulcer (in conjunction with NSAIDs).
Methotrexate	Nausea, stomatitis, mouth ulcers, abnormal liver function tests, hepatic fibrosis.
Azathioprine	Nausea, diarrhoea, abnormal liver function tests, hepatitis.
Mycophenolate mofetil	Nausea, vomiting, diarrhoea, constipation, gastrointestinal ulceration, abnormal liver function tests, hepatitis.
Leflunomide	Stomatitis, diarrhoea, vomiting, abnormal liver function tests.
Sulfasalazine	Nausea, vomiting, diarrhoea (bloody), dyspepsia, abnormal liver function tests, hepatic necrosis, pancreatitis, cholestasis.
Gold	Mouth ulcers, diarrhoea, cholestasis, hepatic necrosis, gold enterocolitis (fever, diarrhoea, megacolon, eosinophilia).
Ciclosporin	Nausea, gum hyperplasia, vomiting, diarrhoea, abnormal liver function tests.
Cyclophosphamide	Nausea, vomiting, stomatitis, diarrhoea, abnormal liver function tests.
Hydroxychloroquine	Nausea, vomiting, diarrhoea.
Colchicine	Nausea, vomiting, diarrhoea, gastrointestinal haemorrhage.
Allopurinol	Nausea, abnormal liver function tests.
Infliximab	Dyspepsia, diarrhoea, constipation, gastrointestinal haemorrhage, hepatitis, cholecystitis.
Adalimumab	Dyspepsia, diarrhoea, constipation, taste disturbance, and oral ulcers.
Etanercept	Dyspepsia, gastrointestinal haemorrhage, pancreatitis, cholecystitis.
Rituximab	Nausea and vomiting during infusion.

Primary biliary cirrhosis (PBC)
PBC is caused by an autoimmune response that destroys small intralobular bile ducts, resulting in cholestasis. The retained bile acids themselves cause damage to hepatocytes and increase expression of HLA antigens on these cells, which enhances the autoimmune response. Antimitochondrial antibodies (AMA) are characteristic of PBC and occur in 95% patients; they are specific for pyruvate dehydrogenase epitopes located on the inner mitochondrial membrane. It is unclear what role AMA plays in the pathogenesis of PBC.

Autoimmune pancreatitis
Can be associated with salivary gland inflammation that can mimic SS and accompany other autoimmune conditions.

CHAPTER 3 **Organ involvement in rheumatological disease** 85

It can result in stricturing of the biliary or pancreatic ducts, and lead to features of sclerosing cholangitis or pancreatic atrophy and exocrine dysfunction. The pancreas is infiltrated with IgG4 secreting plasma cells and IgG4 levels are increased to >135 mg/l in serum.

Risk factors
- RA – associated with ~5-fold risk of GI bleeding.
- DM is associated with pancreatic, stomach and colorectal carcinoma.
- SS is associated with lymphomas, including MALT lymphoma.
- Drug-induced GI disease.

Clinical features
General assessment
Assess nutritional state (e.g. BMI, lean body mass), lymphadenopathy pallor, jaundice (look at sclerae) and nails for clubbing, koilonychia (iron deficiency).

Examine skin
Dermatitis herpetiformis indicates coeliac disease; erythema nodosum occurs in inflammatory bowel disease, Behçet's disease, PAN, sarcoid, and sometimes in other vasculitides; pyoderma gangrenosum may signify co-existing inflammatory bowel disease or vasculitis. Red papules with surrounding atrophy, which evolve to porcelain-white scars, occur in Kohlmeier–Degos syndrome (a cutaneo-intestinal arterio-occlusive syndrome).

Mouth
- Xerostomia (dry mouth) occurs in primary or secondary Sjögren's and typically in sarcoid. Look also for swollen salivary glands and lymphadenopathy. Xerostomia is associated with dental caries.
- Sicca symptoms can be caused by drugs (e.g. diuretics, tricyclic antidepressants).
- Oral ulcers on tongue, buccal mucosa and pharynx can occur in SLE, Behçet's disease (often with genital ulcers), DM, PM, PAN or in association with drugs (e.g. methotrexate, gold, and cyclophosphamide).
- Reduced oral aperture occurs in SSc sometimes making eating (and dental work) difficult.
- Dysphagia may be caused by weakness or incoordination of the skeletal (voluntary) muscle of the pharynx; this may occur in DM/PM and (rarely) as a result of cranial neuropathy in small vessel vasculitis.
- Cervical spine deformity and crico-arytenoid arthritis may affect deglutition in RA.
- Oral fissures (angular cheilosis) and glossitis can reflect iron deficiency or malabsorption, (e.g. SSc).
- Mastication is impaired by temporomandibular joint arthritis in RA and JIA.
- Fissuring of the tongue due to vitamin B12 deficiency.
- Mucositis and white colonies suggestive of candidiasis.

Oesophagus
- Dysphagia may be caused by dysmotility of the smooth (involuntary) muscle of the oesophagus in SSc and by oesophageal strictures or webs (Sjögren's).
- Heartburn or central chest pain, often worse after eating or on bending/lying may occur in GORD. This is common in SSc and SLE (up to 10%), and may also arise from megaoesophagus in Marfan syndrome or EDS. Ischaemic heart disease must be excluded in patients with chest pain.
- Cough, wheezing, and dyspnoea results from aspiration from oesophageal dysfunction, especially in SSc.
- GORD can result in dysphagia due to oesophageal strictures or dysmotility (oesophageal spasm).

Stomach
- Epigastric or left hypochondrial pain may indicate gastritis or gastric ulceration (RA, SLE, CSS).
- Melaena indicates frank blood loss from stomach or small bowel.
- Nausea reflects gastric atrophy (e.g. Sjögren's) or dysfunction, or may be an adverse reaction to drugs.
- A gastric mass may occur in Sjögren's syndrome (lymphoma should be excluded) and CSS.
- Bloating, halitosis, and regurgitation can all reflect delayed gastric emptying, e.g. SSc.

Small intestine
- Weight loss may indicate malabsorption.
- Melaena indicates frank blood loss from stomach or small bowel.
- Abdominal distension or bloating may indicate malabsorption, and/or dysmotility, bacterial overgrowth (especially, SSc, EDS, Marfan syndrome) or ascites (SLE).
- Central abdominal pain, worse 30–60 min after eating, may suggest mesenteric ischaemia.
- Peripheral oedema may occur in a protein-losing enteropathy.
- Colicky abdominal pain may indicate obstruction, pseudo-obstruction (RA, SSc, Kawasaki disease) or intussusception (RA, SSc, SLE). Absolute constipation (no flatus) and faeculent vomiting indicates obstruction.
- Severe abdominal pain with referred pain to shoulder (diaphragmatic irritation) may suggest perforation and/or GI haemorrhage.
- Unrelenting abdominal pain occurs in bowel infarction.
- Steatorrhoea (pale, oily, floating stools) results from fat malabsorption.

Large intestine
- Diarrhoea and/or constipation may both result from dysmotility (SSc, DM, PM, EDS, and Marfan syndromes).
- Pain, which starts in the midline and moves to the right iliac fossa may suggest appendicitis.
- Bloody diarrhoea occurs in the presence of mucosal ulceration or infarction.
- Rectal prolapse occurs with diarrhoea or constipation.

Liver/pancreas/gallbladder
- Pruritis and, in more severe cases, jaundice, occurs in the presence of biliary obstruction.
- Upper abdominal pain, sometimes radiating to the interscapular region, occurs in pancreatitis. Malaise, nausea, and vomiting may accompany pain.
- Haematemesis may be severe and life-threatening in patients with portal hypertension and varices.

Examination of the abdomen
- Distension/asymmetry suggests organomegaly or mass.
- Visible peristalsis with small intestinal dilatation is common in small bowel over-growth or obstruction.
- Telangectasiae (spider naevi) on the chest and upper body (in a non-SSc patient) or caput medusae (rare) indicate cirrhosis.

- Tenderness – guarding, rigidity and rebound tenderness – suggests a 'surgical abdomen'. Local tenderness suggests gastritis/peptic ulcer (LUQ), hepatitis or hepatic congestion or cholecystitis (RUQ), ileocolitis, or appendicitis (RLQ).
- PR examination in suspected appendicitis.
- Perineal ulcers in Behçet's or Crohn's disease.
- Palpate liver, spleen and kidneys, and check for ascites (shifting dullness) in distended abdomen.
- Auscultate for tinkling bowel sounds that may suggest obstruction or pseudo-obstruction sounds in an ileus.

Investigations

Mouth

- Iron studies in patients with angular cheilosis.
- Vitamin B12 and red cell folate in oral ulceration
- WBC (especially neutrophil count) in patients with candidiasis.
- Orthopantomogram to assess TMJ arthritis (usually requested by oral/maxillofacial surgeons).
- Minor salivary gland biopsy may enable a diagnosis of SS or MALT lymphoma associated with SS. Parotid biopsy occasionally necessary to distinguish diabetic sialadenosis, sarcoid and SS.

Oesophagus

- Oesophageal manometry in SSc, SLE, RA, DM, and PM.
- Video-fluoroscopy or fibre-optic endoscopic examination of swallow (FEES) in proximal impaired swallow.
- Barium swallow (SSc, EDS) – use water soluble contrast if at risk of aspiration.
- OGD may reveal reflux oesophagitis, peptic stricture, or Barrett's metaplasia associated with GORD.
- 24-h pH studies with pH catheter or mucosal adherent capsule to assess acid reflux.
- Nuclear scintigraphy can assess volume of reflux in achlorhydric patients (other methods rely on pH drop).
- CXR – air under the diaphragm occurs following perforation of stomach, small or large bowel.

Stomach

- FBC and iron studies if chronic GI bleed suspected.
- Upper GI endoscopy in suspected gastric ulcer/cancer, biopsies for eosinophilic infiltration (CSS) and *Helicobacter pylori* (rapid urease test).
- Nuclear scintigraphic gastric emptying studies (solid and/or liquid phase).

Small intestine

- Malabsorption screen (PTH, iron studies, vitamin B12, red cell folate, vitamins A and E, magnesium, phosphate, and calcium).
- Anti tissue-transglutaminase antibodies (85-95% sensitivity for celiac disease).
- Faecal pancreatic elastase is a measure of exocrine pancreatic dysfunction.
- Albumin and immunoglobulins in suspected protein-losing enteropathy.
- Upper GI endoscopy for: suspected duodenal ulcer, coeliac disease, IBD affecting small bowel, with aspirate and colony count for suspected bacterial over-growth and biopsies for coeliac disease, *Giardia lamblia*, and Whipple's bacillus.
- Glucose-hydrogen breath test for proximal small intestinal over-growth.

- Small bowel follow-through for characteristic 'hide-bound' appearance of small intestine in SSc or presence of diverticulae.
- CT chest, abdomen and pelvis – used to seek solid organ malignancy, lymphadenopathy in risk patients (e.g Sjögren's syndrome, DM), and for pneumatosis cystoides intestinalis.
- CT, conventional angiography of mesenteric arteries in suspected PAN or mesenteric ischaemia.
- MR enteroclysis (filling with contrast medium of small bowel) for suspected intussuception.
- MR angiography or [18]FDG-PET for suspected large vessel vasculitides.
- Video capsule enteroscopy for mucosal abnormalities of the small intestine (telangiectasias, aphthae, ischaemic ulcers, lymphoma).
- Small intestinal manometry for SSc or suspected intestinal dysmotility.

Large intestine

- FBC and iron studies if chronic GI bleed suspected.
- Colonoscopy for bleeding per rectum, where ulceration or ischaemia suspected.
- CT colonography can be used to exclude significant lesions, where colonoscopy is hindered by stricture or high risk.
- Mesenteric angiography (invasive/CT/MR) in suspected ischaemia.
- Anorectal manometry for faecal incontinence.
- Rectal biopsy – for amyloid.

Liver/pancreas/gallbladder

- LFTs – ALT/AST elevated in hepatocellular damage, whereas elevated bilirubin, alkaline phosphatase and gamma GT indicated biliary obstruction. ALT/AST may be elevated in patients with myositis; alkaline phosphatase and gamma GT are acute phase reactants, and an isoform of ALP is also released from bone.
- Elevated amylase reflects acute pancreatitis (SS, PAN, and WG). Can be elevated with salivary disease (SS) or vomiting.
- Infectious hepatitis serology – for hepatitis A, B, C, EBV, CMV.
- Autoimmune hepatitis serology – anti-smooth muscle antibodies and anti-liver-kidney microsomal antibodies accompany autoimmune hepatitis; anti-mitochondrial antibodies (and more specifically anti-pyruvate dehydrogenase antibodies) are associated with PBC.
- Serum IgG4 levels may be helpful in suspected autoimmune pancreatitis.
- HFE genotyping should be performed in individuals with elevated ferritin (without other elevated acute phase reactants) and transferrin saturation >45%.
- USS abdomen – used to visualize liver, including biliary tree, gallbladder, and spleen; and Doppler ultrasound to interrogate portal and hepatic vein blood flow. The view of pancreas is generally inadequate.
- Liver biopsy – generally performed under ultrasound guidance. Biopsy in suspected autoimmune hepatitis and to establish presence of cirrhosis.
- In haemochromatosis, biopsy liver if ferritin >1000 µg/l. Note: Liver biopsy is not essential to confirm the diagnosis of PBC. Do NOT biopsy liver in suspected cases of amyloid.

- Triple phase CT of the abdomen to examine pancreas and portal vasculature.
- Endoscopic ultrasound (EU) for visualization of upper GI mucosa where thickening is present on cross sectional modalities. EU gives good visualization of the pancreas (and for needle cytology of pancreatic masses).
- ERCP for suspected biliary and pancreatic ductal abnormalities.

Treatment
Mouth
- **Ulcers**: review and alter medication, if likely precipitant. Routinely prescribe folic acid 5 mg weekly in patients treated with methotrexate and increase to 5 mg 5 times weekly if mouth ulcers occur. Prescribe benzydamine (Difflam) mouthwash or salicylate gel for symptomatic relief or topical glucocorticoid (e.g. betametasone tablets or triamcinolone paste applied 2–4 times daily) for short courses. Colchicine and, in severe, resistant cases, anti-TNFα agents may be useful for mouth ulcers in Behçet's disease.
- **Oral fissures**: iron supplementation, if required. Prescribe nystatin ointment if fungal infection or short course of hydrocortisone cream for inflammation.
- **Xerostomia**: artificial saliva is available as sprays (e.g. Glandosane, Saliva Orthana, Luborant), lozenges (Saliva Orthana) or gels (e.g. Oralbalance, BioXtra). Note that Luborant is a neutral pH and contains fluoride, and therefore may reduce dental caries. Muscarinic, cholinergic secretagogues may be tried (see SS, p. 254–262).
- **Candidiasis**: if patient uses inhaled corticosteroids, review technique and post-inhaler mouth rinsing. Treat topically with nystatin pastilles suspension qds, miconazole mouthwash or amphotericin lozenges qds. Systemic anti-fungals may be required in resistant cases or in patients with xerostomia (see below).
- **Temporomandibular joint (TMJ) arthritis**: refer to maxillofacial surgeon for assessment and possible TMJ glucocorticoid injection.

Oesophagus
- **Oesophageal dysmotility**: oesophagitis may be reduced with a proton pump inhibitor. Erythromycin or domperidone accelerate oesophageal clearance and gastric emptying.
- **Aspiration**: practical measures, such as raising the head of the bed may reduce nocturnal aspiration. Note: Fundiplication is absolutely contraindicated in patients with oesophageal dysmotility.
- **Barrett's metaplasia**: treat with PPI. Surveillance for the development of oesophageal adenocarcinoma (according to local guidelines), treatment of high grade dysplasia or localized lesions with radiofrequency ablation, mucosal resection, or oesophagectomy.
- **Oesophageal varices**: primary prophylaxis with β-blockers in cirrhosis. There's no evidence of benefit for primary prophylaxis in pre-hepatic portal hypertension. Variceal banding for secondary prophylaxis of bleeding.
- **Oesophageal candidiasis**: check WBC (in particular neutrophils). Treat with systemic anti-fungals (amphotericin, miconazole, fluconazole; NB use ketoconazole only in resistant cases and monitor LFTs carefully).

Stomach
- **Gastritis and gastric ulcers**: minimize use of NSAIDs by optimal use of DMARDs and simple analgesia. COX-2 selective NSAIDs are associated with ~50% risk of severe GI complications compared with non-selective NSAIDs. Risk of GI haemorrhage can be reduced by use of a proton pump inhibitor.
- **Gastric antral vascular ectasia (GAVE)**: treat with argon beam ablation at endoscopy; look for portal hypertension.
- **Delayed gastric emptying** can be improved with domperidone or erythromycin. Botulinum toxin injection into the pylorus can improve emptying in marginal cases.

> **Patients with any of the following risks for NSAID-associated GI disease should be prescribed a proton pump inhibitor:**
> - High dose of NSAID.
> - Prolonged use of NSAID.
> - Age 65 years or over.
> - History of peptic ulcer.
> - Serious comorbidity (RA, CVD, renal/hepatic disease, diabetes mellitus, hypertension).
> - Heavy smoker.
> - Excessive alcohol ingestion.
> - *Helicobacter pylorii* infection.

- **Gastric masses**: treatment depends on the nature of the mass, which is usually determined by biopsy. For malignant neoplasms liaise with oncology and for lymphomas with haematology. Look for and eradicate *Helicobacter pylori*. Occasionally, masses reflect underlying inflammatory disorders and are treated with increased systemic immunosuppression.
- **Severe dysmotility or mega-oesophagus** may require additional routes of feeding into the stomach or intestine such as percutaneous endoscopically placed gastrostomy tube with extension of the enteral tube into the jejunum, or direct placement of a feeding tube into the jejunum in cases of severe GORD.

Small intestine
Mucosal ulceration
This can occur from underlying vasculitis and may respond to immunosuppressive regimens including GCs, azathioprine, anti-TNFα agents, rituximab, or Campath (Alemtuzumab).

Malabsorption
Reversible disease should be treated by appropriate immunosuppression of chronic inflammatory disorders (refer to chapters on individual diseases) or by institution of a gluten-free diet in patients who have co-existing coeliac disease.
- Whipple's disease may be treated with antibiotics; consultation with the Infectious Diseases Team is recommended.
- Patients with calcium malabsorption and secondary hyperparathyroidism require high dose calcium supplements, although if there is severe osteomalacia particularly with fractures, bone pain and muscle disease (deficiency range 25-OHD, high ALP, high PTH, and bone biopsy evidence) 1,25-dihydroxyvitamin D3 therapy should be considered initially. Oral calcitriol is better absorbed than vitamin D3, will heal osteomalacia bone lesions and can be swapped to cholecalciferol after 3 months. The majority of 25-OHD replenishment, however, should be from UV on exposed skin surfaces.

- Vitamin B12 may be supplemented by 3-monthly injections and folic acid by 5 mg daily.
- Creon can be prescribed for patients with exocrine pancreatic insufficiency (e.g. Sjögren's).
- In severe cases of malabsorption, parenteral nutrition is required.

Bacterial over-growth
Low dose oral antibiotics (quinolone, tetracycline, β-lactam) should be cycled with antibiotic free periods between to limit the development of resistant organisms
- Low dose octreotide can stimulate restoration of the migrating motor complex in SSc.
- There is no evidence for benefit of probiotic use in bacterial over-growth.

Pseudo-obstruction
Check and normalize electrolytes, rest bowel (patient nil by mouth), support with IV normal saline/5% dextrose, with appropriate potassium supplementation. A trial of 1–2 mg neostigmine if no contra-indications and with cardiac monitoring. Caecal decompression by percutaneous endoscopically placed colostomy tube or colectomy may be required.

Acute surgical abdomen
Obstruction, small bowel infarction, mesenteric arterial rupture, perforation, appendicitis, toxic megacolon, cholecystitis) – **EMERGENCY:** consult surgical team.
- Meanwhile, institute supportive measures (nil by mouth, IV fluids, IV opiate analgesia, and anti-emetic, IV hydrocortisone for patients treated with GCs (for low/moderate prednisolone doses, approximately double the daily GC dose for the perioperative period; TED stockings).
- Anticipate peritonitis (blood cultures, antibiotics to cover seeding of peritoneal cavity with gut bacteria), hypovolaemic or septic shock (colloid; cross-match blood), and urgent laparotomy (FBC, Cr and electrolytes, LFT, CRP, clotting, ECG, CXR).
- A diagnostic laparoscopy may clarify which patients can be managed expectantly and which require urgent laparotomy). The signs of peritonism may be masked by high dose GC use.

Mesenteric ischaemia
In the presence of vasculitis, this generally requires surgical resection of the involved segment but it may respond to medical treatment with immunosuppression with careful monitoring to pre-empt perforation.

Other conditions
- **Intussusception** may lead to obstruction. Liaise with surgical team.
- **Vasculitis:** treatment of the underlying condition with immunosuppression; see also p. 313.
- **Amyloid:** treatment of AA amyloid requires optimal management of the underlying inflammatory condition. Avoid biopsies of sites where bleeding is difficult to control.

Large intestine
- **Colitis** responds to standard treatment with immunosuppressant medications, such as 5ASA derivatives, GCs, azathioprine, methotrexate, anti-TNFα agents, with additional biological therapy in reserve for severe cases (Rituximab, Campath).

- **Acute surgical abdomen:** appendicitis, toxic megacolon; see above.
- **Constipation** can be troublesome in dysmotility conditions not complicated by bacterial over-growth and malabsorption, and may require a combination of bulk forming and stimulant laxative agents.
- **Diarrhoea** due to dysmotility may be controlled with use of loperamide, as required.
- **Megacolon and giant diverticulae** may require surgical resection.
- **Mucosal telangectasiae:** bleeding point may be treated colonoscopically using argon beam electrocautery.
- **Perineal ulcers:** prescribe topical GCs (e.g. triamcinolone paste applied 2–4 times daily) for short courses). Colchicine and anti-TNFα agents may be useful in Behçet's disease.
- **A defunctioning stoma** may be required for severe perianal disease in Behçet's disease or for faecal incontinence in SSc.

Liver/pancreas/gallbladder
Hepatitis
Consider drugs (including herbal remedies or non-prescription drugs) that could be causing the problem and stop where possible. Treatment with GCs and immunosuppressants may be required for auto-immune features. Note that immunosuppressants, for which transaminitis is an adverse effect (e.g. methotrexate, azathioprine, mycophenoloate mofetil), often result in improvement of LFTs when used to treat autoimmune hepatitis. Close monitoring is required.

Primary biliary cirrhosis
Ursodeoxycholic acid should be prescribed at 13-15 mg/kg/day in 2–4 divided doses for patients with anti-mitochondrial antibodies and a cholestatic pattern of abnormal LFTs. methotrexate, azathioprine, ciclosporin A, and colchicine have all been used to treat PBC, but meta-analyses fail to show efficacy.

Exocrine pancreatic insufficiency
Look for reversible causes (rarely autoimmune pancreatitis) and replace with oral pancreatic enzyme replacement (100 000–200 000 lipase units per day, taken with meals, e.g. creon). Bioavailability improved by use of PPI.

Pancreatitis
Can present as a surgical emergency. Assess severity using Glasgow score and early CT (Balthazar score). Involve specialist team (gastroenterology or surgery).
- Nil by mouth, fluid resuscitation and supportive care for organ dysfunction in the first instance).

Table 3.11 Glasgow Scoring system (severe acute pancreatitis defined by score of 3 or more)

Age	>55 years
WBC	$>15 - 10^9/l$
Glucose	>10 mmol/l
LDH	>600 IU/ml
Urea	>16 mmol/l
Albumin	<32
Calcium (corrected)	<2.00 mmol/l
PO_2	<8 kPa

Other conditions
- **Haemochromatosis:** weekly venesection to maintain ferritin <50 μg/l. Cirrhosis is irreversible.
- **Wilson's disease:** lifelong treatment with penicillamine 1–1.5 g daily; monitor urinary copper; liaise with hepatologist.
- **Cholecystitis:** may require acute cholecystectomy or choecystotomy, and drainage in unwell individuals (see Acute surgical abdomen above).

Resources
Assessment tools
IBD scoring tools should not be used in enterocolitis associated with proven vasculitides as they are not validated in this setting and may be misleading.
- PBC – LFTs generally adequate; Mayo risk score available online: www.mayoclinic.org/gi-rst/maymodel1.html;

Patient organizations
Behçet's Syndrome Society. www.behcets.org.uk
Coeliac UK. http://www.coeliac.co.uk/
National Association for Colitis and Crohn's Disease (NACC). www.nacc.org.uk/content/home.asp

See also:
Spondylarthritis	p. 209
Vasculitis	p. 313
Drugs used in rheumatology	p. 529
SSc	p. 264
Sjögren's syndrome	p. 254

Further reading
Ebert EC. Gastric and enteric involvement in progressive systemic sclerosis. *J Clin Gastroenterol.* 2008; **42**: 5–12.

Gaston JSH. Cytokines in arthritis – the 'big numbers' take centre stage. *Rheumatology* 2008; **47**: 8–12.

Gershwin ME, Mackay IR. The causes of primary biliary cirrhosis: convenient and inconvenient truths. *Hepatology* 2008; **47**: 737–45.

Lindor K. Ursodeoxycholic acid for the treatment of primary biliary cirrhosis. *NEJM* 2007; **357**: 1524–9.

Mody GM, Cassim B. Rheumatologic manifestations of gastrointestinal disorders. *Curr Opin Rheumatol* 1998; **10**: 67–72.

Morgan SL, Baggott JE, et al. Supplementation with folic acid during methotrexate therapy for rheumatoid arthritis. A double-blind, placebo-controlled trial. *Ann Intern Med* 1994; **121**: 833–41.

Nikou GC, Toumpanakis C, et al. Treatment of small intestinal disease in systemic sclerosis with octreotide: a prospective study in seven patients. *J Clin Rheumatol* 2007; **13**: 119–23.

Pagnoux C, Mahr A, et al. Presentation and outcome of gastrointestinal involvement in systemic necrotizing vasculitides: analysis of 62 patients with polyarteritis nodosa, microscopic polyangiitis, Wegener's granulomatosis, Churg–Strauss syndrome, or rheumatoid arthritis-associated vasculitis. *Medicine* 2005; **84**: 115–28.

Schneider T, Moos V, et al. Whipple's disease: new aspects of pathogenesis and treatment. *Lancet Infect Dis* 2008; **8**: 179–90.

Silverstein SB, Rodgers GM. Parenteral Iron Therapy Options. *Am J Hematol* 2004; **76**: 74–8.

Swinkels DW, Jorna AT, Raymakers RA. Synopsis of the Dutch multidisciplinary guideline for the diagnosis and treatment of hereditary haemochromatosis. *Neth J Med* 2007; **65**: 452–5.

Twilt M, Schulten AJ, et al. Long-term follow-up of temporomandibular joint involvement in juvenile idiopathic arthritis. *Arthritis Rheum.* 2008; **59**: 546–52.

Viljammaa M, Kaukinen K, et al. Coeliac disease, autoimmune diseases and gluten exposure. *Scand J Gastroenterol* 2005; **40**: 437–43.

Yazici H, Fresko I, Yurdakul S. Behçet's syndrome: disease manifestations, management, and advances in treatment. *Nat Clin Pract Rheumatol.* 2007; **3**: 148–55.

Yurdakul S, Mat C, et al. A double-blind trial of colchicine in Behçet's syndrome. *Arthritis Rheum* 2001; **44**: 2686–92.

The nervous system

Neurological symptoms occur frequently in outpatient and inpatient rheumatology consultation, with direct consequences of rheumatological disease, such as cervical cord compression in rheumatoid arthritis (RA), nervous system involvement in multisystem disease, and neurological mimics of rheumatological disease, such as early Parkinson's disease or motor neurone disease. The immune system is a key player in both fields and there may be coincidental neuroimmunological and rheumatological disease. Immunosuppressive and other therapies carry with them neurological side effects, and similarly therapies for neurological disorders may occasionally cause side effects that enter the rheumatologist's area. New biological therapies have brought about rapid change.

Risk factors for nervous system involvement

- Smoking.
- Hypertension.
- Hyperlipidaemia.
- Immunosuppression (infection, cancer).
- Anti-phospholipid antibodies.
- Co-existent bone and joint disease.
- Psychiatric co-morbidity and social factors.

Aetiology/pathophysiology: general issues

The large genome wide association studies have increased our knowledge of the molecular mechanisms and pathways behind rheumatological and neuro-immunological disease, and at the current rate new genes are appearing every few months. Functional studies of these genes, mainly in animal models, are starting to ascertain their role in disease. The innate immune system (apoptosis and its clearance, toll-like-receptor activation) has resurfaced as a key component of pathogenesis.

Novel antibodies directed towards cell-surface antigens are being identified and are refining characterization and classification of disease, e.g. the AQ4 target in *Neuromyelitis optica* and Sjögren's myelopathy is a water channel, the regional distribution of disease remains unclear. Voltage-gated potassium channel (VGKC) and *N*-methyl-D-aspartate receptor (NMDA) receptors are important for basic neuronal function and synaptic plasticity. Antibodies directed towards intracellular epitopes may still be pathogenic, if found to cross react with extracellular antigens, e.g. a recent finding has found that ribosomal P antibodies in lupus can recognize a novel neuronal surface antigen.

Gene expression assays on lymphocytes are demonstrating new 'signatures' of disease activity that again may reclassify these disorders in the future and allow tailored drug therapy. It is clear that T cells are also involved in driving inflammation in neurological tissue. Demyelination in multiple sclerosis may be driven predominantly by a recently-defined subset of CD4+ IL-17 secreting T cells (Th17), rather than the Th1 subset. The relevance of these cells in terms of importance in CNS rheumatological involvement, available biomarkers, and alternative therapies is unclear. The biology of B and T cell interaction, memory and regulatory cell 'sub-specialization', and hormonal and epigenetic modification of tolerance, is a fertile research ground.

Cytokines from a wide range of immune cells are important in pathogenesis and therapy; for example, tissues from patients with SLE or Sjögren's exhibit an expression signature reflecting excessive IFNα production and IFNα therapy for melanoma or hepatitis C reliably causes a 'cognitive/depressive lupus syndrome'. Trials of anti-cytokine therapy, notably IL-6 and B cell activating factor are also underway. The cause of anti-TNFα therapy induced demyelination remains purely speculative (non-reduction of CNS TNF and/or increased peripheral T cell reactivity).

History: the approach

The history from the patient and, in most cases, a companion will give the most accurate clues to aetiology, whereas the clinical examination will reveal location(s) of involvement only. Thus, 'a telephone call is more useful than a tendon hammer' (John Garfield). The interrogation of the 'funny turn' in particular requires aggressive cross-examination. Discard terms such as 'stroke' or 'migraine' given by the patient, unless with solid evidence, and attempt to obtain an unbiased, objective temporal description of events. The tempo of symptom onset often provides the most useful part of the history, e.g. sudden (thunderclap), creeping over days to weeks, step-wise, static. Infections involving the nervous system are over represented in immunosuppressed rheumatology patients, and often require sensitive social- and sexual-history taking, as do the possibilities of drug abuse.

Specific aspects of the history should cover the pattern of weakness, headache syndrome, bladder/bowel/sexual function – a new change should ring alarm bells for cord compression or cauda equina syndrome, and are emergencies. Impotence is an early sign of autonomic failure, whereas failure of ejaculation points to the cord. Enquire about hallucinations – visual or olfactory (often indicating organic brain disease); auditory or tactile, psychotic symptoms, depressive symptoms, attention and memory encoding vs retrieval (ask 'what is the worst thing that has happened to you as a result of your poor memory?'), and endocrine factors such as menstruation, shaving, and libido. Screen for sleep disturbance and excessive daytime somnolence, consider sleep apnoea.

'Funny turns'
A witness account is mandatory. Focal and generalized seizures are more prevalent in rheumatological disorders, in particular lupus. A full cardiovascular history is needed including posture during attacks (events lying down in a young person can suggest serious a cardiac cause such as Wolff–Parkinson–White). Medicolegally, such a loaded diagnostic label as epilepsy often requires a neurologist, particularly in the young.

Headaches and facial pain
New headaches require full investigation. Facial pain is best divided into that accompanied by cranial nerve symptoms and signs (a painful opthalmoplegia is often inflammatory), neuralgias (lancinating), trigeminal autonomic cephalalgias, and pure facial pain (sinus/masticatory) – this narrows down a wide list of diagnostic possibilities, for which imaging is generally mandatory.

Neuropathic pain
Mononeuropathies and polyneuropathis can cause peripheral neuropathic pain. Spinal root/dorsal root ganglion, spinal cord, brainstem, thalamus, subcortical and cortical lesions can cause central neuropathic pain. A painful mononeuropathy suggests vasculitis. This symptom deserves full

CHAPTER 3 Organ involvement in rheumatological disease

investigation for a cause, and differentiation from joint pain, osteomyelitis, and complex regional pain syndromes.

Examination: key points

The rheumatologist often has a difficult task due to the patient's frequent co-existing joint disease and pain. The key is to localize the lesion(s) having formulated a prediction to test on the basis of the history. One should ask if the 'hard' signs are sufficient to generate a reasonable explanation and invoke 'soft' signs only towards the end. Involve neurology or neurosurgery teams early if there is doubt. Given the age of the patient, are two separate pathologies likely, or will a unifying cause be most likely? A full systems examination is necessary. Fundoscopy (raised intracranial pressure- tumour; thrombosis; emboli), autonomic assessment (history of erectile failure, postural BP, pupils, referral for tilt testing) and cognitive testing are a physician's most common blind spots. Pattern of weakness, and exaggerated or lost reflexes and sensory signs can distinguish cervical myelopathy from root compression, cauda equina from conus medullaris, and L5 root compression from peroneal nerve palsy, but often investigation will be necessary.

A mini-mental state examination (MMSE) should be performed with any patient who complains (or more likely their companion) of subjective 'memory problems' (a catch-all lay term). A patient who cannot attend (spell WORLD backwards easily, subtract 7 serially from 100, encode an address) will not be able to remember information, but may have intact memory processes. The patient's pre-morbid best cognitive function should be taken to account, as well as a collateral history of rate of decline. Formal neuropsychology or neurological referral is the next step. Functional overlay (non-organic manifestations) must be assumed an elaboration of true organic disease until proved otherwise.

Principles of investigation

Specialist tests should be sought to confirm the examination or where joint deformity precludes accurate examination, but also to rule out important differential diagnoses, e.g. infection and cancer (such as lymphoma), hypertensive encephalopathy, pre-eclampsia, treatable metabolic conditions (e.g. Wilson's disease), and treatable surgical conditions (e.g. normal pressure hydrocephalus, disc disease, abscess). Special investigations should affect management:

Infection

Infective mimics are of the greatest concern in this patient group, many of whom have a dysregulated immune system or are immunosuppressed. Progressive multifocal leukoencephalopathy (PML) and nocardial infection are over-represented in rheumatology patients. For instance, does the patient with valve vegetation, antiphospholipid antibodies, and lupus markers, and microthrombi in the retina and CNS have infective endocarditis or Libman Sacks endocarditis? Does the patient with Wegener's treated with cyclophosphamide, who develops headaches and meningeal enhancement on MR, have meningeal granulomata or bacterial meningitis? MR imaging, blood cultures, laboratory markers, spinal fluid analysis and tissue biopsy – should be vigorously pursued. [See algorithm by Weiner (Warnartz 2003)].

Laboratory tests

The list is beyond the scope of this chapter. Metabolic tests (copper studies in the young with movement abnormalities), endocrine, HIV and hepatitis, cryoglobulins, thrombophilia screen, coeliac antibodies are particularly salient. New serum antibodies (it is helpful to send CSF also and store baseline samples for future available tests in grey cases) include those against the 'cell surface antigens' – a growing list, best directed by phenotype – only those that currently change management (e.g. none for lupus) are listed:

- Anti-aquaporin 4 (AQ4; 'Nmo-Ig' refers to the immunohistochemical pattern of binding) for cord and optic nerve inflammation (neuromyelitis optica or Devic's disease), e.g. longitudinally extensive transverse myelitis (LETM) – in Sjögren's and lupus.
- Anti-VGKC for encephalitis, seizures, amnesia, psychosis often with hyponatraemia (exclude viral encephalitis).
- Anti-nicotinic AChR or voltage gated P/Q type calcium channel (AChR – *Myasthenia gravis*; VGCC – Lambert Eaton myasthenia, often associated with small cell lung cancer) for fatiguable weakness.
- Anti-NMDA for subacute seizures, psychosis, encephalitis, encephalopathy, often associated with teratomata (usually ovary; exclude viral encephalitis). Other paraneoplastic encephalitides are more common: breast, germline testis, small cell lung.
- Anti-basal ganglia antibodies and anti-streptolysin O titre (ASOT) for movement disorder after streptococcal infection [exclude antiphospholipid (APL) antibodies].

Imaging

- MR spine imaging. For cord compression or cauda equina an urgent neurosurgical opinion should be obtained immediately – surgery before 48 h gives the best chance for preservation of sphincter function. MR spine (± biopsy) is also indicated for suspected disc herniation or spinal inflammation, tumours, discitis, and infective endocarditis.
- MR venography (MRV; Figure 3.13) is useful in the investigation of venous thrombosis, idiopathic intracranial hypertension (no longer called 'benign' IH, given visual loss may be permanent).
- MR angiography (MRA) can provide useful clues without the requisite for formal angiography, e.g. vertebral artery dissection.

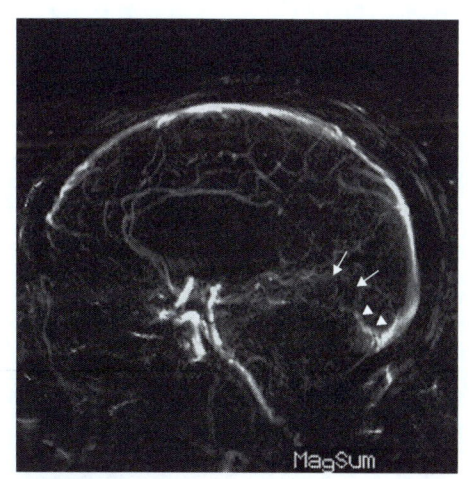

Figure 3.13 Straight sinus thrombosis (phase contrast MRV). Reproduced from the Oxford Handbook of Neurology, Manji et al, 2006, with permission from Oxford University Press.

- Diffusion weighted MR allows abnormalities in water diffusion to be picked up – represents neuronal swelling – used in standard clinical practice to detect early ischaemia or infarct. New or progressive cognitive impairment without focal neurology or acute symptoms may be due to multiple small infarcts and emboli, which should be considered along with infective endocarditis in such patients.
- [18]FDG-PET can be useful in diagnosing and monitoring both GCA and Takayasu's arteritis.
- Diffusion tensor (tractography), MR spectroscopy and functional MR are still chiefly research tools.

Cerebrospinal fluid
Check safe to lumbar puncture (LP) with CT brain if urgent. Measure:
- **Opening pressure.**
- **Microbiology:** gram stain, cell count, culture and sensitivity, including prolonged culture for *Nocardia*, Zielh-Nielson stain and *Mycobacterium tuberculosis* (MTB) culture; PCR for and immunoglobulin against HSV, EBV, VZV, CMV, enterovirus. India Ink stain for *Cryptococcus*. Serology against *Listeria*, *Aspergillus*, *Candida*, *Enterobacteriae*, *Pneumocystis jiroveci*, *Cocciodes*, and HTLV-1 antigens.
- **Biochemistry:** protein, glucose (with paired blood glucose), LDH, ACE.
- **Immunology:** anti-neuronal antibodies (paired serum), oligoclonal bands (paired serum).
- **Cytology:** LP may need to be repeated several times. Includes lymphocyte phenotype.

EEG, video telemetry, electromyography, nerve conduction tests
- **EEG:** establishes encephalopathy, supporting, but not excluding a diagnosis of epilepsy, identifies non-convulsive status epilepticus in coma.
- **EMG:** distinguishes muscle and nerve involvement.
- **NCS:** distinguishes axon vs myelin damage, small vs large fibre and localizing nerve damage.

Visual perimetry and opthalmological assessment
Request for suspected retinal vasculitis, optic neuropathy, endocarditis, CMV retinitis, temporal arteritis (age and ESR>50, abnormalities of the temporal artery on examination and histology; sometimes third nerve palsy) and idiopathic intracranial hypertension (sometimes associated with sixth nerve palsy).

Histopathology
Combined nerve and muscle biopsy provides a greater yield than nerve alone. Skin biopsy is useful in assessing an isolated sensory neuropathy by measurement of intraepidermal nerve fibre density. Biopsy of non-dominant frontal lobe or obvious peripheral lesion in the brain/meninges should be ideally obtained in the workup of possible vasculitis or atypical infection – ask how secure is the diagnosis otherwise?

Miscellaneous
CXR, transthoracic, and transoesophageal echocardiography, tilt testing in an autonomic work up, cardiac CT or MR, 24h ECG, 12-lead ECG for Wolff–Parkinson–White. Carotid ultrasound. Chest-abdomen-pelvis CT, [18]FDG-PET and pelvic and testicular ultrasound in the search for occult malignancy. Sleep studies for obstructive sleep apnoea.

- Cerebral autosomal dominant arteriopathy with subcortical infarcts (CADASIL for NOTCH3 gene) is a differential of MS, APLS, CVAs.

Neurological diagnoses to consider on seeing 'a new patient' in rheumatology

A list of questions to cover blind-spots and an open mind are all that are required to prompt recognition.
- Parkinson's disease can present with stiffness and rigidity, as can the rarer Stiff–Person syndrome (mainly in para-axial muscles – confirm with neurophysiology, check anti-GAD65 antibodies).
- Multiple sclerosis may have an MR scan like antiphospholipid syndrome, and patients may have positive ANA or a transient positive anti-cardiolipin. There is no histopathological report of demyelination in lupus or APLS, but the cases reported as 'lupoid sclerosis' in the early 1970s had false positive syphilis serology, i.e. were probable APLS.
- Restless legs syndrome constitutes a predominantly nocturnal urge to move the legs accompanied or caused by uncomfortable and unpleasant sensations in the legs, relieved by movement. It is seen in 5–10% of the older population, but with greater prevalence in RA, Sjögren's, scleroderma, and fibromyalgia in particular.
- CNS stimulant medication [methylphenidate (Ritalin), and dextroamphetamine] may cause Raynaud's phenomenon and livedo reticularis.

Neurological manifestations of rheumatological diseases

A variety of central and peripheral neurological complications are associated with AICTD and vasculitides (Table 3.12) and drugs used to treat rheumatological conditions are also associated with neurological adverse effects (Table 3.13).

Rheumatoid arthritis (RA)
Cervical myelopathy can present acutely or subacutely. Neuropathy is rare and usually due to entrapment or drugs. A 'pachymeningitis' is rare, usually occurs in long standing disease (high RF) – consider with new headaches, cranial nerve palsies.

Ankylosing spondylitis
Spondylodiscitis including fracture may present with a sudden increase in back pain. A neurosurgical opinion is required as repair may be warranted. Cauda equina may occur insidiously and is less amenable to repair.

Systemic lupus erythematosus (SLE)
Lupus may cause diverse neurological features:
- Psychosis.
- Seizures.
- Encephalopathy.
- Depression.
- Myelitis
- Cognitive impairment (APL antibodies conferring the greatest risk)
- Movement disorder, peripheral nerve disorder, associated *Myasthenia gravis*.

However, attribution to lupus of non-specific neurological symptoms, in particular headache, remains controversial. Structural MR imaging is often normal. CSF lymphocytosis is predictive of a poor prognosis. Test for anti-AQ4 in myelitis.

CHAPTER 3 Organ involvement in rheumatological disease

Antiphospholipid syndrome (APLS)
Stroke predisposition. Sustained elevation of antiphospholipid antibodies, and venous or arterial thrombosis constitute the syndrome; improving imaging studies reveal microthrombi previously missed – diffusion weighted and structural MRI is sufficient in the clinic and ward setting.

Systemic sclerosis
Peripheral neuropathy including autonomic and, in particular, painful trigeminal neuropathy predominates.

Sjögren's syndrome
Sensory polyneuropathy and polyganglionopathy are the most common manifestations, and in the majority of cases precedes the development of sicca symptoms and diagnosis of SS. Use of tricyclics (which dry the mouth), hepatitis C, human T-lymphocyte virus type 1, HIV, and lymphoma must be excluded. It is becoming clear that the severe myelopathy seen occasionally in patients is due to neuromyelitis optica and, hence, antibodies to aquaporin-4 should be tested. Other CNS involvement is rare.

Dermatomyositis, polymyositis and inclusion body myositis (IBM)
IBM is the commonest and least understood. It is characterized by a slow steady progression. CK (lower levels seen in IBM), EMG, and muscle biopsy are the mainstay of investigation.

Sarcoidosis
Cranial neuropathy VII and II are most common. Patients may have episodic meningeal symptoms and chronic m eningitis. Psychosis, epilepsy, neuropathy, and myopathy are recognized. CSF examination, imaging (contrast-enhanced MR essential) and biopsy are the key investigations. Endocrinology collaboration to investigate hypothalamic and pituitary involvement may often helpful.

Takayasu arteritis
Carotid artery stenosis and subclavian steal syndrome are seen secondary to vessel occlusion. Arch angiography and ^{18}FDG-PET are useful in investigation.

Giant cell arteritis
Optic neuropathy and third nerve palsy. All patients require ophthalmological assessment.

Behçet's disease
Vascular-related parenchymal involvement and thrombosis. In the Turkish Neuro-Behçet study group's experience (155 male, 45 females) brainstem involvement occurred in 51% — a common first presentation), followed by cord (14%), then hemisphere. The UK experience is similar. A lymphocytic CSF predicts a recurrent clinical course. Dural sinus thrombosis is also common and hard to diagnose unless specifically considered (raised CSF opening pressure, acellular, MR venography). Peripheral neuropathy is rare, more commonly due to thalidomide therapy.

Primary angiitis of the CNS (PACNS) and benign angiopathy of the CNS
These are rare, and symptoms can reflect focal ischaemia in any part of the brain anatomy. Angiography (beading, segmental narrowing) and a tissue diagnosis should be pursued in combination.

Relapsing polychondritis
A limbic encephalitis has been reported; exclude HSV encephalitis, check anti-VGKC antibodies.

Table 3.12 Anatomical classification of nervous system involvement in rheumatological disease

	Meninges	Brain	Brainstem	Cranial erve	Cord	Root	Nerve	NMJ	Muscle	Thrombosis
Rheumatoid arthritis		•	•		•	••		•		
Ankylosing spondylitis					•					
SLE	•	••	•	•	•	•	•	•		
APLS		••	•		•					••
Systemic sclerosis				•			•			
Sjögren's syndrome					•		•			
DM, PM, IBM									••	
Takayasu arteritis		•	•							•
GCA		•		•						
Wegener's granulomatosis		•		•			••			•
Churg–Strauss, MPA, PAN							••			
Behçet's disease		•	••		•					••
1° angiitis CNS		•	•							
Sarcoidosis	•	•	••	••			•	•		
Relapsing polychondritis	•	•								

•• More common; • less common

Abbreviations: APLS, antiphospholipid syndrome; CNS, central nervous system; IBM, inclusion body myositis; GCA, giant cell or temporal arteritis; DM, dermatomyositis; MPA, microscopic polyangiitis; PAN, polyarteriitis nodosa; PM, polymyositis; SLE, systemic lupus erythematosus.

Table 3.13 Neurological side-effects of drugs used for rheumatological disorders

Side-effect	Drugs
Aseptic meningitis	NSAIDS, trimethoprim, IVIG
Idiopathic intracranial hypertension (IIH)	Glucocorticoids (GCs), especially on withdrawal in children, danazol.
PML	Rituximab (rare reports, FDA warning 2006)
Demyelination	Anti-TNFα
Seizures	Allopurinol (including withdrawal), chlorambucil, cimetidine, ciclosporin, NSAIDs, methotrexate
Headache	NSAIDs, especially at the start of treatment, notably indomethacin, ketoprofen, diclofenac; dipyridamole, ciclosporin, tacrolimus
Psychosis, personality change	Chloroquine, opiates, indomethacin, GCs
Delirium, encephalopathy	Cimetidine and chloroquine, methotrexate
Mania	GCs, ciclosporin
Hallucinations	Ciclosporin
Depression	NSAIDs, GCs, methotrexate, ciclosporin, interferon-α.
Dizziness	NSAIDs, cetirizine
Parkinsonism	Metoclopramide, prochlorperazine, chloroquine, cinnarizine, neuroleptics (particularly if combined with antidepressants), lithium, cyanide, carbon monoxide, other toxins.
Chorea	Cimetidine, metoclopramide, levodopa
Tremor	Cimetidine, ciclosporin, indomethacin, GCs, valproate, caffeine, levothyroxine, bronchodilators
Optic neuropathy	Ibuprofen, indomethacin, D-penicillamine, anti-TNFα, amiodarone, isoniazid, ciclosporin
Ototoxicity	Chloroquine, NSAIDs, salicylates, aminoglycoside antibiotics, furosemide, chemotherapy agents
Dysgeusia	Allopurinol, azathioprine, D-penicillamine, gold salts, salicylates
Muscle cramps	Cimetidine, gold salts, D-penicillamine, statins
Myasthenia	D-penicillamine: chloroquine unmasks myasthenia
Myopathies	Cimetidine, chloroquine (painful), colchicine, steroids (chronic, painless), lovastatin
Myositis	D-penicillamine (painful), zidovudine (AZT). Rhabdomyolysis rarely with statins.
Peripheral neuropathy	Chloroquine, colchicine, gold salts, D-penicillamine, chlorambucil, anti-TNFα, thalidomide, leflunomide, nitrofurantoin, metronidazole, NSAIDs, cimetidine, dapsone, amiodarone

Adapted from 1.3.3 Neurological complications, Ferguson & Hollingworth (2004). Many drugs can affect the levels of immunosuppressive drugs, in particular, ciclosporin and tacrolimus, for which trough levels can be checked. Anti fungal drugs, trimethoprim, erythromycin and the oral contraceptive device are the most common. The following table should not be considered complete, nor an indication that the drug will turn out to be the cause of the symptoms.

Abbreviations: AZT, zidovudine; FDA, US Food and Drug Administration; IVIG, intravenous immunoglobulin G; NSAID, non-steroidal anti-inflammatory drug; PML, progressive multifocal leukoencephalopathy; TNF, tumour necrosis factor.

ANCA-associated vasculitis (AAV) including Wegener's granulomatosis (WG)

Swanson's study of 324 consecutive patients with WG revealed 109 (34%) with neurological involvement: mainly peripheral (mononeuritis multiplex) or cranial neuropathy. CNS involvement was less common.

- There are three patterns: vasculitic, meningeal due to adjacent granulomatous disease, and isolated granulomata in the parenchyma or meninges. Stroke, seizures, and retro-orbital granuloma may be seen.
- Exclude hepatitis B and C.
- In PAN and CSS an epineurial necrotizing vasculitis is seen histologically in >50% cases of neuropathy, often a painful mononeuritis multiplex.
- Vasculitis is the rarest cause of peripheral neuropathy in RA (consider drugs and overlap AICTD).

Treatment

New biological therapies offer hope of true disease modification prior to damage accumulation. Neurosurgeons should be involved early in cases of compressive myelopathy or neuropathy.

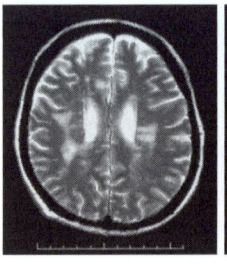

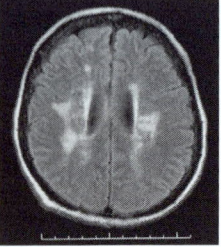

Figure 3.14 (A) A 59-year-old woman with Behcet's syndrome and a spastic paraparesis who developed worsening leg weakness 2 weeks after starting Infliximab (3 mg/kg) T2 (left) and T1-weighted MR images. Reproduced from Zandi and Coles 2007, Notes on the Kidney and its Diseases for the Neurologist, with permission from the BMJ Publishing Group Ltd.

CHAPTER 3 Organ involvement in rheumatological disease

Systemic lupus erythematosus
There is RCT evidence that cyclophosphamide is effective for severe CNS disease. Otherwise pulse methylprednisolone, IVIG, or plasma exchange may give modest effect. rituximab shows the greatest promise in open-label studies, but awaits definitive trial, and mycophenylate is under evaluation.

Antiphospholipid syndrome (APLS) and stroke
The evidence for APLS suggests prolonged warfarin therapy at a target INR of 2.0–3.0 in definite APLS patients with first venous events (including cerebral venous sinus thrombosis), >3.0 if recurrent or arterial events (cerebral infarct). Patients with isolated positive APL antibodies and stroke should be treated as for stroke (see below) unless the antibody persists.

Sjögren's syndrome (see also p. 254)
Unclear. Myelopathy should be treated aggressively (in particular if anti-AQ4 positive) – plasma exchange in the first instance, then long-term azathioprine or mycophenylate, rituximab if refractory.

Dermatomyositis (DM), polymyositis (PM), IBM
The NIH approach for DM and PM is high dose initial GCs (80–100 mg/day for 1 month, halved over 10 weeks to an alternate day regime, then consider high dose azathioprine (3 mg/kg – check TMPT activity, monitor lymphocytes), methotrexate, ciclosporin, or MMF. Therapy for IBM is difficult – add CoQ10 to steroids initially and an exercise programme. For severe disease try IVIG. T cell depletion, with alemtuzumab and anti-TNFα therapy is under evaluation.

Sarcoidosis
One approach is pulse methylprednisolone (1 g IV for 3 days) followed by 0.5–1 mg/kg prednisolone (with methotrexate as the best sparing agent and long-term hydroxychloroquine first line). Beyond cyclophosphamide, infliximab is showing promise. Monitor with imaging, not CSF (remains lymphocytic).

Takayasu's arteritis
Conventional bypass grafts for stenoses. GCs, azathioprine and mycophenylate are used; anti-TNFα therapy shows promise. Accelerated atherosclerosis needs management of conventional risk factors.

Giant cell arteritis.
High dose GCs with prednisolone 60 mg/day until normalization of ESR – may be 6 months to a year. Adjunctive aspirin 100 mg/day may reduce visual loss. 'Rescue' 3 days 1 g IV methylprednisolone, if there are symptoms or signs of visual loss.

Behçet's disease
Controversial. GCs and thalidomide (precautions) are used, with alemtuzumab (Campath-1H) reserved for resistant cases. Venous sinus thrombosis is usually treated with GCs and anticoagulation (heparin then short-term warfarin – duration controversial).

ANCA-associated vasculitides (see p. 330–331)
Heavy induction immunosuppression followed by a maintenance phase. The current best appears to still be initial high dose prednisolone and cyclophosphamide, followed by azathioprine if tolerated.

RA, relapsing polychondritis, systemic sclerosis (SSc)
Extrapolation of extra-nervous system current best treatment suggests that high dose GCs, cyclophosphamide, steroid sparing agents, or appropriate biological therapy may be tried with caution.

Stroke
Stroke deserves a special mention given the high incidence in rheumatological patients, who as a group suffer from accelerated atherosclerosis.
- Primary prevention by aggressive control of hypertension and serum lipids.
- Acute thrombolysis within 3 h of symptom onset with rt-plasminogen activator.
- Stroke units reduce risk of death or dependency in themselves. Neurorehabilitation is disappointingly underfunded and may require a proactive search.
- Anticoagulation for cerebral venous sinus thrombosis with low molecular weight heparin, followed by warfarin (duration controversial).
- Antiplatelet therapy (low dose aspirin and dipyridamole – currently in trials against clopidogrel) – should be given immediately unless contra-indicated. The risks of bleeding must be taken into account in a patient taking NSAIDs.
- Anticoagulation for pre-existing atrial fibrillation and changes to hypertension control generally delayed by 2 weeks – discuss with a specialist. Consider cardioversion in liaison with cardiology.
- Carotid endarterectomy for symptomatic carotid stenosis has most benefit if done early (weeks after symptoms), and for older patients.

Bacterial meningitis
Broad spectrum antibiotics should be administered immediately before LP- benzylpenicillin 2.4 g 4-hourly if not allergic and there is a typical meningococcal rash, cefotaxime 2 g 6-hourly if not. Add vancomycin for suspected S. pneumoniae until sensitivities known and ampicillin 2 g 4-hourly to cover Listeria. If possible, without causing delay, take blood cultures before the first dose. CT before LP to exclude mass effect and look for sufficient CSF space around the brainstem. Give dexamethasone with antibiotics, 10 mg 6-hourly IV for 4 days (first dose with first antibiotic dose), as it has been shown to be beneficial and safe even in areas endemic for MTB.

Encephalitis
Intravenous high dose acyclovir for presumed herpes simplex virus until CSF PCR known to be negative. Consider autoimmune or paraneoplastic encephalitis (send serum and CSF anti-VGKC, anti-NMDAR antibodies, screen for malignancy – small cell lung, germline testis, breast, teratoma).

Headaches and facial pain
Medication overuse headaches are very common and disabling, and can worsen on cessation of the drug, e.g. opiate. Migraine is best treated with a drug to terminate the acute event such as an NSAID, domperidone, or a triptan. Do not treat during aura, or if hemiplegic migraine or any cardio/cerebrovascular disease – consider screening for a patent foramen ovale. If frequent and disabling, a regular night prophylactic agent, such as a β-blocker or tricyclic may be used. Chronic daily headache, tension-type headaches, trigeminal-autonomic cephalalgias may respond idiosyncratically to treatment. Trigeminal neuralgia responds often dramatically to carbamazepine.

Neuropathic pain

Local measures, nerve blocks, epidural injections, transcutaneous electrical nerve stimulation (TENS), cognitive coping strategies, and drugs all have their role. The best drugs are gabapentin, amitryptilline, pregabalin, venlafaxine, carbamazepine, and opiates. Specialist advice is best sought if no progress is made.

Excessive daytime somnolence

Modafenil is useful for truly excessive somnolence (but has cardiovascular and psychiatric side effects).

Restless legs syndrome

Dopamine agonists are the treatment of choice, but require a documented discussion as to the real side effects of impulsive behaviour and gambling in particular and avoided if the patient feels susceptible. Valproate or gabapentin show effect – as a second choice.

Neurorehabilitation

A continence nurse should be involved early in cases of sphincter disturbance with or without cord damage. Intermittent self-catheterization may be required if there is urinary residual or frequent infection. Consider referral to podiatry. Baclofen pumps should be initiated by a specialist centre. It is common sense and increasingly demonstrated in the literature, that keeping an active mind increases ability to function into old age. Exercises to increase 'cognitive reserve' include puzzles, voluntary work, engaging socially.

Psychiatric co-morbidity and psychological therapy

Pain, fatigue and stiffness are common. Cognitive behavioural therapy, if available should be preferred to or added to pharmacological therapy.

Prognosis/natural history

CNS disease in particular is associated with a marked raised mortality, morbidity, and reduction in quality of life. A key message is that baseline CSF and histology secures a diagnosis, and often provides prognostic indicators prior to embarking on new path of therapy.

Monitoring disease activity

Serial clinical assessment, immune parameters (complement, antibodies), MR, and electrophysiology are standard. Serial angiography and CSF is used in primary angiitis of the CNS, but both are of no use in other conditions. There is much research into predictors of flare after biological therapy, e.g. flow cytometric detection of return of B cells after rituximab, serum B lymphocyte stimulator levels.

Other issues

Medicolegal pitfalls

Commonly, failure to recognize treatable conditions that will otherwise result in permanent disability or death, or iatrogenic effects of treatment: life threatening arrhythmia presenting with 'funny turns', nerve entrapment, cord compression, cauda equina, conus medullaris, cerebral venous thrombosis, meningitis in the immunocompromised patient, drug toxicity, Wilson's disease, failure to ascertain suicide risk, and failure to secure a diagnosis before heavy immunosuppression.

Driving

Depending on the type of vehicle driven, there are restrictions after transient ischaemic attack, stroke, fit, and any change of anti-epileptic medication. See the DVLA website for up-to-date guidance.

Resources

Patient information and Internet sites

Neuropsychiatric lupus case definitions. Available at: www.rheumatology.org/publications/ar/1999/aprilappendix.asp

British Hypertension Society. www.bhsoc.org

Stroke Association UK. www.stroke.org

Driving and Licensing authority (UK). www.dvla.gov.uk

Cochrane Neurological Network. www.cochraneneuronet.org

Trigeminal Neuralgia. www.tna-support.org

Neuro-rheumatological trials. http://clinicaltrials.gov/ct2/results?term=nervous+and+rheumatology

ICD10 codes

www.who.int/classifications/apps/icd/icd10online/

Further reading

Akman-Demir G, Serdaroglu P, Tasci B. Clinical patterns of neurological involvement in Behçet's disease: evaluation of 200 patients. The Neuro-Behcet Study Group. *Brain* 1999; **122**:2171–82.

Antel J, Birnbaum G, et al (eds). *Clinical Neuroimmunology*, 2nd edn. Oxford: Oxford University Press, 2005.

Barile-Fabris L, Ariza-Andraca R, et al. Controlled clinical trial of IV cyclophosphamide versus IV methylprednisolone in severe neurological manifestations in systemic lupus erythematosus. *Ann Rheum Dis.* 2005; **64**: 620–5.

Baughman RP, Winget DB, Lower EE. Methotrexate is steroid sparing in acute sarcoidosis: results of a double blind, randomized trial. *Sarcoidosis Vasc Diffuse Lung Dis* 2000; **17**: 60–6.

Bertsias G, Ioannidis JP, et al. EULAR recommendations for the management of systemic lupus erythematosus. Report of a Task Force of the EULAR Standing Committee for International Clinical Studies Including Therapeutics. *Ann Rheum Dis* 2008; **67**: 195–205.

Candalise L, Hughes R, et al. *Evidence-based Neurology*. Blackwell, Oxford, 2007.

Dalakas MC. Immune-mediated mechanisms in inflammatory myopathies. In: Antel J, Birnbaum G, Hartung HP, Vincent A (eds). *Clinical Neuroimmunology*, 2nd edn. Oxford: Oxford University Press, 2005.

Dalmau J, Rosenfeld MR. Paraneoplastic syndromes of the CNS. *Lancet Neurol* 2008; **7**: 327–40.

Drachman DA. Neurological complications of Wegener's granulomatosis. *Arch Neurol* 1963; **8**: 145–55.

Ferguson IT, Hollingworth P. Neurological complications. In: *Oxford Textbook of Rheumatology*, 3rd edn. Oxford: Oxford University Press, 2004.

Fujiki F, Tsuboi Y, Hashimoto K, et al. Non-herpetic limbic encephalitis associated with relapsing polychondritis. *J Neurol Neurosurg Psychiat* 2004; **75**: 1646–7.

Hankey GJ. Clinical update: management of stroke. *Lancet* 2007; **369**: 1330–2.

Hattori N, Ichimura M, Nagamatsu M, et al. Clinicopathological features of Churg–Strauss syndrome-associated neuropathy. *Brain* 1999; **122**: 427–39.

Kidd D, Steuer A, Denman AM, et al. Neurological complications in Behçet's syndrome. *Brain* 1999; **122**: 2183–94.

Kissel JT, Mendell JR. Vasculitic neuropathy. *Neurol Clin* 1992; **10**: 761–81.

Jayne D, Rasmussen N, Andrassy K, et al. A randomized trial of maintenance therapy for vasculitis associated with antineutrophil cytoplasmic autoantibodies. *N Engl J Med* 2003; **349**: 36–44.

Joseph FG, Lammie GA, Scolding NJ. CNS lupus: a study of 41 patients. *Neurology* 2007; **69**: 644–54.

Joseph FG, Scolding NJ. Sarcoidosis of the nervous system. *Pract Neurol* 2007; **7**; 234–44

Lockwood CM, Hale G, Waldman H, et al. Remission induction in Behçet's disease following lymphocyte depletion by the anti-CD52 antibody CAMPATH 1-H. *Rheumatol (Ox)* 2003; **42**: 1539–44.

Manji H, Connelly S, et al. *Oxford Handbook of Neurology*. Oxford University Press, Oxford, 2007.

Matus S, Burgos PV, Bravo-Zehnder M, et al. Antiribosomal-P autoantibodies from psychiatric lupus target a novel neuronal surface protein causing calcium influx and apoptosis. *J Exp Med* 2007; **204**: 3221–34

Mitsikostas DD, Sfikakis PP, Goadsby PJ. A meta-analysis for headache in systemic lupus erythematosus: the evidence and the myth. *Brain* 2004; **127**: 1200–9.

Mohan N, Edwards ET, Cupps TR, et al. Demyelination occurring during anti-tumor necrosis factor alpha therapy for inflammatory arthritides. *Arthritis Rheum* 2001; **44**: 2862–9.

Mori K, Iijima M, Koike H, et al. The wide spectrum of clinical manifestations in Sjogren's syndrome-associated neuropathy. *Brain* 2005; **128**: 2518–34.

Nesher G, Berkun Y, Mates M, et al. Low-dose aspirin and prevention of cranial ischemic complications in giant cell arteritis. *Arthritis Rheum* 2004; **50**: 1332–7.

Ruiz-Irastorza G, Hunt BJ, Khamashta MA. A systematic review of secondary thromboprophylaxis in patients with antiphospholipid antibodies. *Arthritis Rheum* 2007; **57**: 1487–95.

Scadding J. Neuropathic pain. In Warlow C. (ed.) *The Lancet Handbook of Treatment in Neurology*. Elsevier, Amsterdam, 2006.

Scolding N. Neurological involvement in systemic autoimmune and inflammatory diseases. In: Scolding N (ed.) *Contemporary Treatments in Neurology*. Butterworth-Heinemann, Oxford, 2001.

Starosta MA, Brandwein SR. Clinical manifestations and treatment of rheumatoid pachymeningitis. *Neurology*. 2007; **68**: 1079–80.

Siccoli MM, Bassetti CL, Sandor PS. Facial pain: clinical differential diagnosis. *Lancet Neurol*. 2006; **5**: 257–67.

Tokunaga M, Saito K, Kawabata D, et al. Efficacy of rituximab (anti-CD20) for refractory systemic lupus erythematosus involving the central nervous system. *Ann Rheum Dis* 2007; **66**: 470–5.

Vincent A, Buckley C, Schott JM, et al. Potassium channel antibody-associated encephalopathy: a potentially immunotherapy-responsive form of limbic encephalitis. *Brain* 2004; **127**: 701–12.

Vincent TL, Richardson MP, Kworth-Young CG, et al. Sjögren's syndrome-associated myelopathy: response to immunosuppressive treatment. *Am J Med* 2003; **114**: 145–8.

Vital C, Vital A, Canron MH, et al. Combined nerve and muscle biopsy in the diagnosis of vasculitic neuropathy. A 16-year retrospective study of 202 cases. *J Peripher Nerv Syst* 2006; **11**: 20–9.

Warlow C. (ed). *The Lancet Handbook of Treatment in Neurology*. Elsevier, Amsterdam, 2006.

Warnatz K, Peter HH, Schumacher M, et al. Infectious CNS disease as a differential diagnosis in systemic rheumatic diseases: three case reports and a review of the literature. *Ann Rheum Dis* 2003; **62**: 50–7.

Wingerchuk DM, Lennon VA, Lucchinetti CF, et al. The spectrum of neuromyelitis optica. *Lancet Neurol* 2007; **6**: 805–15.

Zandi MS, Coles AJ. Notes on the kidney and its diseases for the neurologist. *J Neurol Neurosurg Psychiat* 2007; **78**: 444–9.

The skin

Skin disease and rheumatological disease regularly co-exist. Knowledge of relevant dermatology for the rheumatologist is essential, as it will aid diagnosis and treatment of rheumatological disease.

Rheumatoid arthritis

Rheumatoid nodules
The most common extra-articular manifestation of rheumatoid arthritis (RA).
- 90% of patients with rheumatoid nodules will be rheumatoid factor (RF) positive.
- **Distribution:** extensor surfaces of the forearm, fingers, occiput, back, and heel.
- **Histology:** granulomas with plasma cells, lymphocytes and histiocytes.
- Methotrexate-induced accelerated rheumatoid nodulosis is well recognized and resolves with cessation of methotrexate. A similar phenomenon has been reported with etanercept.

Rheumatoid cutaneous vasculitis
Incidence of 2–10% in patients with RA, more common in males and RF positive patients.
- Features in order of incidence are: cutaneous ulcers, purpura, nail-fold vasculopathy, non-specific nodular erythema, haemorrhagic blisters, livedo reticularis and erythema elevatum diutinum (red/purple nodules and plaques on extensor surfaces).
- Treatment is with glucocorticoids (GCs) and other immunosuppressants.
- The differential diagnosis of cutaneous ulcers is large.
- Lower leg ulceration in a patient with RA is more likely to be due to venous ulceration. Dermatological advice should be sought before starting systemic treatment for cutaneous ulceration.

Granulomatous dermatitis
This condition is rare, but usually associated with RA, although it can be seen in other autoimmune connective tissue diseases (AICTDs).
- The rash is erythematous to violaceous indurated linear cords (Rope sign).
- Rash is usually symmetrical extending from the axilla to the mid-back, but can occur anywhere.

Cutaneous lupus erythematosus

Cutaneous lupus erythematosus is not synonymous with cutaneous manifestations of systemic lupus erythematosus (SLE). Distinct dermatological patterns of cutaneous lupus exist and the majority of patients with cutaneous lupus do not progress to SLE. Dermatological (American Rheumatology Association; ARA) criteria include malar rash, discoid rash, photosensitivity, and oral ulcers (see Plate 12). It is therefore possible to meet ARA criteria on dermatological signs only. However, some would argue that malar rash and photosensitivity are one and the same. Histology and direct immunofluorescence (IF) are often similar, but not identical in the different types of cutaneous lupus.

Discoid lupus erythematous (DLE)
Well-defined scaly plaques of variable size frequently involving the face. Scarring alopecia, atrophy, and pigmentary changes. Healing occurs with scarring. Can mimic rosacea. Exacerbated by UV light. Chilblain-like lesions often observed on digits. About 35% of patients are ANA positive. Only 6.5% progress to SLE, which is more likely if they are ANA positive. Treatment: sunscreen, topical/intralesional GCs, antimalarials, gold salts, dapsone, thalidomide, and efalizumab.

Subacute cutaneous lupus (SACLE)
Diffuse erythematosus papules and scales or annular polycyclic (ring-like) erythema on neck, trunk, and arms. Exacerbated by UV light. 80% are positive for Ro/SS-A antibodies, 60% are ANA positive. 50% patients fulfil SLE ACR criteria usually on dermatological and serological grounds only. Transformation into SLE with moderate disease activity in 10–15 %. Treatment as for DLE.

Lupus panniculitus/profundus
Deep dermal and subcutaneous nodules with normal overlying skin (although characteristic lupus histology is found in overlying dermis). Heals with lipoatrophy. ANA positive 75%. Uncommonly transforms into SLE.

Acute cutaneous lupus erythematosus (ACLE)
Butterfly erythema. Diffuse erythema/maculopapular rash. Heals without scarring. Oral ulceration. Diffuse non-scarring alopecia. Photosensitivity. Almost always ANA positive and 40–90% of patients are dsDNA positive. Often accompanies flare of systemic disease. Treatment: sunscreen, topical GCs, systemic SLE treatment.

Rare clinical sub-types
Chilblain lupus erythematosus
Peripheral painful nodules; 20% progress to SLE.

Neonatal cutaneous lupus
Transient cutaneous lupus secondary to placental transfer of antibodies.

Bullous lupus erythematosus
Diffuse bullous lesions associated with active SLE.

Lupus erythematosus tumidus
Urticarial plaques on sun exposed areas.

Rowell syndrome.
Erythema multiforme-like lesions. ANA positive – speckled pattern IF, anti-La antibodies and usually RF positive.

Antiphospholipid syndrome (APLS)

Cutaneous findings in this condition have been described with the following frequency:
- Livedo reticularis 24%.
- Leg ulcers 5.5%.
- Pseudovasculitis 3.9%.
- Cutaneous necrosis 2.1%.
- Splinter haemorrhages 0.7%.

Patients with a very similar cutaneous presentation without laboratory evidence of APLS may have Sneddon's syndrome. The pathogenesis of this disease is unclear and the relationship to lupus/APLS is controversial.

Dermatomyositis

Cutaneous features of dermatomyositis (DM) are characteristic and, in well developed cases, diagnostic.
- Classical cutaneous features include heliotrope rash (peri-ocular purple macular rash), eyelid oedema, photosensitivity, erythematosus papules over knuckles (Gottron's papules), linear erythema over fingers,

CHAPTER 3 Organ involvement in rheumatological disease

dilated/tortuous nail-fold capillaries, ragged cuticles, poikiloderma in a photosensitive distribution, cutaneous calcification and erythema of extensor aspect of knees and elbows.
- Non-classical cutaneous features include exfoliative dermatitis, gingival telangiectasia (juvenile DM), flagellate erythema, bullae, erythema nodosum, urticaria, psoarisiform plaques, livedo reticularis, and erythema multiforme.
- SACLE and DM cutaneous signs are often difficult to differentiate. DM often exhibits erythema on the upper eyelids and nasolabial folds, whereas SACLE does not.
- Cutaneous features precede myositis in 30% of cases.
- Amyopathic dermatomyositis (ADM) is being increasingly recognized as a presentation. Progression to classical DM is not inevitable. Patients can have exclusively cutaneous disease for over 5 years.
- A positive ANA is found in 63% of ADM patients, but only 3.5% have myositis-specific autoantibodies (e.g. Jo-1, Mi-2).
- ADM is not a benign condition and is associated with interstitial lung disease in 13% of cases.
- Cutaneous treatment includes sunscreen (UV exposure may exacerbate myositis), topical GCs/calcineurin inhibitors. Systemic GCs and other immunosuppressants are often required.

Localized scleroderma and systemic sclerosis (SSc)

Scleroderma is not synonymous with systemic sclerosis (SSc). Scleroderma is a dermatological sign defined as thickening and induration of the skin caused by new collagen formation with atrophy of pilosebaceous follicles. SSc is also covered in detail elsewhere in this book (p. 264–272). This section will be concerned with cutaneous signs, differential diagnosis, and the dermatological approach to a patient with types of scleroderma.

Cutaneous signs of SSc
Cutaneous systemic sclerosis usually follows three distinct phases progressively.
- **Oedematous phase:** cutaneous oedema, especially fingers. Can be pitting or non-pitting. A minority do not progress beyond this stage.
- **Indurative phase:** increased skin thickening representing increased collagen in the dermis. Skin is shiny and the epidermis is thinned. There is a loss of adenexal structures and the skin becomes hairless and anhidrotic. Pigmentary changes can occur. Typical facial changes of pinched nose and microstomia. Limited cutaneous scleroderma exhibits facial telangiectasia.
- **Atrophic phase:** the dermis and epidermis become thinned. The dermis is adherent to the subcutaneous fat giving the impression that the skin is thickened.

Nail-fold changes
Dermatologists use a dermatoscope to assess nail-fold changes as part of a routine examination. Enlarged loops, haemorrhages, angiogenesis, loss of capillaries, and avascular areas characterize more than 95% of patients with overt SSc.

Raynaud's phenomenon
Capillary nail-fold changes are useful in distinguishing primary Raynaud's phenomenon from secondary Raynaud's phenomenon.

Cutaneous calcinosis
Often digital calcinosis progresses to digital ulcers. A minority of patients have sheets of cutaneous calcinosis over the trunk and limbs leading to extensive ulceration. Can be treated by a carbon dioxide laser and surgery.

Localized scleroderma (morphea)
Localized scleroderma is a skin-limited disease that rarely displays systemic involvement. It is included in this chapter as it is commonly mistaken for SSc.
- There is little evidence to support morphea as part of a spectrum of SSc.
- Morphea can be distinguished from SSc by clinical signs and autoantibody profile.
- Individuals with morphea rarely exhibit Raynaud's phenomenon and do not have nail-fold capillary changes.
- Importantly morphea very rarely progresses to SSc.
- There are a number of recognized subtypes of morphoea, briefly reviewed below.

Plaque morphea
Plaques on trunk, face, and limbs. Well-defined erythematous indurated plaque with violaceous border. Resolves with atrophy and pigmentatory changes.

Generalized morphea
Feature of 13% of patients with morphea. Insidious onset and can progress to involve large surface area. This type of morphea is often mistaken for SSc. Not associated with systemic complications.

Atrophoderma of Pasini and Pierini
Depressed blue-brown macules lacking induration, and inflammatory features found on trunk and proximal extremities.

Linear morphea
Linear morphea often extends to sub-cutaneous tissues and includes the *en coup de sabre* phenotype. Common variant in children. Most likely sub-type to progress to SSc, although still rare. 50% have articular disease.

Deep morphea
Diffuse morphea affecting sub-cutaneous structures. Several clinical variants of which eosinophilic fasciitis is the most common (see p. 310). Eosinophilic fasciitis usually occurs at the extremities primarily with involvement of the fascia. Linear depression along superficial veins (groove sign) often present. Associated with eosinophilia.

The differential diagnosis of scleroderma
There are many scleroderma and scleroderma-like dermatological conditions that mimic SSc and should be excluded. Skin biopsy is recommended in the investigation of scleroderma. The most common of these conditions are described below.

Scleromyxoedema (papular mucinosis)
Waxy papules with marked skin sclerosis on face, neck, and dorsum of hands. Histologically cutaneous mucin depositions. Associated with paraproteinaemia.

Buschke scleredema
Symmetrical indurated skin often on neck extending to face and upper limbs. Deposition of dermal mucopolysaccharide associated with streptococcal infection, diabetes, and paraproteinaemia.

Nephrogenic fibrosing dermopathy
Symmetrical sclerotic plaques over thighs, forearms, and trunk. Patients usually have end-stage renal failure and have had gadolinium radiological contrast administration in the months preceding onset of symptoms.

Porphyria cutanea tarda
Clinically and histologically can be identical to SSc cutaneous disease. A history photosensitivity, blistering, hyperpigmentation, skin fragility, and hypertrichosis should prompt further investigation.

POEMS syndrome
Polyneuropathy, **o**rganomegaly, **e**ndocrinopathy, **m**onoclonal gammopathy, and **s**kin changes. Variable scleroderma-like changes with marked hyperpigmentation.

Diabetes mellitus
Symmetrical, bilateral thickening, and induration of the skin on the dorsum of the fingers with subsequent progressive contractures of finger joints (prayer sign). Oedema and Raynaud's phenomenon not observed.

Stiff skin syndrome
Sclerotic changes over buttocks and thighs from infancy. Recessive and dominant genetic inheritance. Good prognosis with no systemic involvement.

Fibroblastic rheumatism
First recognized as a separate clinical entity in 1980. Cutaneous nodules over the extensors and neck precede a symmetrical destructive polyarthritis. Raynaud's and skin thickening occur. It is differentiated from scleroderma as histology shows reduction in collagen and hyperplastic myofibroblasts. No effective treatment established, although spontaneous resolution is not uncommon.

Other conditions
Rare differentials include:
- Eosinophilia–myalgia syndrome
- Carcinoid syndrome
- Toxic oil syndrome
- Phenylketonuria
- Chronic graft *vs.* host disease;
- Scleroatrophic Huriez syndrome;
- Werner's syndrome.

Treatment of cutaneous SSc and morphea
- Topical GCs.
- Topical imiquimod (toll-like receptor 7 agonist).
- Topical retinoids.
- UVA1 (340–400 nm) phototherapy.
- Carbon dioxide ablation of cutaneous calcinosis.
- Systemic immunosuppressants (particularly methotrexate) are used for severe morphea, but evidence is anecdotal.

Cutaneous vasculitis (see also p. 313)
Cutaneous vasculitis is a common presenting complaint in dermatology. The vast majority of these patients fall into the cutaneous small vessel vasculitis (CSVV) classification of the Chapel Hill Consensus Conference on vasculitis. These patients have no systemic disease, serology is negative, and patients often have a proceeding exposure to drugs or infectious agents. Most patients resolve spontaneously. This section will deal with differential diagnosis of and investigation of cutaneous vasculitis from a dermatological viewpoint.

- Vasculitis is commonly clinically suspected by the presence of palpable non-blanching purpura, but this is not pathognomonic of cutaneous vasculitis.
- An differential diagnosis of purpura includes:
  - platelet disorders;
  - coagulation disorder;
  - dysproteinamias – Sjögren's syndrome, Waldenstrom's cryoproteinnaemias;
  - emboli – fat, crystal, infective;
  - raised intravascular pressure: coughing, venous stasis;
  - loss of dermal support: steroid purpura, senile purpura;
  - inherited collagen disorders;
  - capillaritis (pigmented purpuric dermatoses);
  - solar purpura;
  - scurvy.
- Confusingly, cutaneous vasculitis can present as petechiae, urticaria (urticarial vasculitis), large brown nodules on extensor surfaces (erythema elevatum diutinium), facial asymptomatic plaques (granuloma faciale), suppurative sub-cutaneous nodules of the thighs (erythema induratum) livedo reticularis with gangrene (cutaneous polyarteritis nodosa), and cutaneous ulceration to name, but a few.
- All these dermatological patterns of vasculitis have distinct disease associations and natural history.
- The diagnosis of vasculitis should always be confirmed on histology. The determination of the cutaneous sub-type of vasculitis is usually then made clinically.
- Biopsy should be taken between 12 and 24 h from onset of lesion, either punch biopsy for suspected dermal vasculitis, or deep incisional biopsy for suspected sub-cutaneous vasculitis.
- Direct IF (DIF) can be helpful in suspected Henoch–Schönlein purpura (HSP). Perivascular IgA deposits are characteristic but not exclusive to HSP. A persistent rash or heavy deposition of IgA in the skin is thought to be a prognostic sign for renal disease.
- For other vasculitides DIF is non-specific.

Sjögren's syndrome (SS)
Dermatological manifestations of SS are variable. Many patients have a dry skin, with lichenification present. Annular erythema occurs, and can be raised and almost pustular. Ro-antibody positive patients often exhibit photosensitive polycyclic erythema similar to SACLE. Sweating is often impaired or absent in affected skin. Nail-fold changes occur. A minority of patients have a non-scarring alopecia.

Sarcoidosis
Skin disease occurs in 9–37% of sarcoid patients. It is not uncommon to find cutaneous sarcoid with little systemic involvement. Cutaneous sarcoidosis may appear as macules, papules, patches, plaques, violaceous areas, localized alopecia, ichthyotic areas, psoriaform plaques, subcutaneous nodules, ulcers, and even pustules. There are three main types of cutaneous sarcoid noted.

Lupus pernio
Symmetric, violaceous, indurated plaque-like, and nodular fibrotic lesions that occur on the nose, ear lobes, cheeks, and digits. This pattern carries a greater risk of extensive pulmonary involvement.

CHAPTER 3 **Organ involvement in rheumatological disease** 101

Scar sarcoid
Occurs as the only form of cutaneous sarcoid in 30% of patients. Violaceous palpable hue over scars, tattoos, cosmetic fillers, etc. It is important to examine scars carefully in patients in whom sarcoid is suspected.

Papular sarcoid
Small 2–5 mm papules symmetrically on face with predilection for peri-orbital skin. Dermoscopy reveals a characteristic yellow brown discolouration.

Hereditary periodic fever syndromes
Cutaneous features are not uncommon in this spectrum of systemic disorders

Tumor necrosis factor receptor-associated periodic syndrome (TRAPS)
Migratory macular erythema, conjunctivitis, oedematous dermal plaque. Cutaneous signs usually present before 2 years of age and accompanied by fever.

Familial Mediterranean fever
Charcteristic erysipelas like rash and occasionally cutaneous vasculitis.

Hyperimmunoglobulin D syndrome with periodic fever.
Small erythematous macules, papules, and nodules. Petechiae and purpura are also seen during attacks.

Muckle–Wells syndrome.
Cold-induced non-pruritic urticaria.

Neutrophilic dermatoses
The neutrophilic dermatoses comprise a group of disorders characterized by recruitment of polymorphonuclear leukocytes to various layers of the skin. They often have systemic involvement, usually arthritis.

Pyoderma gangrenosum
Clinical features include painful ulcers with overhanging violaceous edges. Exhibits pathergy. About 40% of patients have arthritis, typically erosive and symmetrical, affecting large and small joints. In 50% of patients the disease is idiopathic. Common associations include haematological malignancy, inflammatory bowel disease and RA.

Acne fulminans
Severe cystic acne accompanied by fever, leukocytosis, and arthritis. Destructive arthropathy can occur with osteolytic lesions around the anterior chest wall. See also section on SAPHO (p. 236–237). May be exacerbated by systemic retinoids. Treatment; systemic GCs.
- Patients with SAPHO can have palmoplantar pustulosis, aseptic discitis, osteitis, synovitis, and enthesitis.
- SAPHO arthropathy can respond to treatment with tetracyclines and NSAIDs.

Sweet's syndrome
Sweet's syndrome (acute febrile neutrophilic dermatosis) is characterized clinically by painful, erythematosus pustules, and plaques with fever.
- Histology shows a dense neutrophilic infiltrate.
- Asymmetric non-erosive large joint arthritis occurs in 10% of cases.
- Associated with upper respiratory tract infection, inflammatory bowel disease, malignancy, RA, and sarcoid.

Behçet's disease
This disease is dealt with in detail elsewhere (see p. 340–341). Mucocutaneous manifestations are the usual presenting feature with oral and genital ulceration. Differential diagnosis includes mucosal and genital ulceration with inflamed cartilage (MAGIC) syndrome. Skin signs include small pustules at the extremities, sometimes with sub-corneal abscesses. Erythema nodosum-like lesions are common. About 55% of patients have a predominantly non-erosive arthritis.

Blind loop dermatosis-arthritis syndrome
Associated with bowel surgery (particularly blind loop formation) and inflammatory bowel disease. Usually, evolves over hours to days with erythema nodosum-like lesions. Rarely pustulates. Associated with non-erosive arthralgia (?enthesitis) and fever. Some evidence may be part of the SpA spectrum of diseases.

Psoriasis vulgaris
Psoriasis is a common disease with 2% of the world's population affected. 90% of patients have plaque psoriasis.

The basic pathology of skin psoriasis involves increased keratinocyte growth, angiogenesis, and lymphocyte migration. Normal keratinocytes have a life cycle of 70 days; for psoriatic keratinocytes this is reduced to 6 days. Psoriasis has recently been classified into separate clinical entities according to phenotype.

Entities of psoriasis

Large plaque psoriasis
Characterized by red scaly well-defined plaques from 5 mm to large areas over the trunk and limbs. Occasionally only have an active edge, with normal skin in the centre of the lesion, termed 'annular' lesions.

Flexural psoriasis
Occurs in axillae and groins. Well-defined, often macular erythema with minimal scale. Fissured and often painful.

Seborrhoeic psoriasis
Similar morphology to flexural psoriasis. Distribution is over nose, cheeks eyebrows, and nasolabial folds. It is often difficult to differentiate between seborrhoeic psoriasis and seborrhoeic dermatitis.

Scalp psoriasis
The scalp is the most common site involved in psoriasis. Varied morphology of lesions from large thick plaques to mild scaling. Distribution is often over occiput, anterior hairline, and posterior auricular. Often asymmetrical.

Guttate psoriasis
Small papules and plaques less than 10 mm occurring mainly over the trunk, but can spread to face and limbs. 70% of patients presenting acutely will have evidence of recent streptococcal infection. Antibiotic therapy can hasten clearance. Some patients progress to chronic plaque psoriasis, but the majority have spontaneous resolution within 3 months, with subsequent flares if infected by streptococcal bacteria.

Acrodermatitis continua of Hallopeau
Erythema and scaling in a distal acral distribution (starting at the fingers and toes, and progressing proximally) often involving the nails and nail folds. Often accompanies other forms of psoriasis and DIP joint disease.

Nail psoriasis
Occurs in 40% of psoriasis patients. Many patients have nail psoriasis exclusively. Thought to be secondary to an enthesitis adjacent to the nail matrix. This may explain why DIP disease and nail psoriasis often co-exist. Nail signs in

psoriasis include pitting, onycholysis (lifting of the nail plate), sub-ungual hyperkeratosis, and oil spots. If there is diagnostic doubt nail biopsy may be helpful.

Generalized pustular psoriasis
Confluent sheets of small pustules over the entire body. This can be provoked by sudden withdrawal of glucocorticoids in patients with classical plaque psoriasis. Patients are often systemically unwell. Dermatological emergency, condition can be fatal.

Erythroderma
Confluent psoriasis affecting 90% or more of the body. Often is macular erythema only and biopsy is required to differentiate between other dermatological disease including eczema and cutaneous T-cell lymphoma. Potentially fatal.

Palmoplantar pustulosis
Pustules on palms and soles of feet that do not spread onto the body. 20% of patients have co-existing plaque psoriasis. Palmoplantar pustulosis is now considered a distinct disease entity separate to psoriasis and is no longer included in the classification of psoriasis.

Table 3.14 Objective measurement tools for psoriasis

Tool	
Psoriasis Area Severity Index (PASI)	A score out of 30; a score of 10 or more being classed as severe.
Dermatology Life Quality Index (DLQI)	A simple 10-question validated Quality of Life questionnaire

The vast majority of research is based on classical large plaque psoriasis. Psoriasis has been shown to affect health-related quality of life to an extent similar to the effects of other chronic diseases such as depression, myocardial infarction, hypertension, congestive heart failure, or type 2 diabetes.

Treatment of psoriasis

Topical treatment
Topical glucocorticoids, retinoids, vitamin D analogues, and coal tar (coal tar extracts, e.g. dithranol). Emollients.

Phototherapy
Ultraviolet B radiation (UVB) (315–280 nm). Many units now use narrow band UVB (nUVB; 311–312 nm) as this has a better side effect profile. Given three times a week for 20–30 exposures.

Photochemotherapy: Psoralen and UVA treatment (PUVA).
- The patient is administered psoralen orally or topically before exposure to UVA (380–315 nm).
- The psoralen sensitises the skin to ultraviolet radiation.
- Burning can occur with only seconds of exposure time.
- Patients must protect themselves with sunblock and UV protective spectacles for 24 h after systemic psoralen administration.
- Although more effective than nUVB patients have a higher risk of subsequent skin cancer, especially if on an immunosuppressant and so is generally not favoured as first line treatment.

Laser
Excimer and pulse dye laser have been shown to improve plaque psoriasis. They are, however, labour-intensive and expensive, and not generally available in the U.K.

Hydroxyurea
An unlicensed application of the drug, but it can be effective in moderate psoriasis. Full blood count and ANA monitoring required.

Fumaric acid esters
Unlicensed in the UK, these are given orally and have good efficacy. Unknown mechanism of action. Gastrointestinal side effects. First line systemic treatment in Germany and Switzerland.

Retinoids
These drugs bind to nuclear hormone receptors in keratinocytes and alter growth and differentiation of the cell.
- The retinoid given in psoriasis is often acitretin.
- Particularly useful in hyperkeratotic psoriasis.
- Synergistic effect with nUVB and PUVA.
- High teratogenicity and potential long half-life mean that it is rarely given to menstruating women.
- Other side effects include dry skin, skin fragility, hepatitis, and dyslipidemia.

Ciclosporin
Used at 2–5 mg/kg. Effective within days and has excellent efficacy. In patients that have received PUVA in the past, the risk of squamous cell carcinoma (SCC) of the skin is 40-fold greater than the general population. After 10 years administration SCC rates are between 100- and 200-fold greater than the general population. Other side effects include renal failure, dyslipidemia, peripheral neuropathy, and gum hyperplasia.

Methotrexate
Used at doses between 5 and 25 mg per week.
- Similar efficacy to ciclosporin, but can take weeks until onset of action.
- Side effects include hepatitis and cirrhosis, nausea, and bone marrow suppression.
- The psoriasis patient population is different to the rheumatoid arthritis population; the psoriasis population have a much higher rate of liver disease prior to methotrexate administration, possibly because of excessive weight and alcohol consumption in this population.
- Pro-collagen III N terminal peptide (PIIINP) assay is used to monitor for hepatic fibrosis routinely in psoriasis patients.

Anti-TNFα therapies
Etanercept, adalimumab, and infliximab are currently licensed in the UK for psoriasis. NICE guidance has been issued for these drugs. Efficacy is similar to ciclosporin and methotrexate. Side effects are described elsewhere (see p. 566)

Anti-T-cell therapies
Alefacept and efalizumab are T cell inhibitors that have good efficacy in skin psoriasis.
- They have no effect on psoriatic arthritis.
- There may be less risk of re-activating mycobacterium tuberculosis (MTB) with these therapies compared with anti-TNFα therapies.
- Efaluzimab can cause thrombocytopenia and regular laboratory monitoring is required.

Anti-interleukin 12/23
Ustekinumab is due to gain a UK licence in 2009. It is the first 'biological' therapy designed specifically for psoriasis. In trials is has achieved a 90% reduction in ® scores in 70%

of patients – a much better rate than is seen with other agents currently available. Safety profile is comparable to placebo. It is effective in psoriatic arthritis.

Further reading

Chen KR, Carlson JA. Clinical approach to cutaneous vasculitis. *Am J Clin Dermatol* 2008; **9**(2): 71–92.

Gerami P, Schope JM, McDonald L, Walling HW, Sontheimer RD. A systematic review of adult-onset clinically amyopathic dermatomyositis (dermatomyositis siné myositis): a missing link within the spectrum of the idiopathic inflammatory myopathies. *J Am Acad Dermatol* 2006; **54**: 597–613.

Griffiths CE, Christophers E, et al. A classification of psoriasis vulgaris according to phenotype. *Br J Dermatol* 2007;**156**: 258–62.

Kaye BR, Kaye RL, Bobrove A. Rheumatoid nodules. Review of the spectrum of associated conditions and proposal of a new classification, with a report of four seronegative cases. *Am J Med* 1984; **76**: 279–92.

Martini G, Foeldvari I, Russo R, et al. Juvenile Scleroderma Working Group of the Pediatric Rheumatology European Society. Systemic sclerosis in childhood: clinical and immunologic features of 153 patients in an international database. *Arthritis Rheum.* 2006; **54**: 3971–8.

Rothfield N, Sontheimer RD, Bernstein M. Lupus erythematosus: systemic and cutaneous manifestations. *Clin Dermatol* 2006; **24**(5): 348–62.

Chapter 4

Rheumatological procedures: injection therapy

Aspiration of joints *106*
Procedure *108*

Aspiration of joints

Aspiration of joints and local injections are commonly performed in rheumatological practice and are used diagnostically, as well as therapeutically. Injections are undertaken for a wide range of soft tissue and joint conditions.

Aspiration is diagnostic and mandatory in patients with suspected septic arthritis. It is also recommended if patients have crystal arthritis or haemarthosis. Aspiration is therapeutic in patients with tense effusions, to remove irritants such as pus, which damages cartilage and to facilitate joint lavage in septic arthritis.

Injectable therapies
- The commonest injected agents are local anaesthetic and steroid therapy. There is evidence to support use of steroids in inflammatory arthritis and osteoarthritis, as well as some soft tissue conditions. However, because steroid injections have been used for many years in routine practice, the evidence base is less robust than for newer therapies, which have been introduced more recently.
- Sclerosants have been used for many years in the treatment of soft tissue and spinal disease, despite a limited evidence base for their efficacy.
- Hyalgan therapy has a role in the treatment of early osteoarthritis, but is not currently supported by National Institute of Clinical Excellence (NICE).
- More novel agents include autologous blood, botulinum toxin, and heparin. However, the evidence base for these therapies is poor and no randomized controlled trials have been published to date.

Route of injection
Injections may be delivered into:
- Joints.
- Tendon sheaths.
- Bursae.
- Muscle.

Injections may also be delivered around nerves to induce nerve blockade. Tendons are structurally hard and injecting substances into tendons is therefore difficult. Dry-needling tendons has a role in the treatment of calcific tendinitis, and plantar fasciitis. Dry needling is believed to induce a local inflammatory reaction, which then is then followed by tissue regeneration.

Complications
Local anaesthetic
Injection of local anaesthetic is relatively safe, but cardiac toxicity limits the dose of anaesthetic, which can be injected.

Steroid therapy
Injection of steroid has a greater number of potential side effects, although many of those reported are rare and by association. Patients should, however, be warned about these prior to the procedure being performed.
- **The risk of sepsis** following injection is estimated to be between 1 in 15 000 and 1 in 50 000 injections. There are no observational studies, and the estimation has been extrapolated from arthroscopic data. Patients who develop a hot, swollen joint after injection should be investigated and treated as those with a *de novo* swollen joint (see chapter 16 p. 446).
- **Tissue atrophy**. Soft tissue atrophy or hypopigmentation can occur after one injection, but is more associated with multiple injections. It is most commonly seen after subcutaneous injection and is irreversible. Anecdotally, it is commoner with longer-acting steroid preparations.
- **Tendon rupture**. There are case reports of tendon rupture following injection of steroid, but it remains to be clarified if these symptomatic tendons may have ruptured anyway.
- **Post-injection flare**. A flare of joint pain may occur in the 24–48 h following injection, and examination confirms a warm and sometime swollen joint in severe cases. Steroid is crystalline and it is likely that small crystalline deposits form in the soft tissues causing transient symptoms. The differential diagnosis is iatrogenic septic arthritis.
- **Osteonecrosis/steroid arthropathy**. There is little evidence to support the development of a steroid arthropathy resulting from repeated steroid injections, and 2-year data in patients receiving knee injections at 3-monthly intervals found no acceleration in cartilage loss compared with the control group.
- **Hypersensitivity**. Hypersensitivity may arise as a result of repeated infection with a more severe inflammatory reaction to repeated injections.
- **Facial flushing**. This is a common side effect and occurs shortly after the injection. It is transient and commoner with larger doses of steroid.
- **Hyperglycaemia in diabetics**. Steroid injections can cause a transient rise in blood sugars, and injections should therefore be planned in advance in brittle diabetics.
- **Suppression of the hypothalamic/pituitary axis**. This is rarely a problem in clinical practice.

Indications for injections
Magnetic resonance (MR) studies have confirmed the efficacy of intra-articular steroid injection in reducing synovitis in rheumatoid arthritis. The effect of the steroid is greater if arthrocentesis is performed prior to administration of the steroid and the joint aspirated to dryness. In osteoarthritis, the largest literature surrounds injections into the knee. It is estimated that around 1 in 4 with osteoarthritis of the knee will respond to an intra-articular steroid injection, but identifying the subgroup who will respond is complex. There is a growing literature supporting the efficacy of steroid into and around soft tissue lesions, although in general this remains an under researched area.

Contraindications to arthrocentesis/injections
There are no absolute contraindications to arthrocentesis or joint or soft tissue injections. However, there are some instanced where special precautions are required.
- **Bleeding diathesis or anticoagulation**. Anticoagulation is not a contraindication to joint or soft tissue injection, but the INR should be checked prior to the procedure and the procedure abandoned if the INR is greater than 3. In patients with an INR lower than this, there is an increased risk of haemarthrosis. It is common practice to apply an ice pack after the procedure to increase vasoconstriction in anticoagulated patients.
- **Prosthetic joints**. Prostheses may become infected, but arthrocentesis carries the risk of introduction of infection

CHAPTER 4 Rheumatological procedures: injection therapy

and should only be undertaken by orthopaedic surgeons in the sterile environment of theatres.
- **Infection of the overlying skin** is a contraindication to arthrocentesis as infection may be introduced into an otherwise sterile joint.
- **No response to previous injection** if there has been no response to a previous injection, the rationale of repeating the procedure should be questioned.

Efficacy of different preparations
The steroid preparations used have a strong glucocorticoid action and less of a mineralocorticoid action, therefore optimizing the anti-inflammatory response. The commonest preparations are hydrocortisone, which is relatively short acting, but may have a slightly weaker glucocorticoid action, and methylprednisolone and triamcinolone, which are both longer acting. The longer-acting preparations are used for large joint injections, and the shorter acting for small joints and soft tissue lesions. See table 4.1 for suggested doses.

Table 4.1 Suggested doses for steroid injections

Depomedrone/-methylprednisolone	80 mg	Knee
	40 mg	Ankle
		Wrist
		Elbow
		Shoulder
		Plantar fasciitis
Hydrocortisone	25 mg	Epicondylitis
	10–25 mg	Carpal tunnel
		Tenosynovitis

Local anaesthetic
Local anaesthetic is useful both diagnostically and therapeutically. In cases where the diagnosis is not clear cut, accurately injected local anaesthetic may abolish symptoms, making a diagnosis more obvious. Local anaesthetic is used for the majority of injections as it reduces the initial pain of a post-injection flare.

Table 4.2 Basic pharmacokinetics of commonly used local anaesthetics

Drug	Onset of action	Duration of action
Lidocaine	1–2 min	1 h
Procaine	1 min	30 min
Bupivacaine	30 min	8 h

While hydrocortisone is easily mixed with local anaesthetic, methylprednisolone forms a visible sediment, as does triamcinolone, although this is less marked than with methylprednisolone. The volume of local anaesthetic depends on the joint to be injected, but normally a volume of 2–4 ml is sufficient. If a number of joints are to be injected at the same visit, the cumulative dose of local anaesthetic should be calculated to ensure toxicity does not occur. The side effects of local anaesthetic include allergy, so patients should be observed for 30 min following injection, and especially in high doses as there is a risk of cardiac toxicity.

Frequency of injections
Soft tissue injections can be repeated after an interval of 3–6 weeks and joint injections may be repeated after a period of 3–4 months. In a patient requiring more frequent injections, for example, in a patient with rheumatoid arthritis, the overall disease management should be reviewed.

Table 4.3 Dose and maximum safe volumes of local anaesthetic

Drug	Strength	Maximum safe dose
Lidocaine	1%	20 ml
	2%	10 ml
Procaine	1%	100 ml
	2%	50 ml
Bupivacaine	0.25%	60 ml
	0.5%	30 ml

Rest
Efficacy in knee injections is improved in patients who rest for 24–48 h after injection. It is reasonable to extend this advice to all who receive soft tissue and joint injections, advising avoidance of heavy manual activities for 2 weeks.

Accuracy of injection
There efficacy of a joint injection is greater if the steroid and local anaesthetic are injected directly into the joint, rather than into the periarticular soft tissues. The accuracy is improved if the injection is undertaken under image guidance, and increasingly, USS is used to increase accuracy of injections.

Procedure

Preparation of equipment
- A number of different needles and syringes are available. Selection of the correct needle length is important and if arthrocentesis is to be undertaken, a narrow bore needle will not allow passage of viscous fluid. If a large volume of synovial fluid is to be aspirated, a container or a number of syringes must be available.
- A sterile universal container is necessary if synovial fluid is to be sent for analysis.
- The steroid and local anaesthetic should be mixed in advance, and the doses and expiry dates checked.
- Once the drugs are drawn up, a clean needle should be attached to the syringe.
- Current recommendation is that gloves be worn during the procedure to protect the clinician against potential infection from bodily fluids. These do not need to be sterile.

Preparation of the patient
- The patient should be warned about the potential complication.
- The procedure should be explained and informed consent obtained.
- The patient should be comfortable, with relaxed muscles around the site to be injected.
- The site of entry should be marked in the skin, either using pressure of the needle sheath or using a pen.
- The skin should be cleaned with an antiseptic. The skin should be allowed to dry before the procedure as it is the drying of the antiseptic, such as alcohol, which kills skin flora.

Administration of the injection
- A no touch technique should be used, so that once the skin has been cleaned, it is not touched again.
- Injections should not be painful. The most uncomfortable part of the procedure should be the needle moving through the skin. The concentration of sensory nerve endings is higher on the skin of the hands and feet, and lower in areas such as the shoulder.
- In the majority of cases, local anaesthetic is not required separately to the skin, but confident introduction of the needle into the correct site will cause little discomfort.
- Once the needle is in place, aspiration should be undertaken to ensure the needle is not in a blood vessel. If it is, the needle should be removed, pressure applied over the puncture site until bleeding has stopped, and the procedure repeated with the needle repositioned.
- If synovial fluid is aspirated, the joint should be aspirated to dryness. If there is concern about the possibility of infection, steroid should not be administered and synovial fluid sent for analysis.
- The local anaesthetic/steroid combination should flow without resistance. If resistance is experienced, the needle tip may be up against bone and small adjustments to the needle position are necessary.
- Once the injection has been administered, the needle may be withdrawn and pressure applied over the site to prevent bleeding. A plaster should be applied if there is no history of allergy to plasters.
- The needle and syringes should be disposed of in a sharps bin.
- The patient should be reassessed after the procedure, and the procedure recorded in the medical notes.

Injection techniques
Shoulder girdle
Glenohumeral joint

The glenohumeral joint is most easily accessed from the posterior approach. From behind, palpate the tip of the acromion and identify the corocoid process. The needle should be inserted perpendicular to the skin, 2.5 cm inferiorly and 2.5 cm medially to the tip of the acromion, with the tip of the needle aiming towards the corocoid process.

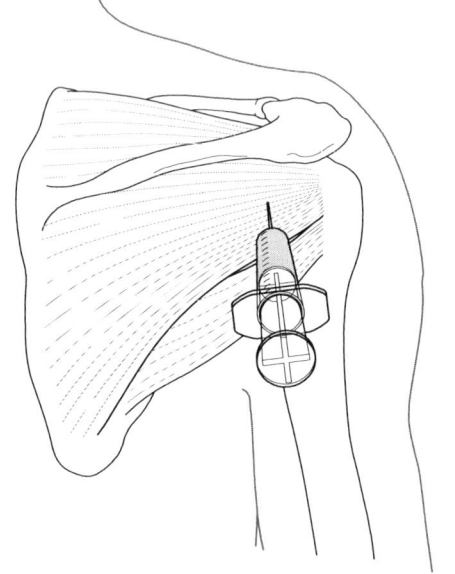

Fig 4.1 Posterior approach to the glenohumeral joint

- The anterior approach requires the needle to be inserted just medially to the corocoid process. The anterior approach is less commonly use than the posterior due to the relative proximity of the large vessels and brachial plexus.
- Needle: 21G, inserted approximately 4 cm.
- Steroid: depomedrone 40 mgB.

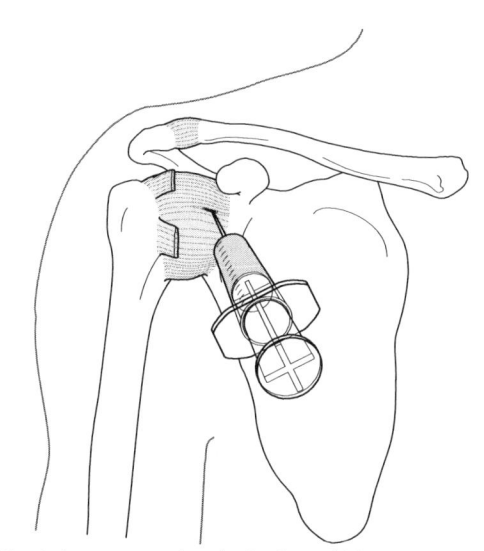

CHAPTER 4 **Rheumatological procedures: injection therapy** 109

Fig 4.2 Anterior approach to the glenohumeral joint

Acromioclavicular joint
- The acromioclavicular joint is identified 1 cm medially from the tip of the acromion. It can be felt to move when the shoulder is shrugged. The patient sits with their arm handing by their side and the needle is inserted at an angle of 30° medially as the joint sits at an angle. This can be a difficult joint to inject, but 'walking' the needle slowly and gently across the acromion can help in identifying the acromioclavicular joint.
- Needle: 25G, inserted 1 cm.
- Steroid: depomedrone 20 mg.

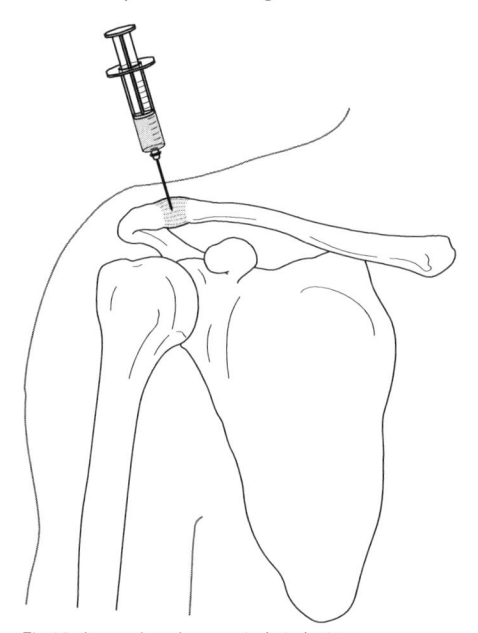

Fig 4.3 Approach to the acromioclavicular joint

Sternoclavicular joint
- The sternocalvicular joint is best accessed with the patient's arm in external rotation. The joint is accessed from a superiolateral approach, with the needle angled down and into the joint.
- Needle: 25G, inserted 1 cm.
- Steroid: depomedrone 20 mg.

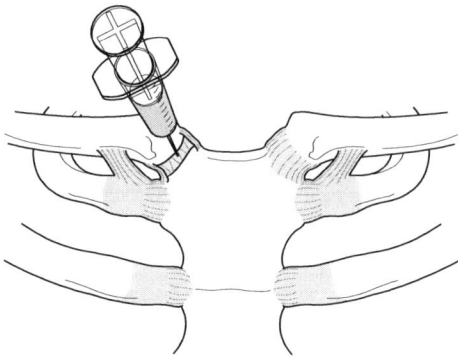

Fig 4.4 Approach to the sternoclavicular joint.

Subacromial space and rotator cuff
- The patient sits with the arm hanging by their side. This opens up the subacromial space between the acromion and humeral head. The lateral edge of the acromion should be palpated and the needle inserted below the midpoint of the acromion.
- Needle: 21G, inserted 3 cm.
- Steroid: depomedrone 40 mg.

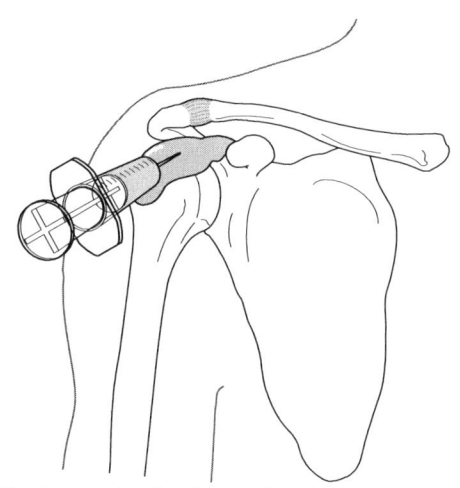

Fig 4.5 Approach to the subacromial bursa

PROCEDURE

The elbow region
The elbow capsule
- The elbow capsule houses the radio-humeral, radioulnar and humero-ulnar joints. The joint is most easily accessed from a lateral approach. The patient sits with the elbow at 90° of flexion. The needle is inserted into the space between the head of the radius and the olecranon process of the humerus, with the needle parallel to the top of the radius.
- Needle: 25G, inserted 2 cm.
- Steroid: depomedrone 40 mg.

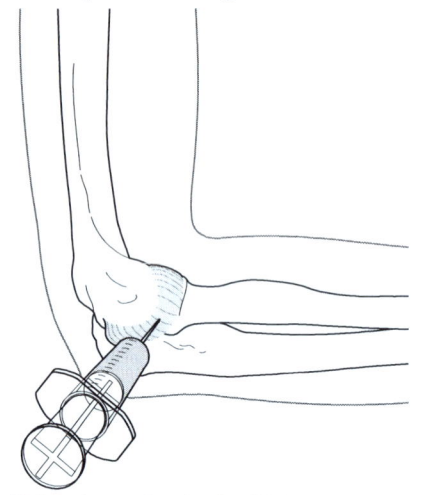

Fig 4.6 Lateral approach to the elbow joint

Lateral epicondylitis
- The patient sits with the elbow at 90° and the arm supported. The lateral epicondyle is palpated and the needle inserted in line with the cubital crease. The steroid combination should be injected in a fan like approach over the bone.
- Needle: 25G, inserted 1 cm.
- Steroid: hydrocortisone 10–25 mg.

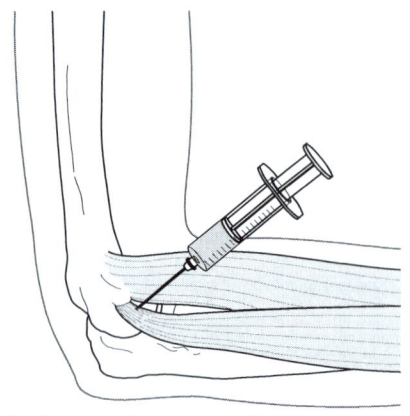

Fig 4.7 Approach for lateral epicondylitis

Medial epicondylitis
- The patient sits with the arm supported and in extension. The medial epicondyle is identified and the needle inserted perpendicular to the anterior facet until bone is touched. The steroid combination should be injected in a fan like approach over the bone.
- Needle: 25 G, inserted 1 cm.
- Steroid: hydrocortisone 10–25 mg.

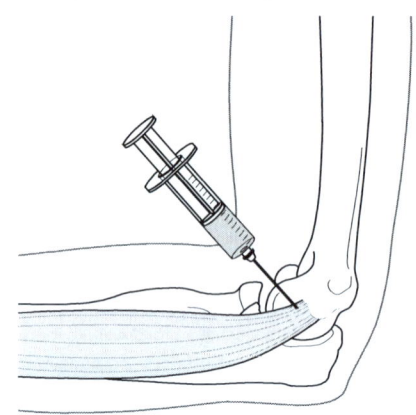

Fig 4.8 Approach for medial epicondylitis

Olecranon bursa
- The patient sits with the elbow flexed to 90°. The area of tenderness is palpated and the needle inserted into the central tenderness.
- Needle: 23G.
- Steroid: hydrocortisone 25 mg.

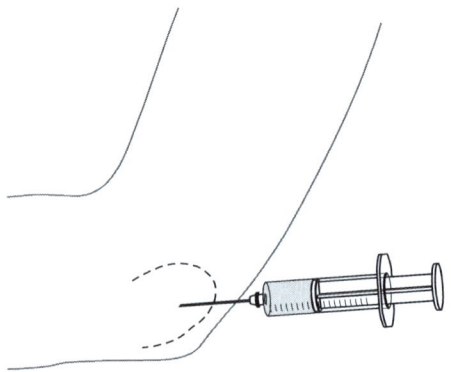

Fig 4.9 Approach for the olecranon bursa

Wrist and hand
Wrist
- The hand is placed palm down, and just proximal to the capitate is a hollow, within the mid carpus bones. The needle is inserted into the hollow.
- Needle: 23G, inserted 2 cm.
- Steroid: depomedrone 40 mg.

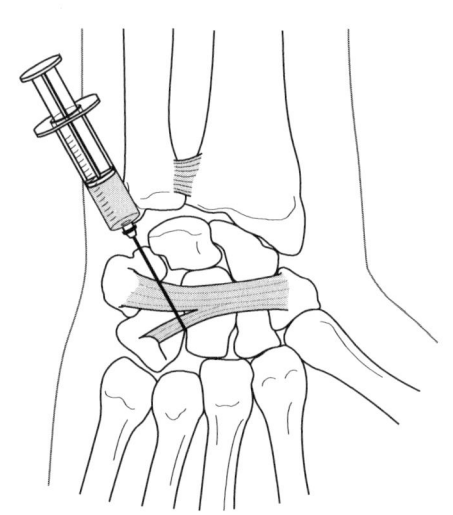

CHAPTER 4 **Rheumatological procedures: injection therapy** 111

Fig 4.10 Approach to the wrist

Distal radioulnar joint
- The hand is placed palm down, and the joint line identified midway between the radial and ulnar styloids. The needle is inserted perpendicular to the skin.
- Needle: 25G, inserted by 1.5 cm.
- Steroid: depomedrone 40 mg.

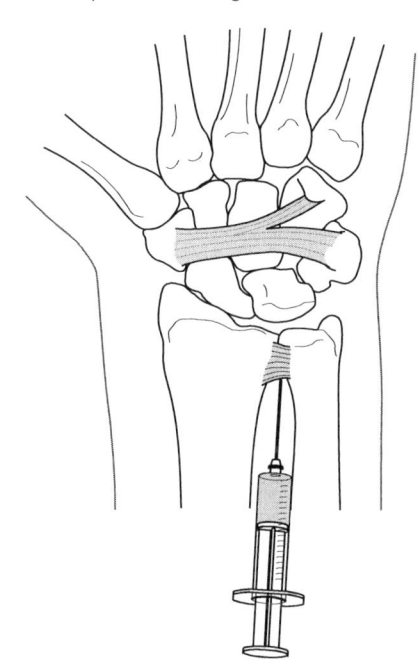

Fig 4.11 Approach to the radioulnar joint

Thumb carpometacarpal joint
- The arm is positioned on the ulnar border of the forearm with the thumb uppermost. The joint space between the trapezium and the metacarpal is easily identified. Traction on the thumb helps to open up the joint space. The needle may be inserted in to the joint.
- Needle: 25G, inserted 0.5 cm
- Steroid: hydrocortisone 10 mg

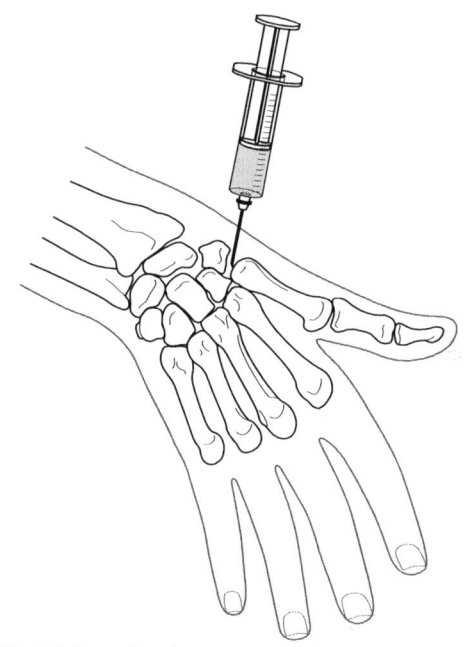

Fig 4.12 Approach to the carpometacarpal joint

De Quervain's tenosynovitis
- The arm is positioned on the ulnar border of the forearm with the thumb uppermost. The abductor pollicus longus and extensor pollicis brevis tendons run together in one tendon sheath. The gap between the tendons is identified and the needle inserted into the gap. As the injection is administered, there may be a swelling as the fluid moves out of the opposite end of the tendon sheath.
- Needle: 25G, inserted 0.5 cm.
- Steroid: hydrocortisone 10 mg.

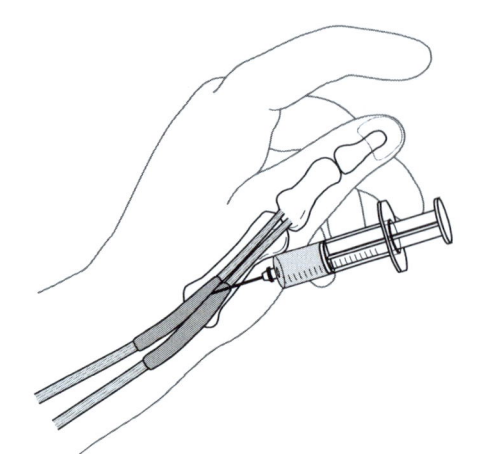

Fig 4.13 Approach for de Quervan's tenosynovitis

Carpal tunnel syndrome
- The hand is placed with the palm facing up. Identify the proximal wrist crease. The palmarus longus tendon should be identified. The needle should be inserted on the ulnar side of the palmarus longus tendon at an angle of 45° with the needle aiming towards the tip of the third (middle) finger. If there is acute worsening of pain and numbness in the distribution of the median nerve, the needle should be removed and repositioned as is within the median nerve. Patients should be warned that the symptoms may deteriorate in severe carpal tunnel due to increase in pressure around the nerve. Local anaesthetic is not normally administered as local anaesthetic may worsen the paraesthesia in the short term.
- Needle: 23G, inserted 1.5 cm.
- Steroid: hydrocortisone 25 mg.

Trigger finger
- A nodule is often palpable at the base of the finger in the flexor tendon sheath. The nodule is directly injected with steroid.
- Needle: 25G, inserted 0.5 cm.
- Steroid: hydrocortisone 10 mg.

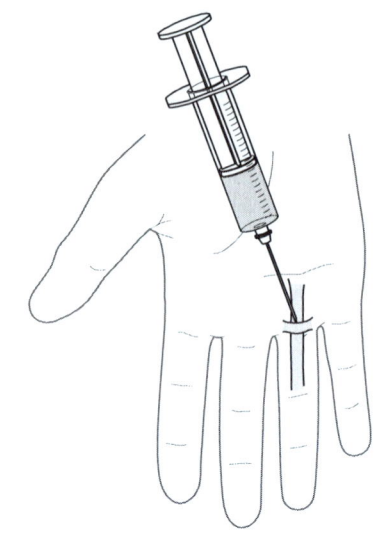

Fig 4.15 Approach for trigger finger

The hip region
The hip
- The hip is a deep joint and should only be injected under radiological guidance.
- Needle 21G, inserted by around 4 cm.
- Steroid: depomedrone 80 mg.

Trochanteric bursitis
- The patient lies on their side with the painful hip uppermost. The site of maximum tenderness is palpated over the greater trochanter. The needle is injected perpendicular to the skin and the steroid and local anaesthetic mixture injected in a fan like approach in the tender region.
- Needle: 21G, inserted 4 cm.
- Steroid: depomedrone 40 mg.

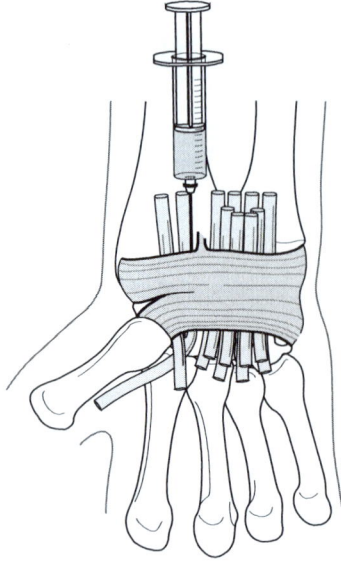

Fig 4.14 Approach to the carpal tunnel

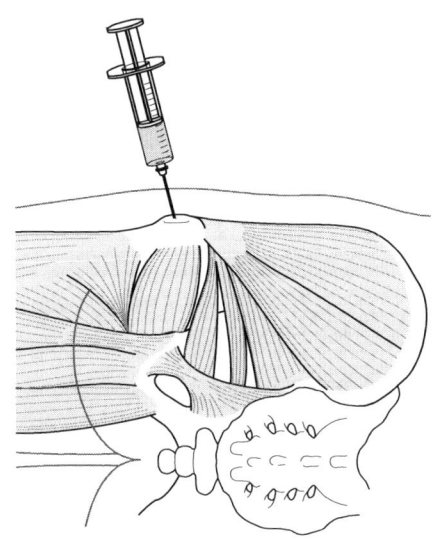

CHAPTER 4 **Rheumatological procedures: injection therapy** 113

Fig 4.16 Approach for trochanteric bursitis

Adductor tendinitis
- The patient lies on their back with the leg abducted and laterally rotated. The origin of the tendon is identified and the needle inserted on to the bone at that point. The steroid is peppered around the origin of the tendon.
- Needle: 23G, inserted 1.5 cm.
- Steroid: hydrocortisone 25 mg

The knee region

The knee
- The patient is positioned on lying on their back with the knee in slight flexion and supported. Either a medial or a lateral approach can be taken. The medial approach requires identification of the midpoint of the patellar and insertion of the needle under the patella and above the femoral condyle. In the lateral approach, the same technique is applied, but from the lateral aspect (see Plate 23).
- Needle: 21G, inserted 3–4 cm.
- Steroid: depomedrone 80 mg.

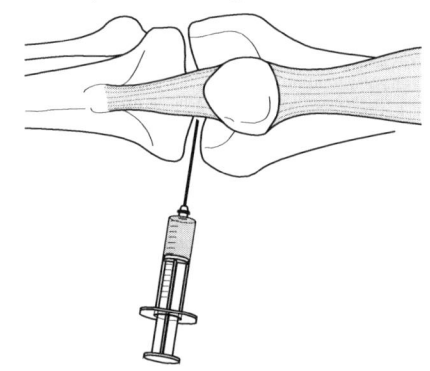

Fig 4.17 Medial approach to the knee

Coronary ligament
- The knee is bent to 90° and the foot of that leg externally rotated. The tibial plateau is palpated to find the area of tenderness, and the needle is inserted on to the plateau.
- Needle: 25G, inserted 2 cm.
- Steroid: hydrocortisone 25 mg.

Medial collateral ligament
- The knee is supported in slight flexion and the medial joint line identified. The area of tenderness is palpated and the needle inserted to the point of tenderness, but not deep enough to penetrate the joint capsule.
- Needle: 25G, inserted 2 cm.
- Steroid: hydrocortisone 25 mg.

Infrapatellar bursa
- The knee is slightly flexed and supported. The deep infrapatellar burse sits beneath the patellar tendon and the needle is inserted beneath the tendon, either from a medial or a lateral approach. It is important not to insert the needle into the patellar tendon.
- Needle: 23G, inserted 2 cm.
- Steroid: hydrocortisone 25 mg.

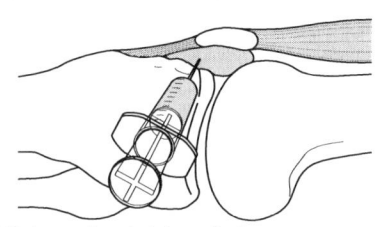

Fig 4.18 Approach to the infrapatellar bursa

Anserine bursa
- The knee is supported in extension. The pes anserine tendon is identified by flexing the knee against resistance. The point of insertion can be palpated on the tibia, and the bursa lies deep to this, and is tender. The needle is inserted into the central area of tenderness, and onto the bone.
- Needle: 23G, inserted 2 cm.
- Steroid: hydrocortisone 25 mg.

PROCEDURE

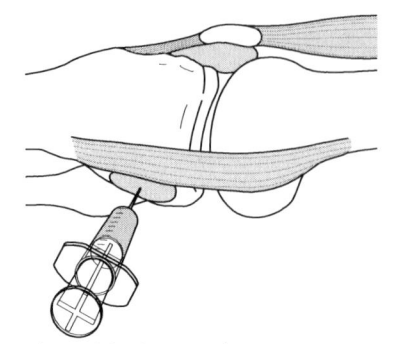

Fig 4.19 Approach for the anserine bursa

Ankle and foot

Ankle mortice

- The foot is supported in neutral. The ankle joint lies between the lateral and medial malleoli, and the ankle joint may be followed laterally, and identified by passively flexing and extending the ankle. The needle is inserted directly into the joint, passing through the capsule.
- Needle: 23G, inserted 2 cm.
- Steroid: depomedrone 40 mg.

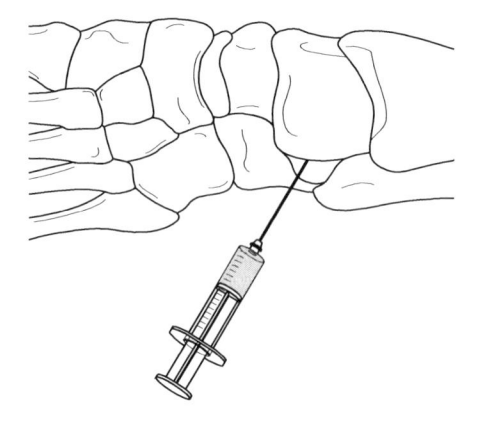

Fig 4.20 Approach to the ankle mortice joint

Subtalar joint and midtarsal joints

- The subtalar and midtarsal joints are difficult to access blindly and should therefore be injected under ultrasound control.

- Needle 25G.
- Steroid: depomedrone 40 mg.

First metatarsal phalangeal joint.

- The patient lies with the foot supported. The joint line can be palpated and identified by passively moving the great toe. The needle is inserted perpendicularly, avoiding the extensor tendon in the midline.
- Needle: 25G, inserted 1 cm.
- Steroid: hydrocortisone 25 mg.

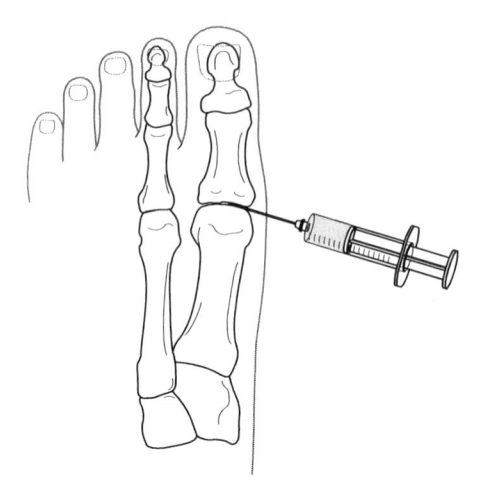

Fig 4.21 Approach to the first metatarsophalangeal joint

The Achilles tendon and bursa.

- The Achilles tendon should not be injected as there is no tendon sheath, and injection may result in rupture. The Achilles bursa sits beneath the Achilles tendon and should be injected under ultrasound control.
- Needle 23G, inserted 2 cm.
- Steroid: hydrocortisone 25 mg.

The peroneal tendons

- The patient lies supine. The two tendons of peroneus longus and brevis share a tendon sheath which can be identified by palpation. The needle should be inserted between the two tendons and the needle slid towards the lateral malleolus. This should ensure the needle is within the tendon sheath.
- Needle: 25G, inserted 1 cm.
- Steroid: Hydrocortisone 25 g.

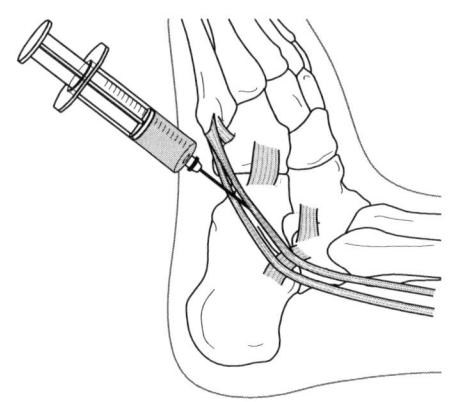

CHAPTER 4 **Rheumatological procedures: injection therapy** 115

Fig 4.22 Approach to the peroneal tendon sheath

Plantar fasciitis
- The patient lies with foot relaxed. The needle should be aimed at the calcaneum, having been inserted either from a lateral approach through the soft tissues, or from the soft part of the sole of the foot.
- Needle: 21G, inserted 2–3 cm.
- Steroid: depomedrone 40 mg.

Caudal (sacral) epidural
Caudal epidurals are performed for low back pain with radicular symptoms. Potential complications include worsening of radicular symptoms, headache, hypotension, infection, the risk of which is similar to that of iatrogenic joint infection, and spinal block.

Procedure
- Informed consent should be obtained.
- The patient should be examined to measure the angle of the straight leg raise. Blood pressure should be measured.
- The patient lies prone with the abdomen supported by a pillow. If patients are uncomfortable lying in this position, it is possible for the procedure to be performed with the patient lying on their side.
- At the top of the buttocks, a small bony protruberance is palpable on the sacrum at S4 and S5 under which lies a sacral hiatus. This should be marked and the skin sterilized with iodine or a similar antiseptic.
- Local anaesthetic, such as 2 ml of 2% lidocaine should be applied to the skin.
- Whilst this is working the epidural solution should be drawn up. This consists of 5 ml of bupivacaine 0.25%, 80 mg of depomedrone and 10 ml of sterile normal saline.
- Using either a 21G needle, or a spinal needle, the needle is inserted through the sacral hiatus at an angle of 45° directed towards the umbilicus. No resistance should be encountered.
- With the needle in the hiatus, the syringe should be detached and the patient asked to cough. This is to ensure the dura has not been perforated. If cerebrospinal fluid is seen, the procedure must be abandoned.
- The epidural should be slowly introduced into the epidural space over a period of a minute of two. The patient may feel a pushing sensation in the low back. The needle is then removed.
- A plaster can be applied to the puncture site.
- Blood pressure should be monitored immediately and then after 15 and 30 min.
- The straight leg raise should be examined again before the patient is discharge.
- The epidural may be repeated, particularly if there has been a response to the previous epidural. It is not clear how often or what the interval should be between epidural injections.

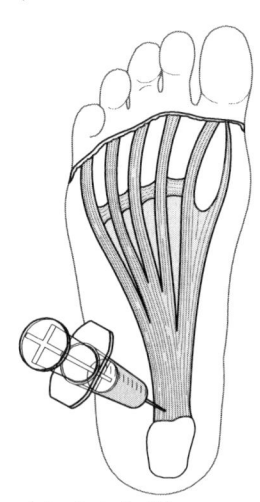

Fig 4.23 Approach for plantar fascilitis

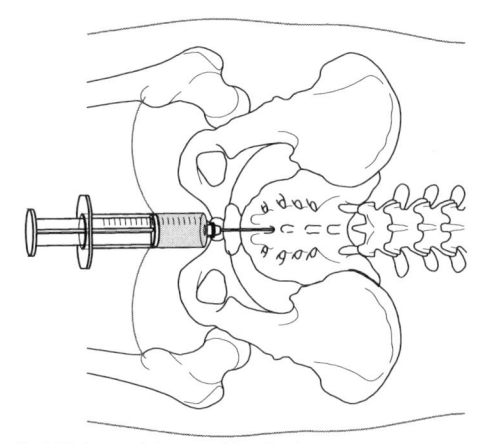

Fig 4.24 Approach for a caudal epidural

Further reading

Dangoisse MJ, et al. Suprasacpular nerve block (using bupivacaine and methylprednisolone acetate] in chronic shoulder pain. *Acta Anaesthesiol Belg* 1994; **45**: 49–54.

Speed CA. Injection therapies for soft-tissue lesions. *Best Pract Res Clin Rheumatol* 2007; **21**: 333–47.

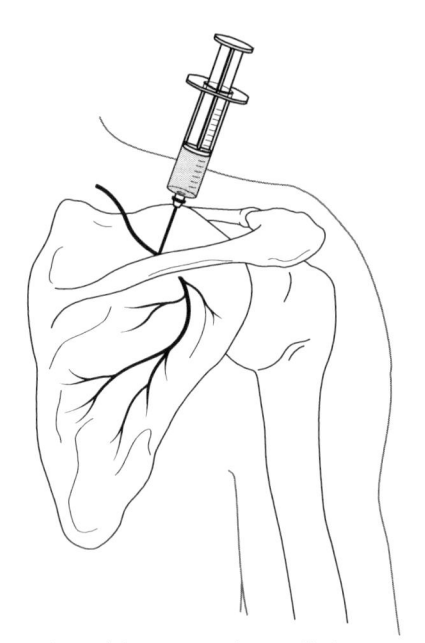

Fig 4.25 Approach for a suprascapular nerve block

Suprascapular nerve block
The suprascapular nerve provides sensory fibres to the acromioclavicular joint and to the shoulder joint.
- The technique involves injecting anaesthetic into the floor of the supraspinatus fossa to block the nerve.
- The solution of 8 ml of 0.5% bupivicaine and 80 mg depomedrone should be drawn up in advance.
- Informed consent must be obtained having explained the potential complications of pneumothorax, and damage to the suprascapular nerve and vessels.
- A sterile, no touch approach should be undertaken.
- The skin is cleaned with iodine or another antiseptic.
- The spine of the scapula is identified and the needle is inserted into the fossa, 1 cm cephalad to the middle of the spine of the scapula and into the floor of the fossa.
- The solution should be injected slowly.
- Patients should be observed for an hour after the procedure.

Chapter 5

Regional musculoskeletal anatomy and conditions

The spine *118*
Cervical spine: regional musculoskeletal conditions *124*
Thoracic spine and chest wall: regional musculoskeletal conditions *128*
Lumbar spine: regional musculoskeletal conditions *130*
The shoulder *136*
The shoulder girdle: regional musculoskeletal conditions *140*
The elbow *146*
The elbow: regional musculoskeletal conditions *148*
The hand and wrist *152*
Hand and wrist: regional musculoskeletal conditions *158*
Pelvis, hip, and groin *164*
Pelvis, hip and groin: regional musculoskeletal conditions *168*
The knee *174*
The knee: regional musculoskeletal conditions *178*
Lower leg and foot *184*
Lower leg and foot: regional musculoskeletal conditions *188*
Conditions of the ankle and hindfoot *190*
Conditions of the mid and forefoot *194*

The spine

The spine is the central axis of the body. The cervical and lumbar vertebrae provide flexibility and the thoracic spine along with the ribs provides a protective cage for the contents of the thorax.

Regional anatomy

The spinal column consists of seven cervical, twelve thoracic and five lumbar vertebrae. It also consists of five fused sacral segments and the fused coccygeal segments. See Figure 5.1.

Bones

The overall structure of each vertebra is similar with some regional variation. Each consists of a vertebral body, which constitutes the anterior element and this is joined via pedicles to the posterior elements. The posterior elements comprise the lamina, the superior and inferior articular processes, the transverse processes, and the spinous processes. The facet joints articulate via a true synovial joint. This is especially relevant in rheumatoid arthritis. The vertebral body consists predominantly of cancellous bone surrounded by a cortical shell. Between them they resist the compressive forces applied to the anterior part of the spinal column. The vertebral body on its superior and inferior surfaces is covered by a layer of cartilage beneath which lies a condensation of bone referred to as the subchondral plate. The subchondral plate is perforated by nutrient arteries which in childhood form end-arterioles

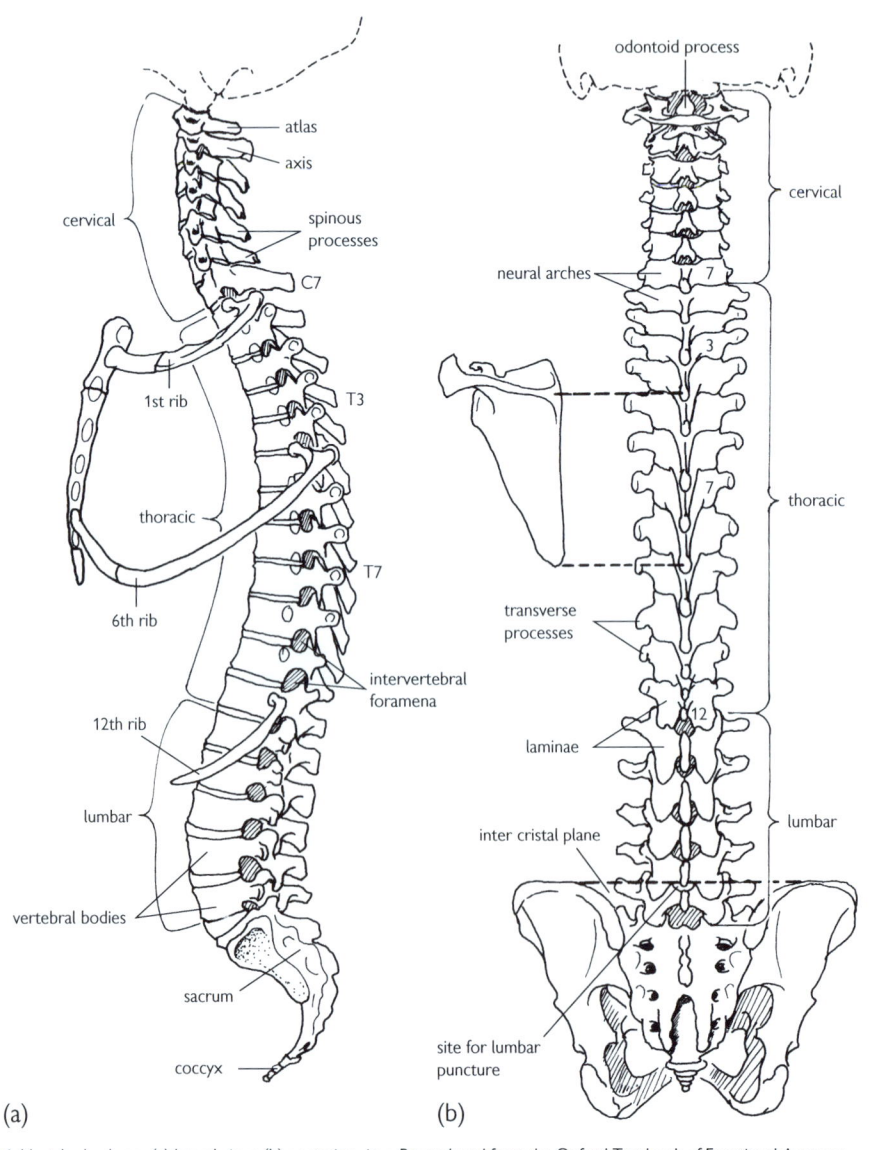

Figure 5.1 Vertebral column: (a) lateral view; (b) posterior view. Reproduced from the Oxford Textbook of Functional Anatomy, MacKinnon and Morris, 2005, with permission from Oxford University Press.

CHAPTER 5 Regional musculoskeletal anatomy and conditions

within the cartilaginous endplate. The loss of vascularity associated with advancing age has been implicated as one of the causes of disc degeneration.

Cervical spine

In the cervical spine the lateral ends of the superior part of the C3–C6 vertebral bodies flare out to form the uncinate processes, which articulate with the under surface of the cervical vertebra cranial to it. The transverse processes have become adapted and contain a foramen transversarium, which accommodates the vertebral artery from the C6 up to the C1 level. The first and second cervical vertebrae are atypical. The vertebral body of C1 is, in fact, part of the C2 vertebra and presents as a cranial projection of the C2 body that is known as the odontoid peg. The C1 vertebra, therefore, is more like a ring than a typical vertebra. The articulations between the skull and the atlas (C1 vertebra), and the C1 and C2 vertebra (axis) are relatively flattened. This allows a significant range of movement particularly with regard to rotation in the transverse plane. The odontoid process on the body of C2 allows identification of this vertebra. The facet joints on this vertebral body articulate with the anterior arch of the atlas on the anterior surface and with the transverse ligament of the atlas on the posterior aspect. The articulations between the other cervical vertebrae are inclined at approximately 45° to the transverse plane. This accounts for the significant degree of flexion that is achievable in the cervical spine.

Thoracic spine

Each thoracic vertebra is larger than that immediately above it. Each has an upper and lower hemifacet joint which articulates with the heads of the ribs. The spinous processes are long in comparison with those of the cervical and lumber spine. The transverse processes bear facets for the tubercles of the ribs. The thoracic vertebral foramena are relatively small. See Figure 5.2.

Lumbar spine

The facet joints in the lumbar region are inclined at approximately 45° to the coronal plane. Pure movements such as flexion, extension, and rotation of the spine are rare in that such movements often elicit a so called coupled movement in another plane. For example, axial rotation of the cervical spine is associated with lateral flexion as a consequence of coupled movement. See Figure 5.3.

Intervertebral discs

The vertebrae are separated anteriorly by intervertebral discs. These constitute a tough outer ring referred to as the annulus fibrosis with a central nucleus pulposus. See Figure 5.4. The annulus consists of concentric rings of collagen fibres, which resist rotational forces within the spine, as well as tensile forces. The nucleus consists predominantly of water that accounts for more than 70% of the nuclear content. It also contains a collagenous matrix, as well as proteoglycans and mucopolysaccharides. The cell content is extremely low and consists mainly of chondrocyte-like cells. The disc is bound superiorly and inferiorly by cartilaginous endplates, which are comprised of hyaline cartilage.

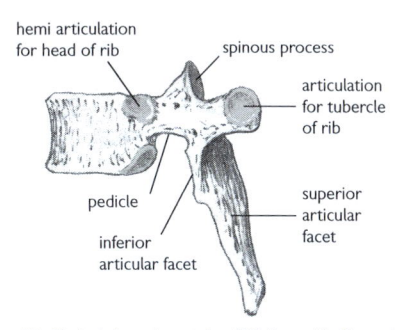

Figure 5.2 Typical thoracic vertebra (T5) from side. Reproduced from the Oxford Textbook of Functional Anatomy, MacKinnon and Morris, 2005, with permission from Oxford University Press.

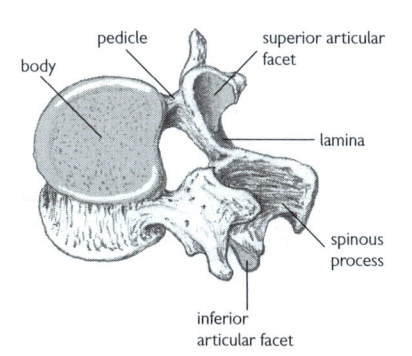

Figure 5.3 Typical lumbar vertebra (L4) from above and the side. Reproduced from the Oxford Textbook of Functional Anatomy, MacKinnon and Morris, 2005, with permission from Oxford University Press.

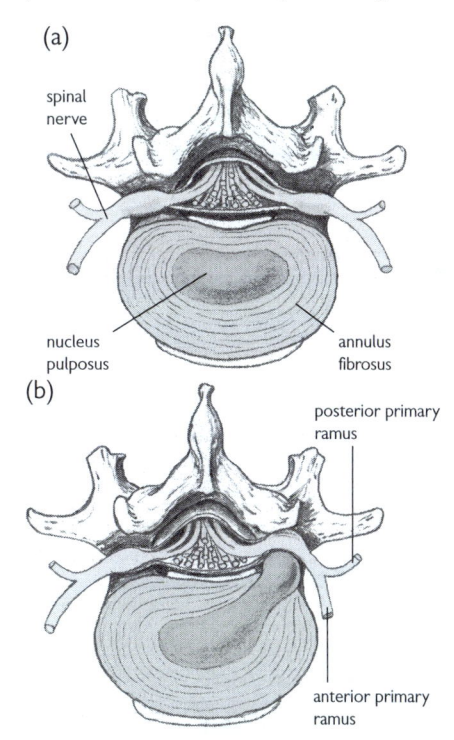

Figure 5.4 (a) Lumbar intervertebral disc viewed from below. (b) Prolapse of nucleus pulposus ('slipped disc'). Reproduced from the Oxford Textbook of Functional Anatomy, MacKinnon and Morris, 2005, with permission from Oxford University Press.

Ligaments

The ligaments of the spine are classified as long or short. The short ligaments include:

- Interspinous ligaments, which attach adjacent spinous processes.
- Intertransverse ligaments, which attach adjacent transverse processes.

- Ligamenta flavum, elastic ligaments, which attach to the laminae of adjacent arches.

The long ligaments include:
- The anterior longitudinal ligament on the anterior surface of the vertebral bodies.
- The posterior longitudinal ligament on the posterior surface of the vertebral bodies.
- The supraspinous ligament, which attaches to the tip of the spinous processes.

The alar ligaments extend from the top and sides of the odontoid peg to the foramen magnum. The cruciate ligament is the name given to the transverse ligament of the atlas.

Muscles

Longus colli and longus capitus extend from the base of the skull to the upper thoracic vertebrae with attachments to the cervical vertebrae and result in flexion of the cervical spine. In the lumbar spine, flexion is primarily achieved by contraction of the psoas muscles, a powerful paravertebral muscle whose origin is the transverse processes of the lumbar vertebrae and insertion is the lesser trochanter of the femur. Lateral flexion is achieved by contraction of the scalene muscles, the origin of which is the transverse processes of the cervical vertebrae, and insertion is the first and second ribs. Extension of the spine arises due to the action of short, deep muscles that attach transverse processes to adjacent spinous processes, more superficial medium length muscles, and longer, superficial muscles including the erector spinae muscles.

Anatomy of the spinal cord

In the adult human, the spinal cord extends from the foramen magnum to its termination at approximately the L1/2 disc space. In the foetus, the cord extends down to the lower lumbar segments, but the termination of the cord migrates cranially due to the greater velocity of longitudinal growth of the spinal column compared with the spinal cord. At birth, the cord terminates at the L1/2 level. As a consequence of this the nerve roots in the cervical region exit almost transversely from the cord whereas distal to the L1 level the nerve roots follow an oblique course until they exit through their respective foraminae. The C1 nerve root exits the spinal cord cranial to the C1 vertebra and this dictates the nomenclature of all the nerve roots thereafter. The C8 nerve root exits the spine cranial to the T1 vertebra and the T1 root, therefore, exits under the pedicle of T1. This pattern is continued in the lumbar spine. For example, the L5 nerve root exits under the L5 pedicle in the L5/S1 exit foramen. This is of particular importance in nomenclature with respect to neural compression.

Spinal tracts

The spinal cord has an ellipsoid cross-section and has a central H-shaped area referred to as the grey matter, which contains the cell bodies. The surrounding white matter contains the ascending and descending columns of nerve fibres. The white matter is divided anatomically into the posterior white column, the lateral white column and the anterior white column.

Afferent impulses usually enter the spinal cord via the first order neurons, whose cell bodies reside in the posterior root ganglion of the spinal nerves. These synapse with second order neurons, which are usually located in the spinal cord. Subsequent synapses are on to third order neurons whose cell bodies reside in the thalamus, although this is a fairly simplistic schema, and in reality several variations and complex patterns exist.

The efferent pathways are divided in to the direct cortical spinal or pyramidal system and the indirect cortical spinal or extra pyramidal system. The pyramidal system originates with cell bodies in the cerebral cortex with fibres extending directly onto the anterior horn cells within the spinal cord. In the extra pyramidal system, the cortical fibres synapse with intermediate neurons located either in the pons, cerebellum, thalamus, or any other number of nuclei. Cells from these intermediate nuclei then project on to the anterior horn cells and this accounts for the reference to this system as an indirect cortical spinal pathway.

Dermatomes

Main nerve roots supplying the lower limb
- Hip:
  - flexion, adduction L2, 3, 4.
- Knee:
  - extension, abduction L4, 5, S1;
  - extension L3, 4.
- Ankle:
  - flexion L5, S1;
  - plantar flexion L4, 5.
- Subtalar joint:
  - dorsiflexion L5, S1;
  - inversion L5.
- Toes:
  - eversion, plantar flexion L5, S1;
  - flexion L5, S1, 2;
  - dorsiflexion S1, 2, 3.

Main nerve roots supplying muscles of the upper limb
- Shoulder:
  - abduction, lateral rotation C5;
  - adduction, medial rotation C6, 7, 8.
- Elbow:
  - flexion C5, 6;
  - extension C7, 8.
- Forearm:
  - supination C6;
  - pronation C7, 8.
- Wrist:
  - flexion and extension C6, 7.
- Fingers:
  - flexors and extensors C7, 8.
- Hand:
  - intrinsic muscles C8, T1.

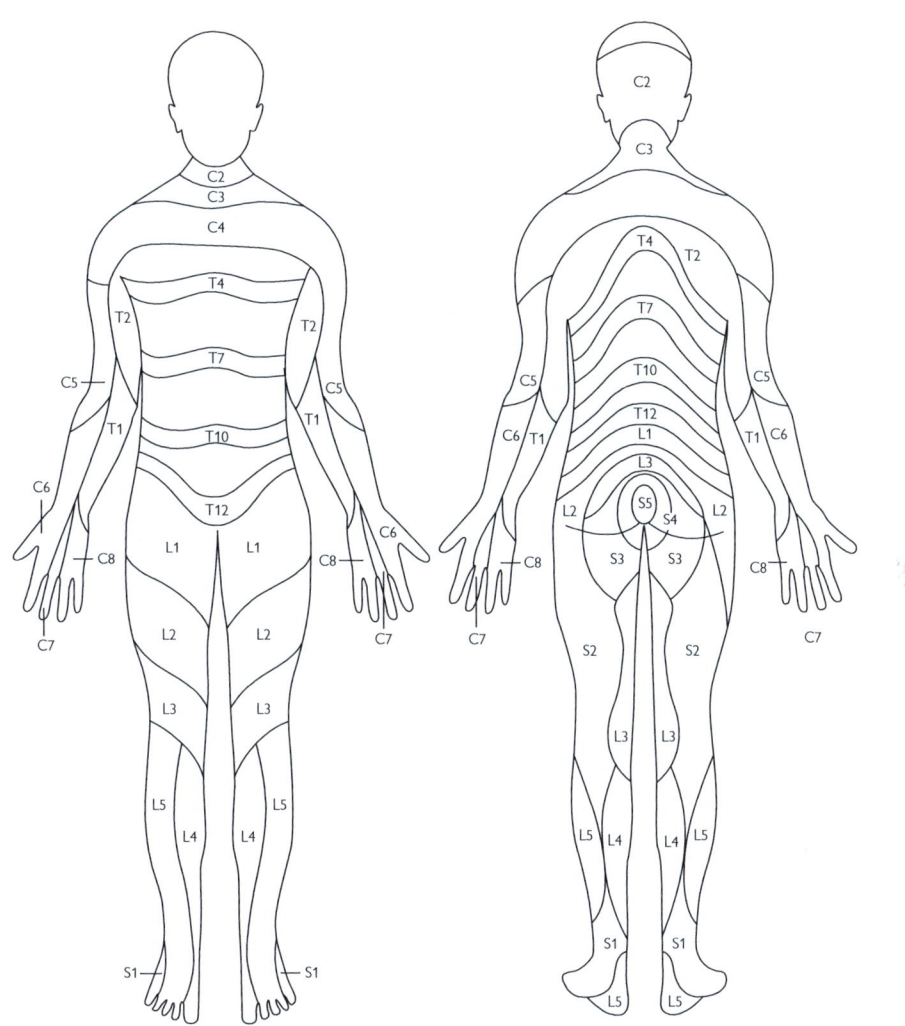

CHAPTER 5 **Regional musculoskeletal anatomy and conditions**

Figure 5.5 Dematome chart. Reproduced from Oxford Textbook of Orthopaedics and Trauma, Bulstrode et al, 2002, with permission from Oxford University Press.

Ascending tracts
The three principle ascending tracts are:
- **Posterior gracile and cuneate tracts:** the gracile tracts transmit fibres from the lower limb and trunk, and the cunate tracts from the upper limb and trunk. They convey proprioceptive impulses and light touch and vibration sensibility.
- **Anterior lateral tract:** afferent fibres from the periphery cross to the contralateral side of the spinal cord and also usually ascend to a variable extent. They may do so for over up to 5 segments. Ten per cent of fibres within the anterior lateral tract synapse in the thalamus and are usually responsible for perception of superficial pain, such as pin prick. Eighty per cent of the fibres in the anterior lateral tract are, in fact spinoreticular thalamic fibres and reach the thalamus after synapsing in the reticular nucleus. These are responsible for deep pain perception such as muscle squeeze. These fibres are laminated with sacral fibres located more laterally and therefore more superficially in the cord.
- **Anterior and posterior spinal cerebellar tracts** are responsible for unconscious proprioception and transmit information from the periphery to the cerebellum.

Descending tracts
- The three principle descending tracts are:
- The lateral cortical spinal tracts, which are formed from the motor decussation in the lower medulla are the principle motor tracts.
- The reticular spinal tracts, which modulate activity of the anterior horn cells, are divided into a lateral and medial reticular spinal tract.
- The lateral vestibular spinal tracts transmit information from the vestibular nucleus of the medulla to the anterior horn cells, and are responsible for trunk and limb musculature posture and balance.

> *Nerve roots supplying reflexes*
> - Biceps C5–6.
> - Brachioradialis C5–6.
> - Triceps C7.
> - Knee L3–4.
> - Ankle S1.

Protective layers of the spinal cord
The spinal cord and nerve roots are lined by the meninges, with a tough protective outer layer called the dura mater. The dura mater consists of a delicate lining, the arachnoid mater, within which is the cerebrospinal fluid. The extradural space lies between the dura mater and the bony skeleton, and contains the interval vertebral venous plexus, which drains the bone marrow contained within the vertebral bodies and communicates with the external vertebral venous plexus via the intervertebral foramena.

Blood supply of the spinal cord
The spinal cord receives its blood supply from the anterior spinal artery and the paired posterior spinal arteries.
- The anterior spinal artery lies in the anterior medial fissure of the spinal cord and is formed by the union of the anterior spinal branches of the vertebral arteries. The artery runs down the anterior part of the spinal cord and at times along its course tapers down to quite a small calibre. It receives contributions from so-called booster or feeder vessels, which usually provide both ascending and descending branches. It is possible therefore for there to be 'watershed' areas of perfusion of the spinal cord, where an ascending vessel meets a descending vessel. The anterior spinal artery supplies the anterior and lateral grey and white matter.
- The paired posterior spinal arteries arise from the posterior inferior cerebellar arteries or the vertebral arteries at the level of the foramen magnum. There are some anastamoses between the posterior spinal arteries, and some scanty anastamoses between these and the anterior spinal artery.
- Radicular arteries are present bilaterally at every level in embryonic life, but most undergo involution during foetal growth. The remaining radicular vessels enter the spinal canal via the intervertebral foramen and run along the spinal roots to eventually penetrate the meninges. They divide into anterior and posterior radicular branches, which subsequently divide into ascending and descending contributions to either the anterior spinal artery or posterior spinal arteries, respectively. These booster vessels may originate from the vertebral artery, the thyrocervical trunk, intercostal vessels, lumbar, or lateral sacral arteries. They vary in number and size and may be as few as two or as many as twelve in number. The arteria radicularis magna of Adamkiewicz usually is present on the left side at the T10 or T11 segment, and supplies much of the thoracic spinal cord. This is susceptible to injury during repair of abdominal aortic aneurysms or corrective surgery of the spine and in most units temporary clamping of the segmental vessels is performed prior to manipulation of the spinal column.
- Anastamotic connections on the surface of the cord exist between the anterior spinal and posterior spinal arteries, as well as the radicular vessels. These anastomoses supply the periphery of the cord and the superficial laminae of the cortical spinal and anterolateral tracts. This may be the basis for 'sacral sparing' following spinal cord injury.
- Venous drainage occurs primarily via the anterior and posterior spinal veins, which drain initially into the internal vertebral venous plexus of Batson. This occupies the spinal canal and is hypothesized to play a role in tumour metastases although this is controversial. The internal venous plexus then drains alongside the nerve roots to the external vertebral venous plexus and then the segmental venous system. In the cervical region this is into the vertebral vein, in the thoracic region into the azygos vein, in the lumbar region into the lumbar veins and in the sacral region into the lateral sacral venous system.

Biomechanics of the spine

Upper cervical spine
- The C0/1 articulation, that is the joint between the occipital condyles and the C1 vertebra, is cup-like in morphology. The occipital condyles articulate with the concave superior articular facets of C1. There are a series of ligaments between this complex. The alar ligaments are the principle limitation to axial rotation. There is a significant degree of flexion and extension between the occiput and C1, which averages about 25°. Lateral bend and axial rotation are each 5° to one side.
- The C1/2 joint is a biconvex articulation. Posteriorly C1 and C2 are joined by the loose atlanto-axial membrane. There is no ligamentum flavum. Flexion and extension of the C1/2 joint averages 20°. Axial rotation is maximal at this level of the cervical spine and measures about 40°. This is of clinical relevance in that patients with cervical spondylosis may experience vertebrobasilar insufficiency because of this significant degree of axial rotation. Patients undergoing C1/C2 fusion, such as those patients with rheumatoid arthritis, also need to be advised that any residual rotation that they have may be lost by fusion surgery.
- Overall, 60% of axial rotation of the cervical spine occurs between the C0–C1–C2 complex.

Lower cervical spine
- The C4/5 and C5/6 segments demonstrate the highest degree of flexion and extension averaging about 20° compared with the other segments, which average approximately 10°. This may explain the increased incidence of disc degeneration at these two levels. Lateral bending averages 10° at the C2/3 level and decreases to 5° at C7/T1 level.
- Axial rotation is maximal at the C4/5 and C5/6 levels and averages 7°.

Thoracic spine
Flexion-extension is maximal at the T10/11, T11/12 and T12/L1 segments. The average is approximately 12° at these lower segments and averages about 4° at the other segments of the thoracic spine. Similarly lateral bending is maximal in the lower thoracic spine and averages about 9°, where as at the other segments is averages 6°.

Lumbar spine
Flexion extension in the lumbar spine is maximal at L4/5 and L5/S1, and averages about 17°. These segments are also subjected to the highest loads and this may explain why they are the most subject to degenerative changes.

CHAPTER 5 Regional musculoskeletal anatomy and conditions

Sacro-iliac joint
The sacro-iliac joint is ankylosed in 76% of patients over 50 years old and its movements are very restricted. It is partly synovial and partly syndesmotic. Some biomechanical studies have demonstrated a maximum of 3mm of anterior translation of the sacrum with respect to the ilium with 1.5° of lateral bend and 6° of axial rotation to each side.

Further reading
Bono C.M, Garfin S.R. (eds). *Spine. Orthopaedic Surgery Essentials.* Lippincott, Williams & Wilkins, 2004.
Fardin D, Garfin S (eds). *Orthopaedic Knowledge Update: Spine 2.* American Academy of Orthopaedic Surgeons, 2002.
McMinn RMH. *Last's Anatomy, Regional & Applied*, 9th edn. Churchill Livingstone, 1994.
White AA, Panjabi MM. *Clinical Biomechanics of the Spine*, 2nd edn. Lippincott, Williams & Wilkins, 2004.

Cervical spine: regional musculoskeletal conditions

Main differential diagnosis of cervical pain
- Cervical vertebral body:
  - fracture, e.g. osteoporotic fracture;
  - tumours, e.g. pathological fracture, metastases;
  - osteoid osteoma;
  - metabolic bone disease, e.g. Paget's disease;
  - osteomalacia.
- Mechanical:
  - non-specific neck pain;
  - whiplash;
  - osteoarthritis of the cervical spine;
  - myofascial pain;
  - scoliosis;
  - diffuse idiopathic skeletal hyperostosis.
- Nerve derived:
  - nerve root compression by herniated disc or osteophyte;
  - thoracic outlet syndrome;
  - spinal cord tumours.
- Inflammatory/infection:
  - spondylarthropathy, rheumatoid arthritis;
  - disciitis, meningitis;
  - crystal, e.g. crowned dens syndrome.
- Referred:
  - from pharynx, larynx, thyroid, lymph nodes, praecordium, pericardium, heart, abdomen, shoulder, gastrointestinal tract.

Mechanical neck pain

The term 'mechanical pain' is used here to describe pain, where no specific pathological condition can be identified and also includes degenerative disease. The exact cause of most cases of mechanical neck pain remains unclear. Neck pain is common in the population. Although the incidence of acute, self-limiting neck pain is unclear, the lifetime prevalence of more chronic pain lasting at least 3 months has been estimated as 71% and is commoner in women than men. Risk factors for neck pain, include whiplash, manual occupations, depression, and age.

History
Pain may be related to a new or different activity, or there may be a history of trauma. Where there is no history of trauma, osteoarthritis, or degenerative disc disease is often found. The commonest site of pain is the posterior surface of the neck, with anterior neck pain rarely arising as a result of musculoskeletal causes. The patient describes a deep, aching pain, with superimposed exacerbations of acute pain described as sharp or shooting in nature. In those patients with upper cervical pathology, pain may be experienced over the back of the head and in lower cervical pathology, shoulder pain may be reported. In general, pain is exacerbated by cervical movements, and is better at rest. Pain that differs from this, for example, with unremitting night pain, should raise suspicion and warrants further investigation.

Examination
When pain arises due to mechanical causes, examination of the cervical spine is often unrewarding. Tenderness in the spinous processes and soft tissues should be sought, although pathology is poorly localized clinically. Examination should exclude both other serious musculoskeletal pathologies and non-musculoskeletal causes from anterior structures in the neck. Movements include flexion, extension, lateral flexion, and rotation. Range of movement is poorly estimated in the cervical spine and restricted movement may occur both as a result of mechanical restriction, with little correlation between movements and underlying pathology. Neurological examination is normal in mechanical causes of cervical pain.

Investigations
Blood tests are unhelpful in the investigations of mechanical cervical pain. Plain radiographs of the cervical spine are difficult to interpret as a number of structures are superimposed upon each other. However, in those with non-degenerative mechanical pain, plain radiographs are usually normal. In those patients with degenerative disease, the radiological findings often do not correlate with the severity of clinical symptoms. The incidence of degenerative change of plain radiographs rises with age, is commonest at the C5–6 level, and occurs at the intervertebral disc and the facet joints. Degenerative changes are found in 50% of those over 30 and are almost universal in those over the age of 50. However, because of the poor correlation of symptoms and radiographic spondylosis, plain films are unhelpful diagnostically, and are indicated only to exclude other pathology. The role of CT and MRI remains to be fully established in the investigation of mechanical neck pain as both potentially detect incidental abnormalities, for example, intervertebral disc disease. Their most useful role is in the exclusion of other pathologies.

Management
Patient education, analgesics, and physiotherapy and exercise are central to management. Tricyclic antidepressants may be helpful in chronic pain and work place assessments should be undertaken if indicated. Facet joint injections and denervation are an option in patients in whom pain is thought to arise from these joints.

Cervical disc herniation

Cervical disc herniation is much less common than herniation of lumbar discs. Most commonly the C5–6 or C6–7 intervertebral discs are implicated. As in the lumbar spine, an annular tear in the annulous fibrosis initiates the herniation of the nucleus pulposus. Central discs herniation may result in spinal cord compression, and posterolateral protrusion arises hours or days after a twisting injury with associated dermatome symptoms.

History
Pain and stiffness are common, but radicular pain may be severe and disabling. Rarely, symptoms and signs of spinal cord compression may occur. Coughing and sneezing typically exacerbate the pain.

Examination
Although neurological symptoms are common, hard neurological signs are less commonly found. Weakness may result from fear of exacerbating pain, but dermatomal sensory loss, myotomal weakness and loss of a reflex warrant further investigation. Determining the level of the neurological defect is vital when interpreting the radiological investigations.

CHAPTER 5 Regional musculoskeletal anatomy and conditions

Natural history
Healing occurs by shrinkage and fibrosis of the extruded material, rather than reabsorption of this material into the disc. Resolution of symptoms may take several months. Herniation of an intervertebral disc predisposes to future osteoarthritis.

Investigations
Although plain radiographs may reveal narrowing of the intervertebral disc space, MRI is the investigation of choice as nerve root compression can be readily visualized. However, radiologically it is difficult to differentiate extruded material from osteophytic bars in the cervical spine.

Treatment
Conservative treatment is usually sufficient, although spinal cord compression requires urgent surgical intervention.

Whiplash
Whiplash is a complex topic, and the term refers to a variable set of clinical signs and symptoms. The onset of symptoms usually follows a minor or moderate rear end collision, and a history of a typical shunt type mechanism is usual. Patients usually present with neck pain, but the underlying pathology is as yet undetermined and probably represents a spectrum of soft tissue injury.

Pathology
Both primate and cadaveric models have been used to investigate the injuries sustained in whiplash, and both demonstrate a significant incidence of tears of the anterior longitudinal ligament. High energy trauma has also been demonstrated to cause failure of the disc.

Mechanism of injury
A biphasic mechanism of injury initially involving flexion of the upper cervical spine with hyperextension of the lower spine occurs within the first 110 ms, and is followed by extension of the entire cervical spine. The response to this trauma is modulated by many factors. Patients who have had a history of prior injury demonstrate greater pain behaviour and the presence of pre-existing degenerative change also predicts a poorer outcome. The position of the head at the time of the collision modulates the clinical presentation, so if the head is rotated at the time of collision there is an increased incidence of pain in the long term. Females seem to have a higher symptoms prevalence compared with males.

Prognosis
At least 45% of patients had persistent symptoms at 2 years after resolution of any claims for compensation. In a prospective study involving 93 patients, 58% of patients had continued symptoms in the long-term with 44% of the overall population having substantial neck pain and stiffness.

The rheumatoid spine

Pathology
Spinal involvement in rheumatoid arthritis is a consequence of the formation of pannus: granulation tissue, which is formed by inflammatory cells leading to the destruction of articular cartilage and to synovial proliferation. As a consequence of articular and ligamentous destruction, the spinal elements may become unstable. The most common site of spinal involvement in the rheumatoid patient is the cervical spine. Three distinct patterns of involvement have been reported:
- **Atlanto-axial instability:** this is the commonest pattern of involvement, reported in up to 50% of rheumatoid spinal disease. Lateral and posterior subluxation can also occur.
- **Basilar invagination (cranial settling):** as a consequence of destruction of the occipitocervical and atlanto-axial articulations the base of the skull can 'settle' onto the cervical spine with consequent invagination of the odontoid peg into the foramen magnum. This can lead to direct compression of the brain stem with consequent myelopathic features or sudden death.
- **Subaxial disease:** subaxial subluxation is the least common pattern and is found approximately 10% of rheumatoid spinal disease. The typical radiographic appearance is of a step-type deformity with multiple levels of anterior subluxation of the cervical spine.

History
- Patients may present with neck pain and/or myelopathic features. A common mode of presentation is with occipital headache and facial pain as a consequence of compression of the greater occipital nerve in patients with atlanto-axial instability.
- Patients may report an audible or even a palpable clunk on attempted movement of the neck.
- Atlanto-axial instability or cervical spine involvement in rheumatoid arthritis is frequently an incidental finding on preoperative cervical spine radiographs undertaken prior to anaesthesia for unrelated procedures. Typically, patients undergoing major lower limb joint replacement surgery are noted at anaesthetic assessment to have atlanto-axial instability.

Examination
Physical assessment of these patients is extremely difficult. As a consequence of their usually long-standing rheumatoid arthritis, they frequently have involvement of all the joints of the appendicular skeleton. Clinical assessment of muscle power is therefore difficult in the context of pain, joint destruction, and muscle atrophy. It is important, therefore, that any assessment of neurological status is made in the context of the patient's normal motor function, which is likely to be compromised as a consequence of their disease. Nevertheless, a careful assessment must be made for any myelopathic signs including:
- Up-going plantar reflexes
- Clonus
- Hyperreflexia
- Gait abnormalities

The classification system of mobility developed by Ranawat is the most widely used amongst spinal surgeons. The subdivisions of the Ranawat classification system are listed in Table 5.1.

Table 5.1 Ranawat classification of cervical rheumatoid involvement

Grade 1	No neurological deficit
Grade 2	Subjective weakness and hyperreflexia
Grade 3a	Objective weakness with definite physical signs of myelopathy but in an ambulant patient
Grade 3b	Objective weakness with definitive signs of myelopathy but in a non-ambulatory patient

Investigations
Plain cervical spine radiography and MRI are essential in assessing the rheumatoid patient presenting with cervical spine pain or instability.

- Frontal, lateral, open mouth and flexion-extension views of the cervical spine should be requested. The most useful of these is the lateral radiograph which will often demonstrate destruction of the odontoid peg by pannus. There may also be widening of the anterior atlantodental interval on the neutral lateral radiograph (the normal value is 3 mm).
- Flexion-extension views allow a dynamic assessment of the stability of the occipitocervical spine see Figure 5.6. The posterior atlantodental interval (PADI) should be greater than 14 mm. A PADI of less than 14 mm has been shown to be a good predictor of subsequent neurological compromise.
- The plain lateral radiograph historically was also very useful in determining the presence or absence of cranial settling. The most widely used radiographic parameter is MacGregor's line. This is a line drawn from the base of the occiput to the tip of the hard palate. Any migration of the tip of the peg more proximal to this line than 4.5 mm suggests a diagnosis of cranial settling.
- MRI has superseded plain radiography in the determination of cranial settling. MRI shows with greater clarity if the odontoid peg has migrated into the cranium. It also images the spinal cord, and will confirm evidence of cord compression or myelomalacic signal change within the spinal cord. The disadvantage of MRI is that a static assessment is provided, so the most important screening test remains flexion-extension views of the cervical spine.
- CT remains an important tool in the preoperative assessment of patients with cervical spine involvement in rheumatoid arthritis. MRI does not adequately visualize the bony architecture which must be fully visualized prior to stabilization and decompression of the cervical spine. CT imaging is particularly useful in assessing the course of the vertebral artery within the C2 lateral masses and aids identification of those patients in whom transarticular screw fixation is not feasible.

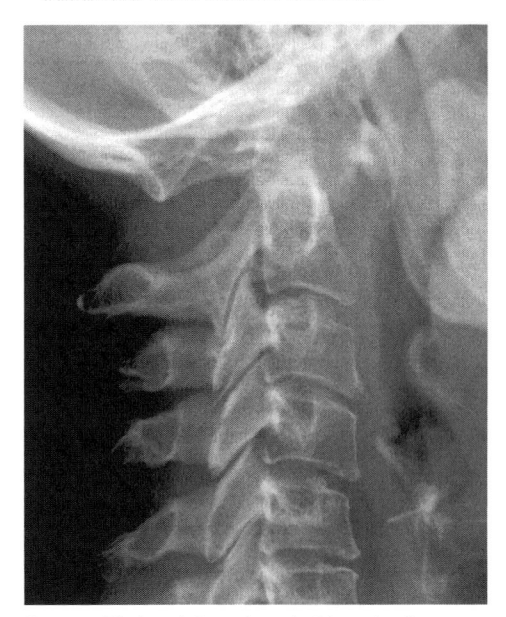

Figure 5.6 This lateral plain radiograph of the neck in flexion demonstrates an increased atlanto-axial distance.

Treatment
Treatment aims to alleviate pain and restore stability of the cervical spine. In patients with severe medical co-morbidities, such as ischaemic heart disease and multi-organ impairment, surgical treatment may be deemed too risky. Immunosuppressed patients carry an increased risk of post-operative complications, such as infection and wound break-down, so the decision to operate on these patients is made on an individual case-by-case basis following consultation between rheumatologist, anaesthetist, and surgeon.

Surgical techniques
- Amongst the earliest techniques described for C1–C2 stabilization were sublaminar wiring techniques as described by Gallie and Brooks. Modern plate and screw techniques allow solid reconstruction of the occipitocervical or atlanto-axial articulations. Coexisting osteoporosis is technically challenging at surgery. Prophylactic surgery prior to neurological deficit remains controversial. There is good evidence to show that those who present with a more advanced neurological deficit have a poorer postoperative outcome in terms of restoration of function. In patients with Ranawat grade 2b disease only 20% of patients showed one grade of improvement following surgery versus 58% of patients with Ranawat grade 3a disease.
- Procedures for pain relief, such as atlanto-axial stabilization for occipital neuralgia, have a success rate of around 80%. Modern stabilization techniques often negate the use of postoperative halo immobilization and often only a cervical collar is required until fusion is achieved. This is obviously a benefit in this population which is usually frail.
- There is recent evidence to show that good results can be anticipated even in those patients who do not achieve a good radiographic fusion, probably because of the lower functional demands of rheumatoid patients.

Intervertebral disciitis
Cervical and thoracic disciitis are less common than lumbar disciitis (see Chapter 16 p. 454, Infection, and lumbar disciitis).

Tumours related to the cervical spine
Tumours of the cervical spine may present in the spinal cord, the meninges, a peripheral nerve, for example, a neurofibroma, or from the vertebral column itself. Metastatic malignancy is commoner than primary malignant tumours. Brachial plexus involvement may result from a Pancoast tumour in the apex of the lung. Presentation is with spinal cord compression, symptoms attributable to local destruction or progressive nerve symptoms.

Torticollis in children
Torticollis is derived from the Latin and literally translates as 'twisted neck'.

Causes
Torticollis may be congenital or acquired.
- The congenital causes may be due to an underlying muscular abnormality, accounting for 80% of congenital torticollis. Causes include a sternocleidomastoid mass, sternocleidomastoid tightness or may occur despite a normal sternocleidomastoid. The remaining 20% of congenital torticollis results from bony abnormalities. These include failure of formation of the upper cervical bones (for example, a congenital hemi-atlas) or due to failure

of segmentation of the upper cervical spine bony elements (such as occurs in Kippel–Feil syndrome). A combination of these bony abnormalities may be present.
- Acquired torticollis is best classified as painful or non-painful. The most common cause of painful acquired torticollis is trauma resulting in atlanto-axial rotatory subluxation. Tumours such as eosinophilic granuloma and osteoid osteoma may cause painful torticollis, and need to be entertained in the differential diagnosis in a child presenting with pain and an abnormal attitude of the head and neck. Inflammatory causes include JIA and post-infectious torticollis. Gastro-oesophageal reflux may be associated with painful torticollis and is referred to as the Sandifer syndrome. The most important differential diagnosis in the older child presenting with a non-painful torticollis is an underlying central nervous system tumour or a syrinx, although the commonest cause is ocular, with the child compensating for weakness of the ocular muscles. Hysterical torticollis is a diagnosis of exclusion.

Clinical presentation
The appearance of the deformity may be variable, but usually the child demonstrates a restricted range of movement of the cervical spine. There may be associated plagiocephaly or facial asymmetry depending on the duration of symptoms. A mass is palpable in the sternocleidomastoid on the ipsilateral side of the head tilt before 6 weeks of life in up to one-third of patients. Torticollis that corrects on covering one of the eyes is due to an underlying ocular cause, and a compensatory manoeuvring of the head and neck.

Investigations
Investigations should include anteroposterior and lateral radiographs of the cervical spine to exclude underlying bony abnormalities. In children presenting with painful torticollis a CT scan should be undertaken to exclude underlying tumour, such as osteoid osteoma. An MRI scan is useful to exclude underlying central nervous system tumours in patients with painless torticollis.

Natural history
The natural history is variable. If there is a sternocleidomastoid mass palpable there is a 50–70% chance of resolution by 1 year. A small sub-group of about 10% of patients require surgical intervention.

Treatment
Treatment is normally conservative with regular follow-up. Orthoses do not seem to be helpful. Exercise and stretching have been demonstrated to yield good results and up to 90% improve with this method. The best results are obtained in patients less than 3 months of age with less successful results in children over 18 months of age.

Indications for surgery
Surgery is indicated in patients with significant head tilt and restriction of movement, where a tight band is palpable in the sternocleidomastoid. Surgery is usually delayed until the patient is over age 1 year and where there has been a failure of non-operative treatment. Surgery may involve a release of the muscle from one or two sites of its attachment, and may involve complete division of the tendon or Z-plasty. Partial or complete muscle resection has also been performed. In general, 90% of patients undergoing surgery have a good result.

Further reading
Clarke CR (ed.). *The Cervical Spine*, 4th edn. The Cervical Spine Research Society/Lippincott, Williams and Wilkins, 2004.

Hildingsson C, Toolanen G. Outcome after soft tissue injury of the cervical spine: Prospective study of 93 car-accident victims. *Acta Orthop Scand* 1990; **61**: 357–9.

Riise T, Jacobsen BK, Gran JT. High mortality in patients with Rheumatoid Arthritis and atlanto-axial subluxation. *J Rheumatol.* 2001; **61**: 357–9.

Roche CJ, Eyes BE, Whitehouse GH. The rheumatoid cervical spine: signs of instability on plain cervical radiographs. *Clin Radiol* 2002; **57**: 241–9.

Santavirta S, Slatis P, Kankaanpaa U, Sandelin J, Laasonen. Treatment of the cervical spine in rheumatoid arthritis. *J BJS(a)* 1988; **70**: 658–67.

Cheung JCY, Wong MWN, Tang SP, Chen TMR, Shum SLF, Wong EMC. Clinical determinates of the outcome of manual stretching in the treatment of congenital muscular torticollis in infants. *JBJS* (a) 2001; **83**; 679–87.

Demirbilek S, Atayurt H. Congenital muscular torticollis and sternomostoid tumour: results of non-operative treatment. *J Pediatr Surg* 1999; **34**: 549–51.

Thoracic spine and chest wall: regional musculoskeletal conditions

Main differential diagnosis of thoracic and chest wall pain

Thoracic vertebral body
- Fracture, e.g. osteoporotic fracture.
- Tumours, e.g. pathological fracture, metastases, osteoid osteoma.
- Metabolic bone disease, e.g. Paget's disease, osteomalacia.

Mechanical
- Osteoarthritis of the thoracic spine.
- Scoliosis.
- Costovertebral joint disease.
- Diffuse idiopathic skeletal hyperostosis.
- Olecranon bursitis.

Nerve derived
- Nerve root compression by herniated disc or osteophyte.
- Pathology of intercostal nerve, e.g. herpes zoster, neuroma.

Inflammatory/infection
- Spondylarthropathy.
- Disciitis osteomyelitis.
- Crystal, e.g. calcium pyrophosphate deposition.

Chest wall lesions
- Rib, e.g. fracture, tumours, osteomalacia.
- Costochondral pathology, e.g. degenerative, rheumatoid arthritis.
- Soft tissue, e.g. intercostal muscle tear, myofascial pain, fibromyalgia, enthesitis.
- Pleural disease, e.g. infection, inflammation, infiltration.
- Breast pathology, e.g. mastitis.

Others
- Scheuermann's.
- Cardiac/praecordial disease.

Thoracic pain is less common that cervical and lumbar pain, and a lower threshold for investigating thoracic pain is therefore warranted.

Scheuermann's disease

Scheuermann's disease was previously called osteochondritis, although this term is now generally avoided. The intervertebral disc protrudes into the adjacent vertebral bodies, at either single or multiple levels in the spine, most commonly involving the thoracic spine. This process results in wedging of the vertebral body and multiple vertebral body involvement results in kyphosis. The cause is unclear but Scheuermann's disease is a risk factor for developing osteoarthritis in later life.

Pathology
Ossification of the vertebral bodies occurs in three places, the primary centre being the middle of the vertebral body and the other, secondary centres being in the upper and lower margins of each vertebral body. The secondary centres are also known as ring epiphyses, and these appear around puberty in the adolescent within the cartilaginous end plates that lie between the developing vertebral body and the intervertebral disc. In Scheuermann's disease, the cartilaginous end plate and ring epiphysis do not develop normally, and the disc protrudes through the cartilage into the vertebral body. The anterior surface is that portion of the vertebral body, which is exposed to the greatest weight-bearing force and is, therefore, that portion most likely to be involved. The disc space narrows anteriorly and wedging of the vertebral body occurs.

History
Pain in the thoracic spine in children aged between 13 and 16 is typical, although this pain is usually self-limiting after a few months. Pain may recur at a later stage as secondary degenerative change develops.

Examination
Examination reveals a tender kyphosis during the 'active' phase of Scheuermann's disease, although this tenderness settles, leaving a pain free kyphosis.

Investigations
Plain radiographs confirm deep notches in the anterior corners of the vertebral bodies. The corresponding epiphyseal rings may also appear irregular. The disc spaces are narrowed, particularly anteriorly. Wedging may be obvious in the anterior portion of the vertebral body and there may be degenerative change later in life. See Figure 5.7.

Treatment
Conservative treatment with analgesia and physiotherapy is the main stay of therapy. Intervertebral grafting is rarely undertaken and only in severe cases.

Thoracic spondylosis

Spondylosis of the thoracic spine presents in a similar fashion to that of the cervical and lumbar spine. Investigations and management are discussed in these sections.

CHAPTER 5 Regional musculoskeletal anatomy and conditions

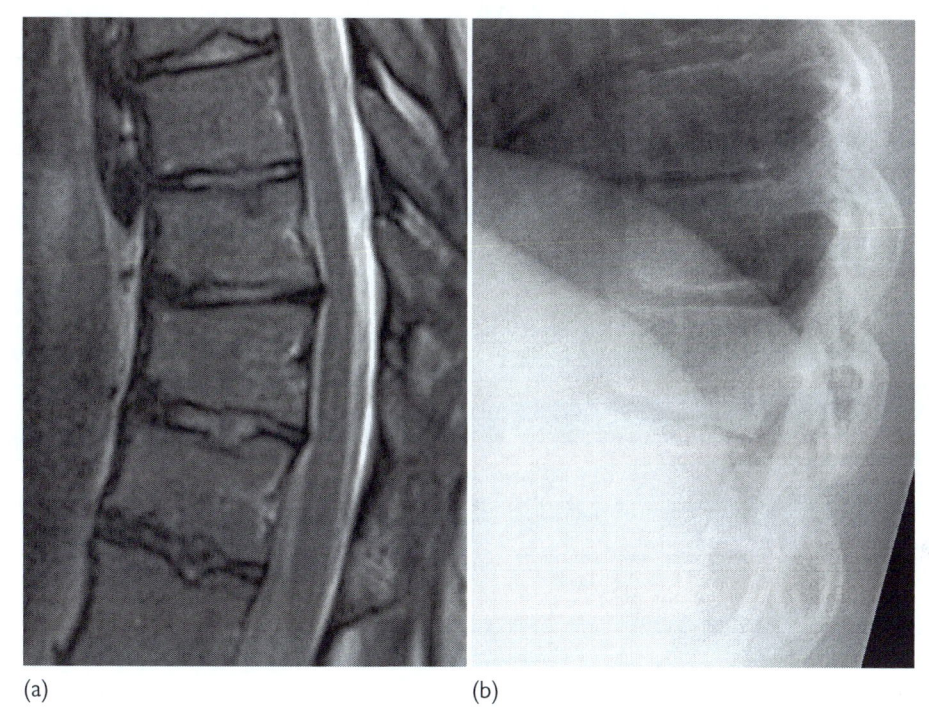

Figure 5.7 This is lateral plain radiograph (a) and a sagittal T2-weighted MR (b) of the lower thoracic spine in a patient with Scheuermann's disease demonstrating anterior wedging and endplate irregularity over three contiguous levels.

Table 5.2 Important features in the history in patients with chest pain

Cardiac pain	• Angina – pain less than 30 mins, usually exertional, typically central and crushing with radiation into arms and jaw. Associated nausea, dyspnoea and sweating.
	• Myocardial infarction is usually more severe and pro-longed.
	• Pericardial disease is typically central sharp pain which may be eased on leaning forward
	• Aortic disease – severe and of acute onset.
Pleural disease	Sharp and exacerbated by inspiration. Pain is superficial. There may be a history of haemoptysis.
Gastrointestinal disease	Retrosternal burning which may be related to eating.
	Peptic disease may radiate to the back
Mediastinal pain	May be intense and radiate to shoulder or may mimic pleural pain.
Musculoskeletal	Insidious in onset, often with a history of recent unfamiliar repetitive activity or upper body. The position of the pain may be localised or diffuse in position and may be exacerbated by specific movements. It may be persistent and prolonged

Musculoskeletal chest wall pain

History
A careful history is important to exclude non-musculoskeletal cause of chest pain. Features of bone pain systemic features and other associated muscu-loskeletal symptoms should be sought.

Examination
Tenderness may be revealed over the costochondral joints in costochondritis, and soft tissue tenderness is common in myofascial pain. Localised rib pathology may reveal bony tenderness over the affected rib. There may be hypomobility of that proportion of the chest wall on deep inspiration. A full medical and neurological exami-nation should be undertaken in all patients with chest pain and thoracic pain.

Investigations
Elevation of serum alkaline phosphastase is suggestive of bone pathology and requires further investigation. Imag-ing is best undertaken with plain radiographs, although isotope bone scintigraphy will detect increased uptake in, metastatic disease, Paget's disease and osteoid osteomas. CT gives more specific bone detail and MRI is indicated in patients with symptoms suggestive of nerve root or cord compression.

Treatment
The treatment should be aimed at the underlying condition. In patients with localised chest wall pain but without significant underlying pathology, reassurance and patient education is central. Physical therapies, simple analgesia and topical or oral NSAIDs may help. Neuralgic pain may respond to amytryptiline and local glucocorticoid with local anaesthetic infiltration may relieve localised tenderness or costochondral pain.

Lumbar spine: regional musculoskeletal conditions

Main differential diagnosis of lumbar pain

Lumbar vertebral body
- Fracture, e.g. osteoporotic fracture.
- Tumours, e.g. multiple myeloma, metastases.
- Metabolic bone disease, e.g. Paget's disease, osteomalacia.

Mechanical
- Non-specific low back pain.
- Osteoarthritis of the lumbar spine.
- Spondylolisis.
- Scoliosis.
- Spinal stenosis.
- Diffuse idiopathic skeletal hyperostosis.
- Hypermobility.

Nerve derived
Nerve root compression by herniated disc or osteophyte.

Inflammatory/infection
- Spondylarthropathy/sacroiliitis.
- Disciitis/osteomyelitis.

Referred
- Retroperitoneal fibrosis.
- Renal disease, e.g. infection.
- Abdominal aortic aneurysm.
- Gynaecological disease.

Others
- Schueurmann's disease.
- Fibromyalgia.

Acute low back pain

Low back pain is extremely common and is estimated to affect 14% of the population at any time. There is a lifetime prevalence of between 58 and 80%. Associated factors include lower social class, work-related injuries particularly in manual occupations, neck pain, and other widespread musculoskeletal pain, and depression. Although back pain is common in all age groups, the highest prevalence is in those in their 5th and 6th decade. The costs of low back pain in the UK are huge with 4.9 billion working days lost per annum, with an estimated cost of £5 billion to the economy in 2005. The average time of work for each episode of low back pain is 19 days according to the Labour Force Survey 2003/4.

History
The onset of pain is acute, and there may be a history of precipitating activity or injury. The pain is improved by immobility and exacerbated by particular actions or movement. There is usually little night pain.

Examination
The aim of examination is to exclude underlying pathologies. Range of movement is generally unhelpful in delineating the underlying cause, as movements are generally restricted by muscle spasm.

Investigations
Investigations are normal in mechanical back pain, and indeed most patients do not require investigations. There is little correlation between low back pain and degenerative change on plain radiographs, and investigations are only indicated if there is doubt about the clinical diagnosis.

Treatment
The natural history of low back pain is that 50% improve after a week, and more than 90% are better at 8 weeks. Treatment is therefore conservative, with analgesia and exercise. Bed rest should be actively discouraged. Early activity helps pain and reassurance should be given that exercise is not causing harm despite pain. Exacerbations of pain are common and there is weak evidence that exercise alone has any impact on the prevention of further episodes.

Chronic low back pain

7–10% of those with an acute episode of back pain have continuing symptoms after 6 months, often with diffuse, non-specific leg pain. There is often an underlying cause identified, such as chronic disc herniation, degenerative disc disease, fibromyalgia, psychological factors, or scar tissue following surgery, although altered chronic pain pathways also contribute to ongoing pain patterns. Altered pain behaviour, with widespread superficial pain, non-anatomical weakness and sensory loss, and restricted straight leg raise on formal testing, but ability to sit with the legs extended all suggest a non-organic cause. Investigations include routine blood tests and imaging to exclude other pathology. Pharmacological options include simple analgesia, non-steroidal anti-inflammatory agents, and tricyclic antidepressants or antiepileptic drugs in those with a neuralgic component. Exercise and physiotherapy encourage physical function, and build on patient education. Local injections can be helpful in some cases, and include facet joints injections, epidurals, and trigger point injections. Back pain programmes involve the full multidisciplinary team, including psychologists, and offer some success in the management of pain, but access to these places is often restricted.

Lumbar spondylosis

The causes of spondylosis are multifactorial, with both genetic and environmental factors playing a role. Predisposing conditions include Schueurmann's disease. The joints most commonly affected are the body to body (central) joint between vertebral bodies, and the posterior intervertebral or facet joints. In the central discs, disc space narrowing is often the first manifestation, with subsequent osteophyte formation. Osteophytes may encroach on the nerve root foramen.

History
Low back pain is common, often exacerbated by activity and often positional, so that particular activities such as putting on shoes and socks cause discomfort. There may be exacerbations of acute pain on a background of more chronic pain.

Examination
The clinical findings are non-specific and there may be some global restriction of lumbar movements. Neurological findings are rare.

Investigations
There is poor correlation between the extent of radiographic abnormalities and the severity of clinical symptoms.

Treatment
Simple analgesics and exercise is indicated for spinal spondylosis, with NSAIDs best reserved for flares. Physiotherapy encourages regular exercise. Targeted injections, such as facet joints injections and epidurals can be repeated in those who find them helpful.

Spondylolysis and spondylolisthesis
Spondylolisis is defined as a defect in the pars intra-articularis, usually of the 5th neural arch, although less commonly the 4th neural arch may be affected. Congenital defects cause the majority of cases, but injury in childhood or adolescence, particularly among those who play sport, is now increasingly recognized. Spondylolysis is a common finding and often of no clinical significance. However, deep low back pain is sometimes described. Spondylolisthesis describes spontaneous displacement of a vertebral body in relation to the vertebral body directly beneath. Usually, the direction of displacement is anterior, but occasionally it may be posterior, termed a retrospondylolisthesis. Underlying causes of spondylolisthesis include congenital malformation, spondylolysis, and posterior facet osteoarthritis. The commonest congenital abnormality is an inadequate posterior intervertebral joint, which normally prevents anterior displacement of the vertebral bodies. Spondylolisis allows separation of the two halves of the neural arch with gradual displacement on the vertebral body, particularly in young adulthood. Osteoarthritis of the posterior facet joint results in thinning of the cartilage, which causes instability of the facet joint and posterior displacement. In both the congenital and spondylolisthesis types, neurological compromise may arise and may be severe, but in the osteoarthritis associated model neurological involvement is rare.

Clinical findings
Spondylolisis is often asymptomatic, and those with symptoms of a spondylolisthesis often depend on the underlying mechanism. Pain may present in young adults or conversely may present in an older population who develop osteoarthritis. Often pain is worse on standing. Examination is often unhelpful, but neurological signs should be sought.

Investigations
Plain radiographs in the oblique view demonstrate abnormalities of the neural arch and the extent of the spondylolisthesis. MRI is the investigation of choice when there are neurological symptoms.

Treatment
Conservative treatment with analgesia and physiotherapy is appropriate, in all but the most severe cases, where spinal fusion may be offered.

Lumbar disc herniation
The L4/5 and L5/S1 discs are most commonly involved in lumbar disc herniation leading to symptomatic radiculopathy. An annular tear facilitates herniation of the nucleus pulposus. Radicular pain arises both due to the compressive affects of the disc protrusion on the involved nerve root and also a chemically mediated inflammatory process.

- The most common site for lumbar disc protrusion is in the posterolateral disc region due to the relative deficiency in the posterior longitudinal ligaments in this region.
- Such protrusions tend to cause compression of the traversing nerve roots. A posterolateral L4/5 disc protrusion could therefore be expected to cause symptoms related to an L5 radiculopathy.
- Less common sites of symptomatic disc herniation include foraminal disc protrusions and far lateral disc protrusions. These far lateral variants tend to compress the exiting nerve root. A far lateral L4/5 disc protrusion could be expected, therefore, to cause symptoms related to L4 nerve root compression.

History
The patient is typically a young adult in the third or forth decade of life. There may be an antecedent history of back pain related to an underlying annular tear. The patient typically reports a sudden onset of severe leg pain in association with their back pain. The distribution of the leg pain may suggest which nerve is involved. S1 radiculopathy manifests as posterior thigh, calf, and heel pain with pain radiating into the lateral border of the foot. Pain related to L5 radiculopathy more typically involves the lateral aspect of the calf and dorsum of the foot. There is frequent overlap of the distribution of pain however.

Examination
The patient may present with a list. L5 radiculopathy may result in dysfunction of the hip abductors and may lead to a Trendelenberg-type gait or a positive Trendelenberg's test. The knee jerk may be absent when the L5 nerve root is involved and in S1 nerve root involvement the ankle jerk may be absent or diminished. Weakness of the tibialis anterior or extensor hallucis longus muscles implicates L5 nerve root compression and weakness of flexor hallucis and ankle eversion suggests S1 compression. The dermatomal alteration of sensibility may also suggest particular nerve root involvement. A particularly important sign is the presence or absence of nerve root tension signs. The most widely used of these is the straight leg raise test where the lower limb is elevated by flexing the hip passively with the knee fully extended. Reproduction of the radicular type pain suggests nerve root compression. Pain aggravated by passive dorsiflexion of the ankle is said to indicate a positive sciatic stretch test and lends further support to the diagnosis of radiculopathy.

Investigations
The currently most widely used investigation is MRI.

- MRI demonstrates the extent and direction of disc protrusion and confirms if there are sequestrated fragments. MRI also allows clear visualization of the cauda equina and has replaced CT myelography as the investigation of choice.
- It is possible to demonstrate disc protrusions on conventional CT, but there is less good soft tissue definition and very large disc protrusions, which occupy most of the spinal canal can be mistakenly interpreted on CT to represent a normal cauda equina.

Treatment
The vast majority of symptomatic lumbar disc protrusions respond to non-operative treatment. Patients should be prescribed analgesics and, where appropriate, non-steroidal anti-inflammatory medication. Strict bed rest should not be enforced and the patient should be encouraged to mobilize as much as comfort allows. Approximately 80% of patients have resolution of their radicular symptoms within 6–8 weeks of initial presentation. In instances where conventional analgesics are not effecting in controlling radicular pain, an epidural steroid injection or selective nerve root block under CT or fluoroscopic guidance usually relieves the leg pain.

LUMBAR SPINE: REGIONAL MUSCULOSKELETAL CONDITIONS

Surgical treatment
Surgical treatment is reserved for:
- Patients with severe intractable pain that does not settle with non-operative treatment, regardless of duration of symptoms.
- Patients with progressive neurological deterioration in the presence of a lumbar disc protrusion. This may be manifested by progressively worsening weakness of tibialis anterior, which if left untreated may result in a permanent foot drop.
- Cauda equina syndrome: this represents compression of the cauda equina elements, which innervate the bowel and bladder, and are responsible for autonomic function. It typically presents with bilateral sciatica, severe back pain, and there may be variable urological problems ranging from increased urinary frequency to overt overflow incontinence. A rectal examination must be performed in any such patient with particular attention paid to the absence of perianal sensibility and loss or diminution of anal sphincter tone. Emergency surgical decompression is required. A large meta-analysis has suggested that the outcome is more favourable in patients who have decompressive surgery within 48 h of presentation with cauda equina syndrome.

Lumbar spinal stenosis

Lumbar spinal stenosis is defined as narrowing of the lumbar spinal canal with consequent symptomatic neural compression. The pathological findings typically include:
- A central or paracentral disc bulge.
- Facet joint hypertrophy, most typically of the medial side of the superior articular facet.
- Buckling of the ligamentum flavum.
- There may also be associated loss of disc height leading to narrowing of the exit foramina.

The overall effect of these pathological changes is narrowing of the space available for the neural elements within the spinal canal.

Classification
Lumbar spinal stenosis can be broadly divided into congenital and acquired forms. There may be idiopathic congenital narrowing of the spinal canal. Congenital lumbar stenosis is also commonly seen in achondroplasia. The most commonly recognized acquired form of lumbar spinal stenosis is degenerative stenosis. It may also occur following previous trauma or secondary to metabolic bone disease such as Paget's disease. Lumbar spinal stenosis may be further classified according to the site of the spinal canal narrowing.
- Lateral recess stenosis refers to narrowing of the space bounded by the lateral edge of the dura and the medial border of the pedicle.
- Central canal stenosis refers to narrowing of the space within the spinal canal available for the cauda equina and the dura itself.
- These two variants frequently co-exist.

History
Lumbar spinal stenosis typically presents in patients in later life and usually in those over the age of 55. It is more

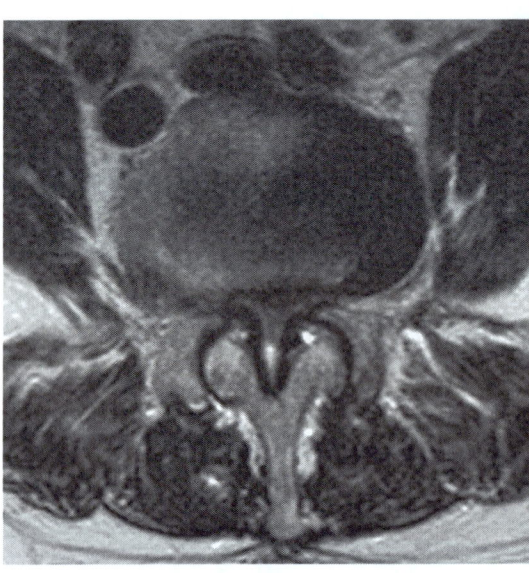

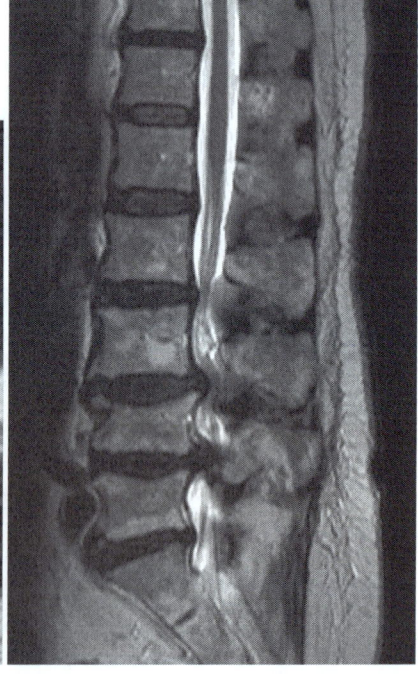

(a) (b)

Figure 5.8 This is a sagittal (a) and axial (b) T1- and T2-weighted MR of the lumbar spine demonstrating spinal stenosis at L3/4 and L4/5 where the CSF is completely effaced around the cauda equina.

common in males. The classical presentation is of neurogenic claudication with the patient reporting limitation of walking distance. On walking the patient typically experiences heaviness, weakness, in coordination, or pain in the lower limbs, which is eased by sitting and resting or by stooping forward.

Examination
Examination is typically normal. Hip examination must be conducted to exclude hip osteoarthritis and the peripheral circulation must be assessed to exclude vascular claudication. The patient typically stands and walks with a stooped forward posture, and has pain which is aggravated by extension of the spine.

Investigations
The gold standard of investigation was conventionally a CT myelogram, which has the advantage of being a dynamic assessment of cauda equina compression. Its principle disadvantage is its invasive nature. It has largely been superseded by MRI, which gives excellent anatomical detail of the soft tissue elements without the need for ionizing radiation or invasive procedure. See Figure 5.8.

Treatment
The natural history of lumbar spinal stenosis is variable. Many studies have demonstrated that progression is not invariable and in one study of patients followed up for 4 years, approximately 40% of patients had no change in their symptoms with 40% showing some degree of improvement. This is relevant when developing management plans.

- **Non-operative treatment:** non-operative treatment is advocated for most patients presenting with mild to moderate lumbar spinal stenosis. Simple analgesia and epidural injections may be effective. These can be repeated if symptomatic relief is obtained for a reasonable length of time.
- **Operative treatment:** surgery involves decompression of the neural elements. This is usually achieved posteriorly either by conventional laminectomy or a laminotomy procedure, which attempts to preserve the midline posterior elements. The aim of the surgery is to remove the ligamentum flavum and the medial side of the facet joint to increase the cross-sectional area of the spinal canal and the lateral recess. Where there is an associated spondylolisthesis the spine may be fused either with or without instrumentation.

Sacroiliac pain
Sacroiliac disease may be inflammatory (see Chapter 7 p. 210) or degenerative.

Sacroiliitis
A history of chronic pain lasting at least 3 months is typical, with early morning stiffness lasting more than 30 min. Pain is often described as buttock pain or proximal posterior thigh pain. Symptoms are normally better with exercise and not improved by rest. Sleep may be disturbed, especially in the early morning. Examination may reveal globally restricted spinal movements, and Schober's test or a modified Schober's test may confirm restriction of spinal movements. Inflammatory markers are often normal, and plain radiographic evidence of sacroiliitis may not be present in early disease. MR is a more sensitive technique for detecting early inflammatory change within the sacroiliac joints, although because the natural history of sacroiliitis remains unclear, it remains to be established how many of those will develop plain radiographic changes in the future.

Degenerative sacroiliac pain
Degenerative sacroiliac pain is rarely the cause of significant symptoms and is often picked up incidentally. However, in those with significant symptoms or doubt about the origin of pain, an image-guided injection targeted to the sacroiliac joint may be beneficial.

Lumbar disciitis
Vertebral osteomyelitis and disciitis usually arise from haematogenous spread, although the exact source of infection may not be clear. The origin of infection may remain obscure.

Clinical features
The symptoms include insidious onset of pain with spinal tenderness on examination. 15% have symptoms and signs of nerve root compression at presentation. Fever is present in less than half of patient.

Investigations
- Inflammatory markers are normally elevated as is the neutrophil count.
- The organism may be isolated on blood cultures.
- MR is the imaging technique of choice and details the abscess clearly.
- Culture of biopsy material is positive in around 50% with *S. aureus* and coagulase negative staphylococci the commonest causative organisms.

Management
- Management is normally conservative with debridement indicated in those with neurological involvement.
- Antibiotics should be continued for 4–6 weeks. Neurological examination should be performed regularly to detect neurological compromise due to spreading infection. Bony fusion often occurs after 1–2 years of infection.

Coccydynia
Coccydynia is the term used to describe pain arising from the region of the coccyx. The commonest clinical presentation of pain is of chronic pain arising from a previous injury, and lasting weeks or even months. Pain is normally self-limiting, and may arise from trauma to the sacro-coccygeal joint or perioseal bruising. Pain is often worse on sitting and sometimes on defaecation. There may be localized tenderness, and clinical examination and radiographs must be performed to exclude other pathologies, such as infection. Plain radiographs may reveal a fracture if there has been sufficient trauma. Treatment is conservative and includes reassurance about the natural history, although local anaesthetic and steroid injection may alleviate symptoms. Rarely, surgical excision is necessary.

Adult scoliosis
Scoliosis is defined as sideward bending of the spine, resulting in a deformity of the spine in the coronal plane. Adult scoliosis is broadly defined into two groups:
- **Idiopathic adult scoliosis:** this represents scoliosis that has been present since adolescence, which has continued to progress into adulthood. The patient may or may not present with superimposed degenerative changes. Adolescent idiopathic scoliosis may continue to progress into adulthood. This is particularly true for curves in the lumbar region which are greater than 50° in magnitude, and where there is significant apical or lateral listhesis. The prevalence of adult scoliosis is approximately 6%. Where there is pre-existing adolescent idiopathic

scoliosis the rate of progression is approximately 1–2° per year.
- **De novo adult scoliosis:** as a consequence of degenerative changes within the spine a deformity arises *de novo* in a previously straight spine. *De novo* scoliosis tends to present in the older age group, typically in patients in their 60s and 70s. The curve progression in the de novo group appears to be more rapid and averages 3–4° per year.

History
- The patient with *de novo* scoliosis typically presents with back pain. This is due to a combination of factors including facet joint degeneration, disc degeneration, and costopelvic impingement when there is a significant kyphotic deformity in association with the scoliosis. The patient may also present with pain secondary to osteoporotic compression fractures or due to muscle fatigue because of the abnormal spinal posture.
- Adult scoliosis patients may also present with spinal claudication or radiculopathy secondary to neural compression. Patients may report progressively increasing deformity and loss of height.

Examination
Examination establishes the degree of rigidity of the curve, as well as the degree of coronal and sagittal imbalance. A careful neurological examination needs to be performed.

Investigations
- Standard scoliosis radiographs including long cassette posterior-anterior and lateral X-rays should be obtained. Bending films aid the assessment of the rigidity of the curves.
- MRI should be performed in all patients presenting with stenotic symptoms or with radicular symptoms, with CT myelograms reserved for those in whom MRI is contraindicated.

Treatment
- Non-surgical treatment should initially be undertaken. Physiotherapy may help with core stability and muscle strengthening. Pain management strategies are crucial and include the use of NSAIDs, as well as epidural steroid injections, facet joint injections and nerve root blocks. Obese patients are encouraged to lose weight, although in this elderly age group weight loss and exercise compliance are often poor.
- Surgical treatment should be reserved for patients who have severe intractable pain that is not controlled by non operative measures. Surgery is also indicated where, uncommonly, there is progressive neurological deterioration. Progression of the deformity is also a relative indication for surgical treatment. Surgery may be fairly minimal, decompressing a single stenotic segment, but in those with progressive disease more extensive surgery to stabilise the spine and provide a solid arthrodesis is necessary. This is often required in a high risk population in whom preoperative assessment and medical optimization is vital. Complications of surgery can be serious and the complication rates are high with pseudoarthrosis demonstrated in up to 28%. There is a significant risk of intraoperative bleeding, graft site morbidity and neurological complications. Infection, wound breakdown and instrumentation failure are not uncommon.

Further reading

Ahn UM, Ahn NU, Buchowski JM, Garrett ES, Sieber AN, Kostuik JP. Cauda equina syndrome secondary to lumbar discherniation. A meta-analysis of surgical outcomes. *Spine* 2000; **25**: 1515–22.

Atlas SJ, Keller RB, Wu YA, Deyo RA, Singer DE. Long-term outcomes of surgical and non-surgical management of lumbar spinal stenosis: 8-10 year results from the Maine Lumbar Spine Study. *Spine* 2005; **30**: 927–935.

Daubs MD, Lenke LG, Cheh G, Stobbs G, Bridwell KH. Adult spinal deformity surgery: complications and outcomes in patients aged over 60. *Spine* 2007; **32**: 2238–44.

Johnsson KE, Rosen I, Uden A. The natural course of lumbar spinal stenosis. *Clin Orthop Relat Res* 1992; **279**: 82–6.

Peul WC, van Houwelingen HC, van der Hout WB, Brand R, Eekhof JAH, Tans JTJ, Thormeer RTWM, Koes BW. Surgery versus prolonged conservative treatment for sciatica. *NEJM* 2007; **356**: 2245–56.

CHAPTER 5 Regional musculoskeletal anatomy and conditions

The shoulder

The shoulder has evolved to provide ability for the hand to reach almost any position relative to the trunk.

Regional anatomy

Movement in the shoulder occurs in four linked articular areas: at the sternoclavicular joint (SCJ), at the acromioclavicular joint (ACJ), at the glenohumeral joint (GHJ), and at the scapulothoracic articulation. Movement at the GHJ can occur in isolation, but movement at the scapulothoracic articulation is accompanied by movement at the ACJ and SCJ joints (See also Plate 1).

Bones

The upper limb is attached to the axial skeleton indirectly, first by the clavicle, which articulates with the sternum at the sternoclavicular joint, and secondly by muscles, which attach the humerus to the scapula.

The clavicle

The clavicle acts as a bony strut holding the shoulder joint away from the chest wall. The anterior aspect of the clavicle is convex medially and concave laterally, and the medial end is bulbous, whereas the lateral end is flattened. It articulates with the sternoclavicular joint at the medial end and the acromioclavicular joint at the lateral end.

The scapular

The scapular has a concave anterior surface and convex posterior surface. The posterior surface is crossed by the spine of the scapular, which increases in height as it crosses from the medial side to the lateral side. At the lateral end of the spine of the scapular it sweeps superiorly and anteriorly above the glenoid, and expands to form the acromion process.

The lateral free edge of the spine is angled posterosuperiorly and arises from the scapular at the same level at which the coracoid process arises from the anterolateral margin of the scapular. When viewed from the lateral side these two processes (spine of scapular posteriorly and coracoid process anteriorly) appear to arise from the region of the neck of the glenoid at the 10'o'clock and 2'o'clock positions, respectively, and account for the 'propellar' appearance of a 'lateral scapular' X-ray view (viewing the lateral aspect of the scapular end-on).

Muscles either take origin from or insert into almost every aspect of the scapular, and hold the scapular in place over the posterolateral chest wall.

Joints of the shoulder

Glenohumeral joint

The head of the humerus lies adjacent to the glenoid and beneath the acromion process, which arches above, with a concave undersurface in both anteroposterior and mediolateral directions. The humeral head is held in place by a combination of ligaments and muscles. The articular surface of the glenoid fossa on the scapula is lined by articular cartilage (the glenoid labrum). See Figure 5.9.

Glenohumeral joint capsule

The capsule is attached around the circumference of the outer edge of the glenoid and envelopes the humeral head, attaching to the anatomical neck of the humeral head, around the rim of the articular surface. The capsule is lined with a synovial membrane.

The sternoclavicular joint

The sternoclavicular joint is a synovial joint between the junction of manubrium and sternum medially and the medial end of the clavicle laterally.

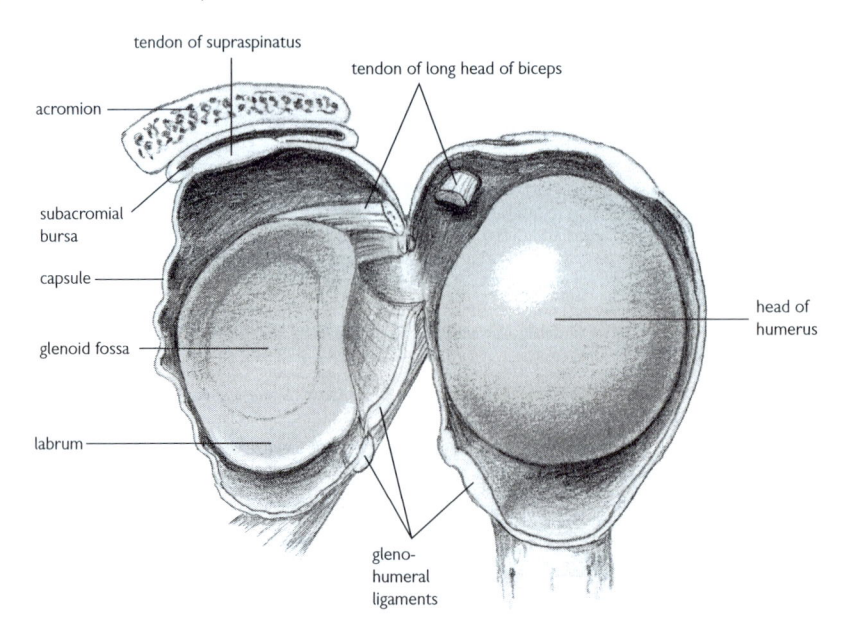

Figure 5.9 Interior of shoulder joint.

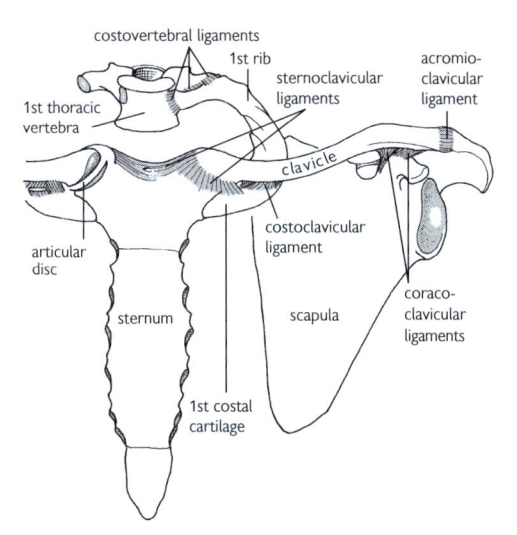

CHAPTER 5 Regional musculoskeletal anatomy and conditions

Figure 5.10 Bones and ligaments of the shoulder girdle. Reproduced from the Oxford Textbook of Functional Anatomy, MacKinnon and Morris, 2005, with permission from Oxford University Press.

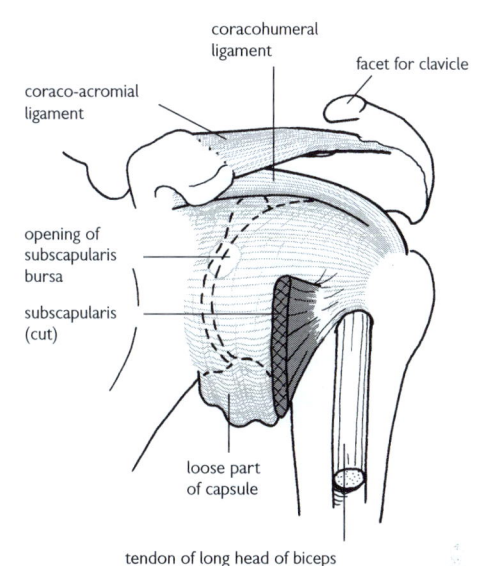

Figure 5.11 Shoulder joint: attachments of the capsule and extrinsic ligaments. Reproduced from the Oxford Textbook of Functional Anatomy, MacKinnon and Morris, 2005, with permission from Oxford University Press.

The acromioclavicular joint

The acromioclavicular joint, a synovial joint, is the articulation between the clavicle and the acromion at the lateral end of the clavicle. The adjacent bones are held together by the circumferential capsule and ligaments. See Fgure 5.10.
- These ligaments of the ACJ are supported by ligaments separate from the joint, which hold the lateral end of the clavicle down.
- These separate ligaments are the coracoclavicular ligaments, which arise from the superior surface of the coracoid and insert into the underside of the clavicle slightly medial to the ACJ.
- One of these ligaments resembles a cone (point of cone is inferior) and is referred to as the 'conoid ligament'.
- The other ligament is more strap-like and trapezoidal in shape, and is known as the 'trapezoid ligament'.

Ligaments

The ligaments comprise the glenohumeral capsule itself and longitudinal condensations which form bands within the substance of the capsule in a consistent arrangement. These bands are the superior, middle, and inferior glenohumeral ligaments, describing the relationship of each to the glenoid. The capsule and ligaments are inelastic, but are lax whilst the humerus is lying adjacent to the thorax, and become taut as the humerus is abducted and externally rotated. See Figures 5.10 and 5.11.

Muscles of the shoulder

The muscles that hold the humeral head in position and which act across this joint can be thought of as either imprecise, but powerful, such as deltoid, pectoralis major, and latissimus dorsi, or precise yet less powerful, as in the muscles of the rotator cuff. See Figure 5.12.
- The deltoid muscle has a wide origin running around from the anterior aspect of the lateral end of the clavicle to the posterior aspect of the acromion. The muscle fibres converge to insert into a prominence on the lateral aspect of the proximal third of the humerus known as the 'deltoid tubercle'. The deltoid muscle is multipennate and different regions can contract independently. Contraction of the anterior fibres aids anterior elevation of the humerus (flexion), contraction of the lateral fibres aids lateral elevation (abduction), and contraction of the posterior fibres aids extension.
- Pectoralis major arises from the sternum, ribs, and medial third of the clavicle, and inserts into the lateral aspect of the intertubercular groove on the anterior aspect of the proximal humerus. It acts as an adductor and internal rotator of the humerus.
- Latissimus dorsi has an expansive origin from the six lower thoracic vertebrae and from the lumbodorsal fascia, which has attachments to the posterior part of the iliac crest, and the sacral and lumbar spinous processes. The muscle fibres converge into a thick tendon, which inserts into the intertubercular groove. The muscle is a powerful adductor, internal rotator and extensor of the humerus.

It is important to remember that isotonic contraction of the deltoid, pectoralis major, and latissimus dorsi muscles will produce the movements mentioned above, but they play a crucial role as stabilizers of the shoulder and achieve this with isometric contraction.

Rotator cuff

This group of muscles comprises subscapularis, supraspinatus, infraspinatus, and teres minor. They each take origin from the scapular and their tendons converge, merge with the lateral part of the glenohumeral capsule, and produce a thick aponeurotic tendon, which drapes over the humeral head from anterior to posterior. The inferior deficiency is compensated for by the inferior glenohumeral ligament.

THE SHOULDER

Table 5.3 Main muscles in the shoulder girdle

Muscle	Action	Innervation
Trapezius	Rotation of scapula	Spinal accessory nerve (XIth cranial)
Latissimus dorsi	Extensor, internal rotator and adductor	Thoracodorsal nerve
Rhomboid major	Adducts scapula	Dorsal scapular nerve
Rhomboid minor	Adducts scapula	Dorsal scapular nerve
Levator scapulae	Scapular elevation and rotation	C3, C4
Pectoralis major	Adduction and int. rotation of humerus	Medial and lateral pectoral nerves
Pectoralis minor	Protracts scap.	Medial pectoral nerve
Subclavius	Depresses clavicle	Nerve to subclavius
Serratus anterior	Protraction of scapular and prevents winging	Long thoracic nerve
Deltoid	Humeral abduction	Axillary nerve
Teres major	Adductor, internal rotator and extensor	Lower subscapular nerve
Subscapularis	Internal rotator and stabilizer of shoulder	Upper and lower subscapular nerves
Supraspinatus	Abductor, ext. rotator and stabilizer	Suprascapular nerve
Infraspinatus	External rotator and stabilizer	Suprascapular nerve
Teres minor	External rotator and stabilizer	Axillary nerve

The movements of the muscles of the rotator cuff are determined by their line of pull across the GHJ.

- The subscapularis runs anteriorly and pulls the humeral head into internal rotation.
- Supraspinatus runs across the superior aspect of the humeral head and, thereby, initiates abduction.
- Infraspinatus and teres minor have a line of pull that runs below the superior pole of the humeral head posteriorly and, therefore, produce external rotation.
- In addition to their individual movements the muscles of the rotator cuff appear to play a role in preventing the humeral head from migrating superiorly out of the glenoid, preventing it from 'impingeing' upon the underside of the acromion.

Biceps
The long tendon of the biceps muscle takes origin from the supraglenoid tubercle and runs laterally, within the joint space between the superior surface of the humeral head and the capsule before turning inferiorly to leave the capsule via the bicipital groove on the anterior aspect of the proximal humerus. The muscle belly of the long head of biceps develops beyond this point and merges distally with the short head, which takes its origin from the coracoid process.

The two heads insert via a tendon into the radial tuberosity on the proximal radius and via an aponeurosis (the lacertus fibrosus) that, ultimately, attaches to the proximal ulnar via the fascia overlying the common flexor muscles of the forearm.

The main muscles around the shoulder their actions and innervation is presented in table 5.3.

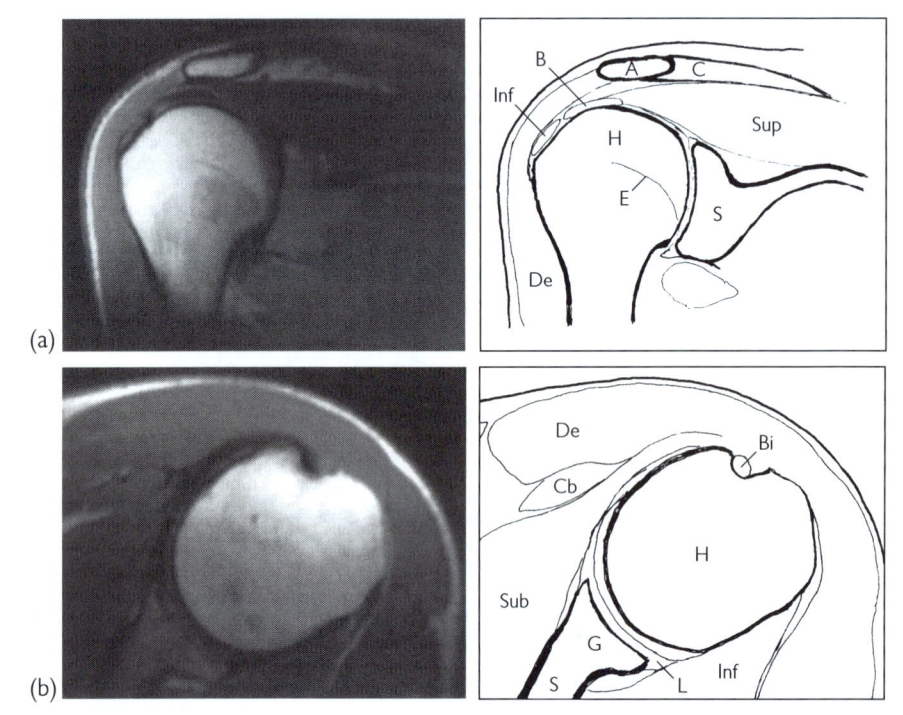

Figure 5.12 MRI of shoulder joint; (a) sagittal plane, (b) horizontal plane. Head of humerus (H), epiphyseal line (E), glenoid labrum (L), glenoid fossa (G) and acromion (A) of scapula (S), clavicle (C), deltoid (De), infraspinatus (Inf), supraspinatus (Sup), subscapularis (Sub), tendon of biceps (Bi), coracobrachialis (Cb). Reproduced from the Oxford Textbook of Functional Anatomy, MacKinnon and Morris, 2005, with permission from Oxford University Press

Bursa

The subacromial bursa is not a true bursa in that it is not a fluid filled space, but is made up of a number of layers of loose areolar connective tissue, enabling the two surfaces to move smoothly against each other.

- The aponeurotic tendon of the rotator cuff lies between the humeral head inferiorly and the acromion superiorly, and its smooth running beneath the acromion is achieved by the friction reducing effects of the subacromial bursa.
- Inflammation within the subacromial bursal tissue will result in all movements of the shoulder being painful.

The MRI apperances of the normal shoulder are visualised in Figure 5.12.

Further reading

Standring S. (Ed.) *Grays Anatomy: the anatomical basis of clinical practice.* Section V. London, 2006.

Last's Anatomy – Regional and Applied. 11th edn.

The shoulder girdle: regional musculoskeletal conditions

> **Main differential diagnosis of shoulder pain**
>
> *Articular*
> - Inflammatory arthritis (GHJ or ACJ).
> - Crystal arthritis.
> - Adhesive capsulitis/frozen shoulder.
> - Glenohumeral instability.
> - Osteoarthritis (GHJ or ACJ).
> - Milwaukee shoulder (also affects periarticular tissues).
>
> *Periarticular*
> - Rototor cuff disease, e.g. tendinopathy or tear.
> - Subacromial bursitis.
> - Calcific tendinitis.
> - Bicipital tendinitis.
>
> *Referred pain*
> - Cervical radiculopathy.
> - Neuralgic amyotrophy.
> - Spinal cord pathology.
> - Subdiaphragmatic pathology.
> - Cardiac ischaemic pain.

Rotator cuff disease

Rotator cuff disease is typically a continuum of pathology ranging from tendinitis and bursitis to partial tearing, to complete tear in one or more of the tendons.

Pathogenesis
The exact mechanism of rotator cuff disease remains disputed, but the current view is that the mechanism is multifactorial, and is influenced by a genetic predisposition, as well as intrinsic and extrinsic factors. Extrinsic factors arise when the tendons sustain mechanical injury through impingement, and intrinsic factors occur where tendon damage and degeneration occurs through changes within the tendon itself.

Extrinsic mechanisms
Mechanical factors include anterosuperior stresses from impingement by the under surface of the anterior acromion, or more rarely posterosuperior stress from the articular side of the supraspinatus tendon and the posterosuperior edge of the glenoid cavity, or anterointernal stress from impingement of the cuff from the coracohumeral interval.

Intrinsic hypothesis
Degenerative change within the supraspinatus tendon increases with age, and more severe degeneration is associated with the development of tendinopathy. Cuff tendinopathy is postulated to result from an imbalance between synthesis and degradation of the tendon, perhaps due to failure to regulate specific matrix metalloproteinase (MMP) enzyme activities in response to repeated injury or mechanical strain.

There is an association of deposition of amyloid within supraspinatus, in patients with chronic degenerative tendinopathy, which accumulates irreversibly over time and ultimately leads to irreversible changes in the structure of the affected tissue.

Spectrum of rotator cuff disease
Stage 1, where oedema and haemorrhage are present is, usually reversible, and affects patients mostly less than 25 years of age.

In Stage 2, fibrosis and tendinitis affect the rotator cuff of patients typically in the 25–40-year age group. Pain often recurs with activity.

Stage 3, with bone spurs and tendon rupture, present in individuals over 40 years of age.

Key features in the history
The history is dependant on both the aetiology, as well as the age of the patient. The commonest presentation includes pain, which is generally activity related and in the younger patient may be acute following an injury such as throwing. A more insidious onset is typical in the older patient with pain and discomfort, and pain on specific movements. Common symptoms include pain on reaching up above the head, reaching behind the back when dressing, or changing gear when driving. There may be sleep interference as rolling on to the shoulder results in pain. A history of weakness may represent a full rotator cuff tear.

Key features on examination
Physical examination involves evaluation of the range of motion, both active and passive, cuff strength testing and special shoulder tests. It should also include assessment of the cervical spine, since shoulder pain may be referred. A painful arc is usual between 70 and 120° of abduction, with pain on both active abduction and when lowering the arm, indicating impingement. Passive movements are normal and often painless. Localized tenderness in the subacromial space is a variable finding. Resisted movements of individual tendons will aid the specific diagnosis.
- Supraspinatus is tested with the arm abducted to 90°, with flexion of 30°, and internal rotation so that the thumb points down to the floor. Resisted abduction is painful. In severe cases, resisted flexion with the arm internally rotated may be less uncomfortable.
- Subscapularis muscle is tested by resisted internal rotation, with either the arm across the abdomen or the arm behind the back.
- Infraspinatus and teres minor are tested by resisted external rotation, although there is some action of supraspinatus.
- Biceps is tested by resisting flexion of the shoulder with the arm in extension (Speed's test) or resisted supination of the arm with the elbow at 90° of flexion (Yergeson's test).
- Impingement is tested by a number of techniques, all of which force the subacromial bursa and rotator cuff against the inferior surface of the acromion. Specific manoeuvres include abduction and forceful internal rotation of the arm with the elbow at 90° of flexion, or the arm is externally rotated from an adducted, flexed, and internally rotated position.
- Bicipital provocation is performed by abduction of the arm to 90° with the palm facing upwards, followed by adduction of the arm across the midline against resistance.

Imaging
- Plain radiography of the shoulder should include three standard views (anteroposterior, lateral scapular or outlet

view, and axial) to provide information on the morphology of the acromion, and to exclude joint degeneration at the GHJ or ACJ, reduction of the subacromial space, etc.
- US and MR are techniques that visualize the soft tissues. US has the advantage of being cheap, non-invasive and is a dynamic investigation, allowing visualization of the structures as they move; however, it is very operator dependent. MR is more expensive and the images are static, but can be interpreted by the treating clinician in the context of the clinical examination. An example of US in a ruptured supraspinatus tendon is seen in figure 5.13.

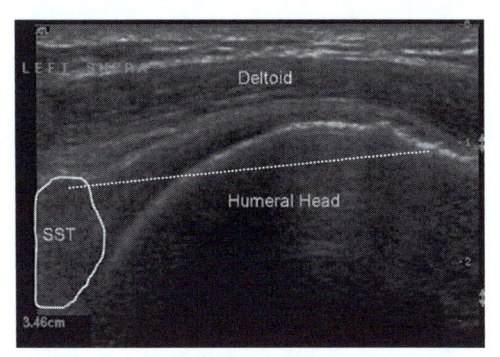

Figure 5.13 A ruptured supraspinatus tendon (SST) tendon is visualized on US, with bunching of the tendon outlined in white, and fibres retracted by 3.46 cm (measured by the dotted line).

Management
- The management of early stage rotator cuff disease (clinical impingement) should be treated conservatively. This involves physical therapy targeted at rehabilitation of the rotator cuff in order to restore its humeral head centring mechanism. This can be aided by pain-relieving measures, such as oral NSAIDs or subacromial glucocorticoid injections, particularly in the presence of bursitis. The duration of conservative management is the subject of controversy, being quoted at anything between 6 weeks and 6 months.
- If conservative management fails, surgical treatment in the form of arthroscopic subacromial decompression is indicated. A high (around 90%) rate of satisfactory results is achieved.
- For symptomatic tears, the threshold for surgery is lower. Partial and small full thickness tears can be successfully treated by decompression alone, although this does not stop the progression of cuff disease. Most cuff tears will progress, either in size or in symptoms. If pain relief and restoration of function is not achieved with rehabilitation, repair of the cuff, by open means or arthroscopic is indicated. A rate of around 95% satisfactory results is quoted in most of the recent outcome studies.

Calcific tendinitis

Epidemiology
Calcific tendinitis of the rotator cuff affects 10% of the population, although it is often asymptomatic.

Clinical presentation
It can present with nagging discomfort in the region of the affected tendon, but it frequently presents with acute onset of severe pain. Distinct phases of development are described, with formative and resorptive phases. The resorptive phase of the condition as the calcium deposits are extravasated into the subacromial bursa is typically very severe and associated with a markedly reduced range of movement. Most will resolve spontaneously.

Management
Initial management would involve analgesia and subacromial glucocorticoid injection. If the pain is not controlled by conservative means, an ultrasound-guided or arthroscopic needling of the lesion releases the calcium and provides immediate pain relief. Once settled, the calcium deposits remain and can be a source of mechanical impingement. In such cases, an acromioplasty can resolve the symptoms.

Frozen shoulder

A frozen shoulder is a painful shoulder condition of insidious onset that is associated with stiffness and difficulty sleeping on the affected side. The term 'adhesive capsulitis' is a misnomer as there are no associated capsular adhesions.

Epidemiology
The cumulative lifetime risk of developing frozen shoulder is about 2%. It commonly presents in the sixth decade with a peak age of 56. It is slightly more common in women than men and the non-dominant shoulder is more likely to be affected.

Aetiology/pathogenesis
The aetiology remains unclear. Histological biopsy confirms synovial inflammation with subsequent reactive capsular fibrosis. A dense matrix of type I and type III collagen is laid down by fibroblasts and myofibroblasts in the joint capsule. Subsequently, this tissue contracts. High expression of growth factors, cytokines, and matrix metalloproteinases is found in capsular biopsy specimens, which have a role in regulating fibroblasts.

Clinical features
Frozen shoulder is characterized by restriction of active and passive movement of the shoulder that occurs in the absence of a known intrinsic shoulder disorder. The disease process particularly affects the anterosuperior joint capsule, the inferior recess and the coracohumeral ligament. The condition is ultimately self-limiting. There are three overlapping phases:
- **Painful freezing phase** (duration 10–36 weeks): pain and stiffness around the shoulder with no history of injury. There is a constant nagging pain, worse at night.
- **Adhesive phase** (occurs at 4–12 months). The pain gradually subsides, but stiffness remains. Pain is apparent only at the extremes of movement and there is global reduction of glenohumeral range of movement.
- **Resolution phase** (takes 12–42 months).

Risk factors
Frozen shoulder can be idiopathic or it may be associated with a number of risk factors:
- **Diabetes mellitus:** the incidence of frozen shoulder in diabetes patients is reported to be 10–36%. The incidence in type 1 and type 2 diabetes is similar. Frozen shoulder in diabetics is often more severe and more prolonged.
- **Dupytren's disease.**
- **Shoulder surgery.**
- **Rarer associations:** hyperthyroidism, hypothyroidism, hypoadrenalism, Parkinson's disease, cardiac disease, pulmonary disease, and cerebrovascular accident.

- **Non-shoulder surgery** such as cardiac surgery has also been associated with secondary frozen shoulder.

Investigations
The diagnosis is essentially clinical. Imaging is used to rule out other pathologies presenting with pain and stiffness, such as degenerative joint disease.
- Plain radiographs are typically normal, although they may show disuse osteopenia.
- MR and US may demonstrate thickening in the joint capsule and the coracohumeral ligament.
- Isotope bone scans may demonstrate an increased uptake of contrast.

None of these investigations are diagnostic.

Treatment
The treatment of frozen shoulder should be tailored to the stage of the disease. It is also important to offer reassurance that the condition will spontaneously resolve, although there may be some residual reduction in the range of movement.
- Treatment in the painful freezing stage will be directed towards controlling pain with analgesia or NSAIDs. The role of glucocorticoid injection and physiotherapy remain controversial, with little evidence to suggest that either significantly shortens the time to resolution of symptoms. Hydrodilatation provides good pain relief and improvement in the range of motion.
- During the adhesive phase, if the stiffness is functionally limiting or pain persists, contracture release is indicated in rare cases. This has traditionally been achieved with manipulation under anaesthesia, although there is a high incidence of iatrogenic damage to the cuff, articular surface, and labrum. The procedure of choice to release the contracture in an arthroscopic arthrolysis. This, combined with continuous interscalene anaesthesia during the early postoperative period, allows early functional restoration.

Shoulder instability

The shoulder is the most mobile joint in the body. Stability on movement is provided both by static (glenoid surface, labrum, and glenohumeral ligaments) and dynamic (rotator cuff and extrinsic muscle balance) mechanisms. Conditions that affect any of these can result in recurrent instability. Shoulder stability can be classified by the direction of the abnormal movement, the severity and by the cause. The Stanmore Classification of Shoulder Instability is based on the characteristics of three main groups:
- **Traumatic structural:** where there is a definite history of trauma, usually anterior and unilateral, resulting in damage to the labrum (Bankart lesion). The treatment is surgical, in the form of a Bankart repair.
- **Atraumatic structural:** it is due to capsular dysfunction due to repetitive microtrauma, usually in a background of increased laxity or structural abnormalities of the articular surfaces. It is not uncommonly bilateral.
- **Habitual non-structural** (muscle patterning): there is no history of trauma, no structural damage to the articular surfaces, but an altered muscle patterning. This can start as a voluntary action (party trick), but becomes uncontrolled. The diagnosis is difficult and sometimes requires EMG studies.

Clinical presentation, however, normally represents a continuum between the three groups.

Investigations
Radiographs can help assess the integrity of the glenoid and humeral head. CT is helpful if a bony lesion is suspected and the radiographs do not demonstrate the osseous architecture adequately. MR arthrography is the investigation of choice (80–90% sensitivity and specificity for labral pathology). In those cases, where aetiology remain uncertain, examination under anaesthesia and diagnostic arthroscopy can be of assistance.

Treatment
Treatment is directed towards the cause of the instability.
- In recurrent dislocations of the traumatic structural group, surgical treatment is indicated. If the damage is to the labrum, a labrum repair resolves the symptoms in over 90% of cases. If the cause is a bony defect, bone grafting of the defect is carried out, either with a coracoid block (Bristow-Latarjet procedure) or an iliac crest graft.
- Atraumatic structural instabilities are amenable to rehabilitation. This involves improving muscle control and proprioception. If this is not sufficient, surgery is used to reduce the volume of the capsule and retighten the glenohumeral ligaments.
- Muscle patterning disorders are rare. Treatment is difficult and requires a specialist multidisciplinary approach, involving a shoulder surgeon, a shoulder physiotherapist and on occasions psychological support.

Arthritis of the shoulder

The shoulder joint is a functional unit composed of several joints: glenohumeral, acromioclavicular, sternoclavicular, scapulothoracic, and subacromial. The first three are susceptible to degenerative joint disease.

Acromioclavicular/sternoclavicular osteoarthritis
Osteoarthritis can happen at either end of the clavicle. On the acromial side osteoarthritis is very common, although not always symptomatic. Sternoclavicular joints rarely become degenerate and osteoarthritis is associated with trauma, instability, and inflammatory arthropathies. The US appearances of an osteoarthritic acromioclavicular joint are demonstrated in Figure 5.14.

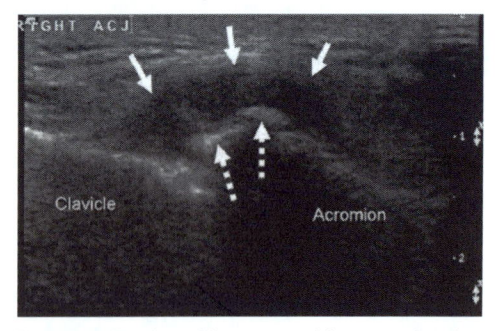

Figure 5.14 Capsular proliferation around the acromioclavicular joint is visualized on US, and is identified here by the solid arrows. The broken arrows demonstrate osteophytes. The joint space is narrowed and obliterated as a consequence and is not clearly seen.

Treatment
Treatment is initially conservative, with activity modification and analgesia. Symptomatic acromio/sternoclavicular osteoarthritis that does not respond to conservative therapy may be treated with excision arthroplasty. At the acromial end, it is usually excised arthroscopically. On the sternal side, an open excision arthroplasty is carried out due to the proximity of big vessels.

Osteoarthritis of the glenohumeral joint
Osteoarthritis of the GHJ is rare and there is normally a predisposing factor, such as trauma, avascular necrosis of the humeral head, or inflammatory disease. The articular cartilage in the GHJ is exposed to less force than weight-bearing joints, making osteoarthritis less common. Typical presentation is of poorly localized shoulder pain with discomfort in the upper arm in an elderly patient. Examination reveals globally restricted movements and the presence of an effusion.

Treatment
- Conservative treatment is normally sufficient with physiotherapy and analgesia.
- Arthroscopic techniques are useful in the younger patient with shoulder symptoms and allow treatment of co-existing soft tissue pathology, for example, subacromial decompression, capsular release, and arthroscopic debridement.
- Severe glenohumeral disease often requires hemiarthroplasty or total shoulder replacement. Both procedures result in significant pain relief, increased range of movement and function. The two types of prosthesis in common use are either surface replacements or traditional stemmed implants. Up to 35% of patients who require a shoulder arthroplasty have rotator cuff tears. These should be repaired at the same time as the arthroplasty to achieve the best results. In general, the results of total shoulder replacement are superior to hemiarthroplasty with better functional results and less pain.

The rheumatoid shoulder
Shoulder symptoms are common in patients with established RA with more than 90% of patients having shoulder pain at 5 years following onset of inflammatory disease. Patients present with symptoms of pain, swelling and a decreased range of motion. Rotator cuff insufficiency is common affecting more than 70% with approximately 30% developing full thickness tears.

Non-surgical management
In early shoulder involvement, there are no significant osseous changes, and treatment is medical, with analgesia, NSAIDs, and overall control of disease activity. Activity modification, intra-articular, or subacromial glucocorticoid injections may also be helpful. Physiotherapy is useful in maintaining and regaining range of motion depending on the stage of the disease.

Surgical management
- Surgical management is indicated when conservative treatment has failed to control pain and maintain function.
- The choice of procedure is determined by the extent of disease in the articular cartilage, bone, and the periarticular soft tissues.
- Synovectomy and debridement are indicated when there is articular cartilage preservation. The procedure can be performed open or arthroscopically with up to 80% gaining a painless range of movement, involving glenohumeral joint synovectomy with a subacromial bursectomy. If rotator cuff disease is present it can be addressed at the time by means of an acromioplasty and release of the coracoacromial ligament.
- Once articular cartilage loss has occurred prosthetic replacement using either a hemiarthroplasty or total joint replacement is usually necessary. The results for rheumatoid arthritis patients are not as good as in patients with osteoarthritis.

Prioritizing of surgical procedures
Although the most symptomatic joint should be treated first, lower limb surgery normally takes priority over upper limb surgery, with upper limb surgery normally deferred until the use of ambulatory aids is no longer required. The elbow takes precedence over the shoulder, as a superior functional result is achieved when the elbow is operated on before the shoulder.

Bicipital tendinitis

Tenosynovitis of the long head of biceps is uncommon and is characterized by pain and tenderness over the long head of biceps in the bicipital groove of the humerus. It may occur in association with degenerative disease of the rotator cuff but in the majority of cases occurs as a result of localized friction from the bone of the humeral bicipital groove. The history is one of localized anterior shoulder pain which is exacerbated by use of the arm. Pain in the bicipital groove is exacerbated by resisted flexion and supination of the forearm.

Treatment
Conservative treatment is normally successful, although a localized glucocorticoid injection is required in more severe cases.

Rupture of the tendon of long head of biceps

Rupture of the tendon of the long head of biceps is not uncommon and often occurs in association with rotator cuff pathology.
- Rupture may be preceded by pain, but is often painless, and presents with bruising and, more characteristically, a 'Popeye' muscle as the muscle belly bulges distally.
- Rupture of the long head does not appear to have any significant adverse effect on function and so nothing more than reassurance is required.
- Avulsion of the distal tendon insertion from the radial tuberosity, however, is a very different situation. This is rare and tends to occur in younger patients and particularly in body builders who overload the tendon insertion. The rupture is painful as it occurs, but the pain quickly settles. The diagnosis is obtained from the history and an inablity to palpate the cord-like structure of the tendon in the antecubital fossa. The distal tendon of the biceps is a powerful supinator of the forearm, as well as elbow flexor, and so surgical repair, by reattachment, is required.

Nerve disorders around the shoulder

Peripheral nerves are highly susceptible to injury from stretch or compression, resulting in nerve ischaemia, oedema and conduction impairment. These changes are proportional to the magnitude and duration of the insult, and eventually lead to irreversible damage.

Suprascapular nerve

Aetiology

The commonest locations of injury include the suprascapular notch, the spinoglenoid notch, and between the spine of the scapula, and the medial tendinous margin of infraspinatus and supraspinatus during extreme abduction and internal rotation of the shoulder. Causes include:
- Trauma – shoulder dislocations, scapular, and clavicular fractures, penetrating trauma, iatrogentic injury during surgery.
- Compression by a mass – commonly a ganglion cyst.
- Repetitive over-use.

Results are especially poor for suprascapular nerve injury secondary to ganglion cyst.

Investigations

Nerve conduction studies and imaging are the most useful techniques. US demonstrates ganglion cysts and other mass lesions, which can be further visualized with CT and MR. MR has the added benefit of identifying changes within supraspinatus and infraspinatus secondary to denervation (atrophy, fatty infiltration, and high signal on T2-weighted images) that appear 3 weeks after injury.

Treatment

Conservative treatment consists of:
- Avoidance of activities that result in irritation and trauma of the nerve.
- Improve flexibility of the surrounding muscles of the GHJ and strengthening of the scapular stabilizing muscles.

Surgical treatment is tailored to the precise underlying cause.
- **Suprascapular notch:** release of the superior transverse scapular ligament for entrapment in the suprascapular notch.
- **Spinoglenoid notch:** release of the spinoglenoid ligament, scapular spine, or medial tendinous margin of the rotator cuff for more distal lesions around the spinoglenoid notch.
- **Ganglion cyst:** US/CT guided aspiration of ganglion cysts. However, this is associated with a risk of recurrence. Arthroscopic or open decompression of the cyst may be required.

Axillary nerve injury

Axillary nerve injuries can present in isolation or as part of a combined brachial plexus injury. Causes include:
- Traction injury to the shoulder (anterior dislocation of the shoulder).
- Closed blunt trauma.
- Penetrating trauma (sharp or blunt).
- Nerve compression due to mass effect (aneurysm, tumour).
- Parsonage–Turner syndrome (neuralgic amyotrophy).
- Quadrilateral space syndrome.

Investigations

Investigations include nerve conduction studies and imaging as discussed for suprascapular nerve disorders. A subclavicular arteriogram may be appropriate if quadrilateral space syndrome is suspected (considered positive if posterior humeral circumflex artery occlusion occurs with less than 60° of abduction).

Spinal accessory nerve injury

The spinal accessory nerve supplies the trapezius muscle.
- It may be injured during trivial surgery, such as lymph node biopsies in the neck. The prognosis for recovery in these cases is poor and can result in significant functional disability and pain. If this is the case, surgical reconstruction with tendon transfers (Eden–Lange procedure) is indicated.
- It is also commonly affected by neurological amyotrophy. This presents with acute onset of severe pain, often at night, followed by weakness and atrophy of the trapezius muscle. It can be bilateral. In contrast with iatrogenic damage, prognosis is good. It tends to resolve spontaneously, although it may take 2–3 years. The treatment is supportive consisting in analgesia and physical therapy. Braces might be helpful, although they are generally poorly tolerated. In cases of incomplete recovery, reconstructive surgery can be considered.

Further reading

Bell S, Coghlan J, Richardson M. Hydrodilatation in the management of shoulder capsulitis. *Aust Radiol* 2003; **47**: 247–51.

Bigliani, L., Morrison, D, April, E. The morphology of the acromion and it relationship to rotator cuff tears. *Orthopaed Trans* 1986; **10**: 228.

Bunker TD Anthony PP. The pathology of frozen shoulder. A Dupuytren-like disease. *J Bone Jt Surg Br* 1995; **77**: 677–83.

Codman EA. *The Shoulder. Rupture of the Supraspinatus Tendon and Other Lesions In or About the Subacromial Bursa*. Boston: Thomas Todd, 1934.

Harvie P, Ostlere SJ, Teh J, et al. Genetic influences in the aetiology of tears of the rotator cuff. Sibling risk of a full-thickness tear. *J Bone Jt Surg Br* 2004; **86**(5): 696–700.

Hawkins RJ, Brock RM, Abrams JS, Hobeika P. Acromioplasty for impingement with an intact rotator cuff. *J Bone Jt Surg Br* 1988; **70**: 795–7.

Hazelman BD. The painful stiff shoulder. *Rheumatol Phys Med* 1972; **11**: 413–21.

Lewis A, Kitamura T, Bayley JIL. The classification of shoulder instability: new light through old windows. *Curr Orthop* 2004; **18**: 97–108.

Massoud SN, Levy O, Copeland SA Subacromial decompression. Treatment for small- and medium-sized tears of the rotator cuff. *J Bone Jt Surg Br* 2002; **84**: 955–60.

Neer CS. Anterior acromioplasty for the chronic impingement syndrome in the shoulder. *J Bone Jt Surg Am* 2005; **87**: 1399.

Neer CS. The surgical management of rheumatoid arthritis. In: Crubbs RL, Mitchell NS (Eds) *The Rheumatoid Shoulder*. Philadelphia: JB Lippincott, 1971; 117–27.

Petersson CJ. Shoulder surgery in rheumatoid arthritis. *Acta Orthopaed Scand* 1986; **57**: 222–6.

Riley GP, Goddard MJ, Hazleman BL. Histopathological assessment and pathological significance of matrix degeneration in supraspinatus tendons. *Rheumatology (Oxf.)* 2001; **40**(2): 293–23.

Titelman RM, Lippitt SB, Rockwood CA Jr, Wirth MA Glenohumeral instability. In: Matsen FA 3rd (Ed.), *The Shoulder*. Volume 2, 3rd edn. Philadelphia: Saunders 2004; 655–794.

Uhtoff HK, Loehr JW Calcific tendinopathy of the rotator cuff: Pathogenesis, diagnosis, and management. *J Am Acad Orthop Surg* 1997; **5**(4): 183–91.

Yamaguchi K, Tetro AM, Blam O, Evanoff BA, Teefey SA, Middleton WD. Natural history of asymptomatic rotator cuff tears: a longitudinal analysis of asymptomatic tears detected sonographically. *J Shoulder Elbow Surg* 2001; **10**(3): 199–203.

Chapter 5 Regional musculoskeletal anatomy and conditions

The elbow

Regional anatomy
The elbow joint comprises both the ulnohumeral articulation and the radiohumeral articulation. The ulnohumeral articulation is a hinge joint, whilst the radiohumeral articulation is a 'universal joint' in that it can both hinge and pivot. It is a synovial joint and its cavity communicates with the proximal radioulnar joint. The function of the elbow, working in conjunction with the shoulder, is to enable positioning of the hand.

Bones
Towards the distal end of the humerus the medial and lateral epicondyles are palpable on either side. They are distinguishable from the adjacent radial head laterally and olecranon posteriorly if the elbow is flexed and extended. Distal to the epicondyles the radial end of the humerus is hemispherical (the capitellum) for articulation with the slightly concave and circular proximal end of the radius. The ulnar end of the distal radius (the trochlear) is pulley-shaped, comprising two rims with a groove between. The trochlear articulates with the olecranon fossa of the proximal ulnar. The olecranon fossa is a concavity from end to end, but convex from side to side and so mirrors the shape of the trochlear. The radial aspect of the proximal ulnar has a concavity for articulation with the rim of the radial head during pronation and supination. See Figure 5.15.

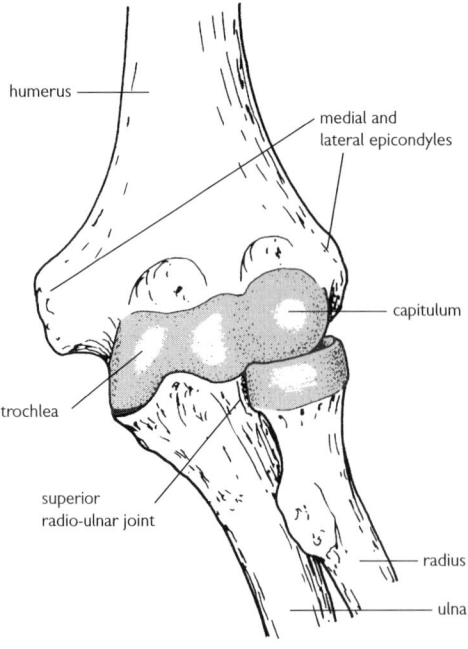

Figure 5.15 Articular surfaces of elbow joint (anterior aspect). Reproduced from the Oxford Textbook of Functional Anatomy, MacKinnon and Morris, 2005, with permission from Oxford University Press.

Joint capsule
The joint capsule encloses the ulnohumeral and radiohumeral articulations, and also the proximal radioulnar joint within a single joint space. An effusion or synovitis can, therefore, produce fluctuant swellings immediately posterior to both the medial and lateral epicondyles of the humerus. Furthermore, swelling can occur around the proximal radius and thereby compress the posterior interosseous nerve. See Figure 5.16.

Ligaments
- On the ulnar aspect two ligaments originate from the lateral epicondyle and diverge to insert onto the olecranon at either end of the lateral aspect of the olecranon fossa. The two divergent ends of these ligaments are joined by a transverse ligament which runs between them.
- On the radial aspect a ligamentous structure arises from the lateral epicondyle and runs distally. As it runs distally it diverges so that one bundle of fibres inserts into the ulnar, at the distal end of the radial side of the olecranon, and the other bundle merges with the lateral aspect of the annular ligament; the annular ligament is attached at either end to the radial side of the ulnar and encircles the radial head.

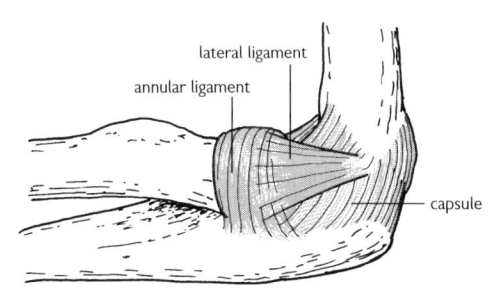

Figure 5.16 Capsule and ligaments of the elbow joint (lateral aspect). Reproduced from the Oxford Textbook of Functional Anatomy, MacKinnon and Morris, 2005, with permission from Oxford University Press.

Bursa
A bursa exists between the posterior surface of the olecranon and the overlying skin. This bursa renders the skin over the olecranon mobile so as to facilitate flexion of the elbow and minimize shearing forces on the deep surface of that portion of skin.

Muscles
Flexion of the elbow is achieved by the combined effects of brachialis, biceps, and brachioradialis.
- Brachialis inserts into the proximal ulnar in the region of the coronoid process, at the distal end of the olecranon fossa.
- The biceps muscle has insertions onto both radius and ulnar. It inserts into the radius via a tendon which inserts into the radial tuberosity and into the ulnar via an aponeurosis (the lacertus fibrosus) that, ultimately, attaches to the proximal ulnar via the fascia overlying the common flexor muscles of the forearm.
- Brachioradialis has a longer lever arm, arguably, than both brachialis and biceps in that it takes origin from the lateral aspect of the distal humerus and inserts via its tendon into the distal radius in the region of the radial styloid.

Extension of the elbow is achieved through the action of triceps, primarily.
- The triceps tendon has a fairly broad insertion into the proximal ulnar, inserting into the olecranon process and the region immediately distal to this.

CHAPTER 5 Regional musculoskeletal anatomy and conditions

- Some flexion and extension of the elbow is also produced by the action of the common flexor and extensor muscles, whose primary actions are on the wrist and hand.

Muscles

Extensor muscles and tendons arising at the elbow
The common extensor origin, from which arises the fused proximal ends of extensor carpi radialis brevis (ECRB), extensor digitorum communis (EDC), extensor digiti minimi (EDM), and extensor carpi ulnaris (ECU) is on the anterior aspect of the lateral epicondyle. The actions and innervation of the extensor muscles are presented in table 5.4.

Table 5.4 Extensor muscles arising from the distal humerus

Muscle	Action	Innervation
Brachioradialis	Elbow flexion	Radial
Extensor carpi radialis longus	Wrist ext. and radial deviation	Radial
Extensor carpi radialis brevis	Wrist ext. and radial extension	Posterior Interosseous
Anconeus	Extends elbow	Radial
Extensor digitorum communis	Extends fingers	Posterior interosseous
Extensor digiti minimi	Extends little finger	Posterior Interosseous
Extensor carpi ulnaris	Wrist ext. and ulnar deviation	Posterior Interosseous
Supinator	Supinates forearm	Posterior interosseous

Flexor muscles and tendons arising at the elbow
The common flexor origin (pronator teres, flexor carpi radialis, flexor digitorum superficialis, palmaris longus, and flexor carpi ulnaris) is from the medial epicondyle. The actions and innervation of the flexor muscles are presented in table 5.5.

Nerves around the elbow

Ulnar nerve
The ulnar nerve runs within the cubital tunnel immediately posterior to the medial epicondyle. The brachial artery, and median nerve lie anterolateral to the medial epicondyle, and the posterior interosseous nerve lies anteromedial to the lateral epicondyle and in close proximity to the anterior part of the radial head and neck.

Table 5.5 Flexor muscles arising from the distal humerus

Muscle	Action	Innervation
Pronator teres	Pronation and elbow flexion	Median
Flexor carpi radialis	Wrist flexion and radial deviation	Median
Palmaris longus	Wrist flexion	Median
Flexor carpi ulnaris	Wrist flexion and ulnar deviation	Ulnar
Flexor digitorum superficialis	Proximal interphalangeal joint flexion	Median

Posterior interosseous nerve
The nerve fibres that comprise the posterior interosseous nerve (PIN) leave the radial nerve in the antecubital fossa, superficial to brachialis, but deep to brachioradialis. The PIN runs away from the superficial radial nerve, having given a branch to the extensor carpi radialis brevis, by passing deeply between the superficial and deep layers of the supinator muscle, which it supplies. On leaving the distal edge of the supinator the PIN branches to supply all remaining extensors and abductor pollicis longus. The terminal branch of the PIN runs along the posterior surface of the interosseous membrane between radius and ulnar (hence, its name) to supply the wrist joint. The muscles supplied by the PIN are presented in table 5.6. The PIN does not have a superficial sensory area of supply and, therefore, a PIN lesion is not accompanied by sensory disturbance of the skin.

Table 5.6 Muscles supplied by the posterior interosseous nerve

Muscle	Action
Externsor carpi radialis brevis	Wrist and radial extension
Anconeus	Extends elbow
Extensor digitorum communis	Extends fingers
Externsor digiti minimi	Extends little finger
Externsor carpi ulnaris	Wrist extension and ulnar deviation
Supinator	Supinates forearm
Abductor pollicis longus	Abducts thumb
Extensor pollicis brevis	Extends thumb MCPJ
Extensor pollicis longus	Extends thumb
Extensor indicis proprius	Extends index finger

Further reading

Standring S (Ed.). *Grays Anatomy: the anatomical basis of clinical practice. Section V.* Churchill Livingstone London: 2006.

Last's Anatomy – Regional and Applied, 11th edn. Churchill Livingstone: 2006.

The elbow: regional musculoskeletal conditions

Main differential diagnosis of elbow pain

Articular
- Inflammatory, e.g. rheumatoid arthritis, crystal arthritis.
- Degenerative.
- Osteochondritis dissicans.
- Traumatic.

Bursitis
Olecranon bursitis.

Tendinopathy
- Lateral epicondylitis.
- Medial epicondylitis.
- Bicipital tendinopathy.
- Triceps tendinopathy.

Nerve entrapment syndromes
- Cubital tunnel syndrome.
- Radial tunnel syndrome.
- Pronator teres syndrome.
- Referred pain.
- Cervical radiculopathy.
- Thoracic outlet syndrome.
- Pancoast tumour.

Bone pathology
- Fracture.
- Infection.
- Tumour.

Others
- Olecranon impingement syndrome.
- Fibromyalgia.
- Regional chonic pain syndrome.

Lateral epicondylitis

Lateral epicondylitis is one of the most common soft tissue conditions in the arm. The term 'tennis elbow' has arisen as a result of a description of the symptoms in the *Lancet* in 1882, then describing 'lawn tennis arm'.

Epidemiology
- A prevalence of 1–3% of the population is estimated for lateral epicondylitis.
- Most of those affected are between the ages of 40 and 60 years.
- Less than 5% are tennis players.
- Risk factors remain elusive and there does not appear to be a link with manual work, although over-use may be a risk factor.

Aetiology
The common extensor tendon origin is the site of insertion of extensor carpi radialis brevis and extensor communis tendons. Although the term 'epicondylitis' implies an inflammatory aetiology, the current hypothesis is that repeated microtrauma causes disruption of the tendon, which in turn results in a degenerative tendinosis.

History
- An insidious onset is usual.
- Pain is localized to the lateral epicondyle or radiates along the extensor tendon.
- Occasionally, a shooting pain is described into the dorsum of the hand.
- Shaking hands or forming a tight grip exacerbates the pain.

Examination
- Tenderness over the lateral epicondyle is typical.
- Pain on resisted wrist dorsiflexion is found with the elbow held in extension.
- Alternatively, pain is precipitated by extending the elbow with the wrist in flexion.
- Resisted supination is painful.
- The elbow demonstrates a normal range of movement.

Investigations
Investigations are not normally required as the diagnosis is clinical.
- Plain radiographs may reveal soft tissue calcification, but are usually normal.
- US detects tendinosis and a periosteal reaction is sometime seen. An example is given in Figure 5.17.
- MR is used preoperatively on occasion to image the soft tissue abnormalities, and may reveal tendon tears, as well as chronic tendinosis.

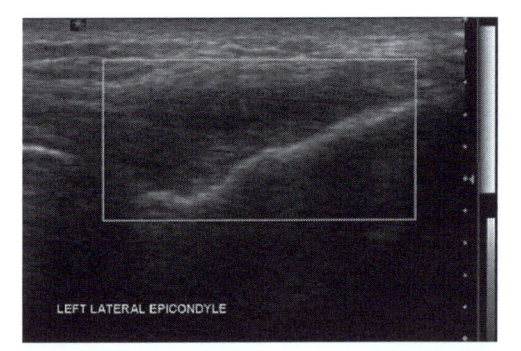

Figure 5.17 The image above was obtained on ultrasound. There is loss of the normal fibrillar pattern of the tendon and hyperaemia was detected using the power Doppler tool. In this case, the cortex of the bone is smooth, although irregularity can be seen in more severe cases.

Treatment
In the majority of cases, lateral epicondylitis is self-limiting within a year and does not require intervention. Treatment is therefore aimed at symptomatic benefit.
- Rehabilitation with strengthening exercises and stretching may be helpful. An elbow clasp reduces movement of the painful tendon, therefore providing short term pain relief, although long-term benefit remains to be shown.
- Topical and oral NSAIDs have been used with some success.
- The role of corticosteroid injection remains controversial, and current evidence is that short-term benefit may be gained by up to three injections, and is superior to conservative management, physiotherapy, strapping, and oral NSAIDs. However, outcome appears better at 12 months in those patients who have not received corticosteroid injections.

- Surgery is occasionally offered to refractory cases, and the extensor origin is stripped from the attachment to the lateral epicondyle and allowed to fall back into place, a technique called a lateral release. Extensive surgery may result in elbow instability. The exact mechanism by which this technique is beneficial remains unclear and there are no long-term outcome studies following surgery for lateral epicondylitis.

Medial epicondylitis

Medial epicondylitis is also known as 'golfers elbow'. It is estimated to be 5-8 times less common than lateral epicondylitis. There may be a history of over-use and the aetiology is thought to be similar to that of lateral epicondylitis.

History

- A history of insidious onset of pain, localized over the medial epicondyle is classical.
- Pain radiates into the forearm and is exacerbated by lifting, gripping, and pronation of the forearm.
- There may be a history of sporting activity or recent increase in repetitive actions.

Examination

- There is tenderness over the medial epicondyle at the point of insertion of the common extensor tendons, and this may extend distally.
- Provocation is achieved by resisted pronation of the forearm, with resisted flexion of the wrist when the arm is extended. Flexion of the fingers, rather than the wrist may provoke pain at the medial epicondyle.

Treatment

As with lateral epicondylitis, symptoms are usually self-limiting and treatment is symptomatic with rehabilitation, and NSAIDs. The role of corticosteroid injection remains even more poorly researched than in lateral epicondylitis.

Bicipital tendinitis

Bicipital tendinitis is rare in the elbow and occurs at the point of insertion of the biceps tendon onto the radius.

History

There is often a history of sport or repetitive movements. Pain is experienced over the bicipital tuberosity of the radius.

Examination

Resisted flexion and supination provoke pain, as does full extension of the elbow.

Treatment

Treatment involved rehabilitation and physiotherapy.

Triceps tendinitis

The pain is experienced behind the elbow over the insertion point of the triceps tendon on the olecranon.

History

There is a history of localized tenderness and pain, and sometimes swelling, usually in men who undertake manual work.

Examination

There may be swelling of the triceps tendon with pain on resisted extension.

Treatment

Conservative treatment and avoidance of heavy manual work often settles the symptoms.

Olecranon bursitis

The olecranon bursa lies behind the olecranon process, is superficial, and is therefore prone to traumatic bursitis and infection. Inflammatory disease, such as gout and rheumatoid arthritis may also result in olecranon bursitis. However, often there is no cause identified.

Traumatic bursitis

- Traumatic bursitis is also known as 'student's elbow'. Pain is present when local pressure is applied, such as resting the elbow on a table or against clothing.
- Pain is well localized, and not provoked by either resisted or passive movements of the elbow.
- Examination reveals localized tenderness over the tip of the olecranon and distension of the bursa may be obvious.
- Traumatic bursitis is self-limiting in the majority of cases.
- Aspiration of the bursa will reveal clear fluid in those cases with a significant swelling and treatment consists of local injection of corticosteroid.
- Rarely, surgical resection is required.

Septic bursitis

Septic bursitis is less common than traumatic bursitis and is often associated with an overlying cellulitis of the skin. There may also be a history of trauma with a skin abrasion providing the site of entry of infection.

- *Staph. aureus* is the commonest organism causing septic bursitis, although streptococcus and *Strep. epidermidis* are also less commonly isolated.
- Localized pain, swelling, and tenderness are the presenting features, and there may be features of systemic sepsis.
- Examination reveals a full range of movement of the elbow, although the bursa is painful and locally tender.
- Aspiration of the bursa should be undertaken for both symptomatic relief and for diagnostic purposes, and a gram stain of the pus and polarized light microscopy undertaken to examine for organisms and the presence of crystals.
- Antibiotic choice should cover gram positive organism pending culture sensitivities.
- Surgical excision and drainage is rarely necessary, either during the cute episode or for repeated infection.

Crystal bursistis

- Gout may present with an olecranon bursitis, and in this situation, tophaceous deposit are sometimes seen.
- Monosodium urate crystals are identified under light microscopy of the bursal fluid.
- When infection has been excluded, the olecranon bursitis may be injected with corticosteroid and treatment of gout should be considered in the appropriate clinical setting.

Osteoarthritis of the elbow

Osteoarthritis of the elbow is unusual in patients who do not have inflammatory arthritis or a history of trauma.

History

- There is often a history of previous fracture, or osteochondritis dissecans.
- There is a slow progression of increasing elbow pain which is exacerbated by use.
- There may be restriction of elbow movement.
- If there are loose bodies within the elbow joint, there may be a history of joint locking.

Examination

- The joint margins are thickened due to osteophyte formation.
- There is restriction of flexion and extension, but rotation may be preserved.
- Coarse crepitation occurs on movement of the joint.

Investigations

Joint space narrowing and osteophyte formation is found on radiographs. Loose bodies may also be seen. See Figure 5.18.

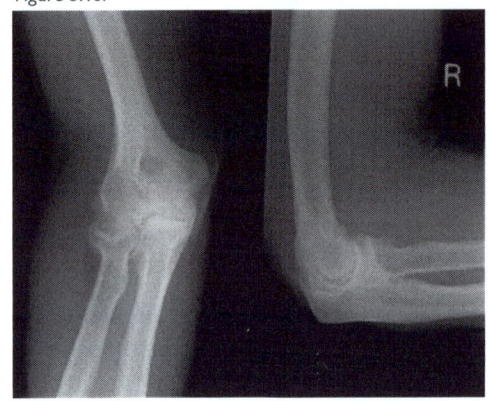

Figure 5.18 Sclerosis, osteophytes and joint space narrowing is evident on this plain radiograph of an osteoarthritic elbow. An effusion can also be detected.

Treatment

In the majority of cases, conservative measures with analgesia and self-management are indicated. Physiotherapy and advice about avoidance of heavy physical work are important.

- If there is a history of locking, arthroscopic removal of loose bodies provides good symptomatic relief.
- If osteoarthritis primarily affects the lateral aspect of the joint, excision of the radial head results in pain relief.
- Rarely, replacement arthroplasty is indicated.

Osteochonditis dissecans

After the knee, the elbow is the most common site of osteochondritis dissecans. Necrosis of part of the articular cartilage occurs, with associated necrosis of the underlying bone. Eventually, this separates from healthy bone resulting in a loose fragment within the joint. This fragment is usually part of the capitulum of the humerus. The cause of osteochonditis dissecans is unclear.

History

There is a history of mild mechanical pain and, following separation of the fragment, there is a history of locking of the joint.

Examination

An effusion can be detected in the early stages and there may be some mild restriction of movement.

Treatment

Treatment is conservative until the fragment results in locking, an indication for surgery.

Olecranon impingement syndrome

This results from a traumatic injury and typically results in posterior elbow pain. Pain is increased by extension of the elbow. There is often a history of clicking or locking in the last few degrees of extension. There may also be crepitus and some restriction of extension. Plain radiographs reveal osteophyte formation.

Nerve entrapment around the elbow

The median, ulnar, and radial nerves may be trapped around the elbow, each giving rise to distinct clinical presentations. Nerve conduction studies are helpful in the investigation of nerve entrapment syndromes.

Radial tunnel syndrome

The deep branch of the radial nerve (posterior interosseus nerve or PIN) may become compressed as it passes through a tunnel formed by fibrous tissue next to the superficial head of the supinator muscle. As this is adjacent to the joint capsule, compression of PIN may occur as a result of synovitis of the capsule. Presentation is usually with lateral elbow pain that radiates into the dorsal aspect of the forearm.

Examination

- Examination reveals local tenderness where the radial nerve crosses the head of the radius.
- Tinel's sign may be positive at this point.
- Provocation of the entrapment occurs with resisted supination of the elbow with the elbow in extension.

If severe, a PIN palsy results, with clinical findings consistent with a more peripheral radial nerve palsy:

- Weak wrist extension due to paralysis of extensor carpi radialis brevis and extensor carpi ulnaris.
- Weak thumb abduction (abductor pollicis longus).
- Loss of thumb extension (extensor pollicis brevis and longus).
- Loss of finger extension (extensor indicis proprius, extensor digitorum communis and extensor digiti minimi).

The diagnosis of a PIN palsy can be difficult if the palsy is partial and the differential diagnosis includes extensor tendon rupture at the wrist. In both cases, those muscles and tendons closest to the ulnar are affected first. The 'tenodesis test' can help differentiate between the two. The extensor tendons are intact if the wrist is passively flexed and the fingers extend due to tension in the extensor tendons. If they do not extend it is likely that the tendons are ruptured.

Treatment of PIN compression is conservative, but decompression of the PIN can be undertaken surgically in those with refractory symptoms or significant motor findings.

The pronator teres syndrome (median nerve entrapment)

Around the elbow, the median nerve can become entrapped as it passes through the two heads of the pronator teres muscle. Presentation is with anterior elbow pain and distal paraesthesia identical to that seen in carpal tunnel syndrome. Treatment consists of conservative measures, including physiotherapy, and NSAIDs, and surgery, is reserved for those who are not responding. Surgery involves release of the humeral head of pronator teres.

Examination
The pain is exacerbated by resisted pronation of the forearm. Weakness of the flexors of the index and middle fingers may result in resting finger extension, the so-called 'papal sign'.

Cubital tunnel syndrome
The ulnar nerve runs in the groove behind the medial epicondyle on its path into the forearm. The main complaint is of pain on the medial side of the elbow with paraesthesia along the ulnar border of the forearm extending into the little and ring fingers. There may be a history of weak grip. Treatment is with activity modification, NSAIDs if severe, and splinting. Surgical techniques involve ulnar nerve transposition or less commonly, medial epicondylectomy.

Examination
There may be tenderness over the ulnar nerve as it lies within the groove behind the medial epicondyle, and there is usually a positive Tinel's test. There is wasting of the intrinsic muscles of the hand in advanced cases

Further reading

Bosworth DM. The role of the orbicular ligament in tennis elbow. *J Bone Jt Surg Am* 1955; **37**: 527–33.

Kraushaar BS, Nirschl RP. Tendinosis of the elbow (tennis elbow). Clinical features and findings of histological, immunohistological and electron micrsopic studies. *J Bone Jt Surg Am* 1999; **81**: 259–78.

Putnam MD, Cohen M. Painful conditions around the elbow. *Orthopaed Clin N Am* 1999; **30**: 109–18.

The hand and wrist

The hand is the body's key functional asset, and for full function and positioning, a normal shoulder and elbow joint is necessary.

Regional anatomy

The anatomy of the wrist, the carpal tunnel, and the hand will be discussed. The osteology of the hand and wrist are visualised in Figure 5.19.

Bones

The wrist

When the wrist is in a neutral position, the wrist and hand are in the same plane as the longitudinal axis of the radius and middle metacarpal. The term 'wrist joint' normally implies the radiocarpal joint, rather than the other articulations of the carpal bones.

The radiocarpal joint is formed by the articulation of the distal radius with the scaphoid and lunate. The triquetrum articulates with the triangular fibrocartilage (TFCC), which is a layer of fibrocartilage of variable thickness attached to the ulnar end of the distal radius and the fovea at the base of the ulnar styloid. The distal end of the ulnar, therefore, does not articulate directly with the proximal carpal row. More distally, further movement occurs at the intercarpal and intermetacarpal articulations.

The distal radius and ulnar also articulate with each other at the distal radioulnar joint. The terms 'radial' and 'ulnar' are preferred to medial and lateral, due to the effect of supination at the elbow on posture of the hand. 'Lister's tubercle' is a bony prominence on the dorsum of the radius, and acts as a pulley for the extensor pollicis longus tendon. The scapholunate interval lies just distal to and in line with Lister's tubercle or dorsal tubercle of the distal radius. Movements of the wrist include palmar flexion, dorsiflexion, ulnar deviation, radial deviation, and circumduction. The intercarpal joints contribute to palmar flexion.

The carpal tunnel

The carpal bones form an upside down arch (as viewed with the wrist in supination) with the flexor retinaculum (= transverse carpal ligament) spanning the arch from the palmar surfaces of scaphoid and trapezium radially to the pisiform, triquetrum, and hamate ulnarly. The combination of arch and spanning 'roof' of the flexor retinaculum produces a tunnel, the carpal tunnel.

The hand

The thumb metacarpal articulates with trapezium. The thumb 'carpometacarpal' joint (CMCJ) and the metacarpals of the fingers articulate proximally with the trapezoid, capitate, and hamate. The thumb has only two phalanges – proximal and distal – and, therefore, only one interphalangeal joint. The fingers have a proximal, middle, and distal phalanx and, therefore, both a proximal and distal interphalangeal joint. The first CMCJ lies between trapezium and the base of the first metacarpal bone. It is a multiplane and very mobile joint allowing thumb extension, abduction, adduction, and opposition with the fingers. Flexion/extension at the first CMCJ is up to 50° of movement and abduction/adduction is up to 70°. The fourth and fifth CMCJs of the

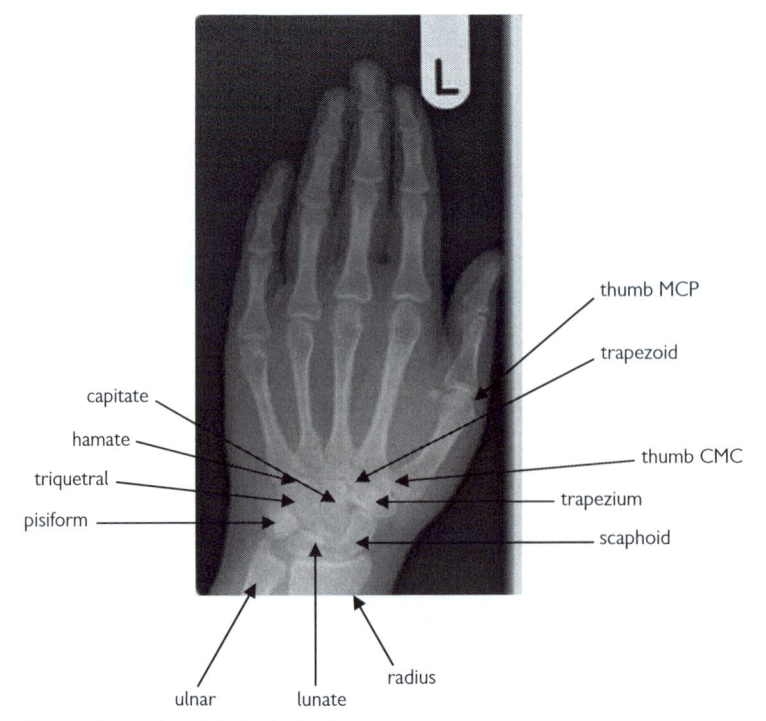

Figure 5.19 Osteology of the hand and wrist.

CHAPTER 5 **Regional musculoskeletal anatomy and conditions**

fingers are more mobile than the second and third, allowing greater opposition with the thumb, and enable the hand to be cupped. The metacarpophalangeal joints (MCPJ) are modified hinge joints. The main function of the MCPJs is to provide flexion/extension of the fingers, with palmar flexion up to 70°, but they also enable the span of the hand to be varied though abduction and adduction. The interphalangeal joints, both proximal (PIPJ) and distal (DIPJ) in the second to fifth digits, and the interphalangeal joint of the thumb are hinge joints. Palmar flexion is up to 120°, and there is not normally significant extension in these joints.

Joint capsules
The wrist joint capsule is bound down to the distal radius and ulnar, bones of the carpus, and bases of the metacarpals, such that, in combination with the intrinsic ligaments between carpal bones, the distal radioulnar joint is a separate cavity from the radiocarpal joint which is also separate from the midcarpal joint. In a normal wrist, therefore, radiographic contrast material injected into any one of these three separate cavities should remain within the cavity into which it is injected. The distal radioulnar joint will develop a communication with the radiocarpal joint if the TFCC becomes perforated either as a result of a traumatic tear, as a result of degenerative breakdown or inflammatory synovitis. The radiocarpal joint will communicate with the radiocarpal joint if either the scapholunate or lunatotriquetral ligaments become perforated. The capsule of the metacarpophalangeal joints is strengthened by the radial and ulnar collateral ligaments on the sides and by the palmar plate on the palmar surface. The capsule attaches to the articular margins.

Ligaments
The ligaments of the hand and wrist are seen in Figure 5.20.
- **Ligaments of the wrist:** these are classified as palmar, dorsal, intrinsic, or extrinsic. Each ligament is named according to the bones to which it attaches, with the most proximal or radial bone attachment being given first, e.g. scapholunate and lunatotriquetral. The palmar capsular ligaments are more numerous than the dorsal and tend to converge distally.
- **Distal radioulnar ligaments:** the dorsal radioulnar and palmar radioulnar ligaments are major stabilizers of the distal radial ulnar joint. They form the dorsal and palmar margins of the TFCC, and the most proximal fibres converge on the ulnar side and attach into the fovea, at the base of the ulnar styloid process. The most distal fibres of the palmar radioulnar ligament form ligaments between the disc of the TFCC and the lunate, and between the disc and the triquetrum.
- **Palmar radiocarpal ligaments:** the palmar radiocarpal ligaments are strong condensations within the palmar wrist capsule and pass from the distal radius to the scaphoid, lunate, and capitate, and form a double V-shaped (one V proximal to the other, rather than side by side) structure with the distal apex on the capitate and the proximal apex on the lunate.
- **Dorsal capsular ligaments:** these are most easily pictured as a Z-shaped structure made up of the dorsal radioulnar ligament, the dorsal radioulnar ligament and the dorsal intercarpal ligament. The main attachments from the proximal end of the Z to distal end of the Z are: distal ulnar, distal radius, triquetrum, and scaphoid and trapezoid (the Z is reversed on the left wrist when looking from the dorsal aspect).

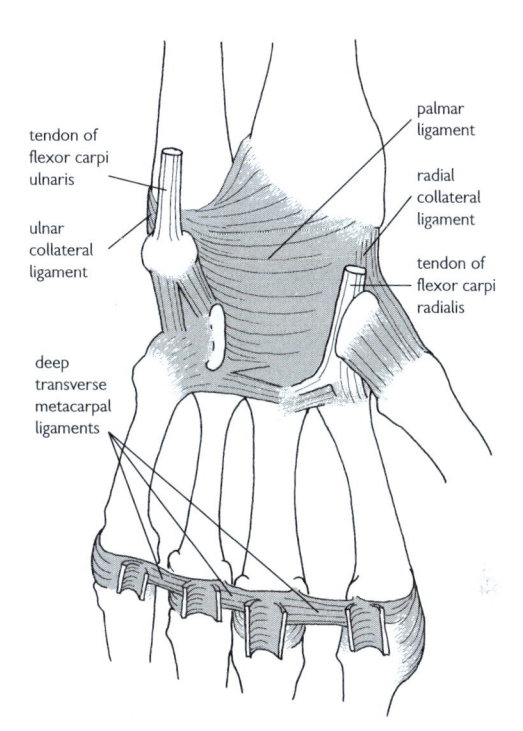

Figure 5.20 Capsule and ligaments of wrist, carpal, and metacarpophalangeal joints. Reproduced from the Oxford Textbook of Functional Anatomy, MacKinnon and Morris, 2005, with permission from Oxford University Press.

- **Ligaments in the digits:** a similar distribution of ligaments occurs in the interphalangeal joints, with collaterals to give longitudinal stability and a palmar plate, which limits extension. The articular surface of the metacarpal head, when viewed laterally, is not spherical, but ovoid, with the top of the oval level with the dorsal cortex of the metacarpal and the bottom of the oval projecting palmar to the palmar cortex of the metacarpal. The collateral ligaments are attached to the side of the metacarpal head closer to the top of the oval and, therefore, are slack when the MCPJ is in extension, but taut when the MCPJ is in flexion. Abduction at these joints, therefore, can only occur when there is slack in the collateral ligaments, i.e. when these joints are in extension; abduction is not possible when these joints are fully flexed. Unlike the MCPJ collateral ligaments, the collateralligaments of the interphalangeal joints remain taut throughout movement, providing a greater degreeof stability and restricting lateral movement. SeeFigure 5.21.

Muscles and tendons
The main muscles of the hand and wrist and their actions are tabulated in Table 5.7.
Extensor tendons. The extensor tendons are bound down to the dorsum of the wrist by the extensor retinaculum. This is a condensation of the fascia of the extensor compartment that forms a strap-like structure. The strap is attached to the distal radius at one end and the distal ulna at the other, and additionally has separate attachments in between such that there are six separate dorsal compartments through which the extensor tendons run.

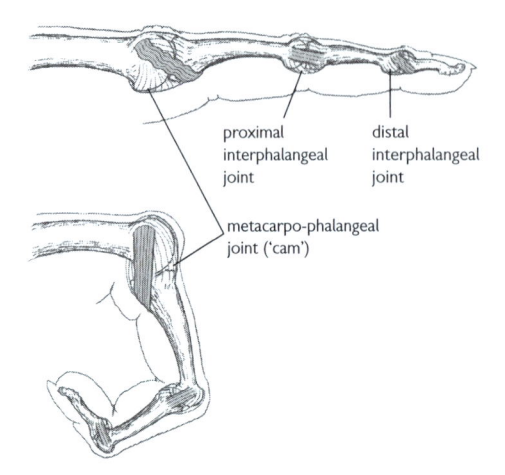

Figure 5.21 Metacarpophalangeal ('cam joint') and interphalangeal joints in flexion and extension. Reproduced from the Oxford Textbook of Functional Anatomy, MacKinnon and Morris, 2005, with permission from Oxford University Press.

Table 5.7 Main muscles of the wrist and hand

Prime dorsiflexors at the wrist	Flexor carpi radialis
	Flexor carpi ulnaris
	Palmaris longus
Dorsiflexors at the MCPJs	Extensor pollicis brevis
	Extensor indicis proprius
	Extensor digitorum communis
	Extensor digiti minimi
Palmar flexors at the MCPJs	Flexor pollicis brevis
	Lumbricals
	Interossei
	Flexor digiti minimi brevis
Flexion of the PIPJs	Flexor digitorum superficialis
Flexion of the DIPJs	Flexor digitorum profundus
Dorsiflexors of the DIPJs and PIPJs	Interossei lumbricals
Flexion of the thumb IPJ	Flexor pollicis longus
Dorsiflexion of the thumb IPJ	Extensor pollicus longus

- The first compartment lies over the radial styloid, on the lateral aspect of the distal radius, and contains the tendons of abductor pollicis longus (APLS) and extensor pollicis brevis (EPB).
- Within the second compartment are the two tendons of the radial wrist extensors [extensor carpi radialis longus (ECRL) and extensor carpi radialis brevis (ECRB)].
- In the third compartment is the extensor pollicis longus tendon, which is prone to rupture in association with fractures of the distal radius.
- The fourth compartment contains the extensor indicis proprius (EIP) tendon and the four tendons of extensor digitorum communis (EDC). Along the floor of this compartment runs the terminal branch of the posterior interosseous nerve (PIN).
- The fifth compartment lies over the ulnar head and contains the extensor digiti minimi (EDM) tendon. This tendon tends to be the first extensor tendon to rupture if the ulnar head erodes through the dorsal distal radioulnar joint capsule. This may occur in either rheumatoid or osteoarthritis.
- The sixth compartment lies over the ulnar aspect of the ulnar head, just dorsal to the ulnar styloid, and contains the tendon of extensor carpi ulnaris (ECU).
- The extensor tendons leave their compartments beneath the extensor retinaculum and diverge to their respective digits where they are held in place by tethers. The main tethers are the saggital bands, which hold the tendons centrally over the dorsal aspect of the MCPJs. The saggital bands are attached to each side of the tendon and run around each side of the base of the proximal phalanx in a palmar direction and attach to each side of the palmar flexor tendon sheath. In addition, the extensor tendons are held by an attachment to the underlying MCPJ capsule. The extensor tendon then separates into three parts, called slips, at the level of the middle of the proximal phalanx. The slips comprise a central slip and two lateral slips.
- The central slip of the extensor tendon inserts into the base of the middle phalanx and extends the PIPJ.
- The two lateral slips diverge to join the lateral bands of the intrinsic muscles at the level of the distal third of the proximal phalanx, where they form the conjoined lateral band.
- The conjoined lateral bands merge at the distal third of the middle phalanx and form a terminal tendon, which inserts into the base of the distal phalanx and extends the DIPJ.
- The intricate weave of the tendons of the long extensors and the aponeurotic expansion of the tendons of the intrinsic muscles form an aponeurosis known as the dorsal aponeurosis (synonymous with dorsal apparatus).
- The action of the central slip is extension of the PIPJ and the action of the terminal tendon is extension of the DIPJ.
- The action of the dorsal aponeurosis at the MCPJ, however, is flexion. This is because the tendons of the intrinsic muscles (interossei and lumbricals) arise palmar and proximal to the centre of rotation of the MCPJ, and then run dorsally to insert into the extensor tendon distal to the MCPJ.
- The intrinsic muscles of the hand are therefore flexors of the MCPJs and, via the extrinsic extensor tendon with which they merge, extensors of the PIPJs and DIPJs.
- Tightness of the intrinsic muscles, as may occur in conditions, such as rheumatoid arthritis, results in PIPJ flexion being more restricted when the MCPJs are in extension than in flexion (if the intrinsic muscles are 'tight' the MCPJs are pulled into flexion and the PIPJs into extension). If the MCPJs are then moved passively into flexion, this has the effect of reducing the tension in the intrinsic tendons and so flexion at the PIPJ may be easier.

Flexor tendons. The flexor tendons of the digits and the median nerve run through the carpal tunnel. Neither the flexor carpi radialis (FCR) tendon and adjacent radial artery, nor the flexor carpi ulnaris (FCU) tendon and adjacent ulnar nerve run through the carpal tunnel. The superficial flexors of the hand are visualised in Figure 5.22.

- The flexor tendons then leave the carpal tunnel, diverge and attach to the digits in the hand.
- The palmaris longus tendon, when present (it is absent in 15% of the population) inserts into the flexor retinaculum, and the palmar aponeurosis. The palmar aponeurosis is a fan-like expansion of fascia in the palm. There are

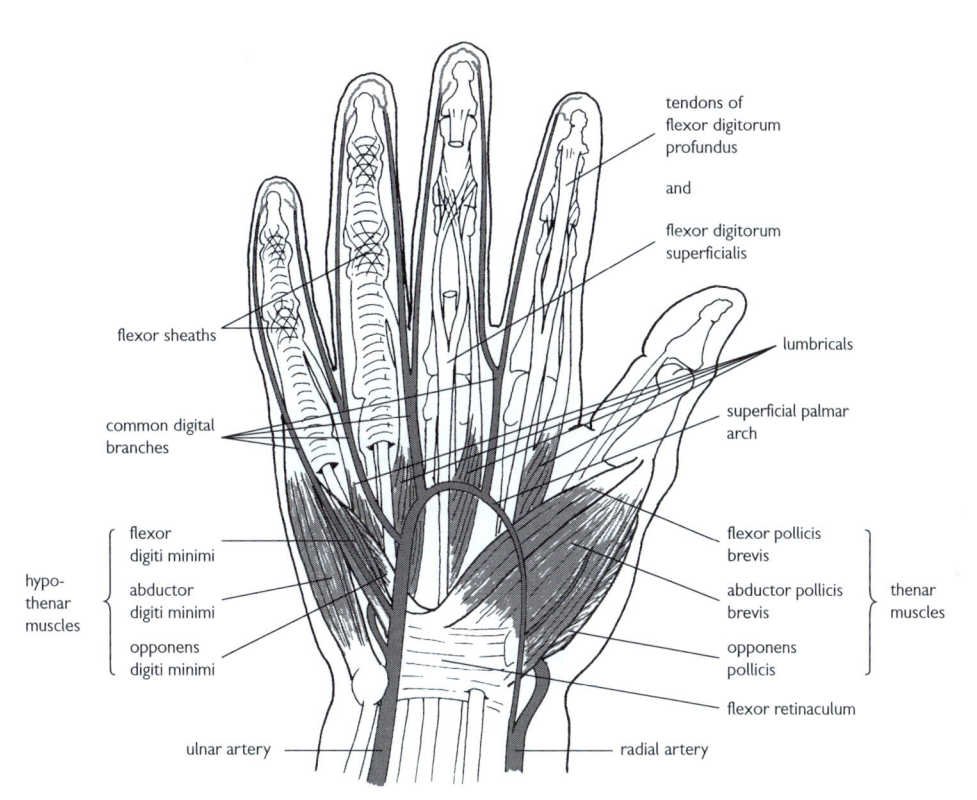

CHAPTER 5 **Regional musculoskeletal anatomy and conditions**   155

Figure 5.22 Superficial aspect of palm. Reproduced from the Oxford Textbook of Functional Anatomy, MacKinnon and Morris, 2005, with permission from Oxford University Press.

longitudinal condensations (bands) running to each digit. In addition, there are transverse fibres and also vertical fibres attaching to the overlying skin. The palmar aponeurosis is, therefore, part of a three dimensional fascial structure known as the 'palmar fascial complex'.
- The flexor tendons and median nerve lie on the radial side of the palmaris longus tendon.
- The flexor tendons, after leaving the carpal tunnel, diverge to their respective digits and are guided along the palmar side of the phalanges by a tunnel. This tunnel comprises the tendon sheath and a series of pulleys that keep the tendon centrally placed. The pulleys occur at intervals and are a series of annular and cruciform retainers that prevent 'bowstringing' of the tendons (i.e. they hold the tendons against the phalanges). The 'A1' (first annular) pulley lies at the level of the MCPJs and is the pulley most commonly involved in 'trigger digits'.

Nerves of the hand
- **Median nerve:** from the antecubital fossa, where it lies to the ulnar side of the radial artery, the median nerve runs deep to the flexor digitorum superficialis (FDS) muscle into the wrist. At the wrist the nerve runs through the carpal tunnel alongside the flexor tendons of the digits. The recurrent motor branch, to the thenar eminence, usually loops back over the distal end of the flexor retinaculum to enter the proximal end of the thenar muscles, but sometimes actually runs through the ligament. The sensory distribution of the median nerve is normally from the palmar aspect of the thumb as far as and including the radial border of the ring finger. This nerve also provides sensibility to the dorsum of the digits distal to the distal interphalangeal joints (sensory supply to the skin of the dorsum of the hand proximal to these points is provided by the radial nerve). In addition, via the recurrent motor branch, the median nerve supplies the muscles of the thenar eminence and the most radial two lumbricals. There is some variation in innervation of the thenar muscles such that the flexor pollicis brevis and opponens pollicis are sometimes innervated by the ulnar nerve. The abductor pollicis brevis muscle is, therefore, the muscle of the thenar eminence most consistently innervated by the median nerve, and, therefore, the muscle to test when assessing the median nerve at the level of the wrist. The anatomy of the carpal tunnel is seen in Figure 5.23.
- **Ulnar nerve:** the ulnar nerve approaches the wrist beneath and to the radial side of the FCU tendon. As the FCU tendon inserts into the pisiform, the nerve runs around the radial side of the pisiform and passes into the palm via Guyon's canal. The ulnar nerve innervates all the small muscles of the hand (apart from those innervated by the median nerve, as previously described) and provides sensibility to the little finger and ulnar border

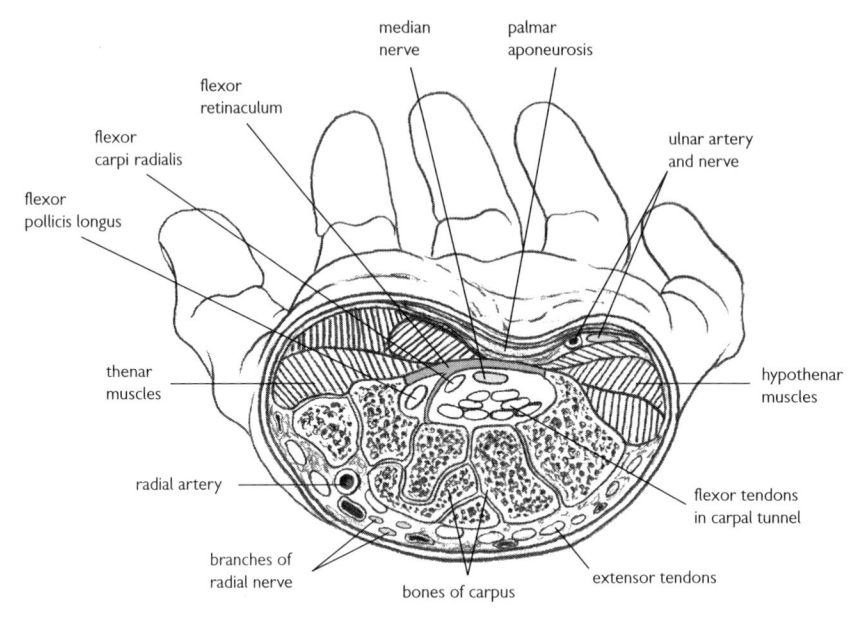

Figure 5.23 Carpal tunnel and contents (tendon shealths not shown); transverse section. Reproduced from the Oxford Textbook of Functional Anatomy, MacKinnon and Morris, 2005, with permission from Oxford University Press.

of the ring finger, on both the palmar and dorsal aspects of the lengths of these fingers. As with innervation of the muscles, there can be some variation in sensory supply in that the ulnar nerve may encroach on median nerve territory by innervating as far as the skin of the ulnar border of the middle finger.

Further reading

Markison RE, Kilgore ES, Hand. In David JH (Eds) *Clinical Surgery*. St Louis: CV Mosby; 1987; **1087**: 2292–353.

McMurty RY. The hand. In: Little AH (Ed.) *The Rheumatological Physical Examination*. Orlando: Grune and Stratton; 1986: 91–100.

McMurty RY, Little AH. The wrist. In: Little AH (Ed.) *The Rheumatological Physical Examination*. Orlando: Grune and Stratton, 1986: 83–9.

Polley HF, Hunder GG. The wrist and carpal joints, metacarpophalangeal, proximal, and distal interphalangeal joints. In: Polley HF, Hunder GG (Eds) *Physical Examination of the Joints*, 2nd edn. Philadelphia: WB Saunders, 1978: 90–148.

Schneider LH. Flexor tendons – late reconstruction. In: Green *et al.* (Eds) *Green's Operative Hand Surgery*, 4th edn. Edinburgh: Churchill Livingstone; 1999: 1909.

Smith RJ. Intrinsic muscles of the fingers: function, dysfunction and surgical reconstruction. *Instruct Course Lect* 1975; **24**: 200–20.

Williams PL, Warwick R, Dyson M, Bannister LH. Joints of the upper limb. In: Williams PL *et al.* (Eds) *Gray's Anatomy*, 37th edn. Edinburgh: Churchill Livingstone 1989: 499–516.

CHAPTER 5 Regional musculoskeletal anatomy and conditions

Hand and wrist: regional musculoskeletal conditions

Main causes of hand and wrist pain

Articular
- Inflammatory arthritis.
- Osteoarthritis.
- Crystal arthritis.

Periarticular
- Tenosynovitis, e.g. De Quervain's, trigger finger.
- Ganglia.
- Tophi/RA nodules.
- Dupytrens contracture.
- Diabetic cheirarthropathy.

Bone
- Fracture.
- Osteochondritis, e.g. scaphoid fracture.

Neurological
- Peripheral nerve entrapment, e.g. carpal tunnel syndrome, PIN entrapment.
- Brachial plexus pathology.
- Thoracic outlet syndrome.
- Cervical radiculopathy.

Conditions associated with osteoarthritis of the hand

See Chapter 12 p. 571(OA). The location of pain can be vital in making a diagnosis. See Table 5.8.

Mucous cyst
This is a sub dermal cyst at the dorsum of the DIPJ. It arises from the joint capsule. Patients must be aware that is a sign of a degenerative joint and not a disease in itself. They can be excised, but carry the risk of recurrence.

Carpometacarpal joint osteoarthritis (CMCJ OA)
This condition exists in up to 70% of people over the age of 60. There is a ratio of 10:1 women to men.
- On clinical examination there is a prominence at the base of the thumb with pain on axially loading, and extending or flexing the thumb.
- Early treatment includes hand therapy with splinting, analgesia, and glucocorticoid injection.
- Surgery involves removal of the trapezium with various procedures to stabilize the base of the thumb. Patients must be told that they will be mobilized for approximately 6 weeks after surgery and that it may take up to 6 months to regain their preoperative hand function.

Scaphoid non-union and advanced collapse (SNAC)
This is a secondary arthritis of the carpus because of a previous scaphoid fracture that has not united.

Scapho-lunate advanced collapse (SLAC)
Damage to the scapho-lunate ligament leads to rotary subluxation of the scaphoid. As a result of this secondary arthritic changes begin in a localized manner at the radio-scaphoid joint and progress to pan-carpal arthritis.

Distal radio-ulna joint disease
The radius and ulna articulate at the distal radio-ulnar joint (DRUJ). The base of the ulna is attached to the radius via the triangular fibrocartilage complex (TFCC). The radius and ulna articulate at the sigmoid notch. The DRUJ and TFCC can be disrupted via trauma, such as a radial fracture malunion, or degenerative and inflammatory conditions.
- Patients may have degeneration or tears of the cartilaginous disc. If the radius loses height, such as in a radial fracture, too much force goes through the relatively longer ulna.
- Patients will often tell you they have pain and clicking on the ulna side of the wrist.
- Two simple tests can be done that indicate ulna-sided pathology include pain on ulna deviation of the wrist with pain on ballotment of the ulna.
- Analgesia and temporary splinting can help alleviate pain, but referral to a hand surgeon is usually recommended. Surgery is complex and often involves long periods of post-operative immobilization.

Table 5.8 Differential diagnosis hand and wrist pain by location

Radial	Osteoarthritis thumb carpometacarpal joint
	Scapho-trapezial-trapezoid osteoarthritis
	Scaphoid fracture, or consequent scaphoid collapse
	De Quervain's disease
	Ganglion
Ulna	Distal radioulnar joint osteoarthritis and instability
	Triangular fibrocartilage complex injury or degeneration.
	Hamate hook fracture and non-union
	Extensor carpi ulnaris (ECU) tendinitis
	Piso-triquetral osteoarthritis
Dorsal	Avascular necrosis of the lunate (Keinbock's disease)
	Ganglion
	Scapho-lunate dissociation
	Scapho-lunate advanced collapse

Tenosynovitis
This is defined as inflammation of the synovial lining of a tendon sheath.

Table 5.9 Causes of tenosynovitis

Proliferative	Erosive, e.g. RA
	Deposition, e.g. amyloid
	Crystalline, e.g. gout, pseudo-gout
	Septic, e.g. bacterial, mycobacterial
Tendon entrapment and stenosing tendonvaginitis	Finger, e.g. trigger
	Radial side of wrist, e.g. De Quervains' disease
	Tendons, e.g. ECU, EPL, FCR

History
There is usually a history of pain and swelling along the line of the affected tendon, usually an extensor tendon, with subsequent loss of function. A careful history will determine an underlying inflammatory or infectious cause.

CHAPTER 5 Regional musculoskeletal anatomy and conditions

Examination
- Soft tissue swelling, which moves as the affected tendon is moved.
- There may be crepitus on movement of the affected tendon through the tendon sheath.
- There may be features of an associated carpal tunnel syndrome.
- Tendon rupture or triggering may be present.

Investigations
The most specific imaging technique is ultrasound, which allows visualization of the synovitis around the tendon and guides accurate placement of an injection into the tendon sheath. Ultrasound will also detect heterogeneity of a tendon indicating degenerative change. See Figure 5.24.

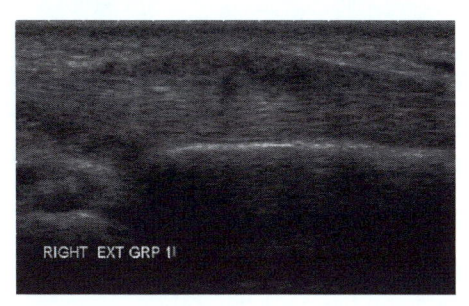

Figure 5.24 There is thickening around the tendon and synovitis around the extensor group 1 tendons, but with no fluid visualized on ultrasound.

Management of tenosynovitis
- In those with an infectious cause, debridement and antibiotic therapy is necessary, with no role for conservative management or glucocorticoid injection (see Chapter 16 p. 459)
- Hand therapy, rest, and splinting are of benefit.
- Medical management aims to prevent tendon rupture.
- Targeted glucocorticoid injections for non-infectious tenosynovitis.
- Surgical steps include synovectomy and trigger finger release with carpal tunnel decompression. Dorsal synovectomy involves a long incision on the back of the hand, followed by bandage or plaster immobilization for 2 weeks. After this period, removal of sutures and hand therapy can begin. Scar massage and occasionally desensitization may be needed.

Specific examples of tenosynovitis
Trigger finger
Trigger finger and thumb are common, and can be primary or associated with diabetes, gout, renal disease, and other rheumatic diseases. The flexor tendon is unable to smoothly slide up and down its sheath, and as a result the finger locks/clicks into a flexed position. It can be very painful to straighten it up.
- On clinical examination the triggering can be elicited and a nodule is often palpated at the distal palmar crease.
- Treatment includes glucocorticoid injection with an approximately 50% success rate.
- If the glucocorticoid injection does not work then surgical release of the trigger finger is performed, usually under local anaesthetic.

- Young babies can have a 'congenital' trigger thumb. Parents may notice that the thumb does not extend. On examination a nodule may be felt at the base of the thumb and it may not be possible to extend the thumb. This is due to a similar pathology and warrants referral to a hand surgeon.

De Quervain's tenosynovitis
De Quervain's tenosynovitis occurs in the first extensor compartment on the back of the thumb. This includes the extensor pollicus brevis (EPB) tendon and abductor pollicus longus (APLS) tendon.
- Pain is the main presenting symptom with triggering a rare finding.
- Flexion of the thumb and ulna deviation of the wrist (Finkelstein's test) causes pain, but is not pathognomonic of de Quervain's tenosynovitis.
- It is common in breast feeding and new mothers due to over-use and positioning of the hands.
- Treatment modalities include glucocorticoid injection and ultimately surgical decompression if this does not work.

Intersection syndrome
Intersection syndrome is a tenosynovitis of the second dorsal compartment of the wrist (This is where the APLS and EPB tendons cross the common radial wrist extensors).
- Patients present with pain and swelling 4 cm proximal to the radial side of the wrist.
- It is more common with repetitive wrist motion especially in sports, such as rowing and weight lifting.
- In the majority of cases rest, splinting, and glucocorticoid injection is sufficient. Occasionally, surgical decompression is necessary.

Extensor carpi ulnaris (ECU) tenosynovitis
This is reactive tenosynovitis in the ECU tendon and it is often initiated by a twisting injury of the wrist.
- It is associated with nocturnal ulna-sided wrist pain and swelling.
- Pain in the sensory branch of the ulna nerve is common. Pain in all motions of the wrist is noted although it is worse in an extensor and ulna deviated position.
- The diagnosis is confirmed when pain is obliterated by injecting local anaesthetic into the ECU sheath.
- Management is the same as intersection syndrome.

Kienböcks disease
This encompasses avascular necrosis of the lunate bone. It involves a degree of wrist degeneration. Reasonable function, however, is maintained. The cause of this condition is uncertain, but is not thought to be related to trauma.

History
- Pain particularly on the dorsum of the wrist.
- Stiffness with subsequent loss of motion.
- Weakness of the wrist with diminished grip strength.
- There is rarely a history of trauma.

Examination
- Tenderness to palpation with occasional dorsal swelling.
- Decreased range of wrist motion.

Investigations
- Radiographs show characteristic increased density of the lunate bone, as well as fragmentation with collapse of the lunate. See Figure 5.25.
- MR may be useful and can help in planning treatment.

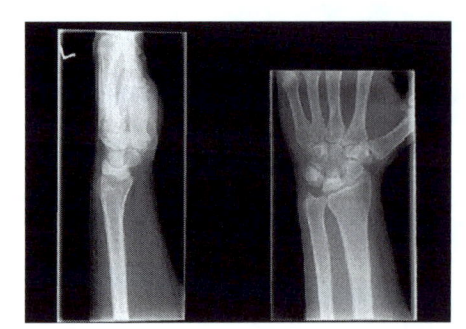

Figure 5.25 On this plain radiograph of a patient with Keinbock's disease, sclerosis of the lunate bone can be seen on both views.

- The disease is staged according to the degree of degeneration, with subsequent secondary changes to the carpal structure and scaphoid bone.

Management
- A short period of physiotherapy with casting or bracing can be attempted, but it is not recommended unless there is quick resolution of symptoms.
- Arthroscopic evaluation may help with diagnosis and can provide pain relief.
- Surgery can be complex and may involve prolonged periods of immobilization after osteotomy.
- Advanced disease can be treated with proximal row carpectomy or arthrodesis. Recovery can often take up to 6 months.

Preisser's disease
- This is a similar condition to Kienböck's, but affects the scaphoid bone.
- It presents with radial and dorsal sided wrist pain.
- There may be an association with previous non-specific wrist trauma but this disease is differentiated from scaphoid fracture and non-union.
- Management is also complex and beyond the scope of this text.

Upper limb nerve entrapment syndromes
The radial, ulna, and median nerves may all be compressed predominantly from the elbow to the wrist. Patients present with a wide range of symptoms starting with occasional paraesthesia, and may progress to sensory loss, muscle weakness, and pain. Severity depends on the degree of compression, as well as duration of compression. It is imperative that the whole limb, as well as the cervical spine is examined when evaluating these patients. Double crush syndrome, as described by Upton and Acoma, is the compression of a nerve at one level, which will make it susceptible to damage at another level. For example, cervical nerve route compression predisposes a patient to carpal tunnel disease.

Median nerve compression
Median nerve compression at the wrist: carpal tunnel syndrome
This is the most common compressive neuropathy in the upper limb and is a term used to describe a broad group of symptoms associated with compression of the median nerve at the wrist. It is generally idiopathic in origin; however, there is an association with rheumatoid arthritis, diabetes, connective tissue diseases, pregnancy, and previous wrist fracture. It occurs most commonly in women in the 30–60-year age groups. The differential diagnosis for this condition includes a cervical radiculopathy, as well as spinal cord lesions and peripheral neuropathies, such as alcoholic and diabetic neuropathies.

History
- Patients often present with a typical history of numbness in the median nerve distribution, particularly in the morning, with pins and needles in a similar distribution.
- They often report that shaking the hand in the morning makes it better.
- Patients initially have pins and needles, and pain in the above mentioned distribution and as time progresses they may well go on to having diminished sensation.
- Patients often present with odd pain shooting up the arms.

Examination
- Examination should include the cervical spine, as well as a neurological examination of the hand.
- There may be diminished sensation in the median nerve distribution with wasting of the thenar muscles.
- Gentle tapping over the median nerve at the wrist in a neutral position often produces paraesthesia in the distribution of the median nerve. (Tinel's test) Holding the wrist in a flexed position will often bring on similar symptoms of tingling (Phalens' test).
- The disease can be divided into mild (sensory deficit only), moderate (sensory and motor deficit), and severe (sensory deficit with motor absence)
- The diagnosis of this disease is generally clinical. However, nerve condition studies may be used as an adjunct.

Management
- Conservative management, such as a Futuro splint and non-steroidal anti-inflammatory drugs often help.
- Injection of local anaesthetic and glucocorticoid into the carpal tunnel have been shown to keep patients symptom-free for at least 1 year in over 50% of cases.
- Injection is best provided by a hand surgeon or rheumatologist as the median nerve is at risk during the injection.
- If conservative treatment has not worked then early referral to a hand surgeon would be recommended. The treatment would include surgical decompression of the carpal tunnel, which can usually be performed under local anaesthetic.

Median nerve compression in the forearm
- The proximal median nerve can be trapped between the ligaments and muscles at the elbow, and proximal forearm, e.g. between the bellies of the pronator teres muscle.
- The anterior interosseous nerve can be trapped in the forearm resulting in diminished thumb flexion and weakness in pronation at 90° of flexion.

History
- Aching pain in the forearm.
- Decreased sensation in the radial three-and-a-half fingers.
- Reduced power in the hand.

Examination
- Sensory deficit in the above-mentioned distribution.
- Negative Tinel's and Phalen's tests.

- The specific provocation test involves flexion of the elbow to 90° with resistance of pronation and supination.
- Nerve conduction studies are often normal.

Management
- This may involve a hand therapist with splinting and strategies to avoid positions that irritate the nerve.
- NSAIDS may help control pain.
- Surgical release will result in a scar that may be prominent and nerve recovery can take up to 6 months.

Ulnar nerve compression
The nerve can be compressed at the elbow (cubital tunnel), usually at an anatomically narrow location. At the wrist (Guyon's canal) there is usually a cause for the compression, such as a ganglion, hamate fracture, direct trauma, or anomalous muscles.

History
- A loss of feeling on the little and ring finger, particularly on the palmar surface and ulna border is typical.
- With involvement at the elbow there can be diminished dorsal sensation.
- Patients often complain of a dull ache down the arm and occasionally above the elbow.

Examination
- Diminished sensation of the above distribution with a positive Tinel's test at the elbow.
- There is intrinsic muscle wasting and weakness with a positive Fromen's test. (Instead of grabbing a piece of paper with a flat thumb, the thumb is bent to grab the paper. This illustrates use of the FPL tendon which is supplied by the median nerve.)
- The provocation test involves persistent flexion at the elbow and recreates the paraesthesiae (Wadsworth test).
- The severity of the disease is graded using the Dellon or modified Bishop system.
- Nerve conduction studies are recommended if there is any doubt regarding the diagnosis.

Management
- Surgical decompression is indicated if conservative treatment fails.
- It is important to tell the patients that there may be a degree of elbow stiffness with a possibility of weak flexor muscles if a sub muscular transposition has been performed.

Radial nerve compression
The nerve is divided into the posterior interosseous nerve (PIN), which is positioned in the proximal third of the forearm, and the superficial branch of the radial nerve, which is predominantly in the distal third, radial aspect of the forearm. The condition must be differentiated from lateral epicondylitis (tennis elbow).

History
- Dull ache in the proximal forearm with extension up the arm at times.
- Entrapment of the sensory branch often causes a sensation of painful water flowing down the arm.
- Complaints of weakness of the hand and wrist.

Clinical examination
- Decreased sensation is not typical.
- A positive Tinels' sign over the course of the nerve.
- Tenderness along the course of the nerve, but not at the common extensor origin at the elbow.

- Symptoms of PIN compression can be elicited by resisted supination with an extended elbow.
- Pressure over the junction of the brachioradialis/extensor carpi radialis tendons, with the forearm in pronation and the wrist in ulna flexion, elicits the pain associated with entrapment of the sensory branch. This entrapment is known as Wartenburg's syndrome.

Management
Management is as for previous entrapment neuropathies.

Thoracic outlet syndrome
This is a diagnosis of exclusion and is not an easy diagnosis to make. The clinical criteria are far more important than special investigations. Aetiology can be subdivided into:
- **Arterial:** this accounts for 1–2% of cases and is usually secondary to a bony protuberance from a cervical rib of other anomaly. The occlusion can be acute or chronic with the development of a collateral circulation. This results in either acute ischaemia or a Raynaud's type phenomenon.
- **Venous:** this accounts for 2–3% of cases and usually occurs in young muscular males, particularly after vigorous exercise.
- **True compression:** this is quite rare and is the result of nerve compression at the C8T1 level, and is always a result of a bony abnormality.
- **Disputed:** this makes up 97% of cases and presents with a variety of symptoms that are often ambiguous. Provocation testing is positive however Doppler, EMG, and radiographs are normal.

History
- Paresthesia usually in the ring and small fingers is classical.
- Shoulder pain, but not upper back pain is experienced.
- Driving, grooming, and lying in bed can all worsen the pain.
- There is an association with depression and anger at a later stage.

Examination
- It is essential to examine the patient fully unclothed to truly appreciate muscle asymmetry and postural abnormality.
- Masses and fullness in the cervical spine and neck region must be looked for, and a thorough neurological examination is important.
- The peripheral nerves must all be evaluated for evidence of compression.
- There are numerous special provocation tests, but the Roos is thought to be the most sensitive and reproducible. The Adson and Halstead manoeuvres can also be performed. The Roos manoeuvre entails 90° of shoulder abduction with external rotation and 3 minute opening and closing (pumping) the hand. This should reproduce symptoms.
- Patients should have plain radiographs and usually have CT/MR and EMG studies, which are often normal.

Management
- Non-operative treatment is the mainstay. It involves postural retraining, as well as physiotherapy. A team approach with a social worker, psychiatrist, and pain specialist is essential.
- Surgery should be performed in specialized centres, but it is not always guaranteed to cure the patient.

Diabetic cheirarthropathy

This condition of the hand is not well understood. It is thought to be as a result of a muscular/tendon imbalance with soft tissue disruption. There is a micro-angiopathy of the dermal and subcutaneous blood vessels. It is more common in Type 1 diabetics (16–42%), and can affect 8–50% of the population.

- Patients will complain of a painless loss of function in the hands.
- On examination there is swelling of the fingers with thick tight and waxy skin. There is initial loss of MCPJ and PIPJ movement but this eventually progresses to DIPJ movement.
- The pathognomonic sign for the disease is the Prayer sign, which is an inability to oppose palmar surfaces.
- Differential diagnosis should include carpal tunnel and Dupuytren's disease, as well as scleroderma.
- Management includes physical therapy with good diabetic control with judicious use of glucocorticoids. Aldose reductase inhibitors have been tried to decrease the effects of this disease.

Soft tissues lesions in the hand and wrist

Small tumours in the hand are common and are usually benign. Their size and possible interference with function should be monitored, and if a proper diagnosis cannot be made then referral is recommended. Tumours include ganglia, implantation dermoid cysts (found along the volar surfaces of the fingers and palms). Malignant tumours such as basal or squamous cell carcinoma, and melanoma are less common. Prompt referral must take place. It is not uncommon for the rheumatologist to diagnose skin cancer.

Ganglion

A ganglion is a cystic myxomatous degeneration of fibrous tissue. Ganglia are extremely common around the wrist joint and often originate from the carpus itself. Ganglia in the proximity of peripheral nerves may cause local irritation. Ganglia generally are not painful, but can be irritating. Large ganglia can interfere with movement. Ganglia generally grow slowly and usually present many months after developing. They are rare in children under 10 years old and often regress in children.

- Dorsal wrist ganglia occur over the scaphoid interval on the dorsal aspect of the wrist.
- Volar ganglia occur over the radial artery and are often quite large.
- On palpation they are cystic and occasionally feel hard. They move underneath the skin and are usually not tender.
- Conservative measures include reassurance, and a watch and wait policy. Ganglia can be aspirated and injected with glucocorticoid, but this does not guarantee removal.
- If the ganglion is significantly painful or interfering with activities of daily living the patient can be referred to a surgeon. It is important to let the patient know that even if the ganglion is excised there is a 20% risk of a recurrence.

Dupuytren's disease

This is a condition of nodular hypertrophy and contracture of the superficial palmar fascia. It is thought be associated with an imbalance of matrix metalloproteinase inhibitors. It is commonly bilateral and is often precipitated by trauma. It is more common in males and usually affects patients over the age of 40, but only presents much later on. There is a hereditary predisposition and an association with diabetes and epilepsy. There is a very small group of people who have what is known as a Dupuytren's diathesis in which the disease progresses rapidly; the patients are usually male. The diathesis is associated with a similar condition on the soles of the feet, as well as Peyronie's disease.

- Patients present with pitting and nodules with thickening of the fascia in the hand. Later on this progresses to deformity at both the metacarpophalangeal and proximal inter-phalangeal joints.
- Patients reports trouble with washing and hygiene of the hands, as well as the finger getting in the way. It is a progressive disease.
- On clinical examination there are bands and nodules on the palmar aspect of the hands with deformity of the joints. Occasionally, there may be pads (Garrods') on the dorsal aspects of the MCPJs and PIPJs. The patient is unable to lay the hand flat on the table (a positive Hueston table top test).
- It is worth having a watchful policy at an early presentation as surgery performed at an immature stage of the disease can worsen it. Referral is recommended when deformity occurs. It must be noted that surgery does not prevent a recurrence of the disease.

Further reading

Clayton ML. Historical perspectives on surgery of the rheumatoid hand. *Hand Clin* 1989; **5**: 111–14.

Finkelstein H. Stenosing tendovaginitis at the radial styloid process. *J Bone Jt Surg Am* 1930; **12**: 509–40.

Green DP. *Green's Operative Hand Surgery*, 5th edn. Philadelphia: Elsevier, 2005.

Hueston JT, Wilson WF. The aetiology of trigger finger. *Hand* 1972; **4**: 257–60.

Jebson PJ, Kasdan ML. *Hand Secrets*, 3rd edn. Philadelphia: Hanley and Balfus, 2006.

Kapoor A, Sibbitt WL Jr. Contractures in diabetes mellitus: the syndrome of limited joint mobility. *Semin Arthritis Rheum* 1989; **18**(3): 168–80.

Kienbock R. Peltier L. Concerning traumatic malacia of the lunate and its consequences: degeneration and compression fractures. *Clin Orthopaed* 1980; **149**: 4–8.

Mackinnon SE. Pathophysiology of nerve compression. *Hand Clin* 2002; **18**: 231–41.

McRae R. *Orthopaedics and Fractures*, 2nd edn. London: Churchill Livingstone, 2006.

Miller MD. *Review of Orthopaedics*, 4th edn. Philadelphia: Elsevier, 2004.

Nagle D J. Evaluation of chronic wrist pain. *J Am Acad Orth Surg* 2000; **8**: 45–55.

Stanley J. Mini-symposium: Rheumatoid Disease of the Hand and Wrist, the rheumatoid wrist. *Curr Orthopaed* 2001; **15**(5): 329–37.

Stanley J. Mini-symposium: Rheumatoid Disease of the Hand and Wrist, degenerative arthritis of the wrist. Curr Orthopaed 1999; **13**(4): 290–6.

Upton ARM, McComas AJ. The double crush in nerve entrapment syndromes. *Lancet* 1973; **2**: 359–62.

Pelvis, hip, and groin

There are a wide range of musculoskeletal and soft-tissue lesions in and around the hip region. However, to understand and appropriately diagnose these conditions, it is important to appreciate the complexity of the anatomy of the hip.

Regional anatomy

Bones (See Figure 5.26)
The pelvic girdle is a ring structure consisting of two paired innominate bones, the sacrum and the coccyx. Each bone is made of three fundamental parts – the ileum, ischium, and the pubis, and each contributes to part of the hip acetabulum. The articulations of the pelvis include the sacroiliac joints and the symphysis pubis anteriorly (secondary cartilaginous joint). The sacroiliac joints are further stabilized by strong posterior and dorsal sacroiliac ligaments, the sacrotuberous and sacrospinous ligaments. The symphysis pubis is reinforced by the suprapubic and arcuate infrapubic ligament. Movement across the joints in the pelvis is minimal, but the essential function of the pelvis is force transmission from lower limb to the trunk.

The hip joint is a multi-axial ball-and-socket synovial joint designed for stability and a wide range of movement. The ileum forms the superior, pubis the anterior and ischium the posteroinferior part of the acetabulum. The femoral head projects superomedially and anteriorly, and forms an angle of inclination with the shaft of the femur (via the neck) at 125–130°. Coxa vara describes an inclination angle less than 100° resulting in shortening of the affected limb, while coxa valga describes an angle greater than 130° resulting in limb lengthening of the affected side.

Stability of the hip joint is afforded by a multitude of factors:

- A substantial bony cup (acetabulum), which is deepened by a fibrocartilaginous labrum and transverse acetabular ligament.
- A fibrous capsule.
- Ligaments.
- Muscles.

Hip joint capsule
This strong fibrous capsule attaches proximally to the acetabular rim and transverse acetabular ligament. Distally, it attaches to the anterior intertrochanteric line and proximal to the intertrochanteric line posteriorly. These capsular fibres take a spiral course from the acetabulum to the intertrochanteric line.

Ligaments of hip joint (See Figure 5.27a)
Hip joint stability is reinforced by ligaments.

Iliofemoral ligament
Reinforces the fibrous capsule anteriorly. It is Y-shaped, and attaches to the anterior inferior iliac spine proximally and the intertrochanteric line distally.

Pubofemoral ligament
It reinforces the inferior and anterior aspect of the fibrous capsule, arises from the obturator foramen margin and passes laterally to insert onto the intertrochanteric line and merges with the medial part of the iliofemoral ligament at its insertion.

Ischiofemoral ligament
It reinforces the posterior part of capsule, arises from ischial part of acetabular rim and attaches medial to the base of greater trochanter.

Muscles (see table for insertion and origins)
Gluteal region
- Gluteus maximus (inferior gluteal nerve).
- Gluteus medius (superior gluteal nerve).
- Gluteus minimus (superior gluteal nerve).
- Short external rotators:
  - piriformis (nerve to piriformis; anterior rami of S1);
  - obturator internus (nerve to obturator internus);

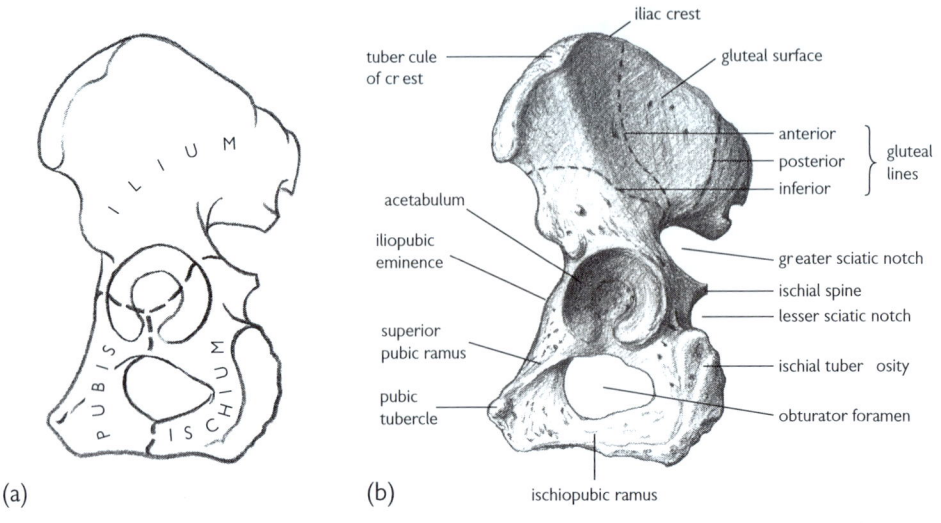

Figure 5.26 (a) diagram of pelvis (lateral view) showin fusion lines wher the three constituent bones (ilumium, ischium, pubis) meet. (b) Lateral aspect of adult pelvis. Reproduced from the Oxford Textbook of Functional Anatomy, MacKinnon and Morris, 2005, with permission from Oxford University Press.

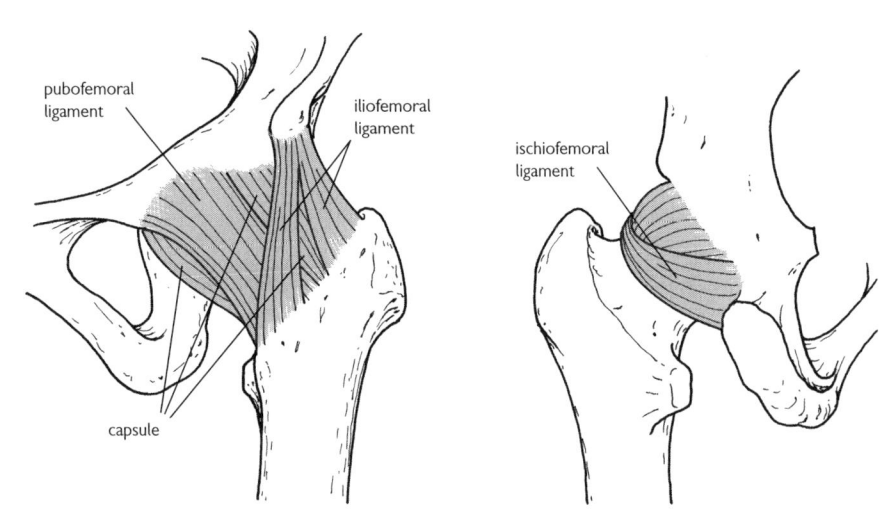

CHAPTER 5 **Regional musculoskeletal anatomy and conditions** 165

Figure 5.27 Inrinsic ligaments of hip joint. Reproduced from the Oxford Textbook of Functional Anatomy, MacKinnon and Morris, 2005, with permission from Oxford University Press.

- superior gemelli (nerve to obturator internus);
- inferior gemelli (nerve to quadratus femoris);
- quadratus femoris (nerve to quadratus femoris).

Anterior compartment of thigh
- Iliopsoas (femoral nerve and anterior rami of lumbar plexus).
- Pectineus (femoral nerve).
- Tensor of fascia lata (superior gluteal nerve).
- Sartorius (femoral nerve).
- Quadriceps femoris (all femoral nerve):
  - rectus femoris;
  - vastus lateralis;
  - vastus medialis;
  - vastus intermedius.

Medial compartment of thigh
- Adductor longus (obturator nerve).
- Adductor brevis (obturator nerve).
- Adductormagnus (obturator and sciatic nerve).
- Gracilis (obturator nerve).
- Obturator externus (obturator nerve).

Posterior compartment of thigh
Hamstrings:
- Semitendinosus (tibial division of sciatic nerve);
- Semimembranosus (tibial division of sciatic nerve);
- Biceps femoris (both tibial and common fibular division of sciatic nerve).

Blood supply to femoral head (See Figure 5.298)
- **Intra-capsular:** branches of obturator artery to head of femur is conveyed via the ligamentum teres femori.
- **Retinacula:** convey branches of the medial and lateral circumflex femoral arteries – the main blood supply to the femoral head.
- **Nutrient arteries:** from branches of the upper perforating arteries of the profunda femoris, conveyed through the marrow cavity.

- **Cruciate anastomosis:** this is a collateral supply posterior to hip joint, and has minimal contribution to arterial supply to the femoral head. From Inferior gluteal artery and 1st profunda femoral perforating artery.

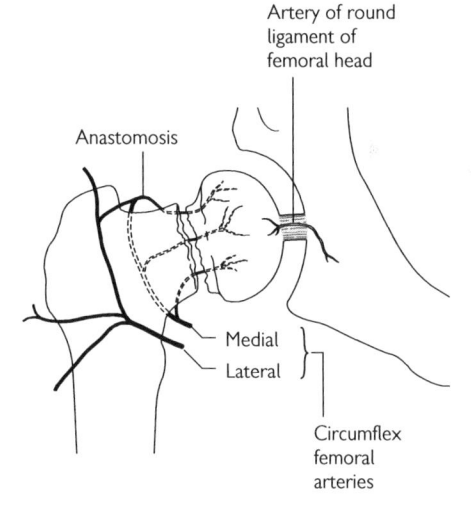

Figure 5.28 Blood supply of the femoral head. Reproduced from the Oxford Textbook of Functional Anatomy, MacKinnon and Morris, 2005, with permission from Oxford University Press.

Functional anatomy
Locking of the hip joint
In the extended position, the hip joint locks. The functional advantage is then the joint can remain in extension (in upright position) without needing muscle contraction.
- Process:
- In an upright position, the body's centre of mass falls behind the hip joint.
- Gravity shifts the hip posteriorly into extension.

- The fibrous capsule (with its spiralling fibres) draws the femoral head into acetabulum with hip extension.
- The iliofemoral ligament tightens and screws the femoral head into the acetabulum with extension.
- The ischiofemoral ligament acts similarly to the iliofemoral ligament, but has a much weaker effect.

As a result, the head of the femur and the acetabulum are tightly engaged, preventing dislocation, and hyperextension of the hip joint.

Range of motion
The motion is in three planes: sagittal, frontal and transverse, with the greatest motion in the sagittal plane.
- **Flexion:** 120° (knee flexed), 90° (knee extended). Iliopsoas and rectus femoris. Smaller contribution from sartorius, tensor of fascia lata (TFL), pectineus, adductor longus, adductor brevis, adductor magnus (anterior part), and gracilis.
- **Extension:** gluteus maximus, semitendinosus, semimembranosus, long head of biceps femoris, and adductor magnus (hamstring portion).
- **Abduction:** normal 45°. TFL, gluteus medius/minimus.
- **Adduction:** normally up to 30°. Adductor longus, brevis and magnus, gracilis and pectineus.
- **Internal rotation:** usually 40°. Gluteus medius and minimus and TFL.
- **External rotation:** up to 45°. Short external rotators (obturator internus and externus, gemelli, piriformis, and quadratus femoris) assisted by gluteus maximus.

Movement limitation of hip joint (Clarkson 2000)
The fibrous capsule and the bony joint configuration itself play a role in limiting hip joint movements. However, in addition to this, the following have additional function in limiting range of motion:
- **Flexion:** by soft tissue apposition, tension of gluteus maximus.
- **Extension:** by iliofemoral and ischiofemoral ligaments, tension of psoas.
- **Abduction:** by pubofemoral ligament and tension of hip adductors.
- **Adduction:** by soft tissue apposition, the lateral band of iliofemoral ligament, tension of iliotibial band and hip abductors.
- **Internal rotation:** Ischiofemoral ligament and tension of external rotators.
- **External rotation:** Iliofemoral and pubofemoral ligament and tension of internal rotators.

Gait
Normal gait consists of two cycles, and the duration of each phase is the same for both limbs thus conferring symmetrical rhythm. By means of pelvic rotation, tilt, and lateral displacement, the displacement of centre of gravity is minimized during normal gait.

During slow walking, the maximum force transmitted across the hip joint is approximately 2.5 times the body weight, and in running this force increases to about 5.2 times the bodyweight during toe-off phase. (van den Bogert et al. 1999)

Stance phase
- **Heel strike:** eccentric contractions of hamstring and gluteus maximus restrains further forward movement of limb, thus allowing heel strike.
- **Loading:** gluteus medius and minimus contract to cause abduction of weight-bearing limb. This prevents pelvic tilt (trendelenburg gait) to the contra-lateral side thus allowing it to swing and maintain centre of gravity.
- **Mid-stance:** during mid and terminal stance, abductors maintain pelvic stability. At the same time, the hip joint moves from a neutral to extended position secondary to the swinging of torso by the contralateral limb.
- **Terminal stance**.
- **Pre-swing:** elastic re-coil of intrinsic foot muscle prepares for toe-off

Swing phase
- Limb goes from weight bearing to non-weight bearing position. Quadriceps contract to limit the degree of knee flexion toe-off.
- Contraction of hip flexors (especially iliopsoas) brings the hip into flexion.
- Adductors play a role in swinging the limb inward, keeping the foot under the pelvis, ready for the next stance phase.
- In late swing/before heel strike, hamstrings contract to decelerate forward swing.

Further reading

Clarkson HM. Musculoskeletal assessment. Joint range of motion and manual of muscle strength, 2nd edn. Baltimore; Lippincott Williams & Wilkins 2000.

Gottschalk F, Kourosh S, et al. The functional anatomy of tensor fascia latae and gluteus medius and minimus. *J Anat* 1989; **166**: 179–89.

McCarthy J, Noble P, et al. Anatomy, pathologic features, and treatment of acetabular labral tears. *Clin Orthopaed Relat Res* 2003; **406**: 38–47.

Moore KL, Agur AMR. *Essential clinical anatomy*, 2nd edn Baltimore; Lippincott Williams & Wilkins, 2002.

van den Bogert AJ, Read L, Nigg BM. An analysis of hip joint loading during walking, running, and skiing. *Med Sci Sports Exerc* 1999; **31**: 131–42.

Pelvis, hip and groin: regional musculoskeletal conditions

Main differential diagnosis of hip pain

Anterior hip pain
- Osteoarthritis of hip.
- Inflammatory arthritis.
- Femoral fracture.
- Iliopsoas bursitis.
- Osteitis pubis.
- Tendonitis (commonly adductor).
- Avascular necrosis of femoral head (see also p. 433).
- Intra-articular pathology (including labral tears, acetabular rim syndrome and femora-acetabular impingement).
- Hernia (inguinal or femoral most commonly).

Lateral hip pain
- Trochanteric bursitis.
- Guteus medius insertional tendonitis/tear.
- Nerve compression (commonly lateral femoral cutaneous nerve).
- Referred pain from lumbar spine.

Posterior hip pain
- Sacroiliitis.
- Ischiogluteal bursitis.
- Referred pain from lumbar spine.
- Vascular insufficiency (Leriche's syndrome).

Bursitis

There are multiple bursae located around the hip, in and around areas subject to friction (between muscle and a bony prominence). Bursitis is commonly an over-use friction phenomenon, but a history of trauma (traumatic bursitis) and infection must be excluded.

Trochanteric bursitis
A common condition in athletes, but also associated with the spondylarthropathies and obesity. It will cause a well localized tenderness to the superolateral aspect of the greater trochanter. Sometimes there may be associated referred pain to the lateral thigh. Hip movement is unaffected except for internal rotation of the hip.

Iliopsoas bursitis
This bursa separates the hip joint from the iliopsoas tendon and may communicate with the joint. More common in sports-related injury requiring extensive hip flexion. Causes deep anterior groin and thigh pain, and may present with large soft tissue swelling lateral to the femoral triangle. Pain is exacerbated with hip extension and resisted hip flexion.

Ischiogluteal bursitis
This is commonly traumatic in nature, occurring after blows to the ischial tuberosity. There is localized tenderness, worse with sitting or lying on it. Sometimes it is hard to distinguish from hamstring injuries.

Diagnosis
Bursitis (especially deep iliopsoas bursitis) is commonly under diagnosed (Johnston et al. 1998). Imaging with US and MR may show fluid collections.

Management
Infection must be excluded. Treatment is usually conservative and consists of rest, NSAIDs, and stretching of the relevant muscles. Glucocorticoid and local anaesthetic injection under imaging guidance can be very useful.

Osteonecrosis (ischaemic necrosis/avascular necrosis) of the femoral head
See also p. 433.

History
- Common in 30–50-year-olds.
- Need to identify the child with Legg–Calve–Perthes syndrome (idiopathic avascular osteonecrosis of the capital femoral epiphysis of the femoral head).
- Identify possible causes – see Table on p. 433.
- Hip/groin pain with possible radiation to knee.

Examination
- May be unremarkable if early stages.
- Antalgic gait with restricted range of motion (especially internal rotation).
- In late stages, significant limb length discrepancy with restricted movement and muscle wasting.

Imaging and diagnosis
- **Radiographs:** degenerative changes, sclerosis, subchondral lucency, collapse of femoral head. See Figure 5.29.
- **MR:** highly sensitive in showing subchondral oedema.
- **Bone scintigraphy:** less sensitive than MR in early stages, phase of disease associated with patterns of photopaenia and excess tracer localization.

Management
- **Conservative measures:** limited weight bearing and/or immobilization. Recent studies suggest a role for bisphosphonates in delaying femoral head collapse.
- Surgical management include core decompression of femoral head or free vascularized fibular grafting in early stages of the disease. Good medium term results have been reported (Urbaniak et al. 1995).
- Advanced diseases will inevitably require surgical intervention, in particular hip joint replacement. Resurfacing hip arthroplasty is gaining increasing popularity in the treatment of painful arthropathy in younger patients.
- In general, there is 70–80% chance of femoral head collapse in patients with confirmed osteonecrosis.

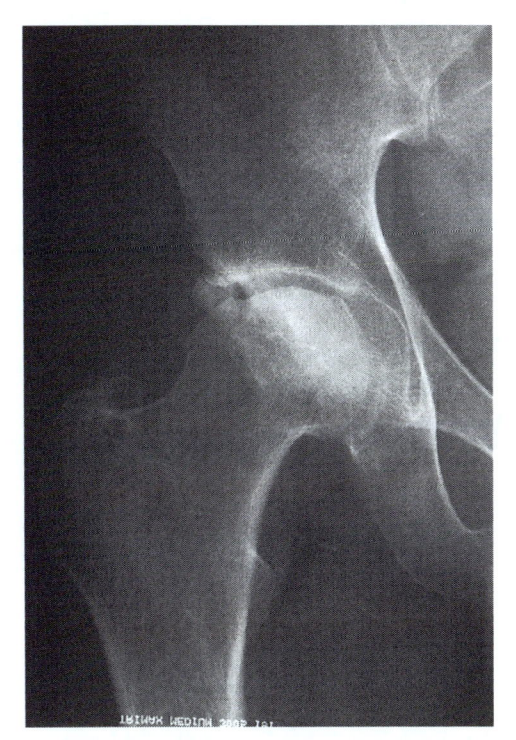

Figure 5.29 Osteonecrosis of the femoral head Ficat stage 3. Ficat stages: Stage 1-2 = anoxia, bone necrosis, microfractures; Stage 3 = segmental collapse; Stage 4 = secondary OA. Reproduced from Oxford Textbook of Orthopaedics and Trauma, Bulstrode et al, 2002, with permission from Oxford University Press.

Labral tears

Although first reported in the late 1950s, it is only in recent times that acetabular labral tears have become a recognized cause for hip/groin pain. Tears occur most commonly in the anterior part of the labrum.

History
- Mechanical hip pain, with sharp and catching sensation on certain movements, and locking.
- Usually groin pain, but may be trochanteric.
- Commonly associated with degenerative disease and in athletes.
- An overwhelming majority of labral tears are associated with structural hip abnormalities. Important to check for acetabular dysplasia and femoroacetabular impingement (FAI).
- Identify history of minor injuries (e.g. twisting, slipping, falling), posterior hip dislocation or recent trauma.

Examination
- **Hip movement** may be unaffected, but may be painful at the extremes.
- **Anterior tear:** acute hip flexion with internal rotation and adduction.
- **Posterior tear:** hyperextension with external rotation and abduction.

Imaging and diagnosis
- Radiographs, CT and MR have not been reliable tools for diagnosis. They are useful for excluding other hip pathologies.
- MR arthrogram has been reported to be a useful tool with high accuracy diagnostic rates. (Czerny et al. 1996).
- Hip arthroscopy has become the gold standard for diagnostic and therapeutic purposes. It allows a comprehensive evaluation of labral anatomy.

Management
- Conservative bed-rest and period of immobilization may be helpful initially, but there are no long-term outcome studies to support such conservative measures.
- Arthroscopic debridement of the lesion has been shown to be successful. Hip arthroscopy is a technically challenging procedure, but in the hands of an experienced surgeon, can produce good outcome.

Femoroacetabular impingement (FAI)

This is the abutment of femoral neck on to the anterior rim of the acetabulum. It is increasingly recognized as a cause of significant hip/groin pain, and strongly implicated as a cause of secondary OA.

FAI can be either *cam* (aspherical contoured femoral head abutting against acetabular rim) or *pincer* (linear abutment of femoral head-neck junction and the acetabular rim) impingement.

Cam impingement has been associated with conditions causing a decrease in femoral head-neck offset.
- Slipped capital femoral epiphysis (SCFE).
- Legg–Calve–Perthes syndrome.
- Acetabular rim syndrome (acetabular dysplasia).
- Malunited femoral neck fractures.

Pincer-type impingements are associated with conditions producing over-coverage by anterior acetabular rim:
- Acetabular retroversion.
- Coxa profunda (increased relative acetabular depth).
- Protrusio acetabuli.

History
- Commonly effects young active adults <50 years old.
- Anterior groin pain.
- Labral tears almost always have co-existing mechanical symptoms (locking, catching, and giving way).
- Elicit history of previous hip disease (SCFE) or surgery.

Examination
- Limp or positive Trendelenburg test maybe present.
- Restricted motion - flexion and internal rotation.
- Anterior impingement test is almost universally positive.

Imaging and diagnosis
- AP and lateral plain radiographs essential.
- Identify femoral abnormalities (pistol-grip deformity, coxa vara and valga) and acetabular abnormalities (os acetbaulare, dysplasia, protrusio acetabuli, and inclination and version of actabulum)
- MRI is now more commonly used, but MR arthrography is becoming the standard investigation. Can help to identify associated labral tears and chondral damage

Management
- **Conservative:** rest, modification of activity and avoiding excessive hip movement. Regular NSAIDs. This usually provides temporary relief.
- **Open surgery** includes hip dislocation and relevant excision osteotomy from the head-neck junction, or resection of the excess acetabular rim causing

the impingement. Any labral tears should be treated with repair or partial resection.
- **Arthroscopic surgery** is becoming popular with favourable results for treatment of FAI. (Sampson 2005). As well as serving as a diagnostic tool, labral debridement, chondroplasty and burr resection of osteophytes can be performed arthroscopically.

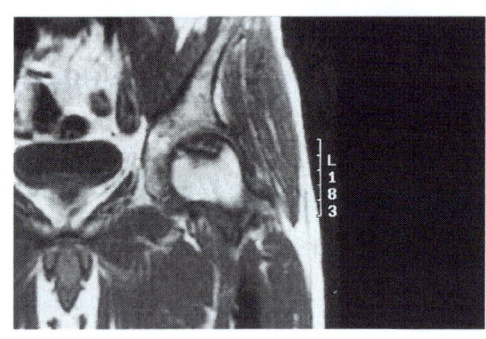

(a)

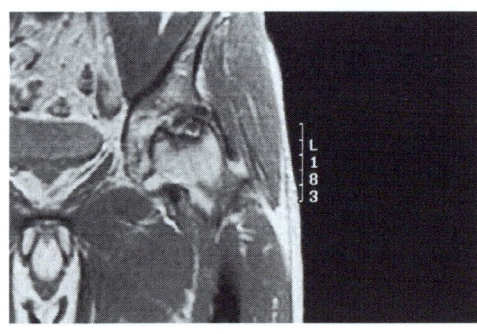

(b)

Figure 5.30 (a) T1 sequence MRI of the hip showing osteonecrosis in the classic superior segment of the femoral head with a hypointense (dark) band outlining the interior extent of the lesion; (b) T2 sequence MRI of the hip showing the hyperintense bright (white) band along the inner rim of the zone of osteonecrosis (dark band noted in (a)). This represents the double-line sign that is diagnostic of osteonecrosis. Reproduced from Oxford Textbook of Orthopaedics and Trauma, Bulstrode et al, 2002, with permission from Oxford University Press.

Acetabular rim syndrome (Klaue et al. 1991)

History
- Usually young active patients (18–35 years old).
- Sharp groin pain.
- Hip locking, catching or giving way.

Examination
- May be normal.
- Positive anterior impingement test.
- Positive apprehension test (extension and external rotation of the hip gives the sensation of instability).

Imaging and diagnosis
- Radiographic appearances constitute the gold standard.
- Incongruent shallow acetabulum.
- Congruent acetabulum with poor femoral head coverage ('short roof').

Management
- Conservative flexibility stretching and pelvic muscle strengthening.
- However, a rotational pelvic osteotomy may be necessary in order to delay onset of OA.

Osteitis pubis

A painful inflammatory process commonly seen in patients with spondylarthropathy and athletes. An infective lesion (osteomyelitis pubis) may present and must be ruled out.

History
- Gradual onset of pain in pubis region.
- Exercise induced symptoms – commonly kicking, striding, or pivoting – in athletes though in 'traumatic' osteitis, as well as SpA-related lesions pain at rest can occur.
- Pain often radiating to medial thigh or up to the abdomen.

Examination
- Point tenderness around pubic symphysis often exacerbated if rectus abdominis contracts.
- Painful passive hip abduction.
- Painful active hip adduction against resistance.

Imaging and diagnosis
- Essential to rule out infection (ESR, CRP, and white cell count may help though low grade acute phase response can be SpA-related. Biopsy and tissue microscopy and culture may be needed.
- Plain radiographs can show widened symphysis, cystic changes and sclerosis in the acute lesion. Old lesions can present with sclerosis and joint irregularity.
- Isotope bone scan (with SPECT) is a sensitive test and will demonstrate increased tracer uptake in the area of the pubic symphysis.
- MR can show inflammatory changes in the bone (e.g. subenthesial osteitis in SpAs) and is increasingly becoming a useful diagnostic tool (Karlsson et al. 1997)

Management
- Treatment begins with rest and NSAIDs.
- Physiotherapy to correct muscular imbalance and maximize functional pelvic stability.
- Use of glucocorticoid injection is controversial.
- If there is extensive osteitis then use of intravenous bisphosphonate can be helpful.
- If there is substantial pelvic instability on weight bearing (Stork-view) radiographs, surgery may be indicated (plating or bone grafting).

Nerve entrapment lesions

Presents with pain and numbness in the affected nerve distribution.

Lateral femoral cutaneous nerve (meralgia paraesthetica)

Commonly due to mechanical entrapment (e.g. tight pants or weight gain) or anatomical entrapment of nerve in origin of the inguinal ligament at the anterior superior iliac spine. Paraesthesia along lateral thigh. (See Fig.5.31).

Ilioinguinal nerve

Can be implicated following surgery (appendicectomy or herniorrhaphy), but also common in athletes following direct trauma or following intensive training of the abdominal musculature. Paraesthesia along upper medial thigh and mons pubis.

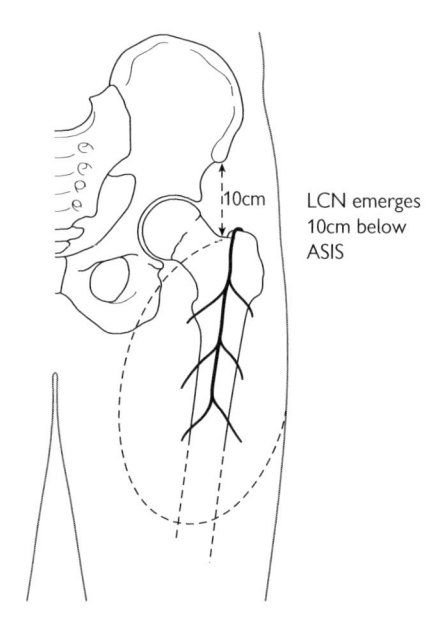

CHAPTER 5 Regional musculoskeletal anatomy and conditions

LCN emerges 10cm below ASIS

Figure 5.31 Usual site of entrapment of lateral cutaneous nerve, and site for injection, just above femoral neck 10cm below anterior superior iliac spine.

Treatment
Rest, NSAIDs, altered training methods. Injection of local anaesthetic can relieve symptoms temporarily, but helps in diagnosis too. Rarely, surgical release or neurolysis may be necessary if pain is refractory. (Westlin 1997)

Tendonitis and enthesitis around the pelvis
Tendonitis arises secondary either due to an acute injury (due to the eccentric contraction of relevant muscle), chronic over-use injury or as part of an inflammatory condition, most usually a SpA condition.

The 'over-use theory' considers that a tendon is subjected to persistent loads resulting in intra-tendinous partial rupture (micro-trauma) of the fibrils and tendon injury. (Curwin et al. 1984). Microscopically, with micro-trauma there is non-inflammatory collagen degeneration with fibre disorientation resulting in abnormal tendon function. Hence the term tendinopathy has been advocated for conditions arising from over-use. (Maffulli et al. 1998).

Enthesitides occur commonly around the pelvis and groin in patients with SpA. Pain and tenderness can be localized or quite diffuse and can mimic tendonitis.

Iliopsoas tendonitis
History of insidious onset of anterior hip pain as a result of repetitive hip flexion. In the acute circumstance, there is an onset of sudden pain caused by flexion against resistance. Pain may be reproducible on certain hip flexion movements especially in runners and kickers.

There may be localized tenderness on palpation of lesser trochanteric region under the gluteal fold, and there may be associated painful snapping in the groin as the tendon moves medially to laterally across the femoral head during hip movements from flexion to extension, respectively. Resisted hip flexion with palpation of the psoas muscle at its insertion point will also elicit pain.

> *Common sites of SpA-related enthesitis around the hip*
> - Posterior superior iliac spine.
> - Anterior superior iliac spine.
> - **Greater trochanter:** often misdiagnosed as bursitis. US or MR imaging can discriminate inflammatory lesions from tenderness associated with referred lumbosacral pain.
> - **Lesser trochanter:** useful place to see erosive enthesitis as a diagnostic aid if SpA diagnosis uncertain.
> - **Adductor tubercle:** difficult to tell sometimes from osteitis pubis. Both lesions can occur in same patient.

Adductor longus
Most frequently injured groin muscle-tendon unit. Primarily affecting football and hockey players, there are associated extrinsic factors (including training methods and types of activity) and intrinsic factors, such as malalignment, muscle strength, and asymmetrical muscular flexibility of the adductor group. (Renstrom, 1992).

There is well localized tenderness over the muscle insertion on the lower pubic ramus. Passive stretching of adductors or resisted adduction elicits pain.

Rectus Femoris
This muscle tendon unit can be damaged at its origin on the anterior inferior iliac spine, often associated with sprinters and in footballers. Pain is elicited with palpation along the muscles insertion and with resisted hip flexion.

Rectus abdominis
Repeated hip flexion, leg raises and abdominal flexion may result in rectus abdominis injury. There is tenderness of the upper pubic ramus and lower abdomen. Pain can be reproduced with patients contracting their abdomen.

Imaging and diagnosis
Plain radiographs are usually normal, but may demonstrate other bony lesions (e.g. degenerative changes or associated bony avulsion fragment), chronic enthesitis or calcified tendinosis in chronic situations.

US and MR may detect more subtle tendon injury or enthesitis inflammation.

Management
The primary aim in treating tendonitis and enthesitis is to relieve pain. As such, the first would be to avoid strenuous and painful activities. Often, simple measures, such as rest, icing, and NSAIDs will relieve symptoms, followed by gentle stretching and physiotherapy regimen. Ultimately, patients who are normally very active will require a period of rehabilitation to normal strength, range of movement, endurance and activity.

Injection of local anaesthetic and glucocorticoid has a role in relieving symptoms, in addition to diagnostic values. Surgical intervention, although uncommon, can be invoked in certain refractory cases of traumatic tendonitis. Procedures include tenotomy, and partial or complete release of the tendon.

Further reading
Curwin S, Stanish WD. *Tendinitis: its etiology and treatment.* Lexington: Collamore Press/DC Heath and Company, 1984.

Czerny C, Hofmann S, Neuhold A, Tschauner C, Engel A, Recht MP et al. Lesions of the acetabular labrum: accuracy of MR imaging and MR arthrography in detection and staging. *Radiology* 1996; **200**: 225–30.

Hungerford MW, Mont MA, Scott R, Fiore C, Hungerford DS, Krackow KA. Surface replacement hemiarthroplasty for the treatment of osteonecrosis of the femoral head. *J Bone Jt Surg Am* 1998; **80**: 656–64.

Ito H, Matsuno T, Kaneda K. Prognosis of early stage avascular necrosis of the femoral head. *Clin Orthopaed* 1999; **358**: 149–57.

Johnston CA, Wiley JP, Lindsay DM, Wiseman DA. Iliopsoas bursitis and tendonitis. *Sports Med* 1998; **25**: 271–83.

Karlsson J, Jerre R. The use of radiography, magnetic resonance, and ultrasound in the diagnosis of hip, pelvis, and groin injuries. *Sports Med Arthrosc Rev* 1997; **5**: 268–73.

Klaue K, Durnin CW, Ganz R. The acetabular rim syndrome. *J Bone Jt Surg Br* 1991; **73**: 423–9.

Lai KA, Shen WJ, Yang CY. The use of alendronate to prevent early collapse of the femoral head in patients with nontraumatic osteonecrosis. A randomized clinical study. *J Bone Jt Surg Am* 2005; **87**: 2155–9.

Maffulli N, Khan KM, Puddu G. Over-use tendon conditions: time to change a confusing terminology. *Arthroscopy* 1998; **14**: 840–3.

Renstrom PAHF. Tendon and muscle injuries in the groin area. *Clin Sports Med* 1992; **11**: 815–31.

Sampson TG. Arthroscopic treatment of femoroacetabular impingement. *Techn Orthopaed* 2005; **20**: 56–62.

Santori N, Villar RN. Acetabular labral tears: results of arthroscopic partial limbectomy. *Arthroscopy* 2000; **16**: 11–15.

Urbaniak JR, Coogan PG, Gunneson EB, Nunley JA. Treatment of osteonecrosis of femoral head with free vascularised fibular grafting. A long term follow-up study of one hundred and three hips. *J Bone Jt Surg Am*. 1995; **77**:681–94.

Westlin N. Groin pain in athletes from Southern Sweden. *Sports Med Arthrosc Rev* 1997; **5**: 280–4.

Chapter 5: Regional musculoskeletal anatomy and conditions

The knee

Regional anatomy
The knee is the largest and most complex synovial joint in the body. It is a modified hinge (condyloid) joint capable of flexion, extension and an element of rotation.

It is made up of two separate joints – the tibiofemoral joint, most commonly referred to as the knee joint; and the patellofemoral joint. The two joints are enclosed within the same synovial cavity in the joint capsule.

Bony anatomy
Tibiofemoral joint
The distal femur, consisting of two condyles, articulates with the flattened tibial plateau to form the tibiofemoral joint. The femoral condyles are markedly convex and are divided by an intercondylar notch, which accommodates the cruciate ligaments.

The tibia plateau condyles are oval and slightly convex. They are separated by the intercondylar eminence, around which the femur rotates and the surrounding intercondylar area to which cruciate ligaments attach.

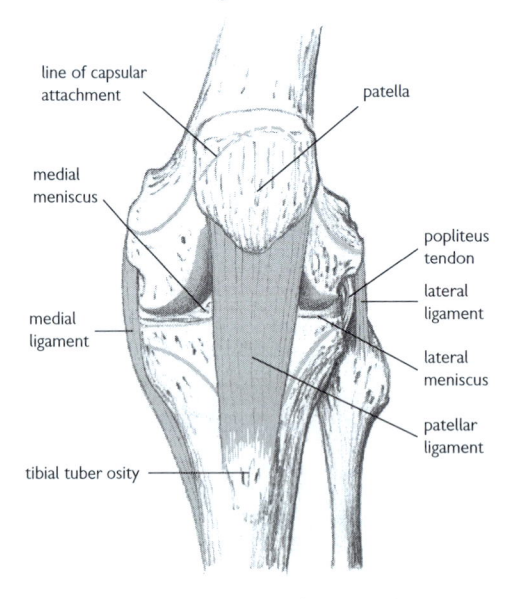

Figure 5.32 Knee joint: anterior view showing capsule attachments and ligaments. Reproduced from the Oxford Textbook of Functional Anatomy, MacKinnon and Morris, 2005, with permission from Oxford University Press.

Patellofemoral joint
The patella is the largest sesamoid bone in the body. It is suspended within the quadriceps and the patella tendon articulating with the concave anterior aspect (the trochlea groove) of the distal femur.
- The under-surface of the patella has the thickest articular cartilage in the body indicating the significant stresses across the joint.
- Primary function of the patella is to increase the lever arm of the quadriceps.

The knee is a potentially unstable joint due to the apposing nature of its bony anatomy. Joint stability is obtained through associated ligaments, menisci, fibrous capsule, and surrounding musculature.

Joint capsule
The knee joint is enclosed by an incomplete fibrous capsule. Anteriorly, the deficiency is completed by the quadriceps femoris tendon, the patellar ligament, and tendinous expansions from the iliotibial band and quadriceps forming the patellar retinaculum. These form an expandable anterior knee space that extends above the upper pole of the patellar as the supra-patellar pouch.

The joint capsule is reinforced by expansions of semimebranosus and biceps femoris tendons, the oblique popliteal ligament and arcuate popliteal ligament, respectively, as well as the medial collateral ligament.

Ligaments of the knee joint (See Figure 5.32)
Medial/tibial collateral ligament (MCL)
The MCL is a broad structure made of two distinct parts:
- The superficial MCL extends from the medial epicondyle of the femur to the anteromedial aspect of the proximal tibia. This part is extracapsular and is predominantly responsible for medial joint stability on valgus stressing.
- The deep MCL attaches to the joint margin reinforcing the joint capsule. It also attaches to the peripheral margin of the medial meniscus.

Lateral/fibular collateral ligament (LCL)
The LCL is a distinct cord-like structure arising from the lateral femoral epicondyle and attaching to the apex of the fibula head.
- The LCL is separate from the capsule and does not reinforce it.
- The LCL prevents lateral opening of the tibia on the femur during varus stressing.

Cruciate ligaments (See Figure 5.33)
Anteroposterior stability is provided by the two cruciate ('cross') ligaments. They are named anterior and posterior in relation to their attachments to the tibia. Although completely contained within the joint capsule the cruciates are enveloped with synovium and are thus described as intracapsular, but extra-synovial structures.

Anterior cruciate ligament (ACL). The ACL runs in an anterior to posterior direction from its attachment near the front of the tibia plateau to its femoral insertion at the posterolateral corner of the intercondylar notch. It consists of two distinct functional bundles:
- **Anteromedial fibres:** tight in flexion; limits anterior translation of tibia on femur.
- **Posterolateral fibres:** tight in extension; limits anterior translation and external rotation of the tibia.

The ACL is an important stabilizer of the knee during pivoting movements. A deficient ACL causes excessive anterior-lateral displacement of the tibia under the femur during activities, such as jumping or rapid deceleration.

Posterior cruciate ligament (PCL). The PCL attaches to the posterior part of the tibial plateau and runs anterosuperiorly to insert into the medial aspect of the intercondylar notch. It restricts anterior translation of the femur on the tibia and prevents hyperextension of the joint.

CHAPTER 5 **Regional musculoskeletal anatomy and conditions** 175

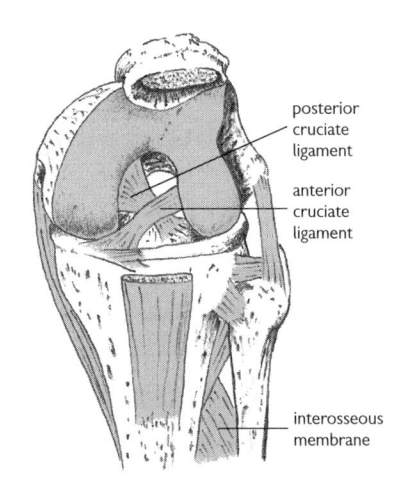

Figure 5.33 Cruciate ligaments, anterior view. Reproduced from the Oxford Textbook of Functional Anatomy, MacKinnon and Morris, 2005, with permission from Oxford University Press.

Menisci (See Figure 5.34)
The menisci are wedge-shaped semi-lunar cartilages situated between the tibiofemoral joint spaces. The medial meniscus is C-shaped and larger than the lateral meniscus, which is more circular.
- Menisci consist of fibrocartilage, which gives them distinctive properties from articular cartilage.
- The medial and lateral menisci are attached at their periphery to the joint capsule, and centrally, via the anterior and posterior horns, to the tibia.
- The peripheral 10–30% and anterior and posterior horns are vascularized giving these areas capacity for repair; otherwise, the rest of the meniscus is avascular.
- Functions of the menisci include:
  - shock absorption;
  - load distribution across the joint surface;
  - reduction of contact stress between articular surfaces by increasing joint congruity;
  - improve stability of the joint by increasing the concavity of the tibia plateau;
  - joint lubrication and nutrition;
  - prevent synovial impingement.

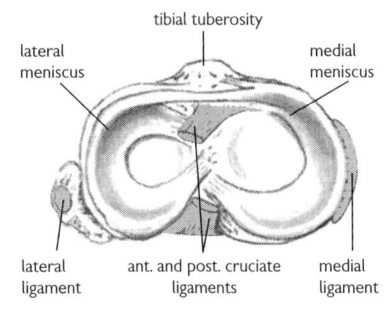

Figure 5.34 Menisci and attachments of cruciate ligaments of left knee viewed from above. Reproduced from the Oxford Textbook of Functional Anatomy, MacKinnon and Morris, 2005, with permission from Oxford University Press.

Bursae of the knee joint
There are several bursae surrounding the knee joint reducing friction between moving structures, such as tendons, bones, ligaments, and skin. The suprapatellar pouch/bursa is not a true bursa, but an extension of the joint capsule. The bursae most susceptible to inflammation include:
- **Prepatellar:** large bursa interposed between the patella and the skin.
- **Infrapetellar:** small bursa located between the skin and patellar tendon.
- **Deep patellar:** bursa located between the tibial tuberosity and the patellar tendon. It is separated from the synovium by and interposing fat pad.
- **Pes anserinus:** located inferior and medial to the knee joint line. It separates the pes anserinus and the tibia.

Alignment of the knee Joint
The normal knee is in slight valgus. The angle between the tibia and the femur is known as the Q angle. In males this is normally 14° and in females 17°.
The Q angle is increased in genu valgum ('knock knees') and decreased in genu varum ('bow leg'). Biomechanics and stability of the patellofemoral joint are determined by the length of the patella tendon and the Q angle.

Muscles around the knee joint (Table 5.10)
Muscles are responsible for movement and stabilization of the joint. Reduced muscle tone may predispose to injury and dislocations of the joint.

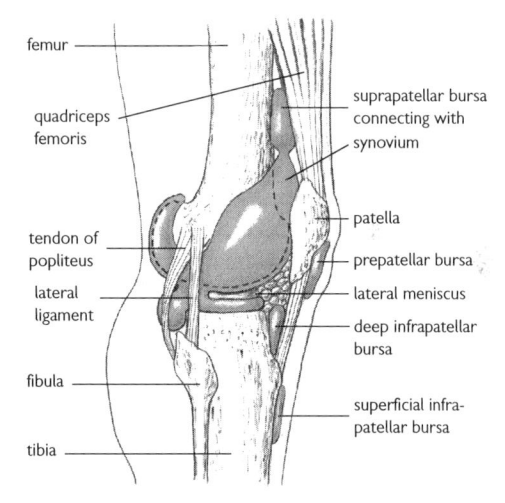

Figure 5.35 Synovial membrane and bursae of knee. Reproduced from the Oxford Textbook of Functional Anatomy, MacKinnon and Morris, 2005, with permission from Oxford University Press.

Table 5.10 Prime muscle movers of the knee

Movement	Muscles
Extension	Rectus femoris, vastus medialis, vastus lateralis, vastus intermedius (quadriceps muscles)
Flexion	Semimembranosus, semitendinosus, biceps femoris (hamstring muscles)
	Sartorius, gracilis, gastrocnemius, adductor magnus
External rotation of tibia	Biceps femoris
Internal rotation of tibia	Popliteus: initiates internal rotation thus unlocking knee when in full extension
	Sartorius, gracilis, semitendinosus. The common tendon insertion of these form the pes anserinus

Lateral aspect knee showing extent of joint and bursae.

Further reading

Aglietti P, Insall JN, et al. Patellar pain and incongruence: 1: Measurements of Incongruence. *Clin Orthopaed Relat Res* 1983; **176**: 217–24.

Amiss AA. Current concepts on anatomy and biomechanics of patellar instability. *Sports Med Arthrosc* 2007; **15**(2): 48–56.

Ellis H. The applied anatomy of examination of the knee. *Br J Hosp Med (Lond)* 2007; **68**(4): 60–1.

Messner K, Gao J. The menisci of the knee joint. Anatomical and functional characteristics, and a rationale for clinical treatment. *J Anat* 1998; **193**: 161–78.

Patel RV, Haddad FS. Technique of knee joint aspiration. *Br J Hosp Med (Lond)* 2007; **68**(6): 100–1.

Rath E, Richmond JC. The menisci: basic science and advances in treatment. *Br J Sports Med* 2000; **34**: 252–7.

The knee: regional musculoskeletal conditions

Patellofemoral instability
Defined by a predisposition for the patella to sublux or dislocate from its normal articulation, the cause of instability is either primary or secondary to a traumatic episode. Women are more prone to primary instability due to increase genu valgum and hence increase Q-angle; greater ligamentous laxity; smaller muscle bulk and shallow trochlear groove.
- Patients complain of sensation of the patella dislocating or moving laterally when performing certain movements. A history of pain may be due to maltracking of the patella, which is apparent on examination.
- Lateral push on the patellar, whilst flexing the knee causes apprehension.
- This is a clinical diagnosis. Plain radiographs may reveal evidence of predisposing anatomical abnormalities and osteochondral defects in traumatic dislocations.
- Acute dislocations are temporarily immobilized following relocation for a short period followed by rehabilitation.
- Surgical intervention to correct predisposing factors is reserved for failed conservative treatment.

Fat pad impingement syndrome (Hoffa's disease)
Acute or chronic impingement of the richly innervated infrapatellar fat-pad between the patella and femur during flexion and extension of the knee.
- The patient describes a long history of anterior knee pain occasionally with associated knee effusion.
- There is tenderness inferior to the patella, but extending beyond the margin of the patellar tendon. The pain is reproduced by straight leg raising.
- MR confirms diagnosis and rules out other pathology.
- Management comprises rest and NSAIDs in the acute stage. Taping of patella may help reduce amount of patella tilt and impingement.
- If conservative measures fail then arthroscopic resection of the fat pad can be helpful.

Patellar tendinosis (Jumper's knee)
Patellar tendinosis is characterized by pain caused by chronic overload of the knee extensor mechanism. This is a common condition seen in athletes that participate in jumping sports and it usually occurs bilaterally. Contrary to initial beliefs, it is not an inflammatory process; tendinosis is a degenerative change or failed healing, with no histological evidence of inflammation. An alternate hypothesis is that the tendinosis is an adaptive process to the loads within the patellar tendon.
- There is patellar tendon pain most commonly at its proximal insertion exacerbated by jumping or hill running. Dispositions include:
  - intrinsic - ligamentous laxity, increase Q-angle, patella height, and gender;
  - extrinsic - frequency of training, level of performance, hardness of underground.
- There is tenderness of the patellar tendon with the knee in full extension, but minimal tenderness when it is flexed and the tendon is taught.
- Differential diagnosis is Osgood–Schlatter's disease; Sinding–Larsen–Johansson Disease; enthesitis (SpAs).

- Depending on duration of symptoms there may be quadriceps atrophy. Symptoms are reproduced on patellar loading.
- Diagnosis is clinical. Confirmation is made with ultrasound scan or MR. Plain radiographs, CT or isotope bone scan are only used when diagnosis is in doubt following initial investigations.
- The management is to rest from sporting activities and NSAIDs in the acute stages.
- Physical therapy to strengthen the quadriceps muscles and stretch the patellar tendon with increasing loads. Patella strapping and soft insoles may help prevent recurrence.
- Peri-tendinous injections of glucocorticoid, autologous blood injection or dry needling of affected using image guidance may resolve recalcitrant symptoms and should be attempted before surgery.
- Surgical intervention is considered for patients that fail to respond to non-surgical measures.

Enthesitis
Inflammation and/or microtrauma of entheses around the knee, particularly at the origin of the patellar tendon (patella inferior pole) and insertion at the tibial tubercle are relatively common lesions associated with SpAs. Lesions can exist without evidence of coincident synovial inflammation in the joint either isolated or in combination with entheseal symptoms elsewhere. Other potential sites of pain from enthesitis around the knee include tendon insertions at medial and lateral femoral condyles [especially psoriatic arthritis (PsA)], gastrocnemius head origins, pes anserinus and quadriceps attachment to the superior patella pole.

History
Well localized pain at anatomical site. Other typical sites coincidentally affected (or previously given potential lifelong predisposition to SpA disease) include heel, Achilles' insertional, alternating buttock (?SIJ) and greater trochanter pains. A history of *inflammatory* back pain should be sought. Patients may have psoriasis (or history of it), Crohn's disease, or recent infection (with *Chlamydia*, *Salmonella* or Campylobacter, for example).

Examination
Tenderness at site may be present, but an absence does not rule out lesions. Swelling is invariably not seen. Resisted activation of muscle/tendon, which inserts at the site may reproduce pain.

Investigations
Ultrasound (US) and MR have recognized patterns in some cases with high signal (osteitis) under entheseal attachment in bone typical. Other traumatic lesions should be excluded.

Treatment
Topical NSAID gel and judicious glucocorticoid injection should be considered. If part of a wider condition (SpA) consideration of immunosuppressing the disease is important (e.g. sulphasalazine).

Prepatella bursitis
Bursae surrounding the knee are susceptible to inflammatory response either from direct or indirect trauma or can

become inflamed spontaneously particularly from crystal-induced inflammation. The prepatella bursa is the most commonly affected bursa. It is commonly caused by acute injury, such as a direct fall onto the knee, or from minor repetitive injury, hence, the moniker of 'housemaid's knee'. It can also represent gout or an acute manifestation of calcium pyrophosphate dihydrate disease (CPPDD; 'pseudogout'). Pyogenic bursitis is common, especially in children with the most common pathogen being *Staphylococcus aureus*.

- A severely swollen prepatellar bursa may be mistaken for septic arthritis. Opening the joint in this case would result in a septic joint.
- Findings include swelling anterior to the patella with erythema and associated with pain in the acute phase or quiescent if chronic.
- Flexion and extension are usually minimally restricted.
- Management: rest and NSAIDs in the acute phase.
- Aspiration and injection of steroid and local anaesthetic; fluid to be sent for polarized light microscopy (?gout or pyrophosphate crystals).
- Traumatic bursitis will often respond to aspiration, steroid injection and compressive dressing.
- Unresponsiveness to conservative management is treated with surgical incision and drainage and complete excision of the bursa.

Infra-patellar bursitis or ('Clergy's knee')
Small bursae located between the patellar ligament and the skin (infrapatellar bursa), and between the ligament and the tibial surface (deep prepatellar bursa).
- There is pain inferior to the lower pole of the patella associated with kneeling or direct pressure. There may also be associated swelling in the area.
- Management is along the same lines as pre-patellar bursitis.
- Differential diagnosis:
  - patellar tendinosis;
  - fat pad impingement syndrome;
  - enthesitis in SpAs.

Anserine bursitis
Pes anserinus is the common insertion for sartorius, gracilis and semitendinosus tendons at the medial proximal tibia. The bursa lies between this and the tibial surface.
- Inflammation of the bursa causes pain along the medial aspect of the knee and tenderness 3–4 cm (2 finger-breadths) below the joint line.
- Anserine bursitis is common in physically active individuals and is attributed to tight hamstring tendons. It is a diagnosis of exclusion.
- An injection of local anaesthetic and steroid helps confirm diagnosis and treat symptoms simultaneously.
- Long-term management is with focused physiotherapy.
- Differential diagnosis:
  - medial collateral strain;
  - meniscal tear;
  - articular cartilage damage;
  - proximal tibial stress fracture;
  - Osgood–Schlatter disease;
  - synovial plica syndrome;
  - enthesitis.

Synovial plica syndrome
Plicae are folds of synovial membrane that divide the knee into different compartments during embryonic development. Incomplete degeneration results in remnant plicae. Medial plica pathology is the most common form. There is repeated trauma/irritation as the plica rubs over the femoral condyle leads to inflammation and fibrosis. Reduced plica elasticity causes impingement of the patella or femoral condyle and wear of articular cartilage. Classically, patients may describe symptoms of snapping, popping, crepitus, or pain at particular degrees of flexion.
- Examination reveals joint line tenderness or tenderness on direct palpation of the plica, whilst flexing and extending the knee.
- The MPP test, as devised by Kim *et al.* is said to be a sensitive method for examination and diagnosing medial patellar plica pathology.
- Essentially the condition is a diagnosis of exclusion. Differential diagnosis includes:
  - meniscus tear;
  - fat pad or synovial fringe impingement;
  - localized synovitis;
  - early patellofemoral degenerative (OA).
- Anterior knee pain in the absence of other causes may be attributed to plica, but presence of plica itself does not imply pathology.
- MR can rule out most other causes of pain, such as meniscal tears. Arthroscopy may help confirm diagnosis and treat problem.
- Conservative management includes rest and NSAIDs.
- Physiotherapy for improved quadriceps strengthening and flexibility.
- Arthroscopic resection is reserved for those with recalcitrant symptoms.

Iliotibial band syndrome (ITBS)
Common over-use injury of the lateral aspect of the knee seen particularly in runners, cyclists and endurance sports.
- Patients describe pain over the lateral femoral condyle caused by friction of the iliotibial tract sliding over the condyle. Pain is caused by either direct attrition of the ITB or inflammation of the interposing bursa.
- Onset of pain usually occurs some time after exercise has commenced. The patient may complain of grating over the area secondary to a chronically inflamed ITB bursa. Genu varum or over-pronation of the feet predisposes to developing ITBS.
- There is tenderness where the ITB slides over the femoral condyle and/or at its insertion into the lateral proximal tibia (Gerdy's tubercule).
- Diagnosis is made from a good history and examination. Confirmation is done with ultrasound or MR.
- **Differential diagnosis**:
  - lateral meniscal tear;
  - discoid lateral meniscus;
  - popliteus tendonitis;
  - patellofemoral pain syndrome.
- Non-operative management includes stretching, tissue massage, orthosis and glucocorticoid injection (under image guidance). In chronic cases excision of the bursa or surgical tenotomy may relieve symptoms after a diagnostic arthroscopy has ruled out other pathology.

Osgood–Schlatter's syndrome (OSS)
Partial avulsion of the tibial tuberosity from its growth plate secondary to repetitive tensile stresses.
- History reflects gradual onset of activity-related pain situated in region of the tibial tuberosity.
- Mostly occurs in athletic adolescent boys between the ages of 12 and 15 years. It can be bilateral in 20–30% of cases.
- There is local swelling and tenderness of the tibial tuberosity. Pain is reproduced by direct pressure on the tibial prominence and pushing off actions.
- In the adult there may be a permanent prominence of the tibial tuberosity.
- OSS is a clinical diagnosis. The ossification centre of the tibial tuberosity appears around 11 years of age, hence, radiographs will not be very useful for diagnosis prior to this. In the adolescent, radiographs may demonstrate a separation of the ossification centre of the tibial tuberosity from the proximal tibia in the early stages and fragmentation in the later stages.
- Radiographs are useful to rule out tibial tuberosity avulsion, infection or tumour. MR may be useful in the future for staging and prognostication of OSS.
- Mild cases can be due to enthesitis, which should be considered in those with psoriasis, juvenile SpA or JAS or enthesitis-related JIA.
- Following an acute phase most symptoms spontaneously subside over a 12–24-month period.
- Treat with rest, ice, and NSAIDs in the acute phase. Activity modification along with focused physical therapy plays a crucial role in managing chronic OSS.
- In 10%, symptoms remain unabated despite conservative management. In these rare cases surgical intervention may play a part.

Differential diagnosis: of anterior knee pain
- Osgood Schlatter's Syndrome (OSS).
- Sinding–Larsen–Johansson syndrome: similar mechanism to OSS, but involving inferior pole of patella.
- Hoffa's/anterior fat pad syndrome.
- Avulsion fracture of tibial tubercle.
- Synovial plica injury.
- Patellar tendonosis.
- Enthesitis inferior patella pole or tibial tubercle (e.g. AS, PsA, JSpA/JAS).
- Proximal tibial periostitis.
- Tumour.

Meniscal injuries
Acute meniscal tears occur when shear forces generated from flexion, compression and rotation of the knee exceeds the menisci ability to resist the force. Attachment of the outer border of the medial meniscus to the capsule means that it is less mobile making it more susceptible to injury. In the older population degenerative tears occur spontaneously usually without a seditious event. There are different types of meniscal tears (see Figure 5.36).

History
The patient may describe a twisting injury to the knee with the foot fixed. The degree and onset of pain is variable and symptoms may be delayed for over 24 h. Other symptoms include restricted range of movement, intermittent locking, giving way and clicking. Meniscal injuries may be associated with ACL or collateral ligament injury. Periphery tears may also be associated with synovial cysts expanding through the joint capsule.

Examination
An effusion is usually present. Joint line tenderness (palpation with the knee flexed at 90°) and pain on squatting are highly sensitive tests for meniscal injury. McMurray's test is positive when pain is reproduced or a clunk is felt as the knee is flexed and rotated (See Plate 2). A new bedside test, the Thessaly test, is suggested to be a more accurate method of diagnosing meniscal injury. (See Figure 5.36).

Investigation and diagnosis
MR scan is the investigation of choice demonstrating the anatomy of the tear. If MR is contra-indicated then an arthrogram may be used to illustrate the lesion.

Management
Depends on severity of the tear and patient symptoms. Conservative management may be appropriate for small or degenerative tears with minimal symptoms. If symptoms are persistent or severe, then arthroscopy is done for partial meniscectomy or meniscal repair. The removal of part of or the entire meniscus predisposes the joint to increase wear rate of articular cartilage.

Differential diagnosis
- ACL tear.
- Articular cartilage damage.
- Osteochondritis dissecans.

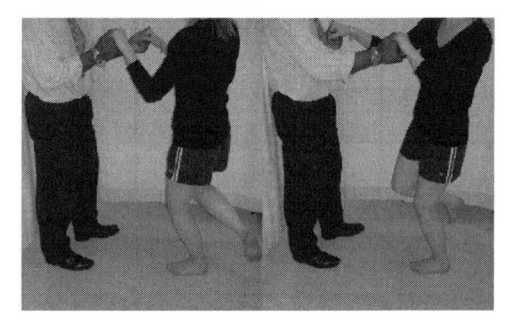

Figure 5.36 Thessaly test: examiner-supported weight-bearing rotation with 20° of knee flexion. A positive test reproduces pain from meniscus tear.

Collateral ligament injury
Injuries to the medial and lateral collateral ligaments occur as a result of a valgus or varus stress, respectively, of the partially flexed knee. Injury may occur from a non-contact or contact mechanism. The different grades of ligament injury are described:
- **Grade I:** local tenderness, but usually no swelling. Pain is reproduced when the ligament is put under stress, but there is no laxity.
- **Grade II:** marked tenderness and sometimes-localized swelling. There is some laxity on straining but there is a distinct endpoint.
- **Grade III:** complete tear of the ligament fibres associated with pain, swelling, and feeling of instability. Complete tear of the MCL may be associated with ACL injury and more commonly with lateral meniscus tear (valgus strain causing compression of lateral compartment). Grade III tear of the LCL usually involves

CHAPTER 5 Regional musculoskeletal anatomy and conditions

the posterolateral complex. This is associated with rotatory instability and requires surgical repair.

Investigation and diagnosis
Diagnosis is clinical, but plain radiographs may show associated bony injury. MRI is helpful in ruling out other soft tissue injury.

Management
MCL injuries routinely are treated conservatively. Patients with grade III injury have been shown to return to sport, as well as those treated surgically. A stabilizing brace is used during the rehabilitation period. Grade I and II LCL injuries are treated conservatively but grade III injuries are treated surgically due to rotational instability.

Differential diagnosis
- Anserine bursitis.
- Patellofemoral syndrome.
- Tibial plateau fracture.

Anterior cruciate ligament Injury
ACL rupture is relatively common particularly in sports involving pivoting and cutting manoeuvres. ACL injury may occur in isolation or in combination with other injuries particularly meniscal tears. There is a higher incidence of ACL rupture in female athletes when compared with males doing similar activities.

History
The majority of ACL tears occur in a non-contact situation when an athlete is landing from a jump, pivoting, or decelerating. An audible 'pop' or feeling that something came out then relocated is described. There is pain limiting any further action and swelling develops over hours.

Examination
In the acute presentation there is swelling of the joint with restricted range of movement. There is widespread tenderness. With subsidence of pain examination will demonstrate a positive Lachman's test (most sensitive and specific test). (See Figure 5.37). The pivot-shift test is diagnostic of ACL deficiency but it is difficult to perform and it is dependent on the ability of the patient to relax. An anterior drawer test is usually positive, but it is the least sensitive of examinations (See Plate 3).

Investigations and diagnosis
Plain radiographs should be done to reveal any associated bony injury, such as an avulsion fracture of tibial spine, or a 'Segond' fracture (anterolateral capsule avulsion). These are pathognomonic of an ACL rupture. If in doubt an MR scan is done to confirm the diagnosis. (See Figure 5.38).

Management
Treatment is dependent on several factors and each patient is considered individually on the merits of conservative and surgical intervention:
- Patient age: more likely to operate if young.
- Degree of instability.
- Associated abnormalities (MCL or meniscal tear) – poorer prognosis if not repaired.
- Patient's level of activity – level of demands placed on the knee (occupation, sports).

Non-surgical management involves physical rehabilitation, the use of braces, and avoidance of aggravating activities. ACL rupture is associated with increased risk of development of osteoarthritis, but there is little evidence at

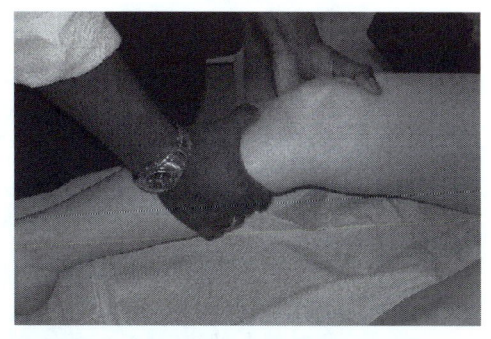

Figure 5.37 Lachmann test. Excessive translation of tibia (upward) from femur suggests ACL deficiency.

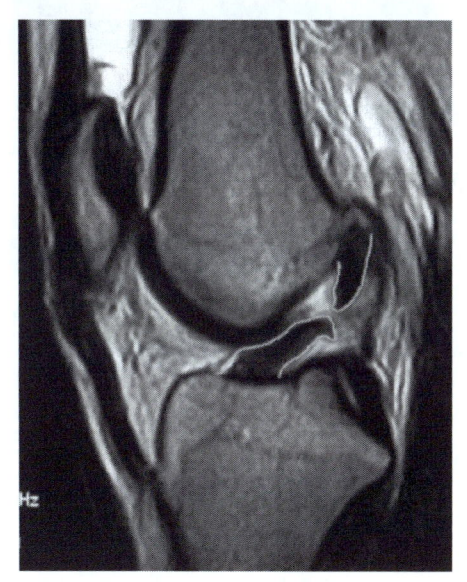

Figure 5.38 MR sagittal image showing ACL tear.

present to show that ACL reconstruction will prevent progression to degenerative joint disease.

Posterior cruciate ligament injury
PCL tears are rarer than ACL injuries and are usually caused by significant direct trauma. Injuries usually occur from direct trauma to the tibia whilst the knee is in a flexed position or from a forced hyperflexion or hyperextension injury. The posterior drawer test is positive. Investigations are the same for ACL injuries.

Management
Isolated PCL tears are treated conservatively with most patients maintaining adequate function. Bony avulsion from the tibial insertion, chronic PCL-related instability, or combination injuries should be surgically repaired.

Baker's (popliteal) cyst (See Figure 5.39)
A cyst developing in the popliteal fossa is usually formed from the egress of fluid from the knee joint through a normal communication to the bursa between semimebranosus and medial head of gastrocnemius. It can also form from a herniation of the synovium through the joint capsule.

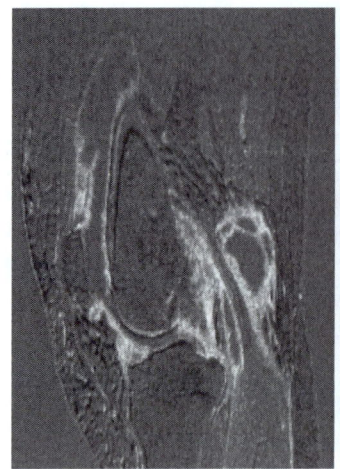

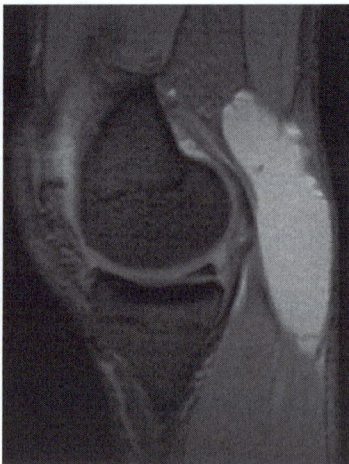

Figure 5.39 Two MR images of popliteal cyst formation. The image on the left is a reconstructed sagittal section from subtraction of identical T1-weighted images taken before and after contrast enhancement. The contrast highlights the complexity of popliteal cyst configuration (as well as showing the extent of suprapatellar pouch synovium). The right-hand image (different patient) shows how large popliteal cysts can be (lateral part of the knee, sagittal section).

In adults it is usually associated with an intra-articular pathology. In association with inflammatory arthritis popliteal cysts can be extensive and lie serpiginously around popliteal structures including the popliteal artery. The prevalence of Baker's cysts in children is low (roughly 6.3% in asymptomatic children undergoing MR of the knee) and it usually does not communicate with the joint or have an associated intra-articular pathology.

Examination
Typically a smooth, painless, non-pulsatile mass is located below the joint line in the popliteal fossa. It is tense with knee in extension.

Investigation and diagnosis
Knee radiograph to characterize joint disease and detect soft tissue mass. US confirms whether the popliteal mass is a pure cystic structure or a complex cyst and/or solid mass with associated vascularity. MR scan demonstrates intra-articular pathology or illustrates any soft tissue pathology, such as rhabdomyosarcoma or pigmented villonodular synovitis. It may also be used to identify the communication between the cyst and the joint cavity.

Management
In children, most cysts spontaneously resolve in 10–20 months. In protracted cases, aspiration and injection with steroid may resolve cysts (note that there is no communication with the joint unlike in adults). In adults, the intra-articular pathology should be addressed (e.g. intra-articular fluid aspirated and steroid injected) and, with time, the cyst should then spontaneously regress. The most common complication of a Baker's cyst is rupture into the proximal gastrocnemius causing a pseudothrombophlebitis syndrome typically causing swelling and discomfort/pain of the lower leg. Skin can be erythematous. This clinically presents similarly to a deep vein thrombosis (DVT).

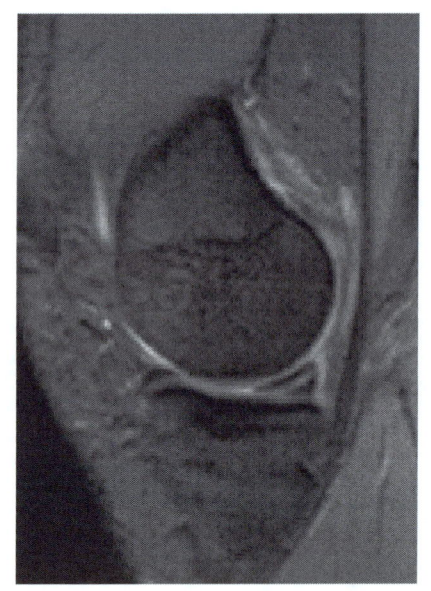

Figure 5.40 Oblique tear in the posterior medial meniscus. See the oblique white (high MR signal) line through the dark wedge shape (the cross sectional appearance of the meniscus).

Differential diagnosis
- Vascular masses (aneurysm or DVT).
- Soft tissue tumours.
- Meniscal cysts; cellulitis.

Further reading

De Maeseneer M, Debaere C, Desprechins B, Osteaux M. Popliteal cysts in children: prevalence, appearance and associated findings at MR imaging. *Pediatr Radiol* 1999; **29**(8): 605–9.

Dupont JY. Synovial plicae of the knee. Controversies and review. *Clin Sports Med* 1997; **16**: 87–122

Gholve PA, Sher DM, Khakharia S, Widmann RF, Green DW. Osgood Schlatter syndrome. *Curr Opin Pediat* 2007; **19**: 44–50.

Hamilton B, Purdam C. Patellar tendinosis as an adaptive process: a new hypothesis. *Br J Sports Med* 2004; **38**: 758–61.

Hirano A, Fukubayashi T, Ishii T, Ochiai N. Magnetic resonance imaging of Osgood–Schlatter disease: the course of the disease. *Skeletal Radiol* 2002; **31**: 334–42.

James SLJ, Ali K, Pocock C, et al. Ultrasound guided dry needling and autologous blood injection for patellar tendinosis. *Br J Sports Med* 2007; **41**: 518–21.

Karachalios T, Hantes M, Zibis AH, et al. Diagnostic accuracy of a new clinical test (the Thessaly test) for early detection of meniscal tears. *J Bone Jt Surg Am* 2005; **87**: 955–62.

Khan KM, Cook JL, Bonar F, et al. Histopathology of common tendinopathies. Update and implications for clinical management. *Sports Med* 1999; **27**: 393–408.

Kim SJ, Jeong JH, Cheon YM, Ryu SW. MPP test in the diagnosis of patellar plica syndrome. *Arthroscopy* 2004; **20**: 1101–3.

Kim SJ, Lee DH, Kim TE. The relationship between the MPP test and arthroscopically found medial patellar plica pathology. *Arthroscopy* 2007; **12**: 1303–8.

Kumar D, Alvand A, Beacon JP. Impingement of infrapatellar fat pad (Hoffa's disease): results of high-portal arthroscopic resection. *Arthroscopy*. 2007; **11**: 1180–6.

Miller TT, Staron RB, Koenigsberg T. MR imaging of Baker cysts: association with internal derangement, effusion, and degenerative arthropathy. *Radiology* 1996; **201**: 247–50.

Scholten RJPM, Opstelten W, van der Plas CG, Bijl D, Deville WLJM, Bouter LM. Accuracy of physical diagnostic tests for assessing ruptures of the anterior cruciate ligament: a meta-analysis. *J Fam Pract* 2003; **52**: 689–94.

Shelbourne KD, Davis TJ, Patel DV. The natural history of acute isolated nonoperatively treated posterior cruciate ligament injuries. A prospective study. *Am J Sports Med* 1999; **27**: 276–83.

Lower leg and foot

Regional anatomy

The tibiofibular articulation
The long bones of the lower leg articulate at three distinct levels:
- The *superior tibiofibular joint* is a synovial joint, reinforced by the anterior and posterior tibiofibular ligaments. The joint cavity may occasionally communicate posteriorly with the bursa deep to the popliteus tendon and the knee joint.
- The *interosseous membrane* slopes steeply from tibia down to fibula.
- The *inferior tibiofibular joint* is a fibrous joint (syndesmosis) reinforced by the interosseous, the anterior and the posterior tibiofibular ligament.

The deep fascia of the leg
The deep fascial envelope of the lower leg is fused to the periosteum of the subcutaneous parts of the tibia, the fibula and their malleoli. Two intermuscular septa pass from its deep surface to become attached to fibula, forming compartments in the leg.

Any further increase in these tight spaces can cause compression and ischaemia of neurovascular and muscular structures (compartment syndrome).

The peroneal (lateral) compartment
This lies between the two intermuscular septa. It contains the plantar flexors and abductors of the foot and ankle – the peroneus longus and brevis muscles; and the superficial peroneal nerve.

The anterior (extensor) compartment
This lies between the anterior intermuscular septum and the tibia. It contains the dorsiflexors or extensors of the foot and ankle – tibialis anterior, extensor hallucis longus, extensor digitorum longus, and peroneus tertius muscles, the deep peroneal nerve, and the anterior tibial vessels.

The posterior (flexor) compartment
This lies between the posterior intermuscular septum and the tibia posteriorly. It contains the plantar flexors in two layers – the gastrocnemius and soleus with plantaris muscles in the superficial layer, which together insert as the Achilles' tendon – the long flexors of the toes, flexor hallucis longus, flexor digitorum longus and tibialis posterior in the deep layer. The neurovascular structures in this layer include the tibial nerve, the popliteal vessels and its posterior branch, and the saphenous veins.

Anatomy of the ankle and foot

The ankle joint
The ankle joint is a synovial hinge joint permitting dorsiflexion and plantar flexion. It is formed between the trochlea tali and the deep socket between the medial and lateral malleoli. The medial (deltoid) ligament and the lateral (anterior and posterior talofibular) ligaments contribute significantly to the stability of the joint.
- The posterior talofibular ligament attaches distally to the posterior tubercle of the talus.
- The talus ossifies from a separate centre and may be mistaken for a fracture; or fail to fuse with the talus to persist as the os trigonum.

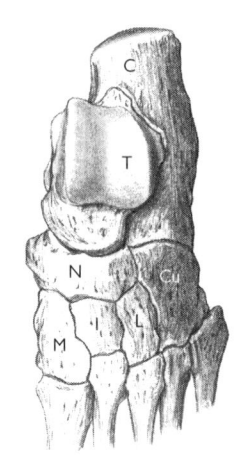

C = calcaneus
T = talus
N = navicular
Cu = cuboid
M = medial cuneiform
I = intermediate cuneiform
L = lateral cuneiform

Figure 5.41 Tarsal bones: dorsal view. Reproduced from the Oxford Textbook of Functional Anatomy, MacKinnon and Morris, 2005, with permission from Oxford University Press.

The hindfoot retinaculae
They are thickened bands of deep fascia at the ankle, which hold the tendons (enclosed in synovial sheaths) of the muscles of the leg and neurovascular bundles close to the joint as they pass into the foot.

Functional compression of the nerves (entrapment syndrome) may occur if there is any increase in the space between the retinacula and underlying bone.

The superior extensor retinaculum
This extends between the triangular subcutaneous area of the fibula and the anterior border of the tibia.

The inferior extensor retinaculum
This is Y-shaped and attaches to the calcaneus laterally, and to the medial malleolus and medial side of foot. Structures passing beneath the extensor retinaculum include:
- The tendons of the extensor digitorum longus.
- Extensor hallucis longus.
- Peroneus tertius.
- Tibialis anterior.
- The anterior tibial vessels.
- Deep peroneal nerve.

Superior and inferior peroneal retinacula
These pass, respectively, postero-inferior to the lateral malleolus and on the lateral surface of the calcaneus.

Structures passing beneath the peroneal retinaculum: The common sheath of the peroneus longus and brevis tendons.

The flexor retinaculum
This stretches from calcaneum to the medial malleolus.

CHAPTER 5 **Regional musculoskeletal anatomy and conditions**

Structures passing beneath the flexor retinaculum: the posterior tibial artery, and nerve and the tendons of the tibialis posterior, the flexor digitorum longus and the flexor hallucis longus.

Regional anatomy of the foot

The arches of the foot

The shape of the foot bones is of a half dome, concave inferiorly. The rim of the half dome consists of the heel, the lateral border of the foot, and the heads of the metatarsals. The skin covering these parts of the foot forms the footprint. The medial non-weight bearing part of the foot forms two arches.

The longitudinal arch

This arch is flat on the lateral side. The talus lies at its summit. The calcaneus is the posterior pillar. The remaining tarsal bones and metatarsals form the longer anterior pillar. This arch is maintained by:

- The plantar calcaneonavicular ligament.
- All the plantar ligaments of the foot.
- The plantar aponeurosis.
- The insertions of the tibialis posterior muscle.

Diminution of the normal longitudinal arch causes 'flat foot' deformity and an exaggerated arch produces 'club foot' deformity.

The horizontal arch

In the region of the tarsometatarsal bones this arch is maintained by the plantar and interosseous ligaments and by the tendon of peroneus longus.

Functional regions of the foot

The foot can be divided into the following three sections:

- The forefoot consists of the five metatarsals and is separated from the midfoot by the tarsometatarsal joint.
- The midfoot contains three cuneiforms, the navicular, and the cuboid, and is separated from the hindfoot by the transverse midtarsal joint.
- The hindfoot consists of the calcaneus and the talus.

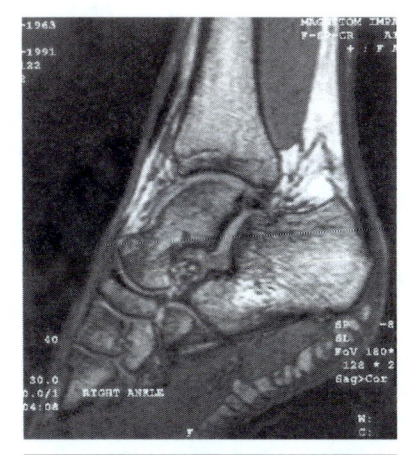

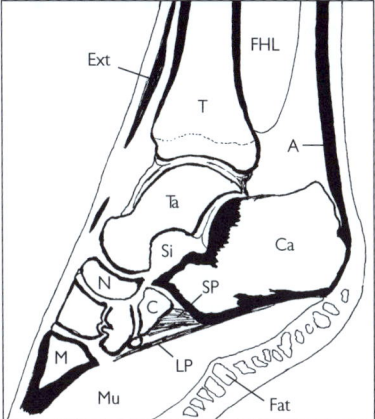

Figure 5.42 MRI of ankle, subtalar, and mid-tarsal joints (sagittal section). T, Tibia; Ta talus; Ca calcaneus; N, navicular; C, cuboid; M, metatarsal; Ext, extensor tendon; FHL, flexor hallucis longus; A Achilles tendon; Si, tarsal sinus containing interosseous ligament; SP, short plantar ligament; LP, long plantar ligament; Mu, muscle of sole; Fat, loculated subcutaneous fat in sole. Reproduced from the Oxford Textbook of Functional Anatomy, MacKinnon and Morris, 2005, with permission from Oxford University Press.

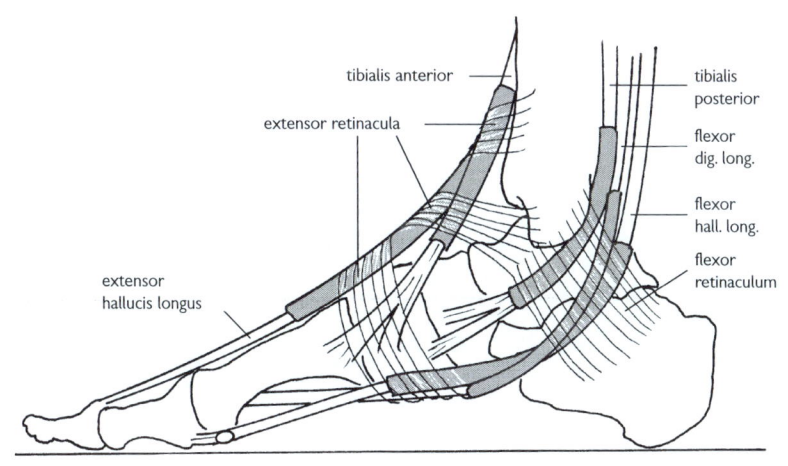

Figure 5.43 Tendons, synovial sheaths, and retinacula on the medial side of the ankle and foot. Reproduced from the Oxford Textbook of Functional Anatomy, MacKinnon and Morris, 2005, with permission from Oxford University Press.

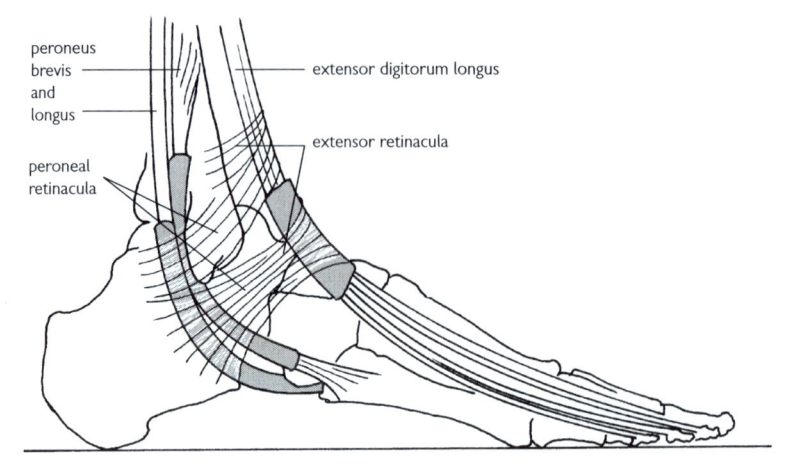

Figure 5.44 Tendons, synovial sheaths, and retinacula on the lateral side of the ankle and foot. Reproduced from the Oxford Textbook of Functional Anatomy, MacKinnon and Morris, 2005, with permission from Oxford University Press.

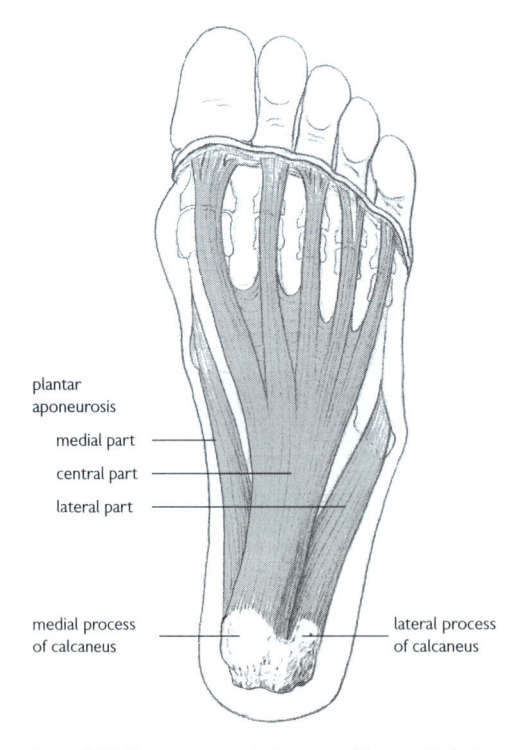

Figure 5.45 Plantar aponeurosis. Reproduced from the Oxford Textbook of Functional Anatomy, MacKinnon and Morris, 2005, with permission from Oxford University Press.

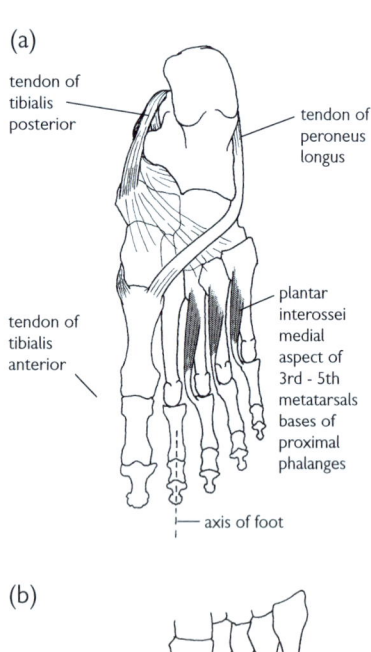

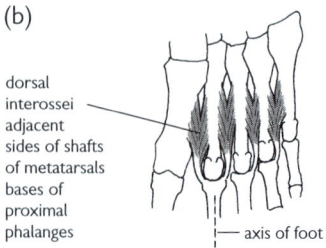

Figure 5.46 Sole of foot muscle layer 4: plantar interossei. Reproduced from the Oxford Textbook of Functional Anatomy, MacKinnon and Morris, 2005, with permission from Oxford University Press.

CHAPTER 5 Regional musculoskeletal anatomy and conditions

Joints

The subtalar joint
The articulation of the calcaneus and talus, the joint is surrounded by its own distinct capsule and does not articulate with other joints.
- Normal range of motion is 5° of inversion and 5° of eversion.
- The subtalar joint provides inversion and eversion of the heel for walking on uneven terrain.

The transverse midtarsal joint of Chopart
Composed of the talonavicular and calcaneocuboid joint the joint permits multi-axial motion, inversion and eversion of the midfoot and forefoot, and to a lesser degree, dorsiflexion and plantar flexion, and abduction and adduction. The bifurcate ligament stabilizes it.

The tarsometatarsal joint of Lisfranc
This joint comprises the interconnected second to fifth tarsometatarsal joints. A complex set of ligaments on their dorsal and plantar aspects provide stability.

The metatarsophalangeal joints
The deep transverse metatarsal ligament and the plantar ligaments stabilize these joints.

The first metatarsophalangeal joint
The joint plays a critical role in normal gait. Under most conditions, 65–75° of dorsiflexion of the hallux on the first metatarsal is required for normal gait and for the hallux to function in propulsion.
Disorders such as hallux valgus and hallux rigidus affect gait adversely by limiting dorsiflexion of the first metatarsophalangeal joint.

The interphalangeal joints
The toe joints are hinge joints stabilized by collateral ligaments and a plantar capsular ligament with a fibrous plate.
Weakness of the lumbricals, which extend the interphalangeal joints, produces 'hammer toe' deformity (extended metatarsal joints and flexed proximal interphalangeal joints).

Fasciae
The plantar aponeurosis, (or plantar fascia) runs from the plantar aspect of the calcaneus to the region of the metatarsal heads. (See Figure 5.4).
- The superficial layer blends with subcutaneous tissue.
- The deep layer joins the deep transverse metatarsal ligament and the flexor tendons.

Bursae
- The retrocalcaneal bursa lies between the calcaneus and the Achilles tendon. This bursa has a synovial lining, which abuts the Achilles fat pad.
- Between the skin and the Achilles tendon is the subcutaneous calcaneal bursa.
- At the plantar aspect of the midcalcaneus is the subcalcaneal bursa.

Os trigonum
The os trigonum may be seen in 3–15 % of feet. It may cause symptoms of pain and tenderness due to impingement in plantar flexion in footballers or ballet dancers.
- The os trigonum can be demonstrated on a plain lateral radiograph of the foot.
- It is important to differentiate this from an old non-united fracture of the normal posterior process seen in 38% of feet.
- The normal ossicle is smooth, well corticated, and has a normally lucent central medulla.
- Chronic impingement causes central sclerosis and cortical irregularity, with pitting and local soft-tissue oedema.
- MR may show changes of osteonecrosis and soft tissue swelling.

Further reading

Balint GP, Korda J, Hangody L, *et al.* Foot and ankle disorders. Best Pract Res Clin Rheumatol 2003; **17**: 87–111.

Romanes GJ. *Cunningham manual of practical anatomy* 1996, 15th edn.

Sinnatamby CS. *Last's regional and applied anatomy*, 10th edn, p. 112.

Lower leg and foot: regional musculoskeletal conditions

Pain can be due to local lesions or referred from the lumbar spine lesions, though the latter is usually posterior and/or lateral in the lower leg.

Differential diagnosis of lower leg pain
- Compartment syndromes.
- Ruptured popliteal cyst.
- Deep venous thrombosis.
- Stress fractures.
- Fibular tunnel syndrome.
- Tibialis anterior tenovaginitis.
- Radicular pain (lumbar disc prolapse, lateral recess stenosis or central lumbar canal stenosis; see p. 132).
- Periostitis.
- Osteitis/bone marrow pain (e.g. Paget's; see p. 418).
- Peripheral neuropathy.
- Erythromelalgia (hot feet/legs, burning pain, erythema; see: www.erythromelalgia.org).
- Myositis (calf muscles).
- Panniculitis (see p. 514).

Compartment syndromes

Increased pressure in confined anatomic compartments of the leg causes compartment syndrome, leading to ischaemia of the muscles and nerves. Unrelieved, pressure causes muscle necrosis and permanent nerve damage. In the lower leg, the anterior compartment syndrome is most commonly affected.

- Acute compartment syndrome is a surgical emergency, and can follow trauma or prolonged surgery in the lithotomy or hemi-lithotomy position, or can complicate deep tissue infection or rhabdomyolysis.
- Acute lower leg extremity compartment syndrome (ALECS) commonly complicates major trauma and appropriate patients should be carefully screened.
- Chronic exertional compartment syndrome occurs during or after exercise and causes diffuse cramp-like pain, which resolves with rest, but recurs with exertion:
  - blood flow scintigraphy suggests ischaemia alone does not account for all cases;
  - causes can be varied and investigations that may be necessary include ^{99m}Tc-MDP and exercise-related blood flow (^{201}Tl-SPECT) scintigraphy and MR or conventional angiography;
  - the diagnosis is easily overlooked and can be confirmed by intra-compartmental pressure monitoring before and during exercise. It resolves with rest
- Pre- and post-operative intracompartmental pressure monitoring confirms efficacy of either open or endoscopic surgical decompression.

Stress fracture of tibia

Stress fractures occur as the result of fatigue failure from repetitive loading below yield strength and are most common in the lower leg. Often there is a focal structural and/or muscle weakness.

Differential diagnoses are osteoid osteoma, chronic sclerosing osteomyelitis, osteomalacia, periostitis, metastases, osteogenic sarcoma, Ewing's tumour.

History
Stress fractures are common in dancers, runners, and jumpers, and occur in older people with osteoporosis. Women athletes with amenorrhoea are particularly at risk of bone fragility. The pain often worsens with exercise.

Examination and investigations
There is local tenderness and swelling. Initially, radiographs are normal, but ^{99m}Tc MDP scintigraphy or CT scanning can be diagnostic. CT is often necessary to differentiate from tumours.

Management
Early recognition is important. Rest is necessary for up to 6 weeks. Exercise in water helps maintain fitness in elite athletes and others. Addressing amenorrhoea is important in premenopausal athletes and osteoporosis investigation prudent in both men and women.

Ruptured popliteal cyst

Acute pain, swelling and skin erythema of the lower leg suggests this. Differential diagnoses: cellulitis and DVT.
- Pedal ecchymosis may discriminate the diagnosis from cellulitis or DVT.
- A history of preceding knee or popliteal swelling is often present. The swelling then often subsides commensurate with the evolution of lower leg swelling.
- Popliteal cysts form as part of inflammatory knee arthritis or secondary to trauma, which induces either an intra-articular knee swelling or fluid accumulating from an extended selling of the semimembranosus bursa.
- Ultrasound to rule out femoral DVT is sensible.
- Adequate analgesia including an NSAID, patient reassurance, limb elevation, and icing is appropriate.
- Some monitoring of the leg and foot is important – compartment syndrome is a recognized complication.
- Although it is not known how effectively glucocorticoid (GC) injected into the knee reduces lower leg swelling (presumably by accessing compartments through the breach in the cyst), an intra-articular GC injection is often undertaken.

Fibular tunnel syndrome

This is an entrapment neuropathy lesion of the peroneal nerve. The common peroneal nerve (CPN) lies on the neck of the fibula, which forms the floor of the 'fibular tunnel'. The tunnel entrance is a musculo-aponeurotic arch derived from soleus and peroneus longus muscles. The CPN is commonly compressed in this tunnel in cases of CPN palsy. In some, however, the nerve follows a more tortuous course higher up where the distal rectus femoris passes adjacent to the lateral head of the gastrocnemius and this has been proposed as a factor increasing the risk of CPN symptoms.
- Post-traumatic CPN entrapment usually occurs after fracture, compression by a walking cast, or sitting cross-legged.
- The patient complains of parasthesias or numbness of the lateral calf and foot. Rarely, a foot drop develops.
- The lesion can be localized by nerve conduction studies.
- Causative factors should be addressed.
- Partial weakness of peroneus longus and brevis is possible and a risk factor for falls.

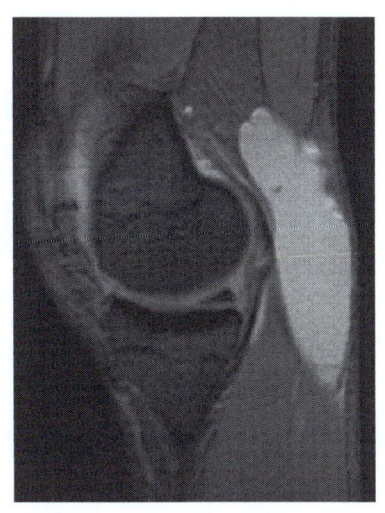

CHAPTER 5 **Regional musculoskeletal anatomy and conditions** 189

Figure 5.47 Popliteal cysts can be large and fluid can accumulate causing high-pressure lesions. Fluid leakage into the calf is a common consequence of large popliteal cyst formation.

- Podiatric, orthotist and/or occupational therapy review is an important part of conservative management so that appropriate foot support is maintained (e.g. splinting).
- Surgical exploration and release of the nerve may be necessary.

Recognized causes of tibial periostitis
- Posteromedial tibial periostitis ('shin splints').
- Sarcoid (see p. 510).
- Psoriatic arthropathy (PsA; see p. 220).
- Polyarteritis nodosa (PAN; see p. 332).
- Primary hypertrophic osteoarthropathy (pachydermoperiostitis).
- Secondary hypertrophic osteoarthropathy (e.g. malignancy, HIV disease).
- Associated with Crohn's disease.
- SAPHO syndrome (see p. 236).
- Syphilis.

Periostitis
A cause of persistent, immobility-related pain of the front or medial aspect of the leg. Pain is often reported with a burning quality and can disturb sleep.
- Can mimic pain from tibial stress fractures.
- Terminology can often confuse. Shin splints is regarded as an outdated term for periostitis of the upper medial tibia now termed medial tibial stress syndrome.
- ^{99m}Tc-MDP scintigraphy can highlight lesions and show lesions elsewhere (e.g. SIJs, periostitis in other leg, PsA/SAPHO).
- Neurophysiology tests may characterize nerve lesions in cases where imaging is negative or show that dual pathology exists (e.g. sarcoid, PAN). However, tests are often negative in small fibre sensory neuropathy in the elderly.
- Treat underlying cause.
- Consider NSAIDs or IV bisphosphonates for periostitis or osteitis, respectively.

Further reading
Anselmi SJ. Common peroneal nerve compression. *J Am Podiatr Med Assoc* 2006; **96**(5): 413–17.
Aoki Y, Yasuda K, Tohyama H, Ito H, Minami A. Magnetic resonance imaging in stress fractures and shin splints. *Clin Orthopaed Relat Res* 2004; **421**: 260–7.
Fayad LM, Kamel IR, Kawamoto S, Bluemke DA, Frassica FJ, Fishman EK. Distinguishing stress fractures from pathological fractures: a multimodality approach. *Skeletal Radiol* 2005; **34**(5): 245–59.
Fottner A, Bauer-Melnyk A, Birkenmeier C, Jansson V, Dürr HR. Stress fractures presenting as tumours: a retrospective analysis of 22 cases. *Int Orthopaed* 2007; Dec 14. Epub ahead of print.
Howard JL, Mohtadi NG, Wiley JP. Evaluation of outcomes in patients following surgical treatment of chronic exertional compartment syndrome in the leg. *Clin J Sports Med* 2000; **10**(3): 176–84.
Kosir R, Moore FA, Selby JH *et al.* Acute lower extremity compartment syndrome in critically ill trauma patients. *J Trauma* 2007; **63**: 268–75.
Meyer RS, White KK, Smith JM, Groppo ER, Mubarak SJ, Hargens AR. Intramuscular and blood pressures in legs positioned in the hemilithotomy position: clarification of risk factors for well-leg acute compartment syndrome. *J Bone Jt Surg Am* 2002; **84-A**: 1829–35.
Ryan W, Malone N, Delaney M, O'Brien M, Murray P. Relationship of the common peroneal nerve and its branches to the head and neck of the fibula. *Clin Anat* 2003; **16**: 501–5.
Viera RL, Rosenberg ZS, Kiprovski K. MRI of the distal biceps femoris muscle: normal anatomy, variants, and association with common peroneal entrapment neuropathy. *Am J Roetgenol* 2007; **189**: 549–55.

Conditions of the ankle and hindfoot

Discrete musculoskeletal lesions of the foot are often to diagnose precisely. Functional examination is not always specific and imaging tends to be less specific in identifying pathology compared with more proximal sites. The foot is a common site for inflammatory arthritides to affect. A knowledge of typical patterns of involvement of structures associated with the Spondylarthropathy conditions (see pp 209–238) – especially psoriatic arthritis – and sarcoid is useful for the rheumatologist. These conditions can affect entheses and periosteum as well as synovial joints and tendons. Involvement of the ankle or subtalar joint is relatively common in CPPDD disease regardless of whether pseudo-gout manifestations are, or have been, present. Gout can affect, in theory, any joint or tendon in the foot but gout frequently causes non-articular tissue inflammation in soft-tissues and if this is diffuse it can be mistaken for cellulitis for example.

Table 5.11

Region of foot	Discrete musculoskeletal lesions
Hindfoot (general)	Ankle or subtalar arthritis
	Osteochondral fracture of talus
	Periostitis (distal lower leg)
	Peroneal tendonitis (lateral)
Medial ankle	Medial ankle impingement syndrome
	Tibialis posterior tendonitis/dysfunction
	Tarsal tunnel syndrome
Lateral ankle	Peroneus longus and brevis tendonitis
	Lateral pre-malleolar bursitis
Anterior ankle	Anterior ankle impingement syndromes
	Dorsal (extensor) tendonitis
	Tibialis anterior tendonitis
Posterior ankle	Posterior ankle impingement syndrome
	Achilles' tendonitis/enthesitis/bursitis
Heel	Plantar fasciitis
	Calcaneal stress fracture
	Tarsal tunnel syndrome (plantar + sole)
Midfoot	Arthritis or enthesitis
	Sinus tarsi syndrome (lateral pain)
	Peroneus tendonitis/enthesitis (lateral)
	Accessory navicular (medial)
	Osteonecrosis of navicular
Toes	Arthritis of MTPJs
	Inter-metatarsal bursitis
	Morton's neuroma
	Metatarsal stress fracture
	Hallux lesions: valgus, rigidus
	Dactylitis

Ankle impingement syndromes

Anterior ankle impingement syndrome
History
Ongoing anterior ankle pain may be present. Enquire for a supination injury or repeated dorsiflexion injury.

Examination
Dorsiflexion of the ankle is painful and restricted. Generalized connective tissue laxity may be present – consider joint hypermobility syndrome and other disorders associated with joint hypermobility. Such patients are at increased risk of recurrent inversion/pronation ankle strains.

Imaging
Look for osteophytes/enthesophytes of the distal tibia and the talar neck on oblique plain radiographs. If ankle effusion is present, MR may demonstrate a 'meniscoid' mass within the lateral gutter of the ankle. Talar enthesophytes can be a part of PsA and DISH, as well as due to simple degenerative changes.

Anteromedial impingement syndrome
History
Presents as anteromedial ankle pain. Ask about previous inversion injury or fracture of the ankle or talus.

Examination
Anteromedial swelling and tenderness may be present. Look for painful restricted dorsiflexion and supination of the ankle.

Imaging
Anteromedial talus osteophytes/enthesophytes may be seen on plain radiography. MR arthrography shows: abnormal appearance of the anteromedial capsule, irregular synovial folding anterior to the tibiotalar ligament and medial malleolus, and presence of tibial osteophytes.

Anterolateral ankle impingement syndrome
History
Presents as anterolateral ankle pain. Ask about previous inversion injury to the ankle.

Examination
Feel for tenderness in the area of antero-inferior tibiofibular ligament and/or anterior talofibular ligament.

Imaging
Plain radiographs may occasionally show small osteophytes on the anterior tibial margin. Increased anterior translation of the talar dome can be seen on stress radiographs in approximately half the cases.

Posterior ankle impingement syndrome.
History
Common in ballet dancers from weight-bearing in maximal plantar flexion, especially when os trigonum is present.

Examination
Tenderness may be elicited behind the lateral malleolus. Passive plantar-flexion is often painful.

Imaging
Plain radiographs may detect os trigonum or trigonal process. MR imaging can demonstrate hypertrophy or tear of the posteroinferior tibiofibular (PITF) ligament, transverse posterior tibiofibular ligament, or the 'tibial slip' running between the PITF ligament and the transverse ligament.

Management of impingement syndromes
Conservative management
Rest, NSAIDs, proper footwear, ankle support aids and physiotherapy is the first line of treatment. Failing this intra-articular glucocorticoid injections (2 or 3 times in 10–14-day intervals) to reduce synovial inflammation.

CHAPTER 5 Regional musculoskeletal anatomy and conditions

Operative management
In failed conservative management arthroscopy with debridement and removal of the hypertrophic synovial tissue, and the osteophytes often provides good results.

Lateral pre-malleolar bursitis
There is often history of the foot being in prolonged periods of plantar-flexed and inverted position (e.g. Muslims during prayer). Ultrasound is often helpful to rule out other soft tissue swelling.
- Differentiate from pre-malleolar fat pad and a ganglion.
- Advise not sitting on the foot.
- NSAIDs and physiotherapy may be beneficial.
- Avoid intra-bursal steroid injections.
- Excised bursa where conservative management fails.

Tarsal tunnel syndrome
Tarsal tunnel syndrome is often under-diagnosed as a cause of foot pain. The posterior tibial nerve and the flexor hallucis and digitorum longus tendons pass behind the medial malleolus under the flexor retinaculum.
- Entrapment of the nerve in this 'tunnel' can occur due to bony deformity after an ankle fracture, a flat foot, inflammation of the tendons, or compression from an ankle synovial cyst.
- Patients present with burning, tingling, and numbness in the distribution of the nerve, notably the toes and distal part of the sole and heel. This is often worse at night. An aching calf at night may also be present.
- Tenderness and swelling may be present around the medial malleolus. A positive Tinnel's sign elicited by percussion of the flexor retinaculum confirms the diagnosis. Reduced vibratory sensation and decreased two-point discrimination may be present on the plantar aspect of the foot and toes.
- In doubtful cases, nerve conduction studies may be used to document delay in conduction of the posterior tibial nerve across the ankle. Denervation on needle sampling is also reliable. MR may be useful in the evaluation of anatomical structures.
- For conservative management use NSAIDs and glucocorticoid injection under the retinaculum between the calcaneum and medial malleolus. Orthotics can reduce abnormal movement of the foot in the gait cycle.
- Treatment of any local cause for compression is appropriate. Occasionally, surgical section of the retinaculum is necessary. In resistant cases, surgical decompression of the posterior tibial nerve may be necessary.

Posterior tibial tendon dysfunction
The posterior tibial tendon suspends the medial arch of the foot. Dysfunction and rupture of the tendon results in acquired unilateral flatfoot, valgus hindfoot, forefoot abduction, and talonavicular subluxation.
- Not uncommon in middle-aged obese women. Associated medial or lateral ankle pain may be present.
- Pes planovalgus results in 'too many toes sign' when the foot is inspected from behind. (More of the lesser toes visible lateral to ankle joint than on the uninvolved side.)
- On palpation, the tendon sheath may be tender and swollen. Specifically look for difficulty in performing a single-limb heel rise. At heel rise there may be pain under the medial malleolus and inability of the valgus hindfoot to invert. Weakness may be noted on resisted active inversion of the fully plantar flexed foot.
- Ask for weight-bearing bilateral anteroposterior and lateral plain radiographs for subtle unilateral pathology.
- US or MR will characterize tendon pathology.
- Local glucocorticoid injection may be appropriate in cases of inflammatory tendonitis, although where there are advanced changes or dysfunction without inflammation, it is best avoided.
- Orthoses and exercise may be useful in the early non-acute phases though there are no robust RCTs of such methods.
- Tenosynovectomy and debridement is needed in acute presentations. Arthrodesis and tendon transfers may be necessary for failed conservative treatment.

Peroneal tendonitis
Both peroneal tendons may be affected. Peroneus longus tendonitis presents as lateral hindfoot pain and cavovalgus foot deformity. The peroneus longus tendon is susceptible to damage at three places:
- At the calcanear trochlear process.
- At the inferior peroneal retinaculum.
- At the cuboid notch, where the tendon sharply changes its direction passing the plantar surface of the foot.

The management should be primarily conservative, but tendon rupture needs surgical treatment.

Sinus tarsi syndrome
In the tarsal sinus lies an arterial anastomosis, three roots of the inferior extensor retinaculum, the cervical ligament, the tarsal canal ligament, and fatty tissue. There is some controversy as to the precise cause and nature of the condition.
- There may be a history of inversion injury or inflammatory joint disease.
- The syndrome consists of lateral foot pain (relieved by injection of local anaesthetics), foot instability (e.g. previous injury or intrinsic hypermobility) and tenderness of the sinus tarsi.
- MRI shows obliteration of fat in the sinus tarsi space.
- Locally administer steroid injection. Chronic cases may warrant synovectomy and reconstruction of the collateral ligament.

Osteochondral lesion of the talus (OLT)
There are a number of synonyms: osteochondral defect, osteochondral fracture, osteochondritis dissecans. There is separation of a fragment of articular cartilage with or without subchondral bone of the talar dome.
- Plain radiographs may demonstrate the fragment and ligament injury is usually detectable in these cases. MR can be used to differentiate avascular necrosis when plain radiographs are negative.
- Non-operative treatment is successful in 45% cases. Excision, curettage and drilling are successful in 85%, excision and curettage in 78%, and excision alone in 3%.
- Mosaicplasty (osteochondral graft transplant) and autologous chondrocyte transplantation are promising methods for the future.

Achilles tendonopathy

Achilles tendonopathy, enthesopathy, and retrocalcaneal bursitis are characteristic features of SpA. Heel pain is often the first manifestation of the disease.

Causes of Achilles' tendononpathy
- Spondylarthropathy.
- Acute or chronic trauma.
- Fluoroquinolone-induced.
- Associated conditions:
  - haemodialysis;
  - hypercholesterolaemia (xanthomas);
  - diabetes.
- Injudicious use of glucocorticoid injection

- In traumatically-induced lesions, 25% of injuries may be missed at the first presentation. The pathological changes described in the tendon may be broadly characterized as tendonosis without inflammation and inflammation of the paratenon (surrounding tendon sheath).
- In cases of rupture, the site is usually in a relatively hypovascular region of the tendon 2–6 cm proximally from the insertion. Rupture may also occur at the enthesis or at the muscle/tendon junction.
- The rupture is unusually painful in fluoroquinolone-induced tendonopathy. Otherwise, especially in chronically developing ruptures, the pain is not severe or is totally absent.
- SpA-related lesions (enthesopathies) are characterized by tenderness over the posterior os calcis, irregularly defined erosions and/or deposition of bone with defined excrescences in the healing stage.
- Examine with patient standing from behind and compare sides. Examine then with patient prone and feet over end of couch. Pathology at muscle-tendon junction, Achilles tendon (cord) and insertion can be palpated. Squeezing the calf plantar-flexes foot if tendon intact.
- US may predict the outcome of achillodynia. Differentiation of full- and partial-thickness tears can be made with 92% accuracy using US and characteristic appearances at the enthesis has been described in SpA-related disease.
- MR imaging frequently shows intra-tendonous changes during fluoroquinolone treatment even in the absence of any clinical signs.
- ^{99m}Tc-MDP scintigraphy highlights enthesopathy at the site and other places in SpA.

Management of Achilles' tendonopathy

Non-inflammatory lesions
Protection of the foot and heel support is appropriate. Surgery is required in the case of complete rupture and provides good results but a rather high (15%) percentage of complications.

Inflammatory SpA-related lesions
NSAIDs and orthotics for heel support. Physiotherapy in recovering cases to avoid shortening of posterior heel structures. Glucocorticoid injections over the enthesis can be considered in isolated enthesitis or where paratenon inflammation exists without intra-tendon substance changes (demonstrable on US).

Retrocalcaneal/subcutaneous calcaneal bursitis

Also known as 'pump bumps', it is rarely a complication of inflammatory joint disease, but is usually caused by irritation of stiff heel counters.
- The overlying skin is usually reddish or hyperkeratotic.
- The management consists of wearing counterless shoes, padding and NSAIDs. Local glucocorticoid injections should be avoided because of the risk of infection.

Plantar fasciitis (PF)

Plantar fasciitis is an enthesopathy of the calcaneal tuberosity. There are both mechanical and autoimmune inflammatory aetiologies. Pure mechanically-induced PF is caused by over-use, repetitive strain, or microtrauma. PF is a common in lesion in spondylarthropathy conditions and chronic musculoskeletal sarcoidosis.
- There is pain and/or stiffness on the plantar heel surface occasionally extending along the proximal sole. Symptoms are often worse with the first few steps of the day.
- Ask about current or previous inflammatory back pain (see p. 210), psoriasis, and pain at entheses elsewhere.
- Tenderness is maximal over the medial calcaneal tubercle. A positive heel squeeze test can discriminate pain from os calcis stress fractures (os calcis squeezed between the heels of your hands from both sides).
- Lateral os calcis radiograph and, if necessary, CT, can help rule out calcaneal stress fracture.
- Characteristic MR, ^{99m}Tc-MDP scintigraphy and US appearances have been described.

Management of PF
Conservative management: rest, night splints, use of soft rubber heel pads, foot orthoses to support of the longitudinal arch, and physiotherapy may all have a role.
- NSAIDs and local GC injection can be considered. Evidence for long-term efficacy of the latter however is lacking.
- US-guided GC injection is no more effective than palpation-guided injection.
- Surgical release of the plantar fascia is rarely required. Healing problems of the overlying skin are relatively frequent. Endoscopic plantar fasciectomy is a recently-developed technique, which probably causes fewer complications compared with open surgery.
- External beam radiotherapy can be helpful in recalcitrant cases.
- A number of alternative treatment modalities have been reported. The efficacy of lithotripsy, botulinum injection, autologous blood injection has not been proven in long-term robust studies compared with GC injection.

Further reading

Irving DB, Cook JL, Menz JB. Factors associated with chronic plantar heel pain: a systematic review. *J Sci Med Sport* 2006; **9**(1–2): 11–22.

Paige NM, Nouvong A. The top 10 things foot and ankle specialists wish every primary care physician knew. *Mayo Clin Proc* 2006; **81**: 818–22.

Wearing SC, Smeathers JE, Urry SR, Henrig EM, Hills AP. The pathomechanics of plantar fasciitis. *Sports Med* 2006; **36**(7): 585–611.

Conditions of the mid and forefoot

Accessory navicular bone
This is present in 4–21% of the population and can be a cause of medial midfoot pain. An accessory navicular is a large triangle or heart-shaped ossicle attached with a cartilaginous or fibrocartilaginous synchondrosis to the navicular bone. It is thought to be a source of symptoms owing to a chronic stress reaction.
- The bone configuration and its involvement in 'bony stress' can be demonstrated on radiographs or CT and bone scintigraphy, respectively.
- An accessory navicular bone may also damage the posterior tibial tendon.
- The management consists of resting from sports activities or surgical excision of the accessory bone.

The Mueller–Weiss syndrome
Osteochondritis/necrosis of the navicular bone. This occurs more frequently bilaterally in adult women. The management is conservative with rest and orthotic foot support as necessary. A failure of conservative therapy can lead to permanent degenerative midfoot arthritis.

Plantar plate disruption
A common cause of metatarsalgia. It occurs frequently in women wearing high-heeled shoes. The second MTPJ is most commonly affected. Diagnosis can be made by MR.

Intermetatarsal bursitis
Overstrain of the MTPJ region often results in bursitis of the intermetatarsal bursae or adventitial bursae beneath the metatarsal heads. Bursitis can also be caused by repetitive trauma, infection, RA, SpA, or gout.

MTPJ synovitis
Pain and/or stiffness across the forefoot or on weight-bearing can denote synovitis of MTPJs though the symptoms are not specific.
- Bilateral forefoot stiffness can occur in RA and psoriatic arthritis notably.
- There may be visible forefoot spreading (look for separation of toes). Toe bases are tender. Squeezing across MTPJs can elicit pain, although this is not a specific test.
- With advanced polyarticular MTPJ synovitis there may be metatarsal head subluxation. Abnormal callus distribution may be evident on the sole of the foot.
- Poly (flexor) tenosynovitis can co-exist with, or mimic, MTPJ synovitis. The usual diagnosis is RA.
- Prior to erosive changes in MTPJs, or joint space loss – both evident in advanced disease on radiographs, US and MR may highlight inflammatory lesion site and distribution.

Morton's neuroma
Morton's neuroma is located most often between the 3rd and 4th metatarsal heads. The neuroma is not a true neoplasm, but is caused by peripheral fibrosis of the compressed inter-digital nerve. Histology of the neuroma is undistinguishable from normal intermetatarsophalangeal nerves.
- The nerve compression can be caused by the metatarsal heads, inter-metatarsal ligaments and bursae.
- The pain presents on the opposing sides of the two toes, accompanied by hypoparaesthesia.
- For differential diagnosis between Morton's neuroma and MTPJ arthritis, local anaesthetics can be given either into the interspaces proximally to the metatarsal head or into the corresponding MTPJ. This 'ex juventibus' effect may show what is the probable cause of pain.
- US or MR can also be used for differential diagnosis.
- Surgical excision of the neuroma may be undertaken in symptomatic cases.

Stress fractures of the metatarsals
These fractures are common in runners, ballet dancers and other sports where there is inadequate shoe support, but they are also found in the middle-aged or the elderly doing sporting activities. Stress fracture also occurs in diabetic osteoarthropathy, and can indicate generalized or regional osteoporosis. Regional cortical-rich bone osteoporosis is a feature of hyperparathyroidism.

Radiologically occult fractures can be detected by MR imaging or bone scintigraphy if clinical suspicion remains when radiographs are normal. With MR and/or bone scintigraphy even the pre-fracture state of stress injury can be diagnosed.

Freiberg's infarction
Probably an osteonecrosis of the second or third metatarsal head, causing secondary osteoarthritis of the adjacent MTPJ. High-heeled shoes, repetitive injury or trauma may be causative factors.

Foreign body granulomas
Granulomas due to thorns, glass, plastic, or wood particles are not rare on the plantar surface of the foot. The foreign bodies can be visualized by US or MR.

Plantar fibromatosis or 'Ledderhose' disease
A benign, but locally often aggressive 'tumour' of the fascia, identical to Dupuytren's contracture of the hand.
- May be tender on palpation. Also there may be a small tender mass palpabale. Fibrous tissue can be palpated at the medial and proximal aspect of the plantar fascia.
- It can be visualized by both US and MR; however, physical examination is often sufficient for a reliable diagnosis.
- The treatment is subtotal fasciectomy, but recurrences are not rare. External beam radiotherapy may arrest progression and prevent the need for surgery.

Sesamoiditis
A painful inflammatory condition caused by repetitive injury to the plantar aspect of the forefoot. Reactive soft-tissue inflammation, such as tendonitis, synovitis, or bursitis often accompanies the condition.

Hallux rigidus
This usually results from OA or PsA changes at the first MTPJ. Loss of motion is due to new growth of bone around dorsal articular surface of first metatarsal head.

Epidemiology
- Most common osteoarthritic joint in the foot.
- Second commonest great toe condition to hallux valgus
- 1 in 40 individuals over 50 years develop hallux rigidus. Females > males (2:1).
- Psoriatic dactylitis/periostitis is also a cause.

CHAPTER 5 Regional musculoskeletal anatomy and conditions

Clinical features
- There is pain or paraesthesia aggravated by standing, walking, and wearing shoes with heels.
- Dactylitis and nail disease may suggest PsA.
- Skin irritation due to pressure from footwear over dorsal exostoses.
- Limitation of motion, especially dorsiflexion though often normal or adequate plantar-flexion.
- Affected feet are often long, narrow and pronated with unstable arches. Feet are frequently hyper-mobile or have an elevated (and long) first metatarsal.

Differential diagnosis
There is a need to rule out 'pseudo-hallux rigidus': Nodular swelling of the proximal flexor hallucis longus (FHL) also limits hallux dorsiflexion. However, in this condition hallux motion is restored when the ankle is plantar flexed.

Investigations
Radiological features include non-uniform joint space narrowing, widening of the first metatarsal head and base of proximal phalanx, subchondral sclerosis and cysts, horseshoe-shaped osteophytes, more osteophyte formation on lateral compared with medial side, sesamoid changes.

Treatment
- Conservative therapy includes moulded stiff orthoses, with rigid bar or rocker bottom shoe.
- Surgical treatment includes cheilectomy for mild to moderate deformity.
- Arthrodesis is the treatment of choice following failed cheilectomy or where advanced degenerative changes are present.
- Implant arthroplasty provides good results. The use of mosaicplasty has been recently reported.

Dactylitis and psoriatic onycho pachydermo periostitis (POPP)

Dactylitis is a common finding in two of the SpA conditions notably – PsA, ReA. Dactylitis is also a feature of AS, USpA, and chronic sarcoidosis. Acute gout involving the whole toe can also cause a dactylitis – although classically the swelling may be more eccentrically-orientated.

In the SpAs dactylitis may be acute, involve one or a number of toes, and is often asymmetrical. More indolent forms of dactylitis can be easily overlooked.

In psoriatic onycho pachydermo periostitis there may be swelling, pain, and stiffness of the toe extremities associated with nail changes. A range of features probably exist. The condition can occur in children.

- Periosteal changes in the great toe in PsA are common and exist 20–50% of patients with PsA.
- Indolent dactylitis of the great toe in PsA associated with periosteal apposition and juxta-articular new bone formation is probably an under-recognized cause of hallux limitus/rigidus.

Further reading

Gehrmann RM, Renard RL. Current concepts review: stress fractures of the foot. *Foot Ankle Int* 2006; **27**(9): 750–7.

Healy PJ, Groves C, Chandrmohan M, Helliwell PS. MRI changes in psoriatic dactylitis – extent of pathology, relationship to tenderness and correlation with clinical indices. *Rheumatology (Ox)* 2008; **47**: 92–5.

Keiserman LS, Sammarco VJ, Sammarco GJ. Surgical treatment of the hallux rigidus. *Foot Ankle Clin* 2005; **10**: 75–96.

Ugolini PA, Raikin SM. The accessory navicular. *Foot Ankle Clin* 2004; **9**: 165–80.

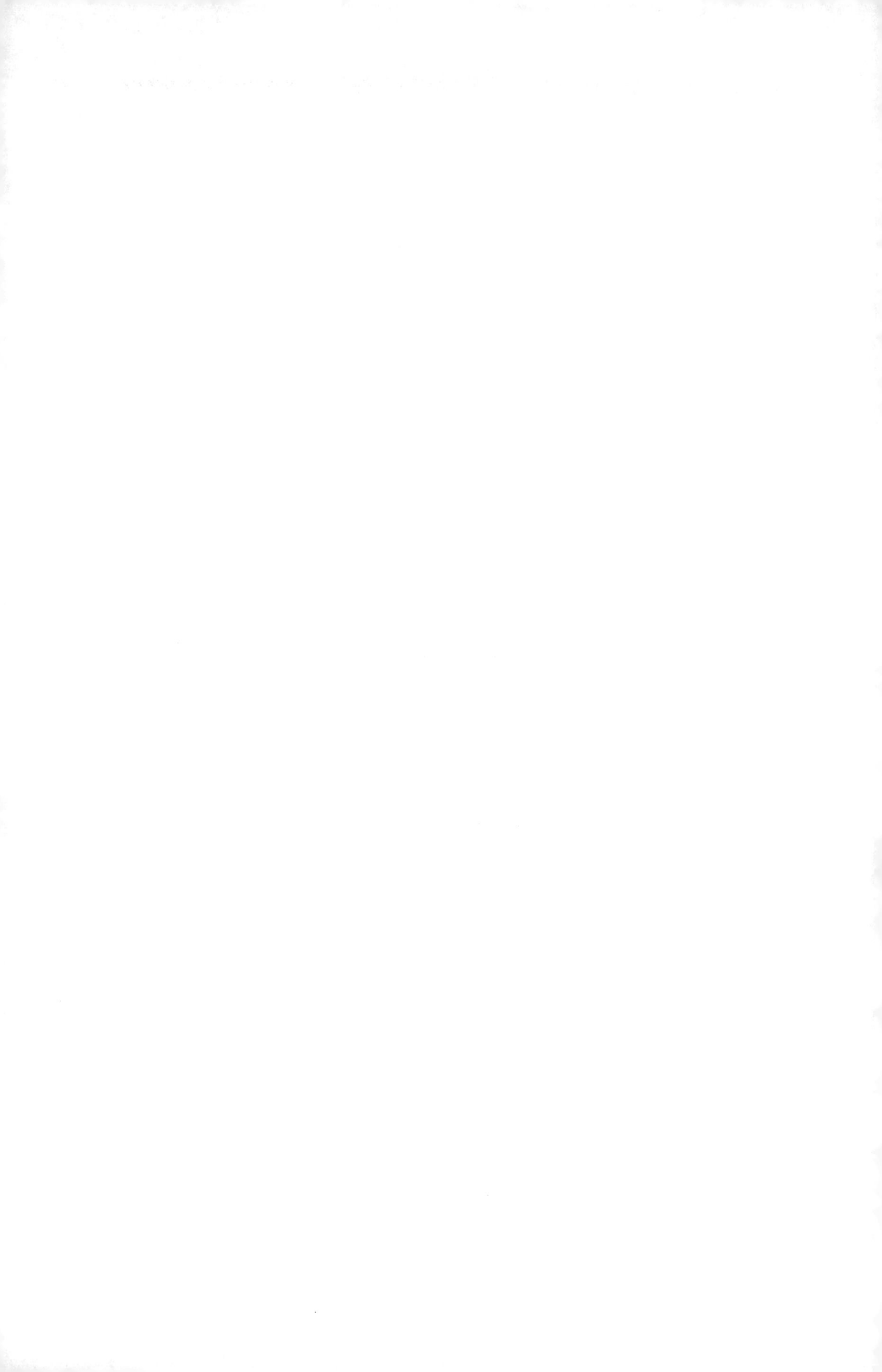

Chapter 6
Rheumatoid arthritis

Guidelines for the management of rheumatoid arthritis *208*

Definition
Rheumatoid arthritis (RA) or, more correctly, rheumatoid disease, is a heterogeneous, multisystem autoinflammatory disorder of unknown aetiology manifest chiefly as synovitis, however, extra-articular involvement is common. The disease is associated with significant disability and premature mortality. As no diagnostic test exists for RA its identification relies on the clinical picture supplemented by laboratory and radiological investigations.

Diagnostic criteria
Due to the heterogeneity of RA and the variable expression of disease, precise categorization of the condition is problematic.
- This complexity is compounded when dealing with early RA or early undifferentiated inflammatory arthritis. This has a profound effect on management as the current paradigm is to capture RA as early as possible in the 'window of opportunity' to switch off the inflammatory process.
- The diagnosis therefore rests upon a constellation of signs and symptoms supported by serological investigation and appropriate imaging.
- Exclusion of other inflammatory arthritides is paramount.
- Classification is based on the American College of Rheumatology 1987 criteria. These criteria were originally devised to classify established disease and therefore do not apply for early arthritis. New diagnostic and classification criteria are therefore required.

Table 6.1 American College of Rheumatology classification criteria for rheumatoid arthritis (1987). Four of the seven criteria must be met. Criteria 1–4 must have been present for at least 6 weeks.

1	Morning stiffness in and around joints, lasting at least 1 h before maximal improvement
2	Arthritis in three of more joint areas. Soft tissue swelling or fluid (not bony overgrowth) observed by a physician. Possible areas include right or left PIP, MCP, wrist, elbow, knee, ankle and MTP joints
3	Swelling (arthritis) of the PIP, MCP, or wrist joints
4	Symmetrical arthritis. Simultaneous involvement of the same joint areas (defined in 2) on both sides of the body. Absolute symmetry not necessary
5	Subcutaneous nodules
6	Positive test for rheumatoid factor
7	Radiographic erosions and/or peri-articular osteopaenia in hand and/or wrist joints

PIP: proximal interphalangeal; MCP: metacarpophalangeal; MTP: metatarsophalangeal.

Epidemiology
RA is the most frequent chronic inflammatory disease of joints and is found ubiquitously.
- Prevalence approaches 1% in the industrialized world and varies with ethnicity. Low figures in certain developing countries may be confounded by age distribution
- Incidence estimated to be 3.4/10 000 in women and 1.4/10 000 in men highlighting the female preponderance (3:1). The gender difference equilibrates in older age groups.
- Hormonal and reproductive factors contribute to the female excess.
- Peak age of onset occurs between 30 and 50 years in females. Incidence increases with age in males
- First-degree relatives have a 2–3-fold increased incidence.
- Monozygotic twins share 30–50% concordance, 4-fold greater than dizygotic twins.
- Uncontrolled severe disease leads to increased mortality, but the expression of RA is heterogeneous, and therefore prognostication, is difficult. Life expectancy is reduced by 3 years in women and 7 years in men.
- Premature mortality is chiefly due to an increase in cardiovascular disease, infections, and respiratory complications.
- Spontaneous remission may occur especially early disease; however, this is less likely once joint damage has developed.
- The direct and indirect costs (including loss of productivity and reduced quality of life) associated with RA are enormous, with indirect costs accounting for up to $2/3$ of the total.

Aetiology/pathogenesis
The aetiology of RA is unknown, but is likely to be multifactorial. Disease is possibly precipitated by an environmental trigger/s or potentially stochastic event occurring in a genetically predisposed individual. No conclusive evidence exists implicating an infective cause such as bacteria or mycoplasma. The potential role of parvovirus B19 is controversial. Cigarette smoking is a risk and severity factor. No other single external environmental factor shows a clear or consistent association with RA.

Genetic
The shared epitope of the HLA-DRB1*04 cluster, present in over 80% of RA patients, shares a highly homologous amino acid sequence at the third hypervariable region of the HLA-DR chain. It is associated with the development of disease and is a severity factor. This sequence is common to most RA patients although disease develops only in a small portion of those with the epitope. Thus, RA is most likely a polygenic disease.

Immunopathology
RA is characterized by destruction of articular cartilage and subchondral bone by invading synovial hyperplasia (pannus). In chronic RA, inflammatory cells accumulate and lymphocytes may organize into discrete aggregates. A diffuse mononuclear cell infiltration or relatively acellular fibrous tissue may also be present.
- Immune dysfunction is central to the pathogenesis with upregulation of pro-inflammatory cells and cytokines (i.e. T cells, B cells, macrophages, dendritic cells, TNFα, IL-1, IL-6, and INFγ) and autoantibody production [rheumatoid factors (RF), anti-citrullinated peptide (CCP) antibodies].
- TNFα and IL-6 appear to be pivotal cytokines in the inflammatory cascade and have pleiotropic effects.

Autoantibodies
Serum-detected RFs are immunoglobulins (usually IgM) with antibody specificity for the Fc region of IgG.
- The distribution and extent of RFs in tissue is less clear. IgA and IgG dimer RFs clearly exist, however.
- Anti-citrullinated antibodies are directed against peptides such as vimentin, fibrinogen and cyclic citrullinated peptide (their specificity determined by their ability to bind citrulline, a modified arginine residue).

- Some patients show evidence of autoimmunity prior to clinical disease with autoantibodies detectable in blood years prior to the onset of clinical disease.

Innate immunity
Initiation of the inflammation may not, however, be autoantibody mediated and may occur via the innate immune system in the synovium.
- This process involves Toll-like receptors (primitive pattern recognition molecules) expressed principally by dendritic cells, which bind to foreign and self antigens. This, in turn, acts upon cells of the adaptive system initiating auto-inflammation. A localized reaction then occurs with influx of inflammatory mediators via activated endothelial cells expressing various adhesion molecules.
- Arthritis associated antigens are subsequently presented to T-helper 1 cell receptors via class II MHC molecules on antigen presenting cells (APCs).
- The shared epitope allows binding of specific peptides and affects antigen presentation.
- T cell co-stimulation is then required for full activation occurring via CD80 and CD86 present on APCs binding to CD28 on T cells.
- Up-regulation of Th1 cells leads to secretion of various inflammatory mediators, which in turn activate B cells, macrophages, fibroblast-like synoviocytes and osteoclasts.

B cells
B cells are most likely involved in the inflammatory process via several mechanisms including:
- Autoantibody production (RFs, anti-CCP antibodies).
- Antigen presentation to T cells (a vicious cycle may develop leading to perpetuation of the autoimmune response).
- T cell co-stimulation, production of pro-inflammatory cytokines.
- Development of immune complexes augments the pro-inflammatory cytokine production via Fc-receptor and complement activation.

Synovial fibroblasts
Local proliferation of the fibroblast-like type B synoviocytes and migration of new macrophage-like type A synoviocytes from the bone marrow and blood into the joint leads to synovial hyperplasia. This mass of type B synoviocytes (pannus) produces pro-inflammatory mediators including cytokines, prostaglandins and matrix metalloproteinases (MMPs), which in turn destroy cartilage and bone.

Erosions
Bone erosions are chiefly caused by osteoclasts.
- Activation of receptor activator of nuclear factor kB (RANK) via its ligand (RANK-L), stimulates osteoclast differentiation from monocyte and macrophage precursors, and leads to maturation and survival of osteoclasts.
- The erosions are seen at the joint margins, where synovium is reflected near the attachment of the capsule. The bone in this area is the so-called 'bare area', which is not protected by a layer of cartilage and is directly attacked by the invading synovium and osteoclasts.

Other factors
Other factors at play in the destructive process include neovascularization, defective apoptosis of synovial cells, deficiency of regulatory T cells, antibodies directed at joint specific antigens such as a RA33. Duplication and redundancy in the inflammatory process is evident as inhibition of various mediators does not necessarily result in down-regulation of inflammation.

The window of opportunity for immunotherapy
In relation to the pathogenesis, a discrete period in early disease (within 3 months of symptom onset), during the acute inflammatory response, may produce a 'window of opportunity' where a disproportionate benefit for intervention exists. Once the chronic phase of disease is established prolonged therapy is most likely required.

Clinical features
The most frequent presentation of RA is inflammation of synovial joints. It is, however, a multisystem disorder and extra-articular features are common

Key features in the history
- Symmetrical polyarthritis predominantly affecting PIPs, MCPs, wrists and MTPs is the most common presentation, however, any synovial joint may be affected (the DIPs are classically spared) leading to pain, stiffness, swelling, and reduced manual dexterity.
- Joint pain onset may be rapid or insidious.
- Joint symptoms are worse in the morning and after periods of immobility (gelling phenomenon).
- Fatigue is common.
- Palindromic rheumatism is a predominantly large joint, migratory arthritis with attacks lasting hours to days. One-third of such presentations eventually develop true RA.
- Classic symptoms of polymyalgia rheumatica (PMR) may herald the onset of RA by weeks to months.
- Neck pain and long tract symptoms may develop if there is significant atlanto-axial subluxation though this is a late feature (C1/C2 cervical spine involvement).
- Constitutional symptoms include fever, malaise, anorexia.

Key features on examination
Arthritis/musculoskeletal
- **Early joint signs:** soft-tissue swelling, tenderness, pain on active and passive movement of joint.
- **The piano key sign:** damped depression of the ulnar head on pressure owing to surrounding synovitis and laxity or disruption of distal radio-ulna ligament.
- **Classic signs of long-standing hand disease:** swan-neck and boutonnière deformities of the fingers, and Z deformity of the thumb, ulnar deviation, and subluxation of the MCP and wrist joints.
- **Rheumatoid nodules** occur in up to 20% especially over pressure areas. Patients are almost always seropositive for RF. The lesion consists of fibrinoid necrosis with the centre surrounded by pallisading histiocytes. Nodules may be exacerbated by MTX.
- **Vasculitic skin lesions** may occur especially in the hands (e.g. nail folds).
- **Muscle weakness** develops secondary to disuse atrophy and asthenia.
- **General mobility** may decline resulting in significant disability and handicap.
- **Hoarseness and vocal cord collapse** may develop with crico-arytenoid cartilage involvement.
- **Late signs in weight-bearing joints:** knee valgus, hindfoot valgus with pes planus and posterior tibial tendon deficiency.
- **Cock-up, over-riding and hammer deformities of the toes** may occur (relatively late signs).

Co-morbidities

Bone
Osteoporosis is common including generalized osteoporosis, periarticular osteopaenia and bony erosions

Haematologic/reticuloendothelial
- Anaemia, leucopaenia, thrombocytosis may occur
- Lymphoma incidence is elevated in RA and is generally accepted to be increased 2-3 fold especially in long-standing disease.
- Lymphadenopathy may occur.
- Felty's syndrome (RF positive RA, splenomegaly and pancytopaenia, most frequently neutropaenia) may lead to recurrent bacterial infections and chronic leg ulcers. Associated with autoimmune hepatitis.

Respiratory system (see also p. 54)
Pulmonary involvement is common including interstitial lung disease, pleurisy, pleural effusions and bronchiectasis.
- Symptoms of lung disease include shortness of breath, wheeze, dry cough and possibly chest pain.
- Caplan's syndrome consists of pulmonary nodulosis and pneumoconiosis (especially coal dust exposure) in patients with RA.

Cardiovascular involvement (see also p. 66)
- Endothelial dysfunction results in cardiovascular disease (increased incidence of ischaemic heart disease and stroke).
- Rarely nodules can form in the heart.
- Pericardial effusion is rarely symptomatic.

Neurological (see also p. 90)
- Signs of compressive neuropathies may develop, the commonest being carpal tunnel syndrome with an equivalent syndrome occurring in the feet (tarsal tunnel syndrome).
- Sensorimotor neuropathy and mononeuritis multiplex is recognized especially when associated with vasculitis.
- Atlanto-axial subluxation may lead to long tract signs.

Ophthalmologic involvement (see also p. 48)
- Scleritis, episcleritis, and scleromalacia perforans (corneal melt) present with various ocular symptoms including pain and blurred vision.
- Sicca symptoms are due to secondary Sjögren's syndrome.

Other
Amyloidosis may complicate longstanding disease. Renal involvement is relatively rare, although membranous glomerulonephritis (GN) is recognized. More common renal lesions in an RA patient might be GN or tubulointerstitial nephritis from the toxic effects of drugs.

Investigations

No pathognomonic test result exists for the diagnosis of RA; therefore, the investigation of polyarthritis is driven by clinical suspicion.

Laboratory
- FBC shows associated anaemia (either normochromic normocytic or mildly hypochromic microcytic) and thrombocytosis.
- Neutropaenia may point to a diagnosis of Felty's syndrome though isolated mild neutropaenia is not an uncommon finding.
- Acute phase response (elevated ESR, CRP).
- The usual iron indices are poorly specific for iron deficiency in the presence of systemic inflammation. A low ferritin <25 µg/l and elevated soluble transferrin receptor values are arguably the most reliable signs of iron deficiency and low erythropoiesis in RA patients.
- Baseline renal, bone biochemistry, and liver function tests (crucial to know baseline results prior to starting pharmacotherapy especially DMARDs).
- Urinalysis is a useful screen for urinary infection and inflammatory renal lesions associated with RA or its therapies.

Immunological tests
- Rheumatoid factors are present in up to 85% of patients, but may be elevated in many other conditions.
- Anti-CCP (cyclic citrullinated protein) antibodies have similar sensitivity to RF (50–60%), but have higher specificity (85–90%).
- Anti-CCP antibodies can be helpful in equivocal, especially RF negative, cases. CCP antibodies are more specific for RA than RF. CCP antibodies might in future be used preferentially for diagnosis.
- ANA is often positive, but usually in low titre.
- Complement levels are normal or high.

Imaging
Radiographs
- Radiographs of hands and feet are mandatory. Ball catcher views can show MCP joint erosions difficult to see on plain AP views. Features may include soft tissue swelling, loss of joint space, periarticular osteopaenia and juxta-articular erosions, but radiographs are frequently normal at presentation.
- With radiographs, bony erosion can be seen, in up to 80% of patients within 2 years of symptom onset. (see Figure 6.1).
- CXR is essential to screen for evidence of RA lung disease especially prior to starting DMARDS (e.g. methotrexate).

Magnetic resonance (MR) imaging and ultrasound (US)
Patients with subclinical disease may have erosions on presentation. Also radiographs can miss erosions.
- MR scanning and high-resolution ultrasound (US) with colour flow Doppler are more sensitive at detecting early erosive disease, subclinical synovitis and small joint effusions compared with radiographs.

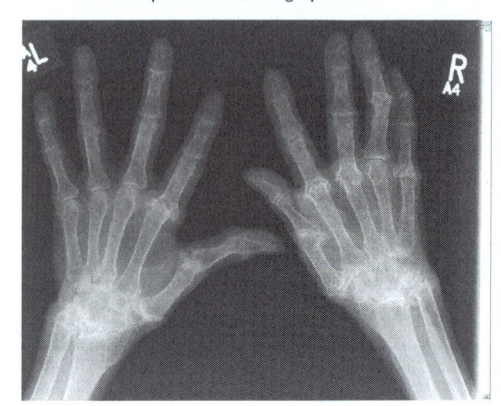

Figure 6.1 Severe erosive rheumatoid arthritis.

CHAPTER 6 Rheumatoid arthritis

- MR with IV gadolinium contrast permits accurate assessment of synovial invasion though discrimination of tissue from fluid can be difficult.

Dual X-ray absorptiometry (DXA) and digital X-ray radiogrammetry (DXR)
DXA software to allow detection of periarticular osteoporosis about the small hand joints is available, but mainly a research tool. DXR is a quantitative methodology for evaluating mineralization in phalanges in the hand and patterns of abnormality associated with RA are recognized compared with reference ranges.

Synovial fluid analysis
- Aspiration and analysis of synovial fluid is not particularly helpful for diagnosis, but analysis can help rule out infection (gram stain and culture), and crystal-induced arthritis (polarized light microscopy).
- Usually the fluid is straw coloured and mildly turbid, and predominantly comprised of neutrophils with the remainder being lymphocytes.
- The fluid glucose level is normal.
- Synovial biopsy can be helpful, but is not currently available in routine clinical practice.

Other investigations
If the diagnosis is unclear, investigation for other causes of polyarthritis is mandatory, such as gout (check urate level), CPPDD (requires metabolic screen, particularly calcium and PTH), SLE (check ANA, ENAs, C3).
- Other tests: thyroid function, creatine kinase, vasculitis screen, serum ACE, complement levels, and infection screen (including parvovirus B19 and mycoplasma).
- Full pulmonary function tests (if suspicious of lung involvement) and high resolution CT scanning in the prone position (pulmonary disease).
- ECG and transthoracic ECHO (cardiovascular involvement – particularly pericardial effusion).
- Nerve conduction studies (neuropathies, e.g. carpal tunnel syndrome, ulna nerve irritation, vasculitis).
- DXA scan (osteoporosis, particularly in post-menopausal women or those who have had fractures).

Investigations to monitor drug therapy (see also p. 529)
Monitoring of drug toxicity involves regular FBC, LFTs, renal function, ESR, CRP, and urinalysis. Hepatitis B and C serology is advisable prior to B-cell depleting treatment.

Special case investigations
- Prior to starting biologic DMARD therapy, especially anti-TNFα agents, Mycobacterium tuberculosis (MTB) should be excluded by thorough history and physical examination, CXR ± tuberculin skin test (see p. 566).
- Patients should be asked about immunity to *Varicella zoster* and tested for antibodies if necessary.

Differential diagnosis
The main differential diagnoses will be psoriatic polyarthritis, inflammatory osteoarthritis, SLE, post-infectious arthritis, and in the elderly, polyarticular CPPDD or gout.

Disease activity assessment
Measurement of different aspects of disease in RA has become important, particularly the assessment of disease activity and the response to treatment. Owing to the heterogeneous nature of RA, various composite indices have been developed to assess disease including the American College of Rheumatology (ACR) Response Criteria, Disease Activity Score (DAS), European League Against Rheumatism (EULAR responses), Health Assessment Questionnaire (HAQ), and the Medical Outcomes Study 36-Item Short Form (SF-36).

Differential diagnosis of inflammatory polyarthropathy

Inflammatory synovitis
- Rheumatoid arthritis
- Spondylarthropathy (incl. psoriatic polyarthritis)
- Post-viral arthritis
- Infectious (e.g. parvovirus B19, Lyme disease)
- Crystal arthritides (e.g. gout and CPPDD)
- Inflammatory osteoarthritis
- Autoimmune Connective Tissue Diseases
- Vasculitis, Sarcoidosis, Behçets disease

Metabolic
- Hyperparathyroidism
- Thyroid disorders
- Haemachromatosis (secondary OA)

Chronic infection
- Infective endocarditis
- Hepatitis B, HIV

Miscellaneous
- Paraneoplastic phenomenon
- Multiple myeloma
- Polymyalgia rheumatica (PMR onset of RA)
- Septic arthritis (usually monoarthrits)

ACR response criteria
- The ACR response criteria are categorical and allow assessment of improvement or change from baseline.
- ACR responses are expressed as ACR20, 50, 70, and 90 indicating 20%, 50%, 70%, and 90% improvement in the respective variables included in the criteria.
- They do not, however, allow assessment of the actual state of disease activity at one time point.
- ACR responses are currently the most widely reported outcomes in clinical trials.

Disease Activity Score (DAS)

American College of Rheumatology response criteria for 20% improvement (ACR20)

20% reduction in the number of tender and swollen joints, plus 20% improvement in 3 of the following 5 parameters:
- Physician global assessment of disease
- Patient global assessment of disease
- Patient assessment of physical function
- Patient assessment of pain
- ESR or CRP

The DAS is a composite index of disease activity
- The DAS is used in clinical trials and is also useful in daily practice as it allows assessment of the actual state of disease activity at any time point.
- DAS-CRP may be used as an alternative to ESR in the calculation of the DAS.

- EULAR response criteria have also been developed, based on the DAS and when measured at two time points the patients clinical response can be assessed.
- EULAR criteria for disease activity are based on the DAS28, allowing a continuous measurement of disease activity.
- Other scores have also been developed that are easier to calculate, such as the simplified disease activity index (SDAI) and the clinical disease activity index (CDAI).

Health status and quality of life measures

Assessment of disability and overall health status is critical in patients with RA. Patient-reported outcomes provide intrinsic knowledge about a patient's symptoms, general health, functional status, satisfaction, preferences for treatment, and quality of life.

Health Assessment Questionnaire (HAQ)
- The HAQ is the most frequently used method to measure functional impairment.
- The HAQ was one of the first self-reported functional status measures and is based on five patient-centred dimensions: disability, pain, medication effects, costs of care, mortality.
- Typically, one of two HAQ versions is used: The Full HAQ, which assesses all five dimensions, and the Short or 2-page HAQ, which contains only the HAQ disability index (HAQ-DI) and the HAQ's patient global and pain visual analog scales (VAS).

Medical Outcomes Study 36-Item Short Form (SF-36)
- The SF-36 is a health-based survey of quality of life.
- Like the HAQ is it patient-derived and objective.
- The SF-36 has been implemented to define disease conditions, to determine the effect of treatment, to differentiate the effect of different treatments, and to compare across conditions.
- SF36 comprises 8 individual subscale scores and physical and mental summary scores.
- Physical component summary includes physical functioning, role-physical, bodily pain and general health.
- Mental component summary includes vitality, social functioning, role-emotional and mental health.

The Disease Activity Score (DAS)

To calculate the DAS28 one requires:
- The number of swollen joints out of 28 (SJC28)
- The number of tender joints out of 28 (TJC28)
- The ESR (measured in mm/hour).
- An assessment of the patient's general health (GH) measured on a Visual Analogue Scale (VAS) of 100 mm

Using these data, the DAS28 can be calculated using the following formula:

DAS28 = (0.56 × sqrt [TJC28]) + (0.28 × sqrt [SJC28]) + (0.70 × ln[ESR]) + (0.014 × GH)

This is not simple, but can easily be calculated using a pre-programmed calculator:
- The DAS28 provides a number on a scale from 0 to 10 indicating the current activity of disease.
- A DAS28 >5.1 means high disease activity.
- DAS28 <3.2 indicates low disease activity.
- Remission is achieved by a DAS28 <2.6.

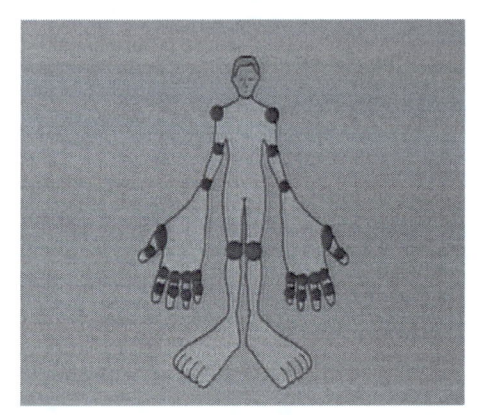

Figure 6.2 Joints utilized in a DAS28 joint count.

Table 6.2 The EULAR response criteria using the DAS28

Current DAS28	DAS28 improvement		
	>1.2	0.6–1.2	<0.6
<3.2	Good response	Moderate response	No response
3.2–5.1	Moderate response	Moderate response	No response
>5.1	Moderate response	No response	No response

Comparing the DAS28 from one patient on two different time points it is possible to define improvement or response.

CHAPTER 6 **Rheumatoid arthritis**

Standards of care developed by The British Society of Rheumatology (BSR) 2005.
Standards of care for RA
Outcome measures
1. Identification of persons with rheumatoid arthritis.
2. Empowering persons with rheumatoid arthritis.

Clinical care of persons with rheumatoid arthritis
3. The multidisciplinary team.
4. Prescription and monitoring of treatments used to manage rheumatoid disease.
5. Annual review.
6. Prevention of steroid-induced osteoporosis.
7. Pain management.
8. Collaboration with orthopaedic surgeons.

Special clinical circumstances
9. Care of young persons with juvenile idiopathic arthritis/rheumatoid arthritis.
10. Pregnancy in persons with rheumatoid arthritis.

Development of patient-centred care
11. Involvement of users and carers.
12. Access to facilities.
13. In-patient management.
14. Out-patient services.

Treatment

Objectives of management
Due to the heterogeneity of RA and the variability of its course no consistent treatment paradigm fits the care plan for all individuals.
- The objectives of management are:
  - the relief of symptoms;
  - slowing of cartilage and bone breakdown;
  - preservation of function;
  - minimizing disability;
  - ameliorating premature mortality;
  - maintaining quality of life.
- The ultimate goal of therapy is the clinical, radiographic, and immunological 'cure', and it appears that long-term remission may be possible in many patients.
- In The UK, standards of care for patients with RA have been published by the British Society of Rheumatology (see Appendix 6.1).
- A multidisciplinary approach is important.

Physical and occupational therapy
Physiotherapists and occupational therapists are key members of the multidisciplinary team. Therapists should be involved early in the care of RA patients.
- Physiotherapy benefits patients in regard to joint movement, function, and muscle strength.
- Physiotherapists' different treatment modalities include heat, ice, wax baths, and hydrotherapy.
- The use of splints are often necessary for joint protection, to reduce joint deformity, and improve hand or finger power and function.
- Adequate rest with graded exercises improve outcome.
- Foot orthoses may be required for deformed feet. Access to podiatry or orthotists is key.
- Occupational therapists should assess patients' disability and offer aids for daily living, such as appropriately fashioned cutlery, taps, long handled combs, etc.

- The role of aerobic exercise is controversial, but there are some studies supporting a role for regular exercise, although promoting weight-bearing activities on hard surfaces regularly would be inappropriate.

Pain relief
The primary initial concern of the patient is relief from pain and, therefore, adequate analgesia is critical. NSAIDs are one of the cornerstones of medical therapy.

NSAIDs
- By decreasing prostaglandin production NSAIDs have analgesic, anti-pyretic and anti-inflammatory effects.
- NSAIDs do not have disease-modifying effects and therefore should not be used in isolation, even if symptoms are greatly improved.
- NSAIDs account for up to 20% of all cases of peptic ulcer haemorrhage and perforation with many being fatal, particularly in the elderly.
- Gastrointestinal side effects (e.g. perforations, ulcers, bleeds) appear to have been reduced with the introduction of the cyclo-oxygenase 2 inhibitors (e.g. Celecoxib, Etoricoxib), although the cardiovascular and renal toxicities are still problematic.
- In the UK, the National Institute for Clinical Excellence (NICE) have recommended the use of COX-2 specific NSAIDs in patients at risk of peptic disease.
- There may be individual responses to different NSAIDs; therefore, a trial of different agents may be necessary to optimize therapeutic effect.

Non-NSAID analgesics
- Simple analgesics, such as paracetamol 1 g tds with or without dextropropoxyphene or codeine, are useful, although side effects are common in the elderly.
- Buprenorphine 3- or 7-day transdermal patches are popular with patients and claims that side effects are less than with oral therapies seem justified.
- There may be substance to data and claims that fish-oils (e.g. cod-liver oil) can have an NSAID-sparing role.

Immunosuppression/disease modifying anti-rheumatic drugs (DMARDs) (see also p. 529)
The pharmacological treatment of RA, especially early disease and undifferentiated early inflammatory polyarthritis, is evolving rapidly.

General points/current approach
- Over the last decade the focus has been to treat RA promptly and aggressively with the most effective medications
- The traditional treatment pyramid ('start low, go slow') has been abandoned.
- Early intervention results in minimum risk with maximum benefit when viewed over the long-term.
- Treatment in the 'window of opportunity' of early RA/ inflammatory arthritis appears to have the greatest impact and early inflammatory arthritis should be considered a medical emergency.
- It is becoming apparent that combination DMARD therapy is more effective than sequential monotherapy.
- The introduction of the 'biologic' DMARDs (e.g. anti-TNFα) has led to a sea change in the treatment of RA and has spearheaded the endeavour for a disease 'cure'.
- Tight control of (the inflammatory component of the) disease has also been found to improve outcomes and

regular assessment of disease activity allows tailored therapy.
- One of the main difficulties is reviewing patients early after symptom onset and, to this end, early inflammatory arthritis clinics are important.
- Strict protocols are required in both primary and secondary care to facilitate referral of appropriate patients.

EULAR and the BSR have published guidelines on the treatment of early RA (See Appendix 6.1 for BSR guide).

DMARDs

DMARD medications are now utilized much earlier in the treatment paradigm of RA due to their efficacy in retarding erosive disease.
- The great challenge is to identify patients most likely to suffer from aggressive disease and institute treatment expediently.
- Due to its tolerability, efficacy, and speed of onset, MTX is regarded as the foundation upon which other drugs are added. It has also become the benchmark drug in clinical trials.
- Many patients are not adequately controlled on DMARD monotherapy, even MTX.
- Combinations of DMARDs have therefore been used to work synergistically without a rise in toxicity.
- A 'step down' approach is favoured, rather than a 'step up' protocol.
- The optimum combination of drugs has not been clearly defined; however, emerging evidence suggests that MTX in combination with glucocorticoids (GCs) and/or other DMARDs such as sulphasalazine (SZP), hydroxychloroquine, and leflunomide is best.
- In practice, rheumatologists use various combinations of DMARDs to achieve the optimal response.
- Ciclosporin, azathioprine, gold salts, and D-penicillamine are now not commonly used owing to the availability of more efficacious and less toxic drugs.
- Cyclophosphamide may be necessary for associated rheumatoid vasculitis.

'Biologic' DMARDs

With greater understanding of the immunological basis of RA novel approaches to treatment has developed. Elucidation of the molecules involved in RA immunopathogenesis has facilitated the development of therapy targeted against specific molecules or molecular interactions. These therapies are termed 'biologic' DMARDs or 'Biologics'.
- Biologics comprise a group of recombinant proteins that include antibodies, cytokines, cytokine inhibitors, and toxins fused with biological 'targeting' segments.
- A number of biologics are now available with many more in development. The most widely used and studied so far have been the anti-TNFα agents (infliximab, etanercept, and adalimumab).
- Infliximab and adalimumab are anti-TNFα antibodies and etanercept is a TNFα receptor fusion protein.
- These biologics produce rapid and sustained amelioration of the signs and symptoms of RA, retard radiological progression, and improve quality of life more effectively than traditional DMARDs.

Table 6.3 EULAR guidelines for early arthritis (see Combe et al. 2007)

	Final set of 12 recommendations on the management of early arthritis based on both evidence and expert opinion
1	Arthritis is characterised by the presence of joint swelling, associated with pain or stiffness. Patients presenting with arthritis of more than one joint should be referred to, and seen by, a rheumatologist, ideally within six weeks after the onset of symptoms
2	Clinical examination is the method of choice for detecting synovitis. In doubtful cases, ultrasound, power Doppler, and MR imaging might be helpful to detect synovitis.
3	Exclusion of diseases other than RA requires careful history taking and clinical examination and ought to include at least the following laboratory tests: complete blood cell count, urinary analysis, liver transaminases, antinuclear antibodies.
4	In every patient presenting with early arthritis to the rheumatologist, the following factors predicting persistent and erosive disease should be measured: number of swollen and tender joints, ESR or CRP, levels of RF and anti-CCP antibodies and radiographic erosions.
5	Patients at risk of developing persistent or erosive arthritis should be started with DMARDs as early as possible, even if they do not yet fulfil established classification criteria for inflammatory rheumatological diseases.
6	Patient information concerning the disease and its treatment and outcome is important. Education programmes aimed at coping with pain, disability and maintenance of work ability may be employed as adjunct interventions.
7	NSAIDs have to be considered in symptomatic patients after evaluation of gastrointestinal, renal, and cardiovascular status.
8	Systemic glucocorticoids reduce pain and swelling and should be considered as adjunctive treatment (mainly temporary), as part of the DMARD strategy. Intra-articular glucocorticoid injections should be considered for the relief of local symptoms of inflammation.
9	Among the DMARDS, methotrexate is considered to be the anchor drug and should be used first in patients at risk of developing persistent disease.
10	The main goal of DMARD treatment is to achieve remission. Regular monitoring of disease activity and adverse events should guide decisions on choice and changes in treatment strategies (DMARDs including biological agents).
11	Non-pharmaceutical interventions such as dynamic exercises, occupational therapy and hydrotherapy can be applied as adjuncts to pharmaceutical interventions in patients with early arthritis.
12	Monitoring of disease activity should include tender and swollen joint count, patient's and physician's global assessments, ESR and CRP. Arthritis activity should be assessed at one to three month intervals, for as long as remission is not achieved. Structural damage should be assessed by radiographs of hands and feet every 6 to 12 months during the first few years. Functional assessment (for example, HAQ) can be used to complement disease activity and structural damage monitoring.

CRP, C reactive protein; DMARD, disease modifying anti-rheumatic drug; ESR, erythrocyte sedimentation rate; HAQ, Health Assessment Questionnaire; MR, magnetic resonance.

- Anti-TNFα therapies are currently expensive and require parenteral (intravenous or subcutaneous) administration [~£10 000 (~12 500 Euros) per year].
- Despite being well tolerated there is an increased incidence of infections and possibly malignancy.
- Up to 30% of patients do not respond to anti-TNFα DMARDs, and a further 30% may lose efficacy with time or develop intolerable side effects.
- Anakinra, an IL-1 receptor antagonist, although effective has fallen out of favour as it is not as effective as anti-TNFα agents.
- Recently rituximab (an anti-CD20 monoclonal antibody) and the T cell co-stimulatory blocker abatacept have been licensed in Europe and N America. Both these biologics have displayed similar efficacy to the anti-TNFα agents.
- The IL-6 receptor antibody tocilizumab has potential for efficacy and is currently being studied in large RCTs.
- Many other biologics are being developed including p38 MAP kinase inhibitors and B-cell modulators.
- In the UK, BSR has issued guidance on the use of anti-TNFα Biologics. Given the cost of biologics to a publicly-funded health system, there are constraints on which patients can be treated with anti-TNFα and Rituximab within the National UK Health Service (see guidance www.nice.org.uk;).
- NICE have issued guidance in the UK on the use of anti-TNFα drugs and rituximab. An unfavourable review of abatacept by NICE will mean that NHS funders are unlikely to allow its' widespread use.
- Two studies have confirmed that remission may be induced with intensive treatment and that therapy may even be withdrawn without recrudescence of disease.
- Further evidence is accruing that a biologic agent may be necessary to maximally inhibit structural damage even if patients respond symptomatically to MTX alone
- The TICORA study showed improved outcomes in patients who were seen regularly and whose treatment was changed frequently in order to maintain a low disease state. When the tight control was stopped the patients deteriorated.
- An inherent risk, however, of intensive treatment is the possibility of over-treating patients with self-limiting and/or milder disease

Glucocorticoids (GCs)
Though very effective at reducing inflammation, long-term toxicity limits the use of GCs. In many patients, however, small doses are required to stabilize the arthritis.
- GCs do have a disease modifying effect.
- Higher doses are occasionally needed for severe flares or extra-articular manifestations.
- Intra-articular GC injections, following joint aspiration, are frequently used with excellent response and minimal side effects.
- Sepsis must be excluded prior to injection.
- Guidelines have been developed for the prevention of GC-induced osteoporosis (see p. 408).

Surgery
- Historically surgery is often required for RA patients, although there is some anecdotal evidence the need for surgery has lessened in recent years.
- Synovectomy and debridement of tissue from 'recalcitrant joints' can be beneficial.
- Arthroplasty invariably results in excellent outcomes for end stage joint disease particularly by reducing pain.
- Tendon reconstructions are being increasingly offered by Orthopaedic Units, to help hand function.
- An alternative to surgical synovectomy is chemical synovectomy with osmium or radiation synovectomy using Yttrium-90 (^{90}Y) colloid. The availability of ^{90}Y from radiopharmaceutical suppliers in the UK and in Europe has become more difficult recently (currently no UK supplier of ^{90}Y and imported products are not UK licensed).

Patient advice/education
- Education is pivotal. Rheumatology practitioners (such as nurse specialists) are indispensable for delivering education (one-to-one or group-led) to patients and their relatives/carers.
- Both patients and their relatives should be informed of the chronic nature of RA, and the importance of rapid disease control in order to improve prognosis.
- This should include discussion regarding co-morbidities and lifestyle modification, such as optimization of weight, healthy diet, exercise, and cessation of smoking.
- Risks of long-term disease should be discussed as some stage. An explanation of the need to screen for various morbidity, such as neck disease, osteoporosis, hyperlipidaemia, over time should be explained.
- The discussion of the concepts of controlling, rather curing disease is important early on.
- In the elderly, those with multiple co-morbidities or polypharmacy the role of making judicious choices of immunosuppressive medication needs to be emphasized.

Prognosis

The prognosis of RA has improved enormously over the last decade with early, intensive use of efficacious medications. However, the natural history of disease is variable.
- Joint destruction and many extra-articular manifestations may be avoided with appropriate intervention.
- Up to 40% of patients presenting to early inflammatory arthritis clinics, however, have self-limiting disease.
- In 75% of patients the disease waxes and wanes over a period of years.
- Pregnancy often relieves the symptoms in the 2nd and 3rd trimester through poorly clarified mechanisms.
- Currently 50% of patients have given up work after 10 years.
- 75% of patients develop at least moderate impairment of function.
- Mortality is increased in RA with cardiovascular disease accounting for up to 45% of deaths, cancer (especially haematological malignancy) 15%, and infections 10%.
- A clearer understanding of the pathogenesis will undoubtedly lead to improved treatment and prognosis.

Poor prognosis patients
Factors that have been found to be associated with aggressive disease include:
- Insidious onset.
- Constitutional symptoms.
- Nodules.
- Female gender.
- Multiple swollen and tender joints at presentation (high disease burden, high DAS).
- RF positivity with high titres (especially IgA RF).

- Anti-CCP antibodies.
- Smokers.
- Presence of the shared epitope.
- High inflammatory markers (ESR, CRP).
- Early bone erosions.
- Poor functionality at 1 year.
- Socially disadvantaged.

Current controversies

Diagnosis and prediction
- The role of MR and US in predicting erosions, disability, and response and/or failure to therapies.
- The role of anti-CCP antibodies.
- Whether composite scores from a combination of clinical, genetic and biomarker data can predict outcome, particularly in relation to specific therapies.

Treatment
- Optimum DMARD regimes at the outset. The role of GCs (e.g. high-dose and tapered as for COBRA or low dose 7.5 mg prednisolone 1–2 years or avoid!).
- Whether chronic inflammatory processes can be permanently and advantageously modified in early disease by early and aggressive Biologic DMARD use.
- The restriction of funding for Biologic therapies in the UK is highly controversial and based only partly on a *clinical* evidence base. Funding is limited by cost-effectivity analyses, which are consistently debated and often disputed. The funding of expensive therapies in wholly or part public-funded Health Systems, however, is not a controversy specific to the UK.

The future

Unprecedented advances occurred over the last decade in the understanding and management of RA and the prospects for the next decade are no less exciting. Areas of intense research include:
- Further clarification of the pathophysiology of RA.
- Genetic influences, including pharmacogenetics and genomics.
- Co-morbidity management.
- Refinement of disease assessment.
- Biomarker identification for prognostication.
- Novel therapeutic targets.

Future treatment options
The following highlight some of rapidly developing areas:
- Emerging cytokine and signalling targets, e.g. IL-15, IL-36 and adipokines, MAP kinases.
- Cell therapies, including T-regulatory cells, haemopoietic, and mesenchymal stem cells.
- Gene therapies.
- Pre-emptive treatment, including vaccination against human cytokines.

Genetic phenotyping
Genetic phenotyping may be used to help identify patients most likely to:
- Respond to treatment.
- Develop adverse events.
- Suffer disease progression.
- Carry risk factors for underlying disease.

Variation has been identified so far in genes coding
- HLA subtypes.
- Folate metabolizing enzymes.
- TNF and TNFα promoter regions.
- Fc receptors.

Resources

Assessment tools
DAS on line: www.das-score.nl

HAQ: See pdf document at www.chcr.brown.edu/pcoc/

Short From 36 (SF-36): www.SF-36.org

Guidelines/NICE (UK)
NICE: www.nice.org.uk; Advice for UK prescribers on Biologic DMARDs.

Guidelines are available for various aspects of RA management from a variety of sources including the BSR, EULAR, and ACR.

Patient organizations
National Rheumatoid Arthritis Society: www.rheumatoid.org.uk

Arthritis Care: www.arthritiscare.org.uk

Internet sites
Arthritis Research Campaign: www.arc.org.uk

British Society for Rheumatology: www.rheumatology.org.uk

American College of Rheumatology: www.rheumatology.org

European League Against Rheumatism (EULAR): www.eular.org

Arthritis and Musculoskeletal Alliance: www.arma.uk.net

www.ncbi.nlm.nih.gov/books/bv.fcgi?rid=eurekah.chapter.1416

Article on RA cytokines. Eurekah Bioscience Coll.

ICD-10 codes
M05   Seropositive rheumatoid arthritis
M06   Other rheumatoid arthritis

Further reading

Bathon JM, Martin RW, et al. A comparison of etanercept and methotrexate in patients with early rheumatoid arthritis. N Engl J Med 2000; **343**: 1586–93.

Boers M, Verhoeven AC, et al. Randomised comparison of combined step-down prednisolone, methotrexate and sulphasalazine with sulphasalazine alone in early rheumatoid arthritis. Lancet 1997; **350**: 309–18.

Breedveld FC, Weisman MH, et al. The PREMIER study: A multicenter, randomized, double-blind clinical trial of combination therapy with adalimumab plus methotrexate versus methotrexate alone or adalimumab alone in patients with early, aggressive rheumatoid arthritis who had not had previous methotrexate treatment. Arthritis Rheum 2006; **54**: 26–37.

Combe B, Landewe R, et al. EULAR recommendations for the management of early arthritis: report of a task force of the European Standing Committee for International Clinical Studies Including Therapeutics (ESCISIT). Ann Rheum Dis 2007; **66**: 34–45.

Goekoop-Ruiteman YP, de Vries-Bouwstra JK, et al. Clinical and radiographic outcomes of four different treatment strategies in patients with early rheumatoid arthritis (the BeSt study): a randomized, controlled trial. Arthritis Rheum 2005; **52**: 3381–90.

Grigor C, Capell H, et al. Effect of a treatment strategy of tight control for rheumatoid arthritis (the TICORA study): a single-blind randomised controlled trial. *Lancet* 2004; **364**(9430): 263–9.

Kennedy T, McCabe C, et al. BSR guidelines on standards of care for persons with rheumatoid arthritis. *Rheumatology* 2005; **44**: 553–6.

Korpela M, Laasonen L, et al. FIN-RACo Trial Group. Retardation of joint damage in patients with early rheumatoid arthritis by initial aggressive treatment with disease-modifying antirheumatic drugs: five-year experience from the FIN-RACo study. *Arthritis Rheum* 2004; **50**: 2072–81.

Maini R, St Clair EW, Breedveld F, et al. Infliximab (chimeric anti-tumour necrosis factor alpha monoclonal antibody) versus placebo in rheumatoid arthritis patients receiving concomitant methotrexate: a randomised phase III trial. ATTRACT Study Group. *Lancet* 1999; **354**: 1932–9.

O'Dell JR, Leff R, et al. Treatment of rheumatoid arthritis with methotrexate and hydroxychloroquine, methotrexate and sulfasalazine, or a combination of the three medications: results of a two-year, randomized, double-blind, placebo-controlled trial. *Arthritis Rheum* 2002; **46**: 1164–70.

Smolen JS, van der Heijde DM, et al. Predictors of joint damage in patients with early rheumatoid arthritis treated with high-dose methotrexate with or without concomitant infliximab: results from the ASPIRE trial.

Quinn MA, Conaghan PG, et al. Very early treatment with infliximab in addition to methotrexate in early, poor-prognosis rheumatoid arthritis reduces magnetic resonance imaging evidence of synovitis and damage, with sustained benefit after infliximab withdrawal: results from a twelve-month randomized, double-blind, placebo-controlled trial. *Arthritis Rheum* 2005; **52**: 27–35.

Van Dongen H, van Aken J, et al. Efficacy of methotrexate treatment in patients with probable rheumatoid arthritis: a double-blind, randomized, placebo-controlled trial. *Arthritis Rheum* 2007; **56**: 1424–32.

Weinblatt ME, Keystone EC, et al. Adalimumab, a fully human anti-tumor necrosis factor alpha monoclonal antibody, for the treatment of rheumatoid arthritis in patients taking concomitant methotrexate: the ARMADA trial. *Arthritis Rheum* 2003; **48**: 35–45.

See also:

Organ involvement and rheumatological disease (p. 408); Glucocorticoid induced osteoporosis (p. 408), Medications/drugs used in rheumatic disease (p. 529)

Guidelines for the management of rheumatoid arthritis (the first 2 years)

1. A diagnosis of RA should be made as early as possible, on the basis of persistent joint inflammation affecting at least three joint areas, involvement of the MCP or MTP joints, or early morning stiffness of at least 30 min duration.

2. In order to identify and treat patients with RA at an early stage, it is necessary for patients with suspected early synovitis to have rapid access to a multidisciplinary team that includes specialists in rheumatology, and includes members from both primary and secondary care in order to provide a seamless service for patients.

3. Access to individual elements of the multidisciplinary service should be available according to patient need.

4. Patients with RA should be provided with a plan of care from diagnosis, which outlines the principles of management including a commitment to training patients to self-manage some aspects of their disease.

5. Specialist rheumatology nurses can provide the ideal support for patients in accessing elements of the multidisciplinary team and in providing important lifestyle advice.

6. RA is a significant independent risk factor for ischaemic heart disease, with the risk related to the severity and duration of inflammation. Control of inflammation should also be accompanied by addressing each patient's other risk factors for ischaemic heart disease, using the established primary care services where appropriate.

7. All patients should have their disease and its impact assessed and documented at onset, prior to starting DMARD therapy. Once established on DMARD therapy, all patients should have a formal assessment of treatment response, or lack of it, in order to justify continuing therapy or changing it. Remission should be defined and documented when achieved, in order to plan reduction or maintenance therapy.

8. Patients with RA should be established on disease-modifying therapy as soon as possible after a diagnosis of RA is established. Disease modifying therapy should be part of an aggressive package of care, incorporating escalating doses, intra-articular steroid injections, parenteral methotrexate and combination therapy, rather than sequential monotherapy, progressing to biologic (anti-TNFα) therapy, when required.

9. Systemic glucocorticoid therapy may have an important early role in establishing control of synovitis or bridging disease control between different DMARD therapies but long-term use is not justified.

10. Patients with RA require assessment of both pain and optimum effective therapy to ensure early symptom control (grade of recommendation A). Long-term use of NSAIDs should be at the lowest effective dose.

11. Current concern over the potential cardiovascular toxicity of coxibs and NSAIDs suggests that such drugs should be avoided in high risk individuals, and used with caution in others who cannot be managed with analgesia, steroid injections, and one or more DMARDs.

12. Patients with RA require early assessment of sleep patterns (grade of recommendation A). Early management of sleep disturbance should include tricyclic agents, behavioural therapy and consider also the use of exercise (grade of recommendation B). Consider the impact of fatigue on quality of life in early RA.

13. The evidence for the effectiveness of complementary therapy is conflicting and no firm recommendations can be made.

14. Timing and format (group/individual/written) of education to meet individual needs must be considered in early disease (grade of recommendation A). Patients should be offered a cognitive behavioural approach to patient education, delivered at the appropriate time in order to promote long-term adherence to management strategies (grade of recommendation C). Patients should be helped to contact support organizations such as National RA Society, Arthritis Care (AC) and the Arthritis Research Campaign (arc).

15. Patients should be encouraged to pace activities and recognize the potential lower, as well as upper limits of physical activity, facilitating a realistic readjustment of the patient's own expectations, guided by members of the multidisciplinary team. Patients should be helped to participate in exercise programmes.

16. Aerobic exercise should be encouraged to help combat the adverse effects of rheumatoid disease on muscle strength, endurance and aerobic capacity, without, in the short-term, exacerbating disease activity or joint destruction.

17. Hydrotherapy should be accessible to maximize positive effects on pain, function and self-efficacy.

18. Transcutaneous electrical nerve stimulation use in RA patient may be effective in pain relief, but trials lack standardization.

19. Heat and cold applications may provide short-term symptomatic relief of symptoms of pain and stiffness. There is no evidence of long-lasting benefit. Paraffin wax baths combined with exercise are beneficial for hands in arthritic conditions.

20. Joint protection, energy conservation and problem-solving skills training should be taught early on in the disease course.

21. Hand function should be maintained and improved with a combination of hand exercises and appropriate devices to improve efficiency of action. OT can be helpful for those experiencing problems at work when these are due to the symptoms of arthritis. Altering work methods, posture, pacing and assistive devices can improve functional ability.

22. When hands and wrists are painful and/or swollen, splints (hand/wrist resting splints and functional wrist splints) should be offered, but the role of splinting at other times remains uncertain.

23. The goals of foot care for patients with RA are to relieve pain, maintain function and improve quality of life using safe, cost-effective treatments, such as palliative foot care, prescribed foot orthoses, and specialist footwear. An annual foot review and assessment is recommended for patients at risk of developing serious complications in order to detect problems early. Foot orthoses are an important and effective intervention in RA.

24. Health professionals should provide opportunities to discuss sexuality and relationship issues where RA affects these. Problems may include pain, dysfunction and changes in relationships, for example dependence and loss of role. Information and help on sexuality and relationship issues should be given backed up with written leaflets and contact details of organizations that can offer support.

Luqmani R, Hennell S, et al., on behalf of the British Society for Rheumatology and British Health Professionals in Rheumatology Standards, Guidelines and Audit Working Group. British Society for Rheumatology and British Health Professionals in Rheumatology Guideline for the Management of Rheumatoid Arthritis (the first 2 years). *Rheumatology (Oxf)* 2006; 45: 1167–9.

Chapter 7

The spondylarthropathies

The spondylarthropathies: disease spectrum (including undifferentiated spondylarthropathy) *210*
Ankylosing spondylitis *214*
Psoriatic arthritis *220*
Reactive arthritis *226*
Enteropathic spondylarthropathy *230*
Juvenile spondylarthropathy/enthesitis-related arthritis *232*
SAPHO (Le Syndrome Acné, Pustulose, Hyperostose, Ostéite) *236*

The spondylarthropathies: disease spectrum (including undifferentiated spondylarthropathy)

The spondylathropathy concept
Spondylarthropathy (SpA) is the term given to a group of conditions characterized by a number of features common to all; particularly inflammation in spinal, sacroiliac, and peripheral musculoskeletal structures, chiefly entheses. The principle SpA conditions are:
- Ankylosing spondylitis (AS).
- Reactive arthritis (ReA).
- Psoriatic arthritis (PsA).
- Enteropathic SpA (ESpA) also termed variably: Enteropathic arthritis, inflammatory bowel disease-related arthritis or Crohn's/UC-related arthritis.
- Juvenile SpA (see p. 232).
- Undifferentiated SpA (USpA).

The concept of SpAs as a linked group of conditions was originally proposed by Wright and Moll (1974) and developed over ensuing years (reviewed in Calin 1998). The three key pathophysiological features common to all SpAs are:
- Axial skeletal inflammation.
- Pathological changes at entheses – the site of insertion of ligaments or tendons into bone.
- An association with HLA B27. Frequency of association depends on ethnic group and disease type (e.g. from about 50% in ESpA to over 95% in AS).

The principle features of the SpAs
- Sacroiliitis.
- Inflammatory neck and back pain:
  - pain with stiffness associated with immobility;
  - waking due to symptoms in the early hours;
  - symptoms easing with movement.
- Enthesopathy
- Dactylitis
- Uveal inflammation (e.g. acute anterior uveitis)
- Aortitis/aortic valve disease
- Skin lesions (psoriasis, balanitis, keratoderma)
- Clinical overlap within the individual and family members
- Familial aggregation
- Urethritis (sterile)
- HLA B27 association

Arguably the least 'comfortable fit' within the SpA group is PsA. A number of different forms of PsA exist, the link with HLA B27 probably being the weakest of the SpA conditions, except perhaps in psoriatic spondylitis. Controversies are discussed on p. 223.

Classification criteria
To accommodate the wide spectrum and degree of overlap of features in SpA conditions, two over-arching classification systems have been developed:
- The Amor criteria (Amor et al., 1990) scores out of 12 features covering 4 domains (symptoms, radiographic and genetic features, and response to treatment).
- The simpler European SpA Study Group (ESSG) criteria are shown below. The two data sets have been validated in many different countries now.
- The two systems have similar sensitivity (85-95%), similar specificity (90-95%) and -ve predictive value (99% both). The Amor criteria may have a slightly higher positive predictive value (73% vs. 60%).

The European Spondylarthropathy Study Group (ESSG) Classification Criteria for Spondylarthropathy
Inflammatory spinal pain
or
Synovitis (asymmetrical or predominantly in the lower limbs)
and one or more of:
*Positive family history
Psoriasis
Inflammatory bowel disease
Alternate buttock pain
Enthesopathy*

± *sacroiliitis**

*Adding sacroiliitis to the core dataset improves sensitivity, but does not change specificity.

Epidemiology
Information about specific conditions is included in the relevant chapter. However, if the SpAs are considered a single condition the prevalence may be about 2% in Caucasians (Braun et al., 1998).

Pathphysiology
Genetic
There is clearly genetic predisposition for SpAs, partly mediated by presence of HLA B27.
- The association of HLA B27 with different SpAs varies with the association with AS the strongest.
- The role of HLA B27 is discussed in the next chapter.

Environmental
- Bacterial triggering of SpA clearly occurs in ReA. The organisms and immunopathological mechanisms are discussed in the chapter on AS.
- Clear links to bacterial triggers in AS, ESpA, JSpA, and USpA have not been substantiated though a substantial body of work investigating the role of *Klebsiella* in triggering AS exists.

Immunopathogenesis
See under 'Ankylosing spondylitis'.

Tissue pathophysiology
Lesions in SpA are present at entheses, in synovium and bone. The latter are varied (e.g. bone oedema as shown on MR in AS, bone erosion at joints and periosteal apposition and whiskering – a hallmark sign in PsA).

The enthesis
- An attachment of a ligament or tendon to bone.
- Enthesitis occurs in all SpAs and it distinguishes SpAs from other arthritides, such as rheumatoid arthritis, which is a synovial-based condition.
- Entheses thus are primarily extra-articular although MR data highlight inflammation at entheses in and around synovial joints in SpAs.
- Where tendons and ligaments insert into metaphyseal bone, entheses are generally rich in fibrocartilage.
- Fibrocartilage-rich tissue is likely to be an adaption to compressive load (Benjamin & Ralphs 1998).
- Fibrocartilage tissue in joints, at entheses, within tendons and periosteum is the focus for recent proposals that this tissue is key in determining the anatomical distribution of disease in the SpAs, although how it relates to autoimmune processes is unknown.

Prognosis and natural history
- SpAs can produce episodic symptoms over a considerable length of time. It is likely that there may be long symptom-free periods.
- Patients diagnosed with SpA may disclose a long history of features suggestive of a chronic SpA condition. Studies documenting this are sparse.
- Early detection of SpA and wider adoption of the ESSG SpA classification into clinical practice may broaden understanding and acceptance of SpAs, and result increasingly to a diagnosis of USpA being made.
- Longitudinal studies will show whether USpA is likely to evolve into an alternate SpA condition.
- Progressive disease in SpAs is recognized, but variable (e.g. substantial proportion in AS; minority in ReA).

Clinical features
Clinical spectrum
The diagnosis of SpA or USpA, applied using broad criteria in the clinic, perhaps reflecting the ESSG or Amor criteria, has a number of uses illustrated by the following:
- **To putatively label PsA-sine-Ps:** where psoriasis is absent, radiographic and other imaging signs may be subtle or absent and where misdiagnosis (e.g. osteoarthritis or Fibromyalgia notably) is best avoided.
- **To label 'limited' SpA:** a number clinical scenarios – some reported in the context of being 'SpA families' – highlight probable limited forms of SpA, such as unilateral sacroiliitis, isolated inflammatory spinal symptoms or dactylitis, (suspicious) recalcitrant or bilateral lateral humeral epicondylitis or plantar fasciitis (see Plate 28).
- **Recognizing early SpA:** undiagnosed inflammatory monoarthritis and oligoarthritis in patients with HLA B27 may represent the first manifestation of a SpA.

Key features in history
- Eliciting the history in early SpA often requires detailed and close questioning (previous relevant symptoms may have been mild, forgotten, or due to other conditions).
- The features of inflammatory back pain are consistent. A high chance of SpA exists where inflammatory back pain is chronic (>3 months) in a young or middle-aged adult with certain features (see Table 7.1).
- A sensitive approach to enquiring about previous (putatively triggering) genital infection is necessary particularly in women, where *Chlamydia trachomatis* infection is often asymptomatic.
- ReA can follow infection with *Campylobacter*, *Shigella* and *Salmonella*, all of which invariably cause diarrhoea.

Table 7.1 Features of inflammatory back pain (IBP) in young adults (<50 years old) that should raise the suspicion of a SpA

Symptom	Features
Chronic pain	>3 months
Morning stiffness	>30 min
Improvement with movement	Symptoms easier or abolished with movement not eased or worsened by rest
Disturbed sleep	Awakening during the second part of the night
Buttock pain	Alternating (?sacroiliitis)

A new classification of IBP has been recently proposed on the basis of these features (Rudwaleit et al., 2006).

Key features on examination
- Spinal mobility may be reduced in all directions. Reduced Schober's test or modified Schober's test.
- Sacroiliitis stress tests may be positive, although they are not specific for sacroiliitis.
- There may be enthesial tenderness especially origin of plantar fascia, insertion of Achilles' tendons, inferior patellar poles, anterior superior iliac spines, and humeral epicondyles.
- Joint synovitis is not always present in USpA (joints may be painful owing to enthesitis alone). If present, synovitis is typically asymmetrical, oligoarticular, and lower limb predominant.
- Synovitis can be monoarticular thus SpA is a differential diagnosis of crystal arthritis.
- A careful search for psoriasis is appropriate. Check posterior hairline, over scalp, in umbilicus, natal cleft.
- Enthesitis in USpA can be mistaken for fibromyalgia tender points by the unwary.

Investigations
For details see individual sections.
In the context of inflammatory spine symptoms, the presence of HLA B27 increases the chance of ultimately diagnosing a SpA.

Laboratory
- ESR and CRP can be raised particularly in severe AS, acute exacerbations (notably ReA and PsA), but are often in the normal range.
- Where inflammatory disease is severe and prolonged, features of anaemia of chronic disease may be evident.
- Persistently elevated serum IgA is a common, but non-specific finding.

Imaging
- Radiographs may be normal, although if there is a long history of suspiciously relevant (previously undiagnosed) symptoms, radiographs may be revealing.
- Ultrasound of entheses can improve an assessment of enthesitis (Lehtinen et al., 1994).

MR
- Using conventional scanning protocols, even using fat-suppression T2-weighted sequences, any signal change in enthesial tissue in SpA may be difficult to detect.
- Bone oedema underlying entheses is often seen however in AS and in SpAs, where clinical features are marked. The cause of the bone oedema is unknown (Figure 7.1).
- Enthesitis and sub-enthesial osteitis have been identified at joints affected by synovitis in patients with SpA.
- Patterns of abnormal bone oedema may be viewed as non-specific, but say, for the spine, if multiple, there should be suspicion of underlying SpA.

Bone scintigraphy
- Whole body ^{99m}Tc-MDP scans can be useful in highlighting the distribution of lesions. Simultaneous tracer localization to Achilles' tendon insertion, origin of plantar fascia, patella ligament insertion, and sacroiliac joint(s), for example, is suggestive of SpA.
- The upper limb lesions associated with SpAs are less well reported in the nuclear medicine literature.
- Isotope bone scans are likely to be insensitive in identifying spinal enthesitis or mild SpA-linked osteitis.
- Aseptic discitis is a recognized lesion seen with bone scintigraphy, but studies linking this (rather non-specific pattern) to a diagnosis of SpA are lacking.

Differential diagnosis

SpAs can present in a wide variety of ways.
- Inflammatory back pain type symptoms in adults can be due to an inflammatory phase of disc degeneration or frank discitis. In the elderly axial skeletal CPPDD disease should be considered.
- Dactylitis can typically occur in sarcoid, as well as SpA. Occasionally, SpA dactylitis can be mistaken for gout dactylitis, but the latter generally involves more eccentric digital swelling.
- Enthesitis almost certainly can occur in chronic sarcoid, as well as in all SpAs.
- If sacroiliitis is confirmed on imaging there are few other conditions to consider and caution in diagnosing 'degenerative' sacroiliac arthritis is advised when PsA is a clinical possibility [PsA associated sacroiliac joint (SIJ) disease can be unilateral and be characterized by subtle SIJ narrowing, sclerosis, and marginal periosteal apposition].

Treatment
Most patients with SpA benefit from a regular NSAID and spinal physiotherapy input.
- Disease-related fatigue and functional impact needs to be recognized and addressed accordingly.
- IBD-related SpA should be treated with NSAIDs cautiously.
- Sulphasalazine is a reasonable first choice therapy for persistent peripheral synovitis/enthesitis.
- There is little evidence for a therapeutic effect of any immunosuppressant on axial SpA disease.
- There no convincing evidence that antibiotics change the course of any SpA in the long-term if it is triggered or aggravated by identifiable disease (e.g. *Campylobacter, Chlamydia*, etc).
- Intravenous bisphosphonates can help axial symptoms, although serial injections may be necessary.
- There is evidence that anti-TNFα therapy can improve USpA symptoms, although long-term studies are lacking.

- An important part of the management of USpA is to keep patients under review for detecting evolution of the disease (e.g. to AS, PsA or IBD-related SpA particularly or involving other SpA features).

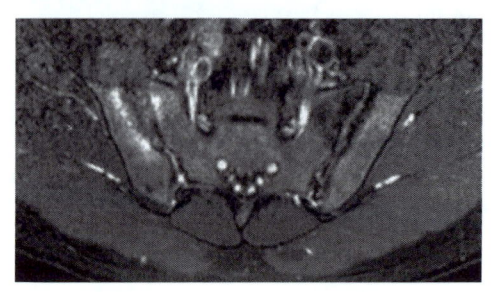

Figure 7.1 USpA. Fat-suppressed T2-weighted MR of SIJs showing sacroiliitis of the right SIJ (high signal) and low signal of juxta-SIJ bone (left SIJ). The right SIJ is acutely inflamed; the left was probably inflamed in the past with current low juxta-SIJ bone signal suggestive of bone sclerosis.

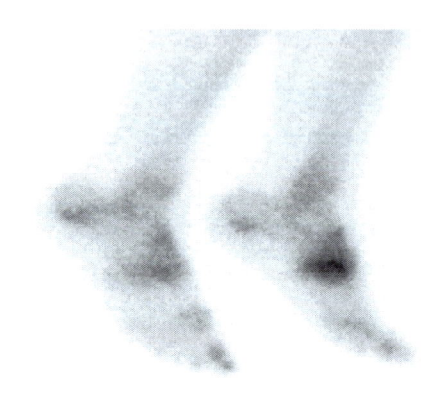

Figure 7.2 Enthesitis and arthritis in the feet in a patient with USpA shown on ^{99m}Tc-MDP scintigraphy. Bilateral plantar fascia origin enthesitis and midfoot disease. Patient developed more characteristic features of PsA ultimately.

Current controversies

There is an overlap of features in the SpAs. This means that patients with one distinct condition may be at increased risk of another. More commonly, features of different conditions can be present in the same person without there necessarily being a full set of clinical features to satisfy (formal or informal) criteria for one SpA or another. The degree to which this occurs is not known precisely chiefly owing to the difficulties of case ascertainment, recall, and a lack of appropriate prospective studies.
- The risk of various features of HLA B27-related disease occurring in patients over time has not been precisely determined. However, it may be useful to explain to patients that, if (for example) they are HLA B27 and have a SpA lesion, they are at risk of their condition evolving in a number of ways. This concept of relapsing and remitting SpA-related features over a lifetime is often poorly understood, but unless appreciated there can be diagnostic difficulties.
- The concept of SpA potentially varying/relapsing can cause confusion. This notably occurs if enthesitis is not recognized as part of the SpA. 'Tennis elbow', plantar

fasciitis, and rotator cuff tendonitis might be diagnosed as distinct problems, rather than SpA-related enthesitis of humeral epicondyle, plantar fascia origin, and deltoid origin, respectively.
- 'Inflammatory' lesions may be present, but not sufficiently severe (or noticeable) for patients to be referred to specialist (or present to their primary care doctor).
- At various times, symptoms may lead to recognition, but then regress or be treated. Patients (particularly the HLA B27+ ones) and their doctors should be alerted to the potential for SpA lesions to 'flare-up' through life.

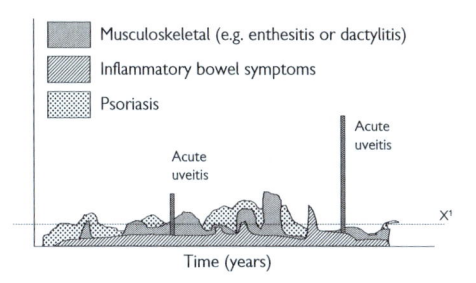

Figure 7.3 An example of features of SpA over time. Schema to show patients how different SpA lesions can relapse and remit, be severe or so mild – even absent (say below the dotted line X^1) - that they are shrugged off or not taken to the doctor.

Resources

Assessment tools
See under Ankylosing spondylitis.

Internet sites
Webpage on Spondylarthritis American College of Rheumatology (www.rheumatology.org/public/factsheets/)

ICD-10 codes
M46.0   Spinal enthesopathy
M76.9   Enthesopathy of lower limb, unspecified
M46.1   Sacroiliitis not elsewhere classified

References

Amor B, Dougados M, Mijiyawa M. Critères de classification des spondylarthropathies. *Rev Rheumat* 1990; **57**: 85–9.

Benjamin M, McGonagle D. The anatomical basis for disease localisation in seronegative spondyloarthropathy at entheses and related sites. *J Anat* 2001; **199**: 503–26.

Benjamin M, Ralphs JR. Fibrocartilage in tendons and ligaments – an adaptation to compressive load. *J Anat* 1998; **193**: 481–94.

Blocka KLN, Sibley JT. Undiagnosed chronic monoarthritis. *Arthritis Rheum* 1987; **30**: 1357–61.

Braun J, Bollow M, Remlinger G, et al. Prevalence of SpAs in HLA B27 positive and negative blood donors. *Arthritis Rheum* 1998; **41**: 58–67.

Calin A. Terminology, introduction, diagnostic criteria and overview. In: The Spondylarthritides. Eds Calin A and Taurog JD. OUP, Oxford 1998; pp3-6.

Khan MA, van der Linden SM. A wider spectrum of spondylarthropathies. *Sem Arthritis Rheum* 1990; **20**: 107–13.

Lehtinen A, Taavitsainen M, Leirisalo-Repo M. Sonographic analysis of enthesopathy in the lower extremities of patients with SpA. *Clin Exp Rheumatol* 1994; **12**: 143–8.

Rudwaleit M, Metter A, Listing J, Sieper J, Braun J. Inflammatory back pain in ankylosing spondylitis. *Arthritis Rheum* 2006; **54**: 569–78.

Schattenkirchner M, Kruger K. Natural course and prognosis of HLA-B27 positive oligoarthritis. *Clin Rheumatol* 1987; **6**(Suppl 2): 83–6.

Van der Linden S, Valkenburg HA, Cats A. Evaluation of diagnostic criteria for ankylosing spondylitis: a proposal for modification of the New York criteria. *Arthritis Rheum* 1984; **27**: 361–8.

Ankylosing spondylitis

Definition
The clinical hallmark of AS is inflammatory spinal pain and stiffness. Pathological changes typically occur at entheses. There are three main classification criteria for AS. The most recent is shown below.

> **Modified New York Criteria for diagnosis of AS**
> See van der Linden 1984.
> *Clinical*
> - Low back pain and stiffness >3 months, which improves with exercise, but is not relieved by rest.
> - Limitation of movement of the lumbar spine in both the sagittal and frontal planes.
> - Limitation of chest expansion relative to normal values corrected for age and sex.
>
> *Radiological*
> - Bilateral sacroiliitis ≥ grade 2 or
> - Unilateral sacroiliitis grade 3 or 4.
>
> AS is diagnosed if a radiological criterion is present with at least one clinical criterion

Epidemiology
- Prevalence in Caucasians about 1%.
- Strong link to HLA B27 (about 95% Caucasians).
- HLA B27 prevalence varies in ethnic groups, although does not always correlate with AS prevalence [e.g. in Native Americans where prevalence of HLA B27 is 18–50%, AS is frequent, whereas in the Fula in Gambia, HLA B27 is highly prevalent (6–68%), but AS is unusual].
- Gender ratio in Caucasians M:F is about 2.5:1.
- Typically develops in late teenage or early adult years.

Pathophysiology
Various theories have been proposed to explain the association of HLA B27 and AS (see below). Uniquely, the HLA B27 molecule itself may be immunogenic and trigger specific lymphocyte reactions.

> **Why AS might be associated with HLA B27**
> - HLA B27 is in genetic linkage with a disease-associated gene.
> - HLA B27 binds and presents 'arthritogenic' peptides.
> - HLA B27 helps select T-cells in the thymus, which can cause disease.
> - The HLA B27 free cysteine at position 67 can be modified leading to 'an altered self'.
> - There is cross-reactivity of antibodies directed at some bacterial proteins and HLA B27.
> - HLA B27 is a receptor for a bacterial ligand.
> - An interaction between HLA B27 and a bacterial superantigen causes non-specific T-cell activation.
> - HLA B27-derived peptides are presented by HLA class 2 molecules to CD4+ T-cells.

Genetic
- HLA B27 is heterogenic. There are >20 allotypes. Most allotypes preferentially predispose to AS, some may not (e.g. B*2706 and B*2709).
- Concordance in MZ B27+ twins is 63%, but 24% in DZ twins, indicating a role for genes other than HLA B27.
- Potentially combinations of certain HLA B27 alleles with polymorphisms in genes encoding for Killer cell Ig-like receptors (KIRs) or Leucocyte Ig-like receptors (LILRs) may predispose to AS (see below).

Environmental
A link to *Klebsiella* has been postulated. Evidence for *Klebsiella* alone triggering AS in all ethnic groups and geographical locations is not persuasive.

Immunopathology
- The HLA B27 heavy chain has a free unpaired cysteine residue; which may lead to abnormal peptide binding or B27 folding, and heavy chain dimerization (*in vitro*). B27 heavy chains can be expressed at cell surfaces in patients with AS.
- HLA B27 heavy chain multimers may be recognized, in the absence of β2-microglobulin, by some lymphocytes.
- There is some evidence for increased numbers of CD57 natural killer cells in the blood of AS patients.
- HLA B27 may be recognized *in vitro* by certain NK cells or other leucocytes through an interaction with specific KIRs or LILRs. The balance of activating and inhibitory B27-recognizing KIRs may be important in generating AS and other HLA B27-related SpAs.
- In early AS, sacroiliitis may be characterized by CD+ T-cells and CD68+ macrophages in the joint and adjacent bone marrow.
- Anatomical site-specific immunopathological data from AS patients is lacking from SI joints and spinal entheses particularly.

Tissue-specific pathophysiology
- Tissue changes associated with disease progression have been illustrated almost exclusively by imaging. MR has been particularly illuminating in this respect.
- In the SIJ, inflammation progresses through fibrosis to ankylosis. Sub-chondral bone inflammation is probably an early associated feature.
- In the spine inflammation precedes calcification and bone formation at entheses. Reactive bone sclerosis at sub-enthesial bone ensues and bony bridges between vertebrae develop (syndesmophytes) (See Plate 34).
- If subenthesial bone inflammation/oedema/pathology is severe, vertebral osteopaenia/osteoporosis occurs.
- Inflammation at entheses both in the spine and peripheries is characterized by enthesial inflammation, sub-enthesial bone oedema/inflammation and ultimately enthesophyte formation.
- Because of the consistent occurrence of inflammation at sites in tendon rich in fibrocartilage (i.e. entheses), it has been postulated that fibrocartilage may be a key target tissue for the immune response in AS.

Natural history
- AS classically progresses from sacroiliitis with inflammatory symptoms ascending the spine leading to spinal ankylosis, kyphosis/stoop and spinal restriction.
- Predicting classical or less extensive disease is difficult in early AS. Osteoporosis, as shown by lumbar spine bone mineral density (BMD) measures might predict progressive disease.
- No known therapy halts or slows the natural history, although it is hoped anti-TNFα therapy may prove to have a disease-modifying role.
- AS can have a considerable socio-economic impact in some, although not all patients.

Associated conditions and co-morbidities
- AS is associated with iritis (40%).
- Cardiac conduction defects, aortic valve (AoV) incompetence and cardiomegaly occur. Anatomic evidence of AoV involvement can be seen in up to 20% AS patients, but few have valvular dysfunction. About 50% patients with isolated AoV incompetence are HLA B27 +ve.
- Frank inflammatory bowel disease or low-grade (often subclinical) disease is commonly associated.
- Although rare, upper lobe lung fibrosis can occur and affected tissue be invaded by aspergillus. Deaths from all pulmonary causes are five times higher in AS compared with normal. This may relate partly to poor thoracic expansion and ventilatory difficulty in the presence of lung infection and cardiac pathology.
- Psoriasis and psoriaform skin lesions occur, arguably more commonly, in men compared with women.

Clinical features
Key clinical features
Delays in diagnosing AS are recognized. Taking a careful history and identifying that chronic inflammatory-type back symptoms in someone <40 years may not reflect a simple mechanical back disorder or a chronic pain syndrome, is probably the most important step in prompting appropriate imaging to be done to make a diagnosis.

Symptoms and signs
- Chronic inflammatory spinal pain in a young adult.
- Fatigue.
- Low back pains radiating to buttocks and posterior thighs.
- History of enthesitis (e.g. plantar fasciitis).
- Positive family history of SpA.
- Spinal movements are symmetrically restricted.
- Tenderness over entheses (particularly pelvis/lower limb).

Key features in the history
- Inflammatory spinal pains are invariable – pains are often associated with stiffness, evolve insidiously, are prominent with immobility, are present on waking, can disturb sleep, and ease with movement.
- Onset after the age of 45 years is very uncommon.
- Fatigue, weight loss, and low-grade fever may occur and appear variable. Fatigue is often scored as the most troublesome symptoms by patients.
- Previous enthesitis (e.g. previous plantar fasciitis) can precede the onset of obvious AS by many years.
- Given HLA B27+ is dominantly inherited there may be familial clustering of HLA B27-related diseases.
- A history of uveitis, psoriasis, inflammatory bowel disease, urethritis may all be relevant.

Key features on examination
- Global restriction of lumbar spine movements in early AS and stiffening of the whole spine as AS progresses. Ultimately completely stiff spine with kyphosis.
- Reduced chest expansion compared to population reference for age/sex (at 4th intercostal space level).
- Peripheral joint synovitis/arthritis is unusual with primary AS (apart from hip and shoulder joints).
- Enthesitis is variable and more prominent in lower limbs. (see Plate 4)
- Associated psoriasis may not be obvious.
- Any evidence of eye signs should prompt a ophthalmology referral to rule out uveitis.
- Cardiovascular and respiratory examination is important with in established AS or those with symptoms.

Investigations
Laboratory
HLA B27 in >90% Caucasians; modest ↑ESR or ESR normal (increases in ESR corresponds to severity of disease (e.g. ↑+ in AS patients with peripheral erosive arthritis); normochromic normocytic anaemia; IgA↑.

Radiographs
In early AS, radiographs of SIJs and spine may be normal. As AS advances sacroiliitis may be become obvious and is usually bilateral. The sequence of sacroiliac changes over time typically consists of:
- Initially, blurring of sub-chondral bone plate.
- Erosions (like postage stamp serrations) and sclerosis of adjacent bone (typically iliac side first).
- Pseudo-widening of the SIJ.
- Gradual interosseous bridging and joint ossification.
- Sclerosis persists or becomes more prominent.
- Bony ankylosis after a number of years. (see Plate 22)

Key radiographic features in the axial skeleton

Features on axial skeleton radiographs in AS patients
- **Early spinal features:** vertebral squaring; small marginal syndesmophytes; erosion/sclerosis at vertebral body corners ['shiny corner' sign/Romanus lesion (severe)].
- **Late spinal features:** ankylosis of vertebral segments (vertebral bodies or posterior segments; ossification of supraspinous and interspinous ligaments.
- **Occurring at any time:** discovertebral junction erosions or destruction; erosion/sclerosis of odontoid or costovertebral joints; posterior spinal subligamentous erosion.
- **Pelvis changes:** sacroiliac pathology (see text); iliac enthesophytes; ischial pole erosions/enthesophytes; symphysis pubis narrowing/sclerosis/erosion and ankylosis (late).

Typical radiographic features in the peripheral skeleton in established AS include:

- **At the hip:** in early disease – a distinctive enthesophyte on the lateral aspect of the femoral head. Eventually, a collar of these enthesophytes can form around the femoral head; diffuse concentric joint space narrowing; bony ankylosis (late).
- **At the shoulder:** concentric joint space loss; superiolateral humeral head erosions (if severe causing a 'hatchet' appearance to the humeral head); erosive acromioclavicular joint (ACJ) and SCJ changes; CA ligament attachment bony proliferation/periosteal changes.
- **Peripheral joints:** periarticular osteoporosis less prominent than in RA; periarticular bone proliferation (fuzzy osteoperiostitis), e.g. at distal humeral epicondyles, patella margins, distal lateral femoral condyles; at attachments of carpal ligaments.
- **At entheses:** erosions, fluffy bone sclerosis and spurs. Changes often seen at plantar fascia origin, insertion of peroneal tendons in midfoot, Achilles' tendon or at lesser or greater trochanters at proximal femur.

Magnetic resonance imaging

- Features of spondylodiscitis on T1- and T2-weighted MR are seen in AS though easy descrimination of AS/SpA-related spondylodiscitis compared with degeneration (Modic lesion) discitis lesions has not been reported.
- The appearance of 'vertebral corner', 'oedema'-type changes on both T1- and T2-weighted sequences is typical in AS. The cause of high signal in vertebral corners on T1-weighted lesions is unknown, but could be fatty change at sites of previous subenthesial osteitis.
- Spinal ligament enthesitis is probably poorly visualized on MR unless lesions are severe or numerous.
- Gd-enhancement appears to add little overall in aiding a diagnosis of SpA or monitoring changes in inflammatory lesions after treatment.
- A number of robust MR scoring tools have been devised to measure and monitor disease in AS. Consensus opinion suggests the 6-discovertebral unit (6-DVU) method devised under the auspices of SPARCC may be of most use.

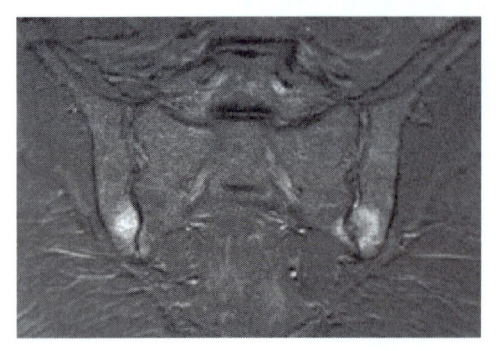

Figure 7.4 Coronal image fat-suppressed sequence MR. High signal (inflammation) on both sides of the lower part of the SIJs.

Differential diagnosis

- **In patients <15 years old:** juvenile AS; juvenile psoriatic arthritis/spondylitis; enthesitis-related arthropathy.
- **In patients 15–50 years old:** mechanical back pain; psoriatic spondylitis; reactive arthritis/spondylitis.
- **In patients >50 years:** as in those 15–40 years old, but also diffuse idiopathic skeletal hyperostosis (DISH).

- DISH can be discriminated from AS (Table 7.2), but doing so using MR is not emphasized in the literature.
- Osteitis Condensans Ilii can mimic sacroiliitis on pelvic radiographs. It usually occurs in nulliparous women and is asymptomatic. Sclerosis occurs on the iliac side of the lower SIJ, but the joint is normal.

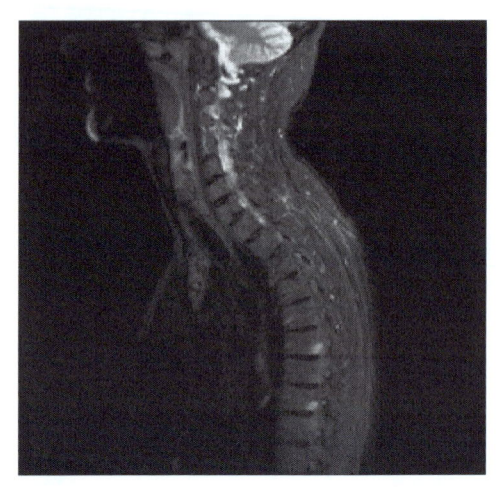

Figure 7.5 T2-weighted sagittal TSp in AS. High signal (in bone ?;osteitis) can be seen in 2 vertebal bodies in the TSp.

Table 7.2 Discriminating AS from DISH

	DISH	**AS**
Usual age on onset	>50y	<40y
TSp kyphosis	±	++
Limitation of spinal mobility	±	++
Pain	±	++
↓ chest expansion	±	++
*Radiographs**		
Hyperostosis	+	+
SIJ erosion**	–	++
SIJ obliteration	±	++
Facet joint obliteration	–	++
Ant. longitudinal ligament	Flowing ossification	±
Syndesmophytes	Florid non-marginal	Usually marginal
Enthesophytes	Often extensive.	Often erosions at base
	Usually no erosions	
Vertebral osteopaenia	Bones often dense	In early disease
HLA B27 (Caucasians)	8%	95%
HLA B27 (Afro-Caribbean)	2%	50%

Adapted from Calin (2004) and Resnick (2002).
*Discriminating DISH from the spectrum of lesions that accompany axial musculoskeletal lesions in psoriatic spondylarthropathy is, by comparison, less well emphasized in the literature.
**Doubt whether SIJ changes may be due atypical AS or DISH, may not be easily resolved by MRI alone. The presence of erosions on SIJ CT (in AS not DISH) may be better discriminatory investigation.

Management

Objectives of disease management

The main key objectives are symptom control, maintaining functional ability and occupational potential, retaining spinal mobility, preventing osteoporosis, and monitoring for extra-musculoskeletal disease.

Physical therapies

- Regular exercises are important in preventing or minimizing deformity. Spinal extension and deep breathing exercises should be done regularly.
- Formal physiotherapy is of value. Posture should be addressed. Group sessions including hydrotherapy may help. Regular swimming is considered the most appropriate aerobic exercise for AS patients.

Control of pain/inflammation

- The responses to NSAIDs vary, but most patients require regular or 'as required' NSAIDs long-term.
- Phenylbutazone (butazoladin) is probably the most effective NSAID for pain/stiffness in AS.
- Although the finding needs substantiating, regular NSAIDs may slow radiographic progression of AS.
- There is a significant side-effect profile from long-term NSAID use.

Immunosupression

- There is some evidence for using sulphasalazine (SZP) in AS with peripheral arthritis though its impact on the spine and peripheral enthesopathy is minimal.
- For AS patients with peripheral arthritis unresponsive to NSAIDs and SZP, methotrexate (MTX) has been used and some benefit reported.

- A single RCT of leflunomide in AS concluded there was no benefit over placebo.
- A Cochrane Review concluded there was inadequate evidence to support MTX use in AS.
- Anti-TNFα therapies have shown efficacy at an acceptable level of toxicity (Table 7.3).
- Infliximab treatment virtually clears spinal inflammation evident by the appearance of osteitis on spinal MR images; it also improves individual productivity lessening adverse physical and emotional factors and loss of workdays (sustained over 6 months).
- Etanercept therapy reduces spinal and SIJ inflammation within 6 weeks of the start of therapy, sustained over 24 weeks, as shown by MR.
- A Markov model of cost-utility over 5y suggests that the high cost of etanercept and infliximab restricts efficient use in all patients with a BASDAI>4.
- Emerging data suggests adalimubab has similar efficacy to other anti-TNFα inhibitors in AS.

Other therapies

Intravenous bisphosphonates may be helpful. Serial monthly pamidronate injections improve symptoms (and BASDAI disease scores) in some patients.

Surgery

- A number of spinal procedures may be useful. These include osteotomy, fusion of unstable segments (caused by spondylodiscitis ± fracture), and laminectomies.
- For AS patients with advanced kyphosis/stoop, spinal osteotomy, generally improving sagittal spinal angle by a mean 20–40° can be effective at improving functional ability, raising eyeline, and may have a role in reducing the risks from poor ventilatory capacity.

Table 7.3 A summary of randomized controlled trials of anti-TNFα therapies in AS

Medication/study	Patients	Design/duration	1e Outcome/response	Comments
Infliximab*				
Braun et al. (2002) 5 mg/kg iv at weeks 0, 2 and 6	35	Randomized placebo-controlled for 12 weeks	18/35 (53%) infliximab treated vs. 3/35(9%) placebo-treated had disease regression by 50% or more (BASDAI)	Small study. 3/35 in the infliximab group had serious side effects
van der Heijde et al. (2005) 5 mg/kg iv at weeks 0, 2, 6, 12, 18	357 screened; 201 infliximab treated and 78 placebo	Randomized placebo controlled for 24 weeks	ASAS20 achieved in 61% infliximab treated patients vs. 19% placebo treated ($p < 0.001$)	Side effects frequent in both groups (82% vs. 72% placebo-treated)
Etanercept**				
25 mg sc ×2/week** Davis et al. (2003) Davis et al. (2005)	277	Randomized placebo-controlled for 24 weeks	ASAS20 achieved in 57% of 138 etanercept vs. 22% of 139 placebo treated pts ($p < 0.001$)	All ASAS components improved. A later study showed sustained improvement in patients over 2 years
Calin et al. (2004)	84	Double blind placebo-controlled for 12 weeks	ASAS20 in 26 (60%) etanercept vs. 9 (23%) pts; $p < 0.001$; CI 17–56%	
Adalimumab				
40 mg sc fortnightly van der Heijde et al. (2006)	315	Double blind placebo-controlled/randomized 2:1 adalimumab:placebo/ 12 weeks	ASAS20 in 58% adalimumab vs. 21% placebo pts ($p < 0.001$)	ASAS40 at 12 and 24 weeks by some patients

*Have been shown in separate studies to reduce attacks of uveitis in AS patients.
**In a later study, 50 mg weekly was shown to be as effective as 25 mg twice weekly.

- Key points of spinal osteotomy are shown below.
- Osteoporotic fractures in the AS spine can be severe and difficult to fix. Surgery is always challenging.
- Intervention criteria/thresholds employed to guide preventive therapy for osteoporotic fractures in AS have not been derived.

Spinal osteotomy in AS: key points
- Surgery and anaesthesia is relatively high risk and challenging. Neurological morbidity can be severe/permanent. Surgery should only be undertaken in specialized centres by experienced staff.
- Technically, osteotomies of lumbar, thoracic or cervical spine vertebrae can, in theory, be considered.
- There are 3 main (posterior approach) techniques (reviewed in Van Royen & De Gast, 1999): opening, closing, or polysegmental wedge osteotomies.
- Closing wedge osteotomy procedures are associated with the lowest incidence of complications.
- The theoretical benefits of improving functional ability, reducing conventional AS-related pulmonary morbidity, general well-being and spinal symptoms in the long-term has not been established in (the almost exclsively retrospective) series of patients reported.

Prognosis
Poor prognostic indicators in early disease
- Polyarticular synovitis.
- High acute phase response.
- Hip involvement.
- Osteoporosis (lumbar vertebrae).

Likely poor prognostic indicators in established disease
- Complete thoracic spine ankylosis.
- Cardiovascular and respiratory disease complications.
- Excessive continual NSAID use.
- Spinal fracture.
- Continued high acute phase response/anaemia.
- Polyarticular synovitis.

Current controversies
Diagnostic issues
- How HLA B27 predisposes to disease.
- How autoimmune processes specifically lead to pathology at entheses and sub-enthesial bone marrow.
- How best to invoke strategies that reduce the delay in diagnosing AS (e.g. triage of chronic back pain patients).
- How best to image SIJs and spine in early AS to make a firm diagnosis (MR of SIJs may be more sensitive in detecting sacroiliitis but classification criteria depend on radiographic changes being present).

Management/treatment issues
- Do NSAIDs slow AS progression (disease-modifying)?
- What role do potent iv bisphosphonates have in controlling pain/inflammation or modifying disease?
- Do oral bisphosphonates have a relevant symptom modifying or disease-progression slowing role?
- Do bisphosphonates reduce fractures in AS?
- Are anti-TNFα medications safe in the long-term? Do they modify disease progression and if so are they equally effective on axial and peripheral disease

Resources
Assessment tools
Self-assessment tools: BASDAI, BASFI, and other assessment tools (e.g. ASQoL, Dougados Functional Index, BASMI, etc) can be downloaded in a number of languages from the ASAS Workshop page link at the ASIF website (www.asif.rheumanet.org).

A reference list of original publications detailing assessments can be reviewed at www.rheumatology.org/publications/abbreviations/index.asp

Guidelines
ASAS guidelines derived by physician consensus based on a Delphi study undertaken by the group. See www.asas-group.org/

NIHCE Guidelines (www.nice.org.uk/) cover the use of anti-TNFα therapies for NHS patients in the UK. These were derived by (chiefly) health economists/clinicians appointed by the UK Government who were cognate of the BSR guidelines.

Patient organizations/information
AS self-help organizations of various countries are listed on the ASIF website (www.asif.rheumanet.org).

Informing licensing authorities about difficult driving may vary between countries. In the UK, where there is significant neck restriction, there is a requirement to inform the DVLA.

Useful information regarding issues of the patient's point of view is summarized in Rogers 2003.

Webpage on Spondylarthritis. See ACR website www.rheumatology.org/public/factsheets/

References
Benjamin M, McGonagle D, Davis JC, van der Heijde DM, Braun J, et al. Sustained durability and tolerability of etanercept in AS for 96 weeks. *Ann Rheum Dis* 2005; **64**: 1557–62.

Boonen A, et al. Employment, disability and work days lost in patients with AS – a cross-sectional study of Dutch patients. *Ann Rheum Dis* 2001; **60**: 353–8.

Boulos P, Dougados M, Macleod SM, Hunsche E. Pharmacological treatment of AS: a systematic review. *Drugs* 2005; **65**: 2111–27.

Bowness P. HLA B27 in health and disease: a double edged sword? *Rheumatology* 2002; **41**: 857–68.

Braun J, Brandt J, Listing J, et al. Treatment of active AS with infliximab: a randomised controlled multicentre trial. *Lancet* 2002; **359**(9313): 1187–93.

Braun J, Pham T, Sieper J, et al. International ASAS consensus statement for the use of anti-TNF agents in patients with AS. *Ann Rheum Dis* 2003; **62**: 817–24.

Calin A. Ankylosing spondylitis. In: Isenberg DA, Maddison PJ, Woo P, Glass D, Breedveld FC (eds) *Oxford Textbook of Rheumatology*, 3rd edn. Oxford: Oxford University Press, 1994: 754–66.

Calin A, Dijkmans BA, Emery P, et al. Outcomes of a multicentre randomised clinical trial of etanercept to treat AS. *Ann Rheum Dis* 2004; **63**: 1594–6000.

Chen J, Liu C, Lin J. Methotrexate for ankylosing spondylitis. *Cochrane Database Syst Rev* 2004; **3**: CD004524.

Davis JC Jr, van der Heijde D, Braun J, et al. Recombinant human tumor necrosis factor receptor for treating AS: a randomised controlled trial. *Arthritis Rheum* 2003; **48**: 3230–6.

Francois RJ, Neure L, Sieper J, Braun J. Immunohistological examination of open sacroiliac biopsies of patients with AS: detection of TNFα in 2 patients with early disease and TGFβ in 3 more advanced cases. *Ann Rheum Dis* 2006; **65**: 713–20.

Keat A, Barkham N, Bhalla A, et al. BSR Guidelines for prescribing TNF-alpha blockers in adults with AS. Report of a working party of the BSR. *Rheumatology* 2005; **44**: 939–47.

Kollnberger S, Bird L, Sun M-Y, et al. Cell surface expression and immune receptor rocognition of HLA B27 homdimers. *Arthritis Rheum* 2002; **46**: 2972–82.

Maksymowych WP, Inman RD, Salonen D, et al. Spondyloarthritis Research Consortium of Canada Magnetic Resonance Imaging Index for Assessment of Spinal Inflammation in Ankylosing Spondylitis. *Arthritis Rheum* 2005; **53**: 502–9.

Resnick DD. Diffuse idiopathic skeletal hyperostosis. In: Resnick DD (ed.) *Diagnosis of Bone and Joint Disorders*, 4th edn. Philadelphia: WB Saunders, 2002, 1476–500.

Resnick DD. Ankylosing spondylitis. In: Resnick DD (ed.) *Diagnosis of Bone and Joint Disorders*, 4th edn. Philadelphia: WB Saunders, 2002, 1023–81.

Rogers FJ. Ankylosing spondylitis – the patient's point of view. In: Calin A and Taurog JD(eds) *The Spondylarthritides*. Oxford: Oxford University Press, pp. 251–65.

Van der Heijde D, Dijkmans B, Geusens P, et al. Efficacy and safety of infliximab in patients with AS: results of a randomised placebo-controlled trial (ASSERT). *Arthritis Rheum* 2005; **52**: 582–91.

Van der Heijde D, Kivitz A, Schiff MH, et al. Efficacy and safety of adalimumab in patients with AS: results of a multicenter, randomized, double blind, placebo-controlled trial. *Arthritis Rheum* 2006; **54**: 2136–46.

Van der Linden S, Valkenburg HA, Cats A. Evaluation of diagnostic criteria for ankylosing spondylitis: a proposal for modification of the New York criteria. *Arthritis Rheum* 1984; **27**: 361–8.

Van Royen BJ, DeGast A. Lumbar osteotomy for correction of thoracolumbar kyphotic deformity in AS. A structured review of 3 months of treatment. *Ann Rheum Dis* 1999; **58**: 399–406.

Wanders A, Heijds D, Landewe R, et al. NSAIDs reduce radiographic progression in patients with AS: a randomized clinical trial. *Arthritis Rheum* 2005; **52**: 1756–65.

Psoriatic arthritis

Definition
PsA is a chronic autoimmune inflammatory arthropathy. In adults, there is no single agreed satisfactory definition encompassing all forms of PsA. Classification of PsA proposed 35 years ago listed the necessary presence of 3 features: inflammatory arthritis, psoriasis and negative rheumatoid factor (Moll & Wright, 1973). In 1984 new criteria expanded the set of potential features classifiable under a diagnosis of PsA, but essentially required the presence of psoriatic skin or nail disease with either a peripheral or axial pattern of disease. The component features of defining 'peripheral' and 'axial' were both restrictive and imprecise, and the criteria were not very user friendly. Criteria did recognize for the first time though the presence of juxta-articular new bone as important.

Subsets of disease were increasingly recognized, although entheseal-predominant disease is a relatively recent determined subgroup.

The clinical spectrum of PsA
- Predominantly DIP Joint involvement
- Arthritis mutilans (digit 'telescoping')
- Symmetrical polyarthritis
- Asymmetrical oligoarthritis
- Spondylitis predominant
- Entheseal predominant

However, subgroups are unstable over time and with treatment, and their definition is dependent on method of detection. The classification of the PsA (CASPAR) study group criteria have been based on observations of 1000 PsA and control patient data, and have high sensitivity (0.91) and specificity (0.99). Criteria were compared against a gold standard of clinician opinion (Table 7.4).

Table 7.4 CASPAR classification criteria for PsA.

Inflammatory articular disease (joint, spine or entheseal) with 3 or more points from the following	
Current psoriasis (2 pts)	Skin or scalp disease judged by a rheumatologist
History of psoriasis	From patient, dermatologist, rheumatologist, or GP
Family history of psoriasis	In first or second degree relative
Psoriatic nail dystrophy	Onycholysis, pitting or hyperkeratosis
Negative rheumatoid factor	By any method except latex
Current dactylitis	Entire digital swelling
History of dactylitis	Recorded by rheumatologist
Radiological evidence of juxta-articular new bone	On hand or foot excluding osteophytes

See Taylor W et al., 2006

The definition of inflammatory joint, spine, or entheseal disease may require some pause for thought and possibly further study. Conventional definitions (e.g. features of synovitis in RA or IBP in AS may not be appropriately transferred given the difference in type of causative lesions.

Epidemiology
- Psoriasis (Ps) affects 3% of the population (North Europe).
- Studies suggest prevalence of PsA in Ps patients is about 40% and in the population up to 1%.
- Estimates suggest that about 20% of patients develop PsA before Ps, in some cases by many years. Old epidemiology data might underestimate PsA prevalence. The new CASPAR criteria, applied in appropriate studies in Primary Care should help clarify the situation.
- There is probably equal sex prevalence with peak presentation between 35–55 years old.

Aetiology and pathophysiology
Genetic
- Polygenic (familial aggregation); high MZ twin concordance; HLA associations found with B13, B16 (B38 and B39), B7, B17, B27, Cw6, DR4, and DR7.
- Susceptibility to PsA may also reside at chromosome 16q, a region overlapping with CARD15, a susceptibility locus for Crohn's disease. There are 3 main mutations. The peptide, located in monocyte, macrophage, and dendritic cell cytoplasm, recognizes certain bacterial components though how immunopathology subsequently develops is uncertain.

Environment
PsA and Ps is triggered, and exacerbated by β-haemolytic streptococci and HIV. Trauma and stress have also been identified as potentiating factors.

Immunopathology
- Information is incomplete. Studies have relied on obtaining material from blood and synovium of affected patients, and relatively little is known about the pathophysiology in enthesial, periosteum, and other bone sites – sites of frequent involvement in PsA.
- In synovium (as in the skin in Ps) there are dilated capillaries and monocyte-rich perivascular infiltrates.
- Th1 cytokines, such as Il-2 and IFNγ are ↑ in skin, but not in synovium; Paired skin and synovial samples show different oligoclonal patterns of TcR usage and T-cells from psoriatic skin transferred into SCID mice can induce psoriasis, but not arthritis. Thus, T-cell recognition patterns may differ in the two tissues and skin, and joint disease might be mediated by different cells.
- Increased TNFα has been detected in skin and joint fluid of patients with PsA.

Prognosis and natural history
- Undoubtedly PsA can be mild and have little impact on functional abilities, even in the long-term; however, progressive PsA impacts substantially on employment social and financial stability and healthcare use/costs.
- Oligoarticular joint disease is associated with a relatively benign prognosis.
- Erosive, deforming arthritis occurs in about 40–60% of PsA patients attending rheumatology clinics.
- Adverse prognostic factors appear to be polyarthritis, greater HAQ, and increase use of DMARDs.

Clinical features

Key clinical features
- Inflammatory joint and/or spinal pains.
- Asymmetric or unilateral symptoms/lesions.
- History of psoriasis or family history of it.
- History of other SpA (or SpA-linked) condition.
- Dactylitis of toes or fingers.
- Enthesitis.
- Ps or psoriaform rash (at any time)

Key features in history
- PsA can present with Ps, long after Ps started or before it, sometimes years before.
- A family history of Ps is not unusual.
- Ps can be mild and ignored by the patient. Direct and repeated questioning about rashes in typical sites for Ps is often helpful (e.g. in ears, umbilicus, posterior hairline, natal cleft, around waist).
- A history detailing all previous musculoskeletal problems, even if seemingly trivial to the patient, may be informative (e.g. previous recurrent heel, groin, pelvic or elbow pains, inflammatory-type back pains, etc).
- Establishing whether there is or has been inflammatory back or neck pain may be relevant.
- PsA lesions may have been triggered by trauma. Be aware of 'injuries' that don't settle satisfactorily.
- Groin and anteromedial thigh pain may be from hip joints, symphysis pubis, or adductor tendons.
- Previous plantar fasciitis and 'tennis elbow' may be relevant to making a diagnosis of chronic PsA.

Key features on examination
Upper limbs
- Asymmetric appearance to small hand joint and finger swelling – may be dactylitis, which is often associated with underlying MCPJ or PIPJ erosions.
- DIPJ changes in advanced PsA can look just like OA, although PsA associated with nail pits and onycholysis.
- Often tender without much swelling at wrists.
- Thumb CMC area is often affected.
- Enthesitis of lateral humeral epicondyles is common.
- Other entheses to check for tenderness: deltoid origin, medial humeral epicondyle.

Pelvis and lower limbs
- In some PsA types synovitis may not obviously accompany pain in the knees, but there may be peri-articular tenderness at entheses (e.g. inferior patella pole and patella ligament insertion).
- Synovial thickening and effusions at the knees can be, but are not always, massive.
- Synovitis and bony tenderness around the hindfoot is common. Tenderness over medial calcaneal tubercle denotes enthesial involvement of plantar fascia origin.
- Midfoot restriction of movement is common.
- Hallux limitus (early) and rigidus (late) can reflect chronic osteo-periostitis of the great toe – a common finding in PsA: indolent dactylitis may be present.
- Nail changes may look non-specific, but extensive subungual hyperkeratosis is typical of Ps-related disease.

Axial skeleton
- Signs in the neck and spine are non-specific, although marked global restriction of movement can occur.
- Common signs of the pelvis include hip joint restriction, tenderness of symphysis pubis (osteitis pubis), sacroiliitis indicated by positive sacroiliac stress tests, and tenderness over entheses particularly greater trochanters, ASISs, and PSISs.

Co-morbidities
PsA is linked to other SpA conditions and SpA-related lesions, such inflammatory bowel lesions (16% in one study) and acute anterior uveitis (<10%).
- Gouty arthritis may occur in 5–7% PsA patients.
- Ps and psoriasis can occur *de novo* or be exaceberbated, in HIV+ people
- Studies that have linked Ps and PsA to coeliac disease have done so on the basis of suboptimal serological testing, although ultimately detailed and appropriate clinco-imaging appraisal of appropriate patient groups has not been done.
- SAPHO syndrome has been proposed by some as a clinical syndrome contiguous with the spectrum of PsA.

Investigations
Laboratory
- ESR and CRP can be normal or only modestly raised.
- Rheumatoid factors (RFs) and anti-CCP antibodies have been described in PsA, but their presence requires very careful scrutiny of diagnosis.

Imaging
Radiographs
Careful evaluation of current and previous radiographs can be enlightening in highlighting bony changes.
- In early PsA radiographic features may be absent.
- In established PsA, radiographic abnormalities may exist where symptoms are minimal or not evident.
- There's a range of radiographic signs in PsA, often mistaken for degenerative disease.
- Axial PsA may be disclosed by radiographs. Without a high index of suspicion, appearances, particularly in the neck, may be confused with degenerative changes.

Ultrasound (US)
- There is increasing experience using US to identify dactylitis and enthesitis.
- Discriminating patterns of soft-tissue abnormality around joints and tendons in RA and PsA may be an achievable, and extremely worthwhile, goal using US.

Typical features on radiographs in patients with PsA
- **General:** enthesophytes; periosteal new bone (often juxta-articular); often no periarticular osteopaenia.
- **Pelvis:** irregular/unilateral sacroiliac changes; hip arthritis; enthesophytes; osteitis pubis.
- **Spine:** syndesmophytes; facet joint arthritis; posterior element new bone formation (enthesophytes and periosteal apposition); spondylodiscitis.
- **Peripheries:** DIPJs: juxta-articular bone; widening joint space; 'flange' osteophytes.
- **Phalanges**: dactylitis; diaphyseal thickening; tuft changes; soft tissue swelling (dactylitis)

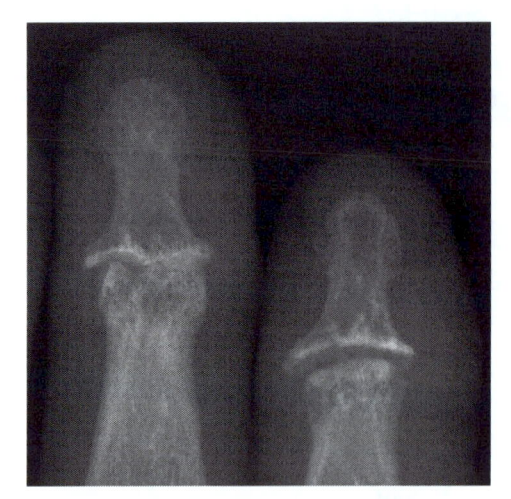

Figure 7.6 DIPJ arthritis in PsA. Flanging of periarticular bone, increased joint width (right), abnormal distal phalanx bone texture changes (in the digit on right with dactylitis) and a paucity of OA features (e.g. subchondral sclerosis, cysts and osteophytes).

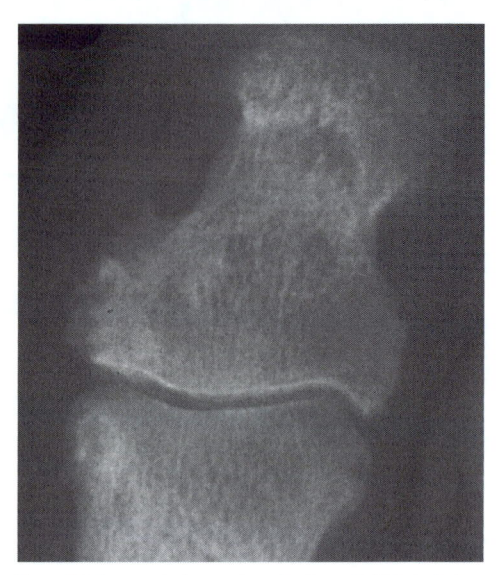

Figure 7.8 Juxta-articular new bone (periosteal whiskering) of the great toe distal phalanx in PsA. Note the relatively normal joint appearance.

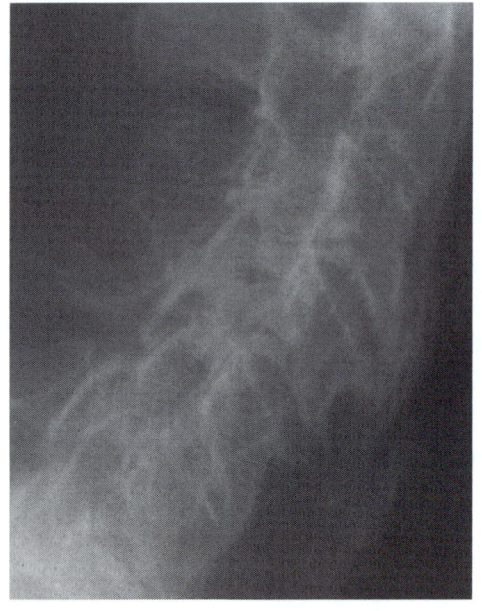

Figure 7.7 PsA neck. Marginal and paramarginal syndesmophytes, florid posterior element periosteal apposition and facet joint involvement.

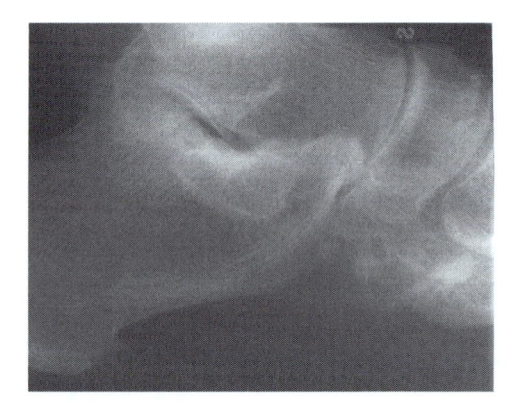

Figure 7.9 Juxta-articular bone at calcaneocuboid joint. A plantar spur can be associated with PsA.

MR
Distinctive patterns of MR abnormality for dactylitis and PsA-related DIPJ arthritis are now recognized, although results need substantiating:
- MR has not yet been shown to discriminate sarcoid from PsA/SpA-related dactylitis.
- MR may not be as useful in identifying inflammatory spinal lesions in PsA as it is in AS.
- MR-identified changes in the nail-bed associated with DIPJ arthritis may be specific for PsA and may be detectable using extremity (0.2T) MR.

Differential diagnosis
- Where there is obvious chronic synovitis in a number of small joints the main differential diagnosis is RA.
- Generalized OA will be the main differential diagnosis of multiple DIPJ involvement. Look for nail pits (associated with PsA not OA).
- Be suspicious of a diagnosis of OA in a patient with Ps (or previous history of it or Ps in first degree relative) in an 'unusual' joint for OA (e.g. ankle or subtalar), where there has been no previous significant trauma.
- Like PsA, all SpAs are characterized by dactylitis, joint and enthesis lesions.
- The enthesopathic/periosteal lesions of PsA can be mistaken for fibromyalgia.

CHAPTER 7 The spondylarthropathies

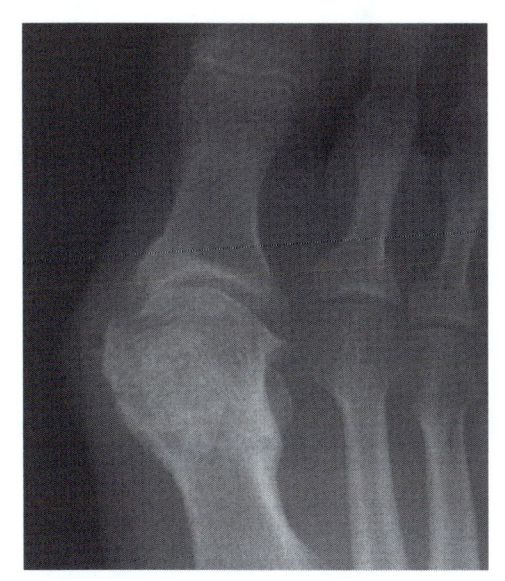

Figure 7.10 PsA toe. Juxta-articular new bone (periosteal apposition) of distal first metatarsal head.

- Chronic sarcoid, like PsA, can involve entheses and periostea particularly around the hindfoot and lower leg (e.g. plantar fasciitis).
- PsA spondylitis can be mistaken for chronic mechanical back (or neck) pain.

Treatment

Objectives of disease management
- To control symptoms and prevent disability through judicious use of NSAIDs and immunosuppressants.
- One-quarter of patients with PsA are dissatisfied with the treatment they receive (see NPF 2002).
- Although PsA is often judged to be indolent, evidence suggests that, lifelong, PsA is associated with significant indices of disability.

Physical therapies
There is little evidence to suggest what role physical therapy plays in PsA.
Hand therapy review for assessing functional impact, and utilizing splinting and joint protection methods.

Control of pain
NSAIDs probably have a variable effect. Trying full dose over 4 weeks and swapping to an alternative if no satisfactory effect occurs is appropriate.

Immunosupression
There is a deficit of therapeutic trials in PsA. This and other suboptimal aspects of the care of PsA patients have been addressed in principle through the aims of GRAPPA, an international group of clinicians convened to work toward facilitating research into PsA.
- Historically the use of therapies in PsA has followed from their established use in patients with RA.
- Though anecdotal evidence for its efficacy can be found, methotrexate (MTX) has not been extensively studied. Studies suffer from low patient numbers, too short follow-up, and other methodological flaws.

- Patients treated with MTX are 9 times more likely to benefit and 5 times less likely to stop treatment compared with patients treated with gold compounds – the latter having shown some efficacy in PsA, given either as auranofin 3 g/day or monthly injections.
- RCT data have shown sulphasalazine, leflunomide, and anti-TNFα therapies can improve PsA symptoms in the short term. Leflunomide and notably anti-TNFα therapies have a significantly improve Ps as well.
- Ciclosporin A, antimalarials D-penicillamine and azathioprine show some efficacy in small, open label studies. Antimalarials can aggravate Ps, however.
- Overall, conventional DMARDs have not shown efficacy in treating axial PsA disease.

Prognosis
- Worse prognosis is associated with polyarticular presentation, high ESR/CRP and IgA and HIV status.
- Persistent dactylitis is associated with erosive disease of underlying small joints.
- HLA B27, B39 and DQw3 are associated with disease progression but DR7 is protective.
- Studies linking synovial fluid constituents to prognosis fail to represent the complete range of PsA subtypes.

Current controversies

Diagnostic issues
- Most controversies probably arise as a consequence of varied case ascertainment in clinical studies.
- Is PsA one condition with many and varied musculoskeletal lesions or are there distinct conditions?
- Can PsA be adequately defined without extensive Primary Care based capture of a broad range of possibly affected patients with and without Ps? Will CASPAR perform appropriately in this respect?
- What is the main lesion in PsA? Enthesitis? Periostitis? Synovitis? A review of the foremost textbook of musculoskeletal radiology would suggest non-articular bone-related lesions are the most frequent across the PsA disease spectrum (see Resnick 2002).
- What is the prevalence of PsA-sine-Ps?
- Is dactylitis always clinically evident?
- What is the *spectrum* of PsA-related spinal disease? For example how commonly is spondylodiscitis or facet joint arthritis a feature of Psoriatic spondylitis?
- Do current diagnostic methods under-estimate Ps-related musculoskeletal disease? In the spine? Current methods of identifying Psoriatic Enthesopathy are suboptimal and there may be diagnostic confusion in patients otherwise thought to have fibromyalgia.
- Does MR discriminate PsA from all phases of OA in DIPJs particularly in early disease?

Management issues
- The role of physiotherapy and whether exercise helps or worsens PsA-related spondylitis in the short-term (symptom modification) and long-term (?accelerated spinal damage).
- What measures should be adopted to gauge results in therpaeutic studies? Should different datasets be used for different disease subtypes?
- Are anti-TNFα therapies cost-effective in PsA in the long-term? Do they prevent radiological progression?

Table 7.5 A summary of the major randomized controlled therapeutic trials in PsA

Drug (reference)	Patient characteristics	RDBPCT* details	Statistically significant results
Sulphasalazine (SZP) Clegg et al. (1996)	221 patients	36-week study. SZP 2 g/day.	SZP significantly effective according to composite pre-defined response measure. High response rate in placebo arm (44%)
Leflunomide (LEF) Kaltwasser et al 2004	190 patients with PsA + psoriasis - all patients having failed DMARD	24-week study. LEF 100 mg/day for 3 days then 20 mg/day	59% LEF vs. 30% placebo responded judged by PsARC
Etanercept (ETN) Mease et al. (2004)	205 patients, 40% on MTX	12-week study. ETN 25 mg × 2/week; sc injection	ACR20 achieved in 59 vs. 12% placebo. PsARC achieved in 72% vs. 31% placebo. Response main tained for 2 years in later analysis Inhibition of radiographic progression at 2 years from later analysis [Mease et al. (2006a)]
Infliximab (INF) Antoni et al. (2005)	200 patients unresponsive to prior treatment	14-week study. INF 5 mg/kg iv regime	ACR20 achieved in 58 vs. 11% placebo PsARC achieved in 77 vs. 27% placebo. Response maintained + inhibition of X-ray progression for 1 year in later analyses
Adalimumab (ALM) Mease et al. (2005b)	313 patients, 50% on MTX	24-week study. ALM 40 mg every 2 weeks	ACR20 achieved in 58 vs. 14% placebo
Alefacept (ALF) human LFA-3/IgG1 fusion protein, which binds CD2 receptors on T cells to block LFA binding on APCs Mease et al. (2006b)	185 patients all on MTX	24-week study, ALF 15 mg im weekly randomized 2:1 vs. placebo injection for 12 weeks. Outcome at 24 weeks (MTX contd only)	ACR20 achieved in 54 vs. 23% placebo.

Table 7.6 New or potential future therapies for PsA

Biologic agent	Notes
Onercept: a recombinant p55 TNF-binding protein, given as a weekly sc injection	Is approved to treat psoriasis. Showed efficacy (ACR20) in a phase 2 study
Efalizumab A recombinant humanized IgG1κ mc antibody, which binds LFA-1/CD11a preventing T-cell-ICAM-1 binding (APCs and endothelium)	Is FDA approved as a once weekly sc injection to treat Ps. A small 12 week RCT in PsA showed a trend for improvement vs. placebo. Concerns about its safety led to a review of reported side effects (Scheinfeld 2006).
Abatacept: Soluble receptor (CTLA-4+IgG-Fc fragment), which blocks T-cell-APC binding	Has been studied in RA and psoriasis. Studies in PsA likely to follow
Anti-Interleukin 12 (p40) antibody	Downregulates Th-1 cytokines in psoriatic skin lesions. Untried as yet in PsA
Anti-Interleukin 15. Inflammatory cytokine active in many inflammatory conditions including Ps	As yet no therapeutic studies in humans. Potentially important molecule to target

Resources

Assessment tools

PsARC (Clegg et al., 1996). Response criteria adapted from a therapeutic study of sulphasalazine in PsA.

Review of assessment tools used in clinical trials (Mease et al., 2005c).

Classification criteria (CASPAR). See Taylor et al. (2006).

Guidelines for physicians

Kyle S, et al. (UK) British Society for Rheumatology (BSR) Guideline for anti-TNFα therapy in PsA. *Rheumatology* 2005; **44**: 390–7 (www.rheumatology.org.uk).

Supplement 2 from Volume **64** (March 2005) of the *Annals of Rheumatic Diseases* contains useful reviews about the clinical and radiographic assessment of PsA.

Patient organizations/information

UK: Psoriatic Arthritis Alliance. Available at: www.paalliance.org

USA: National Psoriasis Foundation. Available at: www.psoriasis.org

The International Federation of Psoriasis Associations. Available at: www.ifpa-pso.org/en/home

ICD10 codes

M07*	Psoriatic and enteropathic arthropathies
M07.0*	Distal interphalangeal psoriatic arthropathy
M.07.1*	Arthritis mutilans
M07.2*	Psoriatic spondylitis
M07.3*	Other psoriatic arthropathies
M09.0*	Juvenile arthritis in psoriasis

References

Antoni CE, Kreuger GG, de Vlam K, et al. Infliximab improves signs and symptoms of PsA: results of the IMPACT2 trial. *Ann Rheum Dis* 2005; **64**: 1150–7.

Clegg DO, Reda DJ, Mejias E, et al. Comparison of sulfasalazine and placebo in the treatment of PsA. A Department of Veterans Affairs Cooperative Study. *Arthritis Rheum* 1996; **39**: 2013–20.

Gladman DD. Psoriatic arthritis. In: Silman AJ, Symmons DPN (eds) *Baillière's Clinical Rheumatology*, International Practice and Research, vol 9. London: Baillière Tindall, 1995, 319–29.

Goupille P, Vedere V, Roulot B, Brunais J, Valat JP. Incidence of osteoperiostitis of the great toe in PsA. *J Rheumatol* 1996; **23**: 1553–6.

Husted JA, Gladman DD, Farewell VT, Cook RJ. Health related quality of life of patients with psoriatic arthritis: a comparison with patients with RA. *Arthritis Rheum* 2001; **45**: 151–8.

Jones G, Crotty M, Brooks P. Interventions for PsA. *Cochrane Database Syst Rev*, CD000212, 2000.

Kaltwasser JP, Nash P, Gladman D, et al. Efficacy and safety of leflunomide in the treatment of psoriatic arthritis and psoriasis: a multinational, double blind randomised placebo-controlled clinical trial. *Arthritis Rheum* 2004; **50**: 1939–50.

Kavanaugh A, Antoni CE, Gladman D, et al. The Infliximab Multinational PsA Controlled Trial (IMPACT): results of radiographic analyses after 1 y. *Ann Rheum Dis* 2006; **65**: 1038–43.

Mease PJ, Antoni CE, Gladman DD, Taylor WJ. PsA assessment tools in clinical trials. *Ann Rheum Dis* 2005c; **64**: 49–54.

Mease PJ, Gladman DD, Kreuger GG. Prologue: Group for Research and Assessment of Psoriasis and Psoriatic Arthritis (GRAPPA). *Ann Rheum Dis* 2005a; **64**: ii1–ii2.

Mease PJ, Gladman D, Ritchlin CT, et al. Adalimumab for the treatment of patients with moderately to severerly active PsA: results of a double-blind randomised placebo-controlled trial. *Arthritis Rheum* 2005b; **52**: 3279–89.

Mease PJ, Kivitz AJ, Burch FX, et al. Etanercept treatment of PsA: safety, efficacy and effect on disease progression. *Arthritis Rheum* 2004; **50**: 2264–72.

Mease PJ, Kivitz AJ, Burch FX, et al. Continued inhibition of radiographic progression in patients with PsA following 2y of treatment on etanercept. *J Rheumatol* 2006a; **33**: 712–21.

Mease PJ, et al. Alefacept in combination with MTX for the treatment of PsA: results of a randomised placebo-controlled study. *Arthritis Rheum* 2006b; **54**: 1638–45.

Moll JM, Wright V. Psoriatic arthritis. *Semin Arthritis Rheum* 1973; **3**: 55–78.

Nash P, Clegg DO. Psoriatic arthritis therapy: NSAIDs and traditional DMARDs. *Ann Rheum Dis* 2005; **64** (Suppl 2): 74–7.

National Psoriasis Foundation. *Benchmark Survey on Psoriasis and PsA 2002*. Available at: www.psoriasis.org/news

Pitzalis C, Cauli A, Pipitone N, et al. Cutaneous lymphocyte antigen positive T lymphocytes preferentially migrate to the skin but not to the joint in psoriatic arthritis. *Arthritis Rheum* 1996; **39**: 137–45.

Resnick D. Psoriatic arthritis. In: Resnick D (ed.) *Diagnosis of Bone and Joint Disorders*, 4th edn. Philedalphia: WB Saunders Co., 2002, 1082–109.

Sheinfeld N. Efalizumab: a review of events reported during clinical trials and side effects. *Expert Opin Drug Saf* 2006; **5**: 197–209.

Taylor W, Gladman D, Heliwell P, et al. Classification criteria for psoriatic arthritis: development of new criteria from a large international study. *Arthritis Rheum* 2006; **54**: 2665–73.

Thune PO. The prevalence of fibromyalgia among patients with psoriasis. *Acta Derm Venerol* 2005; **85**: 33–7.

Reactive arthritis

Definition
No generally accepted diagnostic criteria exist for reactive arthritis (ReA). ReA has historically been used as a broad term applied to a group of non-infectious autoimmune arthritides occurring in association with preceding infection.

Historically, one form of ReA has been known as Reiter's Syndrome (post-chlamydial arthritis). Reiter was a Nazi, involved in eugenics and many understandably believe he should not be credited with the honour of having a condition named after him. Indeed, post-infectious reactive arthritis had been described periodically since the 1500s and Reiter's 1941 paper described a spirochaete-triggered condition and, overall, his paper contributed little to furthering knowledge about reactive arthritis.

- Lyme and viral arthritis are reactive arthritides, but are not generally SpA-like or HLA B27-related (see below) and are not considered here.
- Post-streptococcal arthritis (PSRA) is an heterogenous reactive autoimmune entity. In some patients there are SpA-like features; however, PSRA is not generally considered part of the SpA group of conditions and is not considered further here.
- Up to 1999 there were 32 different terms referring to (SpA-like, HLA B27-associated) ReA in the literature.
- The SpA-like ReA, dealt with here, is either triggered by urogenital or enteric infections.

Epidemiology
Incidence varies in the context of background population frequency of HLA B27 and prevalence of relevant infection. Most estimates are derived from Scandinavia.

- In developed countries (and excluding South Africa), the estimated prevalence of ReA is 0.03–0.1% with an incidence of 5–13/100 000 for post-urethritis ReA and 5–14/100 000 for post-enteric ReA.
- Prior to the evolution of HIV as a relevant influence, urogenital ReA occurred in about 1% of men attending a sexual health clinic with non-gonoccocal urethritis.
- Accumulating reliable epidemiological data is compromised by variable case ascertainment: There are no clear criteria to consistently apply; *C trachomatis* is difficult to diagnose in women owing to difficulty in identifying (the often sub-clinical) genital infection.

Aetiology/pathphysiology
General issues
- Organisms triggering ReA may all persist after infecting humans and altering host immune responses. Each is Gram –ve, invades mucosae, has lipopolysaccharide as part of their outer membrane, exerts intracellular parasitism, and contains virulence factors, which helps them evade host immune responses and survive.
- Bacterial pathogenicity may be enhanced by the presence of HLA B27. See p. 214 for discussion of the role of HLA B27 in SpAs, most relevant for AS and ReA.
- A detailed review of ReA Pathophysiology can be found in Colmegna et al. (2004).

Enteric ReA
- Many different organisms have been found or postulated to trigger ReA.
- Attempts to culture organisms from the joints of ReA patients have failed.
- Components of *Yersinia*, *Salmonella*, and *Shigella* (often lipopolysaccharide) have been detected in ReA joints.
- *Yersinia* and *Salmonella* can persist in gut mucosa and monocytes, which may act as a reservoir and transporter of bacterial components.

Urogenital ReA
- Using a variety of techniques *Chlamydia* has been detected in the joints of ReA patients.
- Chlamydial DNA in ReA joints does not correlate with the immune response and may vary inversely with *Chlamydia*-specific lymphocyte proliferation suggesting impaired T-cell responses may be relevant.
- *C trachomatis* resides in synovial tissue (also primarily enthesial tissue) displaying an aberrant morphology and probably upregulating its *hsp60* gene.
- *Chlamydia* infected monocytes release TNFα and may cause host T-cell apoptosis and can stimulate host cells to release pro-inflammatory soluble mediators (reviewed in Colmegna et al., 2004).

Clinical features
Key clinical features
- ReA generally can affect people at any age, but mean age of onset is between 25 and 35 years.

Table 7.7 The characteristics of Reactive Arthritis (I)

Causative organism*	Incidence of ReA in those infected	HLA B27 frequency	%patients developing ReA within 30 days of infection
Campylobacter jejuni	1–5%**	72%	85%
Salmonella Typhimurium enteritidis, Paratyphi B and C and other Salmonella	1–14%	84%	94%
Shigella S. flexneri/sonnei/dystenteriae	1%	80%	92%
Chlamydia trachomatis	1%	80%	88%
Yersinia enterocolitica O3, O8, O9 or *Yersinia pseudotuberculosis*	5–33%	75%	81%

*Though described as case reports or small series, ReA following *Chlamydia pneumoniae*, *Chlamydia Psittaci*, *Ureaplasma urealyticum* are not included here as extensive data are not available.

CHAPTER 7 **The spondylarthropathies**

- ReA affects a number of musculoskeletal structures, but can also be systemic disease and cause cardiac lesions.
- *Yersinia* ReA may mimic sarcoidosis (both cause periostitis and EN).
- Aortic ring dilatation and incompetence is a rare, late, but important feature.

Key features in history
- Inflammatory-type back or lower limb symptoms within 6 weeks of relevant infection.
- Patients may report toe swelling or refer to 'sausage toe' (?dactylitis).
- A history of enteric symptoms is easy to elicit – diarrhoea usually profuse – except in *Yersinia* ReA where symptoms may be mild.
- Obtaining a full genitourinary history may require sensitive enquiry and an explanation of the relevance of questioning beforehand.

Key features on examination
- Common features: monoarticular joint selling; plantar fasciitis, positive sacroiliac stress tests, enthesitis mainly in lower limbs.
- Keratoderma and pustulosis on palms and soles of feet.
- Balanitis in urogenital ReA.
- EN in *Yersinia* infection – tender subcutaneous swelling or patches of soft-tissue tenderness often in lower limbs often with overlying skin erythema.

Co-morbidities
All SpA features can occur: psoriaform rashes, diarrhoea, uveitis. *Chlamydia* particularly has a number of non-rheumatological co-morbidities including pelvic symptoms, dyspareunia, urethral irritation, and infertility.
- Keratoderma begins on palms or soles as pustules. They become horny crusts and can become confluent. Clinically and microscopically they are difficult to discriminate from pustular psoriasis.
- Circinate balanitis is painless. Erythema of the glans penis occasionally ulcerates.
- Erythema nodosum is associated with *Yersinia*.

Investigations
Laboratory
- ↑ESR, CRP, and IgA. But RF and ANA are negative.
- Urogenital smear – often negative despite suspicion of *Chlamydia* infection.
- Urinalysis can be positive for leucocytes (sterile pyuria).
- Antibodies to relevant organism (>2 SD above upper limit of reference interval IgG + either ↑IgA or ↑IgM) might be suggestive of diagnosis in the presence of inflammatory acute/subacute back pain, oligoarthritis or enthesitis, and evidence or suspicion of recent preceding urogenital or enteric infection.

Table 7.8 The characteristics of reactive arthritis (II)

Clinical features		Outcomes
Peripheral arthritis	Large joint – lower limb synovitis typically non-erosive; dactylitis 16%;	Average duration 4–5 months
		Up to 70% of C trachomatis ReA patients develop recurrent arthritic bouts
		Chronic recurrent arthritis 15–30% on average
		Overall small minority get erosive disease requiring long-term immunosuppressants.
		Increased severity and duration in those HLA B27+
Limb enthesopathy	Heel pain, Achilles' or patella ligament insertional pain (30%)	Unknown. Enthesopathy likely to be part of chronic musculoskeletal condition.
		Increased severity and duration in those HLA B27+
Axial inflammatory symptoms	Sacroiliitis 14–49%; spondylitis 12–26%; pelvic enthesopathy	Increased severity and duration in those HLA B27+
Eye disease	Conjunctivitis (35%); iritis (5%); keratitis; corneal ulceration; episcleritis; retrobulbar neuritis; hyphema.	Conjunctivitis occurs in the majority of *Salmonella*, *Shigella* and *Campylobacter* patients, is often mild and missed.
Gastrointestinal	Diarrhoea; lesions resemble Crohn's/ UC on ileocolonoscopy or biopsy.	Lesions can occur even in post-urethritis ReA (25%).
		The longer the duration of diarrhoea the greater the chance of ReA.
		Gut inflammation can be subclinical with *Yersinia*.
		Chronic ReA following *Salmonella* or *Shigella* infection occurs in 20% and <5% following *Yersinia*
Genitourinary	Urethral pain and discharge; prostatitis; haemorrhagic cystitis; non-specific cervicitis ± bleeding/abdo pain; proteinuria, microhaematuria or aseptic pyuria	Almost exclusively occurs following Chlamydia trachomatis infection though sterile urethritis can occur in some cases of post-enteric ReA.
		Chronic ReA following *Chlamydia* ReA in 17%.
		In post-urethritis ReA about 50% can get abnormalities on urine dipstick testing.
Mucocutaneous lesions	Keratoderma; palmar pustolosis; circinate balanitis (post-C trachomatis); oral ulcers; erythema nodosum (*Yersinia* ReA); hyperkeratotic nails	Mucocutaneous lesions are common in all ReA types.
Cardiac	Aortic valve disease; conduction defects	Symptomatic aortic valve disease rare and a late complication. ECG abnormalities in 14% patients.

- Clinical utility of serum serological tests is modest; chiefly a consequence of suboptimal specificity.
- In enteric ReA, stool culture often unhelpful by the time patients present with musculoskeletal features.
- HLA B27 often positive in severe or chronic ReA cases.
- Consider joint aspiration to rule out infection or crystal-induced monoarthritis.
- Consider screening for HIV, syphilis and gonococcus in patients with evidence of C trachomatis infection.

Imaging
Radiographs
Sacroiliitis: frequently unilateral. Enthesophytes (e.g. plantar fascia or Achilles' tendon insertion) can appear eroded (compared with smooth bone texture as in DISH enthesophytes).

MR
High signal lesions on T2-weighted sequences at SIJs and sites of entheses (peripherally) or showing joint synovitis, but also in spine disease, the corners of vertebrae (Romanus lesions) as per AS.

^{99m}Tc-MDP scintigraphy
Characteristic tracer distribution particularly in lower limbs seen in severe cases. Mild cases often not highlighted by scintigraphy.

Differential diagnosis
- Acute SAPHO, PsA, Sarcoid, ESpA, atypical AS can mimic ReA, particularly where enthesitis is prominent.
- Crystal arthritis, gonococcus arthritis, Lyme disease, and coeliac disease are associated with monoarthritis.

Treatment
Patient information/advice
- If no previous screening then counselling regarding genital testing of sexual partners and HIV testing important where Chlamydia infection suspected.
- Patient information booklets (e.g. arc in the UK).
- Counselling about potential chronicity.

Early disease management
C trachomatis infection should be treated irrespective of symptoms or arthritis. Sexual partners should be traced and treated as well.
- Antibiotics may be useful in urogenital ReA, but weaker evidence exists for enteric ReA.
- An early 3-month treatment course of lymecycline for urogenital ReA can substantially reduce the risk of chronic/recurrent ReA in patients and development of ReA in partners, but in the long-term may not change the natural history of disease.
- Doxycycline for 10 days may be as effective as giving it for 4 months to reduce the effects of ReA.
- Long-term ciprofloxacin provided no benefit to ReA patients in a RCT (Sieper et al., 1999).
- Antibiotics probably make little difference to the outcome of Yersinia ReA.
- Pain control – NSAIDs in full regular dosage and aspirate swollen joints where possible and consider intra-articular glucocorticoid (GC) injection.
- May need to culture joint fluid if infection suspected initially but steroid joint injection useful.
- Input from relevant (eye, sexual health, skin, or gastrointestinal) specialist especially medical ophthalmologist for slit-lamp exam to exclude uveitis.

Immunosupression
- Oral GCs, e.g. 0.25–0.5 mg/kg/day initially; can be used empirically in severe cases. GCs are arguably more effective for the peripheral compared with the axial musculoskeletal lesions.
- In chronic cases, sulphasalazine (SZP; 2 g/day in bd or tds doses) has been shown in a RCT to be effective at controlling ReA (Clegg et al., 1996).
- Although methotrexate (MTX) is used frequently and is associated with some efficacy in ReA, no RCTs exist.
- Chronic ReA has been treated successfully with anti-TNFα. No formal therapeutic trial has been done.

Prognosis and natural history (Table 7.9)
- ReA is usually mild and self-limiting (average duration 3–5 months), although can follow relapsing-remitting or aggressive chronic courses (up to 15%).
- About 75% of cases are in complete remission by 2 years.
- In enteric infection triggered ReA, diarrhoea is usually short-lived though can last a month – self-limiting in the majority of cases.
- Although some enteric infections can persist, chronic troublesome symptoms are unusual.
- In the majority of people, the arthritis is non-erosive. The duration of arthritis varies.
- The presence of HLA B27 is linked to more severe disease, higher likelihood of sacroiliitis, and extra-articular manifestations and persistent arthropathy.
- The greater the number of factors below, the worse the prognosis: male gender; onset <16 years; family history of SpA; hip arthritis; an ESR>30 mm/h; poor NSAID efficacy; stiff lumbar spine; dactylitis

Table 7.9 Long-term (10-20y) prognosis of ReA: arthritis (from Colmegna et al 2004, with permission)

	%of patients with end-point after infection with:			
	Yersinia	Salmonella	Shigella	C trachomatis
Recovered	45	40	20	30
Arthralgia	20	20	NA*	68
Recurrent arthritis	6	22	18	38
Chronic arthritis	4	19	19	17
AS	15	12	14	26
Radiological synovitis	20	14	32	49

*Data not available

Current controversies
Diagnostic issues
- How many other infections can trigger ReA?
- Is infection with any Chlamydia organism or Ureaplasma urealyticum a risk for (SpA-like HLA B27-related) ReA?
- Is mild ReA – manifest for example just by self-limiting inflammatory low back symptoms or enthesitis – under-recognized?

Management and treatment issues
The use of antibiotics remains controversial.
- There may be short-term gains from treatment at

the time of urogenital ReA presentation, but type and duration of antibiotics is debated.
- Do antibiotics alter the long-term outlook of ReA?
- Whether different antibiotics/regimes given for initial enteric or urogenital infection vary in their ability to reduce ReA incidence, severity or chronicity.
- Is MTX more efficacious than SZP in chronic ReA?
- Will leflunomide be efficacious in ReA?
- The role of anti-TNFα needs to be defined in severe chronic ReA.

Resources

Guidelines
The Arthritis Research Campaign (arc). Available at: www.arc.org; Information booklets and other disease-related information for physicians.

Patient resources/organizations
Managing Reactive Arthritis. Article by A Toivanen. Available at: www.rheumatology.oxfordjournals.org/cgi/content/full/39/2/117.

Internet sites
Webpage on Spondylarthritis American College of Rheumatology. Available at: www.rheumatology.org/public/factsheets/

ICD10 codes
M02.1   Post-dysenteric arthropathy
M02.3   Reiter's disease

References

Altman LK. Experts re-examine Dr Reiter, his syndrome, his Nazi past. *Science. New York Times*, March 7th 2000.

Colmegna I, Cuchacovich R, Espinoza LR. HLA B27- associated reactive arthritis: pathogenetic and clinical considerations. *Clin Microbiol Rev* 2004; **17**: 348–69.

Clegg DO, Reda DJ, Abdellatif M. Comparison of sulfasalazine and placebo for the treatment of axial and peripheral articular manifestations of the seronegative spondylarthropathies. *Arthritis Rheum* 1999; **42**: 2325–9.

Kaipanen-Seppanen O, Ano K. Incidence of chronic inflammatory disease in Finland in 1995. *J Rheumatol* 2000; **27**: 94–100.

Keat A. Reiter's syndrome and reactive arthritis in perspective. *N Engl J Med* 1983; **309**: 1606–15.

Pacheco-Tena C, Burgos-Vargas R, Vázquez-Mellado J, Cazarín J, Pérez-Díaz JA. A proposal for the classification of patients for clinical and experimental studies on reactive arthritis. *J Rheumatol* 1999; **26**: 1338–46.

Pope JE, Krizova A, Garq AX, Thiessen-Philbrook H, Ouimet JM. Campylobacter reactive arthritis: a systematic review. *Semin Arthritis Rheum* 2007; Mar 12. Epub.

Press N, Fyfe M, Bowie W, Kelly M. Clinical and microbiological follow-up of an outbreak of *Yersinia pseudotuberculosis* serotype Ib. *Scand J Infect Dis* 2001; **33**: 523–6.

Sieper J, Fendler C, Laitko S, *et al*. No benefit of long-term ciprofloxacin treatment in patients with ReA and undifferentiated oligoarthritis: a 3-month multicenter double-blind, randomised placebo-controlled study. *Arthritis Rheum* 1999; 42: 1386–96.

Enteropathic spondylarthropathy

Definition
The commonest extra-intestinal manifestations of inflammatory bowel disease (IBD) are musculoskeletal. The condition has been variably referred to as enteric arthritis, IBD arthropathy, enteric SpA, Crohn's, or colitis-related arthritis.

Epidemiology
The reports of SpA in IBD have varied owing to definition of SpA and IBD case ascertainment but have suggested:
- SpA prevalence of about 20% in IBD patients.
- Dactylitis, enthesitis, isolated (often asymptomatic) sacroiliitis, and other SpA like lesions all appear to occur in up to 35%.
- Peripheral arthritis prevalence 5–20% in IBD.

Aetiology and pathophysiology
Genetic factors
- Where AS is clearly defined in IBD patients, an association with HLA B27 (50–70% patients) clearly exists.
- HLA B27 frequency may not be increased, however, where there is peripheral arthropathy alone.
- Mutations in the CARD15/NOD2 gene confers susceptibility for Crohn's disease, but not AS.

Environment
- Intestinal bacteria may have an important role in triggering EspA in Crohn's disease.
- Compromised iliocaecal integrity is associated with increased musculoskeletal symptoms in IBD and it has been hypothesized that gut (?luminal/?entero-adhesive) bacteria may play a role in generating arthritis in IBD.

Immunopathology
- The immune response in Crohn's disease suggests CD4 Th1 cells become activated against *normal* gut luminal bacterial flora.
- In Crohn's mucosa there is increased Il-12, Il-6, Il-15, Il-18, TNFα and IFNγ with apoptosis-resistant Th1 cells, activated macrophages and granulomata. There's a paucity of data directly linking enteral immunopathology with immune processes in joints/entheses in ESpA.

Tissue pathophysiology
- The peripheral arthritis in IBD has not been adequately characterized to know whether lesions are predominantly synovitic or enthesitic.
- Axial SpA features in ESpA appear similar to lesions seen in other SpAs though this assertion is based on imaging, rather than direct tissue studies.

Clinical features
Key clinical features
- Various subtypes of IBD-related arthropathy have been described. Incomplete case ascertainment, suboptimal clinical assessments and insufficient confirmatory imaging have hampered clinical pattern recognition studies.
- A careful review of studies suggests SpA features are consistently conspicuous in IBD patients.
- USpA can precede a diagnosis of IBD in 50% patients.
- ESpA symptoms and disease activity do not always correlate well with the activity of the IBD.

> **Key clinical features in ESpA**
> *Musculoskeletal*
> - Inflammatory spinal pain.
> - Alternating buttock pains.
> - Enthesopathy.
> - Anterior chest wall pain.
> - Dactylitis.
> - Peripheral arthritis/arthralgia.
> - Sacroiliitis (most commonly unilateral).
>
> *Non musculoskeletal extra-intestinal*
> - Aphthous stomatitis.
> - Psoriasis.
> - Erythema nodosum.
> - Uveitis.
> - Urethritis/cervicitis.

Key features in history
- In patients without a prior diagnosis of IBD, a history of abdominal pain, recurrent diarrhoea (especially at night), fever, malaise/fatigue, and passing blood per rectum is consistent with a diagnosis of IBD.
- Aphthous ulceration and fatigue are early IBD features.
- As with other SpAs, a history of inflammatory spinal pains, buttock or anterior chest wall pains or previous insertional tendonitis (enthesitis) might point toward ESpA in patients with established IBD.

Key features on examination
Sacroiliitis stress tests (see USpA chapter), and checking for dactylitis and enthesitis are important aspects.

Co-morbidities
All SpA related features can occur in association with IBD and ESpA (e.g. uveitis, psoriasis).
- IBD-related features can occur and include mouth ulcers, erythema nodosum, pyoderma gangrenosum.
- Bone fragility/osteoporosis is a common complication of IBD. Fracture incidence in IBD is markedly higher than the general population.
- Hypovitaminosis-D is common in the general population, associated with GC use and can lead to myalgia, suboptimal calcium absorption from the gut and secondary hyperparathyroidism (SHPT).
- Malabsorption in IBD can include folate, B12, and calcium deficiency. The latter causes SHPT.

Investigations
Laboratory
The interpretation of acute phase response and anaemia requires interpretation of the activity of any IBD. ESpA symptoms can be prominent with relatively little or absent acute phase response.

Tests to rule out malabsorption may be necessary (e.g. B12, folate). Detailed bone biochemistry is sensible (calcium, phosphate, ALP, Vit-D, PTH, Mg). Persistent low Vit-D can cause non-specific musculoskeletal aches.

Imaging
- Pelvis radiographs may show sacroiliitis, osteitis pubis or enthesopathy (although enthesopathic features in ESpA have not been highlighted in the literature).

- Many radiographic features recognized in ESpA are common to all SpAs.
- CT may disclose sacroiliitis in about a third of IBD patients; almost twice the detection rate with radiographs.
- Secondary hypertrophic osteoarthropathy is recognized, although unusual in adults and children with IBD.

Typical features on radiographs in patients with ESpA
- *General*: enthesopathic erosions and enthesophytes.
- *Pelvis*: sacroiliitis, osteitis pubis, destructive hip arthritis (symmetric joint space loss, cystic lesions, but distinguish from osteonecrosis).
- *Spine*: vertebral squaring; marginal and para-marginal syndesmophytes; discitis.
- *Peripheries*: oligoarticular synovitis; radiographic features often lack specificity.

- Discitis presents a diagnostic dilemma. Sterile discitis is a feature of SpAs; however, there is increased risk of septic lesions in IBD. Imaging features might not always distinguish. Biopsy should be considered.

Differential diagnosis
- Vertebral osteoporotic fracture. IBD patients previously treated with GCs are at high risk.
- Inflammatory-type chronic back pain symptoms may occur occasionally with other disorders (e.g. discogenic pain, axial CPPDD disease, etc.).
- Hypovitaminosis-D/osteomalacia (GC-induced or constitutional) and calcium (poor absorption), can cause non-specific musculoskeletal pains.
- Widespread pain in IBD has been reported to be due to fibromyalgia (FM), although studies have not assessed patients for enthesitis. A recent study found no evidence for an association with FM.

Treatment
Objectives of disease management
Liaise closely with a gastroenterologist.
Control pain and consider modifying immunosuppressants if peripheral articular symptoms are severe or disabling or there is erosive/deforming joint disease.

Physical therapies
As with AS, ESpA patients with inflammatory spinal pains may benefit from back physiotherapy, which should be used judiciously where vertebral fracture has occurred.

Control of pain/inflammation
NSAID can aggravate IBD and worsen anaemia.
- Joint fluid aspiration and GC injection is a relatively simple, effective, and overall relatively safe option.
- Serial pamidronate infusions may help ESpA-related spinal osteitis pain and can treat GC-induced osteoporosis. Ibandronate 3 mg iv every 3 months and zoledronate 5 mg iv yearly are untested in this respect.

Immunosupression
In keeping with other SpAs the usual immunosupressants associated with efficacy in ESpA are more beneficial for peripheral compared with axial symptoms.
- GCs, sulphasalazine (SZP), and methotrexate (MTX) may be efficacious. None have been tested in a RCT.

- Azathioprine, although used frequently for severe IBD, and cyclophosphamide, and occasionally for severe IBD, are not recognized as effective for ESpA.
- Mesalazine has weak activity against ESpA, and SZP is not as effective for IBD as mesalazine and has more side effects. If ESpA is the main problem and the IBD in remission, it is reasonable to swap mesalazine for SZP.

Current controversies
Diagnostic issues
- In early ESpA-sine-IBD, which logically would be classified as USpA under ESSG criteria, are there predictors of the development of IBD?
- Uncertainty still remains as to the prevalence of ESpA in IBD. For example, SIJ disease is often asymptomatic. What might the prevalence of isolated enthesitis be?
- The role of MR needs clarification in early diagnosis of ESpA – as is the case in other SpAs.

Management/treatment issues
There are no RCTs of SZP or methotrexate in ESpA. The pharmacological management of ESpA is necessarily complicated by the presence of IBD:
- NSAIDs can aggravate IBD symptomatically or potentially disturb its control by medications;
- Mesalazine, often used by gastro-enterologists for the IBD, is not known to control musculoskeletal features. An intention to use SZP or MTX for the latter requires close liaison with the gastroenterologist.
- The worth of MTX or SZP is tricky to evaluate where GCs might be frequently used for the IBD. GCs will provide a partial therapeutic effect on ESpA lesions.

Resources
Guidelines and patient information
Webpage on SpA: American College of Rheumatology. Available at: www.rheumatology.org/public/factsheets/

ICD10 codes
M07.4*   Arthropathy in Crohn's disease
M07.5*   Arthropathy in ulcerative colitis
M46.9   Inflammatory spondylopathy, unspecified

References
MacDonald TT, DiSabatino A, Gordon JN. Immunopathogenesis of Crohn's disease. *J Paren Enter Nutr* 2005; **29**: S118–25.

Mielants H, Veys EM, Goemaere S, Cuvelier C, De Vos M. A prospective study of patients with SpA with special reference to HLA B27 and to gut histology. *J Rheumatol* 1993; **20**: 1353–8.

Orchard TR, Jewell DP. The importance of ileocaecal integrity in the arthritic complications of Crohn's Disease. *Infl Bowel Dis* 1999; **5**: 92–7.

Orchard TR, Wordsworth BP, Jewell DP. Peripheral arthropathies in inflammatory bowel disease: their articular distribution and natural history. *Gut* 1998; **42**: 387–91.

Palm O, Moum B, Jahnsen J, Gran JT. Fibromyalgia and chronic widespread pain in patients with inflammatory bowel disease: a cross-sectional population survey. *J Rheumatol* 2001; **28**: 590–4.

Palm O, Moum B, Ongre A, Gran JT. Prevalence of AS and other SpAs among patients with inflammatory bowel disease: a population study. *J Rheumatol* 2002; **29**: 511–15.

Resnick D. Enteropathic arthropathies arthritis. In: Resnick D (ed.). *Diagnosis of Bone and Joint Disorders*, 4th edn. Philadelphia: WB Saunders Co, 2002, 1127–55.

Salvarani C, Vlachonikolis IG, van der Heijde DM, et al. Musculoskeletal manifestations in a population-based cohort of inflammatory bowel disease patients. *Scand J Gastroenterol* 2001; **36**:1307–13.

Juvenile spondylarthropathy/enthesitis-related arthritis

Spondylarthropathy (SpA) in children can exist as a discrete clinical entity (e.g. juvenile AS or arthritis associated with psoriasis or inflammatory bowel disease), but it is often not well differentiated. The term enthesitis related arthritis (ERA) was introduced in 1995 as a category in the ILAR classification of childhood arthritis. It defines a type of JIA, which has variously been referred to previously as seronegative enthesitis arthritis (SEA) syndrome or juvenile spondylarthropathy (JSpA).

Definition and classification criteria

The previous classifications of JSpA can be encompassed under the new ERA sub-classification of juvenile arthritis (ILAR classification. See p. 352).

Revised ERA Classification Criteria 2004
Arthritis or enthesitis + at least two of: • Presence or history of sacroiliac tenderness or inflammatory lumbosacral pain. • HLA B27 positive. • Family history of HLA B27-related disease. • Acute anterior uveitis. • Onset of arthritis in a male after his 6th birthday. If any of the following are present then the child is excluded from the category of ERA: • Presence of IgM rheumatoid factor on 2 occasions at least 3 months apart. • Presence of systemic JIA. • Psoriasis or history of psoriasis in child or first-degree relative.

- Although the adult ESSG SpA classification criteria have been applied to JSpA with a sensitivity of about 75% and specificity of over 90%, childhood SpA does not always fit adult disease classification criteria.
- Enthesitis-related arthritis (ERA) may 'capture' for definition the diagnosis of children with undifferentiated and early forms of SpA and includes children who might previously have been considered to have SEA syndrome.
- The overlap in descriptions of classification is illustrated by JPsA, a heterogenous clinical entity. In adolescents JPsA has features typically associated with a SpA – male gender, axial skeleton involvement, HLA B27-associated. In young children, most affected are girls, there is an association with antinuclear antibody and asymptomatic uveitis.

The characteristics of JSpA (/ERA)
• Males > females (up to 9:1). • Late onset age usually > 10 years old. • Family history of SpA. • Axial skeleton involvement – often absent at outset. • Sacroiliitis. • Arthritis of lower limb joints. • Enthesitis – particularly around the knee and foot. • Frequently HLA B27 positive. • Acute uveitis. • Inflammatory bowel disease. • Preceding (few days to some weeks) gut infection (*Yersinia, Salmonella, Shigella, Campylobacter*). • Negative ANA and rheumatoid factor.

JPsA is considered by many a separate entity to JSpA-related (ERA) conditions in children. This is not unlike the situation in adults where some believe PsA sits slightly uneasily within the SpA spectrum of disease. The situation is clearly not clear in adults and children! However, it is accepted that enthesitis/enthesopathy is a lesion associated with psoriasis *in adults*. Whether the presence or absence of enthesitis is a discriminating feature between PsA in adults and children remains to be seen. There are criteria for diagnosing PsA in children, which retain some utility, though do not list enthesopathy among the criteria for diagnosis.

Vancouver 1989 criteria for the diagnosis of JPsA[a]
Definite JPsA Arthritis[b] with typical psoriatic rash *or* Arthritis[b] with 3 of these 4 minor criteria: • Dactylitis. • Nail pitting[c] or onycholysis. • Psoriasis-like rash. • Psoriasis family history (1st/2nd degree relatives). **Probable JPsA** Arthritis[b] with 2 of the 4 minor criteria:

[a]Criteria need not be present simultaneously.
[b]Defined as joint swelling of ≥2 of the following: limited range of motion of joints, pain on movement, or tenderness persisting for at least 6 weeks.
[c]Defined as ≥2 pits on the fingernails at any examination.

Epidemiology

Data on more than 16 000 paediatric patients from two North American disease registries, suggested that of 41% who were registered as having musculoskeletal disease, a third (12% of total) had been diagnosed with a SpA.

- Juvenile AS (JAS) cannot be classified with conventional adult AS criteria (axial disease appears late, reference ranges of metrology indices for age are not available and imaging is often imprecise). Many children with early JAS can be classified under other JIA definitions.
- Based on the percentage of adults who had juvenile onset of adult AS it has been estimated JAS has a prevalence of 12–33/100 000 in Caucasians. In other racial groups, with a higher prevalence of HLA B27, JAS may be present in up to 40–150/100 000.
- JAS occurs in males > females (5:1 to 9:1) mainly late in childhood/adolescent years.
- Reactive arthritis as a distinct entity is recognized, particularly sexually acquired reactive arthritis in teenagers, although no major prevalence estimates exist.
- SpA is the most common non-intestinal manifestation of inflammatory bowel disease (IBD) in children (10–20%). Axial disease occurs only in about 25% of children with both IBD and musculoskeletal manifestations.
- As with adults, juvenile psoriatic arthropathy (JPsA) is a heterogenous entity. Using the 1989 Vancouver criteria for JPsA the prevalence is thought to be about 10–15/100 000 children.
- ILAR definitions of JPsA restrict the diagnosis of PsA in childhood compared with Vancouver.

CHAPTER 7 The spondylarthropathies

Aetiology and pathophysiology

Genetic factors
The frequent finding of SpAs in families suggests a genetic basis for the disease. The relationship between disease and HLA B27 is as striking in children as it is in adults.
- No distinct B27 subtypes have been found to segregate with JAS, or other JSpA or juvenile onset of adult SpA compared with adult disease.
- HLA DR8 is been linked with JAS – it has been found in 39% of AS patients with onset <16 years compared with 20% of those with adult-onset AS.
- The role of HLA B27 in pathophysiology is discussed in the chapter on ankylosing spondylitis.

Environmental
- Preceding infection with *Yersinia enterocolitica* (serotypes 3 or 9 especially), *Campylobacter jejuni*, *Salmonella typhimurium* or *enteriditis*, and *Shigella flexneri* can cause reactive arthritis in children, as well as adults.
- *Chlamydia trachomatis* as a cause of reactive arthritis in adolescents should not be overlooked. They may well be sexually active!
- It is possible many children classified as having ERA may have reactive arthritis.
- There is some evidence that mycoplasma and ureaplasma infections can trigger HLA B27-related reactive arthritis in children and adolescents.
- *Klebsiella* has been linked to JAS as in adults.

Clinical features

Key features in history
Though ERA can occur in younger children, typically in JAS symptoms develop after the age of 10 years and frequently there is a family history of SpA.
- Pain and stiffness of or around one or two often-lower limb joints can indicate JSpA/ERA. Symptoms are unlikely to be specific for ERA, SEA, JAS or JPsA.
- Inflammatory back pain is often not a prominent part of early JAS or JSpAs.
- Heel pain is an important symptom and may indicate enthesitis, although this may occur in any JSpA.
- A family history of psoriasis in a close relative may be a relevant feature when considering a diagnosis of JPsA.
- Recurrent abdominal pain and episodic diarrhoea can denote associated inflammatory bowel disease.
- Reactive arthritis (oligoarticular joint, back or enthesial pains) is often preceded (days to weeks) by enteric symptoms – usually mild, but can be severe and cause acute abdomen in an older child.
- Lumbosacral and/or sacroiliac pain is present in about 25% cases of post-*Yersinia* reactive arthritis.

Key features on examination
Enthesial tenderness perhaps with soft tissue swelling, particularly of knee and foot structures, is the hallmark lesion in children with SpAs.
- Small joint and wrist disease may discriminate JPsA from other JIA subtypes.
- Look for lower limb joint synovitis, dactylitis of the toes, and irritable hips on passive joint movements. (see Plate 21)
- If chronic or severe, enthesitis can lead to bony overgrowth and/or premature closure at epiphyses.
- Psoriasis is often absent in JPsA; may be nail pitting.
- Abdominal tenderness may be non-specific, but inflammatory bowel disease may need excluding.
- Erythema nodosum is associated with inflammatory bowel disease and *Yersinia* infection.
- Detailed ophthalmic examination is important in all JIA and JSpA/ERA patients. Uveitis may be asymptomatic. Unlike in adults, uveitis is not specific for SpA in children.
- Unlike in adults, children with JSpA/ERA have few signs of restricted spinal movement.

Co-morbidities
- Psoriasis, inflammatory bowel disease, uveitis can be associated with any SpA.
- JSpA/ERA might be misdiagnosed as chronic pain syndrome. There may be variable and probably overall suboptimal appreciation of the occurrence of enthesitis as a manifestation of JSpA/ERA in children.
- Arthropathy is the commonest extra-intestinal co-morbidity in inflammatory bowel disease (20% children).

Investigations

Laboratory
- An elevated acute phase response can be detected, although it is often modest, and often in early disease, markers are normal.
- Anaemia is usually mild, and if severe, underlying IBD should be suspected.
- HLA B27 is associated with JAS (the differentiated disease) in about 90% patients.
- RF and ANA are negative.
- Serology for *Yersinia*, *Salmonella*, and *Shigella*, where antecedent gastrointestinal infection are suspected as a cause of reactive arthritis (JSpA/ERA or SEA syndrome also).
- *Yersinia* is seldom identified in stool cultures, but *Salmonella* and *Shigella* can be.

Imaging
- Radiographs are seldom helpful in making a diagnosis in early ERA; nevertheless, it is important to document baseline presence/absence of erosions and spur formation may be present.
- Chronic or severe enthesitis lesions show characteristic enthesial erosions, calcification, hyperostosis, accelerated growth, or premature epiphyseal closure.
- If there are symptoms or signs of SI joint involvement these should be imaged. MRI scans are preferred to avoid radiation to pelvis, and can be helpful, but care must be taken not to over-interpret changes associated with the normal metabolic activity of growing bones.

Differential diagnosis
The differential diagnosis is wide and general principles should be considered.
- A working knowledge of JIA classifications and their overlap is required.
- Establishing the family history with regard to psoriasis is important in linking the arthritis to JSpA and differentiating the condition from ERA (see above).
- Uveitis screening is relevant for all children with arthritis, whatever the likely diagnosis.

Treatment
The management plan for children and adolescents with JSpA/ERA, should be multidisciplinary and address the many facets of disease.

Multidisciplinary approach to managing JSpA: addressing the many patient needs
(see also pp. 352–358)
- Psychological impact of disease.
- Social impact of disease.
- Vocational aspirations.
- Occupational therapy benefits.
- Physiotherapy benefits.
- Judicious use of medications.
- Timely intervention with surgery.

- The mainstay of pharmacological treatment is NSAIDs and judicious use of intra-articular glucocorticoid injections. If arthritis/enthesitis persists then it would be reasonable to consider sulphasalazine (25 mg/kg increased to 50 mg/kg/day if tolerated).
- Methotrexate (10–20 mg/m^2) would offer a second-line option for failure to improve on sulphasalazine.
- Glucocorticoids are used for severe enthesitis, in short courses for 4–6 weeks (oral: 0.5–1 mg/kg/day). Occasional intravenous pulses of methylprednisolone (10–30 mg/kg/day) can be used instead.
- Large RCT trials of sulphasalazine or methotrexate in children with JSpA/ERA are lacking, however.
- There is no evidence that antibiotics significantly affect the severity or course of reactive arthritis in children.
- There is no evidence that one NSAID is superior to another in treating JSpAs/ERA.
- Intra-articular or peri-enthesial glucocorticoid injections are used to treat individual joints. In young children a light general anaesthetic is required (avoids distress, maintains trust, facilitates further investigations/treatment). Older children may tolerate joint injections using good local anaesthesia.
- Methotrexate is an obvious choice for controlling both the joint and skin disease of JPsA.

Prognosis
Identification of factors that might dictate progression of undifferentiated JSpA/ERA or the condition diagnosed as SEA, to a differentiated SpA, is of great importance. The main difficulty in identifying such factors, however, is that axial features can take many years to develop in juvenile disease. Long-term studies of JSpA/ERA are limited.
- Persistent severe disease of at least 5 joints in the first year of disease is a risk factor for progression to AS.
- Early axial symptoms/lesions may define a subset of children who progress to AS (or develop the differentiated form of it from the outset).
- Monitoring of ERA closely is warranted in HLA B27 positive children – long-term problems are more likely.
- Involvement of the hip joint in JAS before the age of 19 years was a significant predictor for the need of hip replacement in studies done many years ago. This underscores the importance of screening for hip disease, and considering treatment with sulphasalazine or methotrexate in adolescents affected.

Resources
British Society for paediatric and Adolescent Rheumatology (BSPAR) www.bspar.org.uk for guidelines on medication and eye screening in childhood arthritis.

Guidelines
Paediatric Rheumatology European Society (PReS). For professionals. Available at: www.pres.org.uk

Patient organizations/resources
PRINTO. Resource for parents of children with rheumatic diseases. Available at: www.printo.it/pediatric-rheumatology/. This is a useful site with information about various paediatric rheumatic diseases and their treatment, weblinks to similar European organizations and individuals who can be contacted by parents of JSpA children.

ICD10 codes
M08.1   Juvenile AS
M08.9   Juvenile arthritis, unspecified

References
Creemers MCW, Franssen MJ, van de Putte LB, Gribnau FW, van Riel PL. Methotrxate in severe ankylosing spondylitis: an open study. *J Rheumatol* 1995; **22**: 1104–7.

Gensler L, Davis JC. Recognition and treatment of juvenile-onset spondyloarthritis. *Curr Opin Rheumatol* 2006; **18**: 507–11.

Heumer C, Malleson PN, Cabral DA, Huemer M, Falger J, Zidek T, Petty RE. Patterns of joint involvement at onset differentiate oligoarticular juveile psoriatic arthritis from pauciarticular juveil rheumatoid arthritis. *J Rheumatol* 2002; **29**: 1531–5.

Pepmueller PH, Moore TL. Juvenile spondyloarthropathies. *Curr Opin Rheumatol* 2000; **12**: 269–73.

Petty RE, Southwood TR, Manners P, et al. International League of Associations for Rheumatology classification of juvenile idiopathic arthritis: second revision, Edmonton, 2001. *J Rheumatol* 2004; **31**: 390–2.

Prieur AM. Spondylarthropathies in childhood. *Ballieres Clin Rheumatol* 1998; **12**: 287–307.

Rosenberg AM, Petty RE. Spondyloarthropathies in children and adolescents. In: Calin A, Taurog JD (eds) *The Spondylarthritides*. Oxford: Oxford University Press, 1998, 113–27.

Saxena N, Misra R, Aggarwal A. Is the enthesitis-related arthritis subtype of JIA a form of chronic reactive arthritis. *Rheum (Ox)* 2006; **45**: 1129–32.

Southwood TR, Petty RE, Malleson PN, et al. Psoriatic arthritis in children. *Arthritis Rheum* 1989; **32**: 1007–13.

Suschke HJ. Die behandlung der juvenilen spondylarthritis umd der reactiven arthritis mit sulfasalzin. *Monats Kinderheilkunde* 1992; **140**: 658–60.

Toll ML, Lio P, Sundel RP, Nigrovic PA. Comparison of Vancouver and ILAR classification criteria for juvenile psoriatic arthritis. *Arthritis Rheum* 2007; **59**: 51–8.

Tse SM, Burgos-Vargas R, Laxer RM. Anti-tumour necrosis factor alpha blockade in the treatment of juveile spondylarthropathy. *Arthritis Rheum* 2005; **52**: 2103–8.

Vesikari T, Iso lauri E, Maki M. Clinical and laboratory features of *Yersinia*, *Campylobacter* and *Salmonella* infections in children. *Klin Padiatr* 1985; **197**: 25–9.

CHAPTER 7 The spondylarthropathies

SAPHO (Le Syndrome Acné, Pustulose, Hyperostose, Ostéite)

Definition
A number of terms have been used to describe a spectrum of features that consistently appear together in patients with acne/skin pustulosis and painful osteopathy particularly of the anterior chest wall. The commonest terms used in the literature are SAPHO, Acquired Hyperostosis Syndrome, pustulotic arthro-osteitis and sternocostoclavicular hyperostosis. Almost 50 synonyms have been used in the literature.
- Some previously-defined conditions may be part of the SAPHO spectrum of disease (e.g. recurrent multifocal osteomyelitis).
- In some publications, 'Synovitis' has been substituted for 'Le Syndrome', although it is unclear how deliberate a change this was in the name or an 'upgrading' of the name in light of features being increasingly recognized as part of the condition (following the early key French description (Chamot et al., 1987).
- The syndrome's original description can probably be credited to Köhler (Köhler et al., 1975).
- There is controversy whether SAPHO is part of the SpA group of conditions. There is reasonable evidence that enthesitis occurs and some evidence of triggering bacteria, but no known association with HLA B27.

Classification criteria
There are no validated classification criteria for SAPHO though diagnostic criteria were suggested in 1988 (Benhamou 1988).

Epidemiology
The condition could be rare, although mild disease and disease characterized by musculoskeletal lesions (not skin) alone is probably under-recognized.

Aetiology and pathphysiology
- SAPHO has been linked to skin lesion infection with *Propionibacterium acnes* in immunocompetent people.
- *P. acnes*, an anaerobe, has been cultured from intervertebral disc and sternal lesions.
- The immunopathology and tissue pathological changes in SAPHO are virtually unknown.

The principle features of SAPHO syndrome
- Anterior chest wall pain.
- Osteitis.
- Enthesopathy.
- Pustular skin lesions.
- Acneiform skin lesions.
- Hydradenitis.
- Hyperostosis.
- Within costal cartilages.
- Ankylosing axial arthritis of anterior chest wall.
- Spondylodiscitis.
- Synovitis.

Clinical features
- The most convincing combination of features are pustulosis or acneiform skin rash (acne fulminans, acne conglobata, or hidradenitis suppurativa) with pains and hyperostosis of anterior chest wall structures.
- Musculoskeletal lesions can occur before the skin lesions and, on the face of it, many lesions are similar to those seen in the SpA.
- Spondylodiscitis can be an associated lesion.

Key features in the history
- Patients often complain of recurrent pains of the anterior chest wall. There may be more persistent pains associated with obvious bony swelling.
- Pains are mainly axial. Synovitis of peripheral joints and limb bony lesions have been described, although are less usual than axial lesions.
- Discogenic back pain can be associated.
- A history of an acneiform or pustular skin rash is typical, but not invariable.
- Patients may often have accumulated different diagnoses or explanations for their symptoms from doctors or other healthcare workers. A chronic pain somatype therefore might be present (e.g. pain amplification, frustration, fatigue, disproportionate disability given an objective review of features, etc.).

Key features on examination
Musculoskeletal
- Bony swelling around manubrium, anterior costal cartilages, and sternum (look for asymmetry).
- Tenderness of bony swellings (above) and tenderness of other anterior chest wall structures, such as over the costoclavicular ligament (?enthesitis).
- Bony swelling and overlying tenderness anywhere else particularly on axial skeletal structures.
- Features of spondylodiscitis: focal or general back stiffness/poor mobility; increased focal spinal pain in forward flexion of segment notably.

Skin
- Most cases and case series have been reported with prominent acne lesions or obvious (palmoplantar or psoriatic) pustulosis.
- Skin lesions may not be concordant with the manifestation or detection of musculoskeletal lesions.
- Hidradenitis may be an associated feature, but has not been a consistent part of all descriptions of the condition in the literature.
- Attempts to link the condition aetiopathologically to just one or two proprionibacterium species (infections or skin lesion 'colonization') might be too restrictive.

Investigations
Laboratory
- Laboratory investigations are invariably normal although modest increases in ESR, CRP, or immunoglobulins can occur. Systemic neutrophilia has been reported.
- There is no known association with HLA B27, but genetic association studies in large well-defined disease populations have not been done.

Imaging
Scintigraphy
- Typical patterns of abnormality have been shown using ^{99m}Tc-MDP scintigraphy. Intense tracer localizing to structures around the upper sternum, viewed also from posterior chest acquisitions, discriminate abnormal scans from false positive images.

CHAPTER 7 **The spondylarthropathies**

- Typical tracer uptake in manubrium and anterior part of the first ribs is referred to as 'the bullhorn sign'. This is thought to be relatively specific for SAPHO.

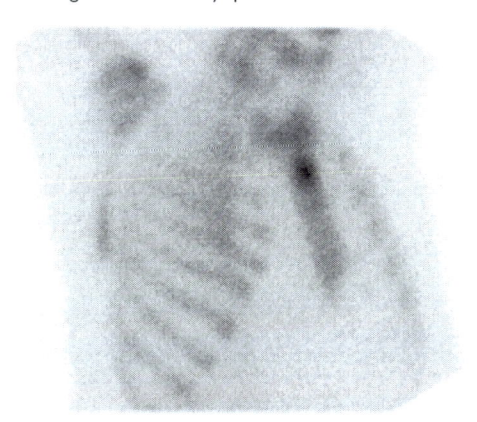

Figure 7.11 ^{99m}Tc-MDP abnormality in SAPHO showing high tracer uptake in manubrium and manubriosternal joint.

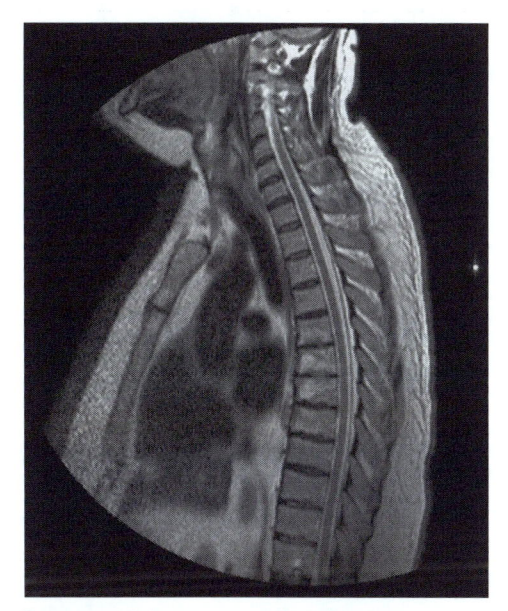

Figure 7.12 MR thoracic spine in SAPHO. Spondylodiscitis at contiguous levels. Note osteitis at manubriosternal joint.

Radiographs and CT
- Hyperostosis lesions are characterized by sclerosing bone remodelling and erosions.
- Radiographs can show abnormal cartilage ossification (e.g. costoclavicular ligament and anterior rib).
- CT may be useful to help discriminate hyperostotic SAPHO lesions from tumours and osteomyelitis.

MR
- SAPHO spondylodiscitis is not easily discriminated from other non-septic causes of discitis with MR.

- MR spine may highlight other SAPHO-associated osteitis lesions. See Figure 7.12.

Biopsy and histology
- Biopsy of bony or spondylodiscitis lesions and culture of material can show *P. acnes* growth.
- Data is derived from a few case reports only. Features seen in osteomyelitis can be present. In one case, epithelioid granulomas were seen.

Differential diagnosis
- Psoriatic arthritis or chronic sarcoidosis where pains are diffuse and suggestive of enthesitis/osteitis or periostitis lesions.
- Osteomyelitis and malignancy where there is clear painful soft-tissue and bone swelling.
- Septic or SpA-associated spondylodiscitis where there is discogenic inflammation.

Treatment
- An explanation of the condition at the outset is exceptionally important especially to those who have had chronic unexplained symptoms or manifold explanations/diagnoses given for their plight.
- NSAIDs, glucocorticoids, and analgesics have been used empirically.
- Antibiotic use, most notably doxycycline, azithromycin, and clindamycin, have been reported as effective in a few cases treated over a number of months.
- Where there is osteitis, particularly if biopsy shows an excessive number of multinucleate osteoclasts or features of increased bone turnover, bisphosphonate treatment may be a logical choice.
- A trial of a potent oral or iv aminobisphosphonate in patients, recruited on the basis of osteitis lesions detected reliably with imaging, is probably warranted.

Prognosis and natural history
SAPHO tends to cause chronic recurrent musculoskeletal symptoms. Descriptions of the condition in the long-term are not available. Reports suggest the condition can persist for >20 years and follow an unpredictable course.

References
Ballara SC, Siraj QH, Maini RN, Venables PJW. Susteained response to doxycycline therapy on 2 patients with SAPHO syndrome. *Arthritis Rheum* 1999; **42**: 819–21.

Benhamou CL, Chamot AM, Kahn MF. Synovitis-acne-pustulosis-hyperostosis-osteomyelitis syndrome (SAPHO): a new syndrome among the spondylarthropathies? *Clin Exp Rheumatol* 1988; **6**: 109–12.

Chamot AM, Benhamou CL, Kahn MF, Beraneck L, Kaplan G, Prost A. Le syndrome acné pustulose hyperostose ostéite (SAPHO). Résultats d'une enquête nationale. 85 observations. *Rev Rheum* 1987; **54**: 187–96.

Dihlman W, Dihlmann SW, Hering L. Acquired Hyperostosis Syndrome – AHYS – (sternocostoclavicular hyperostosis, pustulotic arthro-osteitis, SAPHO-syndrome): Bone scintigraphy of the anterior chest wall. *Clin Rheumatol* 1997; **16**: 13–24.

Köhler H, Uehlinger E, Kutzner J, et al. Sterno-kosto-klavikuläre yperostose, ein bisher nicht beschriebenes Kranksheitsbild. *Dtsch med Wschr* 1975; **100**: 1519–23.

Chapter 8

Autoimmune connective tissue diseases

Systemic lupus erythematosus *240*
Sjögren's syndrome *254*
Systemic sclerosis *264*
Antiphospholipid syndrome *274*
Polymyositis *282*
Dermatomyositis *290*
Juvenile dermatomyositis *298*
Inclusion body myositis *302*
Undifferentiated (autoimmune) connective tissue disease *306*
Mixed connective tissue disease *307*
Overlap syndromes *308*
Eosinophilic fasciitis *310*

Systemic lupus erythematosus

Definition
Systemic lupus erythematosus (SLE) is a systemic autoimmune disease, which is associated with a plethora of autoantibodies including characteristic anti-nuclear antibodies.

Classification
The clinical manifestations of SLE are diverse and a series of classification criteria have been published by the ACR, most recently in 1997 (Table 8.1). Although the classification criteria were not designed as diagnostic criteria, they are frequently applied in this way. SLE may be diagnosed if a patient has four or more criteria, serially, or simultaneously, providing they cannot be attributed to an alternative diagnosis. When considering a diagnosis of SLE, it is important to note that:
- Some classification criteria are highly specific for SLE (e.g. anti-dsDNA antibodies), whereas others are not (e.g. mouth ulcers).
- Several clinical features that are not included in the classification criteria occur commonly in SLE, e.g. alopecia, Raynaud's phenomenon, constitutional symptoms, livedo reticularis, or vasculitic rashes.

Symptoms and signs can occur in any organ system and are often transient; this may lead clinicians to attribute them to a functional disorder.

Epidemiology
The ratio of females to males with SLE is ~ 10:1, with onset most commonly occurring in the second and third decades. In the UK, prevalence is ~45/100 000 for women and ~4/100 000 for men. However, prevalence varies between racial groups and between countries, and most studies indicate that the incidence of SLE is higher in individuals with African or Asian ancestry. It is likely that this reflects both true differences between populations and differences in clinical practice.

Aetiology and pathophysiology
Genetics
The genetic contribution to SLE has been evident from the familial clustering of cases, with a monozygotic twin concordance rate of 24-58% and a sibling recurrence risk (λs) of ~20. A combination of genome-wide linkage and association studies have revealed that genetic susceptibility to SLE is polygenic and probably involves approximately 10 loci. A number of loci have been implicated.

- **X-chromosome:** the preponderance of females with lupus may be attributable to the effects of female sex hormones; an alternative hypothesis is that X-linked TLR7/8 alleles (which encode pattern recognition receptors for nucleic acid) fail to be completely inactivated on one of the two X-chromosomes, leading to excessive IFN production.
- **HLA:** HLA-DRB11501 (DR2) and DRB10301 (DR3) in white Caucasians.
- **Complement C4 (A and B loci):** either complete deficiency or copy number polymorphisms resulting in low levels of C4 production confer degrees of susceptibility.
- **Fc Receptors (FcRγ):** the FcRγIIa R131 allele, which binds human IgG2 poorly, is associated with SLE. The FcRγIIIa F176 allele, which binds human IgG1 and IgG3 relatively weakly, is associated with SLE, particularly lupus nephritis. The T232 alleles of the inhibitory FcRγIIb are associated with SLE in Chinese, Japanese, and Thai patients; this may relate to the relatively low inhibitory activity of the receptor encoded by the T232 allele. Conversely, an FcRγIIb promoter polymorphism is enriched in Caucasian SLE patients.
- **Immunoglobulin receptor homologues (FcRH):** an FcRH3 promoter polymorphism is associated with SLE in Japanese patients; FcRH may modify the behaviour of mature B cells.
- **Protein kinases, phosphatises, and signalling molecules:** SLE is associated with polymorphism in tyrosine kinase 2 (TYK2), interferon regulatory factor 5 (IRF5) and protein tyrosine phosphatase N22 (PTPN22) are associated with SLE.
- **Co-stimulatory/co-inhibitory molecules:** programmed cell death-1 (PD-1) serves to down-regulate lymphocyte activity, particularly in non-lymphoid tissues; a polymorphism in the PDCD1 gene, which encodes PD-1, is associated with SLE in European and Mexican populations. The locus encoding CTLA-4, a negative regulator of

Table 8.1 ACR 1997 Revised criteria for the classification of SLE

Criterion	Comments
Malar rash	
Discoid rash	
Photosensitivity	
Oral ulcers	Oral or nasopharyngeal
Arthritis	NB must be objective synovitis
Serositis	Pleurisy (pleuritic rub/effusion)
	Pericarditis
	*History of pericarditis
	*New pleural thickening
	*Peritonitis
wRenal disorder	*Renal histology indicating immune-complex-mediated glomerulonephritis
	Proteinuria >0.5 g/24 or 3+
	Cellular casts: (RBC/haemoglobin/ granular/tubular/mixed)
Neuropsychiatric disorder	Central or peripheral nervous system involvement or psychiatric condition
Haematological disorder	Haemolytic anaemia or
	Leucopaenia: <4000/µl on ≥2 occasions
	Lymphopaenia: <1500/µl on ≥2 occasions
	Thrombocytopaenia: <100 000/µl
Immunological disorder	Anti-double-stranded DNA antibody
	Anti-Sm antibody
	Antiphospholipid antibodies (either elevated anticardiolipin IgM or IgG or a positive lupus anticoagulant test)
	False positive serologic test for syphilis, positive for at least 6 months
	Positive LE preparation
	*Low levels of complement C3/C4
ANA	Raised titre

*Additional criteria proposed (and widely used) since 1982 publication

CHAPTER 8 **Autoimmune connective tissue diseases**

activated T cells, may be a modest susceptibility factor for SLE; data are inconsistent.
- **Cytokines and chemokines:** polymorphisms of the monocyte chemotactic protein (MCP-1) locus have been suggested to be associated variably with either lupus nephritis or cutaneous vasculitis in SLE. Polymorphisms in the interferon regulatory factor 5 (IRF5) gene have also been implicated.
- **Opsonins:** a promoter polymorphism, which may influence CRP levels, and the G54D allele of mannose binding lection (MBL) have been reported in association with SLE.

It is clear that SLE is clinically and genetically heterogeneous and distinct genetic influences are likely to emerge in different ethnic groups and in association with particular clinical phenotypes.

Environmental

Infectious triggers
- **Epstein-Barr virus (EBV)** has been implicated as trigger by epidemiological studies and in animal models. However, the high prevalence of EBV infection in the population indicates that exposure alone cannot account for the development of SLE. A recent case-control study revealed that EBV-IgA seropositivity was strongly associated with SLE in African Americans and in white Caucasians over the age of 50 years. There was no association of EBV-IgM or EBV-IgG seropositivity with SLE in any groups; this indicates that reactivation of EBV, giving rise to IgA production, may be important. The CTLA-4 promoter gene polymorphism was shown to modify the association of IgA-EBV in the African American population. There is also evidence for molecular mimicry involving EBV in SLE patients. In rodent models, antibodies specific for the EBV antigen, EBNA-1 cross-react with epitopes of the Ro autoantigen.
- **Cytomegalovirus (CMV)** has been implicated with lupus-related vasculitis and thrombocytopaenia in case reports and there is the Carolina Lupus Study suggested a possible association between Anti-CMV seropositivity and SLE in African Americans.
- **Hepatitis C virus (HCV):** chronic HCV infection can mimic SLE. Unsurprisingly, the prevalence of HCV infection in patients diagnosed with SLE has been reported to be elevated (~10%) compared with the background population (~0.13%).
- **Immunization:** several case reports have implicated a variety of immunizations as triggers for lupus onset or flares. The Carolina Lupus Study failed to substantiate any association between SLE and Hepatitis B vaccination. Several studies have indicated that influenza vaccine is safe in patients with quiescent SLE, although it may be associated with a transient increase in autoantibody titres. A small evidence base suggests that vaccination against *Pneumococcus* is also safe.

Non-infectious triggers/promoters
- SLE is more common in women than men and oestrogens exacerbate SLE in murine models. The Nurses' Health Study suggested that use of the oral contraceptive might confer an increased risk of SLE, but other studies have failed to substantiate this or to associate the oral contraceptive with SLE flares; progesterone-only contraceptives may even be protective. Early menarche (age 10 versus 13 years) has been associated with ~4.5 increased risk of SLE. An early menopause is also associated with increased risk of subsequent SLE; this may relate to greater use of hormone-replacement therapy, which is associated with a ~2-fold increase risk of SLE.
- Prenatal exposure to diethylstilboestrol (DES) has been associated with autoimmune disease.
- Hyperprolactinaemia is seen in 20–30% of SLE patients may be involved in pregnancy-related flares. Prolactin has been shown to increase survival and activation of autoreactive B cells.
- Drug-related lupus (DRL) may be caused by a range of agents, several of which induce methylation changes in promoters of genes encoding immunologically active products, e.g. CD70, IL-2. TNFα blockade may also induce production of ANA and a lupus-like syndrome by decreasing the inhibition by TNFα of IFNγ production. Furthermore, case reports indicate that treatment of chronic viral infection with IFN is associated with the induction of SLE.

Drugs implicated in drug-related lupus

Definite

• Hydralazine	Isoniazid.
• Minocycline	Procainamide
• Chlorpromazine	Quinidine
• Methyldopa.	

Probable (for complete list, see Mongey 2008)*

• Allopurinol	Atenolol
• Anti-TNFα agents	Enalapril
• Griseofulvin	Ibuprofen
• IFNα	Lithium
• Nitrofurantoin	Penicillin
• Phenytoin	Prophythiouracil
• Propanolol	Quinine
• Sulindac	Statins
• Sulfasalazine	Tetracyclines

*Where several agents within a class have been implicated, the class is listed instead of individual drugs.

- The influence of smoking as a risk factor for SLE is controversial. Current, rather than previous smoking is associated with anti-dsDNA antibodies and is probably also associated with SLE.
- Exposure to silica. Association reported in humans; murine studies suggest and adjuvant, and pro-apoptotic effect of silica contribute to pathogenesis of SLE.
- Silicone breast implants have received much publicity as potential triggers for AICTDs, but 3 large studies have failed to substantiate this.
- Exposure to organic solvents. Murine studies indicate that trichloroethylene (TCE) elicits lupus-related antibodies in susceptible strains. There are no data showing a relationship between TCE and SLE in humans. Petroleum distillates have been implicated in connective tissue disease, including SLE.
- Pesticides have been suggested as a trigger for SLE, but only 1 of 4 studies has supported this.
- Hair dyes have been associated with SLE in some studies, but this is controversial.
- Dietary factors, such as heavy metals, nightshade vegetables, artificial sweeteners, and a range of other foodstuffs are implicated as risk factors for SLE on many websites, but there is little or no epidemiological evidence to support these claims.

- Ultraviolet light is well recognized as a trigger of cutaneous lupus and, by increasing the load of apoptotic cells, it may also contribute to activation of systemic disease.
- Chronic stress and catastrophic life events have been implicated as triggers of SLE and other autoimmune diseases. It may be relevant that stress is associated with increased release of prolactin, which modifies immune responses.

Environmental factors which decrease risk of SLE
- Sex hormones: progesterone-only contraceptives may be protective.
- Breastfeeding ≥3 babies was associated with protection compared with breastfeeding none; the protective effect may be related to the duration of breastfeeding.
- Alcohol may exert a protective effect; this remains controversial.
- The active metabolite 1,25(OH)$_2$ D3 exerts immunosuppressive properties but the Nurses' Health Study cohort failed to reveal any effect of vitamin D3 supplements on incidence of SLE.
- Omega-3 fatty acids and anti-oxidants delay the onset of SLE in susceptible mice.

Immunopathology (Figure 8.1)

Breaking tolerance
The autoimmune response in SLE results from the failure of tolerance in T and B cells. Failure of central tolerance (thymic selection) and thymic defects have been reported in mice susceptible to SLE. In humans, a diminished thymic output has been reported.
- Aberrant antigen-presenting cell (APC) activity. Intrinsic defects of APCs have been demonstrated in mice susceptible to lupus and these appear to promote presentation of autoantigens to T cells. In humans, it remains difficult to differentiate primary from secondary APC defects. Secondary abnormalities of APC behaviour may result from tissue damage, excessive apoptosis, drugs or microbial infection; viral infections, in particular, have been suspected since SLE patients have been shown to produce large quantities of IFNα. Increased apoptotic activity results in increased clearance and presentation of autoantigens by APC. Immune complexes form between autoantibodies and autoantigen and these, in turn, are ingested by APCs via complement receptors and Fc receptors. Ingestion of immune complexes containing dsDNA causes APCs to release more IFNγ.
- Aberrant T cell activity. Murine models of SLE indicate that primary T cell defects can contribute to initiation of SLE. In humans, a range of abnormal T cell behaviours have been observed, including abnormal signalling and calcium flux, up-regulation of several co-stimulatory receptors and secreted molecules (e.g. CD40L, ICOS, BAFF), which facilitate collaboration with APC and/or B cells and increased expression of molecules promoting T cell survival. Each of these abnormalities could increase the risk of an autoreactive T cell becoming activated and resisting apoptotic death.
- Aberrant B cell activity may reflect both primary and secondary B cell abnormalities. Aberrant T cell activity provides inappropriate 'help' for B cell activation. Plasmablasts (short-lived immunoglobulin-secreting cells) usually remain in the tissue where they were generated, but in SLE patients they are detectable in blood. Excessive production of immunoglobulin-secreting cells leads to the generation of autoantibodies, which are characteristic of SLE.
- Molecular mimicry, e.g. antibodies specific for the EBV antigen, EBNA-1 cross-react with the autoantigen Ro.
- Failure of regulatory T cells.

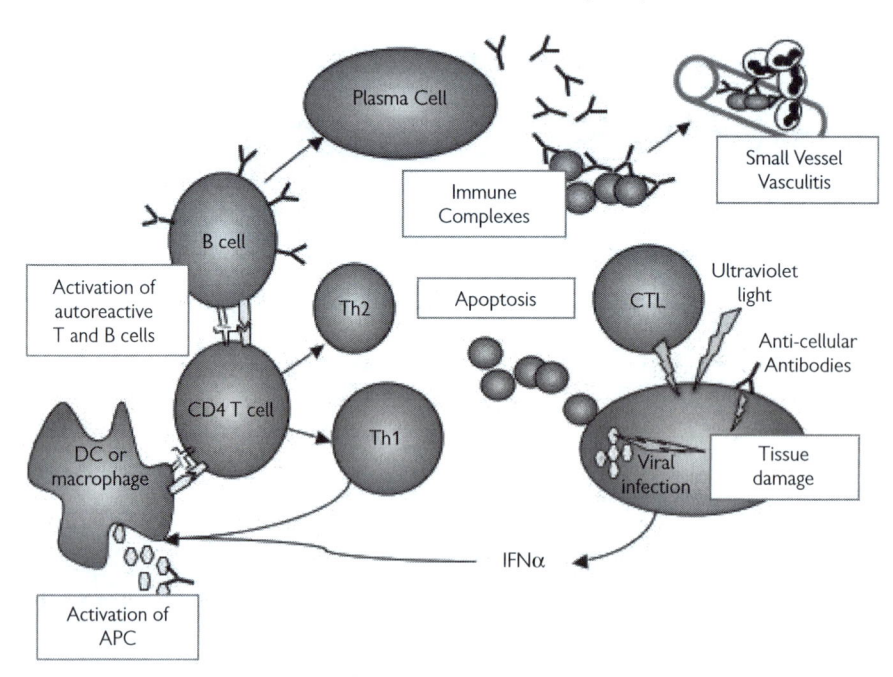

Figure 8.1 Overview of pathophysiology of SLE.

CHAPTER 8 **Autoimmune connective tissue diseases**

- Increased apoptotic activity results in increased presentation of intracellular autoantigens to T and B cells and, hence, generation of autoantibodies and immune complexes. Nuclear autoantigens, including dsDNA, are major targets, hence the characteristic autoantibody profiles associated with SLE. Exposure to ultraviolet light has been shown to increase apoptotic activity and this may trigger a flare of cutaneous (or even systemic) lupus.
- Decreased clearance of apoptotic bodies and/or immune complexes. Primary or secondary deficiencies of proximal complement components, Fc receptors or other receptors for apoptotic remnants are believed to increase inflammatory activity via increased immune complex formation/deposition, and increased availability of cytoplasmic/nuclear antigens.

Effector mechanisms
- Autoantibodies are generated to a range of cellular and soluble autoantigens. Autoantibodies may interfere with the function of their target, e.g. anti-C1q antibodies amplifying the classical pathway of complement activation (Figure 8.2), anti-phospholipid antibodies binding to and activating endothelial cells, neutrophils and platelets, or anti-Ro antibodies altering the electrophysiology of foetal myocytes. Alternatively, antibodies directed at molecules expressed on the cell surface may cause depletion of the cell subset, either via opsonization and phagocytosis of the cell or via antibody-dependent cell-mediated cytotoxicity; this mechanism contributes to leucopaenia, thrombocytopaenia and haemolytic anaemia.

Overview of pathophysiology of SLE

- **Immune complexes** form between autoantibodies and autoantigens. Antigen-presenting cells can ingest immune complexes by Fc receptor-mediated endocytosis; this enhances the presentation of autoantigens to T cells. Furthermore, deposition of immune complexes can occur in any microvascular bed; this may lead to local inflammation, via either the classical pathway of complement activation and/or by activation of immune cells via Fc receptors. Microvascular immune complex deposition is probably responsible for many migratory cutaneous, neurological and musculoskeletal symptoms and signs in SLE, as well as contributing to chronic inflammation, e.g. glomerulonephritis. The vegetations in Libman–Sacks endocarditis have also been shown to contain immunoglobulin and complement components.
- **Th1 responses:** Th1 over-activity in SLE has been demonstrated in several studies. Th1 T cells secrete increased IL-2 and IFNγ. IFNγ causes up-regulation of MHC class II molecules, thereby increasing the potency of antigen-presenting cells as well as stimulating excessive secretion of other Th1 cytokines, e.g. IL-18, by macrophages. In the kidney, IL-18, in turn, up-regulates TNFα and nitric oxide production, which promote apoptosis of renal parenchymal cells. CD4+Th1 cells also promote CD8+ T cells proliferation and survival, and enhance autoantibody production by increased secretion of BAFF.
- **Th2 responses:** although SLE was considered a Th2-mediated disease, recent studies indicate that Th1 cytokines are generally more prominent than Th1 cytokines in SLE. However, several studies indicate that Th2 cytokines are elevated. These may contribute to atopic clinical features present in some SLE patients.
- **Cytotoxic CD8+ T cells** receive 'help' from Th1 CD4+ T cell effectors. The percentage of circulating granzyme B+ CD8+ T cells is related to disease activity in SLE and their killing activity probably contributes to the availability of intracellular autoantigens for ingestion and presentation by antigen-presenting cells.
- **Complement activation** (Figure 8.2) plays many roles in SLE, including enhancement of local inflammatory responses via opsonization, and enhanced antigen presentation, anaphylatoxins and direct cytotoxicity via the membrane attack complex.
- **Endothelial activation** results in increased expression of certain adhesion molecules and chemokines, thereby recruiting certain leucocytes into tissues; activated endothelium also promotes local coagulation more than resting endothelium, and produces vasodilators and mediators of increased vessel permeability. Endothelial damage

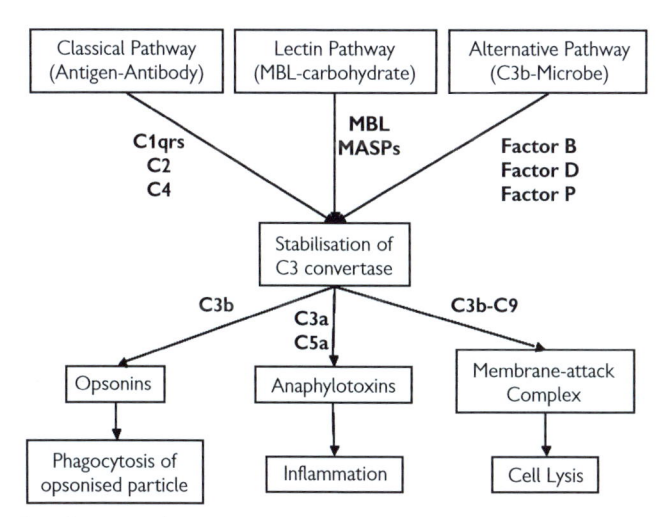

Figure 8.2 Summary of complement cascade.

by inflammatory processes may trigger apoptosis; this triggers local angiogenesis and contributes to the pro-coagulant tendency

Pathophysiology of accelerated cardiovascular disease
Accelerated atherosclerosis, inflammatory and unstable plaques, and an increased thrombotic tendency all probably contribute to the increased incidence of cardiovascular events. Traditional risk factors (with the exception of smoking) are increased in SLE patients, and contribute to endothelial damage and lipid deposition as in the general population. SLE-related non-traditional factors, include many circulating mediators, which may exacerbate endothelial damage [e.g. immune complexes, anti-endothelial antibodies (including anti-HSP antibodies), pro-inflammatory cytokines, oxidized LDLc] and antibodies that may promote thrombosis (antiphospholipid antibodies) or dyslipidaemia (anti-lipoprotein lipase antibodies).

Traditional risk factors
- Hypertension.
- Hyperlipidaemia.
- Diabetes mellitus.
- Smoking.
- Increased BMI.
- Sedentary lifestyle.
- Elevated CRP.

Non-traditional risk factors
- Treatment with glucocorticoids.
- Pro-inflammatory high density lipoprotein (HDL).
- Anti-HSP antibodies.
- Increased oxidized LDLc.
- Circulating immune complexes.
- High systemic inflammatory mediators (e.g. IL-6, TNFα).
- Antiphospholipid antibodies.
- Antibodies to lipoprotein lipase.
- Increased asymmetric dimethylarginine levels.
- Duration of SLE.
- Activity of SLE.

Protective factors
- Treatment with cyclophosphamide.
- Treatment with hydroxychloroquine.
- Management of conventional risk factors.

Risk factors
- Female gender
- SLE in first-degree relative (see above).
- African or Asian ancestry.
- Exposure to environmental agents (see above).
- Risk factors for cardiovascular disease in SLE (see above).
- Risk factors for end-stage renal failure in SLE (see prognosis section below).
- **Risk factors for osteoporosis in SLE:** increasing age, low BMI, elevated CRP or ESR, low exercise levels, high damage (SLICC), renal impairment. Protective factor: hydroxychloroquine. Note: The net effect of corticosteroids on BMD in SLE is unclear, presumably due to the protective effect of decreased inflammation.
- **Risk factors for infection in SLE:** hypocomplementaemia, prednisolone >20 mg daily), cyclophosphamide (ever), splenic hypofunction, mannose binding lectin deficiency (controversial).
- **Risk factors for malignancy in SLE:** age greater than 65 years, smoking; exposure to azathioprine, methotrexate or cyclophosphamide may increase risk of haematological malignancy.

Clinical features

General issues
Fatigue, fever, night sweats, weight loss, lymphadenopathy are all common.

Musculoskeletal
- Polyarthralgia occurs in ~90%, often with early morning stiffness. Arthritis (objective synovitis) occurs in ~10% and deformity is usually due to tenosynovitis; this is known as *Jaccoud's* arthropathy (reducible deformity without radiological erosions).
- Chest pains may occur due to costochondritis.
- Osteoarthritis may coexist with SLE and ~50% fulfil diagnostic criteria for fibromyalgia.
- Spontaneous tendon rupture (usually Achilles or patellar) may occur.
- Myalgia is present in the majority but a myositis occurs in ~5%. Muscle weakness may occur in relation to lupus-related muscle disease, thyroid disease or drugs (especially GCs).

Mucocutaneous (see also p. 98)
The malar or butterfly rash, discoid rashes, photosensitivity, mouth or nasal ulcers and alopecia occur commonly. Less common cutaneous/subcutaneous manifestations include urticaria, splinter haemorrhages, palpable purpura, hyperpigmentation, vitiligo, subcutaneous nodules, calcinosis, pruritis, panniculitis, psoriaform lesions, and leg ulcers.
- Sub-acute cutaneous lupus erythematosus (SCLE) is sometimes diagnosed in patients with widespread recurring, non-scarring annular or papulosquamous lesions, which occur in association with ANA and anti-Ro antibodies. In the absence or renal or other severe systemic features; SCLE is generally recognized as being at the mild end of the spectrum of SLE.

Renal (see also p. 74) (see Plate 35).
The majority of SLE patients will have abnormalities of urinalysis at some stage.
- Nephritic syndrome (~60%): acute renal failure with hypertension and 'active' renal sediment (haematuria, cellular casts and, non-nephrotic range, proteinuria. This normally occurs in patients with proliferative glomerular changes on renal biopsy.
- Nephrotic syndrome (peripheral oedema, hypoalbuminaemia, hyperlipidaemia and nephrotic range proteinuria ≥3.5 g/day) occurs in 10–20% of SLE patients and usually associated with membranous glomerular changes.
- A renal thrombotic microangiopathy may occur as part of APLS and this is associated with more severe hypertension and azotemia than in lupus nephritis without APLS. Renal vein thrombosis may occur in association with APLS or nephrotic syndrome.
- Tubulointerstitial nephritis may present with sterile pyuria, in the absence of haematuria or proteinuria and may cause renal tubular acidosis (RTA) type 1 or nephrogenic diabetes insipidus.

Neurological (see also p. 90)
A wide variety of neurological or psychiatric conditions occur in SLE (Table 8.2). Neurological manifestations occur in the majority of patients, with cognitive dysfunction,

Table 8.2 Manifestations of neuropsychiatric lupus

Central nervous system	Peripheral nervous system
Aseptic meningitis	Guillain–Barre syndrome
Cerebrovascular disease	Autonomic neuropathy
Demyelinating syndrome	Mononeuropathy
Headache	Myasthenia gravis
Movement disorder	Cranial neuropathy
Myelopathy	Plexopathy
Seizures	Polyneuropathy
Acute confusional state	
Anxiety disorder	
Cognitive dysfunction	
Mood disorder	
Psychosis	

mood disorder, headache, cerebrovascular disease and seizures being the most common problems. Attribution of neurological phenomena to SLE is problematic, since this relies on the exclusion of another cause and some conditions, e.g. headache and depression are common in the general population.

Haematological
- Anaemia is present in >70%.and may be normochromic normocytic, hypochromic microcytic (iron deficient?), macrocytic (hypothyroid? vitamin B12 or folate deficient?), autoimmune or microangiopathic haemolytic.
- Lymphopenia is common and correlates with disease activity. Neutropaenia is uncommon, but may occur as a result of drug toxicity.
- Thrombocytopaenia occurs in ~20%, but serious bleeding is uncommon. APLS.
- Lymphadenopathy is common in SLE, but the incidence of non-Hodgkin's lymphoma is increased ~7-fold.
- Functional hyposplenism occurs in ~5% patients with SLE, probably due to blocking of Fc receptors by circulating immune complexes. This results in a susceptibility to infection with Pneumococcus, Meningococcus, Haemophilus influenzae., and occasionally protozoa.

Gastrointestinal (see also p. 82)
Mouth ulcers are common. Mucosal ulceration may occur in the small intestine, occasionally leading to strictures. Oesophageal dysmotility may occur, but is rarely a serious problem. Similarly, hepato- and/or splenomegaly are found in 10–30%, but are rarely serious problems.
- Patients with SLE frequently report episodic abdominal pain, bloating, constipation, and diarrhoea.
- Rare, but serious complications include autoimmune hepatitis, malabsorption, colitis, mesenteric vasculitis, and mesenteric or hepatic artery or vein thrombosis.

Pulmonary (see also p. 54)
Pleurisy occurs in ~50% and pleural effusion in ~25%. Subtle abnormalities of pulmonary function tests are common but significant interstitial lung disease (ILD) occurs in ~20%. Recurrent pneumonia may occur, particularly in patients with splenic hypofunction. Pulmonary embolus is associated with antiphospholipid antibodies. Shrinking lung (related to diaphragmatic dysfunction) and pulmonary hypertension are rare.

Cardiovascular
All layers of the heart may be affected in SLE and accelerated atherosclerosis is the major cause of premature mortality. Pericardial involvement is common, occurring in ~66%; symptomatic in ~33%. Subclinical myocarditis is probably also common, but significant clinical features occur in ~10%. Endocardial lesions are associated with anti-phospholipid antibodies (Libman–Sacks endocarditis). The incidence of subacute bacterial endocarditis may also be increased both by generalized immunosuppression in SLE and by pre-exisitng endocardial lesions. Incidence of MI and stroke is increased between 3- and 10-fold.

Other general issues
- **Sjögren's syndrome** occurs in up to 20% of SLE patients.
- **Thyroid disease:** hypothyroidism occurs in ~6% SLE patients, compared with ~1% of the general population. Hyperthyroidism is not significantly increased.
- **Osteoporosis:** approximately 25% of patients with SLE have densitometry-defined osteoporosis and ~10% suffer fractures.
- **Vitamin D deficiency**: approximately 75% of SLE patients have vitamin D insufficiency (<30 ng/ml) and ~15% have vitamin D deficiency (<10 ng/ml).
- **Osteonecrosis** has been estimated to occur in ~10% of SLE patients and is associated with GC therapy.
- **Infections** are increased in SLE (relative risk of ~1.6 compared with controls overall). UTI, pneumonia, and bacteraemia with unknown source are the commonest types of infection. E. coli is the most frequently isolated organism. CNS infections are uncommon in SLE; organisms include M. tuberculosis, Cryptococcus, Listeria, Klebsiella and Aspergillus. Septic arthritis is also rare in SLE, but most frequently involves the hip and presents with avascular necrosis; Salmonella enteritidis is the most common pathogen in septic joints.
- **Malignancy:** the standardized incidence ratio (SIR) for all malignancies in SLE 1.15. Notable associations include NHL SIR 3.6 and hepatobiliary cancers SIR 2.6.
- **Infertility** is rarely a problem in SLE, but may be associated with active disease, renal failure, or use of NSAIDs, high dose GCs or cyclophosphamide. Miscarriages are associated with antiphospholipid antibodies.

Key features in history
Mucocutaneous involvement
Enquire about malar rash, photosensitivity (adult-onset?), alopecia, other rashes, and unusual mouth or nose ulcers. When urticarial lesions occur, ask if painful/lesions lasting >24 h (probably vasculitic) or itchy, and resolving within 24 h (probably allergic).

Musculoskeletal
Joint pains, swelling, duration of early morning stiffness; muscle pain/weakness; note that a single disproportionately painful, swollen, warm joint may be septic.

Haematological
Enquire about history of thromboembolic disease (DVT, PE and foetal loss), which may indicate APLS. Anaemia may contribute to fatigue and dyspnoea. Enquire about sore throats and infections in patients with neutropaenia (uncommon – note risk of fungal infections) or severe lymphopaenia (consider infection with atypical organisms). Easy bruising/bleeding may be symptoms of thrombocytopaenia. Ask about swollen lymph glands, and fevers and

night sweats; while these all occur in active SLE, their presence should raise suspicion of lymphoma.

Gastrointestinal
Enquire about dyspepsia, nausea, vomiting, abdominal pain or distention, and diarrhoea or constipation.

Pulmonary
Enquire about chest pain (pleuritic or chest wall tenderness), dyspnoea, cough, sputum, haemoptysis, and history of pneumonia.

Cardiovascular
Enquire about chest pains (pericarditic – relieved by sitting forward; angina – central, tight, radiating to L arm or jaw, exertional, associated with dyspnoea), palpitations, ankle swelling, and dyspnoea.

Neurological
Enquire about and clarify the natures of fits, 'funny turns', headache, tingling/numbness, altered mood and difficulty with concentration or memory. An account from a close friend or relative is often revealing. A mini-mental state examination is useful if the presence of significant cognitive dysfunction. Erectile dysfunction may occur with autonomic neuropathy.

Other
- Enquire about dry eyes, mouth, vagina.
- **Raynaud's phenomenon (RP):** classic triphasic (red/white/blue) colour change, but all colours not required for diagnosis of RP; age > 30 years at onset and severe ischaemic pain suggest secondary RP.
- **Lifestyle:** smoking, occupational/recreational history.
- **Drugs**: include history of possible triggering agents for SLE and use of drugs associated with common co-morbidity, e.g. GCs, NSAIDs.
- Past medical history: ask about diseases that may have been a previous manifestation of SLE or which may influence management, e.g. cardiovascular disease, diabetes mellitus, miscarriages, thromboembolic disease, osteoporosis, pleurisy.

Key features on examination

Skin involvement
Look for subtle malar rash, which patients often overlook, discoid lesions, evidence of alopecia, pigmentation, vitiligo, livedo reticularis, and signs of small vessel vasculitis (palpable purpura, urticaria). Circling urticarial lesions facilitates the patient monitoring whether they persist longer than 24 h. Be alert to the presence of evolving lesions, which could indicate skin cancer.

Musculoskeletal
Look for synovitis (consider septic arthritis if one joint disproportionately inflamed or in presence of hip irritability; note that immunosuppression may mask usual signs of septic arthritis), tenosynovitis, Jaccoud's arthropathy (reducible deformities), proximal muscle weakness, muscle tenderness, and fibromyalgia trigger points (see Plate 6).

Renal
BP and urinalysis; haematuria, proteinuria or pyuria (persistent leucouria in the absence of infection) may occur. Enquire about menstruation in women with isolated haematuria. Note that hypertension and azotemia (increased nitrogen-containing compounds in blood – manifest as skin pallor and 'frost' from nitrogen-containing compounds excreted in sweat) are more severe in APLS when thrombotic microangiopathy affects the kidney.

Table 8.3 Mini-mental state examination

Domain	Maximum points
Orientation	
What is the time, date, day, month, year?	5
What is the name of this ward, hospital, district, town, country?	5
Registration	
Name three objects once only. Score 1 point for each correct repetition. Repeat the objects until patient can repeat them accurately (for later recall)	3
Attention and calculation	
Subtract 7 from 100 and then 7 from the result four more times	5
Recall	
Repeat the names of the three objects registered earlier	3
Language	
Name 2 objects (e.g. pen and watch)	2
Repeat phrase 'No ifs, ands or buts'	1
Perform a 3-stage command, e.g. 'With the index finger of your right hand touch your nose and then your left ear'	3
Show the patient the written message 'Close your eyes' (score 1 point if the patient follows the instructions)	1
Ask the patient to write a sentence (score 1 point if it makes sense and includes a noun and a verb)	1
Draw a pair of intersecting pentagons (Score 1 point if accurately copied)	1
Total maximum score	30

Neurological
A basic neurological examination should be performed at diagnosis and at annual review. Otherwise, examination should be performed in response to the development of new symptoms. Include fundoscopy in patients with (early morning?) headache and assess pupillary responses and postural BP drop where the history suggests autonomic neuropathy. A mini-mental state examination (Table 8.3) is useful in patients with cognitive difficulties.

Haematological
- Pallor indicates anaemia. Urobilinogen on urinalysis and, less commonly, jaundice are manifestations of haemolytic anaemia.
- Bruising and bleeding (e.g. from gums) may occur with severe thrombocytopaenia, with a deficiency of clotting factors (?liver failure) or, in the acutely ill patient, as part of disseminated intravascular coagulation. However, note that GC therapy is the usual reason for excessive bruising in SLE patients.
- Livedo reticularis frequently occurs in patients with APLS.
- Lymphadenopathy may merely be a correlate of active disease, but large, unresolving nodes should prompt investigation for lymphoma.

Gastrointestinal
Look for pallor, jaundice, lymphadenopathy, clubbing, spider naevi, signs of nutritional deficiency (low BMI, angular cheilosis, leuconychia, koilonychia) abdominal distention.

CHAPTER 8 Autoimmune connective tissue diseases

A rash suggestive of dermatitis herpetiformis may indicate the co-existence of coeliac disease. Consider partial lipodystrophy and, if present, the distribution (C3 nephritic factor is usually associated with fat loss over face and upper limbs). Check for mouth ulcers and xerostomia (excessive dental caries?). Palpate abdomen for tenderness (surgical abdomen?) and organomegaly.

Pulmonary
Examine for respiratory rate, clubbing, pallor, central cyanosis, chest expansion, costochondral and costovertebral tenderness, stony dull percussion note (pleural effusion), pleural rub, basal inspiratory crepitations (ILD or left ventricular failure), and signs of consolidation in suspected pneumonia.

Cardiovascular
Assess pulse rate and rhythm and blood pressure at each visit. Examine JVP for right heart failure, praecordium for signs of left ventricular pressure or volume overload, and right heart strain; auscultate for murmurs and gallop rhythm. Palpate peripheral pulses and listen for carotid bruit at annual review.

Ophthalmological
SLE is associated with a number of retinal lesions (see p. 48).

Investigations

Recommended lab investigations for annual review

Haematology
- FBC with differential white cell count may show evidence of anaemia of chronic disease (normocytic hypochromic). However, a hypochromic microcytic picture should prompt investigations for iron deficiency and blood loss (peptic ulcers – NSAID use?). A macrocytic picture raises the possibility of hypothyroidism, haemolysis (reticulocytes raise the MCV), excessive alcohol intake, liver disease, and is a normal finding in pregnancy. Thrombocytopaenia and lymphopaenia are common in SLE. Neutrophilia may indicate infection but also occurs with GC treatment.
- Blood film – request to clarify numbers of white blood cell types or of platelets (clumping?), to clarify whether an apparent normocytic normochromic anaemia actually reflects a mixed micro- and macrocytic picture, to seek the Howell–Jolly bodies indicative of hyposplenism, or the helmet cells of microangiopathic haemolytic anaemia, and to quantify reticulocytes in suspected haemolysis (normal <1%).
- ESR classically is elevated in the absence of a raised CRP in patients with SLE. Note that the ESR may be raised due to anaemia and that some SLE patients do exhibit a raised CRP with active disease, most commonly with serositis.

Biochemistry
- Renal function tests. Note that 'normal range' creatinine is not likely to be normal in a patient with low BMI (or low muscle bulk).
- Electrolyte disturbances may arise from renal, endocrine, or neurological involvement or drug toxicity, and may cause neuromuscular or cardiac symptoms.
- Estimated creatinine clearance from Cockcroft–Gault formula:
  Estimated CrCl = [(140 – age) × weight (kg)]/ serum Cr (µmol/L)
  (multiply by 0.85 in women)

Note that this formula is inaccurate in patients with oedema due to nephrotic syndrome.
- Early morning urinary protein to creatinine ratio is probably as accurate as 24 h urine collection for quantifying severity of proteinuria.
- If RTA is suspected, check blood and urine pH (early morning urine sample preferable); pH>5.3 despite metabolic acidosis indicates RTA.
- Also plasma bicarbonate <21 mmol/l in RTA. 24 h urinary calcium measurement may be made if RTA is suspected and to monitor response to treatment. Acid load test (used if plasma bicarbonate >21 mmol/l, but RTA still suspected). For this 100 mg/kg ammonium chloride is administered orally. Urine pH is monitored hourly and plasma bicarbonate at 3 h. In RTA, bicarbonate drops below 21 mmol/l, but urine pH remains <5.3.
- Liver function tests: screen for autoimmune hepatitis, PBC, or drug toxicity.
- CK elevation can suggest myositis.
- Thyroid function tests: hypothyroidism common.
- Bone biochemistry including 25-hydroxyvitamin D and PTH as vitamin D deficiency is common.
- Vitamin B12, folate, and ferritin.
- Fasting lipid profile in patients with any CV risk factor other than the diagnosis (within 10 years) of SLE itself.
- Troponin I – if myocarditis or MI suspected.
- CSF: see under lumbar puncture.

Immunology
- ANA is positive in >95% of patients with SLE (usually by ELISA). Request the more sensitive immunofluorescence ANA assay, if borderline ANA by ELISA.
- Anti-extractable nuclear antigens (ENAs) will usually be checked for when ANA is positive.

Table 8.4 Significance of antibodies to extractable nuclear antigens (ENA) in SLE

ENA	Prevalence in SLE	Clinical Associations
Sm	5% (Caucasian) ~40% (Afro-Caribbean)	Vasculitis, CNS lupus
Ro	~40%	Sjögren's Photosensitivity, rashes, neonatal LE, congenital heart block
La	~15%	Sjögren's
U1RNP	~30%	Raynaud's

ENAs for which antibodies are routinely measured in SLE patients are listed, indicating the prevalence of antibodies and the associated clinical features.

- Anti-histone antibodies in suspected drug-related lupus.
- Anticardiolipin antibodies (measured by ELISA) and lupus anticoagulant (functional test; higher specificity for clinical events in APLS) should both be measured at baseline and annually.
- Other autoantibodies may be positive in overlap AICTD syndromes, e.g. rheumatoid factor (RA), anti-dsDNA (SLE), lupus anticoagulant and APLS, anti-smooth muscle antibodies and anti-liver-kidney microsomal antibodies (autoimmune hepatitis) and anti-mitochondrial antibodies (PBC). Refer to 'The Nervous System and Rheumatological Disease' (p. 90) for autoantibodies associated with autoimmune neurological syndromes.
- Coeliac disease associated antibodies (anti-tissue transglutaminase or anti-endomysial antibodies) should be

considered in patients with malabsorption and/or a rash suggestive of dermatitis herpetiformis.
- Complement C3 and C4 can vary inversely with disease activity in some patients.
- C3 nephritic factor. Request in patients with lipodystrophy (unexplained fat loss) or if C3 is low in the presence of a normal C4.
- Anti-C1 esterase inhibitor. Request if ?angio-oedema.
- Immunoglobulins and both serum and urine protein electrophoresis. Request at diagnosis as part of a screen for neoplasia; repeat annually for patients with SLE-associated Sjögren's.

Other laboratory investigations
- Midstream urine. Request microscopy to look for 'active' renal sediment (e.g. red cell casts), as well as culture/sensitivity.
- Synovial fluid urgent microscopy and culture, if septic arthritis suspected.
- Blood cultures (multiple sets) should be performed whenever bacterial infection is suspected (e.g. possible septic arthritis, endocarditis, meningitis).

Imaging
- CXR is useful at diagnosis as part of a screen for neoplasia, if the diagnosis is unclear. Useful post-diagnosis if new cough or dyspnoea, although may be unnecessary if a high resolution CT chest is planned.
- High resolution (HR) CT chest may reveal honeycombing and ground glass opacities typical of non-specific interstitial (NSIP) associated with AICTDs.
- CT is imaging modality of choice for detecting the thickened bowel of SLE-associated bowel disease.
- Radiographs and Doppler US of joints to exclude erosive joint disease patients with RA pattern synovitis or if septic arthritis is suspected.
- MR head/spinal cord should be performed in patients with clinical focal neurological deficit or with unusual headaches or cognitive defects. See also: 'The Nervous System and Rheumatological Disease' (p. 90).

Histology
- Renal biopsy should be considered in patients with an 'active' renal sediment on urinalysis or isolated proteinuria (+++ or >1 g/l). Liaise with renal team. See: 'The Kidney and Rheumatological Disease' (p. 74) for the classification of histological findings in lupus nephritis (classes I–VI).
- Skin biopsy classically reveals IgG or IgM (± complement) deposition at the dermal/epidermal junction, giving rise to the 'lupus band'. Clinically uninvolved skin usually also shows this deposition 'band'. Macules or papules, which are growing and/or ulcerating, or which show changing and/or irregular pigmentation should be biopsied to exclude skin cancer.
- Sural nerve biopsy should be considered in suspected mononeuritis.
- Muscle biopsy in patients with significantly elevated CK.
- Liver biopsy (usually under US control) if autoimmune hepatitis is suspected.
- Small bowel biopsy if malabsorption suspected (consider infection, coeliac disease, lymphoma, and Whipple's disease).
- Meningeal biopsy or biopsy of non-dominant frontal lobe may occasionally be required.

Other investigations
- **Pulmonary function tests:** spirometry and transfer factor, useful to screen for and monitor interstitial lung disease (ILD), and to screen for pulmonary arterial hypertension (occurs occasionally in SLE).
- **Echocardiogram:** performed to detect pericardial effusion, LVH, reduced LV ejection fraction, valvular lesions (especially in APLS), and as a screening test for PAH.
- **ECG:** useful screen for arrhythmia, ischaemia, LVH.
- **Thiopurine methyltransferase (TPMT) genotype:** checked in some centres prior to prescribing azathioprine, since patients who have reduced/absent TPMT activity may have increased risk of myelotoxicity at the standard doses of azathioprine.
- **Upper GI endoscopy** is required as investigation of possible peptic ulcer disease.
- Ankle/Brachial Pressure Index, Doppler ultrasound, MRA, or conventional angiography to investigate suspected peripheral vascular disease.
- **Carotid ultrasound:** for investigation of carotid bruit or of TIA/stroke.
- **DXA scan** in all postmenopausal women is advisable.
- **Lumbar puncture** is indicated for some central neurological features. Check for raised intracranial pressure prior to LP, with CT brain, if urgent. Measure opening pressure (normal 60–150 mmHg). Send sample to biochemistry for protein (normal 0.2–0.4 g/l), glucose (with paired blood glucose; CSF glucose should be 50–66% of blood glucose) and LDH. Liaise with microbiologist to request gram stain, Ziehl–Nielson stain (for MTB), India ink stain for *Cryptococcus*, culture (request prolonged culture for *Nocardia*), sensitivity, PCR and measurement of antibodies for a microbial agents, which may infect immunosuppressed individuals. Refer to 'The Nervous System and Rheumatological Disease' (p. 90) for further details.
- EEG/EMG/NCS:
- Ocular investigations. Refer to 'The Eye in Rheumatological Disease' (p. 48).

Differential diagnosis
Mainly the other AICTDs and the primary vasculitides, Behçet's disease, cryoglobulinaemia, and hypocomplementaemic urticarial vasculitis. Also:
- Drug-related lupus.
- Hepatitis B, Hepatitis C.
- EBV, CMV, Parvovirus B19.
- Sarcoidosis.
- Whipple's disease.
- MTB.
- Lyme disease.
- Paraneoplastic manifestation of malignancy.
- Periodic fever syndromes.
- Primary immunodeficiency with autoimmune features.

Drug-related lupus
Typical features of DRL are constitutional symptoms, arthralgias/arthritis, myalgia, rashes, serositis, raised ESR, and a positive ANA with elevated anti-histone antibodies, all of which rise weeks to months after introduction of triggering medication. Note that anti-dsDNA antibodies suggest SLE rather than DLE.
To resolve, withdraw the suspected triggering medication and symptoms usually improve within days to weeks.

ANA and anti-histone antibodies may persist for months to years.

Treatment
The objectives of management are to control of disease activity, minimise damage and manage co-morbidity.

Control of SLE disease activity
General principles
- Educate and advise patients regarding nature of SLE and lifestyle issues (see below).
- Management of disease activity in SLE depends on the severity and location of the activity.
- Systemic immunosuppression tailored to control activity in the most sensitive tissue and/or the tissue displaying the greatest activity will usually provide adequate control of less severe manifestations of lupus.
- Clinical scores (SLEDAI, SLAM, BILAG) can be used to assess disease activity. Attribution of a BILAG score of 'A' to an organ system implies that immunosuppression with prednisolone >20 mg daily and/or another agent is required. Attribution of a BILAG score of 'B' to an organ system implies that treatment with prednisolone <20 mg daily, hydroxychloroquine or NSAIDs will be adequate.
- GCs >20 mg daily are particularly useful for gaining rapid control of activity, but their long-term use should be minimized.
- Use topical/local GCs in preference to systemic GCs whenever possible.
- Hydroxychloroquine is associated with reduced flares and reduced accumulation of damage and should be used in the majority of patients – alone for mild cases and in combination for more severe disease.

Management of serious or common scenarios
'Mild spectrum' SLE
Rashes and mild polyarthritis can often be managed with high factor sunblock and antimalarials (e.g. hydroxychloroquine 200 mg bd). Intermittent use of topical GC cream and NSAIDs or simple analgesics may also be used.

'Moderate' SLE activity
- Patients who cannot tolerate antimalarials or, in whom significant disease activity persists, can be treated with azathioprine or mycophenolate mofetil (Table 8.5 provides examples of initiation and monitoring regimes below).
- Methotrexate, ciclosporin, and sirolimus may also be used.
- If the 'conventional' immunosuppressives are either not tolerated or inadequately effective, B cell depletion therapy is often effective (e.g. Rituximab 1 g ×2 over 2 weeks, repeated at 6-month intervals). Note that several weeks elapse before clinical benefit occurs.

Lupus nephritis (see also pp. 75–77)
- Class I lesions do not require specific treatment.
- Class II disease is usually treated with a tapering course of GCs; establish patient on hydroxychloroquine, if tolerated.
- Class III and IV disease: standard treatment consists of induction of remission with a combination of a tapering course of prednisolone (starting at 1 mg/kg/day) and pulses of intravenous cyclophosphamide 0.5–1 g/m^2, given at monthly intervals for 6 months (with oral ondansetron to minimize nausea and mesna to reduce risk of haemorrhagic cystitis, and subsequent bladder malignancy). Patients in remission may be maintained with 3-monthly pulses of cyclophosphamide or, more commonly, azathioprine or mycophenolate mofetil.
- Recent trial data suggests that mycophenolate mofetil (in combination with prednisolone) may be a more effective and less toxic agent with which to induce remission than cyclophosphamide.
- Case reports also indicate that rituximab may be an effective induction and maintenance agent. Success with anti-TNFα agents in class IV lupus nephritis has been reported. However, these agents should be used with caution in SLE owing to their association with the induction of ANA and other lupus-related features.
- In Class V disease mycophenolate mofetil appears to be effective although RCTs are awaited.

Cerebral SLE
Open label trial data suggest that IV cyclophosphamide plus prednisolone is more effective than prednisolone alone or with antimalarials. Successful use of intravenous immunoglobulin and plasma exchange has been reported and Rituximab appears also to be effective in small series. Anti-TNFα agents should generally be avoided due to the risk of SLE exacerbation and their association with exacerbation of demyelination.

Cutaneous SLE/lupus
In cases where cutaneous lupus is the only or dominant feature, topical or intra-lesional treatment with GCs may be used. In resistant cases, the following may be effective: topical tacrolimus, systemic dapsone (check G6PD status; monitor FBC and LFT) or thalidomide (BEWARE teratogenicity and cumulative peripheral neuropathy, thus monitor nerve conduction studies). Methotrexate, efalizumab (anti-CD11a – effective in psoriasis and used in refractory discoid LE) can also be used.

Table 8.5 Initiation and monitoring of azathioprine and mycophenolate

Initiation of azathioprine	Initiation of mycophenolate
Give 50 mg od for 2 weeks	Give 500 mg od for 1 week then 500 mg bd for 1 week
- Check FBC and LFT. If results are satisfactory: 100 mg od for 2 weeks	- Check FBC, Creat U&Es and LFTs. If results are satisfactory then give 750 mg bd for 1 week then 1 g bd for 1 week
- Check FBC and LFT. If results are satisfactory increase in 25 mg increments to 2–2.5 mg/kg/day.	- Check bloods every 2 weeks until stable dose then monthly.
- Check bloods every 2 weeks until stable dose then monthly. Halve doses in TPMT deficiency	

Initiation and monitoring of immunosuppressants such as azathioprine and mycophenolate can often be managed by shared care with local GPs. In these cases, a 'shared care' or monitoring booklet should be provided, in which the patient can collate their blood results. Education and empowerment of patients in this monitoring process greatly improves safety.

Synovitis
Dominant involvement of a single joint should prompt exclusion of septic arthritis. SLE activity restricted to one or two joints may be managed by intra-articular injection. Polyarthritis should be treated systemically as for 'moderate' SLE.

Pregnancy in SLE
Available data suggest that patients with current or historical moderate/severe SLE can be maintained on azathioprine and hydroxychloroquine during pregnancy. Flares may be treated with GCs. Note that a woman on a regular GC dose may need additional GC replacement during labour.
- Note that other medications taken by the patient should be carefully reviewed since many anti-hypertensives are contraindicated (calcium channel blockers appear to be safe).
- The challenges in preparing for pregnancy in SLE are:
  - to maintain control of disease but avoid teratogenic or other harmful effects on the foetus;
  - identification of risk factors for complications;
  - to optimize chances of conception in individuals who may be sub-fertile due to disease or drugs.
- Control of SLE activity at conception is a marker for good control throughout the pregnancy.
- Tetratogenic drugs (e.g. methotrexate, mycophenolate mofetil) must be withdrawn at least 3 months prior to attempts to conceive.
- Azathioprine, hydroxychloroquine, and GCs are relatively safe to use through pregnancy.
- Emerging data suggest that rituximab, in the first trimester, has no major effect on the foetus or neonate; rituximab administered in the third trimester has been reported to cause transient neonatal B cell depletion.
- Risk factors for pregnancy should be clarified, including presence of anti-Ro antibodies, anti-cardiolipin antibodies and/or lupus anticoagulant, history of thromboembolic disease and of previous foetal loss.
- Screening for pulmonary hypertension should include ECHO and pulmonary function tests, with referral for further investigation if these indicate PAH.
- Folic acid and calcium/vitamin D supplementation should be prescribed.
- The chance of conception may be optimized by controlling disease activity and avoiding NSAIDs (may prevent ovulation). Some patients may require referral for assisted conception.

Management of associated morbidity

Cardiovascular disease.
There is currently no standard practice for cardiovascular risk reduction and a dearth of appropriate clinical trials to inform management. However, it is clear that SLE patients are at substantially increased risk.

General principles
- Stop smoking.
- Optimize BP (<140/85).
- Aim for BMI of 22–25.
- Control disease activity, using a minimal dose of GCs.
- Include hydroxychloroquine in treatment regime.
- Use antiplatelet agents in patients with SLE/APLS. The threshold for use of aspirin in other SLE patients is controversial. Generally, the benefits of aspirin outweigh the risks in individuals with a 10 years CVD risk >6%.
- Lipid-lowering is important, but there is no consensus for targets. A pragmatic approach would be to aim for a fasting LDLc <2.6 mmol/L in all SLE patients.
- Given the logistic problem of obtaining fasting lipid profiles, an alternative proposal suggests stratifying patients into the following risk groups:
  - low risk – SLE is the only risk factor for CVD; target total cholesterol <5.2 mmol/l;
  - medium risk – additional risk factors but not in the high-risk group; target LDLc <2.6 mmol/l;
  - high risk – patient has CHD or equivalent condition; target LDLc <2.0 mmol/l.

Osteoporosis (see also p. 395)
SLE is associated with osteoporosis, but also hypovitaminosis-D and secondary hyperparathyroidism. Use DXA data, biochemistry results (including PTH) and absolute fracture risk algorithms (e.g. FRAX) to guide management.
- Keep replete in vitamin D (25-OHD >75 nmol/l) and avoid secondary hyperparathyroidism. Calcium and vitamin D supplements may be needed (use D3 not D2).
- In gross calcium deficiency (indicated by marked secondary hyperparathyroidism plus high ALP, low calcium excretion and serum 25-OHD) rule out coeliac disease.
- In GC-induced osteoporosis (GIO), there is high fracture risk post-menopause, those >65 years, in those with a fragility fracture and where hip of spine T score on DXA is ≤ −1.5) thus prescribe a bisphosphonate.

Other co-morbidities
- **Dyspepsia:** proton pump inhibitors and anti-acids.
- **Constipation:** stool softeners and bulking agents, e.g. lactulose and fybogel. Diarrhoea – loperamide.
- **Malabsorption:** refer to dietician and check tTG antibodies to rule out coeliac disease. Consider using calcium, folate and iron supplements and parenteral administration of vitamin B12.
- **Chronic renal failure:** liaise with renal team - phosphate binders, alfacalcidol, erythropoietin, BP control and, ultimately, dialysis may be required.
- **Hypothyroidism:** replacement therapy.
- **Depression:** SSRIs (e.g. citalopram; fluoxetine may have some efficacy for RP also), amitriptyline, or duloxetine may be useful in patients with coexisting fibromyalgia.
- **Sicca symptoms:** see Sjögren's syndrome, p. 254
- **Interstitial lung disease:** vaccinate against influenza, *Pneumococcus* and *Haemophilus influenzae*; prompt treatment of intercurrent infection.
- **Menopausal symptoms:** generally avoid HRT, since it increases risk of breast carcinoma, thrombosis and accelerates atherosclerosis. However, HRT may be considered in patients with premature ovarian failure (particularly <45 years) or for very troublesome menopausal symptoms. A history of breast cancer or thromboembolic disease is a contraindication to using HRT. The presence of anti-cardiolipin antibodies or a lupus anticoagulant should be considered a relative contra-indication.
- **Hyposplenism:** vaccinate against *Pneumococcus*, *Meningococcus* and *Haemophilus influenzae*, and check antibody titres to confirm successful vaccination. Advise against visiting any endemic malarial zone. Provide prophylactic antibiotics or stand-by antibiotics.

- **Infections:** liaise with infectious diseases team to select appropriate antimicrobial therapy according to current local policies.
- **Bronchiectasis:** physiotherapy to teach lung clearance techniques; vaccination against influenza, *Pneumococcus* and *Haemophilus influenzae*; rotating courses of antibiotics (continuous or covering winter months only).

Multidisciplinary therapy
- Renal physician.
- Dermatologist.
- Dentist and oral medicine specialist.
- Chest physician.
- Gastroenterologist.
- Ophthalmologist.
- Orthopaedic surgeon and vascular surgeon.
- Physiotherapist – exercises to retain mobility and to optimize chest function.
- Occupational therapist. Hand exercises and aids/strategies for overcoming disabilities.
- Dietician – weight reduction, management of hypertension, hyperlipidaemia, renal failure, malabsorption, or functional gastrointestinal symptoms.

Patient advice
- Avoid smoking.
- Avoid exposure to ultraviolet light – use high spf sunblock and skin-shielding clothing.
- For patients with Raynaud's keep core and extremities warm, e.g. put coat on several minutes before leaving house, use thermal gloves and socks in cold temperatures.
- For patients with sicca symptoms maintain careful oral hygiene and arrange regular dental checks.
- Gentle regular aerobic exercise to maintain cardiovascular/respiratory fitness.
- Education regarding cardiovascular risk and importance of regular aerobic exercise and healthy diet.
- Education regarding drug monitoring and important adverse effects (e.g. hydroxychloroquine – regular eye checks; cytotoxic/antiproliferative drugs – monthly FBC, LFTs; report cough or dyspnoea with methotrexate).

Follow up
- Patients with very active disease and/or commencing new therapies may need 1–3-monthly review.
- Six-monthly follow up is recommended for patient with significant disease activity.
- Annual follow-up may be appropriate for patients with mild or quiescent disease.
- BMI, urinalysis, and blood pressure monitoring should be routinely performed in the follow up visits.

At annual review
- Enquire about dyspnoea, chest pains, dental care, smoking, incidence of premature cardiovascular disease in first-degree relatives, fragility fractures, patient-led drug monitoring (e.g. annual eye check for patients on hydroxychloroquine).
- Examination to include assessment of pallor, lymphadenopathy, BMI, BP, peripheral pulses, cardiac and carotid auscultation, chest expansion, and auscultation, GALS examination (or similar musculoskeletal screen), basic neurological examination and urinalysis. A formal activity (SLEDAI or BILAG) or damage (SLICC) score may be performed.

- Laboratory investigations: FBC and differential, ESR, CRP, Creatinine and electrolytes (with estimation of creatinine clearance by Cockcroft–Gault formula), liver function tests, bone function tests including vitamin D and PTH, creatine kinase, thyroid function tests, vitamin B12, folate, ferritin, total cholesterol (low risk group), fasting lipid profile (medium and high risk groups), ANA (and ENA), anticardiolipin antibodies, lupus anticoagulant, complement C3 and C4, immunoglobulin, and protein electrophoresis.
- Consider also DXA scan, ECG, ECHO, lung function tests (including spirometry and transfer factor).

Monitoring lupus nephritis
10-year survival rate is ~70%, but a significant proportion (ranges from 5 to 50% in different series) progress to end-stage renal failure (ESRF) within 5 years. Risk factors for ESRF include:
- Abnormal renal function at presentation.
- Delay between detection of renal disease and first renal biopsy (probably because appropriate treatment is delayed).
- Male.
- Haemotological features of SLE.
- Younger age of diagnosis of lupus nephritis.
- Antiphospholipid antibodies.
- Low socio-economic group.
- African-American or Hispanic ancestry.
- Failure to achieve clinical remission with treatment.
- Flares of lupus nephritis.

Recognizing cardiovascular disease (CVD) risk
CVD accounts for most of the premature mortality in SLE. Incidence of cardiovascular events in SLE is increased between 3–10-fold.

Traditional risk factors
Assess for regularly and address accordingly:
- Hypertension.
- Hyperlipidaemia.
- Diabetes mellitus.
- Smoking.
- Increased BMI.
- Sedentary lifestyle.
- Elevated CRP.

Non-traditional risk factors
- Treatment with GCs. Optimize dose, don't over-treat and use immunosuppressant 'steroid sparing' therapy.
- Pro-inflammatory HDL.
- Anti-HSP antibodies.
- Increased oxidized LDLc.
- Circulating immune complexes.
- High inflammatory mediators (e.g. IL-6, TNFα).
- Antiphospholipid antibodies.
- Antibodies to lipoprotein lipase.
- Increased asymmetric dimethylarginine levels.
- Duration of SLE.
- Activity of SLE.

Protective factors
- Treatment with cyclophosphamide.
- Treatment with hydroxychloroquine.
- Management of conventional risk factors.

Resources

Assessment tools
British Isles Lupus Assessment Group (BILAG) index.

SLE Disease Activity Index (SLEDAI)

Europaean Consensus Lupus Activity Measurement (ECLAM).

SLE Lupus Activity Measure (SLAM).

Systemic Lupus International Collaborating Clinics (SLICC) Damage Index.

For detail of SLEDAI, ECLAM, SLICC with discussion of utility, see Griffiths et al 2005. BILAG, SLICC damage index and references for other activity scores at:

http://www.rheumatology.org/publications/abbreviations/s.asp?aud=prs

Patient organizations
Lupus UK
St James House, Eastern Road, Romford, Essex RM1 3NH. Tel: 01708 731251. www.lupusuk.com

Hughes Syndrome Foundation (antiphospholipid syndrome)
The Rayne Institute, St Thomas' Hospital, London SE1 7EH. Tel: 020 7960 5561. www.hughes-syndrome.org

Internet sites
Neuropsychiatric lupus case definitions. Available at: www.rheumatology.org/publications/ar/1999/aprilappendix.asp;

ICD-10 codes
M32/32.1	SLE/SLE with organ or system involvement
M32.0	Drug-induced SLE
I39*	Libman–Sacks endocarditis
I32.8*	Lupus pericarditis
J99.1	Respiratory disorders in SLE
N08*	Glomerular disorders in SLE
N16*	Renal tubulointerstitial disorders in SLE
M32.8	Other forms of SLE

References

ACR. The American College of Rheumatology nomenclature and case definitions for neuropsychiatric lupus syndromes. *Arthritis Rheum* 1999; **42**: 599–608.

Ahmed M, Berney SM, et al. Prevalence of active hepatitis C virus infection in patients with SLE. *Am J Med Sci* 2006; **331**: 252–6.

Almehed K, Forsblad d'Elia H, et al. Prevalence and risk factors of osteoporosis in female SLE patients – extended report. *Rheumatology* 2007; **46**: 1185–90.

Bernatsky S, Joseph L, et al. The relationship between cancer and medication exposures in systemic lupus erythematosus: a case-cohort study. *Ann Rheum Dis* 2008; **67**: 74–9.

Bernatsky S, Ramsey-Goldman B et al. Malignancy and autoimmunity. *Curr Opin Rheumatol* 2006; **18**: 129–34.

Bijl M, Kallenberg CG. Ultraviolet light and cutaneous lupus. *Lupus* 2006; **15**: 724–7.

Bosch X, Guilabert A, et al. Infections in SLE: a prospective and controlled study of 110 patients. *Lupus* 2006; **15**: 584–9.

Bruce IN. Cardiovascular disease in lupus patients: should all patients be treated with statins and aspirin? *Best Pract Res Clin Rheumatol* 2005; **5**: 823–38.

Camous L, Melander C, et al. Complete remission of lupus nephritis with rituximab and steroids for induction and rituximab alone for maintenance therapy. *Am J Kidney Dis* 2008; **52**: 346-52.

Clarke A. Proposed modifications to 1982 ACR classification criteria for systemic lupus erythematosus: serositis criterion. *Lupus* 2004; **13**: 855–6.

Clowse ME, Magder L, et al. Hydroxychloroquine in lupus pregnancy. *Arthritis Rheum* 2006; **54**: 3640–7.

Costa M, Colia D. Treating infertility in autoimmune patients. *Rheumatology* 2008; **47** Suppl 3: iii38–41.

Croker JA, Kimberly RP. Genetics of susceptibility and severity in systemic lupus erythematosus. *Curr Opin Rheumatol* 2005; **17**: 529–37.

Cross J, Jayne D. Diagnosis and treatment of kidney disease. *Best Pract Res Clin Rheumatol.* 2005; **5**: 785–98.

Danchenko N, Satia JA, Anthony MS. Epidemiology of systemic lupus erythematosus: a comparison of worldwide disease burden. *Lupus* 2006; **15**: 308–18.

Davidson RN, Wall RA. Prevention and management of infections in patients without a spleen. *Clin Microbiol Infect* 2001; **7**: 657–60.

Dooley MA, Aranow C, et al. Review of ACR renal criteria in systemic lupus erythematosus. *Lupus* 2004; **13**: 857–60.

Elliott JR, Manzi S. Induction therapy for active lupus nephritis: mycophenolate mofetil is superior to cyclophosphamide. *Nat Clin Pract Rheumatol* 2006; **2**: 354–5.

Fessler BJ, Alarcon GS, et al. SLE in three ethnic groups: XVI. Association of hydroxychloroquine use with reduced risk of damage accrual. *Arthritis Rheum* 2005; **52**: 1473–80.

Goldstein LH, Dolinsky G, et al. Pregnancy outcome of women exposed to azathioprine during pregnancy. *Birth Defects Res A Clin Mol Teratol* 2007; **79**: 696–701.

Gordon C, Ramsey-Goldman R. Systemic lupus erythematosus. *Best Pract Res Clin Rheumatol* 2005; **19**: 1–859.

Grammer AC, Lipsky PE. B cell abnormalities in systemic lupus erythematosus. *Arthritis Res Ther* 2003; **5**: S22–7.

Holvast B, Huckriede A, et al. Influenza vaccination in SLE: safe and protective? *Autoimmun Rev* 2007; **6**: 300–5.

Griffiths B, Mosca M, Gordon C. Assessment of patients with SLE and the use of lupus disease activity indices. *Best Pract Res Clin Rheumatol.* 2005; **19**: 685–708.

Hall FC, Dalbeth N. Disease modification and cardiovascular risk reduction: two sides of the same coin? *Rheumatology* 2005: **44**: 1473–82.

Huang JL, Huang JJ, et al. Septic arthritis in patients with systemic lupus erythematosus: salmonella and non-salmonella infections compared. *Semin Arthritis Rheum* 2006; **36**: 61–7.

Jara LJ, Vera-Lastra O, et al. Prolactin in human systemic lupus erythematosus. *Lupus* 2001; **10**: 748–56.

Karp DR. Complement and systemic lupus erythematosus. *Curr Opin Rheumatol* 2005; **17**: 538–42.

Lee C, Almagor O, et al. Self-reported fractures and associated factors in women with SLE. *J Rheumatol* 2007; **34**: 2018–23.

Mongey A, Hess EV. Drug insight: autoimmune effects of medications – what's new? *Nat Clin Pract Rheumatol* 2008; **4**: 136–44.

Nagy G, Koncz A, et al. T- and B-cell abnormalities in systemic lupus erythematosus. *Crit Rev Immunol* 2005; **25**: 123–40.

Nived O, Sturfelt G. ACR classification criteria for SLE: complement components. *Lupus* 2004; **13**: 877–9.

Parks GC, Cooper GS, et al. Association of Epstein–Barr virus with systemic lupus erythematosus: effect modification by race, age and cytotoxic T lymphocyte-associated antigen 4 genotype. *Arthritis Rheum* 2005; **52**: 1148–59.

Pyne D, Isenberg DA. Autoimmune thyroid disease in systemic lupus erythematosus. *Ann Rheum Dis* 2002; **61**: 70–2.

Ruiz-Irastorza G, Egurbide MV, et al. Vitamin D deficiency in systemic lupus erythematosus: prevalence, predictors and clinical consequences. *Rheumatol* 2008; **47**: 920–3.

Simard JF, Costenbader KH. What can epidemiology tell us about SLE? *Int J Clin Pract* 2007; **61**: 1170–80.

Stojsnovich L, Stojanovich R, et al. Neuropsychiatric lupus favourable response to low dose i.v. cyclophosphamide and prednisolone (pilot study). *Lupus* 2003; **12**: 3–7.

Tan EM, Cohen AS, et al. The 1982 revised criteria for the classification of SLE. *Arthritis Rheum* 1982; **25**: 1271–7.

Tarjan P, Sipka S, et al. No short-term immunological effects of Pneumococcus vaccination in patients with SLE. *Scand J Rheumatol* 2002; **31**: 211–15.

Westerweel PE, Luyten R, et al. Premature atherosclerotic cardiovascular disease in SLE. *Arthritis Rheum* 2007; **56**: 1384–96.

Sjögren's syndrome

Definition
Sjögren's syndrome (SS) is an autoimmune condition, characterized by dysfunction and destruction of exocrine glands, particularly salivary and lacrimal glands. However, constitutional symptoms are common, multi-organ involvement may occur and SS is associated with an increased incidence of lymphoid malignancy. Primary Sjögren's syndrome (pSS) occurs alone, whereas secondary Sjögren's syndrome (sSS) occurs in the context of another autoimmune disease.

Classification
Developing classification criteria for SS has proved challenging, since the prevalence of symptoms of dry eyes and mouth are common and non-specific. The most widely-used criteria currently are those agreed by the American-European Consensus group (Table 8.6).

Table 8.6 Sjögren's syndrome: classification criteria

I	Ocular symptoms:
	1. Have you had daily, persistent, troublesome dry eyes for more than 3 months?
	2. Do you have a recurrent sensation of sand or gravel in the eyes?
	3. Do you use a tear substitute more than 3 times a day?
II	Oral symptoms:
	1. Have you had a daily feeling of dry mouth for more than 3 months?
	2. Have you had recurrently or persistently swollen salivary glands as an adult?
	3. Do you frequently drink liquids to aid in swallowing dry foods?
III	Objectively dry eyes:
	Positive Schirmer's Test (≤5 mm in 5 min) or Rose Bengal score.
IV	Histopathology:
	Minor salivary gland (MSG) biopsy reveals focus score of ≥1 (see below).
V	Objectively dry mouth (≥1 of):
	1. Unstimulated whole salivary flow ≤1.5 ml in 15 min.
	2. Parotid sialography showing diffuse sialectasias without major duct obstruction.
	3. Salivary scintigraphy showing delayed uptake of tracer.
VI	Serology
	1. Either anti-Ro or anti-La antibodies, or both.
	2. Exclusions: previous head and neck radiation
	3. Hepatitis C infection
	4. Acquired immunodeficiency disease (AIDS)
	5. Pre-existing lymphoma
	6. Sarcoidosis
	7. Graft-versus-host disease
	8. Use of anti-cholinergic drugs

Diagnostic criteria
The American-European classification criteria are used to diagnose SS as follows:

Diagnosis of primary SS
- Presence of 4 of 6 criteria, including either IV (histopathology) or VI serology.
- Presence of 3 of 4 objective criteria (III, IV, V, VI).

Diagnosis of secondary SS
In the presence of a well-defined connective tissue disease, the presence of symptoms of dry eyes or mouth (I or II) plus 2 other criteria from III, IV, and V; note that serology is not used as a criterion, since it may have been used to diagnose the 'primary' connective tissue disease.

Exclusion criteria
History of head/neck radiation, HCV or HIV infection, pre-existing lymphoma, sarcoidosis, graft-versus-host disease or recent use of anti-cholinergic agents.

Despite the European-American consensus, criteria for diagnosing SS remain controversial. Further criteria have been proposed to improve sensitivity and specificity of diagnosis, including a score of IgA+ plasma cells in salivary gland histological sections or measurement of salivary IgA anti M3 muscarinic antibodies.

Epidemiology
The prevalence of SS, diagnosed according to the American-European consensus criteria is ~1% and it is therefore one of the most common autoimmune diseases. The female:male ratio is 9:1 and onset is usually 45–55 years.

Aetiology and pathophysiology
Genetic factors

HLA associations
Several groups have published association of HLA-DR alleles with SS. A recent re-evaluation indicates, however, that the HLA association is with the presence of autoantibodies, rather than with primary SS *per se*. HLA-DR15 appears to be associated with development of anti-Ro antibodies, whereas HLA-DR3 is associated with both anti-Ro and anti-La antibodies. There is tight linkage disequilibrium between HLA-DR and DQ loci and it has been suggested that HLA-mediated susceptibility relies upon expression of a permissive HLA-DQ molecule. Interestingly, secondary SS, in association with RA, is associated with HLA-DR4 rather than HLA-DR3 or 15.

Regulators of complement activation (RCA)
A recent study suggests that certain haplotypes of the RCAα block (encoding complement regulatory genes such as CR1 and MCP) interact epistatically with the HLA haplotype to modify susceptibility to SS. An HLA-DR3 haplotype is known to encode the C4A null allele and to confer a relative deficiency of C4

Interleukin-10
IL-10 promoter polymorphisms have been reported to be associated with primary SS but remains controversial.

Environmental factors

Infectious triggers
- Epstein–Barr virus (EBV) has been proposed to be a trigger for SS, since EBV DNA has been detected in salivary

CHAPTER 8 **Autoimmune connective tissue diseases**

and lachrymal glands. However, there is no evidence that it drives inflammation at these sites.
- Retroviruses are known to infect and modulate behaviour of lymphocytes. An infiltrative sialadenitis (mostly CD8+ T cells) has been described in association with HIV infection. Human T-leukaemia retrovirus-1 (HTLV-1) has also been implicated and may underlie SS in up to 20% of Japanese patients.
- Hepatitis C virus (HCV) infection is associated with sicca symptoms, but this (and HIV infection) is an exclusion to the diagnosis of primary SS

Non-infectious triggers/promoters
- Androgen deficiency has been proposed as a contributing factor in SS, since it leads to altered meibomian gland lipid profiles and tear film instability.
- Microchimerism has been suggested as a driver for chronic aberrant immunological activity in SS. Seeding of foetal leucocytes into the maternal bloodstream occurs during most pregnancies. Two studies have reported male foetal DNA to be detectable in MSG biopsies (but not peripheral blood) of 36–50% SS patients, but in 0–12% controls. However, a third study failed to demonstrate foetal DNA in any of the SS samples.

Immunopathology (Figure 8.3)
B cell over-activity
A decrease in circulating memory CD27+ B cells has been attributed to a combination of B cell trafficking to target tissues. Evidence for excessive somatic mutation and B cell receptor editing in B cells is consistent with antigen-driven (?auto)immune responses. Marked elevation of BAFF, a potential B cell activation/survival factor is implicated in the aberrant B cell behaviour.

T cell over-activity
CD4+ T cells dominate in the lymphocytic infiltrates of salivary glands in SS. Approximately a third of the infiltrating CD4+ T cells also express perforin, which implies that they may have a directly cytotoxic function. Regulatory (CD4+, CD25+, FoxP3+) T cells are rare in the salivary gland infiltrate and their numbers in peripheral blood of pSS are reduced compared with healthy controls; impaired regulation may contribute to T and B cell over-activity.

Ectopic germinal centres
Ectopic lymphoid tissue formation is characteristic of SS. Germinal centres are structures, within secondary lymphoid tissue, in which provision of antigen-specific T cell help to B cells results in activation and proliferaton of B cells, class-switching and somatic hypermutation within the genes encoding the immunoglobulins, and differentiation into plasma cells. Clusters of lymphocytes, resembling germinal centres, are found in the minor and major salivary glands of patients with SS. This suggests that antigens expressed locally in salivary glandular tissue are driving autoimmune T and B cell responses.

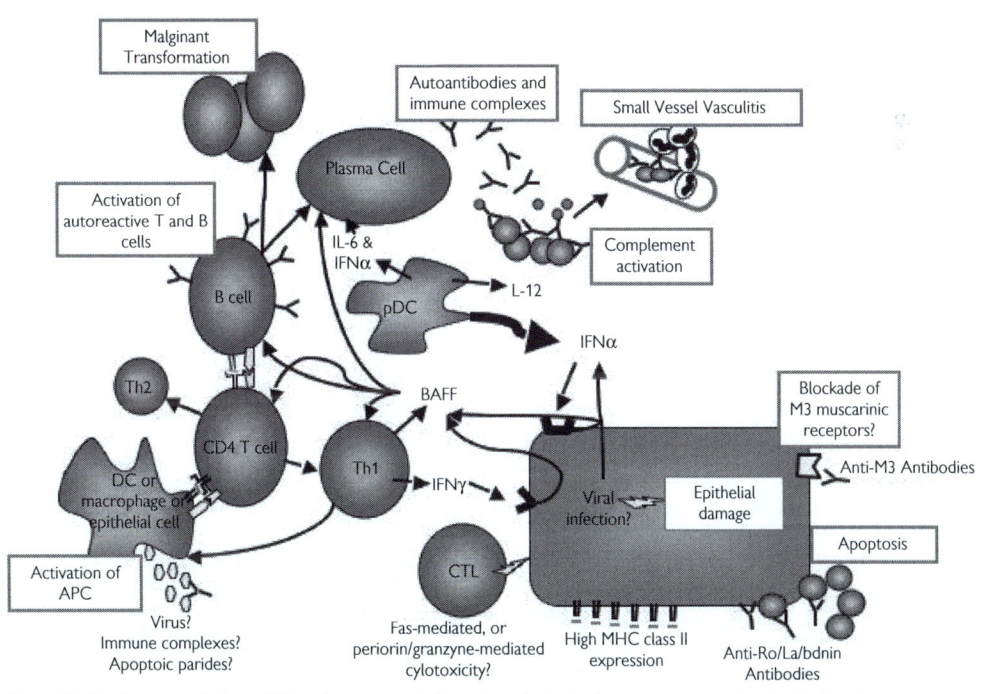

Figure 8.3 The Immunopathology of Sjögren's syndrome. Both innate and adaptive immune systems are involved in the aberrant inflammatory response which leads to the destruction of glandular epithelium in lacrimal and salivary glands. Circulating cells and soluble mediators are also implicated in the systemic features evident in many patients.

Macrophages and dendritic cells
These antigen-presenting cells are present in the salivary gland infiltrates, particularly in the ectopic germinal centres. These cells may ingest and present antigens from apoptotic salivary epithelial cells. Expression of the APC-derived Th1 cytokines, IL-12 and IL-18 have been shown to be elevated in salivary biopsy gland specimens from SS patients, compared with disease controls.

Autoantibodies
Anti-Ro antibodies are present in ~65% and anti-La antibodies in ~50% patients with pSS; these autoantibodies also occur in patients with SLE and SLE/sSS. Ro and La are expressed on blebs on the surface of apoptotic cells and this may contribute to their high immunogenicity. Their role in pathogenesis is unclear. Rheumatoid factors (RFs) and ANA may also occur in SS. Recently, α-fodrin (a molecule involved in apoptosis) and the muscarinic acetylcholine receptor-3 (M3) have been suggested as targets for autoantibodies in SS. The latter has particular appeal since anti-M3 antibodies could cause exocrine glandular dysfunction. The putative association of anti-fodrin and anti-M3 antibodies with SS, and the role of these autoantibodies in pathogenesis, requires further investigation. Autoantibodies specific for calcium channels, α1-adrenoceptors and purinoceptors have all been implicated in the autonomic dysfunction, which may occur in primary SS. However, it is unclear whether any of these autoantibodies has the ability to interfere with the function of their respective targets. Autoantibodies to islet cell antigen 69 (ICA69) have been detected in pSS and studies in animal models of SS indicate that ICA69 may be an important therapeutic target.

Cryoglobulins
Occur in ~15% patients with pSS. They are predominantly comprised of a monoclonal IgM RhF, which binds to polyclonal IgG. Cryoglobulins occur in ~ 35% patients with HCV infection, which itself frequently give rise to sicca symptoms. In the context of pSS, cryoglobulins are an indicator of clonal B cell dysregulation and are a risk factor for developing lymphoma.

Immune complexes
Are deposited in the microvasculature and give rise to purpuric rashes, glomerulonephritis, mononeuritis multiplex, and hypocomplementaemia; all features are associated with an increased risk of lymphoma.

BAFF
BAFF is a membrane-bound molecule, which can be cleaved to a soluble form; it is expressed by monocytes, neutrophils, epithelial cells and, at lower levels, by T cells. It is a critical B cell survival factor and BAFF over-expression, in transgenic murine models, favours the accumulation of low-affinity autoreactive B cells. BAFF can also co-stimulate T cell activation and differentiation. BAFF levels are markedly elevated in patients with SS and may contribute to the development of the disease by promoting auto-reactive plasmablast survival, supporting the development of ectopic germinal centres and by co-stimulating proliferation and cytokine release by CD4+ T cells. Indeed, BAFF levels have been reported to correlate with the titre of serum autoantibodies. The stimulatory, pro-survival effects of BAFF may also contribute to the development of lymphoid malignancies in SS patients.

Cytokines.
IFNα, IFNγ TNFα, and IL-10 are increased in the serum of SS patients. Salivary and conjunctival epithelial cells have been shown to exhibit up-regulated expression of genes stimulated by IFNα, and it is has been proposed that this reflects a viral disease trigger and/or perpetuation by autoantibodies to nucleosomal components. Antigen-presenting cell-derived Th1 cytokines, IL-12, and IL-18 have been detected at increased levels in MSG tissue from patients with pSS, compared with disease controls. However, since both Th1 and Th2 cytokines have been variably reported to be elevated in SS, and it cannot be considered either a predominantly Th1- or Th2-mediated disease. The role of Th17- associated cytokines remains to be clarified.

Apoptosis
Increased apoptosis of salivary epithelial cells has been demonstrated both in humans with SS and in murine models. Ro and La are both present in vesicular structures, which form on the surface of apoptotic cells; this location and increased apoptosis may contribute to their autoantigenicity in SS. α-Fodrin is a candidate autoantigen in SS; it is cleaved from the ubiquitous cytoskeletal protein Fodrin during apoptosis, again implicating excessive or dysregulated apoptosis in SS. Both autoantibodies and T cells may mediate epithelial cell destruction. Autoantibodies may bind to targets, such as the M3 receptor on epithelial cells and fix complement, causing cell death. Direct interaction of T cells with endothelial cells may also trigger apoptosis.

Salivary gland function
It has been assumed that xerostomia is the sequel to salivary acinar destruction. However, correlation between salivary flow rates and histological evidence of acinar atrophy is poor. Furthermore, in murine models of SS, salivary gland hypofunction has been demonstrated prior to tissue destruction. It has been proposed that changes in cytokine levels or other local mediators are responsible for acinar hypofunction.

Aquaporins are a family of water-transporting proteins. AQP1 is expressed on corneal epithelium and AQP 5 on the corneal and lacrimal gland epithelia. Abnormalities in the expression of each of these has been reported in patients with SS, although these findings are still controversial.

Risk factors
- Family history of autoimmune disease: individuals with a first-degree relative with an autoimmune disease have an odds ratio of ~7 of developing SS.
- History of pregnancy confers an odds ratio of ~2 of developing SS.

Clinical features
- **Xerostomia:** dry mouth; dysphagia.
- **Keratoconjunctivitis sicca:** dry eyes, blurred vision, photophobia.
- **Parotid swelling:** often recurrent.
- **Dental caries:** this is accelerated by decreased secretion of alkaline saliva that contains immunologically active molecules
- **Interstitial lung disease** is evident on HRCT chest in up to 30% of SS patients, although this is subclinical in the majority of patients. Lung disease may present with a dry cough or exertional dyspnoea.
- **Dyspareunia:** due to decreased vaginal secretions.
- **Oesophagitis or gastritis:** due to impaired mucosal secretions.
- **Malabsorption:** due to impaired pancreatic or small intestinal mucosal function; elevated amylase has been reported in 25% of patients. Gastrointestinal involvement is usually mild.

- **Interstitial cystitis**.
- **Rashes and skin dryness:** a variety of rashes may occur, including both palpable purpura (small vessel vasculitis) and flat purpura (often associated with hypergammaglobulinaemia), urticaria, and annular lesions. Dryness of the skin (~50% of patients) may result from lymphocytic infiltration of the eccrine glands of the skin.
- **Fatigue:** occurs in ~70% of patients and is often the most debilitating symptom in SS.
- **Inflammatory arthritis:** occurs in ~50% patients with SS; this is rarely erosive.
- **Mononeuritis multiplex**
- **Demyelinating syndromes** occur in ~1% of SS patients.
- **Autonomic neuropathy:** parasympathetic dysfunction has been documented in ~15% of SS patients.
- **Raynaud's phenomenon** occurs in ~30% of SS, but rarely leads to serious sequelae.
- **Purpuric vasculitis** is common, particularly on the legs.
- **Renal tubular acidosis:** sometimes complicated by urolithiasis.
- **Muscle weakness** (rare) may be caused by hypokalaemia in SS-associated RTA.
- **Lymphadenopathy** should prompt suspicion of lymphoma.

Key features in history
Eliciting symptoms of keratoconjunctivitis sicca
- Have you had daily, persistent, troublesome dry eyes for more than 3 months?
- Do you have a recurrent sensation of sand or gravel in the eyes?
- Do you use a tear substitute more than 3 times a day?

Many patients experience dry, gritty, or sticky eyes, and sometimes difficulty opening the eyes in the morning.

Eliciting symptoms of xerostomia
- Have you had a daily feeling of dry mouth for more than 3 months?
- Have you had recurrently or persistently swollen salivary glands as an adult?
- Do you frequently drink liquids to aid in swallowing dry foods? The 'cream cracker sign' refers to the inability to swallow dry foods without sips of fluid.

Also ask the patient about their dental health and ensure that they have regular dental surveillance.

Enquire about smoking history; apart from the general health implications, smoking exacerbates sicca symptoms.

Eliciting symptoms of other exocrine involvement.
Ask about dry hair and skin, vaginal dryness and dyspareunia (problems for ~30%), dyspepsia, abdominal pain, bloating, constipation.

Eliciting symptoms of extraglandular involvement.
Ask about:
- Constitutional symptoms (~70%; fatigue, fever, sweats).
- Pain and stiffness in joints, and the occurrence/duration of early morning stiffness (~30% have inflammatory arthritis).
- Dyspnoea or cough (~25% have abnormal lung function).
- Rashes.
- Cold/blue/white hands (~30%).
- Dysuria, urinary frequency, urgency, or nocturia.
- Rashes.
- Weakness, numbness, or paraesthesiae.

Key features on examination
Keratoconjunctivitis sicca
Palpebral injection of the conjunctiva, manifest as dilated conjunctival blood vessels, particularly around the horizontal meridian of the eye, indicates a response to chronic dryness, most marked at the site of maximal evaporation. Slit-lamp examination (by an ophthalmologist), using Rose Bengal (an aniline dye, which stains damaged corneal or conjunctival epithelium), may reveal filamentary keratitis. Fluorescein staining is used to reveal abnormal break-up of the tear film (time between last blink and appearance of non-fluorescent area in tear film). A positive Schirmer's test is defined as ≤10 mm wetting of a standard strip of filter paper in 5 min, after the end of the paper has been placed in the inferior conjunctival sac.

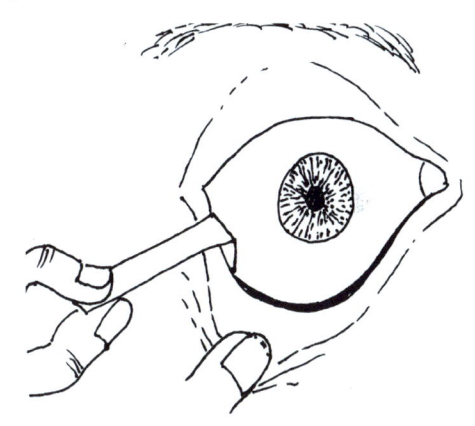

Figure 8.4 Schirmer's Test. Place filter paper in the inferior conjunctival sac, lateral to the cornea, and ask the patient to close their eyes.

Xerostomia
May be evident at the bedside as a reduced salivary pool and/or by a dry, fissured tongue. Accelerated dental caries is a common and important feature.
- Parotid and submandibular salivary glands should be palpated for swelling; nodules raise concern regarding lymphomatous transformation.
- Lymphadenopathy at cervical, submandibular and axillary sites could indicate lymphoma.

Significant interstitial lung disease
May be suggested by fine basal inspiratory crepitations, which fail to clear on coughing.

Rashes
Examine skin, particularly legs, for palpable and impalpable purpura, urticaria, and annular lesions. The skin may also be dry.

Other
- **Weight or BMI:** a drop may indicate lymphomatous transformation or malabsorption.
- **Urinalysis:** blood and protein may indicate UTI or urolithiasis.

Co-morbidities
Lymphoma
About 5% patients with SS eventually develop lymphoma and the relative risk of developing non-Hodgkins lymphoma (NHL) in this group is 44. This may present as

nodular lymphadenopathy, salivary gland enlargement or pulmonary nodules. Histological subtypes of NHL in SS include follicle centre lymphomas, lymphoplasmacytoid lymphomas, diffuse large B cell lymphomas and mucosa-associated lymphoid tissue lymphomas.

Risk factors for the development of lymphoma in SS patients are:
- Presence of autoantibodies.
- CD4+ T cell lymphopenia.
- Monoclonal gammopathies.
- Decrease in serum Ig and disappearance of RF.
- Cyoglobulins.
- Low complement C4.
- Immune complex-mediated disease (e.g. purpuric rash, glomerulonephritis, mononeuritis).
- Nodular lymphoid/glandular swellings.
- Pre-malignant lesions, e.g. myoepithelial sialadenitis.

Other co-morbidities
- Thyroid disease occurs in ~30% of pSS patients.
- Coeliac disease ~15% patients reported to have SS and 12% of SS patients have anti-tissue transglutaminase antibodies, a robust marker for CD.
- Fibromyalgia has been reported in 22% patients with pSS.
- Distal (type 1) renal tubular acidosis. In distal RTA, the distal renal tubules fail to excrete H+ ions and the urine fails to acidify (pH > 5.3, even when the patient become acidotic). Hypokalaemia may manifest as muscle weakness and may predispose to cardiac arrhythmias. Calcium derived from bones buffers the excess H^+ ions. This causes osteomalacia. Renal stone formation may occur as a result of hypercalcuria, hypocitraturia (citrate inhibits precipitation of calcium phosphate), and alkaline urine (which favours calcium phosphate deposition). Urolithiasis itself predisposes the patient to recurrent UTI. Subclinical tubular disease occurs in ~30% of pSS patients.
- Proximal (type 2) renal tubular acidosis has been reported in rarely in SS. It results from failure to reabsorb bicarbonate from the proximal tubule. Hypokalaemia occurs and the urine pH > 5.3, despite systemic acidosis. There may be a generalized proximal tubular 'leak' (glycosuria, aminoaciduria, β2 microglobulin in urine).
- Primary biliary cirrhosis (PBC) has been reported to occur in ~5% of pSS patients.
- Vasculitis may manifest as palpable purpura, glomerulonephritis (usually associated with cryoglobulinaemia) or mononeuritis.
- Depression.
- The coexistence of pernicious anaemia and SS has been reported. The extent of association is unknown.

Investigations

Ocular
- **Schirmer's tear test:** the standard bedside test is described in examination; other variants include Schirmer's test with topical anaesthesia, Schirmer's test with nasal stimulation.
- **Tear break-up time** (see examination section).
- **Lacrimal lysozyme and/or lactoferrin levels:** this provides some qualitative analysis of the lacrimal fluid.
- **Slit-lamp examination** (see examination features).

Laboratory
Haematology
- FBC with differential; mild anaemia of chronic disease occurs in ~25% and leucopenia in ~10%.
- Blood film if lymphomatous transformation is suspected.
- ESR is elevated in the majority.

Biochemistry
- Creatinine and electrolytes (note: hypokalemia may indicate renal tubular acidosis).
- Estimated creatinine clearance.
- Liver function tests.
- Thyroid function tests.
- Bone function tests; consider vitamin D and parathormone levels if malabsorption or RTA suspected.
- CRP is usually normal, unless the patient has an infection.
- Vitamin B12, folate, and ferritin levels if patient is anaemic, or if malabsorption suspected.
- Fasting lipid profile. SS has been reported to be associated with low/normal total cholesterol but with low HDL cholesterol, suggesting an increased risk of cardiovascular disease.
- Lactate dehydrogenase (LDH) if lymphoma suspected.

If RTA is suspected:
- Blood and urine pH (early morning urine sample preferable); pH > 5.3 despite metabolic acidosis in RTA.
- Plasma bicarbonate (<21 mmol/l in RTA).
- 24 h urinary calcium can be checked if RTA is suspected and to monitor response to treatment.
- Acid load test (used if plasma HCO_3^- >21 mmol/l, but RTA still suspected). 100 mg/kg ammonium chloride is administered orally. Urine pH is monitored hourly and plasma HCO_3^- at 3 h; in RTA, HCO_3^- drops below 21 mmol/l, but urine pH remains <5.3.
- β2 microglobulin measurement may be made if a generalized proximal tubular leak is suspected.

Immunology
- ANA, ENA, and RF.
- Complement C3 and C4.
- Immunoglobulins and protein electrophoresis, Bence-Jones protein estimation.
- Cryoglobulins.
- A positive ANA, RF with anti-Ro (in 50–70%) ± anti-La (in 20–50%) antibodies are commonly found.
- Hypergammaglobulinaemia occurs ~80% pSS patients. A monoclonal band and/or low complement C4/C3 are risk factors for developing lymphoma.
- Anti-mitochondrial antibodies – if the clinical features suggest PBC.
- Anti-tissue transglutaminase or anti-endomysial antibodies – if the clinical features suggest coeliac disease. (note: ensure that the patient has normal IgA levels in order to avoid a false negative test).

Microbiology
- Microscopy, culture and (antibiotic) sensitivities (MC&S) of conjunctival swab if a bacterial conjunctivitis is suspected.
- MC&S of an mid-stream urine (MSU) will be needed in patients with dysuria, urinary urgency or blood and/or protein on urinalysis.
- Viral serology is required to exclude HCV and, in appropriate cases, HIV infection.

CHAPTER 8 **Autoimmune connective tissue diseases** 259

Imaging
- Ultrasound (US) and MR can detect infiltrates in the major salivary glands of patients with SS, although such investigations are generally not required.
- Sialography using water-soluble contrast media is used in some centres to assess anatomical changes in the salivary gland ducts.
- Scintigraphy can be used to quantify salivary gland function. Following injection of ^{99m}Tc pertechnetate, the uptake of label by salivary glands can be imaged and the time taken for the label to appear in the mouth measured; both are delayed or absent in patients with SS.
- MR sialography is a sensitive method of assessing changes in minor salivary glands (MSGs), but is not widely used.
- High resolution CT chest will reveal parenchymal abnormalities in ~30% patient with SS, although lung disease is subclinical in the majority.
- Renal and urinary tract US is useful if renal stones are suspected.
- Plain radiographs of hands/feet (or MR or US) may be used to screen for erosive arthritis.

Histology
- MSG biopsy is frequently used to substantiate the diagnosis. A focus score has largely replaced the less sensitive Chisholm classification. (A focus is a cluster of ≥50 lymphocytes; the focus score is the average number of foci in a 4 mm^2 area, assessed from ≥4 salivary gland lobules).
- Parotid gland biopsy provides similar information to the MSG biopsy; lymphoma should be excluded
- Excision biopsies of lymph node(s) should be examined to exclude lymphoma.
- Bladder biopsy (if interstitial cystitis suspected).

Cytology
Urinary cytology may occasionally be indicated in patients with sterile pyuria - ?interstitial cystitis.

Cardiovascular Investigations
- ECG.
- Cardiac ECHO, if clinical examination or ECG indicates new murmur or possible LVH.

Other Investigations
- Pulmonary function tests (spirometry and transfer factor) are abnormal in ~25% patients. Most respiratory disease in SS remains subclinical. However, pulmonary function tests can be used to monitor for significant progression and to determine, which patients require a HRCT chest.
- Nerve conduction studies may be performed on patients with suspected mononeuritis (multiplex)
- MR or CT scanning of brain/spinal cord, along with other appropriate tests are indicated if patients have symptoms suggesting CNS disease.
- Tests of autonomic function may be performed on patients with postural hypotension; these may include beat-to-beat variation or tilt-table tests.

Differential diagnosis
- **Blepharitis** secondary to Meibomian gland dysfunction.
- **Allergic conjunctivitis**.
- **HCV**: this is a common viral infection (prevalence ~2% worldwide), which frequently causes sicca symptoms and cryoglobulinaemia.
- **HIV** can present with sicca symptoms or parotid swelling.
- **Drug-related sicca syndrome**, e.g. tricyclic antidepressants, diuretics.
- **Sarcoidosis** can cause sicca symptoms, arthritis, rashes, and interstitial lung disease.
- **Graft-versus-host disease**.
- **Alcohol abuse** may cause parotid enlargement.
- **Paraneoplastic disease** may present with constitutional and sicca symptoms.
- **Coeliac disease** may also present with constitutional symptoms, oral inflammation and rashes.
- **Fibromyalgia**: fatigue may be indistinguishable from constitutional symptoms/signs of SS and patient may acquire sicca symptoms/signs secondary to medications (e.g. amitriptyline). Fybromyalgia has been reported in 22% of patients with SS.

Disease activity assessment
SCAI   SS Clinical Activity Index
SSDAI   SS Disease Activity Index
PROFAD   Profile of fatigue and discomfort.

Treatment
Objectives of management
- Symptomatic relief of mucosal dryness.
- Improvement of constitutional symptoms.
- Prompt treatment of mucosal infections.
- Analgesia (where relevant).
- Arrest or retardation of underlying autoinflammatory disease.
- Early detection and treatment of lymphoma.
- Reduction of cardiovascular disease. Risk of CV disease is elevated in several chronic inflammatory conditions (e.g. RA and SLE), but it remains to be clarified whether this applies to SS.

General measures
See advice to patients.

Physical therapies
- Artificial tears/ophthalmic lubricants. Short-acting preparations contain polyvinyl alcohol (SnoTears, Liquifilm) or carboxycellulose (Hypromellose, Tears Naturale). Longer-acting preparations contain carbomer gels (e.g. Viscotears, Geltears) or paraffin (e.g. Lacrilube, Lubri-Tears); these are stickier and patients may prefer to use them at night. Some patients are intolerant of preservatives in aqueous drops and preservative-free Liquifilm may be tolerated.
- Mucolytic agents (e.g. acetylcysteine 10%) may be used sparingly for sticky mucus in the eyes.
- Autologous serum (50% in normal saline) eye drops improve objective and subjective measure of ocular surface disease, but this treatment is not generally available.
- Artificial saliva is available as sprays (e.g Glandosane, Saliva Orththa, Luborant), lozenges (Saliva Orthana) or gels (e.g. Oralbalance, BioXtra). Note that Luborant is a neutral pH and contains fluoride, and therefore may reduce dental caries.
- Vaginal lubricant (e.g. KY jelly).
- Skin emollients, e.g. E45 cream.
- Physiotherapy and goal-setting can be helpful for managing constitutional symptoms. Nordic walking for 45 min 3 times a week for 12 weeks has been shown to improve

aerobic capacity and to reduce fatigue and depression. Physiotherapy is also important in the rehabilitation from neurological complications of SS.
- Gluten-free diet (only in SS patients with co-existing coeliac disease).

Pharmacological stimulation of salivary flow
Muscarinic, cholinergic agonists can be used as secretagogues in patients with xerostomia.
- **Pilocarpine:** data from a recent RDBPCT demonstrated that pilocarpine 5 mg qds improves subjective and objective measures of salivary flow. Oral administration of 5% pilocarpine solution is also effective. About ~50% of SS patients respond to pilocarpine (the non-responders may be those with salivary acinar atrophy, but this requires clarification). The main side effects are sweating, flushing, diarrhoea, and urinary urgency; these can be reduced by starting pilocarpine at 5 mg od and gradually increasing the dose.
- **Cevelimine** (licenced in USA and Japan) is a more selective muscarininc agonist than pilocarpine; with greater efficacy at the M1 and M3 receptors, which are prevalent in exocrine glands. Two RDBPCT trials have shown efficacy for 20 or 30 mg tds. The main side-effects (particularly at high doses) are nausea, sweating and headache. Theoretically, the selectivity of cevelimine may result in fewer adverse effects than for pilopcarpine, but this is unproven.

Pain relief
- Simple analgesia (e.g. paracetamol) is first-line.
- NSAIDs should be avoided wherever possible due to increased risk of gastrointestinal (and possibly tubulointerstitial) damage in SS. When unavoidable, NSAIDs should be prescribed with a proton pump inhibitor in SS.
- Opiate analgesia is rarely required in SS.

Conventional Immunosuppression
- Hydroxychloroquine is widely used in Sjögren's. It has been assessed in one small double-blind, placebo-controlled randomized trial (DBPRCT) and a larger retrospective study; both provided some evidence for efficacy (subjective improvement, reduction in acute phase markers and IgG levels).
- Azathioprine was not found to be effective in a single DBPRCT.
- Mycophenolate mofetil has not been subjected to clinical trial in SS.
- Methotrexate (MTX) – a pilot study indicated that MTX was safe, but revealed no objective improvement in sicca features.
- Leflunomide – a pilot study suggested some improvement in acute phase markers and vasculitis.
- Cyclophosphamide – case reports suggest improvement in myelopathy/neuropathy in SS.
- Other immunosuppressives, including ciclosporin or tacrolimus are used empirically.
- Glucocorticoids are used minimally in SS. There is no evidence that they improve sicca features.

Biologic drugs
- **Anti-TNFα treatments** appeared promising following an open-label pilot study of infliximab in pSS, but neither a larger (n = 103) DBPCRCT of infliximab 5 mg/kg nor a DBPCRCT of etanercept in 14 patients showed significant improvement in objective or subjective measures.
- **IFNα:** Phase III studies in pSS of 150U IFNα lozenges tds revealed a significantly increase in the unstimulated (but not stimulated) salivary flow rate and a decrease in sicca symptoms.
- **Rituximab:** given the prominence of B cells in the pathogenesis of SS, it is logical to consider B cell depletion therapy. Reports of small open-label studies of rituximab in SS are promising, suggesting that objective and subjective measures of disease activity may be improved; serial MSG biopsies in one study indicates that rituximab depletes B cells from salivary tissue, as well as from peripheral blood. Rituximab has also been used to successfully treat SS-associated MALT lymphoma. DBPCRCTs are currently being organized.

Other pharmacological therapies/supplements
- Thyroxine to correct hypothyroidism.
- Proton pump inhibitor for dyspepsia.
- Potassium bicarbonate and citrate supplementation in patients with distal RTA.
- Thiazide diuretics may be used to increase proximal tubule bicarbonate reabsorption in RTA.
- Vitamin D3 supplementation if deficient. Note that chewable calcium/Vit D3 preparations are unlikely to be palatable in patients with dry mouth. Dispersible cacit D3 (2 sachets daily) is an alternative.
- Vitamin B12 injection in patients with co-existing pernicious anaemia.
- Treatment of lymphoma. Outcome of patients with low-grade lymphomas in SS is not altered by chemotherapy and patients are managed by observation. High-grade lymphomas are treated with a variety of regimens, including rituximab and cytotoxic agents.

Surgery
Lacrimal ducts may be plugged temporarily or cauterized for permanent occlusion.

Multidisciplinary approach
- Ophthalmologist.
- Dentist.
- Chest physician (if significant ILD).
- Maxillofacial/oral surgeon (MSG biopsy).
- Haematologist (if lymphoma).
- Histopathologist.
- Other specialists (renal physicians, dermatologists, radiologists, urologists).

Patient advice
- Avoid very dry environments. A humidifier in the bedroom/sitting room may be useful.
- Reduce evaporation from eyes by wearing tinted glasses with side panels in bright sunlight or tight fitting goggles during particularly dry/dusty tasks; avoid contact lenses.
- Use lubricants and emollients, e.g. aqueous eye drops, eye ointment overnight, petroleum jelly on lips, skin emollients, vaginal lubricants, and moisturizing hair conditioner. Carry water to sip.
- Stimulate salivary flow using sugar-free pastilles and/or chewing gum.
- Avoid excess alcohol intake and do not smoke.
- Dental care must include careful twice-daily brushing of teeth and regular dental check-ups. The patient should be advised to use acid and sugar-free drinks and sugar-free sweets/gum.

- Seek medical advice if oral, conjunctival, or vaginal infection (including thrush) is suspected.
- Seek medical advice if salivary or lymph glands become swollen.
- An aerobic exercise programme (e.g. swimming lengths or Nordic walking 3 times weekly) should be recommended to patients with fatigue.

Prognosis and natural history
SS is a chronic condition but the majority of cases are mild. Overall, the standardized mortality ratio for SS is ~1.15. However, patients with risk factors for lymphoma (see above) have a less favourable prognosis.

SS patients with non-gastric MALT lymphoma have a 5-year survival of ~90%, despite the fact that ~30% of these are disseminated at diagnosis.

Monitoring disease activity
This is rarely performed in routine clinical practice but scores of disease activity have recently been developed for research purposes (see assessment tools).

Follow-up
- Annual follow-up is acceptable for patients with pSS, with ≤1 risk factor for lymphoma.
- Six-monthly follow-up is recommended for patients with >1 risk factor for developing lymphoma.
- More frequent follow up will also be required following complications such as progressive interstitial lung disease, or vasculitis.

Current controversies
- Role of various putative autoantigens in the pathogenesis.
- Role for T and B cell immunosuppression in management of SS.
- Assessment of activity, including definition of appropriate biomarkers of disease activity.
- Extent of association of SS with cardiovascular disease.

Resources
Nordic walking information. Available at: http://en.wikipedia.org/wiki/Nordic_walking

Assessment tools
VAS: Visual analogue scales for fatigue, sicca symptoms and pain.

SCAI: SS Clinical Activity Index.

SSDAI: SS Disease Activity Index.

PROFAD: Profile of fatigue and discomfort.

SF-36: Short form 36.

Patient organizations
British Sjögren's Syndrome Association. PO Box 10867, Birmingham B16 0ZW. Tel (UK): 0121 455 6532. Email: office@bssa.uk.net

Sjögren's Syndrome Foundation. 6707 Democracy Boulevard, Suite 325, Bethesda, MD 20817, USA. Tel (USA) (toll free): (800) 475-6473.

Internet sites
British Sjögren's Syndrome Association. Available at: www.bssa.uk.nt

Sjögren's Syndrome Foundation. Available at: http://www.sjogrens.com;

Arthritis Research Campaign patient information. Available at: www.arc.org.uk/arthinfo/patpubs/6041/6041.asp

American College of Rheumatology patient information. Available at: www.rheumatology.org/public/factsheets/sjogrens_new.asp?aud=pat

ICD-10 codes
M35.0	Sjögren's syndrome
H19.3	keratoconjunctivitis and keratitis
J99.1	Respiratory disorder in diffuse CTD
G73.7	Myopathy in CTD
N16.4	Renal tubulo-interstitial disorders in CTD

References
Barendregt PJ, van Den Meiracker AH, et al. Parasympathetic failure does not contribute to ocular dryness in primary Sjögren's syndrome. *Ann Rheum Dis* 1999; **58**: 746–50.

D'Arbonneau F, Ansart S, et al. Thyroid dysfunction in primary Sjögren's syndrome: a long-term follow-up study. *Arthritis Rheum* 2003; **49**: 804–9.

Dawson LJ, Smith PM, et al. Sjögren's syndrome – time for a new approach. *Rheumatol* 2000; **39**: 234–7.

Eriksson P, Denneberg T, et al. Urolithiasis and distal renal tubular acidosis preceding primary Sjögren's syndrome: a retrospective study 5–53 years after the presentation of urolithiasis. *J Intern Med* 1996; **239**: 483–8.

Fox RI, Dixon R, et al. Treatment of primary Sjögren's syndrome with hydroxychloroquine: a retrospective, open-label study. *Lupus* 1996; **5**: S31–6.

Gottenberg JE, Busson M, et al. In primary Sjogren's syndrome, HLA class II is associated exclusively with autoantibody production and spreading of the autoimmune response. *Arthritis Rheum* 2003; **48**:2240–5.

Hansen A, Lipsky PE, Dorner T. New concepts in the pathogenesis of Sjogren syndrome: many questions, fewer answers. *Curr Opin Rheumatol* 2003;**15**:563–70.

Jonsson MV, Delaleu N, et al. Impaired salivary gland function in NOD mice: association with changes in cytokine profile but not with histopathologica changes in the salivary gland. *Arthritis Rheum* 2006; **54**: 2300–5.

Klaeger AJ, Cevallos V, et al. Clinical application of a homogeneous colorimetric assay for tear lysozyme. *Ocul Immunol Inflamm* 1999; **7**: 7–15.

Kruize AA, HeneRJ, et al. Hydroxychloroquine treatment for primary Sjögren's syndrome: a two year double blind crossover trial. *Ann Rheum Dis* 1993; **52**: 360–4.

Lodde BM, Sankar V, et al. Serum lipid levels in Sjögren's syndrome. *Rheumatology* 2006; **45**: 481–4.

Luft LM, Barr SG, et al. Autoantibodies to tissue transglutaminase in Sjögren's syndrome and related rheumatic diseases. *J Rheumatol* 2003; **30**: 2613–9.

Mackay F, Groom JR, Tangye SG. An important role for B-cell activation factor and B cells in the pathogenesis of Sjogren's syndrome. *Curr Opin Rheumatol* 2007; **19**: 406–13.

Manoussakis MN, Boiu S, et al. Rates of infiltration by macrophages and dendritic cells and expression of interleukin-18 and interleukin-12 in the chronic inflammatory lesions of Sjögren's syndrome: correlation with certain features of immune hyperactivity and factors associated with high risk of lymphoma development. *Arthritis Rheum* 2007; **56**: 3977–88.

Mariette X, Ravaud P, et al. Inefficacy of infliximab in primary Sjögren's syndrome: results of the randomized, controlled Trial of Remicade in Primary Sjögren's Syndrome (TRIPSS). *Arthritis Rheum* 2004; **50**: 1270–6.

Mavragani CP, Moutsopoulos NM, Moutsopoulos HM. The management of Sjögren's syndrome. *Nat Clin Pract Rheumatol* 2006; **2**: 252–61

Montano-Loza AJ, Crispin-Acuna JC, et al. Abnormal hepatic biochemistries and clinical liver disease in patients with primary Sjögren's syndrome. *Ann Hepatol* 2007; **6**: 150–5.

Nordmark G, Alm GV, Rönnblom I. Mechanisms of disease: primary Sjögren's syndrome and the type I interferon system. *Nat Clin Pract Rheumatol* 2006; **2**: 262–9.

Ono M, Takamura E, et al. Therapeutic effect of cevimeline on dry eye in patients with Sjögren's syndrome: a randomized, double-blind clinical study. *Am J Ophthalmol* 2004; **138**: 6–17.

Patel YI, McHugh NJ. Apoptosis-new clues to the pathogenesis of Sjogren's syndrome? *Rheumatol* 2000; **39**:119–21.

Petrone D, Condemi JJ, et al. A double-blind, randomized, placebo-controlled study of cevimeline in Sjögren's syndrome patients with xerostomia and keratoconjunctivitis sicca. *Arthritis Rheum* 2002; **46**: 748–54.

Pijpe J, Kalk WW, et al. Parotid gland biopsy compared with labial biopsy in the diagnosis of patients with primary Sjögren's syndrome. *Rheumatol* 2007; **46**: 335–41.

Price EJ, Rigby SP, et al. A double blind placebo controlled trial of azathioprine in the treatment of primary Sjögren's syndrome. *J Rheumatol* 1998; **25**: 896–9.

Priori R. Medda E, et al. Risk factors for Sjögren's syndrome: a case-control study. *Clin Exp Rheumatol.* 2007: **25**: 378–84.

Rosas J, Ramos-Casals M, et al. Usefulness of basal and pilocarpine-stimulated salivary flow in primary Sjögren's syndrome. Correlation with clinical, immunological and histological features. *Rheumatol* 2002; **41**: 670–5.

Sankar V, Brennan MT, et al. Etanercept in Sjögren's syndrome: a twelve-week randomized, double-blind, placebo-controlled pilot clinical trial. *Arthritis Rheum* 2004; **50**: 2240–5.

Seror R, Sordet C, et al. Tolerance and efficacy of rituximab and changes in serum B cell biomarkers in patients with systemic complications of primary Sjögren's syndrome. *Ann Rheum Dis* 2007; **66**: 351–7.

Ship JA, Fox PC, et al. Treatment of primary Sjögren's syndrome with low-dose natural interferon-alpha administered by the oral mucosal route: a phase II clinical trial. IFN Protocol Study Group. *J Interferon and Cytok Res* 1999; **19**: 943–51.

Skopouli FN, Jagiello P, et al. Methotrexate in primary Sjögren's syndrome. *Clin Exp Rheumatol* 1996; **14**: 555–8.

Strömbeck BE, Theander E, Jacobsson LT. Effects of exercise on aerobic capacity and fatigue in women with primary Sjögren's syndrome. *Rheumatol* 2007; **46**: 868–71.

Teppo H and Revonta M. A follow-up study of minimally invasive lip biopsy in the diagnosis of Sjögren's syndrome. *Clin Rheumatol* 2007; **26**: 1099–103.

Tsubota K, Kaido M, et al. Diseases associated with ocular surface abnormalities: the importance of reflex tearing. *Br J Ophthalmol* 1999; **83**: 89–91.

Tzioufas A. Update on Sjogren's syndrome autoimmune epithelitis: from classification to increased neoplasias. *Best Pract Res Clin Rheumatol* 2007; **21**: 989–1010.

Valtysdottir ST, Gudbjörnsson B, et al. Psychological well-being in patients with primary Sjögren's syndrome. *Clin Exp Rheumatol* 2000; **18**: 597–600.

van Woerkom JM, Kruize AA, et al. Safety and efficacy of leflunomide in primary Sjögren's syndrome: a phase II pilot study. *Ann Rheum Dis* 2007; **66**: 1026–32.

Venables PJ. Sjogren's syndrome. *Best Pract Res Clin Rheumatol* 2004; **18**: 313–29.

Vitali C, Bombardieri S, et al. Classification criteria for Sjögren's syndrome: a revised version of the European criteria proposed by the American-European Consensus Group. *Ann Rheum Dis* 2002; **61**: 554–8.

Wu Ch, Hsieh SC, et al. Pilocarpine hydrochloride for the treatment of xerostomia in patients with Sjögren's syndrome in Taiwan – a double-blind, placebo-controlled trial. *J Formos Med Assoc* 2006; **105**: 796–803.

Systemic sclerosis

Definition
Systemic sclerosis (SSc) is a multisystem autoimmune disease characterized by widespread microvascular disease, tissue infiltration of mononuclear cells and excessive deposition of extracellular matrix material, particularly collagen.

Classification
Several classification criteria have been established through the years for SSc. In 1980 the American College of Rheumatology (ACR) published consensus criteria for the diagnosis and classification of SSc. This classification is based on the presence one major criterion (sclerosis of the skin proximal to the metacarpophalangeal joints) and two of the three minor criteria (digital pitting scars, sclerodactyly and bilateral pulmonary fibrosis) to establish the diagnosis.
- These criteria require the presence of established disease and do not utilize serological information.
- The most widely used classification is the Le Roy classification of 1988, which divides SSc into limited and diffuse cutaneous systemic sclerosis – lcSSc and dcSSc respectively.
- Roy and Medsger have also proposed a limited SSc category; this will include patients with early SSc, but may also capture patients with autoimmune Raynaud's phenomenon, who do not progress to classical SSc.

Epidemiology
SSc occurs more frequently in women, with a female: male ratio of 3:1. Peak age of onset is between 30 and 50 years. The UK prevalence is ~120 per million with an annual incidence ~4 per million per year. Although there is no racial predilection, the disease may occur more often and most severely in young black women.
- Many environmental agents have been associated with the occurrence of SSc including silica, organic chemicals, e.g. paraffin, vinyl chloride, resin, and toxic oils and drugs, including appetite suppressants, bleomycin, hydroxytryptophan, carbidopa, bleomycin, and cocaine.
- It has been suggested that silicone breast implants may contribute to the development of SSc, but a recent large case-control study and meta-analyses do not support an association.
- Familial clustering may occur and a positive family history is the strongest risk factor identified for SSc and the recurrence rate for first-degree relatives (λr) is 54. However, the absolute risk for each first degree relative is less than 1%. High titres of ANA were present in first-degree relatives of patients with SSc.
- The highest prevalence of SSc has been demonstrated in a genetically isolated population of Choctaw American Indians. In this population, SSc is strongly associated with a polymorphism in the 5'-untranslated region of the FBN1 gene.
- Association studies in other populations have indicated that polymorphism in the genes encoding type I collagen α2 chain (COL1A2) and transforming growth factor (TGF)-β may predispose to SSc.
- Emerging genetic associations with interstitial lung disease (e.g. fibronectin) and with microvascular disease (e.g. bone morphogenetic protein receptor II with primary pulmonary hypertension and activin-receptor-like kinase with hereditary haemorrhagic telangiectasiae) warrant further exploration in SSc.
- HLA associations are weak with SSc overall but anti-centromere antibodies are associated with HLA-DQB1 alleles, and anti-Scl70 antibodies with an HLA-DQB1 and an HLA-DRw11 allele.

The 1988 LeRoy classification of SSc
Diffuse cutaneous systemic sclerosis (dcSSc) ~33%
- Skin sclerosis extending proximal to the elbow and truncal.
- Prominent pruritis and constitutional symptoms.
- Renal, pulmonary (secondary pulmonary arterial hypertension), cardiac and GI involvement.
- Raynaud's often develops after other features.
- Tendon friction rubs.
- Disease activity stable over many years.

Limited cutaneous systemic sclerosis (lcSSc) ~60% (previously CREST: Calcinosis, Raynaud's Esophageal dysmotility, Sclerodacytly and Telangectasias)
- Raynaud's precedes other features.
- Skin involvement restricted – hands, face, forearms and feet.
- Pulmonary arterial hypertension.
- Telangiectasiae.
- Calcinosis.
- Severe gut disease.
- Interstitial lung disease (association with anti-SScl-70).
- Disease progressive in first few years then often stabilizes.
- Associated with anti-centromere antibodies (ACA).

Limited systemic sclerosis
- Raynaud's phenomenon (RP).
- Abnormal nail-fold capillaroscopy.
- SSc-selective antibodies (ACA, anti-Scl-70, anti-RNA polymerase I/III).

Diagnosis based on objective documentation of Raynaud's and one other criterion OR subjective documentation of Raynaud's and BOTH other criteria.

Systemic sclerosis sine scleroderma <2%
- Raynaud's phenomenon visceral manifestations.
- SSc-selective antibodies.
- No skin involvement.

Aetiology and pathophysiology
SSc is a chronic auto-inflammatory syndrome, in which aberrant behaviour of both innate and adaptive elements of the immune system is evident. Endothelial cell dysfunction and damage is prominent. Microvascular damage with vasospasm and vessel dropout, and excessive deposition of extracellular matrix tissue lead to the main clinical manifestations of disease.

Aberrant innate and adaptive immune responses
An aberrant immune response in SSc is most obvious in the florid cutaneous inflammatory infiltrate, which often accompanies early dcSSc.
- The mononuclear infiltrate consists of T cells (mainly CD4+), macrophages, natural killer cells, mast cells and, rarely, B cells.

CHAPTER 8 **Autoimmune connective tissue diseases**

- Oligoclonal expansion of CD4+ T cells in SSc skin lesions has been shown, suggesting local antigen-dependent T cell activation. Activated CD4+ T cells produce IL-4, IL-17 and TGF-β, which stimulate endothelial cells to express HLA and adhesion molecules, promotes PDGF release, fibroblast proliferation, and CTGF secretion, which promotes synthesis of collagen.
- Inflammatory cells (neutrophils, eosinophils, and lymphocytes) are also present in the bronchoalveolar lavage fluid of SSc patients with interstitial lung disease.
- As cutaneous fibrosis progresses, the inflammatory infiltrate recedes, and a similar transition may occur in other tissues.
- It has been noted that graft-versus-host disease often resembles SSc and it has been hypothesized that microchimerism – persistence of alloreactive cells either from maternal blood at birth or from foetal blood at parturition – may drive the chronic (allo)immune response which manifests as SSc.
- Although B cells are scarce in skin infiltrates, an abnormal humoural response is well recognized by virtue of the characteristic autoantibodies associated with SSc (e.g. anticentromere, anti-Scl70, and anti RNA polymerase I/III).
- The role of autoantibodies in pathophysiology is uncertain, but anti-endothelial antibodies may mediate endothelial damage and anti-fibroblast antibodies may contribute to synthesis of matrix constituents.

Endothelial dysfunction and microvascular disease

Vascular tone is determined by the balance between vasoconstrictive and vasodilatory stimuli received by the vascular smooth muscle cells of the tunica media (Figure 8.5). Endocrine, paracrine, autocrine, and neuronal stimuli enable the resistance vessels to respond both to local (ischaemia/inflammation) and systemic (e.g. maintenance of blood pressure) needs.

- Dysregulation of vasomotor tone in SSc may reflect intrinsic abnormalities of endothelial cells or vascular smooth muscle cells, aberrant production of local soluble mediators (e.g. from endothelial cells, platelets, or leucocytes), or neuroendocrine abnormalities.
- Abnormalities suggested in SSc-associated RP include:
  - endothelial cell damage, e.g. by infection, anti-endothelial antibodies, cytotoxic T cells, free radicals;
  - increased contractile response to sudden cooling and to α2-adrenergic agonists; this appears to be mediated by the α2c-adrenoceptors and is associated with increased activity of protein tyrosine kinase;
  - increased levels of endothelin and/or increased density of endothelin receptors;
  - reduction of calcitonin gene-related peptide (CGRP) release from sensory afferent nerve endings (possibly related to ischaemic tissue damage);
  - aberrant activation of platelets and/or coagulation cascade;
  - oxidative stress probably contributes to endothelial cell damage;
  - release of vasomotor mediators from mononuclear cells (e.g. mast cells) in underlying tissue.
- Abnormal vasomotor responses are evident early in the pathophysiology of SSc.

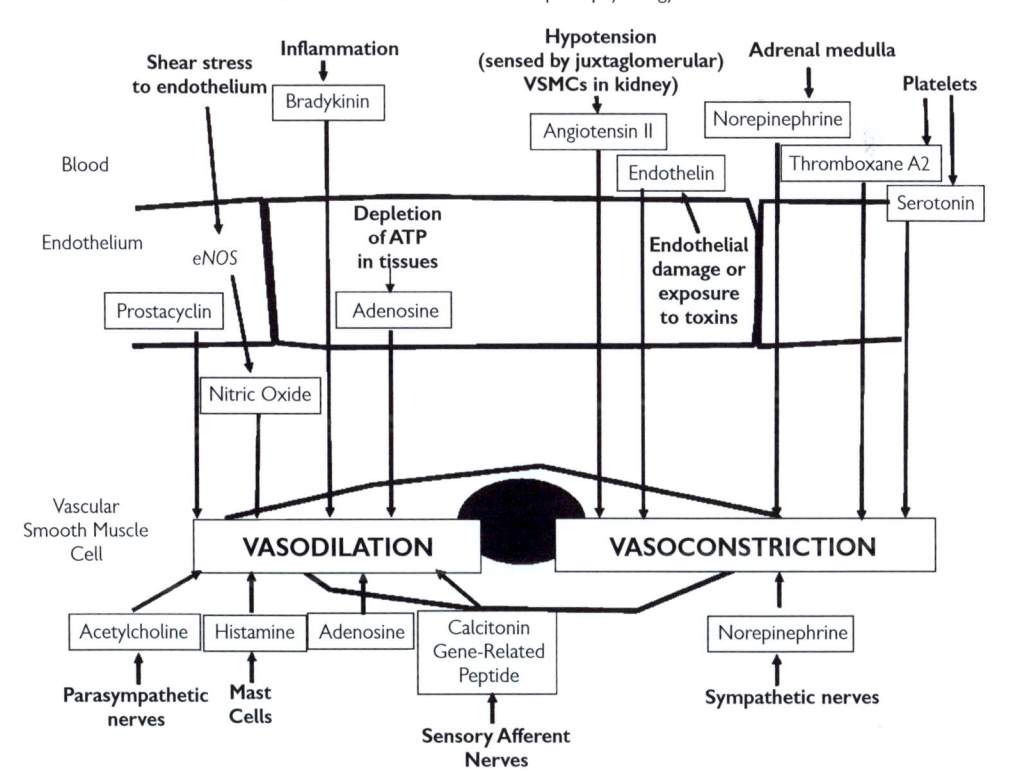

Figure 8.5 Factors influencing vasomotor tone.

- As disease progresses, structural changes in the walls of small and medium sized arteries lead to fixed narrowing and ultimately occlusion of vessel lumens.
- Intimal proliferation and fibrosis is mediated by migration of vascular smooth muscle cells into the intima, their differentiation into myofibroblasts and the deposition of extracellular matrix proteins.
- The combination of this microvascular remodelling with vasomotor disturbance results in ischaemia-reperfusion cycles, which results in tissue damage by free radical formation, endothelial activation (increased adhesion molecules, procoagulant surface) and platelet activation (release of more vasoconstrictive and procoagulant factors).
- Narrowing and eventual occlusion of small arteries leads to digital ischaemia, pulmonary arterial hypertension, renal ischaemia and damage, and probably also dysfunction and damage in the gut and other organs.

Animal models
- Demonstrate that certain genetic and environmental factors can reproduce aspects of the SSc phenotype.
- The tight skin (tsk1) mouse, a model for scleroderma, has duplication within the fibrillin 1 (FBN1) gene, which encodes a major constituent of extracellular matrix.
- Scleroderma can also be induced by bleomycin in a genetically susceptible mouse strain.
- The University of California Davis line 200 (UCD 200) chickens mimic the vascular damage since they develop early endothelial cell apoptosis followed by excessive perivascular collagen deposition.

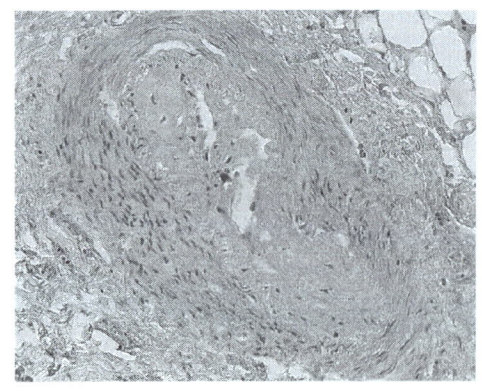

Figure 8.6 Cross-section of a digital artery from a patient with lcSSc showing intimal proliferation and luminal narrowing (with permission from Professor A. Freemont).

Risk factors
- SSc in first degree relative – 54-fold increased risk.
- Males, African-Americans, older age group – generally more severe disease.
- Exposure to environmental agents (see above).
- Anti-centromere antibody is a risk factor for recurrent digital ulceration.
- Anti-Scl-70 antibody is a risk for interstitial lung disease.
- Anti-RNA polymerase III – is a risk for severe skin involvement and scleroderma renal crisis.
- Glucocorticoids in the preceding month are associated with a 24-fold risk of scleroderma renal crisis.

Clinical features
Raynaud's phenomenon
RP is the initial symptom in more than 90% of SSc cases. Transient vasospasm leads to classic colour changes in the digits: white (ischaemia), blue (cyanosis), and red (reperfusion). This is usually triggered by the cold, smoking, or emotional stress. RP usually affects digits, but it can also affect other areas including the tip of the nose, ear lobes, tongue and patellae (see Plate 5).
- Primary RP – affects 10–15% of the general population and is commoner in women.
- RP occurring in the context of an AICTD is secondary and this may be distinguished from primary RP by:
  - onset after age 30 years;
  - severe ischaemic pain;
  - presence of elevated ANA titres;
  - abnormal nail-fold capillary architecture;
  - digital ulceration.

Skin and cutaneous features
Scleroderma typically involves skin tightening and induration, with subsequent thickening and tethering to underlying tissues.
- Scleroderma skin becomes shiny and smooth with loss of hair, sweat glands, and skin creases.
- Sclerodactyly is scleroderma in digits, which results in contractures and loss of function.
- Microstomia results from sclerodermatous changes around the mouth, and can impede access for dental work and, in severe cases, impair eating.
- Sicca syndrome – dry eyes, dry mouth contributing to dysphagia, dyspareunia.
- Telangiectasiae – dilated blood vessels, mainly capillaries and arterioles; these occur commonly on the face and upper trunk and blanch when pressure is applied.
- Calcinosis – calcium deposits in skin and subcutaneous tissue commonly in the hands, legs, and around joints. Calcinotic plaques may become inflamed and often ulcerate, releasing a white chalky material.

Musculoskeletal
Joint pains, stiffness, and reduced range of movement due to the overlying skin tightness are common features.
- Synovitis and muscle weakness may indicate overlap with other autoimmune connective tissue diseases.
- Symmetrical non-erosive arthritis may occur, particularly early on in the disease course.
- Skin and joint capsule fibrosis cause contractures, which restrict joint movement.
- A mild chronic myopathy is common and may be associated with slight elevation of muscle enzymes. Myositis occasionally occurs in SSc.

Gastrointestinal
Gut involvement occurs in about 90% of patients with SSc and is serious in about 50%.
- Initially, this appears to reflect dysfunction of the myenteric nerves, but subsequently atrophy of normal tissue and replacement with fibrous tissue underlie the reduced motility and exocrine insufficiency, which characterizes SSc-bowel disease.
- Oesophageal dysmotility gives rise to dysphagia and heartburn.
- Oesophageal stricture and Barrett's metaplasia occur rarely.
- Gastroparesis leads to loss of appetite and nausea.

CHAPTER 8 Autoimmune connective tissue diseases

- Small bowel dysmotility is associated with postprandial bloating, pseudo-obstruction, and pneumatosis intestinalis.
- Primary biliary cirrhosis occurs in ~3% of lcSSc patients.
- Stasis favours bacterial overgrowth.
- Any exocrine insufficiency can contribute to malabsorption.
- Large bowel dysmotility causes alternating constipation and diarrhoea, pseudo-obstruction, and, occasionally, perforation.
- Anal sphincter dysfunction is common (although rarely discussed) and may lead to faecal incontinence.
- Telangiectasiae occurring in the gastrointestinal tract may lead to bleeding and iron deficiency anaemia. Watermelon stomach (gastric antral vascular ectasia) occurs in ~5% SSc and may be the presenting feature.

Differential diagnosis of RP
AICTD or vasculitis
- Systemic sclerosis.
- Systemic lupus erythematosus.
- Rheumatoid arthritis.
- Cryoglobulinaemia.
- Primary Sjögren's.
- Dermatomyositis/polymyositis.
- Mixed connective tissue disease.
- Giant cell arteritis/Takayasu disease.
- Thromboangiitis obliterans.

Mechanical
- Frost bite.
- Trauma.
- Vibration.

Reduced macrovascular supply
- Atherosclerosis.
- Thoracic outlet obstruction.

Drugs
- Amphitamines.
- Bleomycin.
- Cisplatin.
- Vinblastin.
- β–blockers.
- Cocaine.
- Nicotine.
- Ergot preparation.
- Clonidine.
- Interferon.
- Methysegide.
- Sympathomemetics.

Miscellaneous
- Polycythemia vera.
- Hypothyroidism.
- Carpal tunnel syndrome.
- Paraneoplastic.
- Polyvinyl chloride.

Respiratory
Interstitial lung disease (ILD) occurs in about 80% of patients with SSc, but is clinically significant in about 40%. Pulmonary arterial hypertension (PAH) probably occurs in ~12% patients with lcSSc (estimates vary widely). In dcSScl, the hidebound chest results in a ventilatory defect. Patients with oesophageal dysmotility are at risk from aspiration pneumonia. Pleurisy and pleural effusion may occur, but much less commonly than in SLE.

Cardiac
Pericardial effusions occur, although less commonly than in SLE. Myocardial fibrosis may lead to arrhythmias and/or conduction disturbances. Atrial fibrillation occurs in ~25% and ventricular ectopics/arrhythmias in up to 50%. Coronary artery disease does not appear to be increased compared with the general population. Right heart failure may occur secondary to interstitial lung disease or PAH.

Renal involvement
Scleroderma renal crisis is a serious and potentially fatal complication, which occurs mainly in dcSSc (incidence 10–20%), but can also occur in lcSSc and scleroderma sine scleroderma. Typical features are summarized below. The incidence and outcome of renal crisis has been improved by the use of angiotensin converting enzyme (ACE) inhibitors, but approximately 50% of patients still require dialysis.

Classical features of scleroderma renal crisis
- dcSSc within 5 years of diagnosis.
- Abrupt onset of BP >160/90 mmHg.
- Hypertensive retinopathy grade III/IV.
- Rapid rise in serum creatinine.
- Elevated plasma renin.
- Microangiopathic haemolytic anaemia.
- Hypertensive encephalopathy; often seizures.
- Pulmonary oedema.

Other
- *Hypothyroidism* occurs in up to 40%.
- Carpal tunnel syndrome is often associated with the oedematous/inflammatory early stage of sclerodactyly.
- Trigeminal or glossopharyngeal neuralgia are the most common cranial neuropathies.
- Peripheral and autonomic neuropathies also occur.
- Erectile dysfunction is under-recognized since patients tend not to discuss.

Key features in the history
Raynaud's phenomenon
Classic triphasic (red/white/blue) colour changes, but all colours not required for diagnosis of RP. Historical features suggestive of secondary RP include age >30 years at onset and severe ischaemic pain.

Skin and cutaneous features
Scerloderma skin (e.g. hands, face) feel tight and swollen. There may be noticeable difficulty opening mouth wide or chalky extrusions from skin.
- **Sicca symptoms:** dry gritty eyes, dry mouth, vaginal soreness particularly on intercourse.
- **Digital ulcers:** location, past and present.

- **Gastrointestinal symptoms:** heartburn, bloating, abdominal pain, nausea, vomiting, constipation, diarrhoea, unintended weight loss, faecal incontinence.
- **Cardiorespiratory:** dyspnoea, cough, chest pains.
- **Musculoskeletal:** joint pains, swelling, stiffness; muscle pain/weakness.
- **Neuropathy:** paraesthesiae, numbness, erectile dysfunction.
- **Lifestyle:** smoking, occupational/recreational history (exposure to unusual solvents?).
- **Drugs:** include history of possible triggering agents for SSc and use of drugs associated with common co-morbidity, e.g. NSAIDs.

Key features on examination
Skin involvement
Sclerodacytly, distribution of scleroderma (limbs, trunk, and face?), telangectasiae, calcinosis; microstomia can be assessed by incisor to incisor distance.

Microvascular
Objective demonstration of vasomotor (red/white/blue) disturbance in digits, nose, patellae. Abnormal nail-fold capillary architecture in a patient with RP indicates the presence of an AICTD and, in some centres, is used as a staging examination. Nailfold capillaroscopy can be performed with an ophthalmoscope, using a drop of oil or gel (e.g. KY gel) as a magnifying lens. Digital ulceration, resorption of finger pulps and slow capillary refill indicate digital ischaemia.

(a)

(b)

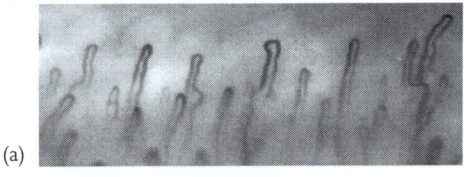

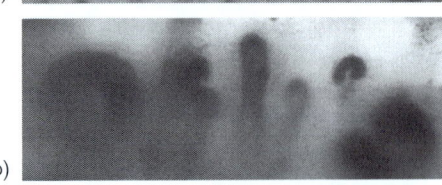

Figure 8.7 Nail-fold capillaries from (a) healthy control subject and (b) patient with SSc showing abnormal widened capillary loops. (with permission from Dr A. Herrick) (see also Plate 9).

Macrovascular
Normal peripheral pulses exclude macrovascular causes of peripheral ischaemia. Check blood pressure to screen for renal involvement.

Other
- Check pulse rhythm and look for signs of right heart strain or failure.
- Chest expansion may be reduced in dcSSc (hidebound chest). Bibasal crepitations suggest ILD.
- Joints – assess range of movement and for synovitis.
- Muscles – look for wasting and reduced power.
- Urinalysis – screen for proteinuria in renal disease.

Investigations
Laboratory investigations for annual review
Haematology
- FBC and ESR may show evidence of anaemia of chronic disease.
- An iron deficiency anaemia may be present in association with peptic ulcers (NSAID use?) or bleeding gut telangiectasiae.
- High platelet count and ESR are features of acute phase response and indicate ongoing inflammation.
- Low white blood cells (WBCs), neutropenia, and/or lymphopaenia and thrombocytopaenia may indicate the presence of an overlap autoimmune connective tissue disease.

Biochemistry
- **Renal function tests** including estimated creatinine clearance from Cockcroft–Gault formula:
  Estimated CrCl = {[140 − age (years)] × weight (kg)}/serum creat (µmol/l)
  (multiply by 0.85 in women).
- **Liver function tests:** screen for PBC or drug toxicity.
- **Creatine kinase:** marked elevation indicates the presence of myositis.
- **Thyroid function tests:** hypothyroidism common.
- **Bone biochemistry** including PTH and vitamin D, since malabsorption is common.
- **Vitamin B12, folate, and ferritin**.
- **Fasting lipid profile:** SSc can be associated with increased risk of cardiovascular disease.

Immunology
- ANA – positive in about 95% of patients with SSc.
- ENAs – will be performed when ANA is positive. See above for associations with anti-centromere, anti-Scl-70 and anti-RNA polymerase III.
- Anti-fibrillarin antibodies (UN3RNP) are measured in some specialist centres and associated with pulmonary arterial hypertension.
- Other autoantibodies may be positive in overlap AICTD syndromes, e.g. rheumatoid factor (RF), anti-dsDNA (SLE), lupus anticoagulant and antiphospholipid antibodies (APLS), anti-mitochondrial antibodies (PBC).
- Coeliac disease antibodies (IgA anti-tissue transglutaminase or anti-endomysial antibodies, but also check Igs to rule out IgA deficiency). Consider in patients with malabsorption (CD and SSc may co-exist).
- Complement C3 and C4, ANCA, cryoglobulins – consider if clinical picture suggests small vessel vasculitis.
- Immunoglobulins and protein electrophoresis, Bence-Jones protein estimation – request at diagnosis as part of a screen for neoplasia.

Imaging
Radiographs
- CXR – useful at diagnosis as part of a screen for neoplasia, if the diagnosis is unclear. Useful post-diagnosis if new cough or dyspnoea, although unnecessary if a high resolution CT chest is planned.
- In cases of suspected pneumoperitoneum, look for air under the diaphragm on CXR.

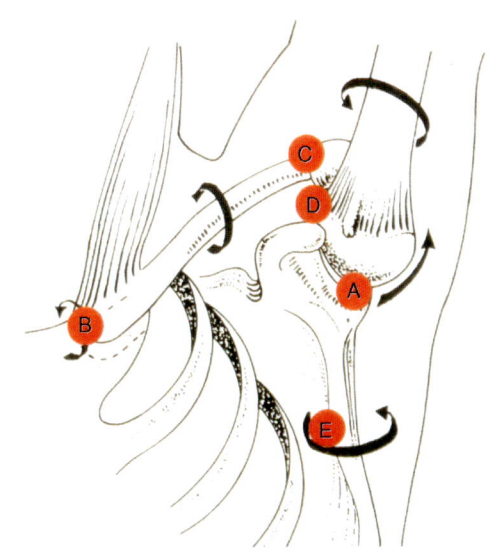

Plate 1 The five functional 'joints' of the shoulder. Involved in arm elevation: depression, glide, rotation and elevation at *glenohumeral joint* (A); rotation of clavicle with rotational shear at *sternoclavicular* (B) and *acromioclavicular* (C) *joints*, translation of humeral head under *coraco-acromial arch* (D) and *rotation of scapula* (E) on thoracic wall.

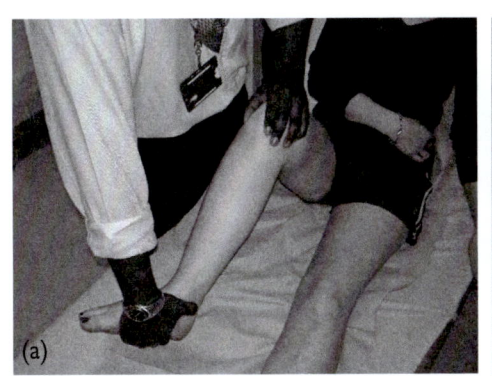

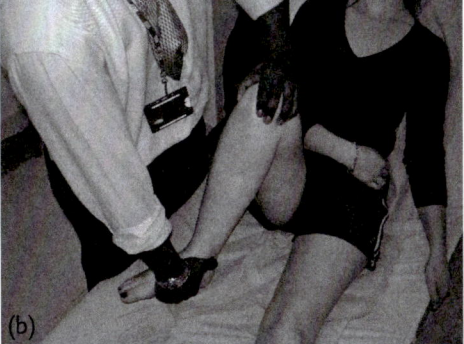

Plate 2 McMurray's test. Rotation of lower leg while flexing at the knee. The test aims to elicit an audible and/or palpable clunk as the damaged meniscus edge obstructs free femoral condylar rotation and flexion on the tibial plateau.

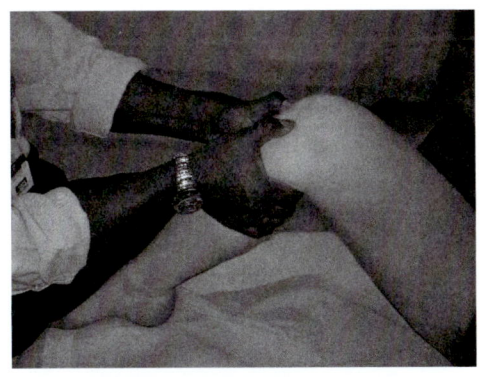

Plate 3 Anterior draw test. Having flexed the patient's knee and immobilised the foot, the examiner draws the tibia forward in the plane of upper leg. Excessive anterior translation of the lower leg can denote anterior cruciate deficiency (important to compare with opposite leg).

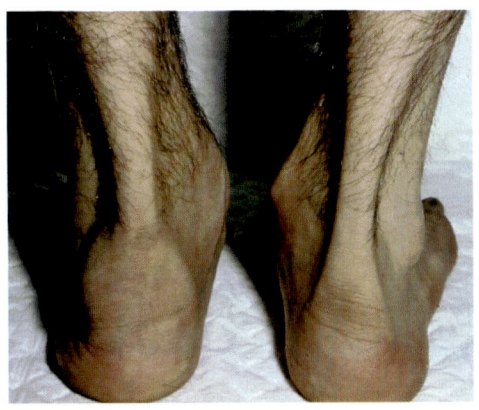

Plate 4 Aggressive left achilles' tendon enthesitis in ankylosing spondylitis (left).

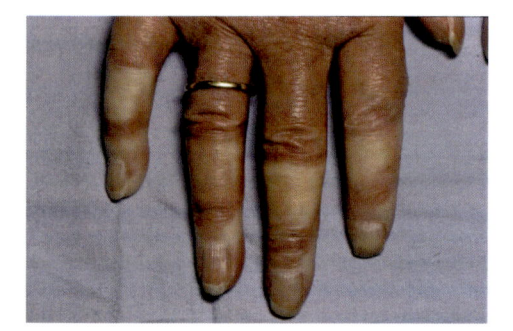

Plate 5 Digital vasospasm in a patient with Raynaud's Phenomenon (RP).

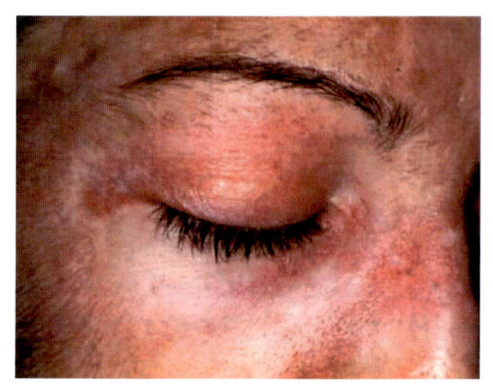

Plate 8 Heliotrope rash in a patient with dermatomyositis.

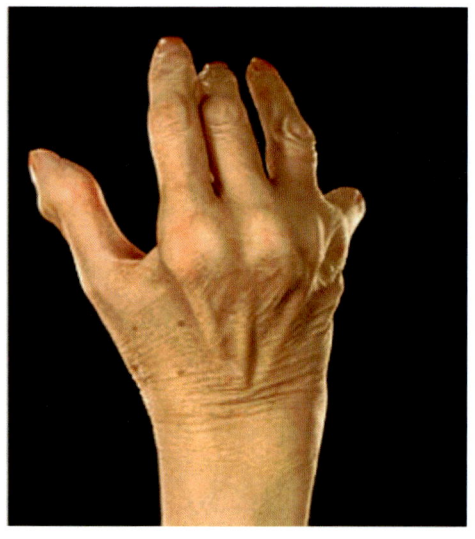

Plate 6 Metacarpophalangeal joint synovitis in SLE.

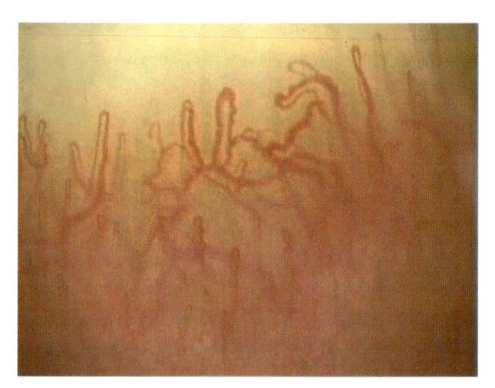

Plate 9 Nailfold capillaroscopy in systemic sclerosis. There is variable size of capillary loops; the larger ones (patent and dilated).compensating for ischaemia from narrowed ones.

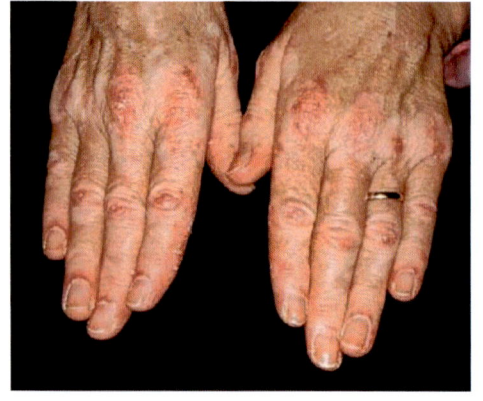

Plate 7 Gottron's papules in dermatomyositis.

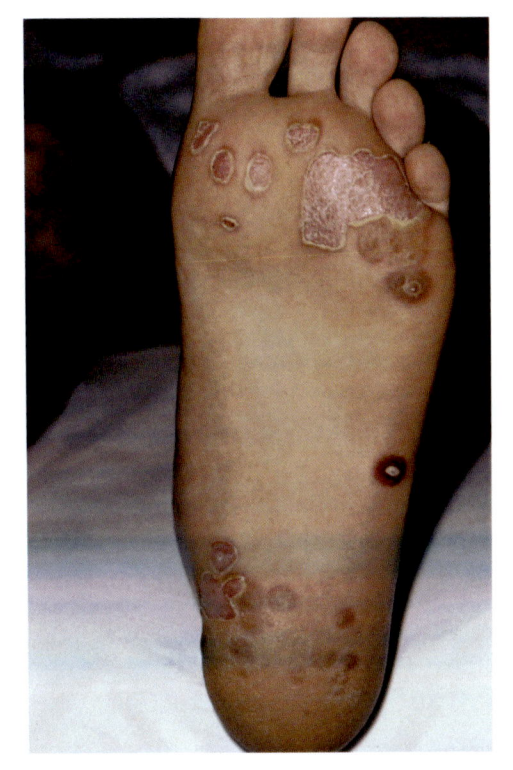

Plate 10 Keratoderma blenorrhagicum in acute reactive arthritis. Macroscopically and histologically some investigators maintain the rash is very similar to psoriasis.

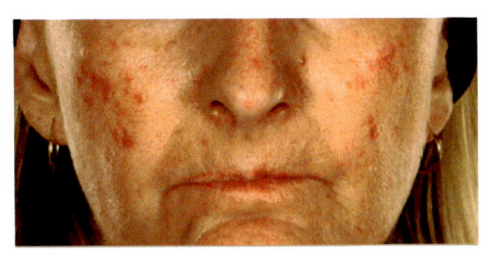

Plate 11 Telangiectasias in systemic sclerosis.

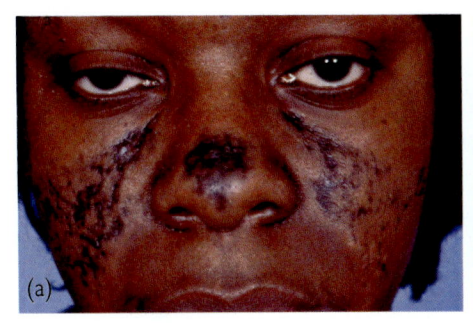

Plate 12 (a) Malar rash in SLE (Afro-Caribbean).
(b) Malar rash in SLE (Caucasian).

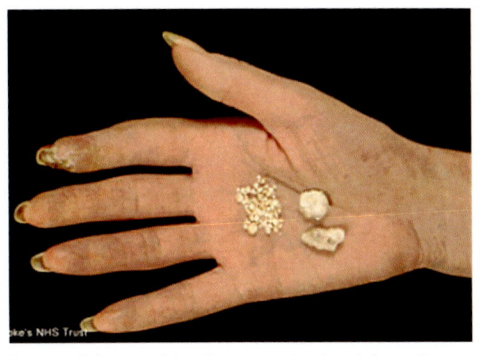

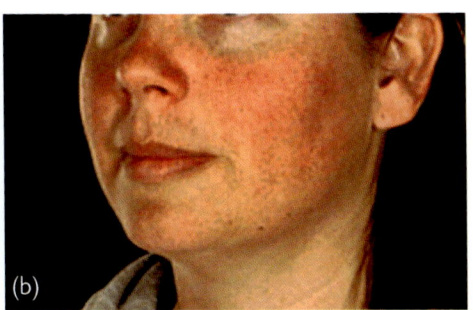

Plate 13 Calcinosis of the skin in systemic sclerosis (note also finger pulp loss).

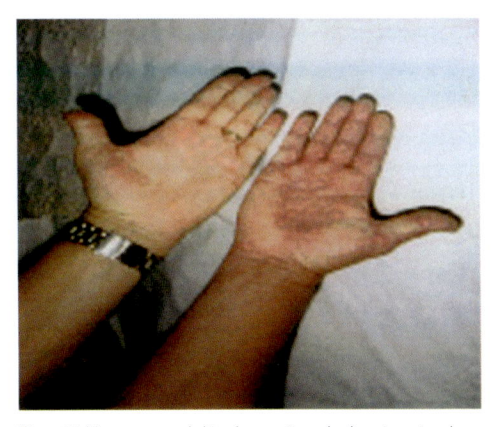

Plate 14 Vasomotor and skin changes in early chronic regional pain syndrome (R hand).

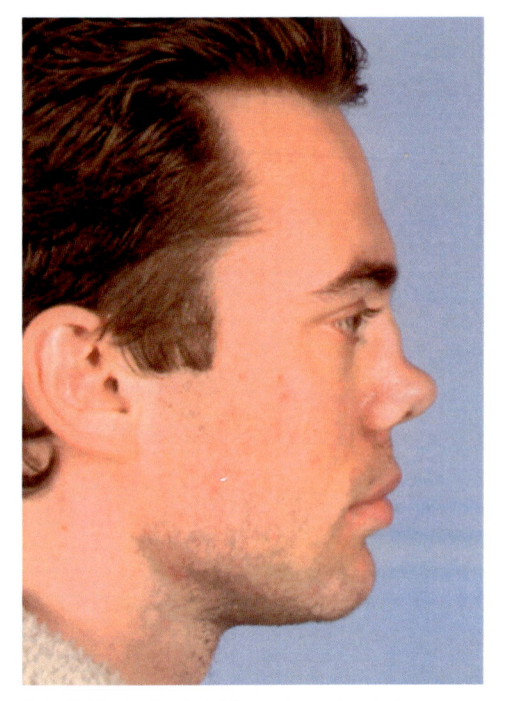

Plate 15 Nasal deformity in Wegener's granulomatosis.

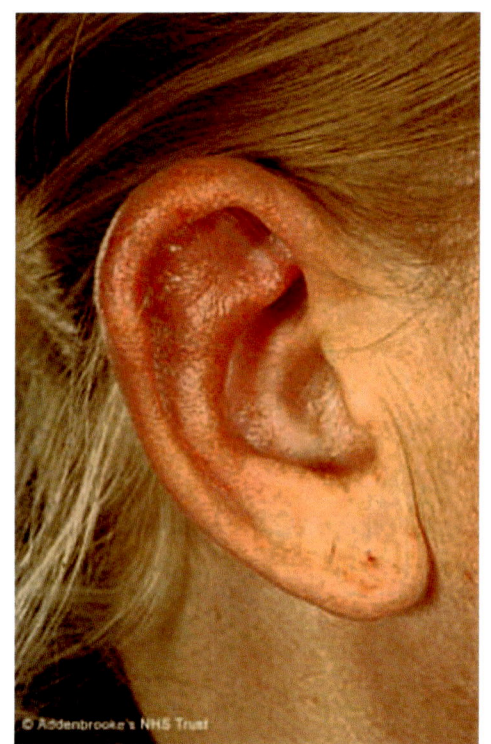

Plate 17 Lobe-sparing chondritis of the ear (relapsing polychondritis).

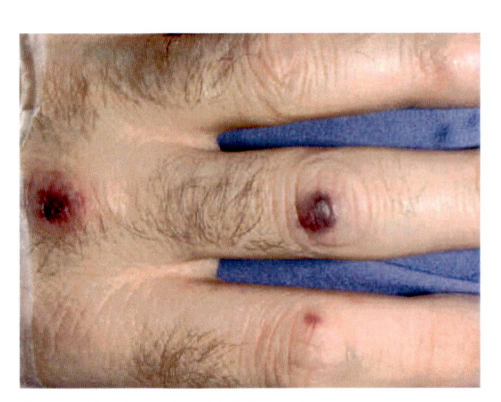

Plate 16 Vasculitic skin rash in Wegener's granulomatosis.

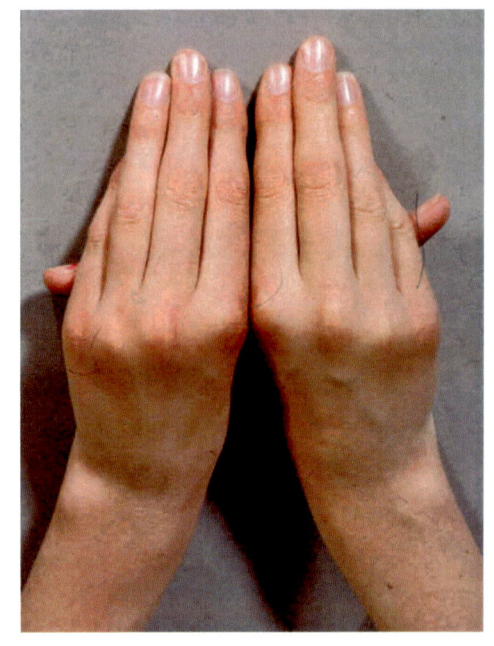

Plate 18 Hypermobility of thumb adduction in Marfan Syndrome.

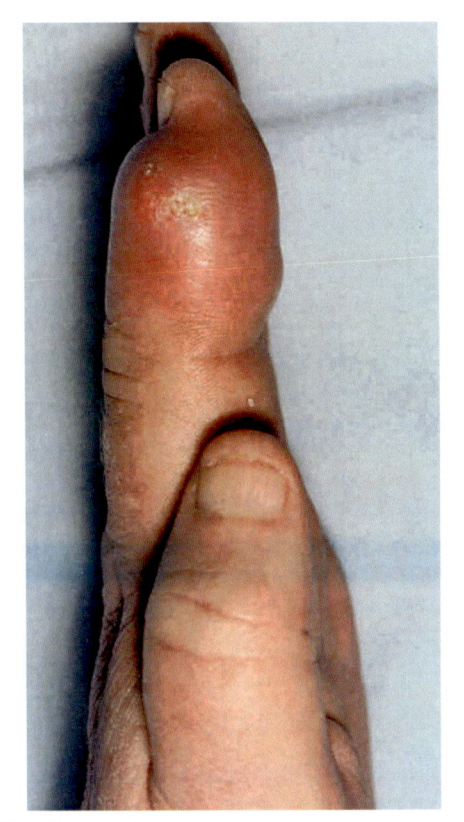

Plate 19 Gout tophus.

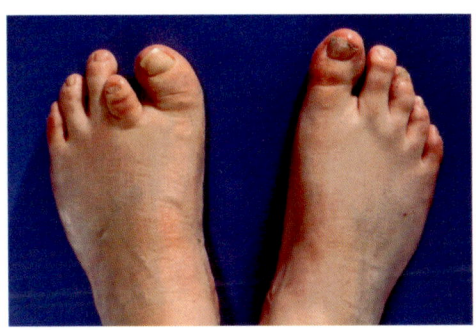

Plate 20 JIA. Left 2nd toe reduced growth due to persistent MTPJ arthritis (note also splaying between base of 1st and 2nd toes on the left from underlying MTPJ synovitis).

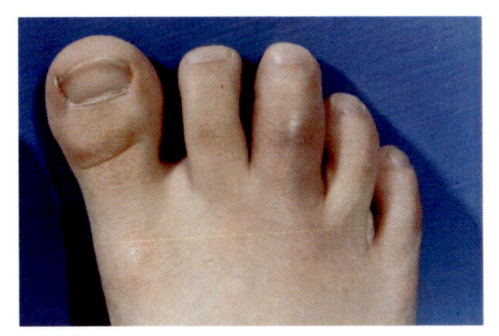

Plate 21 Dactylitis of 3rd toe in juvenile spondylarthropathy (ERA).

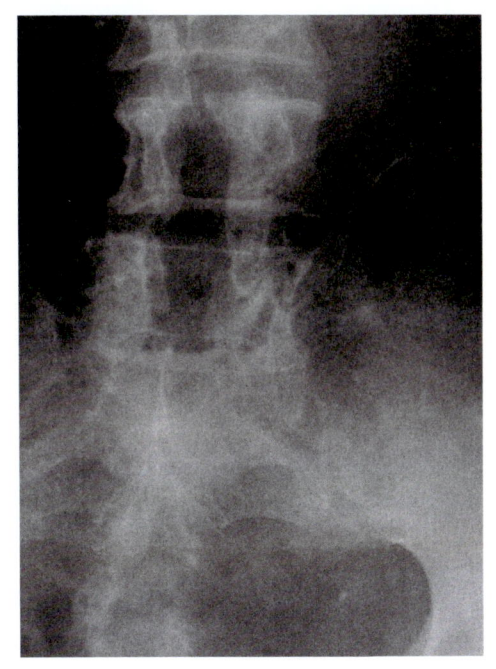

Plate 22 Ankylosed sacroiliac joint in ankylosing spondylitis.

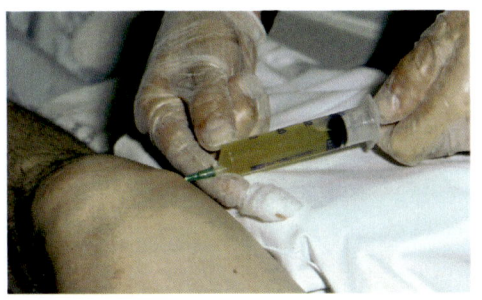

Plate 23 Aspiration of fluid from the knee (lateral approach).

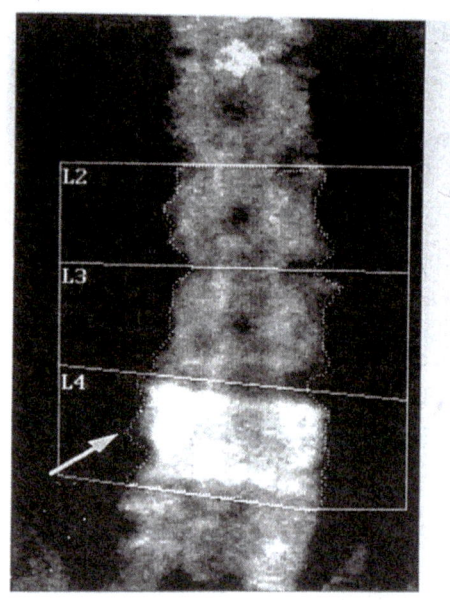

Plate 24 DXA of the lumbar spine. L4 will be omitted from the analysis (Paget's Disease of Bone).

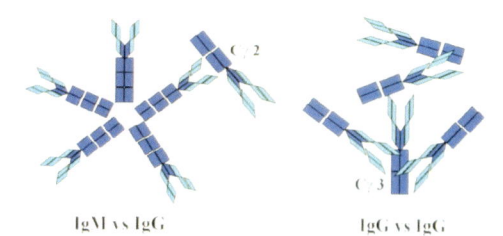

Plate 25 Rheumatoid factors (RFs). In conventional assays only IgM anti-fgG RFs are detected/measured; however, IgG, IgA and mixed RFs also exist.

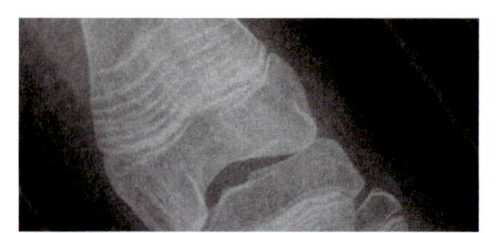

Plate 26 Metaphysis of femur in child with osteogenesis imperfecta (Type I). Sclerotic bands represent courses of intravenous bisphosphonate.

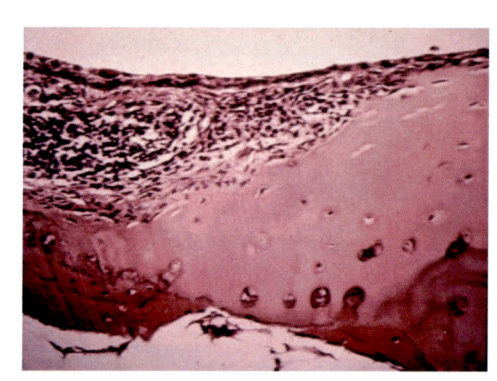

Plate 27 Haematoxylin and eosin stained low power section of synovium encroaching over hyaline (articular) cartilage in rheumatoid arthritis. The synovium (upper left) contains numerous lymphocates, macrophages, fibroblasts and plasma cells.

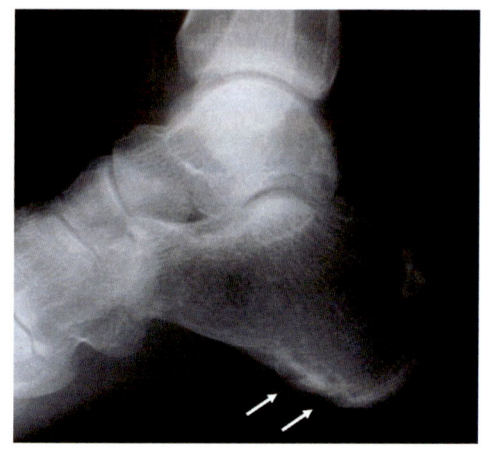

Plate 28 Plantar fasciitis in a patient with HLA B27-positive spondylarthropathy. Patchy lucent-sclerotic appearance at antero-inferior os calcis edge (site of origin of plantar fascia).

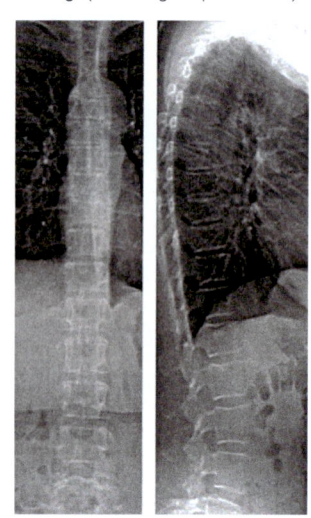

Plate 29 DXA scan. Whole spine lateral images allow an interpretation of vertebral fractures to be made (vertebral fracture analysis [VFA]). Images are dervied with a fraction of the radiation exposure imparted by conventional spinal X-Ray analysis.

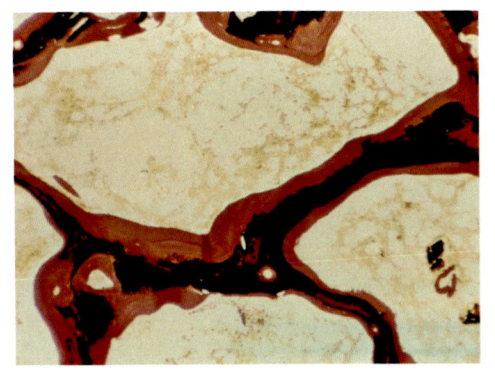

Plate 30 Osteomalacia (Goldner's Trichome). The bone surfaces are covered by large areas of unmineralized osteoid (brown).

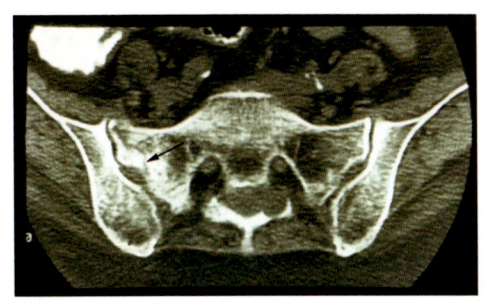

Plate 33 CT scan showing scaral unsufficiency fracture (arrowed).

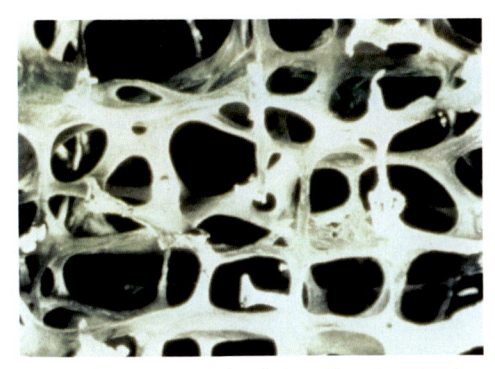

Plate 31 Osteoporosis in trabecular bone. There is a reduced number of bone trabeculae and trabecular connectivity compared with normal.

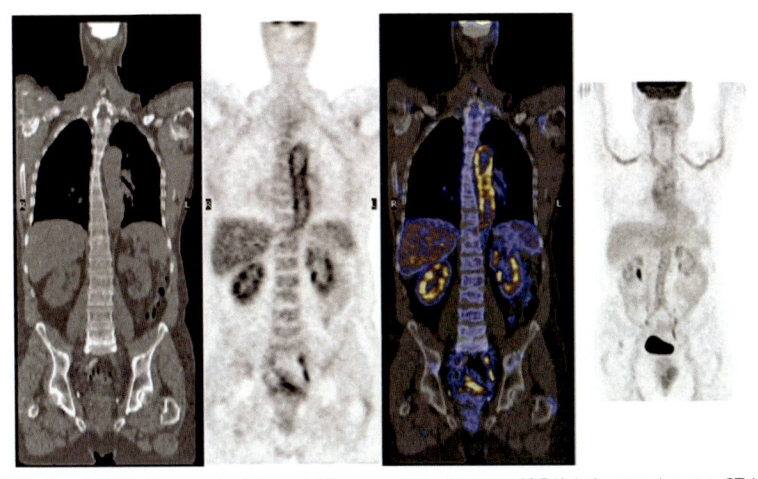

Plate 32 ^{18}FDG Positron Emission Tomography (PET) and CT scan in giant cell arteritis (GCA). Left: coronal section CT; Middle left: contiguous section ^{18}FDG PET showing abnormal tracer accumulating in descending aorta; Middle right: Contiguous CT and PET sections registered (superimposed); Right: (PET scan) image shows additional activity in carotid, and subclavian arteries.

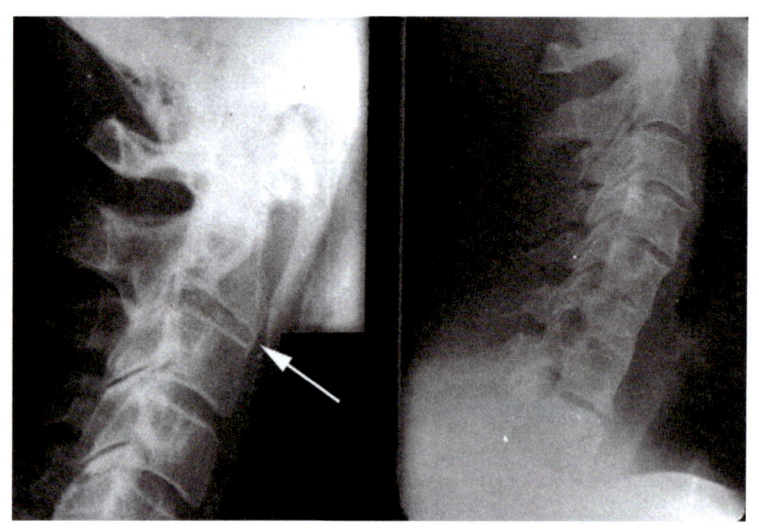

Plate 34 Changes in the cerviical spine in ankylosing spondylitis. Single marginal syndesmophyte in early disease (left, arrowed); more extensive marginal syndesmophytes in advanced disease (right).

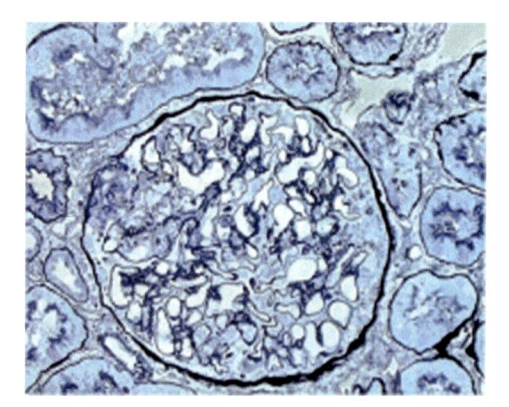

Plate 35 Class IV lupus nephritis demonstrating segmental necrosis and endocapillary proliferation.

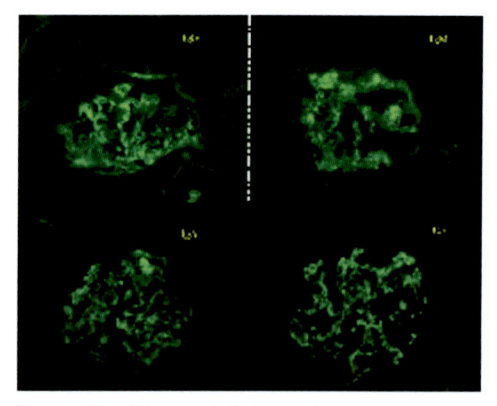

Plate 36 Class IV lupus nephritis immunofluorescene demonstrating deposition of IgG, IgM, IgA and C3, the so-called "full house" appearance.

CHAPTER 8 Autoimmune connective tissue diseases

High resolution CT (HRCT), US, and MR
- High resolution CT of the chest may reveal honeycombing and ground glass opacities typical of nonspecific interstitial (NSIP) associated with AICTDs; may also show patulous oesophagus.
- In cases of aspiration pneumonia, changes will predominantly affect right middle lobe.
- CT abdomen/pelvis may be included with the HRCT chest at diagnosis, as part of a screen for underlying neoplasm.
- US or CT abdomen may be performed to investigate liver disease, or as investigation for abdominal pain/distension; dilated loops of bowel may be evident in dysmotility.
- Barium swallow may be performed to demonstrate oesophageal dysmotility.

Endoscopy
- Upper GI endoscopy is required as investigation of possible peptic ulcer disease, and to monitor Barrett's oesophagus and watermelon stomach.
- Colonoscopy may be required if a colonic neoplasm is suspected.

Other investigations
- Pulmonary function tests – spirometry and transfer factor – are useful to screen for and monitor ILD and pulmonary arterial hypertension (PAH). Lung volumes and transfer factor decrease proportionately in ILD, but isolated or disproportionate drop in transfer factor should prompt further investigations for PAH (see 'The Chest', p. 54).
- The six-minute walk test is useful for monitoring patients with PAH.
- Echocardiogram – to detect pericardial effusion and as a screening test for PAH. In the presence of tricuspid regurgitation an estimated mean pulmonary artery pressure can be obtained. If this value is > 35 mmHg, right heart catheterization is recommended to measure pulmonary artery pressure accurately.
- ECG – useful screen for arrhythmia, ischaemia, LVH; may suggest right heart strain in PAH.
- Bone densitometry should be considered especially in post-menopausal women or if fragility fractures have occurred.

Differential diagnosis
- **Eosinophilia–myalgia syndrome:** myalgia, oedema, thickening and induration of the skin, marked blood eosinophilia; associated with L-tryptophan ingestion.
- **Eosinophilic fasciitis:** tenderness and swelling of the extremities (orange-peel configuration); associated with peripheral eosinophilia (see, p. 310).
- **Primary biliary cirrhosis:** ANA positive, often with rashes and telangectasiae.
- **Primary pulmonary hypertension:** distinguish from scleroderma sine scleroderma.
- **Toxic oil syndrome** (adulterated rape seed oil).
- **Porphyria cutanea tarda.**
- **Radiation exposure:** causes fibrosis.
- **Amyloidosis:** waxy cutaneous infiltration and involvement of viscera (see, p. 496).

Treatment

Objectives of management
- Confirm diagnosis and identify any co-morbidity.
- Initial and annual screening program for complications or associated co-morbidity.
- Modification of microvascular disease.
- Modification of inflammatory disease.
- Management of associated co-morbidity.

Modification of microvascular disease
Several agents have been shown to have effects on endothelial function, proliferative changes in the vessel wall, and/or to be anti-inflammatory or anti-coagulant. These are listed below, since it is likely that they modify the processes underlying the proliferative vasculopathy characteristic of SSc. The best data for clinical efficacy of many of these drugs has emerged from clinical trials of treatment of PAH and, more recently, of digital ulceration. However, further study is required to subject all these agents to appropriate clinical trial, to delineate the efficacy for different microvascular beds and to understand whether drugs synergize in combination.

AVOID glucocorticoids – prednisolone >15 mg per day (and possibly also lower doses) is associated with increased risk of scleroderma renal crisis.

ACE inhibitors and angiotensin receptor blockers
- ACE inhibitors have improved outcome in scleroderma renal crisis (1-year survival 76% in ACE inhibitor treated group instead of 18% in group without ACE inhibitors). It is likely that ACE inhibitors decrease the incidence of renal crisis, but this remains unproven.
- Unfortunately, the recent QUINS study indicates that ACE inhibitors have no effect on the occurrence of digital ulcers or other vascular manifestations of lcSSc over 2–3-year treatment period.
- Angiotensin receptor antagonists may be effective for digital microvascular disease. In an RCT, losartan 50 mg od was superior to nifedipine in reducing frequency and severity of RP attacks.

Endothelin receptor blockers
- Endothelin receptor antagonists (ERA) have demonstrated efficacy for both PAH and digital ulceration in DBRCTs. The non-selective ERA bosentan (125 mg bd) improved 6-min walk and pulmonary haemodynamics in SSc-PAH patients included in two placebo-controlled trials. The open-label extension phase of these studies indicates survival in bosentan group of ~86% at 1 year and 73% at 2 years.
- The selective endothelin receptor A antagonist, sitaxsentan has also been shown to be effective in AICTD-associated PAH.
- The RAPIDS trials in SSc patients with digital ulceration have shown that bosentan does not improve healing of existing ulcers, but that it decreases the incidence of new ulcers by approximately 50%.
- Bosentan and sitaxsentan are licensed to treat PAH and bosentan for SSc with ongoing digital ulcer disease.

Prostanoids.
Continuous intravenous *epoprostenol* is the gold standard of treatment for primary PAH, since it improves exercise capacity and survival and is used in SSc-PAH patients who

deteriorate despite treatment with an ERA. Courses of intravenous *iloprost* are used cyclically to reduce frequency and severity of RP attacks and as salvage therapy for digital ulceration. Further study is required to define the optimal duration and periodicity of these courses. Oral and inhaled preparations of prostanoids are being studied, but current evidence suggests limited efficacy at best.

Other therapies
- **Phosphodiesterase V inhibitors:** Sildenafil 20 mg tds improved 6-min walk distance and pulmonary haemodynamics in a DBPRCT of AICTD-associated PAH. Case reports suggest that it may be also be effective for RP. Sildenafil is licensed as Revatio for use in PAH.
- **Calcium channel blockers:** e.g. nifedipine, are used for RP, but probably provide symptomatic relief only. They should be avoided in patients with SSc PAH.
- **Nitrates:** GTN patches placed on the forearm are sometimes used in severe digital ischaemia.
- **Selective serotonin receptor antagonists (SSRIs):** e.g. fluoxetine have vasodilator activity and have been shown to reduce RP attack severity.
- **Alpha-1 antagonists:** prazosin has been shown to improve RP, but the effect is modest.
- *Anticoagulants* are generally used in patients with PAH. However, risks may outweigh benefit in patients with gastrointestinal telangiectasiae due to risk of GI bleed.
- **Antiplatelet agents:** prostacyclin inhibits platelet activation. Aspirin is rarely used due to increased risk of dyspepsia and GI bleeding. Clopidogrel is an alternative but efficacy in SSc/RP is unknown.
- **Statins** improve endothelial function in a variety of contexts are currently being studied in SSc microvascular disease.

Immunosuppression
- **Mycophenolate mofetil:** retrospective analysis of patients with SSc-ILD suggest improvement; further investigation required.
- **D-penicillamine:** RCT demonstrated lack of efficacy for skin disease.
- **Methotrexate:** Three RCTs together show, at best a minimal effect on skin and ILD.
- **Azathioprine:** appears to be of no/limited efficacy in skin and lung disease.
- **Ciclosporin A:** trial data lacking, but known to cause hypertension and vasculopathy – avoid.
- **Cyclophosphamide:** An RCT in SSc with ILD compared placebo with IV cyclophosphamide (6 pulses) and low-dose prednisolone, followed by azathioprine; there were no significant differences in lung volume or transfer factor between placebo and active groups.
- **Anti-TNFα biologics, rituximab, alemtuzumab:** anecdotal reports only.
- **Imatnib** (tyrosine kinase inhibitor, which inhibits PDGF signalling): case report of efficacy in severe dcSSc.
- **Haematopoietic stem cell transplantation** is being studied in two controlled trials (ASTIS in Europe and SCOT in USA). Treatment-related mortality has fallen to 2.5% from 12.5% reported in 2002, and preliminary reports indicate skin and microvascular disease may be improved.

Management of associated morbidity
See 'Patient Advice' for lifestyle measures.
- **Dyspepsia:** proton pump inhibitors and anti-acids.
- **Dysmotility:** metaclopramide to aid gastric emptying.
- **Constipation:** stool softeners and bulking agents, e.g. lactulose and fybogel.
- **Diarrhoea:** loperamide.
- **Malabsorption:** refer to dietician; oral vitamin D3, and calcium and iron sulphate supplementation and parenteral administration of vitamin B12. Occasionally, parenteral iron and ergocalciferol may be necessary. Total parenteral nutrition is required in a minority.
- **Pruritis:** moisturizers, anti-histamines; tricyclic antidepressants may be helpful.
- **Calcinosis:** surgical removal often successful; assess local blood flow since ischaemic tissue may not heal. Various drugs have been tried, with positive case reports [diltiazem, bisphosphonates, low-dose (1 mg) warfarin, minocycline], but no RCT data are available.
- **Chronic renal failure:** liaise with renal team – phosphate binders, alfacalcidol, erythropoietin, BP control and, ultimately, dialysis may be required.
- **Arthritis** may be treated with NSAIDs and intra-articular glucocorticoids.
- **Aggressive inflammatory disease:** e.g. myositis in overlap syndromes may necessitate systemic glucocorticoids, but ensure the patient is taking an ACE inhibitor and monitor BP and renal function.
- **Hypothyroidisism:** replacement therapy.
- **Osteoporosis:** ensure adequate vitamin D levels, no secondary hyperparathyroidism, and treat with bisphosphonate if T-scores ≤–2.5 if alendronate is not tolerated due to dysphagia/dyspepsia, use monthly oral ibandronate 150 mg or parenteral ibandronate 3 mg every 3 months.
- **Sicca symptoms:** see chapter on Sjögren's syndrome.
- **ILD:** vaccinate against influenza, *Pneumococcus* and *Haemophilus influenzae*; prompt treatment of intercurrent infection; see 'The Chest' in Chapter 3, 'Organ involvement in rheumatological disease'.

Multidisciplinary approach
- Chest physician.
- Specialist PAH unit.
- Gastroenterologist.
- Dentist.
- Renal physician.
- Dermatologist.
- Radiologists.
- Dietician.
- Orthopaedic surgeon.
- Vascular surgeon.
- Physiotherapist – exercises to retain mobility and to optimize chest function.
- Occupational therapist – hand exercises and aids/strategies for overcoming disabilities.
- Speech therapists – for assessing and advising on severe oesophageal dysmotility.

Patient advice
- Avoid smoking.
- Keep core and extremities warm, e.g. put coat on several minutes before leaving house; use thermal gloves and socks in cold temperatures.
- Protect fingers with gloves whenever possible, e.g. dish washing and gardening.
- Seek medical advice with new digital ulcers.
- Maintain careful oral hygiene and arrange regular dental checks.

- For patients with dysphagia – avoid dry abrasive foods.
- For patients with gastrointestinal reflux – avoid eating late in the evening, raise head of bed on blocks.
- For patients with delayed gastric emptying or small bowel dymotility – eat little and often.
- Gentle regular aerobic exercise to maintain cardiovascular/respiratory fitness.
- Hand exercises to maintain range of movement.

Follow-up
- Patients with rapidly-progressive disease, and/or commencing new therapies may need 2–3-monthly review.
- 6-monthly follow-up is appropriate for patients within the first 5 years of disease.
- Annual follow-up may be appropriate for patients without severe organ involvement >5 years post-diagnosis. Urinalysis, blood pressure monitoring should be routinely performed in the follow-up visits.

Prognosis and natural history
lcSSc
- 5-year survival rate reported to be up to 86%.
- PAH is the most frequent cause of death.

dcSSc
- 5-year survival of patients with severe ILD, renal crisis, or cardiac disease each around 50%.
- 5-year survival of dcSSc patients with renal crisis treated with ACE inhibitors approximately 70% (compared with less than 10% in the era before ACE-inhibitors were available).
- Risk of developing severe organ involvement is greatest during the first 5 years of dcSSc.
- 10-year survival of dcSSc who do not develop severe organ involvement within the first 5 years is approximately 80%.

Resources
Assessment Tools – general measures
- Scleroderma-modified health assessment questionnaire.
- Creatinine and creatinine clearance.
- Blood pressure and urinalysis for proteinuria.
- Raynaud's Condition Score – daily self-assessment of RP activity using a 0-10 ordinal scale.
- Rodnan Skin Score.
- Oral aperture.
- Pulmonary function tests: vital capacity to monitor restrictive lung disease; transfer factor to monitor pulmonary vascular disease; 6-min walk distance.
- Echocardiography – estimated mean pulmonary arterial pressure and right heart catheterization.
- Hydrogen breath tests.
- BMI.
- FBC – monitoring for anaemia.

Assessing Raynaud's (condition score)
Circle below the number that best indicates the difficulty you had today with your Raynaud's condition:
No   0 1 2 3 4 5 6 7 8 9 10   Extreme
difficulty   difficulty

Rodnan skin score
For face, neck, anterior chest, abdomen, upper back, lower back, upper arm (L and R), forearm (L and R), hand (L and R), fingers (L and R), thigh (L and R), leg (L and R), foot (L and R), score each of 20 skin regions as follows:
0 = normal
1 = possible thickening
2 = definite thickening but mobile
3 = thickened and tethered
Note: neck and back are sometimes omitted.

Patient organizations
Raynaud's & Scleroderma Association, 112 Crewe Road, Alsager, Cheshire, ST7 2JA, UK. Tel: 01270 872776. Freephone: 0800 9172494 (for UK enquiries only). www.raynauds.org.uk

The Scleroderma Society, 3 Caple Road, London NW10 8AB, UK.
Tel: 020 8961 4912. www.sclerodermasociety.co.uk

ICD-10 codes
M34   SSc
M34.1   CREST syndrome
M34.2   SSc induced by drugs and chemicals
J99.1*   SSc with lung involvement
G73.7*   SSc with myopathy

References
Badesch DB, Hill, NS, et al. Sildenafil for pulmonary arterial hypertension associated with connective tissue disease. *J Rheumatol* 2007; **34**: 2417–22.

Charles C, Clements P, Furst DE. Systemic sclerosis: hypothesis-driven treatment strategies. *Lancet* 2006; **367**: 1683–91.

DeMarco PJ, Weisman MH, et al. Predictors and outcomes of scleroderma renal crisis. *Arthritis Rheum* 2002; **46**: 2983–9.

Denton CP, Humbert M, et al. Bosentan treatment for pulmonary arterial hypertension related to connective tissue disease: a subgroup analysis of the pivotal clinical trials and their open-label extensions. *Ann Rheum Dis* 2006; **65**: 1336–40.

Dziadzio M, Denton CP, et al. Losartan therapy for Raynaud's phenomenon and scleroderma: clinical and biochemical findings in a fifteen-week, randomized, parallel-group, controlled trial. *Arthritis Rheum* 1999; **42**: 2646–55.

Girgis RE, Frost AE, et al. Selective endothelin A receptor antagonism with sitaxsentan for pulmonary arterial hypertension associated with connective tissue disease. *Ann Rheum Dis* 2007; **66**: 1467–72.

Gliddon AE, Dore CJ, et al. Prevention of vascular damage in scleroderma and autoimmune Raynaud's phenomenon: a multicenter, randomized, double-blind, placebo-controlled trial of the angiotensin-converting enzyme inhibitor quinapril. *Arthritis Rheum* 2007; **56**: 3837–46.

Henness S, Wigley FM. Current drug therapy for scleroderma and secondary Raynaud's phenomenon: evidence-based review. *Curr Opin Rheumatol* **19**: 611–18.

Herrick AL. Pathogenesis of Raynaud's phenomenon *Rheumatol* 2005; **44**: 587–96.

Herrick AL, Worthington J. Genetic epidemiology of systemic sclerosis. *Arthritis Res* 2002; **4**: 165–8.

Hoyles RK, Ellis RW, et al. A multicenter, prospective, randomized, double-blind, placebo-controlled trial of corticosteroids and intravenous cyclophosphamide followed by oral azathioprine for the treatment of pulmonary fibrosis in scleroderma. *Arthritis Rheum* 2006; **54**: 3962–70.

LeRoy EC, Black C, et al. Scleroderma (systemic sclerosis) classification, subsets and pathogenesis. *J Rheumatol* 1988 **15**: 202–5.

Korn JH, Mayes M, et al. Digital ulcers in systemic sclerosis: prevention by treatment with bosentan, an oral endothelin receptor antagonist. *Arthritis Rheum* 2004; **50**: 3985–93.

Kuwana M. Potential benefit of statins for vascular disease in systemic sclerosis. *Curr Opin Rheumatol* 2006; **18**: 594–600.

LeRoy EC, Medsger TA, Criteria for the classification of early systemic sclerosis. *J Rheumatol* 2001; **28**: 1573–6.

McLaughlin VV, Shillington A, Rich S. Survival in primary pulmonary hypertension: the impact of epoprostenol therapy. *Circulation* 2002; **106**: 1477–82.

Milio G, Corrado E, et al. Iloprost treatment in patients with Raynaud's phenomenon secondary to systemic sclerosis and the quality of life: a new therapeutic protocol. *Rheumatol* 2006; **45**: 999–1004.

Nietert PJ, Silver RM. Systemic sclerosis: environmental and occupational risk factors. *Curr Opin Rheumatol*. 2000; **12**: 520–6.

Sfikakis PP, Gorgoulis VG, et al. Imatnib for the treatment of refractory, diffuse systemic sclerosis. *Rheumatol* 2008; **47**: 735–7.

Steen VD, Medsger TA. Severe organ involvement in systemic sclerosis with diffuse scleroderma. *Arthritis Rheum* 2000; **43**: 2437–44.

Sunderkötter C and Riemekasten G. Pathophysiology and clinical consequences of Raynaud's phenomenon related to systemic sclerosis. *Rheumatol* 2006; **45**: iii33–5.

Teixeira L, Mouthon L, et al. Mortality and risk factors of scleroderma renal crisis: a French retrospective study of 50 patients. *Ann Rheum Dis* 2008; 67: 110–16.

Tyndall A, Furst DE. Adult stem cell treatment of scleroderma. *Curr Opin Rheumatol* 2007; **19**: 604–10.

Zuber JP, Spertini F. Immunological basis of systemic sclerosis. *Rheumatol* 2006: **45**: iii23–5.

Antiphospholipid syndrome

Definition
Antiphospholipid antibody syndrome (APLS; also known as Hughes' Syndrome) is a systemic autoimmune disease characterized by elevated antiphospholipid (APL) antibodies, and an acquired thrombophilia or clotting tendency.

Classification
The Sapporo preliminary classification criteria, published in 1999, were amended in Sydney and published as the 2006 International Consensus Statement on the Classification Criteria for definite APLS. Note that these criteria are designed to facilitate clinical studies/trials by including a relatively homogenous patient group. The use of the terms 'probable' or 'possible' APLS is appropriate in clinical practice, where thromboembolic disease is associated with antiphospholipid antibodies and no other cause is evident.

Catastrophic APLS is a life-threatening form of the disease, in which at least three different organ systems become involved (objectively) over the course of days or weeks.

Definite APLS
Present if at least one of the **Clinical** criteria and one of the **Laboratory** criteria are satisfied.

Clinical criteria
- **Vascular thrombosis:** arterial, venous or small vessel thrombosis in any tissue or organ (excluding superficial venous thrombosis) – confirmed by appropriate imaging or histopathology.
- **Pregnancy morbidity:** at least one of the following:
  - one or more unexplained deaths of a morphologically normal foetus at or beyond 10th week of gestation;
  - one or more premature births or a morphologically normal neonate before 34th week of gestation due to eclampsia or severe pre-eclampsia or placental insufficiency (see below);
  - three or more unexplained consecutive spontaneous abortions before 10th week of gestation, with hormonal, chromosomal or maternal anatomic causes excluded.

Laboratory criteria
Any must be present on 2 or more occasions at least 12 weeks apart, and must be measured according to the appropriate guidelines).
- Lupus anticoagulant (LA) present in plasma.
- anticardiolipin (aCL) antibody of IgG, and/or IgM isotype in serum or plasma
- anti-β2 glycoprotein-I (β2GPI) antibody of IgG and/or IgM isotype in serum or plasma, present in medium/high titre (e.g. >99th centile).

Comments
- The classification of *Definite APLS* should not be given if the period between the positive (APL) test and clinical manifestations is <12 weeks or >5 years.
- Co-existing risk factors for thrombosis should not prevent classification as *Definite APLS*, but patients should be classified as such in the presence or absence of additional risk factors (see Table 8.7).
- Primary APLS is diagnosed in patients without features of other systemic disease and secondary APLS when patients have features of SLE.
- For histopathologic confirmation of thrombosis, a solid mass, formed *in vivo* and derived from blood constitutents, must be demonstrated in the vessel in the absence of inflammation in the vessel wall.
- Accepted manifestations of placental insufficiency:
  - abnormal foetal surveillance test;
  - abnormal Doppler flow velocimetry waveform or analysis;
  - oligohydramnios;
  - postnatal birth weight <10th centile for gestational age.
- Lupus anticoagulant (LA) must be measured according to guidelines of the International Society on Thrombosis and Haemostasis (see resources).
- Antibodies specific for cardiolipin or β2GPI must be measured using standardized ELISAs.

Table 8.7 Additional risk factors for thrombosis

Age	Males >55 years Females >65 years
Established cardiovascular risk factors	Hypertension
	Diabetes mellitus
	Elevated LDLc
	Reduced HDLc
	Smoking
	FH of premature CVD
	BMI >30 kg/m²
	Microalbuminuria
	Estimated GFR <60 ml/min
Inherited thrombophilia	
Oral contraceptive	
Nephrotic syndrome	
Malignancy	
Immobility	
Surgery	

Epidemiology
High titre aCL antibodies and LA are associated with venous and arterial thromboses, pregnancy losses (mostly mid-trimester), stroke in the under 50s and accelerated atherosclerosis. Approximate figures for prevalence of positive APL tests are provided below. Note that 'prevalence' varies substantially due to variability between studies regarding the titre and persistence of aCL antibodies defined as positive.

Accurate predictions of risk in categories of patients with APL antibodies are impossible with currently available data.
- LA appears to be more strongly associated than with arterial thromboses and thrombocytopaenia compared with aCL antibodies.
- Women who are positive for both aCL antibodies and LA appear to be at increased risk of foetal loss compared with women who are aCL antibody positive alone.

Table 8.8 'Prevalence' of aCL antibodies or LA

	aCL antibodies (IgG/IgM)	LA
Healthy controls	~1.5%	~2%
Pregnant women	<1%	~2%
SLE	~30%	~15%
RA	~20%	
SSc	~19%	~4%
Venous thrombosis	4–24%	1–16%
Stroke <50 years	~30%	~4%

- In patients with definite APLS, the risk of foetal loss is currently ~20%.
- There appears to be an association between LA and pulmonary arterial hypertension (PAH) in Systemic Sclerosis (SSc).

Aetiology and pathophysiology
Genetic
Associations between HLA loci and APLS have been reported. Mice deficient for complement C3, C5 or C5a receptors are resistant to APL-mediated foetal injury.

Environment
Infectious triggers
Many infectious agents have been associated with the development of antiphospholipid antibodies and with clinical manifestations of APLS. These include:
- hepatitis C virus (HCV).
- *Varicella zoster* virus (VZV).
- Cytomegalovirus (CMV).
- Parvovirus B19.
- HIV.
- *Haemophilus influenzae*.
- *Neisseria gonorrhoeae*.

Approximately a third of the cases of catastrophic APLS have clearly been preceded by infections.

Non-infectious triggers/promoters
- **Drugs:** chlorpromazine is associated with the development of aCL antibodies (34%) and lupus anticoagulant (LA, 45%), but the incidence of clinical features is low. A variety of idiosyncratic drug associations with APLS have been reported, including anti-epileptics, anti-hypertensives, anti-arrhythmics, and antibiotics.
- **Trauma** is the second most frequent precipitation factor (after infection) for catastrophic APLS.
- **Vaccination** has been suspected to induce APLS, but there are no data currently to support this.

Immunopathology
Breaking tolerance
Refer to SLE section (AICTD chapter, p. 240) for an overview of mechanisms believed to be involved in breaking tolerance. The generation of antibodies specific for phospholipid/protein cofactor combinations may reflect:
- Exposure of cryptic epitopes within the protein cofactor following binding to the phospholipid target (demonstrated for β2GPI following binding to phospholipid).
- Molecular mimicry. Several microbial pathogens have a component that shares structural homology with the TLRVYK peptide, a peptide shown to induce clinical features of APLS in mice.

Effector mechanisms
Autoimmune APL antibodies include antibodies specific for a variety of phospholipid binding proteins, many of which participate in the coagulation cascade (Fig 8.8). The most important of these protein 'cofactors' are β2GPI and prothrombin, but other cofactors include protein C, protein S, high molecular weight (HMW) kininogen, annexin V, and factor XI. The prolongation of *in vitro* coagulation assays appears to result from the formation of complexes between the APL antibodies, and one or more of the phospholipid-binding proteins that are required for the *in vitro* clotting assay.

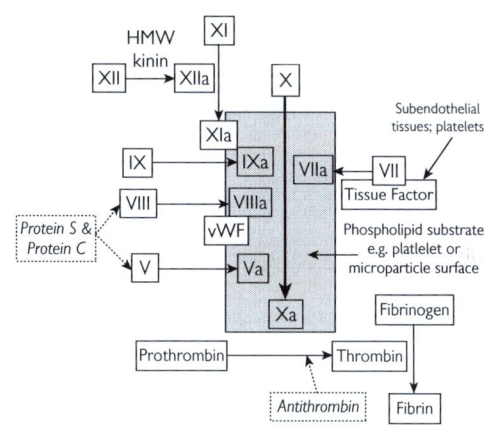

Figure 8.8 Summary of coagulation cascade.
Dotted lines indicate inhibitors. Grey box indicates factors associated with a phospholipid membrane surface.

Promoting thrombosis
Hypotheses regarding the mechanism(s) by which APL antibodies promote thrombosis *in vivo*:
- Activation of endothelial cells to up-regulate adhesion molecules, von Willebrand factor (vWF) tissue factor and tissue plasminogen activator.
- Activation of platelets to release pro-coagulant thromboxane A2.
- Activation of circulating monocytes to increase expression of adhesion molecules and production of pro-inflammatory cytokines.
- Acquired protein C resistance (β2GPI mediates binding of APL to protein C).
- Impaired fibrinolysis.

Hypotheses regarding mechanisms by which APL antibodies impair placental development and function:
- Binding to and interference with annexin V anticoagulant 'shield' on the surface of trophoblast cells.
- Impaired fibrinolysis.
- Defective maturation and invasion of trophoblast cells (partially mediated by reduction in IL-3).
- Activation of complement and promotion of inflammation.

Risk factors
- **LA positive:** high risk of arterial and venous thrombosis (odds ratio [OR] ~10).
- **LA negative**, but persistently aCL antibody positive (i.e. positive in >66% of estimations) – increased risk of venous thrombosis (OR ~3).

- **LA negative and transiently aCL antibody positive** (i.e. positive on at least 2 occasions, but on <66% of estimations) – thrombosis risk is not elevated.
- **Definite APLS:** risk of foetal loss ~20% (reduced from ~50% pre-heparin treatment).
- **SLE plus APL antibodies** ~50% develop definite APLS.
- **LA in SLE patients:** increased risk of coronary artery disease.

Clinical features

Main APLS clinical features
- Arterial thrombosis including:
  - intracranial arterial thrombosis resulting in TIAs, stroke syndromes or multi-infarct dementia;
  - myocardial infarction;
  - renal artery thrombosis;
  - mesenteric arterial thrombosis;
  - digital artery thrombosis.
- Venous thrombosis including:
  - deep venous thrombosis is frequent, sometimes complicated by pulmonary embolus;
  - Budd-Chiari Syndrome (hepatic vein thrombosis);
  - sagittal sinus thrombosis;
  - retinal vein thrombosis;
  - axillary vein thrombosis;
  - renal vein thrombosis;
  - inferior vena caval thrombosis;
  - mesenteric venous thrombosis;
  - adrenal vein thrombosis leading to Addison's disease.
- Maternal pregnancy complications are mainly manifestations of thromboembolic disease, usually DVT or PE. Depression with suicidal ideation is also reported. These complications can start from about 15 weeks gestation.
- Foetal complications arise mainly due to placental insufficiency and include intrauterine growth retardation (usually evident after 20 weeks), oligohydramnios, small placental size, and intrauterine death. Foetal thrombosis is rare and infants born to women with APLS appear to grow and develop normally. A mild verbal processing deficit has been reported in male children of SLE/APLS patients.

Summary of clinical features by body system

Renal
Renal artery stenosis occurs commonly in APLS patients with hypertension. Vasculo-occlusive lesions occur in smaller vessels, as well as result of fibrous intimal hyperplasia in interlobular arteries and thrombotic microangiopathy in microvasculature. Renal vein or inferior vena caval thrombosis are associated with APLS. End-stage renal failure is a rare complication in primary APLS. In patients with SLE, and secondary APLS and renal involvement, immune complex-mediated glomerulonephritis, and glomerular thrombosis both occur.

Neurological
A wide range of features occur including: transient ischaemic attacks, ischaemic stroke, cerebral venous thrombosis, headache, epilepsy, demyelination, cognitive dysfunction, depression, dementia, psychosis, intracranial hypertension, chorea, transverse myelitis, sensorineural hearing loss, transient global amnesia, dystonia, parkinsonism, Guillain–Barre syndrome, amaurosis fugax, and optic neuropathy.

Sneddon's syndrome is defined as the clinical triad of stroke, hypertension, and livedo reticularis. In many cases, there are APL antibodies.

Mucocutaneous
Livedo reticularis is a common feature and ranges from subtle to florid. Splinter haemorrhages are occasionally noted.

Haematological
Thrombocytopaenia is common in APLS, but bleeding is uncommon.

Gastrointestinal
Rare, but serious complications include mesenteric or hepatic artery or vein thrombosis.

Pulmonary
Pulmonary embolus is a well-recognized manifestation of APLS. LA appears to be associated with pulmonary arterial hypertension (PAH) in SSc and perhaps also with PAH in other contexts.

Cardiovascular
Approximately 33% of APLS patients have valvular lesions (Libman–Sacks endocarditis), most commonly on the mitral valve. These pre-exisitng lesions might increase the incidence of subacute bacterial endocarditis. APL antibodies may accelerate atherosclerosis. This, together with the thrombotic tendency, probably contributes to the increased incidence of MI and stroke in APLS.

Musculoskeletal
Avascular necrosis, usually associated with high-dose glucocorticoid use, appears to be increased in patients with APL antibodies.

Key features in history
- **Previous thromboses** (e.g. DVTs, PEs).
- **Obstetric history:** miscarriages, pre-eclampsia, eclampsia, premature delivery, low-birth-weight babies.
- **Haematological:** enquire about history of bleeding (would suggest a different diagnosis) or thromboembolic disease (DVT, PE, and neonatal/foetal loss or premature delivery).
- **Pulmonary:** enquire about exertional dyspnoea, chest pain (pleuritic?), and haemoptysis.
- **Cardiovascular:** calf swelling may indicate a DVT. Ankle swelling may be a manifestation of nephrotic range proteinuria. Hypertension may occur with renal artery stenosis or glomerular disease.
- **Neurological:** enquire about, and clarify the nature of fits, 'funny turns', headache, tingling/numbness, altered mood and difficulty with concentration or memory. See also 'The Nervous System', p. 90
- **Gastrointestinal/Hepatic:** enquire about abdominal pain, diarrhoea (with blood?).
- **Lifestyle:** certain factors increase the risk of thrombosis: Smoking, recent long car journeys, or flights, if DVT/PE suspected. Oral contraceptive use.

Key features on examination
- **Cutaneous:** look for livedo reticularis (may affect a small area only) and other signs of thromboembolism or vasculitis, e.g. splinter haemorrhages
- **Musculoskeletal:** synovitis is not a feature of primary APLS, but may occur as part of associated syndromes in secondary APLS. Avascular necrosis (most commonly of

femoral head) may be associated with irritability of the hip (internal and external rotation).
- **Renal:** BP and urinalysis. Proteinuria (1.5–15 g/24 h) occurs in virtually all cases of APLS nephropathy (microcirculatory thrombosis). Sudden heavy proteinuria should raise suspicion of renal vein thrombosis.
- **Neurological:** a basic neurological examination should be performed at diagnosis and in response to the development of new symptoms. Include fundoscopy in patients with (early morning?) headache and consider a cognitive assessment.
- **Haematological:** pallor indicates anaemia (not usually a feature of APLS). Bruising and excessive bleeding may occur with severe thrombocytopaenia or with a deficiency of clotting factors. However, note that glucocorticoid therapy is the usual reason for excessive bruising in SLE/APLS patients.
- **Gastrointestinal:** palpate abdomen for tenderness and organomegaly.
- **Pulmonary:** examine for respiratory rate, central cyanosis, stony dull percussion note (pleural effusion), pleural rub, signs of right heart strain.
- **Cardiovascular:** assess blood pressure at each visit. Examine for murmurs, right heart strain, peripheral pulses and carotid bruits (in cases with TIA/stroke syndromes).
- **Renal:** blood pressure and urinalysis.
- **Sicca signs** (see Sjögren's disease, p. 254).

Investigations
Laboratory
Anticardiolipin antibodies
Detection of aCL antibodies by ELISA is sufficient to make the diagnosis of APLS in patients with relevant clinical features, even in the absence of LA.

The significance of low titre IgG or IgM aCL antibodies, or of IgA aCL antibodies at any titre is controversial.

Anti β2GPI and other antibodies
β2GPI antibodies can also be measured by ELISA. This assay is less sensitive, but more specific than aCL assays and may be particularly helpful where an infection-associated aCL is suspected.
- Anti-prothrombin antibodies are measured in some centres, but the assay is not widely available.
- ELISAs for other phospholipids (phosphatidyl inositol, phosphatidylethanolamine, and phosphatidylserine) are also sometimes used in specialist centres.

Lupus anticoagulant
A variety of different tests may be employed to demonstrate the presence of an LA (Fig 8.9); however, the principles common to all approaches can be summarized as:
1. Demonstration that a phospholipid-dependent clotting assay is prolonged *in vitro*.
2. Demonstration that this is due to the presence of an inhibitor, rather than the absence of a clotting factor.
3. Demonstration that the inhibitor is phospholipid-dependent and not a specific inhibitor of a single coagulation factor.
    - At least 2 screening tests are used; dAPTT is more sensitive for the detection of APL antibodies utilizing prothrombin as a cofactor, while DRVVT is more sensitive for the detection of antibodies binding to β2GPI.
    - Notify the haematology laboratory if the patient is receiving high or low-molecular weight heparin, since this may cause prolongation of several of the screening assays (dAPTT, DRVVT, dPT).
    - Note that a strong LA can deplete factors VIII and IX, and this may erroneously raise suspicion of a primary factor VIII or IX deficiency.

Other haematology
- FBC may show evidence of anaemia and/or a profound thrombocytopaenia (may suggest an alternative diagnosis, e.g. thrombotic thrombocytopenic purpura [TTP] or haemolytic uremic syndrome [HUS]).
- Blood film to exclude schistocytes (RBC fragments) of microangiopathic haemolytic anaemia (MAHA); this suggests TTP or HUS, rather than APLS.
- Direct Coombs test is usually negative in MAHA.
- ESR may indicate co-existing inflammatory disease.

Biochemistry
- Renal function tests – serum creatinine and estimated creatinine clearance from Cockcroft–Gault formula:

    Estimated CrCl = [(140 − age) × weight (kg)]/ serum Cr (µmol/l)
    (Multiply by 0.85 in women)

    Note that this formula is inaccurate in patients with oedema due to nephrotic syndrome.
- Early morning urinary protein to creatinine ratio is probably as accurate as 24-h urine collection for quantifying severity of proteinuria.
- Liver function tests especially in patients with abdominal pain
- Thyroid function tests: hypothyroidism common.

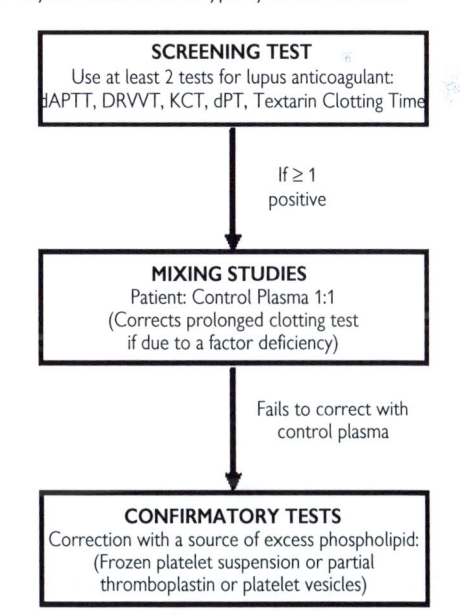

SCREENING TEST
Use at least 2 tests for lupus anticoagulant:
dAPTT, DRVVT, KCT, dPT, Textarin Clotting Time

↓ If ≥ 1 positive

MIXING STUDIES
Patient: Control Plasma 1:1
(Corrects prolonged clotting test if due to a factor deficiency)

↓ Fails to correct with control plasma

CONFIRMATORY TESTS
Correction with a source of excess phospholipid:
(Frozen platelet suspension or partial thromboplastin or platelet vesicles)

(Abbreviations: dAPTT dilute activated partial thromboplastin time; DRVVT dilute Russell'sviper venom time: KCT kaolin cephalin time; dPT dilute prothrombin time)

Figure 8.9 Functional assay use for detecting a LA.

- Bone function tests plus vitamin D and PTH, since vitamin D deficiency is common, particularly in patients with co-existing SLE, who use sunscreen.
- Fasting lipid profile – to detect and monitor co-existing hyperlipidaemia, which adds to the cardiovascular risk of APLS itself.
- Troponin I if myocarditis or myocardial infarction suspected.
- Cerebrospinal fluid (CSF) – see p. 92.

Immunology
- ANA and, if positive, ENA to indicate the likely nature of any associated autoimmune connective tissue disease (AICTD).
- Complement C3 and C4 if co-existing immune complex-mediated disease (e.g. rash, nephritis) is suspected.
- CSF – see p. 92.
- Check a midstream urine if urinanalysis is positive and request microscopy to look for an 'active' renal sediment, as well as culture/sensitivity.
- Blood cultures (multiple sets) should be performed whenever bacterial infection is suspected (e.g. possible endocarditis, meningitis).
- CSF – see p. 92.

Imaging
- Consider obtaining chest radiograph (CXR) if features of pleurisy. Note CXR may be normal in PE.
- Ventilation-perfusion scan in cases of suspected PE with normal CXR.
- CT Pulmonary angiogram – in cases of suspected PE in patients with pre-existing lung disease, if CXR abnormal or to detect pulmonary artery aneurysms.
- MR head/spinal cord should be obtained in patients with clinical focal neurological deficit or with unusual headaches or cognitive defects.

Histology
- Renal biopsy should be considered in patients with an 'active' renal sediment on urinalysis or isolated proteinuria (+++ or >1g/L). Liaise with renal team. See p. 75.
- Skin biopsy may reveal thrombotic microangiopathy. Infiltration of inflammatory cells may also be evident.

Other investigations
- Pulmonary function tests. Spirometry and transfer factor to screen for pulmonary arterial hypertension. See also p. 59.
- Echocardiogram to detect any pericardial effusion, LVH, reduced LV ejection fraction, valvular lesions, and as a screening test for PAH.
- ECG – useful screen for arrhythmia, ischaemia, left ventricular hypertrophy (LVH).
- Ankle/Brachial Pressure index, Doppler ultrasound, MR angiography or conventional angiography to investigate suspected peripheral vascular disease.
- Carotid ultrasound for investigation of carotid bruit or of TIA/stroke.
- Lumbar puncture, EEG and other neurophysiology tests might be necessary (see also p. 90).
- Ocular investigations,– see The Eye, p. 48.

Differential diagnosis

- Behçet's disease - see p. 340.
- Diffuse intravascular coagulation (DIC) with thrombocytopaenia should be considered as a differential diagnosis in catastrophic antiphospholipid syndrome. Clotting assays (PT and APTT) are usually prolonged and fibrin degradation products and D-dimers are markedly raised. The context (sepsis, obstetric complication) is usually helpful in making the diagnosis.
- Deficiency of coagulation regulator, e.g. protein C, protein S, or antithrombin.
- Paraneoplastic manifestation.
- TTP is characterized by fever, MAHA, thrombocytopaenia, renal impairment, and neurological deficits.
- Haemolytic uraemic syndrome (HUS) defined by the triad of MAHA, thrombocytopaenia, and renal impairment. Some forms of HUS are triggered by gastrointestinal infection with a Shigatoxin-producing *E. coli*. Genetic forms of HUS include deficiencies of complement regulatory proteins, e.g. factor H or membrane cofactor protein deficiency.
- TTP and HUS can be distinguished from APLS by presence of MAHA, very low platelet counts, and absence of APL antibodies.
- Sneddon's syndrome, as defined as the clinical trial of stroke, hypertension and livedo reticularis, is often caused by APLS.
- Moya-moya is a rare cerebrovascular occlusive disease characterized by bilateral stenoses of the terminal internal carotid artery, accompanied by abnormalities of the vascular network at the base of the brain; it usually presents with stroke syndromes in children and intracranial haemorrhages in adults.
- Hyperhomocysteinaemia.
- Evan's syndrome – acquired haemolytic anaemia and thrombocytopaenia.
- Pregnancy-related differential diagnoses:
  - HELLP – haemolysis elevated liver enzymes and low platelets is a pregnancy-related hypertensive disorder with underlying thrombotic microangiopathy; defective control of the alternative pathway of complement may be responsible. HELLP is sometimes considered to be a form of pre-eclampsia.
  - Pre-eclampsia – new hypertension and proteinuria during the second half of pregnancy are associated with placental ischaemia; may progress to the convulsive state of eclampsia.

Treatment

Objectives of management
- Prevention of thromboembolic events.
- Management of any associated inflammatory disease.
- Management of associated co-morbidity.
- Maximizing chance of successful pregnancy, whilst minimizing risks to mother.

Prevention of thromboembolic events
Anticoagulation
The evidence base regarding efficacy of antiplatelet and anticoagulant agents is still inadequate. Published RCTs include mainly cases at the low-risk end of the APLS spectrum and it is likely that high-risk APLS patients should be anticoagulated more aggressively than these trial data would suggest (Table 8.9).

Hydroxychloroquine (HCQ)
Several studies have indicated that HCQ reduces thrombotic events in SLE. Further study is required to assess its efficacy in primary APLS, but in view of its relative safety, it is widely used in all categories of APLS.

Risk factors
Additional risks for thromboembolic disease should also be minimized. This includes stopping smoking, treating hypertension, and managing hyperlipidaemia.

HMG-CoA reductase inhibitors (statins)
The pleiotropic effect of statins has been reported to include inhibition of APL-mediated up-regulation of tissue factor expression by monocytes and endothelial cells.

Table 8.9 Recommended therapy for categories of (non-pregnant) patients with aCL antbodies

Category of patient	Recommended therapy
Persistent aCL antibodies. No history of clinical events	HCQ?*
Thrombosis and single positive APL antibody test	Treat as for thrombosis in the general population
APLS (first venous thrombosis)	Warfarin (INR 2.0–3.0) and HCQ
APLS (arterial or recurrent venous thrombosis)	Warfarin (INR 3.0–4.0) and HCQ
APLS (recurrent episodes on warfarin with INR 3.0–4.0)	Low molecular weight or unfractionated heparin or warfarin plus antiplatelet agent

INR: international normalized ratio.
*The APLASA study indicated that patients with persistent aCL antibodies with or without a lupus anticoagulant did NOT benefit from 81 mg aspirin daily.

Management of associated morbidity
Refer to SLE section (AICTDs chapter, pp. 250–251) for management of co-morbidity including: cardiovascular disease, osteoporosis, chronic renal failure, and depression.

Maximizing chance of successful pregnancy whilst minimizing risks to mother

Pregnancy planning
- Repeat aCL antibody testing and check LA to establish whether APL antibodies are persistent.
- In patients with co-existing SLE, optimize disease control on non-teratogenic immunosuppressants (see p. 368–369).
- Postpone pregnancy after a thromboembolic event, especially a stroke.
- Discourage pregnancy in patients with pulmonary hypertension.
- Determine anticoagulant strategy (see Table 8.10).

Anticoagulant strategy
The recommendations below are distilled from a variety of studies and reviews. However, treatment regimes for each scenario remain controversial. HCQ appears to be safe in pregnancy. Either unfractionated heparin or low molecular weight heparin (LMWH) may be given in:
- **Prophylactic doses:** unfractionated heparin 5000–10 000 IU twice daily or LMWH, e.g. enoxaparin 0.5 mg/kg twice daily.
- **Therapeutic doses:** unfractionated heparin 10 000–36 000 IU twice daily or LMWH, e.g. enoxaparin 1 mg/kg twice daily, with monitoring.

Heparin should be suspended for delivery. Stop heparin at least 12 h before an epidural injection for prophylactic regimens and at least 24 h before an epidural for therapeutic regimens. In these patients, heparin should be restarted post-partum, provided there are no haemorrhagic complications and continued for 3 months.

Table 8.10 Recommended therapy for pregnant patient with aCL antibodies

Pregnancy scenario	Recommended treatment
Persistent APL antibodies (LA is higher risk than aCL antibodies), but no previous thrombo-embolism (TE) or adverse obstetric history	Low-dose aspirin? LMWH post-partum?
APLS with adverse obstetric history (no TE history)	Low-dose aspirin ± prophylactic LMWH. LMWH postpartum
APLS with TE history	Stop warfarin as soon as possible post-conception. Use low-dose aspirin and therapeutic dose of LMWH then follow with warfarin postpartum
APLS with recurrent TE disease despite full antithrombotic dose of heparin	Warfarin after organogenesis (weeks 6–12)
Breastfeeding	Warfarin or heparin safe

Anti-inflammatory treatment
Increased leucocyte adhesion and complement activation have been demonstrated in placentae of women with APLS and obstetric complications. Heparins have been shown to reduce both these processes. Glucocorticoids (GCs) appear to be ineffective and can cause significant adverse effects, so should be avoided. HCQ may be beneficial, but there are no outcome data to inform this at present.

Pregnancy monitoring and management
- Blood pressure and urinalysis checked at each antenatal visit at least monthly.
- FBC for patients on heparin to monitor for heparin-induced thrombocytopaenia. This is rare and the risk is lower with LWMH than with unfractionated heparin.
- INR to monitor anticoagulation with warfarin.
- Antifactor Xa activity can be used to monitor anticoagulation with LMWH.
- Frequent ultrasound scans to monitor foetal growth.
- Uterine and umbilical artery Doppler blood flow analysis during second trimester.
- Manage hypertension with calcium channel antagonists.
- Calcium and vitamin D3 (e.g. adcal-D3 2 daily) may be given in pregnant and breastfeeding patients receiving heparin. However, there is no evidence base to indicate whether this reduces the incidence or severity of heparin-induced osteoporosis.
- Activity of co-existing SLE may be treated with systemic GCs, HCQ, azathioprine, or rituximab.
- For severe thrombocytopaenia use prednisolone 30–60 mg daily. This raises platelet count. If effective use this strategy prior to delivery. Other options include intravenous immunoglobulin and early delivery.

Multidisciplinary
- Obstetrician.
- Neonatologist.
- Haematologist.
- Renal physician.
- Dermatologist.
- Chest physician.
- Gastroenterologist.

- Radiologist.
- Ophthalmologist.
- Vascular surgeon.

Patient advice
- Avoid smoking.
- Education regarding cardiovascular risk and importance of regular aerobic exercise, healthy diet, and avoidance of prolonged immobility or oral contraceptive.
- In pregnant women with APLS, the probability of a live birth is ~75–80%, with appropriate management. Risks of pre-eclampsia, premature delivery, thrombosis are increased.

Resources

Guidelines
For guidelines on the identification of LA, see Brandt et al., 1995, in references.

Patient organizations
Hughes Syndrome Foundation (Antiphospholipid Syndrome). The Rayne Institute, St Thomas' Hospital, London SE1 7EH. Tel: 020 7960 5561. Available at: www.hughes-syndrome.org

ICD-10 codes
D68.8 Coagulation defects associated with presence of 'SLE inhibitor'.

O00.0 Spontaneous abortion in abdominal pregnancy

References

Amirlak I, Amirlak B. Haemolytic uraemic syndrome: an overview. *Nephrol* 2006; 11: 21–8.

Belizna CC, Richar V, et al. INsights into atherosclerosis therapy in antiphospholipid syndrome. *Autoimmun Rev* 2007; **7**: 46–51.

Brandt JT, Barna LK, Triplett DA. Laboratory identification of lupus anticoagulants: results of the Second International Workshop for Identification of Lupus Anticoagulants. On behalf of the Subcommittee on Lupus Anticoagulant/Antiphospholipid Antibodies of the ISTH. *Thromb Haemost* 1995; **74**: 1597–603.

Bucciarelli S, Cervera R, et al. Mortality in the catastrophic antiphospholipid syndrome: causes of death and prognostic factors. *Autoimmun Rev* 2006; **6**: 72–5.

Crowther MA, Wisloff F. Evidence based treatment of the antiphospholipid syndrome II. Optimal anti-coagulant therapy for thrombosis. *Thromb Res* 2005; **115**: 3–8.

Erkan D, Harrison MJ, et al. Aspirin for primary thrombosis prevention in the antiphospholipid syndrome. *Arthritis Rheum* 2007; **57**: 2382–91.

Marie I, Jouen F, et al. Anticardiolipin and anti-beta2 glycoprotein I antibodies and lupus-like anticoagulant: prevalence and significance in systemic sclerosis. *Br J Dermatol* 2008; **158**: 141–4.

Miyakis S, Lockshin MD, et al. International consensus statement on an update of the classification criteria for definite antiphospholipid syndrome. *J Thromb Haemost* 2006; **4**: 295–306.

Norris M, Perico N, Remuzzi G. Mechanisms of disease: pre-eclampsia. *Nat Clin Pract Nephrol* 2005; **1**: 98–114.

Petri M. Epidemiology of the antiphospholipid antibody syndrome. *J Autoimmun* 2000; **15**: 145–51.

Ruiz-Irastorza G, Khamashta MA. The treatment of antiphospholipid syndrome: a harmonic contrast. *Best Pract Res Clinical Rheumatol* 2007; **6**: 1079–92.

Salmon JE, Girardi G, Lockshin MD. Antiphospholipid syndrome as a disorder initiated by inflammation: implications for the therapy of pregnant patients. *Nat Clin Pract Rheumatol* 2007; **3**: 140–7.

Sanna G, Bertolaccini ML, et al. Central nervous system involvement in the antiphospholipid (Hughes) syndrome. *Rheumatol* 2003; **42**: 200–13.

Sherer Y, Blank M, Shoenfeld Y. Antiphospholipid syndrome (APS): where does it come from? *Best Pract Res Clinical Rheumatol* 2007; **21**: 1071–8.

Uthman I, Khamashta M. Antiphospholipid syndrome and the kidneys. *Semin Arthritis Rheum* 2006; **35**: 360–7.

Wisloff F, Jacobsen EM, Listol S. Laboratory diagnosis of the antiphospholipid syndrome. *Thrombosis Res* 2003; **108**: 263–71.

Autoimmune connective tissue diseases

Polymyositis

Definition
Polymyositis (PM) is classified as an idiopathic inflammatory myopathy, the other members of the group being dermatomyositis (DM) and sporadic inclusion body myositis (IBM). PM is characterized by subacute onset of proximal muscle weakness and inflammatory infiltrates in skeletal muscle. It may occur in association with other autoimmune connective tissue diseases. There is overlap between the features of PM and DM, and the respective chapters in this text should be read in conjunction. However, there are several key features that distinguish PM from DM, which include:
- Absence of the pathognomonic rash of DM.
- A distinct immunopathological process with characteristic findings on muscle biopsy.
- A lower association with malignancy.

Diagnostic criteria
Diagnostic and classification criteria for the idiopathic inflammatory myopathies remain a subject of much dispute. Bohan and Peter proposed a set of diagnostic criteria for PM and DM in 1975 that have been widely used for many years. This incorporates five major criteria.

> - Symmetrical proximal muscle weakness with or without dysphagia and respiratory muscle weakness.
> - Elevation of serum muscle enzymes, especially CK.
> - Electromyography (EMG) evidence of myositis.
> - Muscle biopsy abnormalities of degeneration, regeneration, necrosis, phagocytosis, and an interstitial mononuclear infiltrate.
> - Typical skin rash of dermatomyositis.
>
> PM is classified as 'definite' in the presence of 4 criteria, 'probable' with three criteria and 'possible' with 2. PM is differentiated from DM by the absence of the rash.

- The classification divides the idiopathic inflammatory myopathies into primary idiopathic DM or PM, Juvenile DM/PM, DM/PM associated with malignancy, PM/DM associated with vasculitis, and DM/PM associated with autoimmune connective tissue disease.
- IBM was identified as a distinct clinical entity several years later and is included in the classification of inflammatory myopathies.
- The above criteria have been criticized for lacking specificity and resulting in over-diagnosis of PM as a result of misclassification of IBM, and other myopathies. The principal concern is that inflammatory infiltrates in skeletal muscle may be present in several other conditions, for example, muscular dystrophies, toxic myopathies and IBM, and these may not be adequately excluded under these criteria.
- Dalakas proposed alternative criteria incorporating more specific muscle biopsy characteristics. However, these criteria have not been validated and have in turn been criticized for being too stringent, with the concern that they would leave many patients with no diagnosis thereby limiting their treatment options (see Table 8.11 in DM section, p. 291).
- The International Myositis Assessment and Clinical Studies (IMACS) Group published guidelines in 2005 for the conduct of clinical trials in myositis. Consensus was reached that a 'definite' or 'probable' diagnosis of PM by Bohan and Peter criteria was sufficient for enrolling patients in trials with the proviso that the muscle biopsy must be consistent with PM, and that all other forms of myopathy must be excluded by clinical, laboratory, genetic, or pathological techniques. However, the limitations of the Bohan and Peter criteria were recognized.
- A large international, multidisciplinary collaborative project has therefore been set up to develop and validate new classification criteria for the idiopathic inflammatory myopathies.

Epidemiology
PM usually affects adults from the 3rd decade onwards with a peak incidence from age 40–60 years. In contrast to DM, PM very rarely affects children. The female to male ratio is 2:1. Data on the frequency of PM in the general population is lacking. US estimates of the annual incidence of PM and DM combined, range from 2 to 10/million.

Aetiology and pathophysiology
PM, DM, and IBM are all characterized by acquired muscle weakness and skeletal muscle inflammation, but differ clinically, histologically, and pathophysiologically.
- PM and DM are autoimmune diseases targeted at as yet unidentified antigens within skeletal muscle. In IBM, inflammatory and degenerative processes are evident.
- The mechanism of muscle damage in PM appears to be predominantly via T-cell mediated cytotoxicity. Muscle biopsy reveals infiltrates of CD8+ cytotoxic T-lymphocytes within muscle fascicles.
- DM is characterized by perivascular infiltrates of CD4+ T cells and B cells, with complement-mediated damage of intra-muscular microvasculature and consequent muscle ischaemia.
- Akin to other autoimmune diseases, PM is thought to arise following exposure to an environmental trigger in genetically predisposed individuals.

Genetic factors
Candidate gene studies have demonstrated HLA-DRB1*0301 and DQA1*0501 to be associated with the development of myositis, especially in patients with anti-synthetase antibodies. Possession of the TNF-308A allele has also been shown to be a risk factor for inflammatory myositis in a UK adult population. PM and DM appear to be genetically different diseases, and work is ongoing to clarify these distinctions.

Environmental
Despite many proposed viral triggers, for example, cocksackie, influenza, parainfluenza, parvovirus and cytomegalovirus, PCR studies have failed to demonstrate evidence of viral genetic material in muscle biopsy samples. Nevertheless, retroviruses, such as HIV or HTLV-1 have been associated with PM and IBM. Similar to retrovirus-negative PM, clonal expansion of subpopulations of CD8 positive (CD8+) T-cells is seen in these patients.

Immunopathology
HLA class I up-regulation
One of the earliest features of PM is ubiquitous expression of major human leucocyte antigen (HLA) class I antigens on muscle fibres, even in areas remote from sites of inflammation. HLA class I is not normally expressed on myofibres

CHAPTER 8 Autoimmune connective tissue diseases

and this widespread up-regulation is typical of PM and IBM, but is not usually seen in other chronic myopathies or dystrophies.

T cell cytotoxicity
CD8+ cytotoxic T cells surround HLA class I expressing myofibres, and contain perforin and granzyme granules, which induce muscle cell necrosis. Subsets of these autoinvasive T cells are clonally expanded, presumably in response to certain antigens present in muscle tissue.

B cell involvement:
B lymphocytes have traditionally been considered to play a less important role in PM than in DM and inflammatory infiltrates in PM typically contain very few B cells. However, autoantibodies are present in 60-80% of patients with PM suggesting involvement of a humoral autoimmune response. Recent studies have supported this, demonstrating large numbers of CD138+ plasma cells in muscle in PM and IBM. In addition, B cell depletion with rituximab has been reported effective in refractory PM.

Endoplasmic reticulum stress
It has been postulated that, in conjunction with T-cell mediated cytotoxicity, there may be concurrent non-immune muscle fibre destruction due to an endoplasmic reticulum (ER) stress response. This could, in part account for the poor correlation between the extent of inflammatory infiltrates on muscle biopsy and the degree of muscle weakness.
- The ER usually processes, folds, and exports proteins, including HLA class I molecules. The stress response occurs due to a discrepancy between the load of proteins in the ER and its ability to process them.
- Major components of the ER stress response pathways are highly activated in myositis. Furthermore, over-expression of HLA class I molecules has been shown to induce an ER stress response in a mouse model.
- ER stress results in accumulation of misfolded HLA glycoproteins and up-regulation of nuclear factor κB and HLA class I molecules, which may perpetuate the inflammatory response. The mechanisms by which this may mediate muscle fibre damage have not been established.

Clinical features

Key features in history
Myopathic muscle weakness
- Insidious onset of weakness over weeks to months.
- Predominantly affects proximal muscles and is typically symmetrical.
- Acute onset with early respiratory muscle involvement is occasionally seen, but is rare.
- Difficulty with activities, such as rising from a chair, climbing steps, and brushing hair.
- Fine motor movements, which rely on distal muscle strength, such as writing, are not usually affected until late in disease.
- Involvement of neck flexors and extensors results in difficulty holding the head up.
- Weakness is typically painless. Myalgia occurs in only around 30% and is rarely severe.
- External ocular muscles are involved.

Key features on examination
Examination should incorporate:
- Evaluation of muscle function by observation of specific activities and direct testing of power against resistance (see below).
- Exclusion of differential diagnoses.
- Assessment for extra-muscular involvement.

Evaluation of muscle function
- Muscle wasting is not usually seen at the outset, but may be evident in long-standing disease.
- On sitting up from supine, the head may lag behind in neck flexor weakness.
- May have difficulty raising the arms above the head.
- May be unable to stand from sitting or rise from a crouching position without using arms to assist.
- Grade muscle power against resistance (see manual muscle testing below).
- Test proximal and distal groups of upper and lower limbs to determine pattern of weakness.

Exclusion of differential diagnoses
The presence of cutaneous features characteristic of dermatomyositis should be excluded.
- Neurological examination is essential. Key features to note include:
  - sensation is normal;
  - deep tendon reflexes are preserved unless muscle atrophy is severe;
  - eye movements are normal (differentiates from myasthenia gravis);
  - fasciculations are not a feature (suggest motor neurone disease).
- Assessment for involvement of other organs.
- Full cardiovascular, respiratory and joint examinations should be performed.
- Fine bi-basal crepitations may indicate ILD.

Co-morbidities
Constitutional symptoms
Fatigue, anorexia, fever and weight loss are seen in around 40%, more commonly in those with anti-synthetase antibodies.

Joint disease
Arthritis is associated with anti-synthetase antibodies. It is typically symmetrical and non-deforming involving wrists, hands, and knees. Arthralgia is common.

Pulmonary disease
- Weakness of chest wall and diaphragmatic muscles can lead to exertional dyspnoea. In severe disease, especially in those with an acute presentation, patients may progress to respiratory failure.
- Pharyngeal and oesophageal striated muscle weakness lead to dysphagia in around 30% of patients with consequent risk of aspiration pneumonia. Dysphonia is a less common manifestation.
- Interstitial lung disease (ILD) affects approximately 30% of patients with PM/DM. Estimates vary widely and are increasing as the sensitivity of diagnostic tests improves.
- ILD is frequently subclinical and in a study screening all newly diagnosed patients with PM/DM, 65% had evidence of ILD. Typical features of ILD include cough and dyspnoea. The spectrum of disease ranges from asymptomatic to severe, rapidly progressive respiratory failure and death.
- Prognosis of ILD is unrelated to the severity of myositis and may develop at any stage, but is present at diagnosis of myositis in most affected patients.
- ILD associated with PM is strongly associated with anti-synthetase antibodies. Over 70% of anti-Jo1 positive patients develop ILD.

- There is no clear guidance as to when and how frequently patients should be investigated for ILD. It has been advocated that all patients should be screened at diagnosis of PM as early intervention may improve outcome.

Cardiovascular disease
- Clinically overt cardiac involvement is relatively rare.
- Subclinical disease affects up to 75% of patients, predominantly manifest as abnormalities on ECG.
- The most common clinically significant cardiac manifestations are myocarditis, arrhythmias, atrioventricular conduction block and congestive cardiac failure. Coronary artery disease is also frequently seen.
- Cardiac involvement is associated with increased mortality and has been reported to be the commonest cause of death in myositis patients.
- A 16 times increased death rate from myocardial infarction has been reported in myositis patients compared to the general population.
- The increased cardiovascular risk may be due to a combination of factors including direct involvement of the heart by the myositis disease process, chronic systemic inflammation and side effects of treatment.

Malignancy
- There is an increased risk of malignancy in DM, but the association with PM is less clearly established.
- Increased incidence of several cancers has been reported in PM, including lung cancer, non-Hodgkin's lymphoma, and bladder cancer.
- However, the overall increased risk of malignancy is modest. Estimated cancer incidence in PM is approximately 1.7–2 times that of the general population.
- The risk of malignancy is greatest within the first year following diagnosis and returns to normal by 5 years.
- Case ascertainment bias as a result of increased surveillance may therefore account for much of the purported association between PM and malignancy. However, it has been reported that cancer risk is increased in years preceding the diagnosis of myositis.

Anti-synthetase syndrome
- Affects up to 30% of patients with PM.
- Clinical features include ILD, constitutional symptoms, Raynaud's phenomenon, mechanic's hands (roughening and cracking of the skin of the fingers), and arthritis.
- Anti-synthetase antibodies are present, most commonly anti-Jo-1. However, similar features may be seen in patients with other antibodies, e.g. anti-PM/Scl.

Associations
PM occurs in conjunction with other autoimmune connective tissue diseases including systemic sclerosis (SSc), systemic lupus erythematosus (SLE), Sjögren's syndrome (SS), rheumatoid arthritis (RA), and mixed connective tissue disease (MCTD). Less commonly, it may be associated with other autoimmune conditions, such as primary biliary cirrhosis and autoimmune thyroiditis.

Investigations
Laboratory tests
General
- FBC may show anaemia or thrombocytosis.
- ESR and/or CRP are elevated in 50%.
- Baseline LFTs and U&E are essential prior to starting immunosuppressive treatments.
- Exclude differential diagnoses: TFTs, bone profile and vitamin D level are essential. LH, FSH, and testosterone may be indicated in males.
- Genetic testing may be helpful in certain cases if an inherited muscular dystrophy or myopathy is suspected

Muscle enzymes
Creatinine kinase (CK) is almost always elevated in active PM and may be as high as 50 times the upper limit of the reference interval.
- Other muscle enzymes [lactate dehydrogenase (LDH), aldolase, aspartate transaminase (AST) and alanine transaminase (ALT)] may also be raised. These are less sensitive than CK, but measurement of two muscle enzymes is advocated when monitoring disease.
- It is imperative to consider other causes of raised muscle enzymes, including muscle trauma, e.g. following intramuscular injections or needle stimulation during EMG (CK may be elevated for up to a month afterwards), exercise, hypothyroidism, and medications.

Auto-antibodies
ANA is positive in up to 80% of cases of PM. 'Myositis-specific antibodies' or 'myositis associated antibodies' are present in around 50%. The former occur solely in myositis but the latter may be seen in other connective tissue diseases in the absence of myositis.
- Myositis specific antibodies are present in around 30% of patients. The three main categories are:
  - Anti-synthetase antibodies. Anti-Jo-1 is the most common. These are directed against aminoacyl tRNA-synthetases and are found in about 20–30% of patients with PM/DM. They are strongly associated with the Anti-synthetase syndrome.
  - Antibodies to the signal recognition particle (anti-SRP), which is required for translocation of proteins into the ER. Anti-SRP antibodies are found almost exclusively in PM and are associated with acute, severe disease with a very high CK and a necrotizing pattern on muscle biopsy.
  - Antibodies to Mi-2, a nuclear helicase, are classically associated with DM, rather than PM.
- Myositis associated autoantibodies include anti-Ro, anti-La, anti-Sm, or anti-RNP, and suggest the myositis is associated with other connective tissue diseases.
- Anti-Ku and anti-PM-Scl occur in patients with overlapping features of myositis and systemic sclerosis.

Imaging
Magnetic resonance (MR) imaging
MR imaging is highly sensitive for muscle inflammation and oedema, and is best demonstrated on fat-suppressed T2-weighted and STIR images. T1-weighted images demonstrate fatty infiltration and muscle atrophy signifying established muscle damage.
- Roles for MRI include identifying a site for muscle biopsy (given that muscle involvement is frequently patchy), distinguishing active myositis from muscle damage and monitoring response to treatment.
- Magnetic resonance spectroscopy (MRS) measures metabolic changes in muscle and is a promising technique for monitoring disease activity, but is not widely available.

Ultrasound (US)
US is less sensitive for muscle inflammation than MR; however, it has the advantages of being cheaper and more easily available. Assessment of muscle blood vessel flow with colour flow Doppler may have a role in monitoring myositis activity.

Histology
- Muscle biopsy is mandatory to confirm the diagnosis and exclude other conditions, which can mimic PM.
- The histological hallmark of PM is endomysial inflammatory infiltrates of CD8+ T lymphocytes surrounding non-necrotic muscle fibres expressing HLA class I molecules.
- A key feature is that the muscle fibres appear histologically healthy. This distinguishes the primary inflammation of PM from inflammation secondary to myofibre damage, which may be seen in other myopathies.
- Muscle pathology can be patchy and repeat biopsy may be required if the first is inconclusive.

Other investigations
Electromyography (EMG)
EMG is abnormal in 90% of patients and is useful for excluding neurogenic disorders and assessing disease activity. However, the findings are non-specific and do not differentiate PM/DM from other myopathies.
- Needle EMG findings include myopathic potentials visible as low-amplitude, short duration polyphasic units on voluntary activation, and increased spontaneous activity manifest as fibrillations, positive sharp waves, and complex repetitive discharges.
- Several muscles should be examined with EMG including the proximal limb and paraspinal muscles as these give the greatest diagnostic yield, and may be the only muscles affected.

Assessment of respiratory muscle function
In the acute setting, if respiratory compromise is suspected, vital capacity should be monitored. Arterial oxygen and carbon dioxide levels may be misleadingly normal. A vital capacity of less than 15 ml/kg is associated with a significantly increased risk of ventilatory failure.

Investigations for interstitial lung disease
- **CXR:** low sensitivity for ILD.
- **Pulmonary function tests:** restrictive pattern with reduced lung volumes, normal or raised FEV1/FVC ratio, and a reduced carbon monoxide transfer factor (DLCO).
- **High-resolution computerized tomography (HRCT)** demonstrates the extent and severity of disease and helps to distinguish active disease, manifest as groundglass shadowing, from the honeycomb appearance of established fibrosis.
- **Bronchoalveolar lavage** may be helpful in assessing disease activity and excluding other causes of ILD.
- **Lung biopsy** is seldom required, but may be prognostically useful.

Investigations for cardiovascular disease
- ECG is mandatory for all patients to detect conduction defects, arrhythmias and evidence of ischaemia.
- Echocardiography may be abnormal in up to 62% of patients with myositis. Left ventricular diastolic dysfunction and mitral valve prolapse are the most common abnormalities.
- Elevation of troponin I is a relatively cardiac specific and is found in suspected myocarditis; however, won't discriminate cardiac lesions.
- Other frequently used markers of myocardial damage, such as troponin T and CK-MB, are less cardiac specific, and may be elevated due to skeletal muscle inflammation.
- Further specialized imaging, e.g. scintigraphy or MR, may be indicated in suspected myocarditis.
- Endomyocardial biopsy is rarely necessary.

Screening for malignancy
An extensive, blind search for malignancy is not recommended. Baseline evaluation at diagnosis of PM should include:
- Thorough history and examination, including lymph nodes, breast and rectal examinations.
- CXR and urinalysis.
- FBC, urea, electrolyte, and creatinine, LFTs, bone profile, and both serum and urine protein electrophoresis.
- Pelvic examination and cervical smear in women.
- PSA in men.
- Consider colonoscopy, mammogram, abdominal and pelvic US, and, if suspicion still high, whole body CT.

There is no clear guidance as to how frequently patients should be screened. However, particular vigilance with annual reassessment is advisable for the first 3 years, especially in older people.

Differential diagnosis

Inclusion body myositis (see also p. 302)
- Onset of weakness is more gradual.
- Has a propensity for involvement of quadriceps and forearm flexors.

Inherited muscular dystrophies
- Particularly limb-girdle muscular dystrophy, dystrophinopathies (Becker and Duchenne), fascioscapulohumeral dystrophy, and dysferlinopathy.
- Ask about family history. Female carriers of dystrophinopathies may develop a milder form with onset of muscle weakness from late teens onwards.
- Pattern of weakness varies, but may mimic PM, although onset tends to be slower.
- A very high CK, more >×100 the upper limit of the reference interval may be a pointer towards dysferlinopathy.
- EMG features may be indistinguishable from PM.
- Muscle biopsy may show inflammatory infiltrates.

Metabolic myopathies (see also p. 293)
- May present with onset of progressive muscle weakness in adult life.
- Ask about exertion-induced myalgia and pigmented urine (myoglobinuria).

Endocrine disorders
- Hypothyroidism induces proximal myopathy and commonly causes an elevated CK.
- Hyperthyroidism, osteomalacia, and parathyroid dysfunction may cause proximal myopathy, but CK is normal.
- Male hypogonadism may cause loss of muscle mass and fatigue.
- Acromegaly and Cushing's syndrome are usually clinically apparent by the time they cause significant muscle weakness.

Drugs
- A full medication history is mandatory.
- Glucocorticoids are an important cause of myopathy.
- Additionally, the following drugs have been reported, amongst others, to cause a myopathy (those marked * are more likely to be painful): lithium, chloroquine-containing drugs*, clofibrate, statins, salbutamol, penicillin, colchicine, D-penicillamine*, sulphonamides, hydralazine, ciclosporin, phenytoin, cimetidine* (muscle cramps), zidovudine, carbimazole, and tamoxifen.
- Compared with PM, in steroid myopathy, the CK is normal and biopsy is consistent with non-inflammatory fibre atrophy. GC-induced myopathy should be considered during GC treatment, especially if there is no response to treatment.
- The myositis occurring with D-penicillamine is not daily dose- or cumulative dose-dependent. It can be life threatening.
- Mild myoarthralgia may be caused by a number of commonly used drugs, e.g. proton pump inhibitors and quinolone antibiotics.
- Alcohol in excess and some illegal drugs (e.g. ecstasy) are associated with severe toxic myopathy occasionally resulting in rhabdomyolysis.

Other
- Neurological diseases: motor neuron disease, spinal muscular atrophy and myasthenia gravis.
- Guillain–Barre syndrome and subacute myelopathy.
- Viral infection, e.g. HIV, HTLV-1 can induce myositis indistinguishable from PM.
- Other types of inflammatory myositis, e.g. eosinophilic myositis, granulomatous myositis, macrophagic myofasciitis.

Pitfalls with interpreting CK results
- The reference range of CK can differ depending on ethnic background. It is generally regarded that people of Afro-Caribbean background have a higher 'normal' reference range CK compared with Caucasians.
- There is allelic variation in the CK gene and post-translational changes that can affect routine CK assays.

> **Key points regarding differential diagnosis**
> *Features that should prompt consideration of alternative diagnoses*
> - Asymmetric pattern of weakness or predominantly distal weakness is more typical of IBM.
> - Muscle pain and tenderness with normal strength is more suggestive of fibromyalgia or polymyalgia rheumatica.
> - Family history of neuromuscular disease. Familial cases of PM have been observed, but are very rare.
> - Slow onset myopathy that evolves over months to years then consider IBM or muscular dystrophy.

- It is important to be aware that production of *macro-CK* can present with elevated routine CK results.
- Macro-CK may be a normal variant but can be associated with malignancy. A screen for tumours may be necessary.
- CK can be elevated secondary to muscle trauma. If modest elevations in CK are thought to arise from trauma, a delay before re-testing is prudent.
- CK can be very modestly (but significantly and persistently) elevated in sarcoid myopathy.

Treatment

Objectives of management
- To improve muscle strength.
- Control extra-muscular complications.
- Avoid treatment related side effects.
- Early identification of malignancy.
- Maintain function and quality of life.

Physical therapies
Exercise and management of muscular function
- Exercise programmes used in conjunction with pharmacotherapy are effective in PM/DM.
- Benefits include improved muscle strength, increased exercise tolerance and prevention of muscle atrophy.
- There is no evidence that exercise worsens muscle inflammation as had previously been suggested.
- Programmes should be tailored to patients' capabilities.
- Passive stretching exercises are utilized for bed-bound patients.
- Oral creatine supplements have been shown to provide additional improvements in muscle function.
- Patients with dysphagia or dysphonia require input from speech and language therapists. Artificial feeding methods are occasionally necessary.

Immunsuppression
There have been very few good quality controlled trials in PM and treatment therefore remains mostly empirical, varying according to individual clinician experience and preference. This was highlighted in a recent Cochrane review (Choy, 2005).
- Glucocorticoids (GCs) are used first-line, often in conjunction with another immunosuppressive agent (usually azathioprine or methotrexate).
- Other immunosuppressants, IVIG, or biological agents are indicated in refractory disease. The approach to therapy is broadly similar for PM and DM; however, PM is more likely to be resistant to treatment.

Glucocorticoids (GCs)
GCs have never been adequately evaluated in a randomized controlled trial (RCT), but are generally accepted as being effective. In retrospective series, muscle weakness improved in up to 88% of those treated. However, up to 50% of patients with PM fail to respond to GCs alone.
- A typical dosing regime: prednisolone 1 mg/kg per day (up to 80 mg daily). Lower doses may be used in milder disease.
- Pulse iv methylprednisolone (1 g/day for 3 days) in acute, severe disease but evidence only in case series.
- After 4–6 weeks, once improvement is seen, the dose is gradually tapered to maintenance of 5–10 mg daily.
- Rapid GC withdrawal may precipitate disease exacerbations. Once dose is reduced to 10 mg, weaning should occur at a maximum of 1mg every 2–4 weeks.
- Patients should be warned about side effects. Prophylaxis against GC-induced osteoporosis (with calcium and vitamin D supplements to avoid secondary hyperparathyroidism and Hypovitaminosis-D) and a bisphosphonate if >65 years, or if the spine, femoral neck, or total hip T-score on DXA scan in –1.5 or less (see p. 408).

- The response to GCs is variable, but tends to be slower than in other autoimmune diseases. Three months may elapse before a demonstrable improvement in muscle weakness is seen.
- In patients who fail to respond to GCs consider:
  - alternative diagnoses;
  - the presence of an unrecognized malignancy;
  - GC-induced myopathy (especially if the CK has fallen but weakness fails to improve or worsens);
  - muscle atrophy with irreversible loss of muscle strength;
  - ongoing active PM (CK may be persistently elevated).
- In GC failure, MR scanning or repeat EMG may be helpful to assess disease activity. In the presence of diagnostic uncertainty the muscle biopsy should be re-examined and further biopsy considered looking for inflammation, alternative diagnoses, or GC-induced myopathy. If the latter is suspected then it is reasonable to try lowering the prednisolone dose and monitoring the muscle strength response.

Other immunosuppressants
Methotrexate (MTX) and azathioprine (AZA) and are the standard second line immunosuppressive agents. They may be commenced from the outset in conjunction with prednisolone, particularly in patients with severe disease or major organ involvement. Alternatively, they may be added later in those who respond poorly to prednisolone, relapse during withdrawal, or experience GC-related side-effects.
- MTX is often preferred as the response is seen more rapidly (AZA may take up to 4–6 months to work).
- When MTX and AZA were compared in a double-blind randomized controlled trial (DBRCT), they had equivalent efficacy but MTX was better tolerated.
- AZA may be preferable in certain patients, e.g. in women of child-bearing age as it is considered safe in pregnancy, or in patients with liver disease or high alcohol intake who are at increased risk of hepatotoxicity with MTX.

Methotrexate
In retrospective series, approximately 75% of patients with PM/DM derived benefit from MTX.
- There has been no RCT comparing MTX with placebo.
- MTX is administered once a week either orally or parenterally. The dose is usually 15 mg/week, increasing up to a maximum of 25 mg/week.
- The risk of side effects is reduced by the concurrent use of folic acid 5 mg per week.

Azathioprine
- There are case series supporting the efficacy of AZA in PM, but the only RCT failed to show a significant benefit over placebo. However, the follow-up period of 3 months may have been too short.
- In a subsequent open study of the same patients, those receiving GCs plus AZA had a better outcome at 3 years than those receiving GCs alone.
- The starting dose of AZA is 50–100 mg per day, increasing by 50 mg at weekly intervals as tolerated up to 3.0 mg/kg/day (maximum dose usually 200 mg/day).

Ciclosporin
Evidence from case reports and small retrospective case series is supportive. A RCT comparing MTX with ciclosporin A (both in conjunction with GCs) in 36 patients with PM/DM demonstrated similar efficacy for the two treatments. Ciclosporin acts more rapidly than azathioprine and may be an appropriate second line agent.

Tacrolimus
Some evidence for efficacy from small case series in refractory PM/DM. Tacrolimus may be particularly effective in ILD associated with myositis.

Mycophenolate mofetil
Appears promising from anecdotal reports in treating refractory disease, although serious opportunistic infections have been reported.

Cyclophosphamide
Several case series have demonstrated limited efficacy in improving muscle strength. Cyclophosphamide is generally reserved for recalcitrant disease unresponsive to other treatments. In a recent series of 17 patients with PM/DM and ILD, 12 showed some improvements in lung disease with cyclophosphamide.

Intravenous immunoglobulin G (IVIG)
Open studies of IVIG in treatment-refractory PM and DM have shown response rates ranging from 75 to 93%.
- There has been a double-blind placebo controlled randomized controlled trial (DBPRCT) demonstrating efficacy of IVIG in refractory DM but none in PM.
- The risk of side effects with IVIG is low but treatment efficacy is of limited duration, usually four to six weeks, and repeated monthly courses are generally required for sustained effect. The usual dose regime is 2g/kg per month (given over 2–5 days) for 4–6 months.

Rituximab
Appears promising based on case reports and small case series in both PM and DM. Rituximab has potential advantages over IVIG in that it is cheaper and may be more likely to give prolonged disease control.

Plasmapheresis
A DBPCRCT in 39 patients with PM/DM showed no significant benefit.

Anti-TNFα
Results from several small case series of patients with PM/DM treated with Infliximab or Etanercept suggested that some patients may benefit. However, in a recent series of 13 patients with refractory PM/DM treated with Infliximab, muscle strength failed to improve in any of the patients and several showed clinical and radiological worsening.

Other
Whole body or total lymphoid radiation have been reported to be effective in small series of treatment refractory patients, but adverse effects are common and the risk of malignancy is a major concern.

Treatment duration
The optimum duration of therapy has not been established. Long-term GCs should be avoided and, in the absence of disease flares, a total of 9–12 months treatment is standard. Immunosuppressants should be continued until patients have been off GCs for >6 months and then withdrawn slowly with close monitoring for relapse.

Prognosis
Data on long-term outcome in PM/DM are limited. Disease course is extremely variable, ranging from mild weakness that improves with GCs to severe, relentlessly progressive muscle failure that is resistant to all therapies.

- Although the majority of patients improve with initial treatment, only a proportion of these achieve long-term clinical remission.
- Approximately a third of patients are refractory to treatment.
- Even those who respond often have significant residual disability or adverse effects from treatment e.g. fractures or osteonecrosis from GC use.
- Mortality is increased in patients with inflammatory myositis, although survival has significantly improved following the introduction of GCs.
- The 5-year survival is currently around 95%, and 10-year survival 85–89%. Common causes of death are cardiac (arrhythmia, heart failure, myocardial infarction), pulmonary (ILD, aspiration pneumonia), malignancy, and infection.
- Poor prognostic factors include:
  - older age;
  - interstitial lung disease;
  - presence of anti-Jo1 antibodies;
  - bulbar muscle weakness;
  - cardiovascular involvement;
  - delayed treatment.

Monitoring disease activity

Improvements in muscle strength should be the principal target of treatment. However, distinguishing active inflammatory disease from established muscle damage is problematic. Combinations of muscle enzymes, EMG and imaging are employed to discriminate but none are definitive.

Muscle strength

Manual muscle testing (MMT) remains the most frequently used method for assessing muscle power.
- IMACS advocated the use of the MMT-8 in assessing outcome in clinical trials. This involves testing eight specified muscle groups against resistance and grading power from 0 to 5 or 0 to 10 using a modified Medical Research Council scale [see IMACS website].
- The total MMT score (sum of the individual muscle scores) is used to serially monitor changes in muscle strength.
- MMT has the advantages of being partially validated with reasonable inter-observer reliability, and is relatively quick and easy to perform.
- Isometric testing, with hand-held dynamometers, may provide more accurate, objective assessment of muscle strength, and is easy to perform in a clinic setting. Computerized dynamometers are also available, but are more time-consuming and are not widely used.

Biochemical monitoring

Muscle enzymes (CK plus one other) should be checked at least monthly during the initial phase of treatment. This is a guide to disease activity and may help predict relapse. However, muscle enzymes may not always correlate with degree of ongoing inflammation, e.g. some treatments may suppress CK with no improvement in weakness.

Imaging

MR, MRS, and US may be helpful, but their role in disease monitoring has yet to be established.

Other measures

Patients should be assessed for the presence of extra-muscular manifestations, which will impact on management decisions. Patient perception of disease, and evaluation of function and quality of life are paramount.

Follow-up

A co-ordinated multi-disciplinary approach should be adopted involving physicians, physiotherapists, occupational therapists, and nurse practitioners with further specialist input as required. Close monitoring with a minimum of 3-monthly assessments is recommended for the first year, reducing in frequency once disease control is established.

Current controversies

- Diagnostic criteria remain a highly contentious area.
- Interaction of immune and non-immune mechanisms in disease pathogenesis.
- Clarifying distinctions between PM, DM and IBM.
- What is the risk of malignancy in PM?
- Role of biologic therapies in myositis.
- Assessment of disease activity and development of robust outcome measures.

Resources

Assessment tools

MITAX: Myositis intention to treat index.

MYOACT: Myositis disease activity assessment.

MDI: Myositis damage index.

SF-36: Short form 36.

Patient organizations

The Myositis Support Group (UK). Available at: www.myositis.org.uk

The Myositis Association (US). Available at: www.myositis.org

Internet Sites

International Myositis Assessment and Clinical Studies Group (IMACS), for manual muscle testing guidelines, grading scheme and score chart, and details of tools for assessing disease activity, damage and patient reported outcomes in myositis. Available at: www.niehs.nih.gov/research/resources/collab/imacs/main.cfm

Dysferlinopathy. See article by Masashi Aoki. Available at: www.ncbi.nlm.nih.gov/bookshelf/br.fcgi?book=gene&partid=1303

ICD-10 codes

M33.2	Polymyositis
M36.0	Dermato(poly)myositis in neoplastic disease
M33.9	Dermatopolymyositis
J99.1	Respiratory disorders in diffuse CT disease

See also:

Dermatomyositis	p. 290
Metabolic myopathies	p. 522
Inclusion body myositis	p. 302

References

Alexanderson H, Dastmalchi M, Esbjornsson-Liljedahl M, Opava CH, Lundberg IE. Benefits of intensive resistance training in patients with chronic polymyositis or dermatomyositis. *Arthritis Rheum* 2007; **57**: 768–77.

Alexanderson H, Lundberg IE. Disease-specific quality indicators, outcome measures and guidelines in polymyositis and dermatomyositis. *Clin Exp Rheumatol* 2007; **25**(6 Suppl 47): 153–8.

Bohan A, Peter JB. Polymyositis and dermatomyositis (first of two parts). *N Engl J Med* 1975; **292**(7): 344–7.

Bohan A, Peter JB. Polymyositis and dermatomyositis (second of two parts). *N Engl J Med* 1975; **292**(8): 403–7.

Bohan A, Peter JB, Bowman RL, Pearson CM. Computer-assisted analysis of 153 patients with polymyositis and dermatomyositis. *Medicine (Baltimore)* 1977; **56**(4): 255–86.

Bunch TW. Prednisone and azathioprine for polymyositis: long-term followup. *Arthritis Rheum* 1981; **24**: 45–8.

Cherin P, Pelletier S, et al. Results and long-term followup of intravenous immunoglobulin infusions in chronic, refractory polymyositis: an open study with thirty-five adult patients. *Arthritis Rheum* 2002; **46**:467–74.

Chinoy H, Salway F, et al. Tumour necrosis factor-alpha single nucleotide polymorphisms are not independent of HLA class I in UK Caucasians with adult onset idiopathic inflammatory myopathies. *Rheumatology (Oxford)* 2007; **46**: 1411–16.

Choy EH, Hoogendijk JE, Lecky B, Winer JB. Immunosuppressant and immunomodulatory treatment for dermatomyositis and polymyositis. *Cochrane Database Syst Rev* 2005; (3): CD003643.

Choy EH, Isenberg DA. Treatment of dermatomyositis and polymyositis. *Rheumatology (Oxford)* 2002; **41**: 7–13.

Chung YL, Alexanderson H, et al. Creatine supplements in patients with idiopathic inflammatory myopathies who are clinically weak after conventional pharmacologic treatment: Six-month, double-blind, randomized, placebo-controlled trial. *Arthritis Rheum* 2007; **57**: 694–702.

Cordeiro AC, Isenberg DA. Treatment of inflammatory myopathies. *Postgrad Med J* 2006; **82**(969): 417–24.

Dalakas MC. Mechanisms of disease: signaling pathways and immunobiology of inflammatory myopathies. *Nat Clin Pract Rheumatol* 2006; **2**(4):219–27.

Dalakas MC. The role of high-dose immune globulin intravenous in the treatment of dermatomyositis. *Int Immunopharmacol* 2006; **6**: 550–6.

Dalakas MC, Hohlfeld R. Polymyositis and dermatomyositis. *Lancet* 2003; **362**(9388): 971–82.

Danko K, Ponyi A, Constantin T, Borgulya G, Szegedi G. Long-term survival of patients with idiopathic inflammatory myopathies according to clinical features: a longitudinal study of 162 cases. *Medicine (Baltimore)* 2004; **83**:35–42.

Dastmalchi M, Grundtman C, et al. A high incidence of disease flares in an open pilot study of infliximab in patients with refractory inflammatory myopathies. *Ann Rheum Dis* 2008.

Fathi M, Lundberg IE. Interstitial lung disease in polymyositis and dermatomyositis. *Curr Opin Rheumatol* 2005; **17**: 701–6.

Hengstman GJ. Advances in the immunopathophysiology of the idiopathic inflammatory myopathies: not as simple as suspected. *Curr Rheumatol Rep* 2007; **9**(4): 280–5.

Hengstman GJ, Brouwer R, Egberts WT, Seelig HP, Jongen PJ, van Venrooij WJ, et al. Clinical and serological characteristics of 125 Dutch myositis patients. Myositis specific autoantibodies aid in the differential diagnosis of the idiopathic inflammatory myopathies. *J Neurol* 2002; **249**: 69–75.

Hengstman GJ, De Bleecker JL, et al. Open-label trial of anti-TNF-alpha in dermato- and polymyositis treated concomitantly with methotrexate. *Eur Neurol* 2008; **59**(3-4):159–63.

Isenberg DA, Allen E, et al. International consensus outcome measures for patients with idiopathic inflammatory myopathies. Development and initial validation of myositis activity and damage indices in patients with adult onset disease. *Rheumatology (Oxford)* 2004; **43**: 49–54.

Lundberg IE. The heart in dermatomyositis and polymyositis. *Rheumatology (Oxford)* 2006; 45 Suppl 4:iv18–21.

Miller FW, Leitman SF, et al. Controlled trial of plasma exchange and leukapheresis in polymyositis and dermatomyositis. *N Engl J Med* 1992; **326**(21): 1380–4.

Miller F, Walsh Y, Saminaden S, Lecky B, Winer J. Randomised double blind trial of methotrexate and steroids compared with azathioprine and steroids in the treatment of idiopathic inflammatory myopathy. *J Neurol Sci* 2002; **199**(Suppl 1): S53.

Mok CC, Ho LY, To CH. Rituximab for refractory polymyositis: an open-label prospective study. *J Rheumatol* 2007; **34**: 1864–8.

Oddis CV, Rider LG, Reed AM, Ruperto N, Brunner HI, Koneru B, et al. International consensus guidelines for trials of therapies in the idiopathic inflammatory myopathies. *Arthritis Rheum* 2005; **52**: 2607–15.

Rider LG, Giannini EH, et al. Defining Clinical Improvement in Adult and Juvenile Myositis. *J Rheumatol* 2003; **30**:603–17.

Sultan SM, Ioannou Y, Moss K, Isenberg DA. Outcome in patients with idiopathic inflammatory myositis: morbidity and mortality. *Rheumatology (Oxford)* 2002; **41**: 22–6.

Vencovsky J, Jarosova K, Machacek S, Studynkova J, Kafkova J, Bartunkova J, et al. Cyclosporine A versus methotrexate in the treatment of polymyositis and dermatomyositis. *Scand J Rheumatol* 2000; **29**(2): 95–102.

Villalba L, Hicks JE, Adams EM, Sherman JB, Gourley MF, Leff RL, et al. Treatment of refractory myositis: a randomized crossover study of two new cytotoxic regimens. *Arthritis Rheum* 1998; **41**: 392–9.

Yamasaki Y, Yamada H, et al. Intravenous cyclophosphamide therapy for progressive interstitial pneumonia in patients with polymyositis/dermatomyositis. *Rheumatology (Oxford)* 2007; **46**: 124–30.

Dermatomyositis

Definition
Dermatomyositis (DM) is an idiopathic inflammatory myopathy characterized by muscle inflammation and cutaneous manifestations. It is part of a heterogeneous group of inflammatory myopathies including polymyositis (PM) and inclusion-body myositis (IBM). DM may present in an isolated form or in association with malignancy or other autoimmune connective tissue diseases.

Epidemiology
DM is a rare disease and only a few epidemiological studies have been published. It has a prevalence of approximately 1 per 100 000 in the North American population and affects all ages. The peak incidence is 40–50 years. There is a female predominance with a ratio of 2:1.

Aetiology and pathophysiology
Genetics
There is still much to learn about the genetics of DM. Recently work had been published demonstrating that HLA susceptibility markers differ in diverse myositis phenotypes and certain genotypes are more closely associated to serology than myositis subtype

Environmental triggers
No clear precipitating triggers identified.

Immunopathology
DM is thought to be a humorally-mediated microangiopathy affecting skin and muscle, where the cellular infiltrate is located in perifascicular regions around blood vessels.
- The trigger of the initial capillary injury is still unknown. It has been proposed that injury results from autoantibody production against an endothelial antigen.
- Complement activation occurs early and has a clear role in the pathology. The terminal complement C5–9 membrane attack complex is detectable in vessel walls before the appearance of an inflammatory cell infiltrate. It is still unclear whether the vasculopathy is primarily complement mediated or secondary to other events.
- Muscle damage probably occurs from ischaemia secondary to capillary damage. The inflammatory infiltrate is composed predominantly of B cells and CD4+ T cells.
- Plasmacytoid dendritic cells are abundant in DM muscle; however, their exact role in the pathogenesis is yet to be confirmed.
- The pro-inflammatory cytokines IL-1 and TNFα are increased in the muscle tissue of patients with DM and may contribute to muscle weakness.

Risk factors
No known risk factors.

Diagnostic criteria
There are no accepted diagnostic criteria for DM.
- Bohan and Peter formulated classification criteria in 1975 defining 5 major criteria for diagnosing both PM and DM:
  - symmetrical muscle weakness;
  - muscle biopsy evidence of inflammation;
  - elevation of serum muscle enzymes;
  - EMG evidence of myositis;
  - cutaneous features of Gottron's papules, heliotrope rash and an erythematous rash in a shawl like distribution (see Plate 7 and 8).
- For a definite diagnosis of DM three of four criteria plus the rash must be present.
- These criteria have never been validated or revised, and criticisms of this system exist, especially as it fails to distinguish PM from IBM (as the latter was not recognized until the 1980s) and the criteria were formulated prior to testing for myositis specific autoantibodies (MSAs).
- More recent diagnostic criteria based on histopathologic change have been proposed by Dalakas. These have not been formally validated.

Clinical features
Key features in history
Musculoskeletal
- Symptoms can start insidiously – typically difficulty with everyday tasks, such as rising from a chair, climbing stairs, lifting objects, brushing their hair, or shaving.
- Myalgia is not a common complaint.
- Dysphonia can be noticed by relatives.
- Patients usually have fatigue and can complain of joint pains – usually small joints.

Key features on examination
Musculoskeletal
- DM presents with varying degrees of muscle weakness, which develops insidiously over weeks to months, but acutely in rare cases.
- DM, like PM, primarily affects the proximal muscles and is generally symmetrical. Testing power in trapezius, deltoids, biceps brachii, quadriceps, and hip stabilizers is essential. Strength is scored out of five using the Medical Research Council (MRC) scale (in which zero is the lowest score and five the highest). There are no sensory deficits and reflexes may be absent in severe weakness.
- Distal muscle involvement occurs late in the disease and fine motor movements may then be affected.
- Facial muscles remain normal and the extra-ocular muscles are never affected as compared to myasthenia gravis where frequent involvement of facial and oculobulbar muscles occurs.
- The neck extensor muscles may be involved causing head drop and pelvic stability can be lost.
- With advanced disease dysphagia, aspiration, and respiratory muscle weakness can occur.

Dermatological clinical features
The characteristic rash in dermatomyositis accompanies or precedes muscle weakness. Common cutaneous manifestation of DM include:
- A heliotrope rash (violaceous to dusky erythematous rash on eyelids occasionally with oedema). It is rarely seen in other autoimmune connective tissue disorders.
- Gottron's papules are found over the metacarpophangeal joints and proximal interphalangeal joints. These are slightly raised violaceous papules and plaques. Papules may also be found overlying the elbows, knees, or feet. These may appear scaly and psoriaform.
- An erythematous rash on the face, neck and anterior chest (V sign) or back and shoulders (shawl sign).
- Nail-fold changes of periungal telangiectasia, cuticular hypertrophy, and small haemorrhagic infarcts.

Table 8.11 Pathological features of polymyositis (PM) and dermatomyositis (DM).

Criterion	PM Definite	PM Probable	Myopathic DM Definite	Myopathic DM Probable	Amyopathic DM definite
Myopathic muscle weakness	Yes	Yes	Yes	Yes	No
EMG findings	Myopathic	Myopathic	Myopathic	Myopathic	Myopathic or non-specific
Muscle enzymes	High (up to 50 times normal)	High (up to 50 times normal) or normal	High (up to 50 times normal)	High	High (up to 10 times normal) or normal
Muscle-biopsy findings	Primary inflammation, with the CD8+ T-cell/HLA class-1 complex and no vacuoles	Ubiquitous HLA class-1 expression, but no CD8+ T-cell infiltrates or vacuoles	Perifascicular perimysial or perivascular infiltrates with perifascicular atrophy	Perifascicular perimysial or perivascular infiltrates with perifascicular atrophy	Non specific or diagnostic for DM (subclinical myopathy)
Rash or calcinosis	Absent	Absent	Present	Not detected	Present

PM, polymyostitis; DM, dermatomyositis; EMG, Electromyography; HLA, Human Leucocyte Antigen.
Adapted from Dalakas and Hohlfeld 2003, with permission.

- A photosensitive rash characterized by an erythematous to violaceous psoriaform dermatitis.
- Calcinosis of the skin or muscle. It is commoner in juvenile DM. Calcinosis cutis occurs over bony prominences and can lead to ulceration and infection.
- Amyopathic dermatitis (DM-sine-myositis), where muscle strength is normal, but there is skin disease. However, muscle MR and biopsy is often abnormal.

Co-morbidities
Systemic and other clinical features
DM is a multisystem disorder. Extra-muscular involvement may be present in up to 50% of patients.
- Systemic features include fever, weight loss, anorexia, and fatigue.
- Pulmonary disease occurs in up to 30% of patients and includes ILD. The strongest predictor of ILD is anti-Jo-1 antibody; however, ILD may occur in its absence.
- Respiratory muscle weakness can lead to hypoventilation and respiratory compromise.
- Arthritis is found in up to 25%. It is symmetrical and non-deforming. Usually, the small joints are involved, and patients complain of pain and morning stiffness.
- Oesophageal disease is present in up to 50% of patients and manifests as dysphagia. Striated muscle involvement of the pharynx or proximal oesophagus leads to proximal dysphagia. This correlates with severity of muscle disease and is steroid responsive. Distal dysphagia suggests involvement of non-striated muscle. It tends to be more common in those with an overlap disorder. Dysphagia often indicates a poor prognosis.
- Cardiac involvement may occur in up to 50% of patients causing conduction defects, arrhythmias, pericarditis, and valvular heart disease. Only a small percentage of those with cardiac involvement are symptomatic.

Malignancy
There is an association between DM and cancer. The reported rate is 20–25% in adults >45 years old.

- The association with other inflammatory myopathies is less clear and the associated reported rates are lower.
- There is no correlation between the severity of the myopathy and occurrence of malignancy.
- Malignancy may not be obvious. Clinical examination of abdomen, pelvis, breast, and rectum and for lymph nodes is important (see below).
- The most common malignancies in decreasing order of frequency are:
  - ovarian
  - lung;
  - pancreatic;
  - non-Hodgkin lymphoma;
  - stomach;
  - colorectal.
- In Asian populations there is a higher incidence of nasopharyngeal carcinoma.
- Malignant disease may occur before the onset, concurrently or after the onset of myositis.

Overlap syndromes
Reports estimate that between 11–40% of patients with PM or DM have an associated autoimmune connective tissue disease. DM has most commonly been described in association with systemic sclerosis (SSc) and MCTD.

Investigations
Laboratory
Blood tests are important to assess the severity of disease, to help guide treatment, and to monitor for the complications of the disease and/or treatment.
- Initial investigations should include urinalysis, faecal occult blood assessment.
- FBC/CBC may show evidence of anaemia of chronic disease or thrombocytosis with active inflammation.
- Abnormalities in renal function may be seen in overlap syndromes (e.g. SLE).
- LDH, AST, and ALT may be elevated.

- Baseline tests are important to guide the feasibility of therapeutic options (e.g. methotrexate).
- ESR and CRP are usually elevated, but if normal do not rule out a diagnosis of myositis.
- Creatine kinase (CK) can be increased up to 50 times the upper limit of the reference interval, although it can be normal CK can also be low in those with advanced disease and significant loss of muscle mass.
- Myoglobin in serum and urine rises with active disease and can be detected in 70–80% of patients. Serum myoglobin levels increase earlier than CK and normalize faster. Myoglobinuria is less common.
- Vitamin D levels to exclude low vitamin D as a contributory cause for muscle weakness.
- Testosterone and LH in males to rule out hypogonadism – can cause fatigue and reduced muscle mass.

Autoantibodies
ANA is positive in 80% of patients with inflammatory myositis (either PM or DM).
- Autoantibodies associated with DM can be divided into two groups: Myositis-specific autoantibodies (MSA) and Myositis-associated autoantibodies (MAA).
- The three main groups of MSAs are:
  - anti-aminoacyl transfer-RNA (tRNA) synthetase autoantibodies. Anti-Jo-1 antibody (against histidyl-tRNA synthetase) is the commonest occurring of the six autoantibodies in this group. These MSAs characterize 'Antisynthetase Syndrome' (myositis, interstitial lung disease, arthritis, mechanic's hands and Raynaud's phenomenon);
  - anti-signal recognition peptide (SRP). These occur almost exclusively in PM;
  - anti-Mi-2. Directed against the helicase family of proteins. This antibody has a frequency of 20% in DM and is more common in DM than in PM.
- More recently, a specific autoantibody (anti-CADM-140) has been identified in patients with clinical amyopathic DM. The target antigen remains unknown. It may be associated with a subset of DM with cutaneous manifestations and ILD but no muscle symptoms.
- Anti-p155 antibody has also recently been reported in DM. The target antigen is a transcriptional intermediary factor and, thus far, has a frequency of 20% in DM especially in cancer-associated disease.
- MAAs correlate with myositis overlap syndromes. Anti-U1 RNP defines mixed connective tissue disease (MCTD). Anti-Ku and anti-PM-Scl characterize PM/SSc overlap syndrome.

Imaging
Radiographs, mammography, US and CT
Given the association of DM with malignancy, CXR is essential. An indiscriminate search for malignancy is not recommended.
- The use of ultrasound (US) and CT will need to be considered depending on clinical assessment and the need to focus on identifying any potential malignancy.
- MR demonstrates areas of muscle inflammation by evaluating the presence or absence of muscle oedema.
- The most commonly used MR modalities for skeletal muscle imaging include T1- and T2-weighted, proton density, and STIR sequences.
- T1-weighted images help to differentiate skeletal muscle from fat, while T2-weighted images and STIR are useful for the detection of oedema.
- MR imaging identifies an appropriate area for muscle biopsy, as muscle involvement may be patchy.

Histology
When the diagnosis is suspected on clinical grounds a definitive diagnosis can be confirmed on histology. Muscle is the preferred tissue though in some cases skin biopsy can be helpful.
- On haematoxylin and eosin the cellular infiltrate is seen in perifascicular regions around blood vessels.
- Myofibre necrosis and regeneration and perifascicular atrophy are characteristic in DM.
- Using appropriate immunohistochemistry stains, complement C5–9 and immune complexes are detectable in vessel walls.
- The inflammatory infiltrate consists of primarily B cells, macrophages, and CD4+ T cells.
- In PM the inflammatory infiltrate is endomysial, consists primarily of CD8+ T cells and there is no evidence of immune deposits.
- In muscular dystrophy the inflammatory cell infiltrate is endomysial, but is limited to areas adjacent to necrotic muscle fibres.

Other investigations
Electromyography (EMG)
EMG can distinguish myopathic from neuropathic weakness and it has a role in targeting a site for muscle biopsy.
- Characteristic EMG changes show evidence of increased membrane irritability manifest as:
  - increased insertional activity and spontaneous fibrillations;
  - abnormal myopathic low amplitude short duration polyphasic motor potentials;
  - complex repetitive discharges.
- EMG abnormalities support the diagnosis of DM, but are not diagnostic.

Respiratory investigations
There is an association of DM with lung pathology (ILD or thoracic muscular weakness).
- Measuring peak flow is an easy bedside test to monitor for deterioration if spirometry is not easily available.
- Formal lung function with spirometry and diffusion capacity should be performed at time of diagnosis.
- Additional investigation is based on risk and age appropriate screening tests (such as mammography).

Differential diagnosis
Mimics of DM should be considered. Although rare, paraneoplastic syndromes should be considered, but also:

Drug or toxic myopathies
A number of drugs, including glucocorticoids (GCs), cause proximal myopathy.
- Additionally, the following drugs have been reported, amongst others, to cause a myopathy (those marked * are more likely to be painful): lithium, chloroquine-containing drugs*, clofibrate, statins, salbutamol, penicillin, colchicine, D-penicillamine*, sulphonamides, hydralazine, ciclosporin, phenytoin, cimetidine* (muscle cramps), zidovudine, carbimazole, and tamoxifen.
- Compared with DM, in steroid myopathy the CK is normal and biopsy is consistent with non-inflammatory fibre atrophy. GC-induced myopathy should be considered during GC treatment, especially if there is no response to treatment.

CHAPTER 8 Autoimmune connective tissue diseases

- The myositis occurring with D-penicillamine is not daily dose or cumulative dose-dependent. It can be life threatening.
- Mild myoarthralgia may be caused by a number of commonly used drugs, e.g. proton pump inhibitors and quinolone antibiotics.
- Alcohol in excess and some illegal drugs (e.g. ecstasy) are associated with severe toxic myopathy occasionally resulting in rhabdomyolysis.

Endocrine myopathies
Hypothyroidism mimics inflammatory myopathy. Distinguishing features are the subacute onset of muscle weakness and abnormal thyroid function tests.

Metabolic myopathies
Caused by disorders of carbohydrate and lipid metabolism, they can be distinguished from DM clinically by the intermittent nature of the attacks of acute muscle pain and tenderness, usually induced by exertion.

Infectious myositis
Viral and parasitic infections may cause diffuse muscular involvement with a subacute or chronic course.
- Bacterial myositis tends to be localized and has a fulminant presentation.
- Myositis can be the presenting feature of HIV disease. In HIV-positive patients, infections causing muscle disease include MTB and microsporidia.

Muscular dystrophies
These conditions are an inherited group of progressive myopathic disorders where an increase of CK, electodiagnostic studies, and biopsy findings may be similar to DM. They can be distinguished from DM, however, by the positive family history and relatively early insidious onset and slow progression.

Other inflammatory myositis
- In chronic sarcoid some evidence for muscle inflammation is not uncommon with raised CK fairly typical. Indeed, in biopsy studies, there is evidence for sarcoid granulomata in a substantial number of patients with the diagnosis. However, many patients are asymptomatic and have no obvious or mild muscle weakness.
- Myasthenia gravis can present insidiously, often with variable weakness during the day (fatiguability is a key feature, which may be more noticeable in its effect towards the end of the day).

Other conditions
An appreciation of some conditions that can present with widespread pain, and either frank or perceived weakness is important. The following should always be considered in these cases: Guillain–Barre syndrome, myelopathic lesions, extensive SpA-related polyenthesopathy (usually psoriasis-related), and fibromyalgia.

Pitfalls with interpreting CK results
- The reference range of CK can differ depending on ethnic background. It is generally regarded that people of Afro-Caribbean background have a higher 'normal' reference range CK compared with Caucasians.
- There is allelic variation in the CK gene and post-translational changes that can affect routine CK assays.
- It is important to be aware of that production of *macro-CK* can present with elevated routine CK results.

- Macro-CK may be a normal variant, but can be produced in association with malignancy. A screen for tumours may be necessary.
- CK can be elevated secondary to muscle trauma. If modest elevations in CK are thought to arise from trauma, a delay before re-testing is prudent.
- CK can be very modestly (but significantly and persistently) elevated in sarcoid myopathy.

Disease activity assessment and monitoring
Clinical assessment should be based on evaluating changes in several muscle groups and these same groups should be tested at each review. Muscle strength represents one of the most sensitive parameters for monitoring disease activity, and needs to be scored between zero and five for standardization. Isokinetic testing with dynamometers, if available, are more sensitive than physical examination and can be used to measure and monitor muscle strength objectively (e.g. using a Cybex dynamometer).

Treatment
Objectives of management
The goals of treatment are to improve muscle strength, prevent muscle loss, improve skin disease, avoid glucocorticoid-induced myopathy by using judicious doses of GCs, and prevent extra muscular manifestations. Treatment should begin immediately following diagnosis.

Physical therapies
Early rehabilitation and physiotherapy (PT) are necessary to prevent contractures and improve muscle function.
Exercise regimens should be tailored to the severity of weakness. Wheelchair or bed-bound patients should still receive passive range of motion exercises, and may benefit from heat and massage prior to therapy

Non-pharmacological skin management
- Patients should be advised regarding protection from the sun and the importance of applying broad sunscreens
- There is no effective medical treatment for calcinosis and controlled trials are lacking. Aluminium hydroxide antacids, diltiazem, probenecid, and colchicine can be trialled but often provide less than ideal results. Surgical therapy may be required for localized calcific deposits that interfere with joint function or are painful, but is usually a last resort
- If the deposits are infected or discharging than surgical intervention is required

Immunosuppression
Glucocorticoids (GCs) are used initially and are used first line to establish disease control. A number of immunosuppressants can be used in a 'steroid-sparing' role (second-line agents). It is logical to commence the second-line agent at the outset to reduce the cumulative dose of prednisolone.

Glucocorticoids (GCs)
The usual initial dose of prednisolone is 1 mg/kg per day up to a maximum dose of 80mg/day.
- In more severe cases pulse methylprednisolone may be given at 1 g/day on 3 consecutive days. There is nothing in the literature on lower doses of pulse methylprednisolone, but individual factors need to be taken into account such as age, co-morbidities, etc.
- High dose oral GCs are continued for up to 6 weeks then should be tapered, but in light of clinical progress and use of GC-sparing drug use.

- Complications of GC therapy inevitably occur with the high doses and long duration of treatment necessary. Ensuring patients are replete in vitamin-D (25OHD) and avoiding secondary hyperparathyroidism, if necessary with supplements, is important.
- A regular bisphosphonate is recommended (UK Royal College of Physicians Guidelines 1999/2000) for all patients ≥65 years old treated with GCs and for younger patients with hip or spine T-score (DXA scan) ≤−2.5).

Azathioprine (AZA)

Azathioprine (AZA) is usually initiated at a dose of 50 mg/day. If tolerated the dose may be increased to 150–200 mg/day to a maximum of 2.5 mg/kg/day.
- Before beginning AZA, screening for low thiopurine methyltransferase activity is recommended.
- AZA is preferable to methotrexate (MTX) in those with associated ILD, heavy alcohol use or underlying liver disease, where MTX is relatively contra-indicated.

Methotrexate (MTX)

Methotrexate is administered in doses of 15–25 mg/week with folic acid 5 mg/week the day after MTX.
- It is often preferred to AZA due to its favourable dosing regimen and earlier benefit.
- At doses greater than 15 mg/week subcutaneous or intramuscular administration should be considered.

GC, AZA, and MTX Therapy duration

There are no clear guidelines on the optimal duration of therapy. A typical course of GCs lasts 9–12 months and the 'steroid-sparer' continued for longer.
- Once remission has been achieved the 'steroid-sparer' should be tapered with a view to cessation after a further 6 months.
- Response to treatment is variable – with some patients showing improvement within weeks, while others take months.
- When cutaneous findings are refractory to systemic treatment topical tacrolimus or antimalarial therapies, such as hydroxychloroquine may be of benefit.
- Failure of DM to respond to GCs with AZA or MTX requires treatment with third line agents (see below). However, limited evidence for the efficacy of treatments given for resistant DM exists.
- Failure to respond also prompts reassessment of the diagnosis.

Intravenous immunoglobulin (IVIG)

There have been two small controlled trials, one of which was a double-blind randomized controlled-trial (RCT) involving exclusively patients with DM. Improvement in both muscle and skin became noticeable after the first infusion.
- The benefit of IVIG is usually short-lived. Repeat infusions are needed although there have been reports of patients having sustained responses for up to 3 years.
- The usual IVIG regime is 2 g/kg/monthly for 4–6 months. In the acute setting IVIG may be used in a dose of 0.5–2 g/kg daily for 3–5 days.
- There is no evidence for relative efficacy of the different IVIG preparations.

Plasmapheresis

Plasmapheresis has no proven efficacy compared with placebo in double-blind RCTs.

Anti-CD20 chimaeric monoclonal antibody (Rituximab)

In a number of small case series, improvement in muscle strength has been seen with Rituximab as early as 4 weeks after the initial infusion with cutaneous disease improving within 12 weeks. The optimal dose has yet to be determined. Rituximab is more likely to lead to prolonged disease control than IVIG.

Other immunosuppressive therapeutic options
- Ciclosporin has the same efficacy as MTX and is useful in those cases with ILD, and in combination with MTX for refractory DM.
- Tacrolimus has been used in those with refractory inflammatory myositis complicated by ILD, there have been small case series reported indicating efficacy of tacrolimus in improving muscle strength and respiratory function. Applied topically, it is effective on cutaneous lesions.
- Mycophenolate mofetil has been used with some success in resistant myositis, evidence is emerging of it's efficacy on both the myositis and dermatological features. It has a slow onset of action. Doses of 2 g daily are effective and it is useful as a steroid-sparing agent.
- Cyclophosphamide can be effective though given the side effect profile its use should be reserved for those with aggressive disease or associated severe ILD.
- Anti-TNFα therapies have been used with mixed results in DM. Convincing data that they are efficacious overall is lacking.
- AZA and MTX combination therapy is a further option, but treatment-related morbidity is a risk.

Relapse (of muscle or skin disease)
- Relapse after definite disease control requires either an increase or recommencement of prednisolone at the lowest dose required to establish disease control.
- If the relapse is severe, pulse methylprednisolone therapy (of up to 1 g daily for 3 days) or high dose oral GCs (1 mg/kg to a maximum 80 mg) should be used.
- Immunosuppressant dose should be maximized and if disease control is still not achieved, agents for refractory disease should be used.
- Reconsideration of the diagnosis or iatrogenic causes of myopathy (steroid) should be assessed

Other issues regarding treatment with immunosuppression

Owing to use of high dose GCs and immunosupression, patients are at risk for opportunistic infections.
- Vigilant monitoring is required at each review for signs and symptoms of infection.
- Pneumocystis jiroveci prophylaxis with co-trimoxazole should be considered in patients requiring high dose GCs and immunosuppressants.

Patient advice
- All patients should be advised regarding healthy lifestyle including no smoking and moderate alcohol intake.
- Patients should be advised about the risk of infections and taught how to measure their own temperature.
- Live vaccinations should not be given. Yearly influenza vaccine should be given (and pneumococcal vaccine status brought up to date) for those on immunosuppressants.

- Advice about: the treatments, GC-induced osteoporosis, and the need to be vigilant about possible evolving malignancy need to be given.

Other
Patients with dysphagia and/or dysphonia should be referred to a speech therapist for advice regarding dietary guidance (considering aspiration risk).

Prognosis
Serum CK does not predict the course of disease or response to treatment, but should be used as a guide for management decisions. The clinical and laboratory features associated with a poor prognosis include:
- Older age at onset.
- Severe weakness at presentation.
- Dysphagia.
- Respiratory muscle weakness.
- Interstitial lung disease.
- Associated malignancy.
- Calcinosis.
- Presence of anti-Jo-1 antibody.
- Anti-SRP antibodies.

Current controversies
Aetiological hypotheses and diagnostic issues
- There is still much to be learnt about the pathogenesis of DM – the genetic, environmental factors, and the exact role of MSAs. With further understanding, specific immunotherapies can be formulated.
- The exact incidence of DM is difficult to ascertain, as there are few published epidemiological studies and previous data are based on old studies using unvalidated diagnostic criteria.
- No formally validated classification criteria or assessment tools are available for clinical use.
- The direct relationship of inflammatory myositis to malignancy is still not understood, although there does appear to be a causal relationship.
- Controversy exists regarding the extent of screening for malignancy in a new diagnosis of DM.
- The role of muscle US in evaluating extent and location of inflammation.

Therapy issues
- The superiority of high-dose GC versus immunosupressant plus high-dose GC initially.
- There is a lack of high quality RCTs with therapeutic agents in DM making decisions regarding appropriate first and second line therapy less clear.
- There are no trials comparing AZA with MTX as steroid-sparing agents in DM. Decisions are based on patient profile and physician preference.
- There is a lack of international or national guidelines on management of DM.

Resources
Assessment tools
Muscle strength testing using Medical Research Council (MRC) scale graded from zero (which is the lowest) to five (the highest).

HAQ questionnaire widely used generic instrument assessing self-reported patient-orientated outcome measures.

Guidelines
No published society guidelines.

Patient organizations
www.myositis.org.uk

Other Internet sites
Arthritis research campaign website provides useful information about arthritis for health professionals and patients. Available at: www.arc.org.uk;

American College of Rheumatology website has extensive resources including information on conditions for members and patients. Available at: www.rheumatology.org/

ICD10 codes
M33.1   Dermatomyositis;
M36.0   Dermato(poly)myositis in neoplastic disease;
M33.9   Dermatopolymyositis.

See also:
Polymyositis	p. 282
Metabolic myopathies	p. 522
Eosinophilia myalgia syndrome	p. 520
Inclusion body myositis	p. 302

References
Bohan A, Peter J. Polymyositis and dermatomyositis (Part 1). *NEJM* 1975; **292**: 344–7.

Bohan A., Peter J. Polymyositis and dermatomyositis (Part 2) *NEJM* 1975; **292**: 403–7.

Briani C, Doria A, Sarzi-Puttini P, Dalakas M. Update on idiopathic inflammatory myopathies. *Autoimmunity* 2006; **39**(3): 161–70.

Buchbinder R, Forbes A, Hall S, et al. Incidence of malignant disease in biopsy-proven inflammatory myopathy. *Ann Intern Med* 2001; **134**: 1087–95.

Callen J. Dermatomyositis. *Lancet* 2000; **355**: 53–7.

Cherin P, Pelletier S, Teixeira A. Results and long term follow up of intravenous immunoglobulin infusions in chronic refractory polymyositis: an open study with thirty-five adult patients. *Arthritis Rheum* 2002; **46**: 467–74.

Chinoy H, Salway F, Fertig N, Shephard N. In adult onset myositis, the presence of interstitial lung disease and myositis specific/associated antibodies are governed by HLA Class II haplotype, rather than myositis subtype. *Arthritis Res Ther* 2006; **8**: R13.

Choy E, Hoogendijk J, Lecky B. *Cochrane Database Syst Rev* 2005; **3**: CD003643.

Cordeiro A, Isenberg D. Treatment of inflammatory myopathies. *Postgrad Med J* 2006; **82**: 417–24

Dalakas M. Polymyositis, dermatomyositis, and inclusion-body myositis *NEJM* 1991; **325**: 1487–96.

Dalakas M, Hohlfeld R. Polymyositis and dermatomyositis. *Lancet* 2003; **362**: 971–82.

Dalakas MC, Illa I, Dambrosia JM. A controlled trial of high- dose intravenous immune globulin infusions as treatment for dermatomyositis. *NEJM* 1993; **329**: 1993–2000.

Dinh HV, Mc Cormack C, Hall S, Prince HM. Rituximab for the treatment of the skin manifestations of dermatomyositis: a report of 3 cases. *J Am Acad Dermatol* 2007; **56**: 148–53.

Efthimiou P, Schwartzman S, Kagen L. Possible role for tumour necrosis factor inhibitors in the treatment of resistant dermatomyositis and polymyositis: a retrospective study of eight patients. *Ann Rheum Dis* 2006; **65**: 1233–6.

Greenberg.A gene expression approach to study perturbed pathways in myositis. *Curr Opin Rheum* 2007; **19**: 536–41.

Greenberg S. Proposed immunologic models of the inflammatory myopathies and potential therapeutic implications. *Neurology* 2007; **69**: 2008–19.

Iannone F, Scioscia C, Falappone PC. Use of etanercept in the treatment of dermatomyositis: a case series. *J Rheumatol* 2006; **33**: 1802–4.

Kuo G, Carrino J. Skeletal muscle imaging and inflammatory myopathies. *Curr Opin Rheumatol* 2007; **19**: 530–5.

Levine TD. Rituximab in the treatment of dermatomyositis: an open-label pilot study. *Arthritis Rheum* 2005; **52**: 601–7.

Mastaglia FL, Phillips BA. Idiopathic inflammatory myopathies: epidemiology, classification, and diagnostic criteria. *Rheum Dis Clin N Am* 2002; **28**: 723–41.

Medsger TA, Dawson WN, Masi AT. The epidemiology of polymyositis. *Am J Med* 1979; **48**: 715–23.

Mimori T, Yoshitaka I, Nakashima R, Yoshifuji H. Autoantibodies in idiopathic inflammatory myopathy: an update on clinical and pathophysiological significance. *Curr Opin Rheum* 2007; **19**: 523–9.

Neri R, Mosca M, Stampacchia G, et al. Functional and isokinetic assessment of muscle strength in patients with idiopathic inflammatory myopathies. *Autoimmunity* 2006; **39**(3): 255–9.

Noss EH, Hausner-Sypeck DI, Weinblatt ME. Rituximab as therapy for refractory polymyositis and dermatomyositis. *J Rheumatol* 2006; **33**: 1021–6.

Saito E, Koike T, Hashimoto H, et al. Efficacy of high dose intravenous immune globulin therapy in Japanese patients with steroid resistant polymyositis and dermatomyositis. *Mod Rheum* 2008; **18**: 34–44.

Therapeutic Guidelines Rheumatology. 2006 *Rheumatology Expert Group*. North Melbourne: Therapeutic Guidelines Ltd.

Juvenile dermatomyositis

Definition
Juvenile dermatomyositis (JDM) is one of a number of juvenile idiopathic inflammatory myopathies (JIIMs). JIIMs are rare and JDM is by far the commonest. There is a decreasing occurrence in juvenile polymyositis, amyopathic dermatomyositis, overlap myositis and inclusion body myositis (IBM). The reader is referred to more detailed texts for further information on these other rare JIIMs (Compeyrot-Lacassagne & Feldman, 2007). JDM differs from the adult form in a number of ways:
- Vasculitis is frequent and often severe.
- Calcinosis is common, especially in the recovery phase.
- Polymyositis is uncommon.
- Malignancy is very rare.

Diagnostic criteria
The diagnosis is based on the characteristic JDM rash and proximal muscle inflammation. The diagnostic criteria were originally proposed by Bohan and Peter and have not been superceded (Bohan, 1975).
- In paediatric patients a diagnosis of JDM requires the presence of the pathognomonic rash and two of the other criteria.
- Polymyositis is considered probable with three of the criteria (no rash).
- Muscle appearances on MR may be sufficiently reliable to become part of the diagnostic criteria for JDM in future (Brown et al., 2006).

Diagnostic criteria for juvenile dermatomyositis

Cutaneous lesions consisting of heliotrope (lilac) discolouration of the eyelids with periorbital oedema and an erythematous scaly rash over the dorsal aspects of the metacarpophalangeal and proximal interphalangeal joints (Gottron's sign)

+ any 2 from:
- Symmetrical and progressive proximal muscle weakness (± dysphagia or respiratory muscle involvement).
- Elevation of the serum level of one or more of the following skeletal muscle enzymes: creatine kinase (CK), aspartate aminotransferase (AST), lactate dehydrogenase (LDH) or aldolase (ALD).
- Electromyographic (EMG) demonstration of the characteristics of myopathy and denervation.
- Muscle biopsy documenting histologic evidence of necrosis and inflammation.

Epidemiology
A survey in the UK in 1995 suggested an incidence of 1.9 per million children below the age of 16 years. In the USA, between 1995 and 1998, data suggested an incidence of 3.2 per million children below 17 years. There does not seem to be an ethnic difference. Mean age of onset was 6.8 years in the UK survey with 5:1 girls to boys.

Aetiology and pathogenesis
Genetic
- HLA-DQA1*0501 is associated with JIIM in several ethnic groups.
- HLA-DMA*0103 and HLA-DMB*0102 alleles are more frequent in JDM.
- Maternal microchimaerism (the persistence of maternal blood cells transferred by the placenta during foetal development) has been implicated and might induce a graft-versus-host type response.

Environment
Moderately high frequencies of infectious symptoms are found at onset suggesting an infectious trigger.

Clinical features
Key features in the history
Most children present with insidious onset disease, whereby the rash precedes obvious muscle weakness by months.
- A few children present with an acute onset illness characterized by fever, prostration, rash, and profound weakness.
- Diagnosis is frequently delayed, and the rash is attributed to infection or allergy.
- Muscle pain and arthralgia are common.
- Subtle signs of muscle weakness must be sought in the history, such as:
  - a refusal to use the potty (difficulty getting up from squatting);
  - a refusal to use the school bus (difficultly with the high first step);
  - struggling to brush hair.
- Sometimes the child's actions are put down to behavioural problems, particularly as the children are often in pain and become increasingly frustrated.

Key features on examination
Skin
The first sign of the rash is often swelling of the eyelids and supraorbital areas.
- A heliotrope hue to upper eyelids evolves.
- A mild eruption on the face follows, typically extending down the nasolabial folds.
- An erythematous or violacious maculopapular eruption appears over the extensor surfaces of the PIP joints, elbows, and knees.
- The erythematous plaques over the PIPJs (Gottren's papules) can atrophy.
- Nail cuticles become erythematous owing to periungual vasculitis (the nail-fold capillary vessels show thickening, tortuosity, dropout, and thrombosis seen under the microscope).

Muscles and joints
- One characteristic suggestive sign of muscle weakness is difficulty with prolonged elevation of the head whilst supine.
- An inability to do an unassisted sit up and Gower's sign (an inability to rise from the floor without using the hands to 'climb up' the legs) are reliable signs of truncal and proximal leg muscle weakness, respectively.
- Dysphagia (palatal muscle weakness) is common with more severe presentations and a nasal speech pattern may develop. These children are at risk of aspiration pneumonia.

- Weakness of respiratory muscles and impaired ability to increases the risk of aspiration pneumonia.
- About 60% of JDM patients have inflammatory arthritis, two-thirds having an oligoarticular pattern of arthritis and a third, polyarticular.
- Many children have a flitting or migratory arthralgia.
- In insidious onset disease, joint contractures can develop and need to be discriminated from any limitation of joint movement owing to arthritis.

Other
- Co-existent fibrosing alveolitis may be under-diagnosed. Chest auscultation and simple spirometry should be undertaken.
- Visceral vasculitis occurs in a minority of children, with abdominal pain, GI bleeding, and perforation.
- Dystrophic calcification occurs in about 40%, often within 6 months of onset of the disease.
- Calcinosis is seen as superficial plaques or nodules, or as deep tumorous deposits in muscle or in the inter-muscular fascial plane.
- Subcutaneous calcinosis can erupt sometimes discharging in ulcerated skin lesions. It may occur during the healing phase of the disease.
- Lipodystrophy – generalized or partial loss of subcutaneous fat; occurs in a minority of children.

Investigations
Laboratory
- Creatine kinase (CK) may be raised, although this is not essential to make the diagnosis. Its detection depends on at what stage of the disease it is measured.
- LDH, ALT, and AST are enzymes derived from both liver and muscle. γGT– a specific liver enzyme – is not elevated in myositis.
- ESR is not a good marker of muscle inflammation and is often normal even in active disease.
- ANA is not always positive but anti-tRNA antibodies have been described (e.g. Jo-1).
- Von Willebrand factor, a marker of endothelial cell activation, may be useful for monitoring vasculitic complications.

Imaging
- Mild myositis as demonstrated by MR scanning (using fat-suppressed T2-weighted sequences) may be present without elevation of muscle enzymes.
- A CXR and pulmonary function testing with a check of transfer factor and then if necessary HRCT chest should be done if there is respiratory compromise. Discriminating thoracic muscle weakness from intrinsic lung disease as a cause of dyspnoea is key.

Differential diagnoses
- The presence of Raynaud's phenomenon should raise the suspicion of mixed connective tissue disease (MCTD) or SLE as alternative diagnoses.
- Post-infectious myositis (influenza A&B, cocksackie B) causes a raised CK, but usually lasts just 3–5 days.
- Metabolic myopathies and inflammatory myositis accompanying other autoimmune connective tissue diseases - such as Systemic Sclerosis (SSc) – need to be considered.

Disease activity assessment
Commonly used and validated tools for assessing disease activity are the Childhood Health Assessment Questionnaire (CHAQ), Manual Muscle Testing (MMT), Childhood Myositis Assessment Scale (CMAS), Myositis Disease Activity Assessment Tool (MDAAT), and both physician and patient global assessments of disease and skin activity. Most tools are available at the NIH website (see Resources below).
- Measurement of height, weight, and pubertal status should be done regularly.
- The CMAS assesses function, as well as muscle strength, and is validated for use in children with JIIMs to serially measure the child's proximal muscle power.
- Nail-fold capillaries should be examined for infarcts.
- Contractures, arthritis, and calcinosis assessed.
- Serial MR scans of proximal muscle may be helpful in assessing ongoing inflammation in the absence of other markers of activity.

Treatment
Objectives of treatment
Induction of remission of the inflammatory disease, prevention of loss of muscle bulk and strength, controlling skin disease, and minimizing the side effects of immunosuppression long-term. Ensuring adequate growth and development, maintaining progress at school, and social development through the input of a multidisciplinary care team is of obvious importance.

Physical therapies
Dedicated paediatric physiotherapy is a key component of retaining muscle strength once the inflammatory muscle disease is controlled on medication.

Immunosuppression
- High dose glucocorticoids (GCs) are given (prednisolone 2 mg/kg/day in 3 divided doses) for about 6 weeks. Dose is tapered slowly depending on response.
- If there is a poor response to oral GCs, or in the presence of dysphagia, dysphonia, pulmonary disease or gastrointestinal vasculitis, pulse intravenous methylprednisolone is given.
- Children need to remain replete in vitamin-D (deficiency may evolve as children will be advised to avoid exposure of skin to the sun because of the photosensitive skin rash).
- Secondary hyperparathyroidism should be avoided by remaining vitamin-D replete and keeping dietary calcium intake adequate.
- If DXA scanning suggests very low Z scores where fragility fractures have also occurred, then a bisphosphonate needs to be considered to protect against GC-induced osteoporosis.
- Immunosuppression, with methotrexate (MTX) 15 mg/m^2 by subcutaneous injection, is often introduced early as a 'steroid-sparing' strategy, despite limited published evidence for its effect.
- Cyclophosphamide, IVIG, azathioprine and ciclosporin have been used for GC and MTX resistant disease, or where there is intolerance to MTX. There is notable trial activity in this area (see IMACS and PRINTO).
- Anti-TNFα is being used increasingly for persistent disease and in one notable series, infliximab has shown to be effective in refractory JDM (see Riley et al., 2008).
- Rituximab (anti-CD20) trials in JDM are being undertaken under the auspices of the International Myositis Assessment and Clinical Studies (IMACS) group.
- Topical tacrolimus may be useful adjunctive treatment for the JDM rash.

Patient advice

The JDM rash is photosensitive. It is critical to advise children and their parents that the child needs to protect the skin from the sun: wear UVA/UVB sunblock on areas affected by the rash, but also other exposed surfaces, and wear a hat with a brim or at least a peaked cap.

Natural history and prognosis

The disease has a high mortality if left untreated (from historical accounts before glucocorticoid use).
- Most children are ill for a number of years.
- A cohort of 65 patients were followed up over a median of 7.2 years (Huber, 2000): 37% had a monocyclic course, going into permanent remission after about 2 years of activity and 63% had a continuous or polycyclic course. A significant minority had significant growth impairment.
- The duration of JDM and severity from calcinosis may associate with TNFα genotype allelic variation.

Resources

Assessment tools

Health assessment tool (CHAQ) score is found on the BSPAR website (www.bspar.org.uk;) or from www.niehs.nih.gov/research/resources/collab/imacs/diseaseactivity.cfm, where other assessment tools can be found.

The (abbreviated) Cutaneous Assessment Tool. See Huber et al., 2008.

Muscle strength testing: Manual Muscle Test (MMT). Available at: www.niehs.nih.gov/research/resources/collab/imacs/diseaseactivity.cfm;

Myositis Disease Activity Assessment Tool; see also www.niehs.nih.gov/

Patient information

The Myositis Association. Available at: www.myositis.org

Myositis Support Group (UK). Available at: www.myositis.org.uk/r

Arthritis Research Campaign. Various resources, but see www.arc.org.uk/news/arthritistoday/123_4.asp

Physician information

Paediatric Rheumatology International Trials Organization (PRINTO). Information about current and previous studies in JDM. Available at: www.printo.it

International Myositis Assessment and Clinical Studies (IMACS) group studies (see, for example, www.edc.gsph.pitt.edu/rimstudy/referphys.html)

ICD10 codes

M33.0   Juvenile dermatomyositis

References

Compeyrot-lacassagne S, Feldman BM. Inflammatory Myopathies in Children. *Rheum Dis Clin N Am* 2007; **33**: 525–53.

Bohan A, Peter JB. Polymyositis and dermatomyositis (part 1 of 2). *N Eng J Med* 1975; **292**: 34–7.

Brown VE, Pilkington CA, Feldman BM, Davidson JE. An international consensus survey of the diagnostic criteria for juvenile dermatomyositis (JDM). *Rheumatology (Oxford)* 2006; **45**: 990–3.

Huber AM, Lachenbruch PA, et al. Alternative scoring of the cutaneous assessment tool in juvenile dermatomyositis: results using abbreviated formats. *Arthritis Care Res* 2008; **59**: 352–6.

Huber AM, Lang B, LeBlanc CMA, et al. Medium and long term functional outcomes in a multicenter cohort of children with juvenile dermatomyositis. *Arthritis Rheum* 2000; **43**: 541–9.

Riley P, McCann LJ, et al. Effectiveness of Infliximab in the treatment of refractory juvenile dermatomyositis with calcinosis. *Rheumatology* 2008; **47**: 877–80.

See also

Dermatomyositis (adults), see p. 290
Idiopathic juvenile osteoporosis; see p. 35

Inclusion body myositis

Definition
Sporadic inclusion body myositis (IBM), first described in 1967, is characterized by both inflammation and abnormal accumulation of proteins within muscle forming distinctive inclusions. It was originally considered a variant of polymyositis but is now recognized as a clinically and pathologically distinct entity within the group of idiopathic inflammatory myopathies. Debate is ongoing as to whether IBM arises as a primary immune-mediated disease or whether muscle inflammation occurs secondary to degenerative processes.

Diagnostic criteria
The diagnostic criteria of Griggs (see Griggs et al., 1995, and Griggs et al., 2006) are widely accepted:

Clinical features
- Duration of illness >6 months.
- Age at onset >30 years.
- Slowly progressive muscle weakness affecting arms and legs. May have a selective pattern and be asymmetrical. Patients must have at least one of:
  - finger flexor weakness;
  - wrist flexor > wrist extensor weakness;
  - quadriceps muscle weakness.

Laboratory features
- Creatine kinase (CK) <×12 the upper limit of the reference interval.
- EMG – myopathic or mixed pattern. May be both short and long duration motor unit potentials.

Muscle biopsy
- Inflammatory myopathy characterized by:
  - endomysial mononuclear cell infiltrate and invasion of non-necrotic muscle fibres (predominantly by CD8 positive [CD8+] T cells);
  - myofibre necrosis and regeneration;
  - HLA class I expression in otherwise morphologically healthy muscle fibres.
- Vacuolated muscle fibres.
- Either:
  - intracellular (within muscle fibres) ubiquitin-positive inclusions and amyloid deposits;
  - nuclear and/or cytoplasmic 15–20 nm tubulofilamentous inclusions on electron microscopy.

Definite IBM:
All diagnostic biopsy features present. No other clinical or laboratory features are mandatory.

Probable IBM
Characteristic clinical and laboratory features, but incomplete biopsy criteria.

Epidemiology
IBM is the most common inflammatory myopathy in people aged over 50 years old. It is more common in northern European, white North American and Australian populations. Prevalence estimates vary from 4.9 to 10.7 per million in these areas. However, the true frequency is probably higher as IBM has traditionally been under recognized and misdiagnosed as polymyositis or other diseases. In contrast to polymyositis (PM) and dermatomyositis (DM), there is a male predominance in IBM.

Aetiology and pathophysiology

Genetic factors
- HLA-DR3 is present in 75% of cases.
- Other alleles within the autoimmune 8.1 HLA ancestral haplotype (HLA-A1, B8, DRB3*0101, DRB1*0301, DQB1*0201) are also associated.
- Familial forms of IBM are seen but are extremely rare.

Environment
It has been speculated that viruses may trigger inflammation in IBM. IBM, like PM, may develop in the presence of HIV and HTLV-1 infection. It is noteworthy that the clonally activated CD8+ T cells in these patients are retrovirus specific.

Pathogenesis
The aetiology of IBM is unknown. It is likely that ageing and environmental factors play a contributory role in genetically predisposed individuals.
- IBM is characterized by both inflammation and muscle degeneration; however, it is unclear which of these is the primary pathological process.
- An immune basis for IBM is favoured by the substantial overlap of pathological features with polymyositis. Both involve ubiquitous expression of HLA class I antigens on muscle fibres, which are surrounded and invaded by CD8+ cytotoxic T cells. Subsets of these autoinvasive CD8+ T-cells are clonally expanded, presumably in response to specific antigens expressed by myofibres.
- However, a key-differentiating feature of IBM is the formation of vacuoles and abnormal accumulation of amyloid-like proteins within muscle fibres. These degenerative changes have similarities to those seen in Alzheimer's disease and analogous disease mechanisms have been suggested, with abnormal protein processing as a primary pathogenic event. This could potentially mediate cell damage by triggering the endoplasmic stress response, which additionally induces up-regulation of MHC-1 expression and thus may perpetuate muscle inflammation (see PM for further explanation of these pathological processes).

Clinical features

Key features in history
- Presentation is usually after the age of 50 years, although symptoms may develop from the age of 30 years onwards.
- Insidious onset of muscle weakness over >6 months.
- Mean time from symptom onset to diagnosis is 6 years.
- Weakness involves both proximal and distal muscles, may be asymmetrical and is usually painless.
- Frequent falls are a common presenting feature as a result of the predilection for quadriceps involvement.
- Loss of manual dexterity. The finger flexors are affected early, particularly flexor digitorum profundus and flexor pollicis longus.
- Patients complain of difficulty manipulating small items, e.g. a pen or keys, and problems grasping and lifting.
- Dysphagia occurs in up to 60% of patients, but is rarely a presenting symptom.
- Dyspnoea – respiratory muscle weakness can develop.

CHAPTER 8 Autoimmune connective tissue diseases

Key features on examination
- Look for selective atrophy of quadriceps and forearm flexors – muscle wasting may be prominent.
- Neck flexors may be affected in more advanced disease.
- A weak grip may be detectable on shaking hands.
- Might be unable to stand from sitting unaided.
- Facial weakness is quite common (in contrast with PM).
- Extra-ocular muscles are spared.
- Reflexes may be absent if muscle atrophy is severe.
- Muscle power in proximal and distal groups should be graded against resistance using the MRC scale (see IMACS website for guidance on manual muscle testing).

Co-morbidities
IBM may occasionally associate with autoimmune connective tissue diseases, but less commonly than PM/DM.

Differential diagnosis
The differential is wide (see PM pp. 285–286 or differential diagnosis of progressive muscle weakness). Conditions more likely to be confused with IBM include:
- Polymyositis (PM).
- Motor neurone disease: look for fasciculations.
- Hereditary vacuolar myopathies, e.g. myofibrillar myopathies, hereditary inclusion body myopathy.
- Muscular dystrophies: ask about family history

Key points
Features favouring a diagnosis of IBM over PM
- More gradual onset of weakness, over months to years, rather than weeks to months.
- Age of onset over 50 years and male sex.
- Early involvement of quadriceps, but also distal muscles, particularly finger flexors.
- Asymmetrical muscle weakness.
- Normal or only mildly elevated CK.
- Absence of autoantibodies.
- Failure to respond to steroids and other immunosuppressants.

Investigations
Laboratory
- CK can be normal or moderately elevated, usually less than 10 times the upper limit of normal.
- Autoantibodies, including myositis-specific autoantibodies, are found in IBM. However, they are not a characteristic feature, and are more commonly associated with PM or DM.

Imaging
MR imaging may demonstrate the characteristic selective involvement of quadriceps and forearm flexors. Early muscle inflammation may be detectable before clinically significant weakness develops.

Histology
Muscle biopsy is essential for definitive diagnosis of IBM.
- Quadriceps is the best site to sample unless atrophy is very severe.
- Characteristically there is a triad of histological findings: inflammatory infiltrates, rimmed vacuoles, and abnormal protein accumulation, evident as amyloid deposits and filamentous inclusions (see diagnostic criteria).

- Other features include cytochrome oxidase negative fibres and ragged red fibres due to abnormal mitochondria.
- Muscle biopsy findings in early IBM are sometimes indistinguishable from those seen in PM.

Other
Electromyography (EMG)
Findings may be similar to the other inflammatory myopathies and are therefore not diagnostic. EMG typically demonstrates increased spontaneous activity in conjunction with myopathic features manifest as low-amplitude, short duration potentials on voluntary activation. However, long duration potentials may co-exist in some patients with IBM, potentially leading to confusion with neurogenic disorders such as motor neurone disease.

Treatment
Objectives of treatment
- Improve muscle strength.
- Maintain swallowing, prevent aspiration pneumonia.
- Preserve mobility, function, and quality of life.

Physical therapies
- Exercise programmes have been shown to improve muscle strength and function.
- Creatine supplements may be helpful.
- Knee-locking braces and ankle-foot orthoses may help to prevent falls.
- Strategies to treat dysphagia include cricopharyngneal myotomy, bougie dilatation, and botulinum toxin.

Immunosuppressive therapies
There are no established effective treatments for IBM; therefore, therapy is empirical and varies between centres.
- Despite the evidence for an ongoing inflammatory process in IBM, trials of glucocorticoids, and other immunosuppressants have been disappointing.
- In view of the limited therapeutic options, many advocate an initial trial of prednisolone plus another immunosuppressive agent for 3–6 months.
- Methotrexate, azathioprine, mycophenolate, ciclosporin, cyclophosphamide, and others have been trialled but with limited success.

Glucocorticoids (GCs)
Most patients derive no benefit from treatment with GCs. Stabilization of symptoms has been reported in some cases, although this is seldom maintained and may simply reflect the natural history of the disease. Interestingly, although GCs reduce muscle inflammation, the degenerative changes and muscle weakness continue to progress.

Intravenous immunoglobulin (IVIG)
In 3 double-blind studies of IVIG, improvements in muscle strength overall were minimal and not sustained. However, IVIG may be considered on an individual case basis as it may be helpful in some patients. IVIG has been used successfully to treat dysphagia.

Antithymocyte globulin
A 12-month randomized, open trial in 10 patients showed promising results.

Other
Interferon-β and etanercept have proved relatively ineffective in clinical trials. A trial of the T-cell depleting antibody alemtuzumab is ongoing.

Surgery

Tendon transfers to maintain pincer grip are worth considering, e.g. extensor carpi radialis to replace atrophied flexor tendons.

Prognosis

IBM typically follows a gradually progressive course with slow, inexorable decline in muscle function. However, up to 50% of patients experience 3–6-month periods of temporary stabilization of symptoms making response to therapeutic trials difficult to interpret. The majority of patients require a wheelchair by 10 years from symptom onset. More rapid functional decline may be seen in older people.

Resources

Assessment tools

MITAX   myositis intention to treat index
MYOACT   myositis disease activity assessment
MDI   myositis damage index
SF-36   short form 36
Studies to validate these tools in IBM are ongoing

Guidelines

There are no current therapeutic guidelines for sIBM.

Patient organizations

The Myositis Support Group (UK). Available at: www.myositis.org.uk

The Myositis Association (US). Available at: www.myositis.org

Internet sites

International Myositis Assessment and Clinical Studies Group (IMACS) for manual muscle testing guidelines, grading scheme and score chart and details of tools for assessing disease activity, damage and patient reported outcomes in myositis. Available at: www.niehs.nih.gov/research/resources/collab/imacs/main.cfm

ICD-10 codes

M60.8   Other myositis

See also

Polymyositis	p. 282
Dermatomyositis	p. 290
Metabolic myopathies	p. 522
The nervous system	p. 90

References

Cherin P, Pelletier S, Teixeira A, Laforet P, Simon A, Herson S, et al. Intravenous immunoglobulin for dysphagia of inclusion body myositis. *Neurology* 2002; **58**: 326.

Dalakas MC, Sonies B, Dambrosia J, Sekul E, Cupler E, Sivakumar K. Treatment of inclusion-body myositis with IVIg: a double-blind, placebo-controlled study. *Neurology* 1997; **48**: 712–16.

Dalakas MC. Sporadic inclusion body myositis--diagnosis, pathogenesis and therapeutic strategies. *Nat Clin Pract Neurol* 2006; **2**(8): 437–47.

Griggs RC, Askanas V, DiMauro S, Engel A, Karpati G, Mendell JR et al. Inclusion body myositis and myopathies. *Ann Neurol* 1995; **38**: 705–13.

Griggs RC. The current status of treatment for inclusion-body myositis. *Neurology* 2006; **66**(2 Suppl 1): S30–2.

Lindberg C, Trysberg E, Tarkowski A, Oldfors A. Anti-T-lymphocyte globulin treatment in inclusion body myositis: a randomized pilot study. *Neurology* 2003; **61**: 260–2.

Needham M, Mastaglia FL. Inclusion body myositis: current pathogenetic concepts and diagnostic and therapeutic approaches. *Lancet Neurol* 2007; **6**: 620–31.

Tawil R, Griggs RC. Inclusion body myositis. *Curr Opin Rheumatol* 2002; **14**: 653–7.

Walter MC, Lochmuller H, Toepfer M, Schlotter B, Reilich P, Schroder M, et al. High-dose immunoglobulin therapy in sporadic inclusion body myositis: a double-blind, placebo-controlled study. *J Neurol* 2000; **247**: 22–8.

Undifferentiated (autoimmune) connective tissue disease

Definition
People with undifferentiated autoimmune connective tissue disease (UAICTD/UCTD) have features suggestive of autoimmune disease, but do not fulfil any individual classification criteria. A minority of patients subsequently develop a more defined condition [e.g. rheumatoid arthritis (RA), systemic lupus erythematous (SLE), Sjögren's syndrome]; however, stable UCTD should be considered a distinct clinical entity.

Preliminary classification criteria
- Signs and symptoms suggestive of an AICTD, but not fulfilling the criteria for any defined AICTD.
- Positive ANA.
- Disease duration of at least 3 years.

Patients with shorter follow-up should be defined as having early UCTD, including patients who will develop a specific AICTD and patients with transitory disease.

Clinical features
No specific signs or symptoms exist for UCTD. Most commonly patients suffer from:
- Arthritis/arthralgias (if small joints consider RA, SLE, and sarcoid; if ankles exclusively consider sarcoid).
- Raynaud's phenomenon.
- Sicca symptoms (xerostomia and xerophthalmia).
- Dyspepsia and heartburn.
- Low grade fevers.
- Myalgias.
- Serositis.
- Fatigue.
- Weight loss
- Photosensitive rash.

Neurological and renal disease is virtually absent.

Investigations
The most frequent abnormalities include:
- Anaemia.
- Leukopaenia – particularly lymphopaenia.
- Thrombocytopaenia.
- ANA (positive in up to 90%).

Interestingly, up to 80% of patients with UCTD have a single autoantibody specificity (most commonly anti-Ro or anti-RNP), which remains stable over time. New autoantibody specificity should prompt a review to consider evolution of the disease.

Antibodies with greater diagnostic value include:
- Anti-CCP antibodies (RA).
- Anti-dsDNA and anti-Sm antibodies (SLE).
- Anti-centromere antibodies (lcSSc).
- Anti-topoisomerase 1 [Scl-70] (dcSSc).

Anti-thyroid antibodies have been associated with rash in UCTD.

Differential diagnosis
In early disease the well-characterized AICTDs may present incompletely; therefore, the differential diagnosis includes:
- SLE.
- Sjögrens syndrome.
- RA.
- Systemic sclerosis.
- Primary biliary sclerosis.
- MCTD.
- Polymyositis (PM).
- Sarcoidosis.
- Antiphospholipid syndrome.

Treatment
The major clinical manifestations dictate therapy and management decisions should not be influenced by the predicted definite diagnosis. Symptomatic treatment is usually sufficient and includes:
- NSAIDs.
- Low dose glucocorticoids (GCs).
- Antimalarials (e.g. hydroxychloroquine).
- DMARDs.

Prognosis
Overall, UCTD is a mild condition. Patients require careful monitoring for the evolution of disease to a more specific AICTD (in up to 25%); however, clinicians should not be hasty in making a definitive diagnosis as the undifferentiated nature usually persists.
- Overall resolution of disease is less common than evolution.
- Evolution to SLE is not uncommon and occurs within 5 years of disease onset. Predictors for the development of SLE include:
  - young age at onset;
  - ethnicity (African-American);
  - alopecia;
  - serositis;
  - presence of specific autoantibodies (e.g. dsDNA, Sm, phospholipid);
  - low C3 and C4;
  - photosensitive and discoid rash;
  - cardiac complications.

Data are sparse on predictors for the development of other AICTDs. It's important that where insidious evolution of internal organ disease is a possibility that relevant monitoring is undertaken – even sometimes on minimal clinical evidence for symptoms. Examples of this include monitoring KCO and RVSP for asymptomatic pulmonary hypertension if there is anti-centromere antibody (SSc-sine-scleroderma), and monitoring urinalysis and urine microscopy for nephritis if there are raised DNA antibodies (SLE). No obvious triggers have been identified for disease progression.

Mixed connective tissue disease

Definition
First described in 1971, MCTD has clinical features of SLE, SSc, PM, and RA, but clinical features occur in association with U1RNP autoantibodies. Some debate has appeared periodically in the literature as whether a condition has specific clinical features and should be defined essentially on the basis of the presence of a single autoantibody.

Classification criteria
Several exist, but that of Alarcon-Segovia is the most widely used.

Serologic criteria
Anti-RNP antibodies at a haemagglutination titre >1:1600.

Clinical criteria
- Swollen hands.
- Synovitis.
- Biologically or histologically proven myositis.
- Raynaud's phenomenon.
- Acrosclerosis (with or without proximal SSc).

If the serological criterion and at least three of the five clinical criteria are present then a diagnosis of MCTD can be made. However, a patient with sufficiently elevated anti-RNP titres in combination with swollen hands, Raynaud's phenomenon, and acrosclerosis with or without proximal SSc, must also have either synovitis or myositis to meet the criteria for diagnosis.

Epidemiology
- Incidence remains unknown.
- Disease of the 2nd-4th decades of life.
- Mean age of onset 35 years (10 years in children).
- More common in women (80%).

Pathophysiology
MCTD is associated with HLA-DR4 or HLA-DR2 genotypes. Vascular changes similar to SSc are seen however less fibrosis is present (see individual chapters for a detailed description of the relevant immune mechanisms for each 'subcategory' of MCTD.

Clinical features
Symptoms seldom occur simultaneously and years may elapse before one can be confident of the diagnosis. The commonest manifestations in early disease include:
- Raynaud's phenomenon (75–100%).
- Arthralgia/arthritis.
- Hand oedema/sclerodactyly (extension proximally is not a feature).

Other early symptoms include
- Fatigue;
- Myalgias/mild myositis;
- Serositis;
- Low-grade fever.
  Less common manifestations include:
- Dysphagia and reflux symptoms.
- Sicca symptoms.
- Alopecia.
- Rash (telangiectasia, erythema nodosum, discoid lesions).
- Florid myositis.
- Acute arthritis.
- Dyspnoea.
- Pleuritic pain.
- Aseptic meningitis.
- Digital gangrene.
- High fever.
- Acute abdomen.
- Trigeminal sensory neuropathy.
- Lymphadenopathy.

Malar rash and dermatomyositic rash are more frequent in children. Significant renal and central nervous system disorders are uncommon. A propensity exists for the development of pulmonary hypertension and an SSc type vasculopathy.

Investigations
Laboratory
- High titre ANA in a speckled pattern.
- The presence of U1 RNP antibodies is the *sine qua non* of MCTD.
- FBC: anaemia of chronic disease, thrombocytopaenia.
- Hypergammaglobulinaemia.
- Hypocomplementaemia and cryoglobulinaemia (present in up to one-third, but not associated with renal or other organ involvement).

Other
- Nail-fold capillaroscopy reveals capillary dilatation and capillary loss.
- Cardiac transthoracic ECHO and pulmonary function tests are necessary to monitor for pulmonary hypertension.
- Oesophageal manometry abnormalities (up to 85%).

Treatment
Depends on disease manifestation. Raynaud's phenomenon is treated along standard lines (see pp. 269–270).
Other medications utilized include:
- NSAIDS.
- Proton pump inhibitors.
- Low dose glucocorticoids.
- DMARDS (e.g. hydroxychloroquine and MTX).

Prognosis
In the early phase of disease the features of a single condition (usually systemic sclerosis or SLE) predominate over the 'overlap' features. Invariably, all patients will fulfil criteria for another AICTD at some stage. Pulmonary hypertension is the major cause of death in MCTD.

Overlap syndromes

Definition
An overlap autoimmune connective tissue disease occurs when 2 or more autoimmune rheumatological or connective tissue diseases are present simultaneously in the same individual. The following are considered established overlap syndromes:
- 'Rhupus': SLE/RA.
- Sclerodermatomyositis.
- Scleromyositis.
- MCTD (considered separately).

Other 'overlaps' may be classified as subsets of defined CTDs including:
- SLE/myositis.
- RA/myositis.
- SLE/APS.
- RA/vasculitis.
- SLE/vasculitis.

Clinical features
Disease presentation is varied and comprises features of individual AICTDs in an overlapping fashion (see appropriate sections of the book for full descriptions of the specific AICTDs). The following gives a brief overview of the recognized overlap AICTDs.

Rhupus
- Criteria met for a diagnosis of both RA and SLE.
- Rheumatoid factor sero-positive, erosive, symmetrical polyarthritis usually pre-dates the onset of the clinical features of SLE.
- Autoantibodies of both disorders are present, such as IgM-RF; ANA, Anti-DNA, Anti-Ro.

Sclerodermatomyositis or scleromyositis
- Features of SSc with myositis ± skin manifestations.
- Dermatological change occurs over years and is not severe (absence of digital ulceration, trunk or face involvement, only mild telangiectasia).
- High titre ANA.
- PM-Scl antibodies.
- Anti-U1 RNA absent.

Treatment of overlap syndromes
- Treatment follows the symptoms and severity of disease.
- Therapeutic modalities are those used in the individual AICTDs (see Rheumatoid arthritis, Systemic lupus erythematosus, Systemic sclerosis).

Prognosis
Prognosis is variable and depends upon the extent of organ involvement, the responsiveness to treatment and any intervening complications.

Resources (for UCTD, MCTD, and Overlap syndromes)

Specific assessment tools and guidelines do not exist for UCTD, MCTD, and Overlap syndromes. The quality and breadth of information on a crude search engine screen is of variable quality. Readers are referred to individual scientific and clinical reports where greater detail is required.

ICD-10 codes
M35.1   Other overlap syndromes
M35.8   Other specified systemic involvement of connective tissue
M35.9   Systemic involvement of connective tissue, unspecified

References

Alarcon-Segovia, D, Cardiel, MH. Comparison between 3 diagnostic criteria for mixed connective tissue disease. Study of 593 patients. *J Rheumatol* 1989; **16**: 328.

Bodolay E, Csiki Z, Szekanecz Z, Ben T, Kiss E, Zeher M, et al. Five-year follow-up of 665 Hungarian patients with undifferentiated connective tissue disease (UCTD). *Clin Exp Rheumatol* 2003; **21**: 313–20.

Mosca M, Neri R, Bombardieri S. Undifferentiated connective tissue diseases (UCTD): a review of the literature and a proposal for preliminary classification criteria. *Clin Exp Rheumatol* 1999; **17**: 615–20.

Mosca M, Tani C, Neri C, Baldini C, Bombardieri S. Undifferentiated connective tissue diseases (UCTD) *Autoimmun Rev* 2006; **6**: 1–4

See also
SSc (p. 264)
SLE (p. 240)
RA (p. 197)
PM (p. 282)

Eosinophilic fasciitis

Definition
Eosinophilic fasciitis (Schulman syndrome) was first described in 1974 as a disorder characterized by peripheral eosinophilia and fasciitis (manifest clinically as symmetrical swelling, induration, and thickening of the skin and subcutaneous tissue of the extremities). It differed from the related condition systemic sclerosis (SSc) in that fascia was involved, rather than dermis, the digits were spared and Raynaud's phenomenon was absent. More recently, the syndrome has been broadened to include elevation of the erythrocyte sedimentation rate (ESR) and hypergammaglobulinaemia.

Diagnostic criteria
The diagnosis rests on the clinical, laboratory, and biopsy findings. Specific criteria have not been developed.

Epidemiology
- Very rare.
- Caucasian > Afro Caribbean.
- Females > males (although data vary).
- Mean age of onset 40–50 years.
- Can occur in children who are more likely to suffer from persistent disease.

Aetiology and pathophysiology
The aetiology of eosinophilic fasciitis is unknown. It has been shown that fibroblasts from affected patients produce excess collagen *in vitro* and up-regulation of TGF-β and type 1 collagen mRNA has been seen. A cytotoxic immune response to an environmental or infectious agent is possible as CD8 positive (CD8+) T lymphocytes and macrophages have been found in the fascial inflammatory infiltrate. *Borrelia burgdorferi* has been implicated as an inciting agent.

Clinical features
- A history of significant physical activity precedes the onset in 50% of patients.
- Skin changes occur sub-acutely and progress through several phases in the following order:
  - blotchy skin erythema initially;
  - non-pitting oedema (most commonly of the lower extremities);
  - peau d'orange with hyperpigmentation;
  - skin tightness with woody induration.
- Inflammatory arthritis mainly affects hands and wrists (up to 40% cases).
- Joint contractures are common especially in the upper limb.
- Carpal and tarsal tunnel syndrome symptoms.
- Restrictive lung disease (extra-thoracic) and pleural effusions.
- Venous guttering (linear depressions; 'groove' sign). Not common in the initial stages, but with progression of the skin lesion, veins become tethered within the connective tissue. Elevation of a limb then drains the veins causes guttering at the site of vein.
- Crucially, there is an absence of gastrointestinal, pulmonary parenchymal, and cardiac involvement, and no Raynaud's phenomenon.

Co-morbidities
Eosinophilic fasciitis is frequently associated with haematological abnormalities, including malignant lymphoproliferative diseases and, rarely, as a paraneoplastic phenomenon (e.g. colorectal adenocarcinoma). It has also rarely been associated with autoimmune thyroiditis.

Investigations
It is worth noting that laboratory changes and the clinical manifestations do not necessarily correlate well. Peripheral blood eosinophilia is not necessary for the diagnosis.

Laboratory
- Peripheral blood eosinophilia in 64% (variable over time even in the absence of specific therapy).
- Hypergammaglobulinaemia in 75% cases (polyclonal increase in IgG).
- FBC may reveal thrombocytopaenia, haemolytic anaemia, pernicious anaemia, leukaemia, and aplastic anaemia.
- In doubtful cases, given the association with haematological malignancy, bone marrow aspiration (and trephine if necessary) should be considered.
- The majority have a raised ESR.
- ANA positive in one-third.
- Creatinine kinase (CK) and aldolase normal.

Imaging
Gadolinium-enhanced MR may reveal fascial enhancement consistent with acute inflammation and/or deep fascial thickening.

Histology
Deep fascial biopsy, which includes skin, fat, fascia, and superficial muscle is required for the definitive diagnosis. Biopsy features include thickening of collagen bundles of the superficial muscle fascia with infiltration of lymphocytes, eosinophils and plasma cells.

Other investigations
- EMG can show evidence of underlying myositis.
- Pulmonary function tests show restrictive pattern in those with severe truncal tissue involvement.

Differential diagnosis
The average time taken from the first symptoms to diagnosis has been found to be 9 months due to the rarity and limited awareness of the condition. The differential diagnosis includes:
- Hypereosinophilia syndrome.
- Systemic sclerosis.
- Polymyositis.
- Churg–Strauss vasculitis.
- Eosinophilia-myalgia syndrome.
- Toxic oil syndrome.

Treatment
Physical therapies
Occupational and physiotherapy are helpful, especially for minimizing the development and impact of joint contractures.

Immunosuppression
Glucocorticoids are the mainstay of treatment. The initial dose of prednisolone is 20–60 mg/day, which is then tapered over months.

- Prolonged courses of GCs may be required to reduce the oedema, skin thickening, and joint contracture.
- Eosinophilia usually resolves rapidly following GC treatment. Disease onset in childhood is less likely to respond to GCs.
- Although most patients respond to GCs alone, second line agents are often required including ciclosporin, methotrexate, azathioprine, hydroxychloroquine, and cyclophosphamide.
- Recently, anti-TNFα has been used in recalcitrant disease.
- Photochemotherapy has also been utilized for severe skin involvement.

Prognosis

Early institution of treatment has been found to improve the outcome, yet the disease may remit spontaneously. Oedema usually resolves within 1 month of GC treatment. However, 6 months may elapse before maximal skin softening and improvement in contractures occurs. Residual sclerodermatous-type skin changes may persist indefinitely despite treatment. Raised ESR and immunoglobulin levels may remain abnormal for 12 months or more. Aplastic anaemia is a rare, but often fatal complication.

Factors predicting persistent disease include:
- Young age at onset (<12 years of age).
- Morphea-like skin changes.
- Truncal involvement.

Resources

Assessment tools
None available

Patient resources

Articles

http://www.emedicine.com/derm/topic119.htm;
http://www.medicinenet.com/eosinophilic_fasciitis/article.htm;

Guidelines
None available

ICD-10 Codes
M35.4   Diffuse (eosinophilic) fasciitis

References

Bischoff L, Derk CT. Eosinophilic fasciitis: demographics, disease pattern and response to treatment: report of 12 cases and review of the literature. *Int J Dermatol.* 2008; **47**: 29–35.

Endo Y, Tamura A, Matsushima Y, Iwasaki T, Hasegawa M, Nagai Y, Ishikawa O. Eosinophilic fasciitis: report of two cases and a systematic review of the literature dealing with clinical variables that predict outcome. *Clin Rheumatol.* 2007; **26**: 1445–51.

Shulman LE. Diffuse fasciitis with hypergammaglobulinemia and eosinophilia: a new syndrome? *J Rheumatol* 1974; **1**: 46.

Chapter 9

Vasculitis

Introduction *314*
Giant cell arteritis *318*
Polymyalgia rheumatica *320*
Takayasu arteritis *322*
Wegener's granulomatosis *324*
Churg–Strauss Syndrome *326*
Microscopic polyangiitis *328*
Treatment of ANCA-associated vasculitis *330*
Polyarteritis nodosa *332*
Cryoglobulinaemia *334*
Primary central nervous system vasculitis *336*
Cogan's syndrome *338*
Behçet's disease *340*
Henoch–Schönlein purpura *342*
Kawasaki disease *344*
Relapsing polychondritis *346*
Thromboangiitis obliterans *348*

Introduction

The vasculitides are group of generally rare conditions characterized by inflammation of blood vessels. The conditions have some common features which will be described here, but for greater detail refer to the individual diseases.

Definition and classification

The vasculitides can be classified on the basis of size of vessel involved (Table 9.1), and whether they are primary (or idiopathic) or secondary to a known cause such as infection or connective tissue disease.

The ACR in 1990 developed classification criteria for seven types of vasculitis; these are given with the individual diseases (Fries et al., 1990). The major criticism of the ACR criteria is that they did not include MPA or ANCA. They were derived using patients with known vasculitis and not tested against patients with other conditions.

The Chapel Hill Consensus Conference (CHCC) in 1994 produced definitions for the major types of systemic vasculitis. The CHCC included MPA, but not ANCA. They were not designed for use as classification criteria.

There has until recently been a lack of consensus as to how to reconcile these two systems. A European group has recently produced an algorithm for using both these systems for the classification of the AAV (Table 9.2) (Watts et al., 2007).

Epidemiology

- Overall, the vasculitides are diseases of the extremes of age.
- Kawasaki disease and Henoch–Schönlein purpura occur in childhood, whilst GCA occurs in those aged >65 years.
- The other types of vasculitis are all much rarer, but also tend to occur in older people.

Clinical features

Key features on history

In the early stages, the symptoms can be non-specific and a high index of suspicion is required to achieve an early diagnosis. Age is an important discriminating feature. Takayasu arteritis (TA) is rare aged over 40 years, whilst GCA is most common aged >65 years.

Symptoms suggestive of vasculitis include:

Systemic
Fever, weight loss, myalgia, arthralgia.

ENT
Epistaxis, nasal crusting, deafness, sinusitis (all especially suggestive of WG).

Pulmonary
- Cough, haemoptysis (especially WG or MPA), dyspnoea, and wheeze.
- Late onset asthma is suggestive of CSS.

Cutaneous
Purpuric rash, ulcers.

Neurological
- Peripheral neuropathy (especially CSS or PAN).
- Headache – especially located in the temple, new onset or of a different character to previous headache. Suggestive of GCA.

Vascular
- Jaw claudication is suggestive of GCA.
- Limb claudication is suggestive of TA or GCA.
- Carotidynia (tender carotid arteries) suggests carotid involvement.
- Difficulty in obtaining blood pressure readings.

Key features on examination

Cutaneous
Purpuric rash, ulcers, digital gangrene.

Musculoskeletal
Synovitis.

Neurological
- Motor or sensory neuropathy.
- Mononeuritis multiplex.

Table 9.1 Classification of the vasculitic syndromes according to vessel size and ANCA

Dominant vessel	Primary	Secondary
Large arteries	Giant cell arteritis Takayasu arteritis	Aortitis associated with RA, infection (e.g. syphilis, TB)
Medium arteries	Classical PAN Kawasaki disease	Hepatitis B associated PAN
Small vessels and medium arteries	Wegener's granulomatosis* Churg-Strauss syndrome* Microscopic polyangiitis*	Vasculitis secondary to rheumatoid arthritis, systemic lupus erythematosus, Sjögren's syndrome, drugs, infection (e.g. HIV)
Small vessels	Henoch-Schönlein purpura Cryoglobulinaemia Cutaneous leucocytoclastic angiitis	Drugs Hepatitis C associated Infection

* Diseases most commonly associated with ANCA and a significant risk of renal involvement, and most responsive to immunosuppression with cyclophosphamide. Adapted from Scott & Watts (1994).

Table 9.2 Names and definitions of vasculitides adopted by the Chapel Hill Consensus Conference on the Nomenclature of Systemic vasculitis

Large vessel vasculitis

Giant cell (temporal) arteritis

Granulomatous arteritis of the aorta and its major branches, with a predilection for the extra cranial branches of the carotid artery. Often involves the temporal artery. Usually occurs in patients older than 50 and often is associated with polymyalgia rheumatica.

Takayasu arteritis

Granulomatous inflammation of the aorta and its major branches. Usually occurs in patients younger than 50

Medium-sized vessel vasculitis

Polyarteritis nodosa† (classic polyarteritis nodosa)

Necrotizing inflammation of medium-sized or small arteries without glomerulonephritis or vasculitis in arterioles, capillaries, or venules

Kawasaki disease

Arteritis involving large, medium-sized, small arteries, and associated with mucocutaneous lymph node syndrome. Coronary arteries are often involved. Aorta and veins may be involved. Usually occurs in children

Small vessel vasculitis

Wegener's granulomatosis‡

Granulomatous inflammation involving the respiratory tract, and necrotizing vasculitis affecting small to medium-sized vessels (e.g. capillaries, venules, arterioles, and arteries). Necrotizing glomerulonephritis is common

Churg–Strauss syndrome‡

Eosinophil-rich and granulomatous inflammation involving the respiratory tract, necrotizing vasculitis affecting small to medium-sized vessels, and associated with asthma and eosinophilia

Microscopic polyangiitis† (microscopic polyarteritis)‡

Necrotizing vasculitis, with few or no immune deposits, affecting small vessels (i.e. capillaries, venules, or arterioles). Necrotizing arteritis involving small and medium sized arteries may be present. Necrotizing glomerulonephritis is very common. Pulmonary capillaritis often occurs.

Henoch–Schönlein purpura

Vasculitis, with IgA-dominant immune deposits, affecting small vessels, i.e. capillaries, venules, or arterioles). Typically involves skin, gut, and glomeruli, and is associated arthralgia or arthritis

Essential cryoglobulinaemic vasculitis

Vasculitis, with cryoglobulin immune deposits, affecting small vessels (i.e. capillaries, venules, or arterioles), and associated with cryoglobulins in serum. Skin and glomeruli are often involved

Cutaneous leucocytoclastic angiitis

Isolated cutaneous leucocytoclastic angiitis without systemic vasculitis glomerulonephritis

*Large vessel refers to the aorta and the largest branches directed towards the major body regions (e.g. to the extremities and the head and neck); medium-sized vessel refers to the main visceral arteries (e.g. renal, hepatic, coronary, and mesenteric arteries); small vessel refers to venules, capillaries, arterioles, and the intraparenchymal distal arterial radicals that connect with arterioles. Some small and large vessel vasculitides may involve medium-sized arteries, but large and medium sized vessel vasculitides do not involve smaller than arteries. Essential components are represented by normal type; italicized type represents usual, but not essential, components.
†Preferred term.
‡Strongly associated with antineutrophil cytoplasmic antibodies.
From Jennette et al. (1994).

Vascular
- Tender non-pulsatile temporal arteries. Suggestive of GCA.
- Absent peripheral pulses, bruits.
- Difficulty in obtaining blood pressure measurement

ENT
Nasal bridge collapse. Suggestive of WG or RP.

General investigations
Investigation is directed at establishing the diagnosis and assessing the extent and severity of organ involvement.
- FBC anaemia, leucocytosis, eosinophils (eosinophilia suggestive of CSS).
- Acute phase response (ESR and CRP).
- Liver function.

Assessment of organ involvement
In all patients
- Urinalysis (proteinuria, haematuria, red cell casts), should be performed urgently in all patients in whom systemic vasculitis is suspected.
- Renal function (creatinine clearance, quantification of protein leak if present using either 24-h protein excretion or urine protein/creatinine ratio).
- CXR may show infiltrates, haemorrhage, granuloma (especially WG, CSS, MPA).
- Liver function.

Where appropriate
- Nervous system (nerve conduction studies in all four limbs, biopsy).

Table 9.3 Relationship between vessel size and response to induction treatment

Dominant vessel	Corticosteroids alone	Cyclophosphamide and corticosteroids	Other treatments
Large arteries	+++	–	+
Medium arteries	+	++	++*
Small vessels and medium arteries	+	+++	+
Small vessels	+	+/–	++*

*Includes plasmapheresis, anti-viral therapy for hepatitis B-associated PAN and HCV associated cryoglobulinaemia, and IVIg for Kawasaki disease. Adapted from Scott & Watts (1994).

- Cardiac function (ECG, echocardiography).
- Gut (celiac axis angiography).

Biopsy of an affected organ should be obtained where possible to confirm diagnosis prior to treatment.

Serological investigations
- ANCA. A cANCA pattern on indirect immunofluorescence and PR3 by ELISA are together strongly associated with WG (>90%). pANCA and MPO is suggestive of MPA or CSS. Preferably both indirect immunofluorescence and ELISA for PR3/MPO should be performed in all patients.
- ANA.
- RF (may be positive in cryoglobulinaemic vasculitis or systemic rheumatoid vasculitis).
- Anticardiolipin antibodies (usually negative, but if positive consider anti-phospholipid syndrome).
- Complement (low in cryoglobulinaemic vasculitis).
- Cryoglobulins (suggestive of cryoglobulinaemic vasculitis).

Differential diagnosis
This is from vasculitis mimics (e.g. malignancy, cholesterol embolism, atrial myxoma, calciphylaxis) or infection (especially subacute bacterial endocarditis).
- Blood cultures.
- Viral serology (HBV, HCV, HIV, CMV).
- Echocardiography (two-dimensional and/or transoesophageal).

Disease assessment
- Severity of involvement of target organs should be carefully assessed.
- Where appropriate scoring systems should be used. A number of scoring systems are available. The Birmingham Vasculitis Activity Score is widely used in clinical trials.
- Active uncontrolled disease is associated with cumulative organ damage, which should be assessed using the Birmingham Vasculitis Damage Index (VDI).
- General health function can be assessed using the SF-36 or HAQ.

Patient advice
This applies to patients with any type of vasculitis.

General
- Potentially serious multisystem condition, requiring immunosuppressive therapy and lifelong follow-up.
- Attention to cardiovascular risk.
- Stop smoking.
- Healthy balance diet.
- Regular exercise.
- Vaccination (influenza and pneumococcal).
- Male and female infertility is a recognized complication of cyclophosphamide therapy. These patients should be counselled about the possibility of infertility following cyclophosphamide.

Treatment
Intensity of initial immunosuppression depends on extent and severity of organ involvement. Treatment can be divided into stages: induction, consolidation, and maintenance of remission. Where there is evidence of threatened vital organ involvement treatment should be started urgently.

For specific details see each individual disease.

Resources
Guidelines
BSR guidelines on treatment systemic vasculitis.

EULAR recommendations for the management of large vessel vasculitis.

EULAR recommendations for management of medium and small vessel vasculitis.

Patient organizations
Vasculitis Foundation. Available at: www.vasculitisfoundation.org

Stuart Strange Trust. Available at: www.vasculitis-uk.org

References
Bacon PA, Luqmani RA. Assessment of vasculitis. In: Ball GV, Bridges L (eds) *Vasculitis*. Oxford: Oxford University Press, 246–54.

British Society for Rheumatology. Vaccinations in the immunocompromised person. Guidelines for the patient taking immunosuppressant, steroids and the new biologic therapies. London: BSR, 2002. Available at: www.rheumatology.org.uk

De Groot K, Rasmussen N, Bacon P, et al. Randomised trial of cyclophpsphamide versus methotrexate for induction of remission in early systemic antineutrophil cytoplasmic antibody associated vasculitis. *Arthritis Rheum* 2005; **52**: 2462–8.

Fries JF, Hunder GG, Bloch DA. et al. The American College of Rheumatology 1990 criteria for the classification of vasculitis. Summary. *Arthritis Rheum* 1990; **33**: 1136–6.

Jayne D, Rasmussen N, Andrassy K, et al. A randomised trial of maintenance therapy for vasculitis associated with antineutrophil cytoplasmic auto antibodies. *N Engl J Med* 2003; **349**: 36–44.

Jennette JC, Falk RJ, Andrassy K, et al. Nomenclature of systemic vasculitides. Proposal of an international consensus conference. *Arthritis Rheum* 1994; **37**: 187–92.

Lapraik C, Watts RA, Scott DG. BSR & BHPR guidelines for the management of adults with ANCA associated vasculitis. *Rheumatology* 2007; **46**: 1615–16.

Mukhtyar C, Guillevin L, Cid M, et al. EULAR recommendations for the management of large vessel vasculitis. *Ann Rheum Dis* 2008 (in press).

Mukhtyar C, Guillevin L, Cid M, et al. EULAR recommendations for the management of primary small and medium vasculitis. *Ann Rheum Dis* 2008 (in press).

Scott DGI, Watts RA. Classification and epidemiology of systemic vasculitis. *Br J Rheum* 1994; **33**: 897–9.

Watts RA, Lane SE, Hanslik T, Hauser T, Hellmich B, Koldingsnes W, Mahr A, Segelmark M, Scott DG. Development and validation of a consensus methodology for the classification of the ANCA-associated vasculitides and polyarteritis nodosa for epidemiological studies. *Ann Rheum Dis* 2007; **66:** 222–7.

Watts RA, Scott DGI, Overview of the inflammatory vascular disease. In: Hochberg MC, Silman AJ, Smolen JE, Weinblatt ME, Weisman MH (eds) *Rheumatology*. New York: Mosby, 1583–91.

Giant cell arteritis

Giant cell arteritis (temporal arteritis) (GCA) is the most common of the systemic vasculitides and is characterized by involvement of large vessels particularly the extra-cranial branches of the aorta. There is a close relationship with polymyalgia rheumatica (PMR).

Definition
The Chapel Hill Consensus Conference defined GCA as: Granulomatous arteritis of the aorta and its major branches, with a predilection for the extra cranial branches of the carotid artery. *Often involves the temporal artery. Usually occurs in patients older than 50 and often is associated with polymyalgia rheumatica.*

Classification criteria
The ACR in 1990 developed classification criteria, which are widely used in clinical trials. They have a specificity of 91.2% and sensitivity of 93.5%. There are no validated diagnostic criteria.

ACR criteria for classification of GCA
1. **Age at onset > 50 years:** development of symptoms or findings beginning aged 50 years or older.
2. **New headache:** new onset or new type of localized pains in the head.
3. **Temporal artery abnormality:** temporal artery tenderness to palpation or decreased pulsation, unrelated to atherosclerosis of cervical arteries.
4. **Increase in ESR:** ESR > 50 mm/h by Westergren method.
5. **Abnormal artery biopsy:** Biopsy specimen with artery showing vasculitis characterized by a predominance of mononuclear infiltration or granulomatous inflammation.

Note: for purposes of classification a patient shall be said to have giant cell arteritis if at least 3 of these 5 criteria are present (Hunder et al., 1990).

Epidemiology
- Incidence in people aged > 50 years 10–33/100 000/year.
- There is a female preponderance.
- Peak age onset >75 years, very rare < 50 years
- More common in populations of Scandinavian descent. Occurs much less frequently in other ethnic groups such as Japanese or Afro-Caribbeans.

Aetiology
The aetiology is unknown. There is an association with HLA DRB*0401. Although infectious triggers have long been suspected, no clear associations have yet been confirmed.

A proposed hypothesis suggests that the arterial wall dendritic cells become activated and then recruit CD4+ lymphocytes, which become clonally expanded producing IL-2 and IFN-g. Macrophages produce PDGF, which stimulates intimal arterial thickening. Monocyte- macrophages become multinucleate giant cells.

Clinical features
In the early stages, the symptoms can be non-specific and a high index of suspicion is required to achieve an early diagnosis.

Key features on history
Systemic
- Fever, weight loss.
- Myalgia, arthralgia. Morning stiffness across the shoulder and hip girdles is suggestive of co-existent PMR.

Headache
The characteristic feature is new onset or change in character from previous headache. The headache is located typically in the temples.

Visual disturbance
- This may occur suddenly without warning and may be bilateral.
- Transient visual loss may be a warning, of impeding acute visual loss, which may be profound.
- Ophthalmoplegia is a rare occurrence.

Jaw claudication
Pain on eating is characteristic, but uncommon symptom.

Arm or leg claudication
This is uncommon. Leg claudication is more likely to be due to atherosclerosis in the elderly. Arm claudication is an uncommon feature of atherosclerosis

Key features on examination
Vascular
- The temporal arteries may be tender, thickened, and non-pulsatile.
- Bruits may be audible over affected arteries, especially in the carotid and supraclavicular regions.

Eye
Signs anterior ischaemic optic neuropathy. Formal slit lamp examination by an ophthalmologist may be required. The optic disc may be pale with profound loss of acuity to counting fingers or less.

Investigations
- FBC microcytic anaemia, thrombocytosis.
- Acute phase response (ESR and CRP). These are both usually raised in active GCA. Rarely patients may present with a normal ESR or CRP

Serological investigations
ANCA, ANA, RF, Anticardiolipin are usually negative

Temporal artery biopsy
A biopsy of the temporal artery should be obtained where possible.
- A negative biopsy does not exclude the diagnosis because the lesions are focal in nature and may be missed due to sampling error. Bilateral biopsies should not routinely be performed.
- A biopsy should be obtained as speedily as possible, but if delayed more than 2 weeks may not show changes of active vasculitis, but changes consistent with previous vasculitis.

Imaging
Ultrasound
Ultrasonography of the temporal arteries shows a characteristic halo sign in active disease. Ultrasonography should

only be performed by experienced operators and its role in the routine assessment of patients with suspected GCA is uncertain.

^{18}FDG-PET scintigraphy
^{18}FDG-PET scintigraphy is a useful method of demonstrating disease active in large vessels, such as the aorta and its major branches. The technique is too insensitive to demonstrate the temporal arteries. PET scanning has a role in the assessment of disease activity, but its role in the assessment of relapse or remission remains to be determined (see Plate 32).

Angiography
Angiography is not usually required to make the diagnosis. The role of MRA of the temporal arteries remains to be established. Where extra-cranial large vessel involvement is suspected MRA or contrast angiography should be considered.

Differential diagnosis
Takayasu arteritis (TA) in the younger patient. Other forms of systemic necrotizing vasculitis may rarely present with vasculitis affecting the temporal arteries.

Disease assessment
ESR and CRP are a guide to disease activity, but may be normal in relapse particularly in patients on corticosteroids.

Prognosis
Untreated GCA is associated with a significant risk of permanent blindness risk. This is greatly reduced by the early introduction of corticosteroids. The risk of the second eye being involved in a patient with profound visual loss is 70% within 1 week unless treated. The risk of blindness occurring in patients on corticosteroids is very low.

Pathology
Granulomatous necrotizing vasculitis affecting large vessels especially the extracranial branches of the aorta. There is destruction of the internal elastic lamina with giant cells and granuloma formation. The lesions are focal and careful examination of adequate biopsy is required.

Patient advice
General
Potentially serious condition, requiring glucocorticoid therapy with a risk of blindness

Treatment
Observational studies support the use of high dose glucocorticoids in GCA.

- In patients without ocular symptoms oral corticosteroids starting at 0.7–1 mg/kg (maximum dose 60–80 mg). Steroids should be started as soon as the diagnosis is suspected, as there is a risk of blindness, which is significantly reduced by the use of early corticosteroids. The headache should resolve rapidly (<48 h) with the introduction of steroids.
- A recent randomized study suggested that use of IV methylprednisolone (15 mg/kg) for 3 days in addition to oral prednisolone 40 mg/day permitted more rapid steroid taper.
- In patients with ocular symptoms IV methylprednisolone 1 g daily for 3 days should be used in addition to oral corticosteroids.
- Oral corticosteroids should be tapered quickly aiming for 10 mg/day at 6 months.
- Low dose aspirin reduces the risk of thrombosis.

Relapsing disease
Minor relapse can be treated with an increase in prednisolone dose to the last effective dose.

Refractory disease
- Use of azathioprine or methotrexate should be considered in patients with relapsing disease or who are resistant to corticosteroids. However, a randomized trial of methotrexate showed no benefit in either reduction of relapse rate or reduction of steroid dosage.
- The role of biologic agents such as infliximab remains to be determined.

Resources
Guidelines
EULAR recommendations for the management of large vessel vasculitis (Mukhtyar et al., 2008).

Patient organizations
Vasculitis Foundation. www.vasculitisfoundation.org

ICD-10 coding
M31.5 Giant cell arteritis with polymyalgia rheumatica
M31.6 Other giant cell arteritis

References
Hunder GG, Bloch DA, Michel BA, et al. The American College of Rheumatology 1990 criteria for the classification of Giant Cell Arteritis. *Arthritis Rheum* 1990; **33**: 1122–18.

Mazlumzadeh M, et al. Treatment of giant cell arteritis using induction therapy with high-dose glucocorticoids: a double-blind, placebo controlled, randomised prospective clinical trial. *Arthritis Rheum* 2006; **54**: 3310–18.

Mukhtyar C, Guillevin L, Cid MC, et al. EULAR recommendations for the management of large vessel vasculitis. *Ann Rheum Dis* 2008 (in press).

Polymyalgia rheumatica

Polymyalgia rheumatica (PMR) is an inflammatory condition of the elderly characterized by proximal shoulder and hip girdle pain and morning stiffness. It commonly co-exists with giant cell arteritis.

Diagnostic criteria
Several sets of diagnostic criteria have been proposed, the most useful are given in the Table 9.4. New criteria are being developed by consensus, but are still being validated.

Table 9.4 Diagnostic criteria for PMR

	Bird et al. (1979)	Jones & Hazleman (1981)
Age (years)	>65	
Onset	<2 weeks	
Duration		>2 months
Pain location	Bilateral shoulder pain and stiffness	Shoulder and pelvic girdle
Morning stiffness	>1 h	Present
Tenderness	Upper arms	
Systemic symptoms	Depression, weight loss	
ESR	>40 mm/h	>30 mm/h, or CRP >6 mg/l
Response to glucocorticoids		Prompt and dramatic
Requirements to fulfil criteria	If any 3 criteria are present, sensitivity is 92% and specificity 80%	All criteria

Epidemiology
- PMR is more common than GCA.
- GCA occurs in 4–31% of PMR patients and PMR is present in 1–66% of GCA patients.
- The incidence like GCA is highest in Scandinavia 68–112/100 000 persons aged >50 years.
- Prevalence rates of up to 1:30 in person aged >65 years have been reported.
- There is a female preponderance.
- The peak age of onset >75 years, very rare < 50 years.

Aetiology
The aetiology is unknown. No clear HLA associations for pure PMR have emerged and it is likely because of the overlap with GCA that similar HLA associations will be observed.

Polymorphisms in a number of other genes (e.g. ICAM-1, IFN-γ, VEGF, IL-1 and endothelial nitric oxide synthase have been described, suggesting a polygenic aetiology.

The striking association with age and disease onset suggests that immunosenescence may be important, with possible breakdown in immune tolerance or increased susceptibility to infectious triggers.

Numerous infections have been implicated in small studies but none so far has emerged following rigorous case control studies.

Clinical features
In the early stages, the symptoms can be non-specific and a high index of suspicion is required to achieve an early diagnosis.

Key features on history

Systemic
Fever, weight loss.

Musculoskeletal
Typically, there is a proximal myalgia affecting the shoulder and hip girdles. There may be local tenderness, but there should not be muscle tenderness. This may be of acute onset, and is associated with significant morning stiffness.

Headache
New onset or change in character of headache suggests co-existent giant cell arteritis.

Arthritis
A peripheral arthritis may occur, but this is suggestive of elderly onset rheumatoid arthritis.

Key features on examination

Musculoskeletal
- There may be muscle tenderness proximally, but this should not be major feature. Weakness is not a feature of PMR; if present suggests an inflammatory myopathy.
- The presence of a small joint synovitis suggests elderly onset rheumatoid arthritis.
- Temporal artery tenderness suggests co-existent GCA.

General investigations
Investigation is directed at establishing the diagnosis and excluding malignancy.
- Acute phase response (ESR and CRP): these are both usually raised active PMR. Rarely patients may present with a normal ESR or CRP.
- CK: this should normal. A raised CK suggests an inflammatory myopathy.
- Renal, liver, bone, and thyroid function: FBC, PSA, Igs, electrophoretic strip, chest X-ray may be needed to exclude malignancy.

Serological investigations
- RF: a positive RF is suggestive of elderly onset RA, especially if anti-CCP antibodies are also present.
- ANCA, ANA: anticardiolipin antibodies are all negative.

Detection co-existent GCA
The optimum method of detecting co-existent GCA is uncertain. Routine temporal artery biopsy has a very low detection rate. Biopsy of symptomatic patients improves the detection rate.

Imaging
^{18}FDG-PET scan
^{18}FDG PET scanning is a useful method of demonstrating associated GCA with large vessel arteritis. The technique is too insensitive to demonstrate the temporal arteries. A PET scan may detect a previously unsuspected malignancy.

Ultrasonography
- Ultrasonography of the temporal arteries may demonstrate co-existent GCA. The halo sign is characteristic.
- Ultrasonography of the shoulders and hips may reveal evidence of bursitis or synovitis, but similar appearance may occur in elderly onset RA.

MR

MR of the shoulders and hips may reveal evidence of bursitis or synovitis, but similar appearance may occur in elderly onset RA.

Differential diagnosis

The relatively non-specific presentation of PMR makes the differential wide. There is no diagnostic test. A low threshold must be observed for further investigation. The major differential is malignancy, elderly onset RA, polymyositis, myxoedema, cervical spondylosis, bilateral shoulder capsulitis, and fibromyalgia.

Disease assessment

Response criteria and an activity score for PMR have been developed, but as yet are not widely used.

Prognosis

- PMR generally has a good prognosis.
- There is an overlap with GCA and, therefore, there is a risk of permanent blindness in untreated patients. This is greatly reduced by the early introduction of corticosteroids. The risk of blindness occurring in patients on corticosteroids is very low. The majority of patients require corticosteroids for 18–24 months.

Patient advice

General

- Potentially serious condition, requiring glucocorticoid therapy for 18–24 months.
- There is an association with GCA and, therefore, there is a risk of blindness if associated with GC324A.

Treatment

Prednisolone is the mainstay of treatment.

Newly diagnosed patients

- In patients without symptoms of GCA oral glucocorticoid starting at 15 mg/day.
- There should be a very rapid (< 48 h) response. If there is not a rapid response the diagnosis should be questioned.
- Oral corticosteroids should be tapered quickly aiming for 7.5 mg/day at 6 months.
- Adjunctive low dose weekly methotrexate reduces the risk of relapse and reduces exposure to corticosteroids.

Relapsing disease

Minor relapse be can treated with an increase in prednisolone dose to the last effective dose.

Refractory disease

- Use of azathioprine or methotrexate should be considered in patients with relapsing disease or resistant to corticosteroids. However, a randomized trial of methotrexate showed no benefit in either reduction of relapse rate or steroid dosage.
- Infliximab appears to have no role in the treatment of newly diagnosed PMR.

Follow-up

- Initially every month until stable and then every 3–6 months as patient's condition dictates. Follow-up is required.
- ESR and CRP are a guide to disease activity, but may be normal in relapse particularly in patients on corticosteroids.

Resources

Assessment tools

EULAR response criteria for PMR.

Patient organizations

Vasculitis Foundation. www.vasculitisfoundation.org

Arc leaflet. Available at: www.arc.org.uk/

ICD-10 codes

M31.5   Giant cell arteritis with polymyalgia rheumatica
M35.5   Polymyalgia rheumatica

References

Bird HA, Esselinckxx W, Dixon A StJ, Mowat AG, Wood PH. An evaluation of criteria for polymyalgia rheumatica. *Ann Rheum Dis* 1979; **38**: 434–9.

Jones JG, Hazleman BL. Prognosis and management of polymyalgia rheumatica. *Ann Rheum Dis* 1981; **40**: 1–5.

Leeb BF, Bird HA, Nesher G, Andel I, Hueber W, Logar D, et al. EULAR response criteria for polymyalgia rheumatica: results of an initiative of the European collaborating polymyalgia group. *Ann Rheum Dis* 2003; **62**: 1189–94.

Mahr AD, Jover JA, Spiera RF, Hernandez-Garcia C, Fernandez-Gutierrez B, LaValley MP, et al. Adjunctive methotrexate for treatment of giant cell arteritis. *Arthritis Rheum* 2007; **56**: 2789–97.

Salvarani C, Macchioni P, Manzini C, Paolazzi G, Trotta A, Manganelli P, et al. Infliximab plus prednisone or placebo plus prednisone for the initial treatment of polymyalgia rheumatica: a randomized trial. *Ann Intern Med* 2007; **146**: 631–9.

See also

Giant cell arteritis

Takayasu arteritis

Takayasu arteritis (TA) is a rare systemic vasculitis of unknown aetiology, characterized by a large vessel vasculitis.

Definition
The Chapel Hill Consensus Conference defined TA as: Granulomatous inflammation of the aorta and its major branches. Usually occurs in patients younger than 50.

Classification criteria
The ACR in 1990 developed classification criteria, which are widely used in clinical trials.

> **ACR classification criteria for Takayasu arteritis**
> 1. **Age < 40 years old:** development of symptoms or signs related to Takayasu arteritis at age < 40 years.
> 2. **Claudication of extremities:** development and worsening of fatigue and discomfort in muscles of one or more extremity while in use, especially the upper extremities.
> 3. **Decreased brachial arterial pulse:** decreased pulsation of one or both brachial arteries.
> 4. **BP difference >10 mmHg:** difference of >10 mmHg in systolic blood pressure between arms.
> 5. **Bruit over subclavian arteries or aorta:** Bruit audible on auscultation over one or both subclavian arteries or abdominal aorta.
> 6. **Arteriogram abnormality:** arteriographic narrowing or occlusion of the entire aorta, its proximal branches, or large arteries in the proximal upper or lower extremities, not due to atherosclerosis, fibromuscular dysplasia, or similar causes; changes usually focal or segmental.
>
> Note: for purposes of classification a patient shall be said to have Takayasu arteritis if at least 3 of these 6 criteria are present. The presence of any 3 or more criteria yields a sensitivity of 90.5% and specificity of 97.8%. From Arend et al. (1994).

Epidemiology
- Incidence 1–2/million/year in most populations studied.
- The prevalence in a Japanese autopsy series was 1 in 3000 cases.
- Most series report a female preponderance (80–90%).
- Occurs aged <50 years with a median age of onset of 25–30 years.

Aetiology
The aetiology is unknown. TA has been linked to infection, but no clear organism as yet been identified. Autoimmunity is suggested by the presence of anti-endothelial antibodies. TA has been associated with HLA B52 and DR4, but no consistent overall association has emerged.

Clinical features
The occurrence of stroke in a young person especially when associated with a high ESR or CRP should heighten suspicion of TA.

Key features on history
Systemic
Fever, weight loss.

Musculoskeletal
Myalgia, arthralgia are common at presentation.

Cardiovascular
- The most common symptoms at presentation are absence or asymmetry of peripheral pulses.
- Claudication of arm or legs (occurs in 50%). Transient visual disturbance (scotoma, blurring, or diplopia; 12%).
- Transient ischaemic attacks and stroke are uncommon at presentation.

Key features on examination
Cardiovascular
- Blood pressure inequality between arms and legs. This should be done in all 4 limbs. Brachial/subclavian artery involvement may make measurement of blood pressure in the arms difficult or impossible. In severe cases, intra-arterial measurement may be necessary.
- Hypertension new onset (28%) cases and 58% have evidence of renal artery stenosis.
- Vascular bruits most often heard over the carotid arteries.
- Carotidynia (tenderness over carotids) is rare, but characteristic.

Neurological
Evidence of previous stroke.

General investigations
- FBC anaemia is common.
- ESR and CRP are elevated.

Imaging
Angiography
Percutaneous intravascular contrast angiography has been the gold standard investigation for the diagnosis of TA. Localized narrowing or irregularity of the lumen is the earliest lesion detectable, and may develop into stenosis and occlusion. The characterisitic finding is the presence of skip lesions, where stenosis or aneurysms alternate with normal vessels. The angiographic appearances have been classified into five types. Angiography is invasive and provides information on luminal anatomy, and cannot study changes in the vessel wall (Table 9.5).

Table 9.5 Angiographic classification of TA

Type	Site of involvement
I	Branches of aortic arch
IIa	Ascending aorta, aortic arch and its branches
IIb	Ascending aorta, aortic arch and its branches and thoracic descending aorta
III	Thoracic descending aorta, abdominal aorta and/or renal arteries
IV	Abdominal aorta and/or renal arteries
V	Combination of Types IIb and IV

From Moriwaki et al. (1997).

Magnetic resonance angiography
MRA can provide high resolution imaging of anatomical features, including mural thickening, luminal changes, and aneurysm formation.

18FDG-PET
^{18}F-FDG is taken up by metabolically active cells, including sites of inflammation. Uptake can be visualized in the walls of inflamed large vessels (>4 mm). Small studies suggest

^{18}FDG-PET is useful in the assessment of active disease and response to treatment, but the exact role remains to be determined.

High resolution Doppler ultrasound
High resolution Doppler ultrasound provides a non-invasive method of assessing disease especially in the carotid and subclavian arteries. The role remains to be evaluated.

Serological investigations
ANCA, ANA, RF, and anticardiolipin antibodies are all typically negative in TA.

Differential diagnosis
This is from other types of vasculitis especially in giant cell arteritis in the older patient.

Disease assessment
Severity of involvement of target organs should be carefully assessed. ESR and CRP may be helpful in assessing disease activity and response to treatment, but are unreliable in some patients. May be normal in patients with progressive disease.

Prognosis
- **Mortality:** the overall mortality rate is low at around 3% in the USA.
- **Remission** can be achieved in the majority of patients using corticosteroids, but 73% of patients in a recent US series required additional immunosuppressants to achieve or maintain remission. Relapse occurred in 96% of patients in a recent US series.
- **Restenosis** is common after initially successful angioplasty.

Pathology
Granulomatous necrotizing vasculitis affecting large vessels. There is adventitial thickening, cellular infiltration of the tunica media, with local destruction of the vascular smooth muscle. The intima becomes fibrosed, which leads to stenosis.

Patient advice
Potentially serious multisystem condition, requiring immunosuppressive therapy and life-long follow-up.

Treatment
There are no randomized controlled trials of treatment in TA.

Initial therapy
- Oral corticosteroids start at 1 mg/kg (maximum dose 60–80 mg) and taper quickly; aim for 10 mg/day at 6 months.
- Immunosuppression with methotrexate or azathioprine should be started at the same time as oral corticosteroids.
- Control hypertension.

Relapsing disease
Relapse is treated with increased in prednisolone dose and optimization of immunosuppression.

Refractory disease
Consideration should be given to the use of other immunosuppressive agents, such as mycophenolate mofetil and biological agents, such as infliximab. There is limited data for the latter, but open studies are encouraging.

Surgery
Stenotic lesions may be treated surgically, either with bypass procedures or stenting. Stenting should be considered for renovascular hypertension. Revascularization should only be considered if stenotic or occlusive lesions are leading to haemodynamic compromise, or aneurismal lesions, which may rupture. There is a high restenosis rate of 20–30%.

Resources
Assessment tools
The BVAS and VDI can be used to assess activity and damage.

Guidelines
EULAR recommendations for the management of large vessel vasculitis.

Patient organizations
Vasculitis Foundation. www.vasculitisfoundation.org
Stuart Strange Trust. www.vasculitis-uk.org

ICD-10 code
M31.4   Aortic arch Syndrome (Takayasu arteritis)

References
Arend WA, Michel BA, Bloch DA, et al. The American College of Rheumatology 1990 criteria for the classification of Takayasu arteritis. *Arthritis Rheum* 1990; **33**: 1101–7.

Maksimowicz-McKinnon K, Clark TM, Hoffman GC. Limitations of therapy and a guarded prognosis in an American cohort of Takayasu arteritis patients. *Arthritis Rheum* 2007; **56**: 1000–9.

Andrews J, Mason JC. Takayasu's arteritis-recent advances in imaging offer promise. *Rheumatology* 2007; **46**: 6–15.

Liang P, Tan-Ong M, Hoffman GS. Takayasu arteritis: vascular interventions and outcomes. *J Rheumatol* 2004; **31**: 102–6.

Mukhtyar C, Guillevin L, Cid MC, et al. EULAR recommendations for the management of large vessel vasculitis. *Ann Rheum Dis* 2008 (in press).

Moriwaki R, Noda M, Yajima M, Sharma BK, Numano F. Clinical manifestations of Takayasu arteritis in India and Japan-new classification of angiographic findings. *Angiology* 1997; **48**: 369–79.

Wegener's granulomatosis

Wegener's granulomatosis is a rare systemic vasculitis of unknown aetiology, characterized by involvement of the upper airways with granuloma formation.

Definition
The Chapel Hill Consensus Conference defined Wegener's granulomatosis as:
> Granulomatous inflammation involving the respiratory tract and necrotizing vasculitis affecting small to medium sized vessels (e.g. capillaries, venules, arterioles and arteries). *Necrotizing glomerulonephritis is common.*

The ACR in 1990 developed classification criteria, which are widely used in clinical trials. There are no validated diagnostic criteria.

> **ACR criteria for classification of Wegener's granulomatosis**
> 1. **Nasal or oral inflammation:** development of painful or painless oral ulcers or purulent or bloody nasal discharge.
> 2. **Abnormal chest radiograph:** chest radiograph showing the presence of nodules, fixed infiltrates or cavities.
> 3. **Urinary sediment:** microhaematuria (>5 red cells per high power field) or red cell casts in urinary sediment.
> 4. **Granulomatous inflammation:** histological changes showing granulomatous on biopsy inflammation within the wall of an artery or in the perivascular or extravascular area (artery or arteriole).
>
> For purposes of classification, a person shall be said to have Wegener's granulomatosis if at least 2 of these 4 criteria are present. The presence of any 2 or more criteria yields a sensitivity of 88.2% and specificity of 92.0%. (Leavitt et al., 1990).

Epidemiology
- The incidence in Europe is 10/million/year.
- The prevalence in Europe is 190/million.
- In most studies there is a male preponderance (Figure 9.1).
- The peak age of onset 65–74 years.
- In Europe WG is more common at higher latitudes than MPA.
- Occurs most frequently in white Caucasians and is much rarer in other ethnic groups.

Aetiology
The aetiology is unknown, but like many autoimmune conditions is generally believed to result from an environmental trigger interacting with a genetically predisposed host.

Genetic factors
Familial cases are rare and there are no clear HLA associations. HLA-DPB*0401 has been associated in some studies. Numerous cytokine and signal transducer gene polymorphisms have been studied, but again no clear associations have emerged. No infectious triggers have been identified.

In vitro and animal studies support the idea that PR3-ANCA is has a pathogenic role in the induction of vasculitis. PR3-ANCA interaction with neutrophils primed with TNFα or IL-1 results in their degranulation, generation of oxygen radicals, endothelial damage, and leucocyte recruitment.

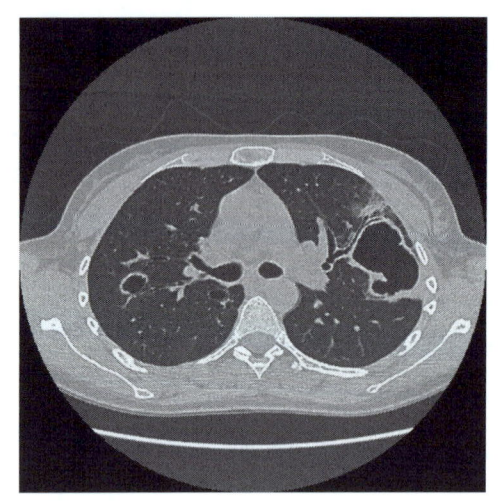

Figure 9.1 CT thorax from patient with WG showing extensive pulmonary cavitation

This finally results in intravascular lysis of neutrophils and necrotizing vasculitis.

Clinical features
Key points on history
In the early stages, the symptoms can be non-specific and a high index of suspicion is required to achieve an early diagnosis.
Symptoms suggestive of WG include:

Systemic:
Fever, weight loss, myalgia, arthralgia.

ENT
Epistaxis, nasal crusting, deafness, sinusitis.

Pulmonary
Cough, haemoptysis, dyspnoea.

Cutaneous
Purpuric rash, ulcers (see Plate 16).

Peripheral neuropathy

Key features on examination
Skin
Purpura, ulcers.

Arthritis

Eye
Scleritis, proptosis is suggestive of a retro-orbital mass.

ENT:
Nasal collapse, suggestive of destructive sino-nasal disease (see Plate 15).

General investigations
Investigation is directed at establishing the diagnosis and assessing the extent and severity of organ involvement.
- FBC anaemia, leucocytosis, eosinophils (an eosinophilia is suggestive of CSS).
- Acute phase response (ESR and CRP).
- Liver function.

Assessment of organ involvement

In all patients

- Urinalysis (proteinuria, haematuria, red cell casts), should be performed urgently in all patients in whom systemic vasculitis is suspected.
- Renal function (creatinine clearance, quantification of protein leak if present using either 24-h protein excretion or urine protein/creatinine ratio).
- CXR may show infiltrates, haemorrhage, granuloma.
- Liver function.

Where appropriate

- Nervous system (nerve conduction studies in all four limbs, biopsy).
- Cardiac function (ECG, echocardiography).
- Gut (celiac axis angiography).
- Skin (biopsy).

Biopsy of an affected organ should be obtained where possible to confirm diagnosis prior to treatment

Serological investigations

- ANCA. A cANCA pattern on indirect immunofluorescence and PR3 by ELISA are together strongly associated with WG (>90%). Preferably both indirect immunofluorescence and ELISA for PR3/MPO should be performed in all patients.
- ANA, RF, anticardiolipin antibodies, complement will be negative.
- Cryoglobulins to differentiate from cryoglobulinaemic vasculitis.

Differential diagnosis

This is from other types of vasculitis (especially MPA, CSS, PAN), vasculitis mimics (e.g. malignancy, cholesterol embolism, atrial myxoma, calciphylaxis) or infection (especially SBE).

- Blood cultures.
- Viral serology (HBV, HCV, HIV, CMV).
- Echocardiography (two dimensional and/or transoesophageal).

Disease assessment

- Severity of involvement of target organs should be carefully assessed.
- Where appropriate scoring systems should be used.
- Active uncontrolled disease is associated with cumulative organ damage which should be assessed using the Birmingham Vasculitis Damage Index (VDI).
- General health function can be assessed using the SF-36 or HAQ.

Prognosis

- Untreated WG has very high mortality (82% at 1 year). This has been substantially improved following the introduction of prednisolone and cyclophosphamide.
- Mortality with current treatment regimens is 18% at 5 years.
- Poor prognostic factor include age >65 years at presentation, renal disease, pulmonary haemorrhage.
- 50% chance relapse at 5 years.

Pathology

Biopsies of affected organs show a granulomatous necrotizing vasculitis affecting medium and small vessels. In the kidney the typical appearance is a focal segmental necrotizing vasculitis.

Patient advice

Potentially serious multisystem condition, requiring immunosuppressive therapy and life-long follow-up.

Treatment

For the general approach to treatment for Wegener's granulomatosis and ANCA-associated vasculitis, see p. 330.

Resources

Assessment tools

The BVAS and VDI should be used to assess disease activity and damage.

Patient organizations

Vasculitis Foundation. www.vasculitisfoundation.org

Stuart Strange Trust. www.vasculitis-uk.org

Coding ICD-10

M31.3   Wegener's granulomatosis

References

Birck R, Schmitt W, Kaelsch IA, van Der Woude FJ. Serial ANCA determinations for monitoring disease activity in patients with ANCA-associated vasculitis: systematic review. *Am J Kidney Dis* 2006; **47**: 15–23.

Jennette JC, Falk RJ, Andrassy K, et al. Nomenclature of systemic vasculitides. Proposal of an international consensus conference. *Arthritis Rheum* 1994; **37**: 187–92.

Lamprecht P, Holl-Ulrich K, Gross W. Wegener's granulomatosis: pathogenesis. In: Ball GV, Bridges L (eds) *Vasculitis*, 2nd edn. Oxford: Oxford University Press 2008: 391–402.

Leavitt, RY, Fauci AS, Bloch DA, et al. The American College of Rheumatology 1990 criteria for the classification of Wegener's granulomatosis. *Arthritis Rheum* 1990; **33**: 1101–7.

Luqmani RA, Bacon PA. Assessment of vasculitis. In: Ball GV, Bridges L (eds) *Vasculitis*, 2nd edn. Oxford: Oxford University Press 2008: 297–306.

See also

Churg–Strauss syndrome	p.326
Microscopic polyangiitis	p.328

Churg–Strauss Syndrome

Churg–Strauss Syndrome (CSS) is a rare systemic vasculitis of unknown aetiology, characterized by late onset asthma with peripheral and tissue eosinophilia.

Definition
The Chapel Hill Consensus Conference defined Churg–Strauss Syndrome as
Eosinophil-rich and granulomatous inflammation involving the respiratory tract and necrotizing vasculitis affecting small to medium-sized vessels associated with asthma and eosinophilia.

Classification criteria
The ACR in 1990 developed classification criteria, which are widely used in clinical trials. They have a specificity of 99.7% and sensitivity of 85.0%. There are no validated diagnostic criteria. Lanham in 1984 produced criteria that have not been validated.

ACR criteria for classification CSS
1. **Asthma:** history of wheezing or diffuse high pitch rales on expiration.
2. **Eosinophilia** >10% on white cell differential count.
3. **Mononeuropathy or polyneuropathy:** development of mononeuropathy, multiple mononeuropathies, or polyneuropathy (i.e. glove/stocking distribution) attributable to systemic vasculitis.
4. **Pulmonary infiltrates, non-fixed:** migratory or transient pulmonary radiographs (not including fixed infiltrates), attributable to a systemic vasculitis.
5. **Paranasal sinus abnormality:** history of acute or chronic paranasalor tenderness or radiographic opacification of the paranasal sinuses.
6. **Extravascular eosinophils:** biopsy including artery, arteriole, or venule showing accumulations of eosinophils in extravascular areas

For purposes of classification, a person shall be said to have Churg–Strauss Syndrome if at least 4 of these 6 criteria are present. Masi et al., 1990.

Lanham criteria for Churg–Strauss syndrome
1. **Asthma**.
2. **Peripheral blood eosinophilia** $>1 \times 10^9$l.
3. **Systemic vasculitis** involving two or more extra pulmonary organs.

Note: biopsy evidence of granuloma is not required (Lanham et al., 1984).

Epidemiology
- The incidence in Europe is 2/million/year.
- In most studies there is a male preponderance.
- The peak age onset is 65–74 years.
- Occurs most frequently in white Caucasians, is much rarer in other ethnic groups.

Aetiology
The aetiology is unknown. Allergy is a common feature to all patients. Tissue injury is due to toxic eosinophil and neutrophil degranulation products. Eosinophils are activated and markers of eosinophil activation mirror disease activity.

HLA-DRB4 has recently been reported to be associated with CSS.

Churg–Strauss Syndrome has been associated with the use of leukotriene inhibitors. The association is now believed to be an unmasking of previously undiagnosed Churg–Strauss syndrome, rather than precipitation of *de novo* vasculitis.

Clinical features
Key points on history
In the early stages, the symptoms can be non-specific and a high index of suspicion is required to achieve an early diagnosis. There is typically a history of adult onset asthma that has become more difficult to control, requiring oral corticosteroids. Cardiac involvement is more common than in WG or MPA.

Symptoms suggestive of CSS include:

Systemic:
Fever, weight loss, myalgia, arthralgia.

Pulmonary
Cough, wheeze, dyspnoea. Upper respiratory tract symptoms occur in 50–60%. Asthma is virtually universal.

Cutaneous
Purpuric rash or cutaneous granulomata occur in up to 50%.

Neurological
Peripheral neuropathy or mononeuritis multiplex occurs in up to 76%.

Cardiac
Dyspnoea, cardiac failure, arrthymia, due to endomyocardial disease occurs in 47%.

Renal involvement
Occurs in 50%.

Key features on examination
Cutaneous
Purpuric vasculitic rash or palpable granulomata.

Musculoskeletal
Arthritis.

Ophthalmic:
Scleritis (uncommon <5%).

ENT
Nasal polyps.

Neurological
Mononeuritis multiplex; sensory or motor neuropathy.

General investigations
Investigation is directed at establishing the diagnosis and assessing the extent and severity of organ involvement.
- FBC anaemia, leucocytosis, eosinophil count $>1.5 \times 10^9$ is particularly suggestive of CSS.
- Acute phase response (ESR and CRP).
- Liver function.

Assessment of organ involvement

In all patients
- Urinalysis (proteinuria, haematuria, red cell casts). This should be performed urgently in all patients in whom systemic vasculitis is suspected.
- Renal function (creatinine clearance, quantification of protein leak if present using either 24-h protein excretion or urine protein/creatinine ratio).
- CXR may show infiltrates, haemorrhage, granuloma.
- Liver function.

Where appropriate
- Nervous system (nerve conduction studies in all four limbs, biopsy).
- Cardiac function (ECG, echocardiography).
- Gut (celiac axis angiography).
- Skin (biopsy).

Biopsy of an affected organ should be obtained where possible to confirm diagnosis prior to treatment

Serological investigations
- ANCA. About 50% of patients are ANCA positive typically MPO-ANCA.
- ANA, RF, anticardiolipin antibodies, complement, cryoglobulins are normal or negative.

Differential diagnosis
This is from other types of vasculitis (especially WG, MPA, PAN), vasculitis mimics (e.g. malignancy, cholesterol embolism, atrial myxoma, calciphylaxis) or infection (especially SBE). Infection should be excluded.

Differentiation needs to be made from other causes of hypereosinophilia such as the hypereosinophilic syndrome, eosinophilic leukaemia and chronic parasitic infection.

Disease assessment
- Severity of involvement of target organs should be carefully assessed.
- Where appropriate scoring systems should be used. A number of scoring systems are available. The Birmingham Vasculitis Activity Score is widely used in clinical trials.
- Active uncontrolled disease is associated with cumulative organ damage which should be assessed using the Birmingham VDI.
- General health function can be assessed using the SF-36 or HAQ.

Prognosis
- 1-year survival rate is 83.2% and 5-year survival is 68.1%.
- Poor prognostic factor include age > 65 years at presentation, renal disease, pulmonary haemorrhage.

Pathology
Granulomatous necrotizing vasculitis affecting medium and small vessels typically with an eosinophilic infiltrate.

Patient advice

General
Potentially serious multisystem condition, requiring immunosuppressive therapy and lifelong follow-up

Treatment
Intensity of initial immunosuppression depends on extent and severity of organ involvement. Treatment can be divided into stages: induction, consolidation and maintenance of remission. The EUVAS trials on which the treatment approach is based were conducted in WG and MPA, but the treatment approach is similar.

Resources

Assessment tools
The BVAS and VDI should be used to assess disease activity and damage.

Patient organizations
Vasculitis Foundation: www.vasculitisfoundation.org
Stuart Strange Trust: www.vasculitis-uk.org

ICD-10 coding
M30.1   Polyarteritis with lung involvement (Churg–Strauss). Allergic granulomatous angiitis.

References
Lanham JG, Elkon KB, Pusey CD, Hughes GR. Systemic vasculitis with asthma and eosinophilia: a clinical approach to the Churg–Strauss syndrome. *Medicine (Baltimore)* 1984; **63**: 65–81.

Luqmani RA, Bacon PA. Assessment of vasculitis. In: Ball GV, Bridges L (eds) *Vasculitis*. Oxford: Oxford University Press, 2008: 297–306.

Masi AT, Hunder GG, Lie JT, et al. The American College of Rheumatology 1990 criteria for the classification of Churg–Strauss Syndrome. *Arthritis Rheum* 1990; **33**: 1094–100.

Specks U. Churg–Strauss Syndrome. In: Ball GV, Bridges L (eds) *Vasculitis*. Oxford: Oxford University Press, 2008: 429–38.

Microscopic polyangiitis

Definition
The Chapel Hill Consensus Conference defined microscopic polyangiitis as a:
Necrotizing vasculitis, with few or no immune deposits, affecting small vessels (i.e. capillaries, venules, or arterioles). Necrotizing arteritis involving small and medium sized arteries may be present. *Necrotizing glomerulonephritis is very common. Pulmonary capillaritis often occurs.*

Classification criteria
The ACR 1990 classification criteria did not include microscopic polyangiitis. There are no validated diagnostic criteria

Epidemiology
- The incidence in Europe is 3–8/million/year.
- Peak age onset 65–74 years.
- More common at lower latitudes in Europe.
- Occurs most frequently in white Caucasians, is much rarer in other ethnic groups.

Aetiology
MPO is a 140 KDa protein composed of two heterodimers. The gene is located at 17q21.3. Myeloperoxidase (MPO) comprises 5% of neutrophil proteins and is present in the cytoplasmic granules. The precise function of MPO is uncertain, the enzyme may catalyse the H_2O_2 dependent oxidation of halides that can kill microbes. Alternatively MPO may protect digestive enzymes from oxidative denaturation by removing H_2O_2 from the phagocytic granule.

The mechanisms involved in ANCA-induced neutrophil activation are not clearly understood. In a rat model MPO-ANCA are pathogenic. Immunization with a human MPO led to development of anti-MPO antibodies and a systemic vasculitis.

Clinical features
In the early stages, the symptoms can be non-specific and a high index of suspicion is required to achieve an early diagnosis. There may be an indolent course for several months before diagnosis.

Key features on history
Systemic
Fever, weight loss, myalgia, arthralgia are present in 56–76% of patients.

Pulmonary
Cough, haemoptysis, dyspnoea. Haemoptysis especially in a patient with renal failure suggests MPA or anti-GBM disease.

Renal
Renal involvement is often asymptomatic, but is present in virtually all patients.

Cutaneous
Purpuric rash.

Neurological
Peripheral neuropathy.

Key features on examination
Cutaneous
Purpura are present in 40%. Other lesions include digital ischaemia, ulcers, livedo reticularis.

Neurological
Mononeuritis multiplex, sensorimotor neuropathy are present in up to 60%.

Pulmonary
Interstitial lung disease occurs as a consequence of recurrent haemorrhage.

General investigations
Investigation is directed at establishing the diagnosis and assessing the extent and severity of organ involvement.
- FBC anaemia, leucocytosis, eosinophils (eosinophilia is suggestive of CSS).
- Acute phase response (ESR and CRP).
- Liver function.

Assessment of organ involvement
In all patients
- Urinalysis (proteinuria, haematuria, red cell casts). This should be performed urgently in all patients in whom systemic vasculitis is suspected.
- Renal function (creatinine clearance, quantification of protein leak if present using either 24-h protein excretion or urine protein/creatinine ratio).
- CXR may show infiltrates, haemorrhage.

Where appropriate
- Nervous system (nerve conduction studies in all four limbs, biopsy).
- Cardiac function (ECG, echocardiography).
- Gut (celiac axis angiography).
- Skin (biopsy).
- Pulmonary function tests may show increased gas transfer indicative of alveolar haemorrhage.

Tissue biopsy
Biopsy of an affected organ should be obtained where possible to confirm diagnosis prior to treatment.

Serological investigations
- ANCA: A pANCA pattern on indirect immunofluorescence and MPO by ELISA are together associated with MPA (75%).
- Anti-GBM: negative in MPA, their presence indicates the occurrence of anti-GBM disease (Goodpasture's syndrome).
- ANA, RF: anticardiolipin antibodies are typically negative.
- Complement.
- Cryoglobulins.

Differential diagnosis
This is from other types of vasculitis (especially WG, CSS, PAN), vasculitis mimics (e.g. malignancy, cholesterol embolism, atrial myxoma, calciphylaxis) or infection (especially SBE). Other causes of a pulmonary-renal syndrome should be considered such as anti-GBM disease (Goodpasture's syndrome).
- Blood cultures.
- Viral serology (HBV, HCV, HIV, CMV).
- Echocardiography (two-dimensional and/or transoesophageal).

Disease assessment
- Severity of involvement of target organs should be carefully assessed.
- A five factor score has been developed to guide prognosis.

Five factor score
Proteinuria >1 g/24 h
Serum creatinine >140 µmol/l
Gastrointestinal involvement
Cardiomyopathy
CNS involvement
1 point for each of these items present (from Guillevin et al., 1996).

Prognosis
- Overall mortality with current treatment regimens is 18% at 5 years.
- There is a risk of relapse of 50% at 5 years.
- Poor prognostic factor include age > 65 years at presentation, renal disease, pulmonary haemorrhage.

Prognosis based on FFS

FFS	5ª year survival (%)	relative risk
0	88.1	0.62
1	74.1*	1.35
≥2	54.1**	2.40

*P < 0.005; **p < 0.0001 compared with FFS = 0 (Gayraud et al., 2001).

Pathology
The typical renal biopsy appearance is a focal segmental necrotizing glomerulonephritis. Extracapillary crescents are present in most renal biopsies and involve 60% of glomeruli. Glomerular sclerosis is associated with more severe disease.

Patient advice
General
- Potentially serious multisystem condition, requiring immunosuppressive therapy and lifelong follow-up.
- Attention to cardiovascular risk.
- Stop smoking.
- Healthy balance diet.
- Regular exercise.
- Vaccination (influenza and pneumococcal).
- Male and female infertility is a recognized complication of cyclophosphamide therapy. These patients should be counselled about the possibility of infertility following cyclophosphamide.

Treatment
Intensity of initial immunosuppression depends on extent and severity of organ involvement (see p. 330). Treatment can be divided into stages: induction, consolidation, and maintenance of remission.

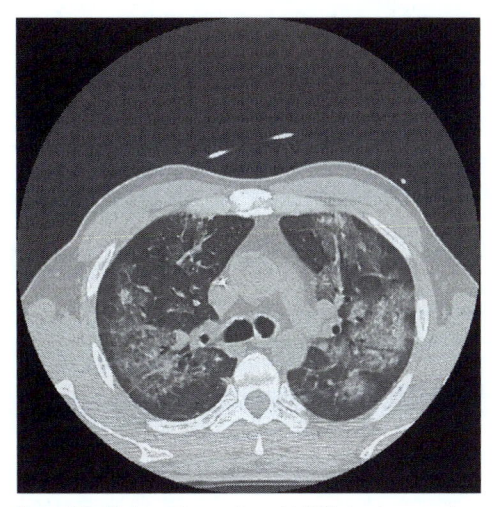

Figure 9.2 CT thorax from patient with MPA showing extensive pulmonary haemorrhage.

Resources
Assessment tools
The BVAS and VDI should be used to assess disease activity and damage.

Patient organizations
Vasculitis Foundation: www.vasculitisfoundation.org
Stuart Strange Trust: www.vasculitis-uk.org

Coding ICD-10
M31.7   Microscopic polyangiitis

References
Gayraud M, Guillevin L, Le Toumalin P, Cohen P, Lhote F, Cassusus P, et al. Longterm follow up of polyarteritis nodosa, microscopic polyangiitis and Churg–Strauss syndrome: analysis of four prospective trials including 278 patients. *Arthritis Rheum* 2001; **44**: 666–75.

Guillevin L, Lhote F, Gayraud M, et al. Prognostic factors in polyarteritis nodosa and Churg–Strauss syndrome. A prospective study in 342 patients. *Medicine (Baltimore)* 1996; **75**: 17–28.

Guillevin L, Pagneux C, Teixeira L. Microscopic polyangiitis. In: Ball GV, Bridges L (eds) *Vasculitis*. Oxford: Oxford University Press, 2008: 2355–364.

Luqmani RA, Bacon PA. Assessment of vasculitis. In: Ball GV, Bridges L (eds) *Vasculitis*. Oxford: Oxford University Press, 2008: 297–306.

See also
Wegener's granulomatosis	p. 324
Microscopic polyangiitis	p. 334

Treatment of ANCA-associated vasculitis

Treatment
Intensity of initial immunosuppression for the ANCA-associated vasculitides (WG, CSS, MPA) depends on extent and severity of organ involvement. The principles of treatment are the same for all the AAV. Treatment can be divided into stages: induction, consolidation and maintenance of remission. The EUVAS trials on which the following treatment approach were conducted in WG and MPA but the approach is the same for CSS.

Induction
- Non-organ/life-threatening: oral corticosteroids combined with either methotrexate, mycophenolate mofetil or cyclophosphamide.
- Oral corticosteroids start at 1 mg/kg (maximum dose 60–80 mg) and taper quickly aim for 10 mg/day at 6 months.
- Creatinine <500 µmol/l corticosteroids and cyclophosphamide. CYC can be given either PO (1.5–2.0 mg/kg/day) or IV (15 mg/kg, max 1 g). CYC should be continued until 3 months after remission is achieved and then change to azathioprine.
- Creatinine >500 µmol/l consider use of plasma exchange in addition to corticosteroids and CYC.
- Regular monitoring of WBC is necessary.
- Consider Septrin prophylaxis against pneumocystis carinii, PPI against gastric ulceration, Mesna against haemorrhagic cystitis, prophylaxis against osteoporosis.
- Pulmonary haemorrhage consider plasma exchange.

Maintenance treatment
Once remission has been induced and consolidated then maintenance treatment should be started this is typically after 3–6 months of therapy.
- Azathioprine should be used for maintenance in place of cyclophosphamide for a further 18–24 months. Methotrexate or mycophenolate mofetil are acceptable alternatives in patients intolerant of azathioprine.
- Taper oral prednisolone.
- Consider Septrin to reduce relapse rate (NB avoid with methotrexate).

Relapsing disease
Minor relapse can treated with an increase in prednisolone dose, and then gradual taper and optimization of other immunosuppression. Major relapse is treated with cyclophosphamide as for induction.

Refractory disease
Disease refractory to full dose cyclophosphamide and prednisolone is rare. More commonly, optimal doses are not tolerated or a prolonged relapsing course with high cumulative exposure to cyclophosphamide and prednisolone occurs, and is an indication for other agents. Experimental agents include deoxyspergualin, rituximab (anti-CD20).

Prevention and detection of toxicity secondary to immunosuppressive therapy.
- Mesna should be considered in patients receiving IV CYC. The risks of bladder cancer are directly related to the cumulative dose of CYC. The risk with modern low dose regimens is unknown.
- Pneumocystis jiroveci (formerly carinii) infection. Immunosuppressed patients are at risk of Pneumocystis jiroveci infection. There is no RCT data; observational studies support the use of prophylaxis with trimethoprim/sulfamethoxazole 960 mg 3× weekly.
- Osteoporosis see guidelines for prevention of corticosteroid-induced osteoporosis.
- Cervical intraepithelial neoplasia. Secondary malignancies are associated with immunosuppressive therapy. Patients receiving treatment with cytotoxic drugs should be considered for an annual cervical smear for the first 3 years after CYC treatment
- Annual cervical smear yearly for the first 3 years after CYC treatment.
- Mycobacterium infection. Patients receiving therapy for systemic vasculitis are at an increased risk of reactivation of TB or new infection, therefore, a detailed history, examination, and chest X-ray should be undertaken to assess the risk of TB.

Follow-up
- Every 3–6 months as patients condition dictates. CSS is a relapsing condition and lifelong follow up is required. 6-monthly urinalysis lifelong is necessary to detect bladder malignancy secondary to CYC
- ANCA measurements are not closely associated with disease activity. Treatment should not be escalated solely on the basis of an increase in ANCA. An increase should be taken as a warning of possible impending relapse. Treatment withdrawal in patients with persistently positive ANCA is associated with relapse.

Table 9.6 Categorization of treatment according to extent and severity of disease

Clinical subgroup	Constitutional symptoms	Typical ANCA status	Threatened vital organ function	Serum creatinine (µmol/l)	Treatment Induction
Localized/early systemic	Yes	Positive or negative	No	<150	Methotrexate or cyclophosphamide
Generalized	Yes	Positive	Yes	<500	Cyclophosphamide
Severe	Yes	Positive	Yes	>500	Cyclophosphamide/plasma exchange/methyl prednisolone

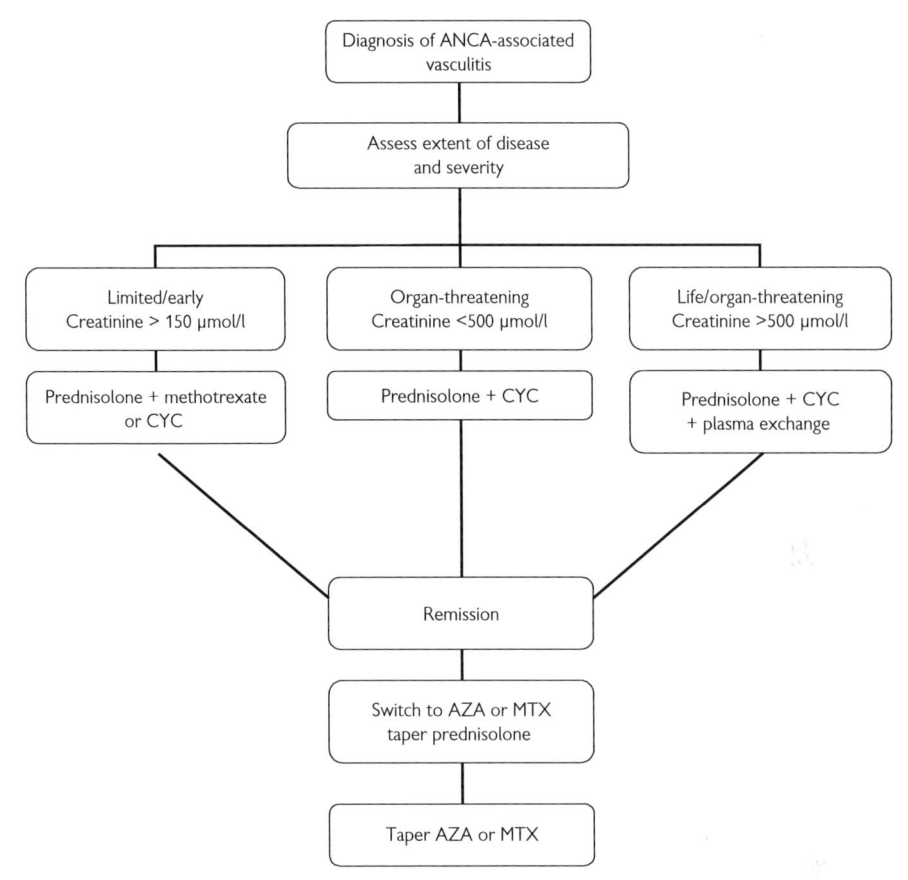

```
                    ┌─────────────────────────────┐
                    │ Diagnosis of ANCA-associated│
                    │         vasculitis          │
                    └──────────────┬──────────────┘
                                   │
                    ┌──────────────┴──────────────┐
                    │    Assess extent of disease  │
                    │         and severity         │
                    └──────────────┬──────────────┘
        ┌──────────────────────────┼──────────────────────────┐
┌───────┴────────┐        ┌────────┴────────┐        ┌────────┴────────┐
│ Limited/early  │        │ Organ-threatening│        │Life/organ-threatening│
│Creatinine >150 │        │Creatinine <500  │        │Creatinine >500  │
│    µmol/l      │        │     µmol/l      │        │     µmol/l      │
└───────┬────────┘        └────────┬────────┘        └────────┬────────┘
┌───────┴────────┐        ┌────────┴────────┐        ┌────────┴────────┐
│Prednisolone +  │        │Prednisolone + CYC│       │Prednisolone + CYC│
│methotrexate    │        │                 │        │+ plasma exchange │
│   or CYC       │        │                 │        │                 │
└───────┬────────┘        └────────┬────────┘        └────────┬────────┘
        └──────────────────────────┼──────────────────────────┘
                          ┌────────┴────────┐
                          │    Remission    │
                          └────────┬────────┘
                          ┌────────┴────────┐
                          │Switch to AZA or │
                          │MTX taper        │
                          │prednisolone     │
                          └────────┬────────┘
                          ┌────────┴────────┐
                          │Taper AZA or MTX │
                          └─────────────────┘
```

Figure 9.3 Algorithm for the management of ANCA-associated systemic vasculitis (from Lapraik et al., 2007).

Resources

Guidelines
- BSR and BHPR guidelines on treatment systemic vasculitis for the management of adults with ANCA associated vasculitis.
- EULAR recommendations for the management of small and medium sized vessel vasculitis.

References

Birck R, Schmitt W, Kaelsch IA, van Der Woude FJ. Serial ANCA determinations for monitoring disease activity in patients with ANCA-associated vasculitis: systematic review. *Am J Kidney Dis* 2006; **47**: 15–23.

De Groot K, Rasmussen N, Bacon P, et al. Randomised trial of cyclophosphamide versus methotrexate for induction of remission in early systemic antineutrophil cytoplasmic antibody associated vasculitis. *Arthritis Rheum* 2005; **52**: 2462–8.

Jayne D, Rasmussen N, Andrassy K, et al. A randomised trial of maintenance therapy for vasculitis associated with antineutrophil cytoplasmic auto antibodies. *N Engl J Med* 2003; **349**: 36–44.

Jayne DR, Gaskin G, Rasmussen N, et al. Randomised trial of plasma exchange and high-dosage methylprednisolone as adjunctive therapy for severe renal vasculitis. *J Am Soc Nephrol* 2007; **18**: 2180–8.

Lapraik C, Watts RA, Scott DG. BSR & BHPR guidelines for the management of adults with ANCA associated vasculitis. *Rheumatology* 2007; **46**: 1615–16

Mukhtyar C, Guillevin L, Cid M, et al. EULAR recommendations for the management of small and medium sized vessel vasculitis. *Ann Rheum Dis* 2008 (in press).

Polyarteritis nodosa

Polyarteritis nodosa (PAN) is a rare medium vessel vasculitis that is often associated with HBV infection.

Definition
The Chapel Hill Consensus Conference defined polyarteritis nodosa as:
   Necrotizing inflammation of medium-sized or small arteries without glomerulonephritis or vasculitis in arterioles, capillaries, or venules.

Classification criteria
The ACR in 1990 developed classification criteria that are widely used in clinical trials. There are no validated diagnostic criteria.

> **ACR (1990) classification criteria for PAN**
> 1. **Weight loss:** loss of 4 kg or more of body weight since the illness began, not due to dieting or other factors.
> 2. **Livedo reticularis:** mottled reticular pattern over the skin of portions of the extremities or torso.
> 3. **Testicular pain or tenderness:** pain or tenderness of the testicles, not due to infection, trauma, or other causes.
> 4. **Myalgias, weakness, or leg tenderness:** diffuse myalgias (excluding shoulder or hip girdle) or weakness of muscles or tenderness of leg muscles.
> 5. **Mononeuropathy or polyneuropathy:** development of mononeuropathy, multiple mononeuropathies, or polyneuropathy.
> 6. **Diastolic BP >90 mmHg:** development of hypertension with diastolic BP >90 mmHg.
> 7. **Elevated blood urea or creatinine:** elevated BUN >40 mg/dl or creatinine 1.5 mg/dl, not due to dehydration or obstruction.
> 8. **Hepatitis B virus:** presence of hepatitis B surface antigen or antibody in serum.
> 9. **Arteriographic abnormality:** arteriogram showing aneurysms or occlusion of the visceral arteries, not due to arteriosclerosis, fibromuscular dysplasia, or other non-inflammatory causes.
> 10. **Biopsy of small or medium vessel:** histological changes showing the presence of sized artery containing PMN granulocytes or granulocytes and mononuclear leucocytes in the artery wall.
>
> Note for purposes of classification a patient shall be said to have PAN if at least 3 of these 10 criteria are present. The presence of any 3 or more criteria yields a sensitivity of 82.2% and specificity of 86.6% (from Lightfoot et al., 1990).

Epidemiology
- Classical polyarteritis nodosa as defined by the CHCC is very rare with an annual incidence of <1/million
- HBV PAN occurs with an incidence of 77/million in HBV endemic areas
- The incidence of HBV PAN is falling due to increased vaccination against HBV and screening of blood products for HBV infection. The commonest cause is now drug abuse.

Aetiology
In areas endemic for HBV up to 95% of cases are associated with HBV infection. PAN usually develops within 12 months infection and hepatitis is mild before development of PAN. Familial cases are rare and there are no clear HLA associations.

Key features on history
In the early stages, the symptoms can be non-specific and a high index of suspicion is required to achieve an early diagnosis

Systemic
Fever, weight loss, myalgia, arthralgia.

Cutaneous
Rash.

Neurological
Peripheral neuropathy – motor or sensory neuropathy.

Testicular pain

Key features on examination
Features of HBV pain are similar to those observed in non-HBV PAN apart from more frequent GIT involvement, extra-glomerular renovascular disease with malignant hypertension and orchitis in HBV-PAN.
   Testicular tenderness (orchitis) occurs in:

Hypertension
Which may be malignant, occurs in 31%.

Cutaneous
Livedo reticularis, a mottled reticular pattern over the extremities.

Neurological
Mononeuritis multiplex is the most common pattern of neurological involvement (83.5%).

General investigations
Investigation is directed at establishing the diagnosis and assessing the extent and severity of organ involvement.
- FBC anaemia, leucocytosis, eosinophils (eosinophilia suggestive CSS).
- Acute phase response (ESR and CRP).

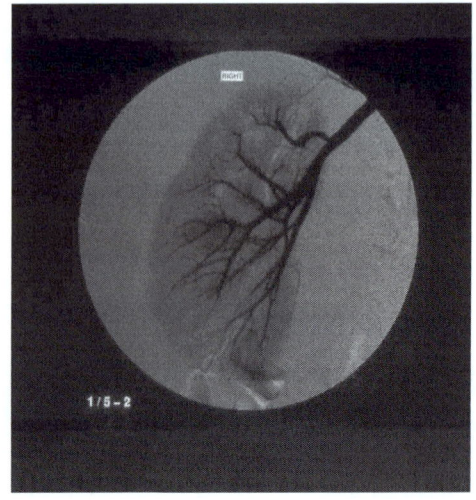

Figure. 9.4 Angiogram showing microaneurysms and segmental cortical infarction.

- Liver function. Abnormalities suggest presence of HBV or HCV infection.

Assessment of organ involvement
In all patients
- Urinalysis (proteinuria, haematuria, red cell casts). This should be performed urgently in all patients in whom systemic vasculitis is suspected.
- Renal function (creatinine clearance, quantification of protein leak if present using either 24-h protein excretion or urine protein/creatinine ratio).
- Liver function (including markers of viral infection such as HBV and HCV).
- Nervous system (nerve conduction studies in all four limbs, biopsy).
- Cardiac function (ECG, echocardiography).
- Angiography should be performed if PAN is suspected. Angiography will show the typical microaneurysms and/or stenosis in the celiac axis and renal vasculature.
- Skin (biopsy).

Biopsy of an affected organ should be obtained where possible to confirm diagnosis prior to treatment

Serological investigations
- ANCA. PAN with or without HBV infection is not associated with ANCA.
- ANA, RF, anticardiolipin antibodies, complement. Cryoglobulins are negative or normal.

Differential diagnosis
This is from other types of vasculitis (especially MPA, CSS), vasculitis mimics (e.g. malignancy, cholesterol embolism, atrial myxoma, calciphylaxis), or infection (especially SBE).
- Blood cultures.
- Viral serology (HIV, CMV).
- Echocardiography (two-dimensional and/or transoesophageal).

Disease assessment
- Severity of involvement of target organs should be carefully assessed.
- Where appropriate scoring systems should be used. A number of scoring systems are available. The Birmingham Vasculitis Activity Score is widely used in clinical trials.
- Active uncontrolled disease is associated with cumulative organ damage which should be assessed using the Birmingham Vasculitis Damage Index (VDI).
- General health function can be assessed using the SF-36 or HAQ.

Prognosis
- HBV-PAN has a good prognosis with 60% survival at 10 years.
- HBV-PAN treated with anti-viral therapy has a 6% relapse rate.
- PAN tends not to be a relapsing remitting disease.
- Poor prognostic factor include age >65 years at presentation, gastrointestinal involvement.

Pathology
- Necrotizing vasculitis affecting medium and small arteries, the lesions are focal. The inflammation is characterized by fibrinoid necrosis and a pleomorphic cellular infiltrate. With predominant macrophages and lymphocytes.

Patient advice
- Potentially serious multisystem condition, requiring immunosuppressive therapy and lifelong follow-up.
- Association with HBV infection.

Treatment
- Treatment of non-HBV PAN: the principles, as for other types of vasculitis, are based on immunosuppression. Treatment can be divided into stages: induction, consolidation and maintenance of remission. For details see p. 334.
- HBV associated PAN should be treated with antiviral therapy: there are no controlled trials as the condition is rare. The current preferred protocol is Lamivudine (100 mg/day) combined with plasma exchange to remove immune complexes. This is accompanied by a short course of corticosteroids. Seroconversion from HBeAG to HBeAB is usually achieved. And is associated with a decreased risk of relapse.

Resources
Assessment tools
The BVAS and VDI should be used to assess disease activity and damage.

Guidelines
EULAR recommendations for the management of small and medium-sized vessel vasculitis.

Patient organizations
Vasculitis Foundation: www.vasculitisfoundation.org
Stuart Strange Trust: www.vasculitis-uk.org

ICD-10 coding
M30.0   Polyarteritis nodosa

References
Guillevin L, Mahr A, Callard P, Godemer P, Pagnoux C, Leray E, et al. Hepatitis B virus associated polyarteritis nodosa: clinical characteristics, outcome and impact of treatment in 115 patients. *Medicine* 2005; **84**: 313–22.

Jennette JC, Falk RJ, Andrassy K, et al. Nomenclature of systemic vasculitides. Proposal of an international consensus conference. *Arthritis Rheum* 1994; **37**: 187–92.

Lightfoot R, Michel B, Bloch D, et al. The American College of Rheumatology 1990 criteria for the classification of polyarteritis nodosa. *Arthritis Rheum* 1990; **33**: 1088–93.

Pagnoux C, Cohen P, Guillevin L. Vasculitis secondary to infections. *Clin Exp Rheumatol* 2006; **24** (Suppl. 2): S71–81.

Watts RA, Scott DGI. Overview of the inflammatory vascular disease. In: Hochberg MC, Silman AJ, Smolen JE, Weinblatt ME, Weisman MH (eds) *Rheumatology*. 1583–91.

See also
Microscopic polyangiitis

Cryoglobulinaemia

Cryoglobulinaemic vasculitis is a rare medium/small vessel vasculitis that is often associated with hepatitis C virus (HCV) infection.

Definition
The Chapel Hill Consensus Conference defined cryoglobulinaemic vasculitis as:

> Vasculitis, with cryoglobulin immune deposits, affecting small vessels (i.e. capillaries, venules, or arterioles), and associated with cryoglobulins in serum. *Skin and glomeruli are often involved.*

Aetiology
There is a strong association between HCV infection and essential mixed cryoglobulinaemia, with 80–90% of such patients positive for anti-HCV antibodies. Type II cryoglobulins with a monoclonal IgM-kappa is most typically associated with cryoglobulinaemic vasculitis. Circulating HCV RNA has been found in the peripheral blood of patients with cryoglobulinaemia. HCV has been identified within cutaneous vasculitis lesions and has been selectively concentrated together with specific antibody in cryoprecipitates.

The exact mechanism of formation of cryoprecipitates is unknown. However, HCV virions and non-envelope core proteins form cold insoluble immune complexes. There is strong evidence of a clonal B cell expansion.

Clinical features
In the early stages, the symptoms can be non-specific and a high index of suspicion is required to achieve an early diagnosis. Renal disease is common.

Meltzer's triad (purpura, arthralgia, weakness) is present in < 40%.

Key features on history
Systemic
Fever, weight loss, myalgia, arthralgia.

Cutaneous
Rash, purpura, Raynaud's phenomenon.

Neurological
Subacute, gradual onset may be either symmetric or asymmetric peripheral neuropathy, acute mononeuritis multiplex.

Musculoskeletal
Arthralgias or arthritis.

Key features on examination
Cutaneous
Purpura (less often: urticaria, livedo, exanthem, acral necrosis, leg ulcers).

Neurological
Polyneuropathy is present in 40-70% (distal, symmetrical or asymmetrical, motor and/or sensory polyneuropathy, acute mononeuritis multiplex).

Muscle weakness
Proximal muscle weakness.

General investigations
Investigation is directed at establishing the diagnosis and assessing the extent and severity of organ involvement.

- FBC anaemia, leucocytosis, eosinophils (eosinophilia suggestive CSS).
- Acute phase response (ESR and CRP).
- Liver function.

Assessment of organ involvement
In all patients
- Urinalysis (proteinuria, haematuria, red cell casts). This should be performed urgently in all patients in whom systemic vasculitis is suspected.
- Renal function (creatinine clearance, quantification of protein leak if present using either 24-h protein excretion or urine protein/creatinine ratio).

Cryoglobulin detection
Cryoglobulins are proteins that precipitate in the cold. Samples for cryoglobulin detection must be kept warm during transport to the laboratory.

Where appropriate
- Nervous system (nerve conduction studies in all four limbs, biopsy) electrophysiological variables may be altered in up to 80% of patients.
- Cardiac function (ECG, echocardiography).

Biopsy
Biopsy of an affected organ should be obtained where possible to confirm diagnosis prior to treatment. Cryoglobulins may be detected tissue biopsies especially renal biopsy specimens.

Viral serology
HCV, HBC, HIV, and CMV serology.

Serological investigations
- ANCA, ANA, anticardiolipin antibodies are negative.
- RF is present in 70%.
- Complement. Hypocomplementaemia is present in 90% and is a useful distinguishing feature from ANCA associated vasculitis in which complement levels are normal.

Differential diagnosis
This is from other types of vasculitis (especially WG, MPA, CSS), vasculitis mimics (e.g. malignancy, cholesterol embolism, atrial myxoma, calciphylaxis), or infection (especially SBE).

Disease assessment
- Severity of involvement of target organs should be carefully assessed.
- Where appropriate scoring systems should be used. A number of scoring systems are available. The Birmingham Vasculitis Activity Score is widely used in clinical trials.
- Active uncontrolled disease is associated with cumulative organ damage, which should be assessed using the Birmingham Vasculitis Damage Index (VDI).
- General health function can be assessed using the SF-36 or HAQ.

Prognosis
Relapsing remitting disease requiring maintenance anti-viral therapy.

Pathology
The characteristic lesion on renal biopsy is a membranoproliferative glomerulonephritis with intracapillary thrombi, which contain cryoglobulin precipitates. This distinguishes it from ANCA-associated vasculitis.

Patient advice
- Systemic vasculitis associated with HCV infection.
- Relapsing remitting disease requiring long-term treatment with anti-viral therapy.

Treatment
- Severe or life-threatening disease should be treated with steroids, cyclophosphamide +/− plasma exchange.
- Less severe disease (arthralgia, purpura, neuropathy) with IFN-alpha, ribivirin +/− plasma exchange.
- Interferon and ribivirin is effective. Ribivirin alone is ineffective.
- The role of anti-CD20 therapy remains to be determined.
- Because of the relapsing nature of disease maintenance anti-viral therapy is necessary.

Resources
Assessment tools
The BVAS and VDI should be used to assess disease activity and damage.

Guidelines
EULAR recommendations for the management of small- and medium-sized vessel vasculitis.

Patient organizations
Vasculitis Foundation: www.vasculitisfoundation.org
Stuart Strange Trust: www.vasculitis-uk.org

ICD-10 coding
D89.1 Cryoglobulinaemia

References
Galli, M, Invernizzi F, Monti G. Cryoglobulinaemic vasculitis. In: Ball GV, Bridges L (eds) *Vasculitis*. Oxford: Oxford University Press, 2008: 529–44.

Mukhtyar C, Guillevin L, Cid MC, et al. EULAR recommendations for the management of medium and small vessel vasculitis. *Ann Rheum Dis* 2008 (in press).

Pagnoux C, Cohen P, Guillevin L. Vasculitis secondary to infections. *Clin Exp Rheumatol* 2006; **24** (Suppl. 2): S71–81.

Primary central nervous system vasculitis

Primary central nervous system vasculitis (PCNSV) is a rare vasculitis of unknown aetiology affecting the brain and spinal cord.

Epidemiology
- The annual incidence is 2.4/million in Olmsted County (USA).
- The mean age at diagnosis was 47 years.
- The condition is more common in females (3:2).

Diagnostic criteria
(i) Recent history or presence of an acquired neurological deficit unexplained by other causes.
(ii) Evidence of vasculitis in a CNS biopsy specimen.
(iii) Cerebral angiogram with changes characteristic of vasculitis.

Diagnosis requires i) and ii) or iii) (Calabrese & Mallek, 1988). These criteria have not been validated.

Aetiology
The aetiology is unknown.

Clinical features
Key feature on history
Neurological
- Headache: present in 63% at presentation.
- Altered cognition: occurs in 50%.
- Stroke: persistent deficit occurs in 40% with 28% having a transient ischaemic attack.
- Visual symptoms occur in 42%, with field defects in 21%, diplopia in 16%, loss visual acuity in 11%.
- Nausea and vomiting occur in 25%.

Systemic
These are relatively uncommon with fever occurring in 9%.

Key features on examination
Neurological
- Focal neurological deficit.
- Paraparesis or quadriparesis in 7%.
- Visual field defects occur in 21%
- Decreased visual acuity in 11%.
- Papilloedema in 5%.

General investigations
Investigation is directed at establishing the diagnosis and assessing the extent and severity of organ involvement.
- FBC is typically normal.
- Acute phase response (ESR and CRP) are infrequently elevated.
- Liver function.

Serological investigations
ANCA, ANA, RF, anticardiolipin antibodies, complement, cryoglobulins are normal or negative.

Cerebral spinal fluid
Abnormalities in the CSF are found in 88% of patients. The white cell count is typically mildly elevated with an increase in total protein. RBCs are found in 79%.

Imaging
Cerebral angiography
- Angiographic changes are found in multiple vessels usually bilateral (90%).
- Involvement of small vessels is more common than large vessels. Large vessel involvement alone is uncommon.
- Conventional angiography is probably more sensitive for detecting intracranial vasculitis than MRA.

Magnetic resonance angiography
Involvement of both large and small vessels is typically seen, with multiple vessel abnormalities.

Magnetic resonance imaging
- Cerebral MRI is abnormal in 97% of patients.
- The most common lesion is cerebral infarction seen in half of patients, the majority of patients have multiple infarctions often bilateral and involving the cortex and subcortex.
- Intracranial haemorrhage is unusual (<10%).
- Gadolinium-enhancing lesions can be seen in one-third of patients.

Brain biopsy
- CNS biopsy is necessary to make a definitive diagnosis and is positive in two-thirds of patients.
- Histology may show a granulomatous vasculitis, with or without acute necrosis. A lymphocytic pattern may be seen.

Electroencephalography
There are no specific features. Findings include dysrhythmias, epileptogenic changes, and delta waves.

Differential diagnosis
This is from other types of vasculitis (e.g. PAN or SLE). Infection needs to be excluded especially *Varicella zoster*, CMV, etc. Hypercoagulable states may mimic PCNSV.

Prognosis
- PCNSV is associated with increased mortality compared with the general population. Poor prognosis is associated with the following at presentation neurological deficit, cerebral infarction, cerebral infarction, and large vessel involvement.
- Cerebral infarction is frequent cause of death.
- Relapse in a quarter of patients followed for a mean of 13 months.

Pathology
There is evidence of transmural vessel inflammation with involvement of the leptomeningeal and parenchymal vessels. Fibrinoid necrosis may be present.

Patient advice
General
Potentially serious neurological condition, requiring immunosuppressive therapy and lifelong follow-up.

Treatment
There are no controlled trials to guide therapy.

Induction
High dose corticosteroids are necessary
- Oral corticosteroids start at 1 mg/kg (maximum dose 60–80 mg) and taper quickly aim for 10 mg/day at 6 months.
- Consider pulse IV steroids in severe cases.
- In patients with a poor prognostic outcome consider use of cyclophosphamide.
- Cyclophosphamide may be given either orally or intravenously (see p. 562 for details).

Maintenance
Maintenance therapy is with oral corticosteroids with a tapering dose of prednisolone. The majority of patients require treatment for less than 18 months.

Relapsing disease
Relapse is treated with an increase in prednisolone dosage and the introduction of other immunosuppressive agents, such as cyclophosphamide or azathioprine.

Refractory disease
Refractory disease may require treatment with novel agents such as mycophenolate mofetil or biological agents, but there is at the present time little evidence to support their use.

Follow-up
As dictated by clinical condition.

Resources
Patient organizations
Vasculitis Foundation: www.vasculitisfoundation.org

References
Calabrese H, Mallek JA. Primary angiitis of the central nervous system: report of 8 new cases, review of the literature, and proposal for diagnostic criteria. *Medicine (Baltimore)* 1988; **67**: 20–39.

Salvarani C, Brown RD, Calamia KT, *et al.* Primary central nervous system vasculitis: analysis of 101 patients. *Annl Neurol* 2007, epubl.

Cogan's syndrome

Cogan's syndrome (CS) is a rare inflammatory disease of unknown aetiology, characterized by involvement of the eye and inner ear.

Epidemiology
- CS occur mainly in young adults with peak incidence in the 20s.
- The incidence and prevalence is unknown.
- There is no gender predominance.

Aetiology
The aetiology is unknown, but like many autoimmune conditions is generally believed to result from an environmental trigger interacting with a genetically predisposed host. Infection has long been suspected as a trigger, but not proven. The eye and the ear are both capable of mounting a vigorous response to infection, trauma, or toxins. In an experimental model of autoimmune keratitis in rats transfer of corneal specific T cells produces a severe keratitis. Similarly transfer of activated T cells can induce vestibular inflammation in animal models.

Clinical features
Key points on history
The combination of ocular and vestibular symptoms in a young adult should raise a suspicion of CS.

Ocular
- The predominant complaint is of ocular pain, redness, and photophobia.
- Blurred vision, tearing, diplopia, a sensation of foreign body, or visual field defects occur frequently.

Vestibular auditory
Sudden onset vertigo, nausea, vomiting, tinnitus, and hearing loss. Attacks are similar to Meniere's disease.

Vascular
Symptoms of vasculitis depend on the territory and size of vessel involved. Any size of vessel may be involved. Large vessel vasculitis akin to Takayasu arteritis is most common.

Neurological
Neurological involvement is uncommon in CS, but features include meningitis, encephalitis, psychosis, and seizures.

Musculoskeletal
Non-specific arthralgias and myalgias.

Systemic
Fever, weight loss, fatigue.

Key features on examination
Ocular
- Slit lamp examination is necessary to observe interstitial keratitis, which occurs in 70%. The earliest findings are faint corneal infiltrates which are 0.5–1 mm in diameter.
- Other frequent manifestations are conjunctivitis (35%), iridocyclitis (30%), episcleritis/scleritis (30%).
- Less commonly papillitis, posterior uveitis.

Vestibular auditory
Hearing loss occurs in 95%, ataxia (45%), nystagmus (30%), oscillopsia (15%).

Cardiovascular
Aortitis occurs in 10% with severe aortic regurgitation. Pericarditis, arrhythmias.

General investigations
Investigation is directed at establishing the diagnosis, and assessing the extent and severity of organ involvement.
- FBC anaemia, leucocytosis, with relative lymphopaenia.
- Acute phase response (ESR and CRP).

Assessment of organ involvement
In all patients
Urinalysis (proteinuria, haematuria, red cell casts), should be performed urgently in all patients in whom systemic vasculitis is suspected.

Ophthalmic examination
Slit lamp examination is necessary to examine the anterior chamber and cornea. Fluorescein angiography is useful to assess retinal vasculitis or retinochoroiditis.

Audiometry
- 95% of patients have hearing loss, with relative sparing of the middle range.
- Brainstem-evoked responses are abnormal in patients with cochlear damage.
- Caloric responses are abnormal with vestibular injury.

Serological investigations
- ANCA. ANA, RF, anticardiolipin antibodies are typically negative.
- Complement.
- Cryoglobulins.

Differential diagnosis
This is from other types of vasculitis, which may cause scleritis or uveitis (Wegener's granulomatosis, polyarteritis nodosa, Behçet's disease). CS should be considered in any patient presenting with ocular inflammation and evidence of audiovestibular dysfunction.

Disease assessment
Severity of involvement of target organs should be carefully assessed.

Prognosis
There is an initial flare, which may last several weeks to months, followed by a chronic slowly progressive phase.
- Ocular outcomes are good. Blindness occurs in <5% of eyes.
- Deafness is a frequent and debilitating outcome occurring in up to 54% of patients. Corticosteroids may improve the outcome.
- Vestibular manifestations improve for most patients.
- Large vessel vasculitis with aortic incompetence can be associated with a poor prognosis.

Pathology
- Corneal biopsies may show plasma infiltrate and lymphocytes in the deeper layers of the cornea with scarring and neovascularization.
- The histology of vessels is similar to that seen in GCA, with an inflammatory infiltrate, intimal proliferation, disruption of the internal elastic lamina, and multinucleate giant cells.

Patient advice
Rare inflammatory disease of the eye and ear requiring treatment with steroids and possibly immunosuppressive therapy.

Treatment
- Glucocorticoids are the mainstay of treatment for acute flares, and recurrences of ocular and auditory inflammation.
- Keratitis and anterior uveitis usually respond to topical glucocorticoids
- Posterior scleritis and retinitis require oral glucocorticoids.
- Audiovestibular disease requires high dose oral glucocorticoids (prednisone 1–2 mg/kg/day).
- Resistant disease requires immunosuppression with methotrexate; ciclosporin, azathioprine, tacrolimus, and cyclophosphamide have all been tried.

Resources
Patient organizations
Vasculitis Foundation: www.vasculitisfoundation.org

References
Grasland A, Pouchout J, Hachulla E, Bletry O, Papo T, Vinceneux P, and the Study Group for Cogan's syndrome. Typical and atypical Cogan's syndrome: 32 cases and review of the literature. *Rheumatology* 2004; **43**: 1007–15.

Mazlumzadeh M, Matteson EL. Cogan's syndrome: an audiovestibular, ocular, and systemic autoimmune disease. *Rheum Dis Clin N Am* 2007; **33**: 855–74.

Behçet's disease

Behçet's Disease (BD) is a systemic vasculitis of unknown aetiology involving veins and arteries of all sizes, characterized by oro-genital ulceration and ocular involvement.

Diagnostic criteria

The International Study Group diagnostic criteria are widely used, but have not been formally validated.

> **International Study Group diagnostic criteria for Behçet's disease**
> Recurrent oral ulceration (aphthous or herpetiform) observed by a physician or the patient at least three times over one 12-month period.
> And two of the following:
> - Recurrent genital ulceration.
> - Eye lesions: anterior uveitis, posterior uveitis, cells in the vitreous by slit lamp examination, or retinal vasculitis.
> - Skin lesions: erythema nodosum, pseudofolliculitis, papulopustular lesions, or acneiform nodules in post-pubescent patients not on steroids.
> - Positive pathergy test.

Epidemiology

- The highest prevalence rates are in Turkey (8–38/10 000) and Japan (10/10 000).
- More common around the Mediterranean littoral, the Silk Route, and Japan.
- BD has been described in every ethnic group, but is rare in white Caucasians, and black Africans.
- Males and females are affected equally, but males tend to have more severe disease.
- Onset before puberty and after the age of 60 is uncommon.

Aetiology

- The aetiology is unknown; however, there is likely to be a strong genetic component, as the frequency varies considerably between different ethnic groups. Although often considered to be autoimmune in aetiology, there are few features of classic autoimmunity in BD.
- There is an association with HLA-B51, which is not found in other autoimmune diseases.
- There is a state of immune hyper-reactivity as evidenced by the pathergy reaction. There is overproduction of pro-inflammatory Th1 type cytokines.
- No clear infectious cause has yet been identified.

Clinical features

In the early stages, the symptoms can be non-specific and a high index of suspicion is required to achieve an early diagnosis. BD is multisystem and not all features will occur at presentation; therefore, a detailed past history is required, particularly with regard to genital ulceration, skin and eye involvement.

Key features on history

Oral ulcers

- These occur in 97–99% of patients and are frequently the first manifestation.
- They may occur many years before development of other manifestations.
- Oral ulceration can be minor, major or herpetiform. Minor ulcers are small, shallow, multiple ulcers. They constitute 90% of BD oral ulcers. They heal in 15 days. Major ulcers are large 1–3 cm in diameter and are slow to heal.

Genital ulcers

- These begin as papules or pustules that ulcerate quickly and tend to become infected.
- In men they occur typically on the scrotum and scar on healing.
- In women vaginal ulcers may go unnoticed, until they become infected. Formal gynaecological examination should be performed in all women suspected of BD.

Skin lesions
Skin involvement is common in BD but can be non-specific.

Pathergy

- This is a non-specific hyper-reactivity in response to minor trauma. It is characteristic of BD. A history of pathergy is often available with development of papules or pustules at the sites of venepuncture or intravenous cannulation.
- Pathergy most commonly occurs in patients from the Middle East, Far East, and the Mediterranean littoral.

Eye

- Eye involvement is the most serious manifestation of BD, and is a common cause of blindness and should be sought in all cases.
- The overall prevalence of eye involvement is 50%. It occurs frequently within the first 3 years and rarely after 5 years.

Nervous system

- Headaches are common feature of BD and may represent dural sinus thrombosis.
- Parenchymal lesions in the brain stem are the most common lesions seen in the CNS.

Vascular disease

- BD can involve both large arteries and veins. Venous involvement is more common (37%).
- Deep venous thrombosis of the legs is common. Arterial lesions are mainly aneurysmal and can rupture.
- Pulmonary artery involvement presents with recurrent haemoptysis, due to rupture into a bronchus.

Musculoskeletal

- Arthralgias and arthritis occur in 50%. It is usually mono or oligo-articular.
- Knee, ankle and wrist are the most common sites. It lasts a few weeks and is not destructive. The sacroiliac joints and axial skeleton are spared.

Gastrointestinal

- Lesions of BD occur throughout the GI tract and are histologically indistinguishable from inflammatory bowel disease.
- They are chronic, multiple deep ulcers associated with chronic inflammation and occasionally granulomata.

Key features on examination

X-ray
Chest radiography may show pulmonary artery aneurysms.

Differential diagnosis
- This is from other types of vasculitis. The key feature is the occurrence of oro-genital ulcers as there are very few other conditions in which this is a predominant feature.
- Oral ulcers must be differentiated from other causes of oral ulceration such as benign aphthous ulcers, viral infection, and inflammatory bowel disease. The oral ulcers of BD tend to be more frequent and multiple. Genital ulcers especially in the absence of oral ulcers need to be distinguished from herpetic ulcers or other viral ulcers, inflammatory bowel disease.
- MAGIC syndrome is an overlap between relapsing polychondritis and Behçet's disease. Mouth and genital ulcers with inflamed cartilage (MAGIC).

Prognosis
- Young males have an increased mortality.
- Ocular involvement can lead to blindness in 5–10%.
- Major vessel involvement (arterial or venous) is associated with mortality in 1–3% of patients.

Pathology
Histological examination of oral ulcers shows a lymphocytic and monocytic infiltrate in the basal layer and dermis with erosion of the epidermis.

Patient advice
General
Potentially serious multisystem condition, requiring immunosuppressive therapy and lifelong follow-up.

Treatment
Oro-genital ulceration
- Patients with minor aphthous like lesions may respond well to topical corticosteroids. Major and persistent lesions may require oral corticosteroids. Secondary infection should be treated with appropriate antibacterial or antifungal agents.
- Genital ulcers are often painful and a local analgesic gel may be required. Topical corticosteroids are usually necessary and may be applied using a gel. An asthma inhaler may be a convenient way of delivering topical steroids to relatively inaccessible regions.
- Colchicine and thalidomide are effective in controlling ulceration.

Ophthalmic
- Oral corticosteroids are used, but there are no controlled trials.
- Azathioprine in an RCT is effective at controlling ocular disease compared with placebo.
- Other drugs that are used include ciclosporin, interferon alpha, and tacrolimus.

Resources
Guidelines
EULAR recommendations for the management of Behçet's disease: report of a task force of the European Standing Committee for International Clinical Studies Including Therapeutics (ESCISIT).

Patient organizations
Behçet's Syndrome Society: www.behcets.org.uk

American Behçet's Disease Association: www.behcets.com

References
Hatemi G, Silman A, Bang D, Bodaghi B, Chamberlain M, Gul A, et al. EULAR recommendations for the management of Behçet's disease: report of a task force of the European Standing Committee for International Clinical Studies Including Therapeutics (ESCISIT). *Ann Rheum Dis* 2008 (in press).

International Study Group for Behçet's Disease. Criteria for diagnosis of Behçet's disease. *Lancet* 1990; **335**: 1078–80.

Henoch–Schönlein purpura

Henoch–Schönlein purpura (HSP) is an acute small vessel vasculitis occurring predominately in childhood. The classical triad is arthritis, palpable purpura, and abnormal renal sediment.

Classification
The CHCC defined HSP as:

> Vasculitis, with IgA-dominant immune deposits, affecting small vessels i.e. capillaries, venules, or arterioles). Typically involves skin, gut, and glomeruli, and is associated with arthralgia or arthritis.

Criteria
The ACR in 1990 developed classification criteria, which are widely used in clinical trials. There are no validated diagnostic criteria. Criteria for childhood HSP have recently been developed.

ACR classification criteria for Henoch–Schönlein purpura
1. **Palpable purpura:** slightly elevated purpuric rash over one or more areas of the skin not related to thrombocytopaenia.
2. **Bowel angina:** diffuse abdominal pain worse after meals, or bowel ischaemia, usually bloody diarrhoea.
3. **Age at onset <20 years:** development of first symptoms at age 20 years or less.
4. **Wall granulocytes on biopsy:** histological changes showing granulocytes in the walls of arteries or venules.

Note: for purposes of classification a patient shall be said to have Henoch–Schönlein purpura if at least 2 of these 4 criteria are present. The presence of any 2 or more criteria yields a sensitivity of 87.1% and specificity of 87.7% (from Mills et al., 1990).

Classification criteria for childhood HSP
Palpable purpura in the presence of at least one of:
- Diffuse abdominal pain
- Any biopsy showing predominant IgA deposition
- Arthralgia or arthritis
- Any haematuria and/or proteinuria.

From Ozen et al. (2006).

Epidemiology
- The peak age of onset is 5–7 years.
- The annual incidence is 135–180/million children aged 0–14 years.
- HSP is rare in adults (>16 years) with an incidence of 13/million.
- HSP is commoner in children of Asian and Caucasian origin than Afro-Caribbeans.
- Slightly more common in boys (1.2:1.0).

Aetiology
The aetiology is unknown. Report of associations with streptococci, mycoplasma, Bartonella, and viruses suggest an infectious aetiology, but no clear association has emerged. Seasonal peaks in incidence have been reported, but no consistent pattern has emerged in the various population studied.

A number of HLA associations have been reported including HLA B35 and DRB1*01 with nephritis. HSP nephritis and IgA nephropathy have been associated with deficiencies in C2 and C4, and with deletion of C4 genes.

Clinical features
Key features on history
Cutaneous
A rash is present in all cases, but is not always the presenting feature.

Gastrointestinal
- Abdominal pain, related to meals and suggestive of mesenteric ischaemia.
- Bloody diarrhoea.
- Nausea and vomiting.

Musculoskeletal
- Arthralgias with or without joint swelling may precede the rash by several days in up to 25% of cases, and occurs in 83% of children.
- The typical pattern is oligoarticular involving the legs.

Renal
- Nephropathy may present with gross haematuria lasting for a few days. In children renal involvement is usually only detected on urinalysis.
- Renal involvement occurs in up to 80% of adults and one third of children.

Other
Rarer manifestations include orchitis (9%), seizures 2% and (1%) duodenal obstruction (1%), intussusception (2%).

Key features on examination
Cutaneous
- Palpable purpura, most common over the posterior aspects of the legs and buttocks. The arms and trunk are less commonly involved.
- The rash is usually petechial or purpuric with macular and papular elements. Urticarial or vesicular lesions may be occasionally seen.
- Adults may develop skin necrosis particularly in dependent areas.

Musculoskeletal
Inflammatory synovitis most commonly affecting the lower limb joints, in an oligoarticular pattern.

Gastrointestinal
Diffuse abdominal tenderness, which may be sufficiently severe to mimic an acute abdomen. HSP can be complicated by intussusception in children and this must be considered with referral to paediatric surgery if suspected (palpable mass, bloody stool, signs of obstruction).

Renal
Rare. Features of nephrotic syndrome with peripheral oedema.

General investigations
The majority of children with a classical presentation do not need investigation to establish the diagnosis. It is imperative to perform a urinalysis for blood and check the blood pressure with an appropriately sized cuff. If there is any doubt of the diagnosis then further investigations

are required. In adults, the following investigations should be performed since the condition is much less common and usually more severe
- FBC and film. Anaemia (only if severe GI or renal haemorrhage), leucocytosis. Exclude idiopathic thrombocytopenic purpura and leukaemia.
- Coagulation screen normal.
- Acute phase response (ESR and CRP).
- Blood culture to rule out meningococcal septicaemia.

Assessment of organ involvement
In all patients
- Urinalysis (proteinuria, haematuria, red cell casts), should be performed urgently in all patients in whom HSP is suspected.
- Renal function (creatinine clearance, quantification of protein leak if present using either 24-h protein excretion or urine protein/creatinine ratio).
- Blood pressure.

Serological investigations
- ANA, ANCA, RF should all be negative. A positive ANA or ANCA suggests the presence of a connective tissue disease or other vasculitis.
- Complement levels are normal.

Biopsy
A renal biopsy should be considered in both children and adults if there is significant proteinuria or haematuria that persists (in children > 1 year).

Pathology
- IgA-dominant immune deposits are observed in the walls of small vessels and in the renal glomeruli.
- The cutaneous lesions of HSP show a small vessel vasculitis with involvement of the capillaries, post capillary venules and non-muscular arteries. There is often leucocytoclasis. The appearances are difficult to distinguish from leucocytoclastic (hypersensitivity) vasculitis or other small vessel vasculitis. IgA deposits are present in the skin lesions of HSP and may be a distinguishing feature.
- In the kidney the earliest lesion is focal or diffuse proliferative glomerulonephritis. The appearances may be indistinguishable from IgA nephropathy. Immunofluorescence reveals diffuse mesangial IgA deposition.

Differential diagnosis
The classical triad of palpable purpura, arthritis, and gastrointestinal involvement makes the diagnosis relatively easy in children. In adults, other types of vasculitis should be considered, especially in those who are ANCA or ANA positive.

Prognosis
- Overall, prognosis is determined by the extent of renal involvement.
- Most patients have a good prognosis and the illness is self-limiting, resolving within 2–3 weeks. Up to 50% of children have recurrences typically purpura and abdominal pain. Haematuria and proteinuria may persist for up to 1 year in 50% of children.

- Chronic renal failure develops in <5% of children and is associated with hypertension, nephritis or nephrotic syndrome at presentation.
- Renal failure is more common in adults.

Patient advice
- Self-limiting acute vasculitis, prognosis is generally good, with a low risk of recurrence.
- Risk of significant renal involvement is low but urine samples should be tested and blood pressure checked (by GP) initially weekly and then monthly for a year. Return if proteinuria occurs or haematuria does not resolve

Treatment
Most patients do not need specific therapy, as the condition is self-limiting. NSAIDs help arthralgia, but should be avoided in those with significant renal involvement.
The role of corticosteroids is controversial.
- Several RCTS have shown that in children the routine use of corticosteroids early in the disease process does not alter the progression to severe nephritis or GI complications (Huber et al., 2004; Ronkainen et al., 2006). In these studies oral prednisolone was used at a dose of 1–2 mg/kg/day tapering rapidly over 2–4 weeks. Prednisolone is, however, effective in reducing the severity of abdominal pain and arthralgias. Patients with severe abdominal should therefore probably receive corticosteroids. Rule out intussusception prior to treatment
- There are no RCTs to guide therapy in patients with rapidly progressive or established glomerulonephritis and these patients should receive immunosuppressive therapy with prednisolone combined with cyclophosphamide initially with maintenance azathioprine. For details see p. 562.
- Treatment of adults has been less well studied, but follows the same principles as childhood disease.

Resources
Internet resources
www.vasculitisfoundation.org

ICD-10 code
D69.0   Allergic purpura

References
Huber AM, King J, McKaine P, Klassen T, Pothos M. A randomised placebo controlled trial of prednisolone in early Henoch-Schönlein purpura. *Bio Med Central* 2004; **2**: 7.

Mills JA, Michel BA, Bloch DA, Calabrese LH, Hunder GG, Arend WP. et al. The ACR 1990 classification criteria for the classification of Henoch–Schönlein purpura. *Arthritis Rheum* 1990; **33**: 1114–21.

Ozen S, Ruperto N, Dillon MJ, et al. EULAR/PReS endorsed consensus criteria for the classification of childhood vasculitides. *Ann Rheum Dis* 2006; **65**: 936–41.

Ronkainen J, Koskimies O, Ala-Houhala M, et al. Early prednisone therapy in Henoch-Schönlein purpura: a randomized, double-blind, placebo-controlled trial. *J Pediatr* 2006; **149**: 241–7.

Saulsbury FT. Henoch-Schönlein purpura in children. Report of 100 patients and review of the literature. *Medicine (Baltimore)* 1999; **78**: 395–409.

Kawasaki disease

Kawasaki disease (KD) is an acute small and medium vessel vasculitis occurring in childhood with a predilection for the coronary arteries. Previously known as 'mucocutaneous lymph node syndrome'.

Diagnostic criteria
Criteria have been developed by the Japanese Kawasaki Research committee.

Diagnostic criteria for Kawasaki disease
1. **Fever persisting for 5 days**
2. **Bilateral conjunctival congestion**
3. **Oromucosal**
   - Reddening of lips.
   - Strawberry tongue.
   - Diffuse injection of oral and pharyngeal mucosa.
4. **Polymorphous exanthem**
5. **Peripheral extremities**
   - Initial stage:
     - reddening of palms and soles;
     - indurative oedema.
   - Convalescent stage: membranous desquamation from fingertips
6. **Acute non-purulent cervical lymphadenopathy**

At least five items are required for a diagnosis of KD. If coronary aneurysms are noted on 2D echocardiography or coronary angiography then 4 items are sufficient (from Kamiya, 1984).

Epidemiology
- In Japan the annual incidence is 150/100 000 children aged <4 years.
- 50% are aged <2 years.
- Onset age >10 years is rare.
- KD occurs worldwide, but is most prevalent in Japan and East Asia.
- In the UK the incidence is 14.6/100 000 in Indian Subcontinent Asians and 4.6/100 000 in White Caucasians.

Aetiopathogenesis
The aetiopathogenesis is unknown. An infectious aetiology has long been suspected. Cyclical epidemics have been observed especially in Japan supporting the notion that there is an infectious cause. So far no specific organism has been identified.

KD is similar to scarlet fever and toxic shock syndrome, and it has been suggested that KD is caused by toxin producing bacteria with superantigen activity. The acute phase of KD is associated with production of inflammatory cytokines, including TNF-alpha, IL-1B, and y-IFN with induction of endothelial injury via ELAM-1 and ICAM-1.

Pathology
Coronary arteritis begins with oedema in the media with a lymphocytic and macrophage infiltration. This spreads to cause a panarteritis involving all layers of the vessel wall. Around the twelfth day the artery begins to dilate, abnormal blood flow leads to thrombus formation and vascular occlusion. Inflammatory cell infiltration continues for 3–4 weeks and then resolves, leaving scarring.

Clinical features
Key features on history
Systemic
- Acute febrile illness lasting at least 5 days, unresponsive to NSAIDS/paracetamol.
- Cervical lymphadenopathy, may be unilateral.

Mucocutaneous
- Swelling of hands and feet, red palms and soles.
- Truncal rash.

Musculoskeletal
Acute polyarthralgia.

Cardiac
Angina, dyspnoea.

Key features on examination
The child is miserable.

Mucosal
- Bilateral conjunctival congestion, suffused without exudates.
- Erythema and fissuring of lips and oropharynx.
- Strawberry tongue.
- Non-purulent cervical lymphadenopathy.

Cutaneous
- Indurative oedema of hands and feet, erythema palms and soles.
- Polymorphous exanthema, perineal accentuation.
- Desquamation fingers and toes in convalescent period only.

Musculoskeletal
- Polyarthritis (less common).
- Irritability and aseptic meningitis are frequent, abdominal pain and diarrhoea, hydrops of gall bladder, and hepatomegaly rarer.

Cardiovascular
- Heart murmurs mitral regurgitation most common. Valvular heart disease occurs in 1% patients.
- Gallop rhythm.
- Faint heart sounds, suggestive of pericardial effusion. Pericarditis occurs in 13% patients.
- Peripheral artery aneurysms (1%).

General investigations
Investigation is directed at establishing the diagnosis, and assessing the extent and severity of organ involvement.
- FBC mild anaemia, leucocytosis with a left shift, thrombocytosis in the second week of illness.
- Acute phase response (significantly raised ESR and CRP).
- Elevated liver enzymes, hypoalbuminaemia.
- Urinalysis sterile pyuria, proteinuria.

Assessment of organ involvement
Cardiac
- **Electrocardiography:** prolonged PR/QT intervals, abnormal Q waves, low voltage, ST-T changes, dysrhythmias

- **Echocardiography:**
  - dilatation of coronary arteries;
  - coronary artery aneurysms are shown in 10–20% of patients;
  - pericardial effusion.
- **Angiography:**
  - coronary angiography enables accurate definition of coronary artery abnormalities and the severity of valvular lesions;
  - angiography should be performed in patients with cardiovascular involvement because there is a risk of progression to ischaemic heart disease especially in patients with giant aneurysms.

Serological investigations
- ANA, ANCA, RF all negative.
- Complement levels are normal.

Differential diagnosis
Conditions to be considered/excluded: Erythema multiforme/Steven's Johnson, scarlet fever, toxic shock syndrome, systemic JIA, measles, reactive arthritis.

Prognosis
- Generally good.
- The recurrence rate is 3.3%.
- Mortality is very low 0.1–0.2% and is due to acute myocardial infarction.
- 50% of coronary aneurysms regress at 2 years.
- KD is now the commonest cause of acquired cardiac disease, and may cause premature adult atherosclerosis.

Patient advice
- Potentially serious acute vasculitis, prognosis is generally good, with a low risk of recurrence.
- Risk of development of coronary aneurysms.

Treatment
Acute phase
- Aspirin high dose 80–100 mg/kg per day in divided doses for 14 days.
- Intravenous immunoglobulin (IVIg) 400 mg/kg for 4 days. When given within the first ten days the rate of aneurysm formation is reduced to 5% overall, and 15% for giant aneurysms.
- The combination of high dose aspirin and IVIg has been shown in an RCT to prevent coronary artery aneurysm formation (Neuberger et al., 1986, 1991, 2000).
- The optimal dose and timing of IVIg remains controversial and single doses of IVIg 2 g/kg has been show to be effective.
- Intravenous corticosteroids have been show in a recent RCT to confer no additional benefit when used in conjunction with IVIg.

Convalescent phase
- Aspirin 3–5 mg/kg for 6–8 weeks in those without coronary abnormalities.
- Aspirin should be continued in patients with coronary abnormalities until they have resolved.
- Anti-coagulation with warfarin should be considered in those with giant aneurysms.
- Other therapies.
  - Plasma exchange, TNF-alpha blockade with infliximab and cytotoxic therapy have all been used successfully but there is not controlled trial data to support their use.

Follow-up
- All children should have a repeat 2D echocardiography in the convalescent phase (4–6 weeks) regardless of initial echocardiography in accute phase.
- Regular 2D echocardiography is required in patients with coronary aneurysms to document regression.
- Management should be in conjunction with a paediatric cardiologist.

Resources
Patient organizations
Kawasaki disease foundation: www.kdfoundation.org

ICD 10 code
M30.3 Mucocutaneous lymph node syndrome (Kawasaki).

References
Kamiya T. *Research committee on Kawasaki disease.* Tkio: Ministry of Health and Welfare, 1984.

Newburger JW, Sleeper LW, McCridle BW, et al. Randomised trial of pulse corticosteroid therapy for primary treatment of Kawasaki disease. *N Engl J Med* 2000; **356**: 663–75.

Newburger JW, Takahashi M, Beiser AS, et al. A single infusion of gamma globulin as compared with four infusions in the treatment of acute Kawasaki syndrome. *N Engl J Med* 1991; **324**: 1633–9.

Newburger JW, Takahashi M, Burns JC, et al. The treatment of Kawasaki syndrome with intravenous gamma globulin. *N Engl J Med* 1986; **315**: 341–7.

Relapsing polychondritis

Relapsing polychondritis (RP) is a rare condition characterized by inflammation and destruction of cartilage.

Definition
Relapsing polychondritis is a rare condition characterized by recurrent episodes of inflammation and destruction of cartilage.

Diagnostic criteria
The following diagnostic criteria have been proposed.

> **Diagnostic criteria for relapsing polychondritis**
> - Recurrent chondritis of both auricles.
> - Non-erosive seronegative inflammatory polyarthritis.
> - Nasal chondritis.
> - Inflammation of ocular structures (conjunctivitis, keratitis, scleritis, episcleritis, uveitis).
> - Chondritis of the respiratory tract involving laryngeal and/or tracheal cartilage.
> - Cochlear and/or vestibular damage causing sensorineural hearing loss, tinnitus and/or vertigo.
>
> To establish a diagnosis of RP, patients must have one of the following:
> - At least three of the above clinical criteria.
> - One or more of the above clinical criteria in conjunction with cartilage biopsy confirmation.
> - Chondritis at two or more separate anatomical locations with response to steroids and/or dapsone.
>
> (From Michet et al., 1986).

Epidemiology
- The incidence in Rochester County, USA is 3.5/million.
- Males and females are affected equally.
- The peak age of onset is 50 years.
- More common around the Mediterranean littoral, the Silk Route, and Japan.
- RP has been described in every ethnic group.

Aetiology
The aetiology is unknown, but like many autoimmune conditions is generally believed to result from an environmental trigger interacting with a genetically predisposed host. Familial cases are rare.

There is an association with HLA-DR4. No infectious triggers have been identified. There is frequently a co-existent autoimmune disease.

Antibodies to type II collagen are found.

Clinical features
Initial symptoms may be non-specific with fever, weight loss and fatigue.

Key features on history
Cartilage inflammation
Auricular inflammation is present in almost all patients (85%). This involves the cartilaginous part of the pinna and spares the non-cartilaginous lobe (see Plate 17).

Musculoskeletal
Joint pain is a common feature. This can involve both large and small joints and the axial skeleton.

Respiratory
Dyspnoea with stridor is suggestive of tracheal involvement. Respiratory involvement is the most serious complication of RP. Up to 50% of patients have respiratory involvement.

Ophthalmic
Painful red eyes with blurred vision suggest scleritis or episcleritis.

Cutaneous
Skin involvement is common with purpura.

Key features on examination
Cartilage inflammation
- The pinna becomes red, painful, swollen. Inflammatory episodes last a few days or weeks.
- The pinna becomes floppy and loses its rigidity.
- There may be inflammation of the middle ear and audiovestibular structures.
- Nasal chondritis occurs in 50% of case, presenting with pain, erythema, swelling, stuffiness. The nasal bridge is destroyed and collapses.

Respiratory
- Tenderness over the trachea and thyroid cartilage.
- Larynx and racial inflammation leads to hoarseness, dry cough, dyspnoea, wheeze, and stridor.
- Damage to laryngeal and epiglottis may lead to upper airway collapse, which will require emergency tracheostomy.

Ophthalmic
There are recurrent episodes of episcleritis or scleritis, conjunctivitis, keratitis, and uveitis. Slit lamp examination may be required.

Cardiovascular
Uncommon, but is cause of death in RP patients, the most common involvement being complete heart block, aortic valve rupture, and acute aortic regurgitation.

Mucocutaneous
- Skin involvement is common. Purpura, papules, aphthosis, pustules, Biopsy may show a leucocytoclastic or lymphocytic vasculitis.
- MAGIC syndrome is an overlap between RP and Behçet's disease. Mouth and genital ulcers with inflamed cartilage (MAGIC).

General investigations
The diagnosis is usually made on the characteristic clinical features. Investigation is directed at establishing the diagnosis and assessing the extent and severity of organ involvement. There is evidence of inflammation.
- FBC anaemia, leucocytosis (to exclude co-existent haematological disease).
- Acute phase response (ESR and CRP).
- Liver function.

Imaging
CT
Fast sequence CT scanning can visual dynamic airway collapse.

Assessment of organ involvement
- Severity of involvement of target organs should be carefully assessed. In particular evidence tracheal involvement with pulmonary function tests including inspiratory and expiratory flow-volume curves.
- Biopsy of inflamed areas may confirm the diagnosis bit is not specific.

Serological investigations
- ANCA, ANA, RF, Anticardiolipin antibodies. These are usually negative unless there is co-existent autoimmune disease.
- Complement levels are normal
- Cryoglobulins are not detected

Differential diagnosis
This is from other types of chondritis and perichondritis. Infection may lead to perichondritis. Wegener's granulomatosis and lethal midline granuloma may lead to nasal destruction.

Prognosis
- The course is usually relapsing remitting. Mortality is low at 6% at 8 years.
- There is a risk of myelodysplasia.
- Most patients develop some disability with hearing or visual impairment, speech impediment

Pathology
Biopsy of the ear shows perichondritis with the presence of mononuclear cells and occasional polymorphonuclear leucocytes at the fibrochondral junction.

Patient advice
General
Potentially serious multisystem condition, requiring immunosuppressive therapy and lifelong follow-up.

Treatment
- There are no randomized controlled trials in RP. NSAIDs only are adequate for patients with mild chondritis.
- Laryngotracheal involvement requires corticosteroids at high doses (prednisolone 0.5–1.0 mg/kg). Long-term maintenance therapy may be required to control inflammation.
- Immunosuppression with methotrexate, azathioprine, leflunomide and ciclosporin has been reported to be effective in controlling chronic inflammation.
- The role of TNF-alpha blockade is still to be determined, but encouraging responses have been described.
- Acute airway obstruction refractory to medical treatment may require tracheostomy. Patients with tracheal collapse may be managed with stents.

Follow-up
RP is a relapsing condition and lifelong follow-up is required.

Resources
Patient organizations
www.vasculitisfoundation.org

Relapsing polychondritis support group. www.polychondritis.com

ICD-10 coding
M94.1   Relapsing polychondritis

References
Gergely P, Poor G. Relapsing polychondritis. *Best Prac Res Clin Rheumatol* 2004;**18**: 723–38.

Michet C, McKeena CH, Luthra HS, O'Fallon WM. Relapsing polychondritis. Survival and predictive role of early disease manifestations. *Annl Intern Med* 1986; **104**: 74–8.

Staats BA, Utz JP, Michet CJ. Relapsing polychondritis. *Semin Resp Crit Care Med* 2002; **23**: 145–54.

See also
Wegener's granulomatosis
Behcet's syndrome

Thromboangiitis obliterans

Thromboangiitis obliterans (TAO - Buergher's disease) is a rare thrombo-occlusive vasculopathy of medium and small arteries, characteristically occurring in young males smokers with distal leg ischaemia.

Classification and diagnostic criteria
There are no validated diagnostic or classification criteria.

The diagnosis is very likely in young smokers with distal lower limb ischaemia. In addition, the diagnosis should be considered in patients with at least two of the following three symptoms:
- Superficial thrombophlebitis.
- Arterial upper limb involvement.
- Raynaud's phenomenon.

The following must be excluded
- Diabetes mellitus.
- Atheroma.
- Embolism.
- Entrapment syndrome.
- Auto-immune disease.
- Myeloproliferative syndrome.
- Hypercoagulability states.

The occurrence of one symptom makes the diagnosis possible (from Puechal & Fiessinger, 2007).

Epidemiology
- In Europe and the USA, TAO accounts for 0.5-5% of patients with arterial disease, whilst in Japan up to 16% of such patients are affected.
- Males are affected much more frequently than women up to 10:1.
- Clinical onset is age <40 years.

Aetiology
There is a strong link with smoking, most patients being heavy smokers. Rechallenge after stopping smoking results in a recurrence of symptoms, suggesting that some component of tobacco is a key factor. A genetic component has been proposed, as TAO is more common in Ashkenazi Jews than non-Ashkenazi Jews in Israel. No association with HLA has been demonstrated. Impaired endothelium-dependent vasorelaxation in peripheral vasculature has been described in both affected and non-affected limbs. No clear evidence for autoimmunity has been found.

Clinical features
Key points on history
TAO usually presents with distal limb ischaemia in a young, male smoker.

Systemic
Systemic symptoms uncommon in TAO.

Ischaemia of legs
- Claudication of the foot is an early feature; diagnosis is often not made until rest pain and ulceration has developed;
- Rest pain is continuous and the patient has to sleep with feet hanging down.

Ischaemia of arms
Arm ischaemia occurs in 40–50% of cases, Allen's test is positive in 63%.

Superficial thrombophlebitis
- Superficial thrombophlebitis occurs in 40–60% of cases; deep venous thrombosis is suggestive of an alternative diagnosis;
- Migratory superficial thrombophlebitis in a young person is very suggestive of TAO.

Musculoskeletal
Arthralgias are not uncommon (15%), transient single joint inflammation. Wrists and knees are the most common joints. These may precede the onset of ischaemia by 10 years. The arthritis is not erosive.

Neurological
Neurological involvement and cerebral ischaemia is very rare.

Key features on examination
- Upper limb ischaemia. Allen's test. Place both thumbs to occlude the radial and ulnar arteries of one hand. The examiner releases the radial artery, but not the ulnar artery. If the radial artery distal to the wrist is patent, there is rapid return of colour to the hand (negative test). If the artery is occluded the hand will remain pale. The procedure can be repeated with the ulnar artery.
- Trophic changes, which may progress to gangrene.
- Superficial thrombophlebitis.

General investigations
Investigation is directed at establishing the diagnosis and excluding other causes of distal arteriopathy.
- FBC is normal, but excludes are myeloproliferative disorder.
- Elevated acute phase response (ESR and CRP) suggests a systemic vasculitis. They are normal or only marginally elevated in the absence of extensive trophic change.
- Modest hyperlipidaemia is compatible with TAO.
- Diabetes mellitus should be sought, as DM is an exclusion criterion for TAO.
- Thrombophilia screening is necessary to exclude a hypercoagulable state.

Serological investigations
ANCA, ANA, RF, anticardiolipin antibodies, complement levels, cryoglobulins will be negative or normal. Serology for HBV and HCV will be negative.

Differential diagnosis
This is from atherosclerosis and other forms of inflammatory vasculopathy.

Imaging
Angiography
There is no specific appearance of TAO. Angiography will reveal involvement in clinically uninvolved limbs.

The artery proximal to the lesion appears smooth and non-atherosclerotic. Small- and medium-sized vessels are involved in a segmental and bilateral pattern.

Disease assessment
Severity is assessed by the presence of rest pain and trophic changes.

Prognosis
- The course is relapsing and remitting with long periods of remission.
- Life expectancy is normal with up to 85% 25-year survival reported (Ohta et al., 2004)
- Overall, prognosis is determined by abstinence from smoking, with relapse being association with resumption of smoking.
- Progressive and recurrent amputations may be needed. The risk of amputation is strongly associated with continuation of smoking with 2.73 times increased risk. In smokers (Sasaki et al., 2000)

Pathology
- TAO is characterized histopathologically by a cellular and inflammatory thrombus formation primarily in distal extremities. Fibrinoid necrosis of arterial wall is not observed and the structure of the vessel wall is preserved. These features distinguish TAO from the systemic arteritides and atherosclerosis, in which there is fibrinoid necrosis in the former, and disruption of the internal elastic lamina and media in the latter.
- In the acute phase arterial and venous lesions are characterized by an association of inflammation and thrombus formation.

Patient advice
General
- Stop smoking.
- Attention to cardiovascular risk.
- Healthy balance diet.
- Regular exercise.

Treatment
- Cessation of smoking is the main stay of treatment and means of support should be proved to achieve this.
- Local care of trophic wounds is important.
- Prostacycline derivatives are effective, but must be given continuously often for several weeks.
- In an RCT of 152 patients of Iloprost IV daily compared with placebo plus aspirin, after 21–28 days of infusion with Iloprost 85% of patients had healed lesions or abolished pain compared with 17% receiving aspirin alone (Fiessinger et al., 1990). These results were maintained to 6 months and the amputation rate was lower in the Iloprost group 6% versus 18%).
- Oral Iloprost appears to be less effective.
- Revascularization is rarely possible due to the diffuse distal nature of the vascular disease.
- Experimental therapies include gene transfer using VEGF gene transfer; stem cell transplantation.

Resources
Information and support
Vasculitis Foundation: www.vasculitisfoundation.org

ICD-10 coding
I73.1

References
Fiessinger JN, Schaffer M. Trial of Iloprost versus aspirin treatment for critical limb ischaemia of thrmoboangiitis obliterans: the TAO study. *Lancet* 1990; **335**: 555–7.

Ohta T, Ishioashi H, Hosaka M, Sugimoto I. Clinical and social consequences of Buergher's disease. *J Vasc Surg* 2004; **39**: 176–80.

Puechal X, Fiessinger JN. Thromboangiitis obliterans or Buergher's disease: a challenge for the rheumatologist. *Rheumatology* 2007; **46**: 192–9.

Chapter 10

Juvenile idiopathic arthritis

Juvenile idiopathic arthritis: overview *352*
Oligoarticular juvenile idiopathic arthritis *358*
Rheumatoid factor (RF) negative polyarticular JIA *359*
Rheumatoid factor (RF) positive polyarticular JIA *360*
Systemic onset JIA *362*
Juvenile PsA *364*

Juvenile idiopathic arthritis: overview

Long-term studies have shown that juvenile idiopathic arthritis (JIA) is not as benign as previously thought, with approximately 50% of adults suffering from persistent inflammation and disability (Packham, 2002). There has been a shift towards early aggressive treatment to limit inflammation and achieve a normal lifestyle, since there is some evidence for a better long-term prognosis with this approach. The development of drugs such as the anti-cytokine agents for disease resistant to conventional treatment has greatly improved disease management.

Definition

JIA is defined as arthritis (swelling or limitation of motion of the joint accompanied by heat, pain or tenderness) of unknown aetiology beginning before the 16th birthday and persisting for at least 6 weeks where other known conditions are excluded. Historically, there have been a number of classifications, but the most recent by The International League of Associations for Rheumatology (ILAR) has widely been accepted. It was revised in 2001. The importance is primarily in classification for research purposes, but is also a useful clinical tool. With further research into the genetics and cytokines involved in JIA, classification will no doubt be revised further. We will deal with JIA as a whole in this chapter. Subsequent chapters will discuss specific subtypes separately.

The ILAR classification of JIA

Systemic onset arthritis (systemic onset JIA)

Arthritis with or preceeded by daily fever of at least 2 weeks duration that is documented to be quotidian* for at least 3 days, and accompanied by one or more of the following:
- Evanescent, non-fixed, erythematous rash.
- Generalized lymph node enlargement.
- Hepatomegaly and/or splenomegaly.
- Serositis**.

Exclusions: a–d (see below).

*Quotidian fever is defined as a fever that rises to >39°C once a day and returns to <37°C between fever peaks.
**Pericarditis and/or pleuritis and/or peritonitis.

Oligoarthritis (oligoarticular JIA)

Arthritis affecting one to four joints during the first 6 months of disease. Two subcategories are recognized:
- **Persistent oligoarthritis:** affects no more than four joints throughout the disease course.
- **Extended oligoarthritis:** affects a total of more than four joints after the first 6 months of disease.

Exclusions: a–e (see below).

Polyarticular JIA (RF negative)

Arthritis affecting five or more joints during the first 6 months of disease. Tests for rheumatoid factor (RF) are negative.

Exclusions: a–e (see below).

Polyarticular JIA (RF positive)

Arthritis affecting five or more joints during the first six months of disease; two or more tests for RF at least 3 months apart are positive.

Exclusions: a–e (see below).

Juvenile psoriatic arthritis (JPsA)

Arthritis and psoriasis (Ps) or arthritis and at least two of the following:
- Dactylitis†.
- Nail pitting¶ or onycholysis.
- Psoriasis in a first degree relative.

Exclusions: b–e (see below).

†Swelling of one or more digits, usually asymmetrical extending beyond the joint margin.
¶Minimum of 2 pits on any one or more nails at any time.

Enthesitis-related arthritis (ERA)

(See Juvenile SpA/ERA, Chapter 7 on p. 232)

Arthritis and enthesitis, or arthritis or enthesitis with at least two of the following:
- Sacroiliac (SIJ) tenderness and/or inflammatory lumbosacral pain (at rest with morning stiffness, improves on movement).
- The presence of HLA-B27 antigen.
- Onset of arthritis in a male >6 years of age.
- Acute (symptomatic) anterior uveitis.
- History of AS, ERA, sacroiliitis with inflammatory bowel disease, reactive arthritis or acute anterior uveitis in a 1st degree relative.

Exclusions: a, d, e (see below).

Enthesitis: tenderness at the insertion of a tendon, ligament, joint capsule, or fascia to bone.

Undifferentiated arthritis

Arthritis that doesn't fulfil inclusion criteria for any category or is excluded by fulfilling criteria for >1 category.

Exclusion criteria

(a) Ps/history of Ps in the patient or 1st degree relative.
(b) Arthritis in HLA-B27+ male starting after 6th birthday.
(c) AS, enthesitis-related arthritis, sacroiliitis with inflammatory bowel disease, Reiter's syndrome or acute anterior uveitis or a history of one of these disorders in a first degree relative.
(d) The presence of IgM RF on at least two occasions more than 3 months apart.
(e) The presence of systemic JIA in the patient.

Epidemiology

JIA has an incidence in the UK of 1 in 10 000 and a prevalence of 1 in 1000 (similar to that of diabetes) with a female predominance (Symmons, 1996). It is described in all races and geographic areas, but large regional variations exist. The aetiology remains unknown.

Aetiology and pathophysiology

There is good evidence that T-cells play an important role with recruitment to the joint by up-regulation of adhesion molecules on synovial endothelium and retention in the joint of activated cells.
- The pattern of cytokine expression is of the Th1 type.
- Pro-inflammatory cytokine levels in the joint are high. From T-cells: TNFα, Interferon γ, IL2, macrophage inhibitory factor (MIF). From monocytes: TNFα, IL1, IL6, IL8, IL12.

- Regulatory T-cells and anti-inflammatory cytokines (IL4, IL10 and TGFβ) appear reduced.
- A number of HLA class I and class II antigens are found in association with sub-types of JIA.
- HLA-A2 with early onset oligoarthritis in girls. Twin and sibling studies lend weight to genetic susceptibility.

Environmental
The notion that an infectious agent triggers JIA is attractive, but as yet unproven. There appears to be interaction between microbes and the immune system triggering JIA in a susceptible child.

Clinical features
Key features in the history
It goes without saying that the history will be taken from both the child (if old enough), and the parent or carer.
- Sensitivity is required in the young person who might want to consult with you on his or her own, and/or with their parent/carer.
- The child or young person's functioning at home and at school is critical to the assessment. What can they do for themselves? What do they need help with that they used to be able to do? Do they use any aids or appliances? This can be assessed using the Children's Health Assessment Questionnaire (CHAQ), which is helpful in clinical assessment and is critical for research purposes and in assessing response to therapy (see p. 4).

Key features on examination
'Every joint, every time'.
- Since children may not be able to express where there is pain and stiffness, it is critical that every joint is examined on every contact with the clinician.
- All too often a child is subjected to a knee aspiration for presumed sepsis, when careful examination would have revealed toe dactylitis or a swollen ankle.
- It is helpful in the infant/small child to examine the ankle from behind, whilst the child is standing.
- Examine small children on their parents lap with ready access to distracting toys. Perform a PGALS (paediatric gait, arms, legs, spine) examination for screening and hone in on affected joints for detailed examination (DVD available from ARC) (see p. 11).
- Perform a careful systematic examination at the initial assessment (rash, nail changes, mouth ulcers, hepatosplenomegaly, respiratory, or cardiac findings, weakness, scalp/hair changes, etc.).

Co-morbidities
Co-morbidity can arise as a result from JIA- associated lesions in extra-articular organs, from long-term complications of the conditions or their treatment.
- Most complications of JIA can be avoided with early diagnosis and aggressive control of disease.
- Complications and co-morbidities include poor dentition, osteoporosis, and growth failure (disease severity and GC use associated), infections secondary to immune suppression, VZ in particular, blindness owing to anterior uveitis, amyloidosis and macrophage activation syndrome (haemophagocytosis) (see Plate 20).
- Psychosocial problems with depression, anxiety, loss of schooling/education and peer interaction can be a particular problem in adolescents.

- Disability accumulates from a multitude of effects but specific musculoskeletal disability can arise from leg length discrepancy (overgrowth of growth plates around affected joints), postural scoliosis (secondary to leg length discrepancy) and joint contractures (fixed loss of extension commonly).

Investigations
No investigation is diagnostic of JIA. The diagnosis is made clinically with consistent investigation findings.

Laboratory
- FBC/CBC: haemoglobin may be low (normocytic normochromic, or microcytic commonly). White cell count normal/mildly raised (with normal differential). Platelets commonly mildly raised.
- Erythrocyte sedimentation rate (ESR) and C-reactive protein (CRP) are often mildly raised.
- Antinuclear antibody (ANA) if consistently raised suggests an increased risk of associated iritis.
- RF, dsDNA and HLA B27 are helpful in classification.
- Serology for suspected viral or bacterial triggers if history suggestive of reactive arthritis and for *Varicella zoster* titres to check immunity (as may subsequently consider immunosuppressants).

Imaging
- Radiographs of affected joints are usually normal in early arthritis. They can show joint effusions, peri-articular osteoporosis, soft tissue swelling or surprises, such as evidence of trauma, osteomyelitis, malignancy.
- Ultrasound (US) examination can show joint effusion and synovitis (especially where clinical examination is difficult, such as the hips).
- Magnetic resonance (MR) shows joint anatomy and shows early changes in cartilage. Gadolinium enhancement may be more sensitive in detection of synovitis compared with routine T2-weighted sequences.
- In young children, good preparation by a play specialist is essential to obtain good images. A general anaesthetic may be necessary.

Other
Arthrocentesis should be performed if septic arthritis is suspected. Straw coloured fluid with a high white cell count, but no organism cultured is typical of JIA.

Differential diagnosis
The differential diagnoses for all subtypes of JIA are similar and their key features are listed in the table below.

Disease activity assessment and monitoring
Combinations of measures are employed including joint counts, pain measures, acute phase measures, and global assessments.
- Active joint score – those joints with tenderness, and/or pain and/or swelling, with swelling being the most objective of these parameters, but difficult to detect in neck, hip, shoulder, temporomandibular joint (TMJ). The restricted joint count measures joints with a limited range of movement and may count joints with previously active disease.
- Pain may reflect current active disease or joint damage from previous disease activity and should be routinely monitored. Simple methods utilize a visual analogue scale (e.g. as part of the CHAQ).

Condition	Features
Septic arthritis	Usually (but not invariably) single joint; fever and systemically unwell. Severe joint pain. Inability to weight-bear. Raised ESR and CRP. Leucocytosis. Arthrocentesis with stain, culture and antigen testing prudent. Tuberculous – typically chronic monoarthritis eventually causing severe destruction.
Osteomyelitis	Fever. Severe bone pain extending beyond joint margins. Local swelling and/or erythema; pseudoparalysis – young infants and children stop using a limb, although they may not be able to say it hurts. Maintain a low index of suspicion in neonates or immunocompromised children, as easily missed. Bone scan or MR scan helpful. Under 18 months highly likely to extend to the joint and include a septic arthritis; radiograph changes seen late (weeks).
Reactive and post-infectious arthritis	Secondary to infection with enteric organisms. Asymmetric oligoarticular pattern. Viral infections (rubella, measles, mumps, parvovirus, varicella, hepatitis) and vaccinations can cause a short-lived reactive arthritis responsive to NSAIDs.
Rheumatic fever	Diagnosis made on the presence of two major criteria (carditis, polyarthritis, chorea, erythema marginatum, subcutaneous nodules) or one major and two minor criteria (arthralgia, fever) plus evidence of group A streptococcal infection (throat swab or rising titres). Raised ESR or CRP, prolonged PR interval on ECG, raised or rising ASOT or anti DNAseB antibody tests are supportive. The arthritis is often migratory and short-lived.
Lyme disease	Weeks to months after infection with *Borrelia burgdorferi*. History of tick bite may or may not be elicited. Large joint oligoarthritis (typically knee), usually lasting days to weeks completely resolving for weeks before recurring in the same joint or elsewhere. *Erythema migrans* – spreading pink rash following the bite. Lethargy and general malaise with fever. Neurological or cardiac abnormalities also occur. Diagnosis is made on serological testing.
Trauma	In young infants and children a history of trauma may not be elicited. Consider non-accidental injury if evidence of trauma without a history or inconsistent history.
Mechanical	Mechanical musculoskeletal pains occur after activity or later in the day. Diagnoses include: joint hypermobility syndrome, Perthe's disease, slipped capital femoral epiphysis, spondylolysis, and spondylolisthesis
Pain syndromes	Non-inflammatory and non-mechanical pain should be considered such as pain amplification, chronic pain syndrome (localized or generalized), Chronic regional pain syndrome (1 or 2).
Inflammatory bowel disease	Arthritis may be the first presenting symptom of IBD. Weight loss/faltering growth. Mouth ulcers/anal skin tags. Family history of HLAB27 associated conditions.
Systemic diseases	Rickets. Haemaglobinopathies. Haemophilia. Diabetes mellitus. Hyperparathyroidism. Glycogen storage disorders.
Malignancy	Symptoms suggestive of malignancy include night pain, non-articular bone pain, back pain, systemically unwell, weight loss, pallor, bruising. *Investigations:* raised ESR in presence of low/normal platelets, raised LDH, abnormal blood film. Where there is suspicion do a bone marrow aspirate or specific imaging. Differentials include leukaemia, lymphoma, neuroblastoma, Ewings sarcoma, and bone tumours.
Autoimmune connective tissue disease	Systemic lupus erythematosus (SLE). Juvenile dermatomyositis (JDM). Henoch Schönlein purpura (HSP). Sarcoid: polyarthritis, rash, uveitis, hepatosplenomegaly, malaise, boggy large joints and tendon sheath effusions with minimal pain, serum ACE positive in only 50%. Diagnosis on biopsy.

- ESR and CRP are relatively insensitive to disease activity, although a persistently elevated ESR and platelet count over 6 months is associated with later erosions.
- Physician global assessment score is used, measured on a 10-cm visual analogue scale
- Parent and patient scored global assessment of overall well-being is valuable.

Disease damage
Radiographic appearances are relatively insensitive measures of change in JIA unless there is a severely aggressive RF positive polyarthritis or psoriatic JIA (JPsA). In adults US or MR scans can show cartilage damage before the appearance of erosions, but as yet there is no evidence for this in children.

Function and quality of life
The Child Health Assessment Questionnaire (CHAQ) is a validated measure of function, which is not specific to children with JIA but has been shown to be sensitive to change in this group.
- Global measures of 'quality of life', which indicate an individual's 'well-being', and includes physical, psychological, and social factors have been developed for children. They include health-related quality of life (HRQOL) measures (e.g. PedsQL), which has a generic and a rheumatology module to it.

Core set outcome variables for JIA
The Paediatric ACR score was developed in 1997 by Giannini to standardize assessments and allow for outcomes to be measured in clinical trials. These variables can be routinely monitored in paediatric rheumatology clinics, as they are quick and easy to carry out.

> **Paediatric ACR score: core set outcome variables for children being treated for JIA**
> - Physician global assessment of disease activity [10-cm Visual Analogue Scale (VAS)].
> - Parent/patient global assessment of overall well-being (10-cm VAS).
> - Functional ability (CHAQ).
> - Number of joints with active arthritis.
> - Number of joints with limited range of motion.
> - ESR.

Treatment

Objectives
Medical management of JIA has changed in recent years with an overriding principle of early and aggressive treatment to suppress inflammation and prevent progression to the complications detailed above. To this end, intra-articular glucocorticoids (GCs) are used early, with progression to methotrexate as the first line disease modifying anti-inflammatory drug (DMARD) and the use of biological therapy where necessary.

Multidisciplinary team
A multidisciplinary team working effectively together best manages all children with JIA.
- A paediatric rheumatology nurse specialist for disease and medication education, and co-ordination of care.
- Physiotherapy to help reverse the effects of the disease once it is under control (encourage full range of joint motion and strengthen atrophied muscles).
- Occupational therapy (OT) to assess and provide appliances where necessary to encourage independence, and school liaison to ensure teachers are aware and encouraging activity with guidance.
- Orthotist (or podiatrist).
- Ophthalmology liaison.
- Dentist, orthodontist, maxillofacial surgeon where necessary.
- Informed musculoskeletal radiologist.
- Orthopaedic surgery for an opinion on the role of timely joint surgery.
- Social worker where needed to help address impact on family financially (Disability Living Allowance).
- Psychologist and play specialist to help with issues around impact of disease on child/adolescent/family, issues of compliance, difficulties with needle phobia, imaging, joint injections, etc.
- Dietician to optimize nutrition, advise, and supervise calcium and vitamin D supplementation.
- In addition, transition to adult services, addressing sexual health issues and liaison with the general practitioner are critical. Further detail in this chapter will concentrate on medical management.

Pain relief
Non-steroidal anti-inflammatory drugs (NSAIDs)
NSAIDs are used for the initial treatment of pain, inflammation, and stiffness.
- Gastrointestinal side effects are common to all, but they are usually well tolerated in children. Gastroprotective medication may be required if symptoms occur.
- There are few comparative data to aid prescribing NSAIDs, and choices are usually made on the tolerability of the formulation and dosage schedule.
- Ibuprofen syrup is commonly used at a dose of 10 mg/kg/dose tds or qds (up to 6x day in systemic JIA), since it is palatable and well tolerated. The disadvantage is the dosing schedule.
- Naproxen was compared with piroxicam in a multicentre double-blind crossover study in 47 children with JIA, and no significant difference in clinical variables or patient preference was found (Williams, 1986).
- A dispersible formulation of piroxicam is available and naproxen syrup can be obtained if ordered specifically.
- Naproxen, diclofenac and tolmetin (not available in UK) were compared in a single-blind cross-over trial in 28 children with (RF) seronegative JIA with clinical improvement in all three and increased adverse events in diclofenac (Leak, 1988).
- Meloxicam (selective COX-2 inhibitor) has been shown to be effective in JIA, but no comparative studies have been carried out.

Immunosupression
Glucocorticoids
Intra-articular GC injections are a well-established treatment in JIA and are used early to gain rapid control of joint inflammation, solely in oligoarticular disease, and as an adjuvant in polyarticular disease.
- Indications will be described further under the types of JIA, but in general, those children with no systemic symptoms can have up to a maximum of 10 injections.
- It will depend upon the individual and the number/type of joints to be injected as to whether this done under general or local anaesthetic, but in general those under 12 should be offered a general anaesthetic.
- Children over 12 may manage with local anaesthesia and access to entonox or sedation with midazolam.
- Triamcinolone hexacetonide at a dose of 1 mg/kg for large joints, 0.5 mg/kg small joints, is the GC of choice having been shown to give better results than triamcinolone acetonide, betamethasone, and methylprednisolone acetate.
- Pulsed intravenous (IV) methylprednisolone at a dose of 30 mg/kg/day on 3 consecutive days (maximum 1 g daily) and repeated 1 week later as necessary is valuable for achieving rapid control of symptoms in polyarticular or systemic onset JIA.
- IV GC regimes may result in less cumulative GC dosage than an oral GC regime alone. If GCs are required to maintain disease control they should be given at the lowest possible daily (or alternate daily) dosage. If systemic GCs are required, a disease-modifying agent should be started for longer-term disease control.

Methotrexate
Methotrexate (MTX) is the first-line disease modifying anti-rheumatic drug (DMARD) for the vast majority of children with JIA.
- MTX is safe, reliable and effective in at least 60-70% of children treated for JIA, although the maximal benefit may not be evident for 9–12 months.
- Evidence suggests that a dose of 15 mg/m^2/week is optimal (range 10–20 mg/m^2/week).
- Subcutaneous (sc) MTX is superior in terms of bioavailability and tolerance compared to oral MTX (at the higher doses). Oral MTX may be sufficient for relatively mild disease.
- Oral MTX is available in tablet or syrup forms. Parents should be discouraged from crushing tablets and mixing with food because of the risk to the parent of handling cytotoxic medication. For some children refusing medication, however, this is the method of last resort.
- Appropriate counselling is required prior to commencing methotrexate and immunity to chickenpox should be known. There may be time to recommend immunization with *Varicella zoster* (VZ) vaccine in children known to be VZ IgG negative, but this will require delaying MTX or GCs for 6–8 weeks post-vaccination.

- Children >12 years often need two doses of VZ vaccine, 4–6 weeks apart to seroconvert, delaying treatment still further.
- If the child is susceptible to chicken pox, parents need clear instructions on consulting following a chicken pox contact for consideration of VZ immunoglobulin or acyclovir treatment.
- Concurrent immunosuppression with GCs increases the risk of complicated VZ infection substantially.

Information to be discussed before starting MTX

- Avoid all live vaccinations.
- Seek advice from paediatric rheumatology team if VZ contact and non-immune.
- Seek advice from paediatric rheumatology team if acutely unwell with intercurrent infection (missing a dose may be advised).
- Monitor FBC and LFT monthly initially, then 6–8-weekly when stable (ESR /CRP for disease monitoring).
- Ensure adequate contraception.
- Minimize alcohol intake.
- If prescribed other medications ensure prescriber is aware of MTX treatment (potential interactions).
- Side effects of MTX (nausea, vomiting, mouth ulcers, anorexia, alopecia, transient rise in ALT, leucopenia) and occur in about 20% of children.
- Folic acid has been shown to benefit adults, although there is no evidence for benefit in children. Dose regimes include 1 mg/day (except on day of MTX) or 5mg/week, syrup or tablet formulations available.
- Switching from oral to sc MTX may resolve nausea. Most families learn to administer sc MTX at home.

Other DMARDS

Sulphasalazine (SZP) can be beneficial for ERA. Hydroxychloroquine confers little benefit alone, but is used in combination with MTX, particularly for juvenile systemic lupus erythematosus (SLE).

Anti-TNFα treatment

In those children who fail to respond adequately to MTX (and have ongoing swollen joints or require ongoing GCs), or who are unable to tolerate MTX, it is now common practice to use anti-TNFα therapy.

- UK National Institute of Clinical Excellence (NICE) guidance for the use of etanercept in JIA advises that etanercept should be reserved for children with JIA where MTX has failed (at a dose of 20 mg/m^2/week by sc injection for 3 months).
- Etanercept is the only licensed anti-TNFα to treat JIA in children, and studies show impressive benefits [74% achieved JRA30 (Lovell, 2000)] at a standard dose of 400 μg/kg twice a week.
- Nevertheless, long-term follow up of Etanercept treatment is lacking and all children should be registered on a Biologics Registry (in the UK – www.bsparreg.org).
- Side effects include injection site reactions, headaches, urticaria, abdominal pain, nausea, and vomiting.

Infliximab is a chimeric monoclonal anti-TNFα, which is given by iv infusion every 4–12 weeks.

- In a small non-randomized, open-label study of 24 JIA patients Infliximab was shown to have equivalent efficacy to, but increased side effects compared with, etanercept (Lahdenne, 2003).
- Infliximab (unlicensed in UK) may be useful in children with compliance issues or side effects to etanercept.
- Adalimumab is a humanized monoclonal antibody to TNFα given by sc injection every 2 weeks. Adalimumab has showed some efficacy in polyarticular JIA in preliminary studies (Lovell, 2004).
- Anakinra, a recombinant IL-1 receptor antagonist, injected daily, is also showing promising results in JIA with response documented in 58% of patients after 4 months treatment.

Autologous stem cell transplantation

This still experimental treatment is used only as a last resort in children with an intolerably poor quality of life because of the high morbidity and mortality associated with treatment. Intensive immunosuppression to remove autoreactive lymphocytes is followed by rescue therapy with haematopoietic stem cells – data are published on 34 children within nine centres in Europe. Eighteen children (53%) achieved complete drug-free remission and a 15% mortality rate was reported.

Surgery

Orthopaedic operations are required infrequently. Access to the expertise of a paediatric orthopaedic surgeon is important. Indications for surgery may include:

- Poor jaw growth (micrognathia and overbite possibly requiring maxillofacial surgery).
- Joint deformity and destruction requires joint replacement surgery as in adults.

Prognosis

Available long-term outcome studies reflect historical treatment regimes and make for sober reading – 40% of children with JIA take their arthritis with them to adulthood (Packham, 2002) and between 30–56% have severe functional limitations.

- Unemployment is 3× higher in JIA patients compared with controls despite excellent educational results.
- Poor prognostic indicators include polyarticular/ systemic onset, poor disease control in the first 6 months, presence of autoantibodies (ANA and RF), and rapid development of erosive changes.

Resources

Assessment tools

CHAQ (see www.arc.org.uk); PGALS (joint examination of young children); HRQoL; PedsQL; Paediatric ACR score. British society for paediatric and adolescent rheumatology www.bspar.org.uk for eye screening guidelines.

Guidelines

British Society for Paediatric and Adolescent Rheumatology. UK guidelines on medication, link to NICE guidelines, CHAQ and scoring available. www.bspar.org.uk

Paediatric Rheumatology European Society: www.pres.org.uk

NICE. Guidance on the use of etanercept for the treatment of juvenile idiopathic arthritis, March 2002, Ref. N0070. www.nice.org.uk

Arthritis Research Campaign: http://www.arc.org.uk/arthinfo/medpubs/6535/6535.asp
www.arc.org.uk/arthinfo/emedia.asp#pGALS

Patient information

Paediatric Rheumatology International Trials Organization. www.printo.it/ (good information for families and resource for research activity).

Arthritis Research Campaign. www.arc.org.uk – useful patient information.

ICD10 codes
M08   Juvenile arthritis
M08.0   Juvenile RA
M08.2   Juvenile arthritis with systemic onset
M08.4   Pauciarticular juvenile arthritis

References

Gylis-Morin VM, Graham TB, Blebea JS, et al. Knee in early juvenile rheumatoid arthritis: MR imaging findings. *Radiology* 2001; **220**: 696–706

Lahdenne P, Vahasalo P, Honkanen V. Infliximab or etanercept in the treatment of children with refractory juvenile idiopathic arthritis; an open label study. *Ann Rheum Dis* 2003; **62**: 245–7.

Leak AM, Richter MR, Clemens LE, et al. A crossover study of naproxen, diclofenac and tolmetin in seronegative juvenile chronic arthritis. *Clin Exp Rheumatol* 1988; **6**: 157–60.

Lovell DJ, Giannini EH, Reiff A, Cawkwell GD, et al. Etanercept in children with polyarticular juvenile rheumatoid arthritis. *N Engl J Med* 2000; **342**: 763–800.

Lovell DJ, Ruperto N, Goodman S, et al. Preliminary data from the study of adalimumab in children with juvenile idiopathic arthritis. *Arthritis Rheum* 2004; **50** (Suppl): S436.

Packham JC, Hall MA. Long-term follow-up of 246 adults with juvenile idiopathic arthritis: functional outcome. *Rheumatology (Oxf)* 2002; **41**: 428–35.

Packham JC, Hall MA. Long-term follow-up of 246 adults with juvenile idiopathic arthritis: functional outcome. *Rheumatology* 2002; **41**: 1428–35.

Petty RE, Southwood TR, Manners P, et al. International League of Associations for Rheumatology classification of juvenile arthritis: second revision, Edmonton, 2001. *J Rheumatol* 2004; **31**: 390–2.

Ravelli A, Martini A. Juvenile idiopathic arthritis. *Lancet* 2007; **369**: 767–79.

Symmons DP, Jones M, Osborne J, et al. Pediatric rheumatology in the United Kingdom: data from the British Pediatric Rheumatology Group National Diagnostic Register. *J Rheumatol* 1996; **23**: 1975–80.

Williams PL, Ansell BM, Bell A, et al. Multicentre study of piroxicam versus naproxen in juvenile chronic arthritis, with special reference to problem areas in clinical trials of nonsteroidal anti-inflammatory drugs in childhood. *Br J Rheumatol* 1986; **25**: 67–71.

See also
Juvenile SpA/ERA

Oligoarticular juvenile idiopathic arthritis

Oligoarticular JIA (oligo-JIA) is the commonest type of JIA and occurs in over 50% of JIA cases. Some oligo-JIA cases 'extend' over time to involve >4 joints evolving >6 months after onset.

Epidemiology
Early onset persistent oligoarthritis is characterized by onset less than 6 years of age, female predominance, asymmetric arthritis, uveitis, and ANA positivity.
- Oligo-JIA is common in European and North American Caucasians, rare in Asian, Arab, and African children.
- Persistent oligo-JIA is associated with HLA A2 and Class II HLA alleles DR8, DR5, and DR6. Extended oligo-JIA, by contrast, is associated with DR1.
- The differential diagnosis is detailed in the JIA chapter. A septic arthritis is the primary differential. Rarely, a haemangioma can cause joint swelling and pain.

Clinical features
Key features in the history
Typically children complain about a single swollen joint usually of the lower limb, which causes stiffness and limited movement.
- Often children report less pain than expected. Thus, the differential of septic arthritis is relatively easily made.
- The joint swelling is often noted by a parent before the child is thought to be in pain or complains of pain, and is sometimes revealed by an episode of minor trauma.
- The child is otherwise well with an unremarkable history and often no past history to note.
- A family history of psoriasis should be sought.
- Any preceding infection is important, particularly an episode of infection suggestive of a streptococcal sore throat, diarrhoea, or tick bite.

Key features on examination
Physicians often find more affected joints than parents have identified.
- It is important to carefully examine all joints – synovial swelling, warmth, effusion, and limitation without much tenderness are hallmark features.
- Knee and ankle are most commonly affected. Hips, neck, and TMJ are not affected initially.
- Look for nail dystrophy or nail pitting, and hidden psoriasis present in scalp or umbilicus. Look for enthesitis tenderness or swelling (more likely ERA, especially in male >6 years) and dactylitis (psoriasis).
- Wrist and upper limb involvement, symmetrical joint involvement and an ESR >20 mm/h are predictive of extended oligo-JIA.
- Asymmetrical increased growth and muscle atrophy of the involved limb is characteristic.
- Involved joints mature faster than their opposite. A valgus knee is common in untreated disease.
- Asymmetric jaw opening can develop with unilateral temporomandibular (TMJ) involvement (usually in extended oligo-JIA).

Co-morbidities
Uveitis
The most serious complication for children with oligo-JIA is blindness from uveitis (iridocyclitis).
- Uveitis is diagnosed in up to 30%, is associated with positive ANA, and is insidious and asymptomatic.
- The iris and ciliary body are principally involved resulting in deposition of cells in the anterior chamber, and formation of synechiae or band keratopathy.
- Slit-lamp examination is critical early in the diagnosis of Oligo-JIA and regular check-ups are necessary.
- Most children develop uveitis within the first 5–7 years of onset of arthritis. The course can be relapsing or chronic and does not parallel the course of arthritis.
- Treatment is with topical GCs and mydriatics, and close monitoring to judge benefit.
- In uveitis resistant to topical treatment, systemic GCs and DMARDs, usually MTX, are used initially.
- Ciclosporin and azathioprine can also be used. There are anecdotal reports on the benefits of infliximab in cases resistant to MTX.

Conditions related to growth and skeletal development
See also JIA chapter.

Leg length discrepancy is commonly seen in children with persistent knee inflammation. A heel insert can be used in the shoe to address asymmetry and prevent secondary mechanical symptoms developing.

Investigations
Laboratory
FBC/CBC, ESR, and routine biochemistry are typically normal. ANA is present in up to 70–80% of young girls.

Treatment
Initial treatment: intra-articular GC injection with NSAIDs. Joint injection can be safely repeated after 3–6 months and up to 3× in a year in the same joint, but if required more frequently than this, MTX is advisable.

Prognosis
About 50% of children with oligo-JIA will have persistent disease or functional joint problems 10 years later (often the children whose disease extends to a polyarticular form). In 50% the arthritis will remit.

Monitoring
Very young children should be monitored regularly since they often do not recognize or are unable to communicate their problems. School age children should be able to alert their parents to any problems and can be discharged when in remission. They should be expected to return promptly if symptoms recur.

See also
Juvenile idiopathic arthritis: overview

Rheumatoid factor (RF) negative polyarticular JIA

Oligo-JIA denotes <5 joints and Polyarticular JIA more joints with a more symmetrical distribution. There is nothing magical about '5' joints. This group may include those with extended oligo-JIA who simply extended earlier than average. This classification, therefore, results in a rather heterogeneous group.

Epidemiology
RF negative polyarticular JIA (RF – ve poly-JIA) makes up 25% of all JIA in Europe and the US. Mean age of onset is 6.5 years, with two peaks at toddler to pre-school and pre-adolescent. Girls are more frequently affected than boys (ratio about 3:1). There are no consistent HLA types associated.

Clinical features
Three distinct subsets are recognized.
- The first resembles early onset oligoarthritis with more joints affected earlier. Thus it is asymmetrical, onset <6 years, female>male, ANA positive and high risk of uveitis (seen in 20–40%).
- The second comprises symmetrical synovitis of large and small joints; onset 7–9 years; elevated ESR; PIPJs are affected more than MCPJs initially; tenosynovitis around wrists and ankles is common. The outcome is variable.
- The third is known as 'dry synovitis'. There is negligible joint swelling, but stiffness, flexion contractures, and normal or slightly raised ESR. It often responds poorly to treatment and can follow a destructive course.

Investigations
An improvement in US technology has lead to it's emergence as a very useful investigation tool, valuable in confirming joint effusions, synovial hypertrophy, tendon pathology, and early erosions. There are few published data on its use in children and young people. MR scans with gadolinium enhancement are very valuable where there is diagnostic uncertainty.

Treatment
NSAIDS are commenced immediately. A short course of systemic GCs (either oral or intra-venous) is commonly used for rapid symptomatic relief with the aim to taper it quickly. Intra-articular GCs can be used for specific joints, which are particularly symptomatic or remain troublesome. A DMARD should be started immediately or within a few weeks of diagnosis, since remission is highly unlikely to occur with NSAIDs alone. The only exception would be in cases of diagnostic uncertainty where reactive arthritis is possible. Methotrexate is the DMARD of choice.

Prognosis
Overall remission rate at 10 years is 23%, with remissions most frequently occurring within 5 years of onset. This is worse than oligo-JIA, but better than RF positive Polyarticular JIA (Oen, 2002).

Monitoring
It is prudent to monitor radiographs on a yearly basis in those children with active disease. Joint space narrowing and erosions develop commonly in carpal bones. Cervical spine ankylosis can be seen.

Complications
Growth disturbance is common and proportional to the degree and duration of inflammation. Mandibular hypoplasia secondary to TMJ involvement is common.

Resources
See after section Juvenile idiopathic arthritis: overview

See also
Juvenile idiopathic arthritis: overview

Rheumatoid factor (RF) positive polyarticular JIA

About 5% of JIA cases have multiple joints affected and are rheumatoid factor (RF) positive (RF + poly-JIA). Rheumatoid factor (RF) needs to be seen on two occasions 3 or more months apart. However, RFs occur in the healthy population (1%), thus the diagnosis should not be made on RF alone!

Epidemiology
There are no population-based surveys. Hospital based surveys suggest an incidence of 0.25–1.8 per 100 000. Age of onset is around 9–12 years (female:male 6–12:1). There may be a higher incidence in Native North American, Canadian, Aboriginal, African American, Caribbean, and Latin American people compared with Caucasian populations.

Genetics
As with adult RA, RF + poly-JIA associates with HLA DR4, and its subtype DRB*0401 and DW4.

Clinical features
Typically a symmetrical polyarthrits of the small and large joints often affecting the wrists, MCP, and PIP joints.
- Rheumatoid nodules may be palpable around the elbow or in other areas of friction (in about 10%).
- Tenosynovitis, low-grade fever, hepatosplenomegaly and lymphadenopathy, serositis, and pericardial effusions may be seen.
- The differential diagnosis includes SLE and sarcoid.
- Uveitis is uncommon, but keratitis and dry eyes are occasionally seen.

Investigations
Laboratory
As in the adult form, anaemia of chronic disease, neutrophilia, thrombocytosis, and raised inflammatory markers are hallmarks of the disease.
- Urinalysis, U&E, LFT should be normal.
- ANA, ENA, dsDNA are negative and help to distinguish RF + Poly-JIA from autoimmune connective tissue diseases, all of which may be RF positive.
- A substantial proportion has circulating antibodies against cyclic citrullinated peptide (Ravelli, 2007).

Imaging
Radiographs of affected joints should be taken at baseline.

Treatment
Good disease control is the primary aim and is critical in attempting to prevent the many complications of chronic inflammation on the growing child.
- Osteoporosis, growth failure, poor nutrition, differential growth problems, delayed puberty are all potential consequences of persistent disease activity.
- Early use of immunosuppressants (particularly subcutaneous methotrexate) is warranted.
- It is important to discuss sexual health, fertility, contraception, and planned pregnancy with adolescents.

Prognosis
Only 6% of RF + poly-JIA patients achieved remission at 10 years (Oen, 2002). There is a high risk of ongoing erosive disease and need for joint replacement surgery. Such children need good careers advice.

Resources
See after section Juvenile idiopathic arthritis: overview

References
Oen K, Malleson PN, et al. Disease course and outcome of juvenile rheumatoid arthritis in a multicentre cohort. *J Rheumatol* 2002; **29**: 1989–99.

Ravelli A, Martini A. Juvenile idiopathic arthritis. *Lancet* 2007; **369**: 767–79.

See also
Juvenile idiopathic arthritis: overview

Systemic onset JIA

All types of JIA have both arthritis and the risk of joint destruction in common, but it is the extra-articular manifestations of systemic onset JIA arthritis, which makes it unique. Systemic onset JIA makes up 5–10% of all JIA. George Frederick Still described the disease as a distinct entity in children in 1897 (Still, 1897).

Classification and diagnosis
See under Juvenile idiopathic arthritis: overview

Epidemiology
Incidence varies from 0.49–1.3 per 100 000 children at risk. There is some evidence that incidence is decreasing, and some evidence of seasonality (peaking in spring and autumn) suggesting an infectious trigger, but this is by no means clear.
- The disease is equally common in males and females, with an average age of onset of 5 years, but wide variability.
- Systemic onset JIA occurs in all ages and in adults is termed 'adult onset Still disease'.

Aetiology and pathophysiology
Unknown. At the outset the systemic features of fever and rash mimic infection, but no infectious agent can be found. There is only limited evidence for a genetic link in the disease.

Clinical features
Daily high spiking fevers are the most important criterion for diagnosis. Almost always fevers are present at the outset of the illness.
- The fever pattern is a single high spike in the afternoon or evening, falling to baseline or below.
- Double temperature spikes are also seen. This typical quotidian (or double quotidian) pattern may only become obvious once treatment with NSAIDs is started.
- The rash is present in more than 90% of cases at the outset. It is a non-fixed erythematous rash, evanescent with fever and appearing as salmon-pink macules 2–10 mm in size that may coalesce.
- The Koebner phenomenon is exhibited and it can resemble urticaria with mild pruritus.
- The liver is mildly enlarged and 30% of children have mild splenomegaly.
- There is generalized lymphadenopathy in 50% with small, freely mobile, painless nodes.
- Serositis – typically pericarditis with or without effusion is usually mild and asymptomatic.
- Myocarditis occurs infrequently and there is rarely cardiac compromise. Pleuritis and peritonitis can occur.
- Arthritis is only present at onset of the disease in about a third of patients (symmetrical and polyarticular).
- Arthritis will often develop within the first few months if not at the outset. Knees, wrists, ankles, and C-spine are commonly involved.

Clinical complications
Macrophage activation syndrome
Alternatively described as secondary haemophagocytic lymphohistiocytosis. Characterized by:
- Fever, hepatosplenomegaly, bruising and coagulopathy, encephalopathy (dizzy, lethargy, disorientation).
- Haemoglobin, WBC, platelets fall.
- ESR is elevated.
- Increased triglycerides and liver transaminases.
- Extremely high ferritin.

This life-threatening condition may be triggered by changes in medication or viral infection.

Secondary amyloidosis
Rare if inflammation controlled.

Joint pathology
High probability of arthroplasty in chronic severe form (57% after 10 years follow-up). Synovial cysts occur more commonly than other forms of JIA and lymphodema of unknown cause may occur.

Investigations
Routine laboratory tests, serology and specific imaging is important where Systemic-onset JIA is being considered.

Abnormal results from investigations arranged when considering a diagnosis of systemic onset JIA
- Anaemia (usually of chronic inflammation, may also be GI blood loss secondary to medication).
- Leukocytosis with neutrophilia.
- Thrombocytosis.
- ESR often >100 mm/h.
- CRP elevated.
- Fibrinogen, immunoglobulins, and complement C3 and C4 raised.
- Autoantibodies including ANA, ANCA negative.
- Ferritin is high [if very high consider macrophage activation syndrome (MAS)].
- LDH low/normal. If raised consider malignancy.
- Imaging – US of joints helpful if synovitis present. Radiographs usually normal at baseline.
- Transthoracic echocardiogram for pericarditis/myocarditis and effusion.

Differential diagnosis
Many children present systemically unwell with fevers and rash. The primary differential diagnosis then includes infectious disease and malignancy.
- There are no pathognomonic laboratory test results for systemic onset JIA.
- Investigations are aimed at ruling out other diagnoses.
- If leukaemia remains a possibility, a bone marrow aspiration/biopsy must be performed.
- Kawasaki disease (fever, rash, joint pains) must be considered in younger children, as well as other vasculitides and fever syndromes (see p. 344).

Treatment
Treat with NSAIDs initially.
- Ibuprofen at 60 mg/kg/day (6 divided doses), indometacin at 1–2 mg/kg/day (2 divided doses).
- Glucocorticoids (GCs) are used for systemic symptoms (e.g. intravenous methylprednisolone 30 mg/kg/day for three consecutive days, repeated as required).

- Pulse methylprednisolone may result in lower cumulative doses of GCs over time compared with high dose oral prednisolone.
- Oral prednisolone can be given at doses of 1–2 mg/kg/day in 2–3 divided doses initially.
- Disease modifying anti-rheumatic drugs (DMARDs) should be started early.
- Subcutaneous methotrexate is the usual first line DMARD.
- Cyclophosphamide and ciclosporin can be used for severe cases or where methotrexate has failed or children are intolerant of it.
- Anakinra, a recombinant IL-1 receptor antagonist, is under study and preliminary reports suggest 79% of systemic onset JIA patients responding (Verbsky, 2004).
- Anti IL-6 antibody (MRA) is theoretically beneficial and requires further study.

Natural history and prognosis

Three disease courses are described:
- **Monocyclic:** remits completely (11%).
- **Polycyclic:** relapses with intervals of remission some lasting several years (34%).
- **Unremitting:** about 55% who never go into remission and suffer long-term disability.

Resources

See after section Juvenile idiopathic arthritis: overview

References

Lomater C, Gerloni V, Gattinara M, Mazzotti J, Cimaz R, Fantini F. Systemic onset juvenile rheumatoid arthritis; A retrospective study of 80 consecutive patients followed for 10 years. *J Rheumatol* 2000; **27**: 491–6.

Still GE. On a form of chronic joint disease in children. *Med Chir Trans* 1897; **80**: 47.

Verbsky JW. White AJ. Effective use of the recombinant interleukin-1 receptor agonist anakinra in therapy resistant systemic onset juvenile rheumatoid arthritis. *J Rheumatol* 2004; **31**: 2071–5.

See also

Juvenile idiopathic arthritis: overview
Kawasaki disease

Juvenile PsA

Psoriatic arthritis in children has only recently been recognized as a distinct condition within the JIA spectrum. Juvenile PsA (JPsA), as in adults, may pre-date psoriasis by many years (may be 15 years or more) and for this reason the condition has been under-diagnosed.

Classification
See the ILAR classification; see Juvenile idiopathic arthritis: overview (see p. 352).

Note: male >6 yrs and HLA-B27 +ve are excluded, as are those with enthesitis, sacroiliitis, or a spondyloarthropathy.

Epidemiology
Prevalence figures are difficult to estimate because of changes to the classification of the condition.
- The annual incidence of JPsA is in the order of 0.23–0.4 per 100 000 children.
- JPsA represents 2–15% of all children with JIA (Symmons, 1996).
- There is a female preponderance of 2:1 and mean age of onset is 6 years old (but children as young as 1 year old may be affected).

Clinical features
Asymmetric arthritis of both large and small joints is characteristic of JPsA.
- Sacroiliitis occurs in a very small minority.
- In many ways, the presentation is similar to oligo-JIA with onset in early childhood, female preponderance and the occurrence of asymptomatic chronic uveitis.
- Unlike in oligo-JIA dactylitis is frequent, and both small and large joints are involved.
- Dactylitis represents the combination of arthritis and tenosynovitis, and the clinical picture is one of swelling extending well beyond the margins of any joint capsule.
- JPsA dactylitis is usually asymmetrical and frequently involves the second toe.
- In 33–67% of children arthritis predates psoriasis. Careful examination of the hairline, behind the ears, the naval, groin, and natal cleft should be undertaken.
- Examination of the nails for pitting, splitting of the free edge, salmon pink subungual discolouration, and subungual hyperkeratosis.
- Asymptomatic uveitis occurs in up to 20% of children with JPsA in a pattern similar to that seen in oligo-JIA. Screening is therefore important.

Investigations
As with other forms of JIA. Specific scanning protocols and appearances of JPsA-related dactylitis using MR and US are not well developed.

Treatment
The management of JPsA is similar to the management adopted for oligo-JIA or polyarticular JIA, and is dependant on the extent of joint involvement. Since the prognosis is worse for JPsA than it is for oligo-JIA, immunosuppression is usually started early in the disease course. Methotrexate is the first-line choice.

Prognosis
The ILAR classification differs from previous classification systems and, therefore, there are few data on long-term follow-up and prognosis in this condition. From one case series, about 40% of JPsA children have persisting active disease, progressing to a polyarthritis, at 7-year follow-up, and 8% were severely functionally limited (Roberton, 1996).

References
Roberton DM, Cabral DA, Malleson P, Petty RE. Juvenile psoriatic arthritis: Followup and evaluation of diagnostic criteria. *J Rheumatol* 1996; **23**:166–70.

Symmons DP, Jones M, Osborne J, et al. Pediatric rheumatology in the United Kingdom: data from the British Pediatric Rheumatology Group National Diagnostic Register. *J Rheumatol* 1996; **23**: 1975–80.

Chapter 11

Pregnancy and the rheumatic diseases

Pregnancy and the rheumatic diseases 366

Pregnancy and the rheumatic diseases

- Most rheumatic diseases are associated with normal fertility. However some diseases, such as lupus, are associated with autoimmune ovarian failure. Additionally, severe disease may require treatment with regimes including high dose glucocorticoids or cyclophosphamide therapy, which may reduce fertility.
- Most rheumatic diseases that are well controlled prior to conception do not deteriorate in pregnancy, providing that the patient continues with appropriate disease-modifying therapy.
- Some patients with inflammatory disease experience disease remission during pregnancy.
- Postpartum flare is common in all the rheumatic diseases.

Rheumatoid arthritis

Effect of pregnancy on disease
- Significant improvement in disease activity is reported in 75–95% of pregnant women with RA, with full remission reported in only 16% in one series.
- The improvement starts in the first trimester and continues throughout pregnancy, with most women reporting the best disease control in the last trimester.
- In up to a quarter of pregnancies, there is no improvement or deterioration in symptoms.
- Flares in the postpartum period are common.
- It is unclear why the majority of women improve in pregnancy and, although immunoregulation, cytokine expression, HLA antigens, microchimerism and innate immunity have all been postulated to play a role, the exact mechanism remains elusive.
- Pregnancy does not appear to impact on the long-term outcome of joint damage.
- New onset RA is 3–5× more common in the postpartum period.

Effect of disease on pregnancy
- Patients with rheumatoid arthritis do not have reduced fertility. However, high disease activity may result in menstrual cycle disturbance or anovulatory cycles due to high dose glucocorticoid therapy.
- It remains unclear if RA is associated with an increased risk of miscarriage/spontaneous abortion.
- Pre-eclampsia is more common in patients with RA.

Effect of disease on the foetus
There is no association between poor foetal outcome and severity of RA, although prematurity and low birth weight have been reported in patients with RA.

SLE

Effect of pregnancy on disease
- It remains unclear if pregnancy results in an increased risk of flares in women with lupus as the data are conflicting. Increased frequency of flares may reflect withdrawal of therapy during pregnancy.
- Flares can occur during pregnancy or in the immediate postpartum period, and are usually mild and respond to low dose glucocorticoids, hydroxychloroquine, and or azathioprine
- Poor disease control at conception is the best predictor of disease flares in pregnancy, while conversely, good control reflects a lower risk of flares.

Complications of lupus
- **Hypertension:** a quarter of lupus pregnancies are associated with hypertension. Hypertension is associated with renal disease and glucocorticoid use, and results in an increased risk of intrauterine growth restriction, and a higher rate of Caesarean section.
- **Lupus nephritis:** renal disease is associated with a poor foetal outcome and increased risk of maternal complications. Active renal disease is a contraindication to pregnancy. Improved disease control is mandatory before embarking on pregnancy, and disease remission is recommended for at least 6 months prior to conception. Differentiating between pre-eclampsia and lupus nephritis with onset during pregnancy may be challenging, but autoantibodies, evidence of complement consumption and clinical evidence of disease activity may be useful in assessment. Complement levels rise in normal pregnancy and in pre-eclampsia. A positive urinary sediment with cell or casts makes lupus nephritis more likely than pre-eclampsia. HELLP (haemolysis, elevated liver enzymes, low platelets) makes pre-eclampsia more likely but these features may also be features of active lupus. Pre-eclampsia may be exacerbated by glucocorticoid therapy, but is the acute treatment of choice in patients with lupus nephritis.
- Pulmonary hypertension in lupus is rare, but has an associated mortality of 50% in pregnancy.

Effect of disease on pregnancy
- Lupus is not known to affect fertility. However, there is an association with increased foetal and maternal complications in patients undergoing fertility treatments such as IVF.
- Premature delivery is common in patients with lupus, and occurs in up to 55%. Foetal outcome (IUGR, prematurity, and foetal loss) in women with lupus nephritis is better in women with normal renal function, well-controlled blood pressure, and no significant proteinuria at conception.

Effect of disease on the foetus
- Pregnancies in SLE patients are associated with a greater risk of stillbirth, abortion, and premature delivery than in the general population.
- The risk is increased in women who have previously experienced foetal loss, have active renal disease at conception, maternal hypertension, and the presence of antiphospholipid antibodies.
- The prevalence of Ro and La antibodies in SLE patient is 35%, but transmission of IgG antibodies across the placenta occurs in about 5% of mothers between weeks 16 and 32 gestation, and may result in neonatal lupus from week 16.
- Presentation includes cutaneous lupus, complete heart block, cytopaenia, hepatic and other manifestations. Resolution typically occurs within the first 6 months of life.

- Complete congenital heart block (CHB) is diagnosed when foetal bradycardia is detected between 18 and 28 weeks. Monitoring involves serial Doppler echocardiography.
- Incomplete congenital heart block may progress *in utero* or post-delivery, and carries a 20% mortality rate. Permanent pacemakers are required by 67% of complete CHB survivors.
- Dexamethasone may reverse first and second degree heart block, but is ineffective in complete heart block.
- Half the cases of neonatal lupus will occur in pregnancies where the woman has not been diagnosed with a connective tissue disease, but who often develop Sjögren's syndrome or lupus in the next 10 years.
- The risk of intrauterine growth restriction is increased in pregnancies in women with SLE, particularly those with hypertension, active lupus, and co-existing APLS as significant predictive factors.

Antiphospholipid syndrome

Effect of disease on pregnancy

- It remains unclear whether APLS is associated with infertility. In those undergoing fertility treatment, there is an increased risk of thrombosis during ovarian induction as well as later in pregnancy.
- Normal pregnancy results in an increased thrombotic tendency from conception to 6 weeks following delivery. APLS further increases the risk of arterial and venous thrombosis, but a better foetal outcome is reported in women taking low dose aspirin who have had an early miscarriage.
- Pre-eclampsia results in multiple placental infarcts and placental insufficiency. In APLS pre-eclampsia may occur early and before 20 weeks. Although supportive treatment is indicated initially, delivery of the foetus is the definitive treatment in both cases.
- HELLP is also commoner in patients with APLS.

Effect of disease on the foetus

- Recurrent foetal loss is also one of the criteria when diagnosing APLS, and the presence of both lupus anticoagulant and anticardiolipin antibodies is associated with the highest risk of foetal loss.
- Foetal loss in early pregnancy in women with APLS can be due to failure of the placenta to implant, the effect of antiphospholipid antibodies on anionic phospholipids or the effect of B2-glycoprotein on trophoblasts. Thrombosis in APLS is also thought to have a role in pregnancy loss due to uteroplacental insufficiency from multiple placental thromboses and infarcts.
- The use of aspirin and heparin in pregnancy probably reduces miscarriages by an antithrombotic mechanism, as well as by preventing pathological apoptosis and anti-complement effects.
- Anticoagulation with heparin, rather than low dose aspirin is indicated in women with recurrent miscarriages, thromboembolic events or stillbirth.
- A good predictor of adverse pregnancy outcome is Doppler ultrasound examination during the second trimester and an abnormal uterine artery wave form is one predictor of foetal or neonatal death.
- Non-autoimmune causes of thrombocytopenia include normal pregnancy, where thrombocytopenia is mild and affects 9%. However, in mothers with APLS, neonatal thrombocytopenia is recognized to occur due to the transmission of anti-platelet antibodies across the placenta. Thrombotic complications in the neonate are rare.
- Intrauterine growth restriction of the foetus is more common in women with APLS.
- Premature delivery is common in patients with APLS.

Sjogren's syndrome

Effect of disease on pregnancy

- Sjogren's syndrome normally presents in older women, although normal fertility is reported in those women of childbearing age.
- If disease is well controlled and stable at conception, the outcome of pregnancy is generally favourable, as long as treatment with maintenance therapy is continued during pregnancy.

Systemic sclerosis

Effect of pregnancy on disease

- Systemic sclerosis does not usually progress during pregnancy, but pulmonary hypertension should be excluded as a cause of breathlessness in women in later pregnancy, a commonly reported symptom in normal advanced pregnancy.
- Women with pre-existing pulmonary hypertension should be discouraged from pregnancy due to the high mortality of around 50%, which is seen in women with any cause of pulmonary hypertension.
- Symptoms of Raynaud's phenomenon and skin involvement may improve in pregnancy, although skin disease may deteriorate postpartum.
- Hypertensive renal crises are commoner in women with a diagnosis of systemic sclerosis made in the last 5 years, and can mimic pre-eclampsia or eclampsia. ACE inhibitors offer protection against renal crises and are used in pregnancy despite the risk of foetal malformation, and only after counselling.
- Renal crises in a previous pregnancy does not exclude a further pregnancy, but hypertensive control is vital prior to conception.

Effect of disease on pregnancy

- Normal fertility has been reported in women with systemic sclerosis.
- Premature delivery is common in patients with systemic sclerosis.

Spondyloarthropathy

The effect of pregnancy on disease

- The majority of cases improve in pregnancy, especially those with small joint involvement.
- A quarter of patients with primarily spinal involvement experience a flare of their symptoms.
- Uveitis often improves during pregnancy.

Effect of disease on pregnancy

- The spondyloarthropathies are not known to directly impair fertility.
- Postpartum flares are common.

Vasculitides

Effect of pregnancy on disease

- Women of childbearing age are rarely affected by the vasculitides, so there is little data for pregnancy in women with vasculitis.

- In all of the vasculitides, disease control should be maximal prior to conception due to poor foetal outcomes and maternal mortality.
- Pre-eclampsia and renal vasculitis need to be differentiated from each other.

Effect of disease on pregnancy
- The vasculitides are not known to directly affect fertility.
- Premature delivery is common in patients with vasculitis.

Takayasu's arteritis
- Takayasu's in pregnancy may be complicated by pre-eclampsia, antepartum haemorrhage, stroke (thrombosis and bleed), and sepsis.
- Renal involvement may be difficult to differentiate from pre-eclampsia.

Beçhet's vasculitis.
Women with Beçhet's disease carry an increased risk of thrombosis due to both the disease and pregnancy itself. Central venous thrombosis may occur and should be treated with heparin.

Wegener's granulomatosis
- Wegener's granulomatosis may present during pregnancy. In those with established disease, the commonest time for flares is in the first or second trimester, or postpartum. Glucocorticoids and azathioprine have been used successfully in pregnancy.
- Cyclophosphamide is more toxic and is rarely recommended in pregnancy, but has been used successfully in the third trimester.

Churg–Strauss vasculitis
Churg–Strauss vasculitis is associated with flares in pregnancy and during the postpartum period.

Drug treatment in patients with rheumatic disease in pregnancy
In every individual case, the risk/benefit ratio of exposure to drugs and the risk of disease flare should be undertaken.

Non-steroidal anti-inflammatory drugs
NSAIDs cross the placenta and are associated with relative safety in early pregnancy, although there have been report of oral cleft, cardiac, and gastric defects along with an increased risk of miscarriage. In late pregnancy, there is a well established association with premature closure of the ductus arteriosis. Impaired renal development, oligohydramnios, and foetal haemorrhage have been reported in late pregnancy, and NSAIDs should therefore be avoided from 32 weeks of pregnancy. There is a sparcity of data for COX-11 inhibitors and these agents should therefore be avoided in pregnancy.

Glucocorticoids
Glucocorticoids are considered to be safe in pregnancy. Prednisolone is mainly metabolized, so very little crosses the placenta in doses up to 20 mg daily. However, high doses of glucocorticoids are associated with an increased risk of pre-eclampsia, pregnancy–induced hypertension, gestational diabetes, infection, and premature rupture of membranes.

Hydroxychloroquine
Hydroxychloroquine crosses the placenta, raising a theoretical possibility of foetal toxicity. However, there appears to be no increased risk of foetal malformation in a number of small observational longitudinal studies. Even though hydroxychloroquine is excreted in breast milk, there appear to be no long-term sequelae in infants.

Methotrexate
Methotrexate crosses the placenta and high dose in pregnancy is associated with a specific pattern of foetal abnormalities, involving the cranium, central nervous system, and limbs. The risk in women prescribed low dose methotrexate, however, is less clear, and although a higher risk of spontaneous abortion has been reported than in controls (20%), the data are conflicting with regard to congenital abnormalities. As a consequence of this, current recommendations are that methotrexate is stopped 3–4 months prior to conception. Methotrexate is also contraindicated in women who are breastfeeding as methotrexate is excreted into breast milk.

Sulphasalazine
Both sulfasalazine and its metabolite sulfapyridone cross the placenta. Although there are reports of an increase in oral cleft, cardiac, renal, and neural tube defects, the main bulk of the evidence does not support this, and the risk of teratogenicity is low. Sulfasalazine is also present in breast milk and caution is therefore advised in women who breastfeed.

Leflunomide
Leflunomide has been shown to be teratogenic in animals, although exposure in early pregnancy in humans has not been reported to result in abnormalities. However, because of the potential to cause severe foetal abnormalities, the drug should be discontinued, and women either wait 2 years for elimination of the drug, or undergo cholestyramine chelation and wait for a further 3 months before embarking on a pregnancy. Drug levels should be checked in this instance. Leflunomide should also be avoided in breast feeding mothers.

Azathioprine
There is a well established good safety profile in pregnancy. Immunosuppression in infants has been reported.

Ciclosporin
There is an association with intrauterine growth restriction, although whether this relates to drug treatment or maternal disease is unclear.

Mycophenolate mofetil
Digital and corpus callosum abnormalities are recognized foetal abnormalities in pregnancies exposed to mycophenolate mofetil, and therefore this drug should be avoided.

Anti-tumour necrosis factor agents
Although patients are counselled not to become pregnant whilst being treated with anti-TNF therapies, there have been successful pregnancies when either parent has been treated with anti-TNF therapy. It remains unclear if anti-TNF therapies cross the placenta or into breast milk, and the effect this may have on the foetus. Although the total number of pregnancies exposed to anti-TNF therapy is low, the incidence of abnormalities appears no higher than that expected in the general population.

Anakinra
There are no data to support safety or raise safety issues in pregnancy or lactation in either animals or humans.

Rituximab
There are no data in pregnancy or lactation, and pregnancy should therefore be avoided.

Abatacept
There are no data in pregnant humans, although in animal studies no increased teratogenicity is reported. Pregnancy should be avoided in pregnancy.

Cyclophosphamide
Cyclophosphamide therapy is contraindicated in the first and second trimesters of pregnancy, but has been used successfully in the third trimester in severe disease. Therapy is associated with premature, irreversible, ovarian failure, but is less likely in women under the age of 26, and those with a lower cumulative dose. Premature ovarian failure due to cyclophosphamide therapy is reported as between 11 and 59%. Although there has been interest in preserving fertility in this subgroup, there are no data to support the use of the combined oral contraceptive pill, although gonadotrophin-releasing hormone may be promising in this situation.

Role of multidisciplinary team
Physiotherapy input in pregnant patients is important for advice about maintaining muscle strength and stability around joints where ligaments are subjected the hormonal influences resulting in increased joint laxity. Occupational therapists may have significant input into self-management for the mother and care of the child. Review of maternal needs may cover appropriate splinting, and household and work needs both during pregnancy and postpartum. Functional problem areas, which may be covered include modification of suitable baby equipment, and childcare techniques, for example, when feeding and or carrying the infant.

Tools
The lupus activity index in pregnancy (LAI-P) has been validated and a version of BILAG-2004 for use in pregnancy is currently being developed.

Patient advice
Counselling patients about the need for improved disease control prior to conception, potential complications to both mother and foetus, and the risk of flares in the post-partum period should be discussed. Screening for complications should be undertaken regularly during pregnancy, and the risks and benefits of drug therapies, both in pregnancy and whilst breastfeeding, discussed.

Monitoring in pregnancy
Monitoring of both mother and foetus should be undertaken regularly. In the mother, disease activity and disease complications such as renal involvement should be sought. Additionally, close monitoring for complications of pregnancy, such as thrombo-embolic disease and pre-eclampsia, particularly in those patients with SLE, APLS, vasculitis, and systemic sclerosis, should be undertaken. In the foetus, close monitoring to detect IUGR, foetal abnormalities and abnormalities in uterine blood flow waveform should be regularly performed.

Resources
Internet sites
Systemic lupus erythematosis and pregnancy. Available at: http://www.uklupus.co.uk/fact13.html and http://www.uklupus.co.uk/preg.html

Rheumatoid arthritis and pregnancy. Available at: http://www.rheumatoid.org.uk/article.php?article_id=83 and http://www.arc.org.uk/arthinfo/patpubs/6060/6060.asp

Ankylosing spondylitis and pregnancy. Available at: http://www.asresearch.co.uk/pregnancy.htm and http://www.nass.co.uk/life.htm

Systemic sclerosis and pregnancy. Available at: http://www.patient.co.uk/showdoc/40002313/

ICD-10 codes
O00 to O99

See also
Chapter 19 p. 531 Drug therapies
Chapter 8 p. 240 SLE, antiphospholipid syndrome

References
Barrett JH, Brennan P, Fiddler M, Silman AJ. Does rheumatoid arthritis remit during pregnancy and relapse postpartum? Results from a nationwide study in the United Kingdom performed prospectively from late pregnancy. *Arthritis Rheum* 1999; **42**: 1219–27.

Boumpas DT, Austin HAIII, Vaughan EM, Yarboro CH, Klippel JH, Balow JE, Risk for sustained amenorrhoea in patients with systemic lupus erythematosis receiving intermittent pulse cyclophosphamie therapy. *Ann Intern Med* 1993; **119**: 366–9.

Brucato A, Doria A, Frassi M, et al. Pregnancy outcome in 100 women with autoimmune diseases and anti-Ro/SSA antibodies: a prospective controlled study. *Lupus* 2002; **11**: 716–21.

Buyon JP, Clancy RM. Neonatal lupus syndromes. *Curr Opin Rheumatol* 2003; **15**: 535–41.

Farquharson RG, Quenby S, Greaves M. Antiphospholipid syndrome in pregnancy a randomized, controlled trial of treatment. *Obstet Gynecol* 2002; **100**: 408–1342: 1219–27.

Gayed M, Gordon C. Pregnancy and rheumatic diseases. *Rheumatology* 2007; **46**: 1634–40.

Golding A, Haque UJ, Gile JT. Rheumatoid arthritis and reproduction. *Rheum Dis Clin N Am* 2007; **33**: 319–43.

Gordon C. Pregnancy and autoimmune diseases. *Best Pract Res Clin Rheumatol* 2004; **18**: 359–79.

Iijima T, Tada H, Hidaka Y, et al. Prediction of postpartum onset of rheumatoid arthritis. *Ann Rheum Dis* 1998; **57**: 460–3.

Kong NC. Pregnancy of a lupus patients – a challenge to the nephrologist. *Nephrol Dial Transplant* 2006; **21**: 268–72.

Mok CC, Wong RW. Pregnancy in systemic lupus erythematosus. *Postgrad Med J* 2001; **77**: 157–65.

Ostensen M, Forger F, Nelson JL, Schuhmacher A, Hebisch G, Villiger PM. Pregnancy in patients with rheumatic disease: anti-inflammatory cytokines increase in pregnancy and decrease post partum. *Ann Rheum Dis* 2005; **64**: 839–44.

Ostensen M, Villiger PM. The remission of rheumatoid arthritis during pregnancy. *Semin Immunopathol* 2007; **29**: 185–91.

Petri M, Allbritton J. Fetal outcome of lupus pregnancy: a retrospective case-control study of the Hopkins Lupus Cohort. *J Rheumatol* 1993; **20**: 650–6.

Ruiz-Irastorza G, Khamashta MA, Gordon C, et al. Measuring systemic lupus erythematosis activity during pregnancy: validation of the lupus activity index in pregnancy scale. *Arthritis Rheum* 2004; **51**: 78–82.

Yee CS, Farewll V, Isenberg DA, et al. Revised British Isles Lupus Assessment Group 2004 Index: a reliable tool for assessment of systemic lupus erythematosis activity. *Arthritis Rheum* 2006; **54**: 3300–5.

Chapter 12

Osteoarthritis and related disorders

Osteoarthritis *372*
Osteoarthritis-related disorders *380*

Osteoarthritis

Osteoarthritis (OA) is a mechanically driven, but biochemically-mediated disease of synovial joints.

Definition

In clinical practice, as in epidemiologic studies, OA is diagnosed where there is joint pain, together with characteristic radiographic changes, in the absence of an alternative cause. Surprisingly, one of the most useful definitions of OA is to be found on Wikipedia:

... Osteoarthritis (OA), also known as degenerative arthritis or degenerative joint disease, and sometimes referred to as 'arthrosis' or 'osteoarthrosis'), is a condition in which low-grade inflammation results in pain in the joints, caused by wearing of the cartilage that covers and acts as a cushion inside joints. As the bone surfaces become less well protected by cartilage, the patient experiences pain upon weight bearing, including walking and standing. Due to decreased movement because of the pain, regional muscles may atrophy and ligaments may become more lax. OA is the most common form of arthritis. The word is derived from the Greek word 'osteo' meaning 'of the bone', 'arthro' meaning 'joint', and 'itis' meaning inflammation, although many sufferers have little or no inflammation ...

A more unwieldy, but widely quoted definition is from the American Academy of Orthopaedic Surgeons (1995):

... Osteoarthritis diseases are a result of both mechanical and biologic events that destabilise the normal coupling of degradation and synthesis of articular cartilage chondrocytes, extracellular matrix and subchondral bone. Although they may be initiated by multiple factors such as genetic developmental, metabolic, and traumatic factors, osteoarthritis diseases are manifest by morphologic, biochemical, molecular and biomechanical changes of both cells and matrix which leads to a softening, fibrillation, ulceration and loss of articular cartilage, sclerosis and eburnation of subchondral bone, osteophytes and subchondral cysts. When clinically evident, osteoarthritis diseases are characterised by joint pain, tenderness, limitation of movement and variable degrees of inflammation without systemic effects.

Classification

The American College of Rheumatology (ACR) criteria were developed to differentiate OA from other, especially inflammatory, arthritides in specialist practice. Epidemiological studies usually classify occurrence of OA on the basis of radiographic changes alone. However, the presence of pain in addition to osteophytes or joint space narrowing is now generally accepted.

Spondylosis

The term given to the (degenerative) process causing reduced intervertebral disc space. Synovial facet joints are typically secondarily affected by an OA process; however, primary OA of facet joints can occur. The degree to which costovertebral and costotransverse joints are affected by OA is not well documented.

The ACR classification criteria for OA

Hand OA

Pain, aching or stiffness in the hand[a] and 3 of the following:
- Bony swelling of ≥2 distal interphalangeal (DIP) joints.
- Bony swelling of 2 or more of 10 selected joints*.
- <3 swollen metacarpophalangeal (MCP) joints.
- Deformity of 2 or more of 10 selected joints*.

Knee OA: using history and examination

Pain in the knee[a] and 3 of the following:
- Age >50 years.
- Morning stiffness <30 min.
- Crepitus on active motion.
- Bony tenderness.
- Bony enlargement.
- No palpable warmth of synovium.

Hip OA: using history, examination and laboratory findings

Pain in the hip[a] and:
- Internal rotation ≤15° and either ESR ≤45 mm/h or hip flexion ≤115° if ESR unavailable.

Or
- Internal rotation >15° with pain, morning stiffness ≤60 minutes, >50 years old.

[a]On most days of the previous month.
[b]Right and left 2nd and 3rd proximal interphalangeal joints, 2nd and 3rd DIPJ, and 1st carpometacarpal joints.

Patterns of OA

Primary
- Nodal (hand).
- Erosive (hand).
- Generalized (hand + knee/hip).
- Diffuse idiopathic skeletal hyperostosis (DISH).

Secondary
- Localized (e.g. fracture, infection).
- Diffuse (e.g. secondary to rheumatoid arthritis).
- Calcium pyrophosphate dihydrate (CPPDD) deposition.
- Metabolic (e.g. haemochromatosis; ochronosis).
- Neuropathic [e.g. tabes dorsalis, diabetes mellitus (DM)].
- Bone dysplasias.

Epidemiology

OA is the commonest arthropathy, typically affecting joints most exposed to mechanical load, including the hand, knee, hip, and 1st MTP joints.

- The prevalence of radiographic changes alone in anyone >50 years old is notable: hip 8%; hand 15%; knee 30%. About 50% of these people will have pain over a 1-year period.
- Robust UK incidence data is lacking. Incidence data from the United States of America shows an age- and sex-standardized incidence for symptomatic knee OA of

160–240 per 100 000 patient-years, rising to 1% in those over age 70 years.
- This compares to 47–88 per 100 000 patient-years for hip OA (compared to 10–30 per 100 000 in Sweden) and 100 per 100 000 patient-years for hand OA.
- Serial radiographic surveys, including the Framingham, Goteberg, and Tecumseh cohorts show higher rates of incident radiographic change alone, from 2.7 to 11.9%, depending on the joint and definition used.
- The number of joint replacement operations (and probably the prevalence and incidence of underlying OA) are increasing in the UK, due to demographic population changes and the NHS evolving from a supply limited to a demand led service.
- In 2007, 137 000 hip and knee replacements were performed in England and Wales, contributing to a cost of over £3 bn per annum for OA management.
- In general, Caucasians have a high rate of OA with lower rates in Afro-Caribbean and Asian populations, which is thought to be primarily genetically determined.
- OA prevalence might be modified by environmental factors, e.g. the higher prevalence of knee OA in indigenous Chinese population thought to be influenced by the tendency to squat.
- The prevalence of OA probably peaks around 70-year-old; however, a recent study in the very elderly (85–97 years of age) suggests all who survive to this age develop radiographic change of one or more joint. Function is often well preserved.
- There is a female preponderance of up to 2:1 for knee and hand OA, but a less consistent gender difference for hip OA.
- Occupational and mechanical factors are relevant. For example, knee bending and obesity are important factors determining knee OA; farming is associated with hip OA and occupations where there is intensive use of a precision grip, a risk for hand OA.

Aetiology and pathophysiology

Most OA can be classified into primary or secondary variants. Secondary OA occurs earlier with more predictable severity in a damaged joint e.g. after cruciate ligament injury in the knee or congenital hip dysplasia. Primary OA is more contentious, but there is some evidence for both genetic and environmental contributions.
- The prevailing dogma is that that OA is a failure of compensation for an imbalance within the degradative and reparative connective tissue processes within the whole joint, leading to failure of the joint.
- However, while biochemical markers suggest a degree of synthetic activity of type II collagen and other matrix components in OA models, and sometimes subjects, there has been no clear demonstration of meaningful reconstruction of cartilage damage once established.
- The caveat to the above comes from anecdotes reporting improved joint space on non-weight-bearing films. However, this is more likely to represent a lack of apposition of weight-bearing surfaces, rather than cartilage regeneration. Similarly, recent work on surgical joint distraction has only demonstrated fibrocartilage, not true hyaline cartilage, formation.
- Overall, it seems plausible that the degree of connective tissue matrix turnover in normal joints may not be structurally relevant and, therefore, that decompensation of matrix turnover is not the most universally relevant model of OA.

Genetic factors
The genetic associations observed so far have been small and rarely replicated in more the one cohort.
- Some genetic associations might explain a minority of disease (e.g. ADAM12 for knee OA, frizzled related protein 3 in hip OA).
- Large collaborative studies, such as arcOGEN (funded by Arthritis Research Campaign) and TREAT_OA (funded by The European Union FP-7 programme) are likely to provide a definitive estimate of the genetic effects on OA within the next 5 years.

Environment
Damage to structures in and around the joint that result in altered joint biomechanics, whatever the cause, has a consistent effect on promoting the development and progression of OA.
- Early changes include reduced muscle power and ligamentous changes. This has led to the recent suggestion that entheseal changes may be central to the pathophysiology of OA. However, no longitudinal epidemiological studies with high-resolution imaging have addressed this hypothesis.
- Although there has been no definitive demonstration of the sequence of initiation of pathological processes in OA, other hypotheses include:
  - the central importance of subchondral bone changes as an initiating factor;
  - the widespread assumption that cartilage changes are the earliest event;.
  - the widespread acceptance that osteophytes are a reaction to early changes within the joint.
- There is evidence that cartilage becomes less elastic, at least in part due to the accumulation of advanced glycosylation end-products and reduced matrix fluid pressurization.
- Finally, chondrocytes are sensitive to mechanical loading. This provides a potential link between altered loading and joint pathology.

Celular, matrix, and immunobiology
Mechanical stress is required for joint maintenance, but pathological stresses may lead to microtrauma and inflammatory changes. Although there are far fewer 'features of inflammation' compared with the inflammatory arthritides, inflammation is found in OA.
- Arthroscopic and histological studies together with high-resolution musculoskeletal ultrasound (US) have suggested that low-grade inflammation is an important feature of OA.
- Also, recent magnetic resonance (MR) imaging studies have suggested that changes consistent with inflammatory lesions have are consistently identified in OA joints (e.g. joint fluid and increased bone marrow signal).
- In OA, inflammation is characterized by raised levels of IL-1 and TNF-α in the joint and activation of inducible nitric oxide synthase and cyclo-oxygenase 2. These changes are associated with changes in expression of matrix metalloproteinases (MMPs) and tissue inhibitors of MMPs (TIMPs), favouring excessive proteolysis.

Risk factors
The most clinically relevant way to consider the risk factors for OA is whether they are constitutive (and therefore cannot be modified) or potentially modifiable.

Constitutive risk factors
Age, gender, race, familial factors, genetically determined osteophytic response/evolution, congenital, and/or developmental deformities.

Potentially modifiable risk factors
Obesity, joint malalignment, or previous injury, co-existent inflammatory arthritis, adjacent muscular weakness, occupational factors, hormonal status (e.g. HRT is protective) and bone mass (high baseline bone mass and greater loss in OA).

Clinical features
OA can present with one or more affected joints. It is always important to assess pattern and extent of disease, including hand (distal/proximal interphalangeal/1st carpometacarpal joints), knee, and hip involvement.

Key features in history
There are consistent features to the history associated with severity and duration of disease.
- In early/mild disease there is typically joint use-related pain and pain can be episodic.
- In late/severe disease there may be refractory or pain disturbing sleep at night.
- Early morning stiffness is usually short-lived or absent. Any such stiffness clearly involves affected joints, rather than being generalized.
- There is usually impairment of function especially when OA involves the major weight bearing joints.
- Ideally history-taking should be by appropriate open questioning to allow the patient to encapsulate the problem from their perspective.
- Screening questions from The GALS assessment (see p. 9) might be expected to unmask an OA in all but the most trivial symptomatic cases:
  - Do you have any pain or stiffness in your arms, legs, neck, or back?
  - Do you have any problems with washing or dressing?
  - Do you have any problems with stairs or steps?
- Problems identified from the initial history can be explored further with respect to affected joints:
  - Did you have pain most days last month?
  - Do you get pain with using the joint (e.g. when standing or walking for a knee or hip)? If so, how far can you walk?
  - Is the joint stiff in the morning? For how long?
  - Do you get pain at night?
  - Does pain affect your work/leisure activities?

Eliciting a history of risk factors
Some risk factors will have relevance to development of OA in all joints, whereas other risk factors will be joint-specific.
- For knee OA ask about previous injuries or meniscal ('cartilage') problems or operations in the past, and occupational overuse (e.g. Do you do bend your knees or lift heavy weights repeatedly at work?).
- Ask if there is a family history of OA. If the patient is unsure, ask about hip or knee replacement operations, and if their relatives' hand deformities included the DIP or MCP joints.
- Hormonal status has some relevance. Ask (a postmenopausal female) when they last menstruated and whether they're taking HRT.

History to help guide therapeutic decisions
Knowledge of previous disease and full assessment of gastrointestinal and cardiovascular risk factors is required in any patient being considered for treatment with non-steroidal anti-inflammatory drugs is important.

Depression
Depression commonly co-exists with OA, as with other painful arthropathies, and may require separate assessment and treatment (e.g. initially with the HADS questionnaire tool).

Key features on examination
Signs of generalized OA are often found in those presenting with a single painful joint, so while initial examination may focus on the presenting problem, examination of all potentially involved joints should be undertaken, including hands, knees, and hips.
- Index joint examination should be as per the REMS model: look, feel, move, and assess function.
- Observe any wasting of surrounding muscles; bony enlargement of the articular margins, including Heberden's nodes (DIPJ). These may be red (known as 'hot Heberden's') at presentation (See Figure. 12.1).
- Also observe Bouchard's nodes (PIPJ) occurring at PIPJ and OA of the 1st carpometacarpal joints typically gives squaring. Valgus/varus deformities, especially at the knee and ankle, can be seen; as can use of sticks or orthoses; uneven wear of shoes.
- OA can result in cool effusions (especially knee).
- There are few OA-specific signs from examination of joint movement, but crepitus, and pain on movement or weight-bearing is typical.
- Restriction of extension and internal rotation is an early feature of hip OA.
- In small hand joint OA, finger flexion can be reduced and associated with fixed flexion deformities. Active and passive movement ranges are usually the same unless severe intra-capsular inflammation restricts active movement.
- Functional assessment should include writing and assessment of walking (often the latter previously examined by the observant clinician who uses the arrival of the patient in the clinic as an opportunity to scrutinize).

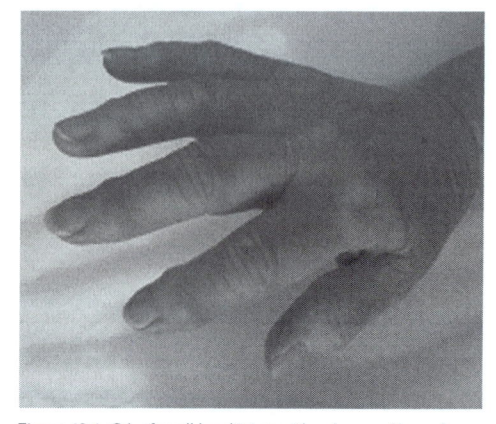

Figure 12.1 OA of small hand joints with a degree of loss of digital extension owing to bony deformities: Heberden's and Bouchard's nodes.

CHAPTER 12 **Osteoarthritis and related disorders** 375

Investigations
A typical clinical presentation where referral for consideration of surgery is not required would not usually require investigation. The high age-associated prevalence leads to OA being a common coincidental diagnosis in patients with other arthropathies.

Laboratory
OA is typically not associated with high acute phase response, although a modest elevation in ESR is consistent with the diagnosis.
- Tests may be necessary to discriminate other arthritides (or assess for their presence). Both RF and anti-CCP antibodies may be useful in this respect.
- Endocrine and metabolic tests might be indicated where OA is thought to be secondary or CPPDD arthritis a possibility [e.g. transferrin saturation (>50%) and very high ferritin in haemachromatosis; elevated parathyroid hormone in primary hyperparathyroidism].
- Polarized light microscopy of aspirated joint fluid should be examined for CPPDD and gout crystals. Other calcium-containing crystals might be detected if pathology support is sufficiently expert.

Imaging
Radiographs
Where radiographs are indicated, appropriate films to request are:
- **Hand:** anteroposterior (AP) view (See Figure. 12.2).
- **Knee:** weight-bearing AP, lateral, and patella skyline view (photon beam parallel to articular side of patella and can be done at varying degrees of knee flexion) (See Figure. 12.3).
- **Hip:** supine AP pelvis view with 10° internal hip rotation. Consider lateral or false profile view if AP not diagnostic, but clinical features suggestive of articular disease, i.e. reduced painful extension or internal rotation on passive movement (See Figure. 12.4).
- **Characteristic changes on plain radiographs:** include osteophytes, joint space narrowing, and subchondral changes: sclerosis and cysts.

Radiographic variants
- **Erosive osteoarthritis:** a more destructive variant characterized by more profound disruption to joint anatomy. Needs to be discriminated from psoriatic arthritis and CPPDD arthritis though extensive involvement of small hand joints in CPPDD disease is unusual.
- Secondary collapse of the femoral head in advanced hip OA.

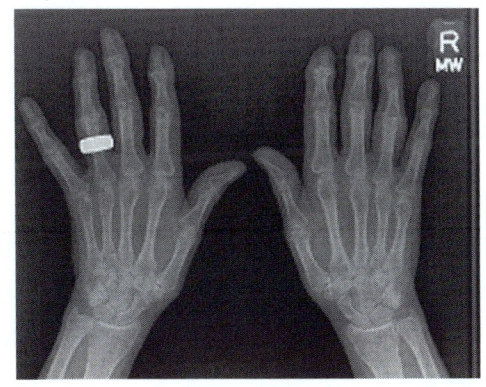

Figure 12.2 Generalized small hand joint OA involving DIP and PIP joints (AP view).

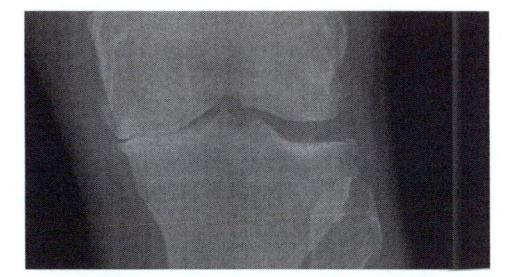

Figure 12.3 Weight-bearing AP knee radiograph showing characteristic loss of medial compartment tibio-femoral joint space loss in advanced OA.

Other imaging
Experience using US to characterize changes in OA joints is increasing in some units. MR is mainly employed to assess internal joint derangement, particularly where surgical intervention is planned, and assess osteonecrosis in appropriate situations.
- High resolution musculoskeletal US can be useful if

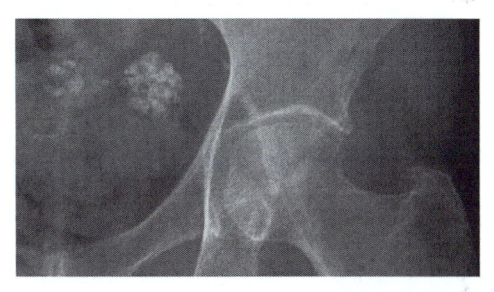

(a)

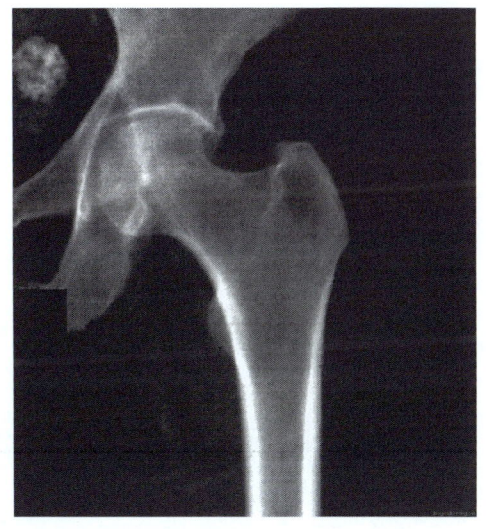

(b)

Figure 12.4 (a) Plain radiograph of left hip joint, and below it, (b) a high-resolution Dual Energy X-ray Absorptiometry image (iDXA, GE Healthcare), showing joint space narrowing.

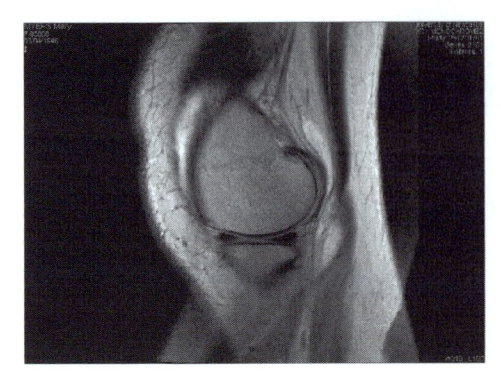

Figure 12.5 3T MRI showing delayed gadolinum uptake in OA cartilage.

co-existent inflammatory arthritis is being considered and the sonographer is experienced in examining joints.
- MR is important in a knee affected by OA if planning arthroscopy particularly if additional meniscal damage is a possibility (e.g. knee locking, giving way on weight bearing and positive examination tests; see p. 178–183) See Figure 12.5.
- Situations where MR of the hip is indicated include confirmation and staging of osteonecrosis of the femoral head if appearances are unclear on radiographs, ruling out a labral tear (may need contrast-enhanced MR) and assessing inflammatory changes (if US not available) if intra-articular glucocorticoid injection is being contemplated.
- Characteristic patterns of tracer localization on bone scintigraphy, particularly for knee OA, are reasonably predictive of the need for arthroplasty.
- In community studies, where high-resolution dual energy X-Ray Absorptiometry (DXA) images have been acquired, images can be scored for the features of osteoarthritis.

Differential diagnosis

The main differential diagnosis of OA is with inflammatory arthritis, although the two commonly co-exist.

Psoriatic arthritis (PsA)

Erosive OA must be differentiated from PsA (p. 220). Erosive OA does not exhibit new bone formation within erosions, exhibits less juxta-articular new bone formation in advanced disease and involves less extensive inflammatory entheseal changes on ultrasound.

Gout

Gout can involve DIPJ, but it is more inflammatory than OA, usually asymmetrical in its distribution and associated with eccentric soft-tissue swelling.

CPPDD disease

Chondrocalcinosis may be a feature of knee OA, where it is regarded as an epiphenomenon. CPPDD can present as pseudogout in a single joint or oligoarticular distribution, or mimicking RA occurring in a symmetrical distribution especially in elderly females.

Rheumatoid arthritis

If there is hip or knee destruction, then examination of the hands and wrists should establish if changes are likely to be secondary OA related to RA. If there is any doubt laboratory investigations should be used.

Disease activity assessment

Often not used in clinical practice, but extremely helpful for monitoring impact of OA over time. The following are validated questionnaire and assessment tools.
- VAS: Visual Analogue pain score.
- HAQ: Health Assessment Questionnaire.
- SF-36: Short Form 36.
- EQ-5D: EuroQol.
- WOMAC: Western Ontario & McMaster Universities OA Index.
- Harris hip score (used in orthopaedic practice).

Treatment

Objectives of treatment

Given the biomechanical influence on OA and the lack of therapies with a disease-modifying effect, non-pharmacological treatments, and simple analgesia with paracetamol should be regarded as the core treatments. In the UK, the evidence was recently reviewed by the National Institute for Health and Clinical Excellence for their clinical guideline (NICE, 2008). Core objectives of disease management are:
- Relief of pain.
- Improved function.
- Slow progression of structural change.

Non-pharmacological therapy

Involve the multi-disciplinary team, including occupational therapy, physiotherapy, and podiatry, as appropriate.
- Education about the disease and effective treatments (see resources below).
- Exercise therapy should include both aerobic conditioning and strengthening exercise. Compliance and cost effectiveness are improved by delivery in groups, which may be combined with other measures.
- Weight loss advice for all who are overweight or obese.
- Foot orthoses for all with significant abnormal lower limb biomechanics, e.g. wedge orthoses for ankle valgus, corrective bracing for knee valgus/varus.
- Aids and devices: a stick for use in contralateral hand for knee or hip OA; consider thumb splint for 1st carpometacarpal joint OA; a home assessment may be required where activities and participation limited.
- Hot and cold packs can be helpful for acute exacerbations of joint pain.
- Transcutaneous electrical nerve stimulation may be appropriate for some patients with refractory pain.
- Acupuncture can give additional, short-lived pain relief as adjunctive therapy.
- Manual therapy such as manipulation can be considered for hip OA.
- Complementary therapies are used extensively by patients with OA:
  - There is considerable, if somewhat inconsistent, evidence for glucosamine sulphate 1500mg daily in helping pain and loss of function in knee OA, and possibly slowing radiographic change (although the latter has not been replicated in independent studies). The only trial in hip OA did not show any benefit.
  - Chondroitin sulphate also has some supporting evidence for symptomatic benefit in hip and knee OA. One study has shown benefit from combining

glucosamine and chondroitin in a pre-specified subgroup with moderate to severe knee OA.
- The side effect profile of glucosamine and chondroitin is excellent (although there are case reports on the potentiation of warfarin with glucosamine).
- Avocado/soybean unsaponifiables, a Chinese herbal preparation (SKI306X), and rosehip extracts, were also recommended by a recent Cochrane review.
- A comfrey extract ointment and several different ginger preparations have single RCT evidence showing effectiveness on symptoms.

Pharmacological therapy
Oral analgesics
- Paracetamol (up to 1 g qds) is preferred as first line analgesia, because of its favourable safety profile.
- Opioids, such as codeine or dihydrocodeine, or higher strength opioids may be needed.

Non-steroidal anti-inflammatories (NSAIDs)
- NSAIDs (including 'Coxib' NSAIDs) provide additional symptomatic benefit in some patients.
- Gastrointestinal and cardiovascular risks must be considered before use NSAIDs. They should be avoided in patients with established ischaemic heart disease or cerebrovascular disease, and used with caution in those with risk factors for these conditions.
- Conventional NSAIDs should be used with gastroprotection when risk factors exist, such as previous peptic ulceration or current aspirin use.

Topical treatments
- Certain topical NSAID preparations are effective, but many of the widely available preparations have absent or negative evidence of effectiveness.
- Capsaicin can be effective, especially for hand OA, but has a high rate of skin reactions.

Intra-articular injections
- Glucocorticoid injections can give short-term relief (2–3 weeks) in knee OA and as long as 3–4 months in hip OA (where fluoroscopic or US guidance are required for their delivery).
- There is little compelling evidence for the efficacy of intra-articular Hyaluronan. In view of their high cost, further high quality studies are needed to establish their role.

Disease modifying OA drugs (DMOADs)
There are currently no universally accepted disease-modifying OA drugs. Single studies have suggested efficacy for a number of agents and toxicity has prevented development of others. This is a very active research area. Potential DMOADs include:
- Diacerein (hip).
- Doxycycline (knee).
- Licofelone (knee).
- Strontium ranelate.
- Bisphosphonates.
- Matrix metalloproteinase inhibitors.

Surgery
- Hip and knee arthroplasty are established effective treatments for end-stage disease, with an effect size of more than 2- and 10-year arthroplasty survival of over 90% (although arthroplasty has never been subjected to randomized controlled trial).
- Articular hip resurfacing is becoming increasingly available and has potential advantages for younger patients, as less bone is excised and revision is technically less demanding. However, no long-term data is available.
- Arthroscopy should be restricted to those with likely meniscal/ligament pathology.

Clinical tips (extracted from UK NICE OA guidelines)
- Exercise should be a core component of therapy, irrespective of age, co-morbidity, pain severity, and disability. Exercise should include local muscle strengthening and general aerobic fitness.
- Interventions to effect weight loss should be a core treatment for the obese and overweight.
- People with biomechanical joint pain or instability should be considered for assessment for bracing/joint supports/insoles as an adjunct to core therapy.
- Accurate verbal and written information should be offered to enhance understanding of OA and its management, and to counter misconceptions, such as that OA inevitably progresses and cannot be treated.
- Individual self-management and group programmes should emphasize the recommended core treatments, especially exercise.
- Full dose paracetamol (1 g tds/qds) should be tried before other analgesics or anti-inflammatories.

Prognosis and natural history
OA is a condition with a variable course. Those affected usually present with one painful joint, and this episode often improves or resolves. A minority of patients develop progressive disease and require total joint replacement surgery. Those who present with severe pain and advanced disease will usually require operative intervention and there is evidence that early surgery helps to prevent the functional deterioration that otherwise occurs. Over time, other joints become involved, so that single joint OA often becomes generalized and episodes of pain affect different joints over time in individuals with generalized OA.

Monitoring disease activity
This is not routinely undertaken, but there are validated tools for research active units and trials (see below).

Current controversies
- Site and nature of the initial insult in OA.
- Extent of matrix turnover and decompensation.
- Role of glucosamine sulphate.
- Efficacy of disease modifying OA therapy.
- Cardiovascular risk attributable to OA.

Resources on OA
Assessment tools
OMERACT
An organization originally set up to define outcome measures for rheumatoid arthritis clinical trials recommended a core set of outcome measures for OA trials in 1997. This included both generic and disease specific assessment tools.

Generic tools
Instruments developed to assess health status and quality of life in other conditions: HAQ, SF-36 and EQ-5D. Download pain tools including Visual analogue scale and

SF-36 are available from http://www.painworld.zip.com.au/articles/pain_tools.html

Disease specific tools
These tools have been developed and validated to a varying degree in OA.
- WOMAC is probably the best validated tool for assessment of knee and hip OA. It measures 3 domains: pain, stiffness, and function, using either visual analogue, numerical rating scale or Likert scales.
- Lequesne index. Robust tool, but has some overlapping item options leading to some scoring ambiguity.
- Knee OA outcome score (KOOS) was developed for surgical assessment and outcome.
- Australian/Canadian Hand OA Index (AUSCAN). This tool is analogous in structure and rigour of development to WOMAC, but is for hand OA.

Priority scoring tools
There are various tools that have been used for assigning priority for patients to undergo total hip or knee replacement surgery. These include the New Zealand, NIH, Ontario, and Western Canada criteria. They include a combination of pain, and functional and radiographic assessment, often with a degree of subjective assessment of overall disease state or requirement for surgery. They are not suitable for determining who should receive surgery.

Resources

Guidelines
NICE Guideline CG59. OA: the care and management of adults with osteoarthritis. Implementation tools: http://www.nice.org.uk/CG059#implementation.

OA Society International (OARSI) recommendations for the management of hip and knee osteoarthritis. http://www.oarsi.org/index2.cfm?section=Publications_and_Newsroom&content=Indexes

EULAR evidenced based recommendations for the management of hip and knee OA.

MOVE consensus: evidence-based recommendations for the role of exercise in the management of OA of the hip or knee.

Patient organizations (UK)
Arthritis Care. Head Office: Arthritis Care, 18 Stephenson Way, London NW1 2HD. Telephone 020 7380 6500. E-mail: Info@arthritiscare.org.uk

Internet sites
Arthritis Care: http://www.arthritiscare.org.uk/.

Arthritis Research Campaign (excellent patient and professional resources): http://www.arc.org.uk/arthinfo/patpubs/6025/6025.asp.

Patient information: http://www.patient.co.uk/showdoc/23068795/, or http://www.cks.library.nhs.uk/patient_information_leaflet/osteoarthritis.

Clinical knowledge summaries: osteoarthritis: http://www.cks.library.nhs.uk/osteoarthritis;

NHS direct: basic patient information and access to out of hours advice: http://www.nhsdirect.nhs.uk/articles/article.aspx?articleId=268

Wheeless' Textbook of Orthopaedics. Available at: http://www.wheelessonline.com/ortho/osteoarthritis.

ICD 10 codes

Nodal/generalized OA
M15.0	Primary generalized (osteo)arthrosis
M15.1	Heberden's nodes (with arthropathy)
M15.2	Bouchard's nodes (with arthropathy)
M15.4	Erosive (osteo)arthrosis
M15.9	Generalized osteoarthritis

Hip OA
M16.0–16.9 Hip OA codes ('coxarthrosis').

Knee OA
M17–17.9 Knee OA codes ('gonarthrosis').

Hand OA
M18–18.9 1st CMC joint (and subcodes)

References

Altman RD & Gold G. *Atlas of individual radiographic features in osteoarthritis*. OARSI: 2007. Available at: http://www.oarsi.org/index2.cfm?section=Publications_and_Newsroom&content=atlas

Brandt KD, Doherty M, Lohmander LS. *Osteoarthritis*, 2nd edn. Oxford: Oxford University Press, 2003.

Dickson J, Hughes R, Marsh D. *Royal: the New Science of Osteoarthritis – from Bench to Bedside*. London: Royal Society of Medicine Publications, 2008.

Doherty M, Jones A, Cawston T. Osteoarthritis. In: Maddison PJ, Woo P, Isenberg D, Glass D (eds) *Oxford Textbook of Rheumatology*, 3rd edn. Oxford: Oxford University Press (in press).

Jordan KM, Arden NK, Doherty M, et al. EULAR recommendations 2003: an evidence based approach to the management of knee osteoarthritis: report of a Task Force of the standing committee for international clinical studies including therapeutic trials (ESCISIT). *Ann Rheum Dis* 2003; **62**: 1145–55.

NICE Guideline CG59. *Osteoarthritis: the Care and Management of Adults with Osteoarthritis*. London: HMSO, 2008. Available at: http://www.nice.org.uk/guidance/index.jsp?action=byID&o=11926 (accessed 28 March 2008).

Moskowitz R, et al. *Osteoarthritis: Diagnosis and Medical/Surgical Management*, 4th edn. Philadelphia: Lippincott Williams & Wilkins, 2007.

Roddy E, et al. Evidence-based recommendations for the role of exercise in the management of osteoarthritis of the hip or knee--the MOVE consensus. *Rheumatology* 2005; **44**: 67–73.

Zhang W, Moskowitz RW, Nuki G, et al. OARSI recommendations for the management of hip and knee osteoarthritis, part I: critical appraisal of existing treatment guidelines and systematic review of current research evidence. *Osteoarthritis Cartilage*. 2007; **15**: 981–1000.

Zhang W, Moskowitz RW, Nuki G, et al. OARSI recommendations for the management of hip and knee osteoarthritis. Part II: OARSI evidenced-based, expert consensus guidelines. *Osteoarthritis Cartilage* 2008; **16**: 137–62.

Osteoarthritis-related disorders

Diffuse idiopathic skeletal hyperostosis
Diffuse idiopathic skeletal hyperostosis (DISH, Forestier's Disease) is a condition where calcification of the anterior spinal ligament occurs across at least 4 contiguous vertebrae leading to bony excrescences with an appearance that has been likened to dripping wax.
- There are no robust European epidemiological data. DISH affects 6–12% of the adult population in the USA, increasing to 28% of those over 80 years of age. There is a male preponderance 2:1.
- Aetiology unknown (hence, 'idiopathic'), although an association has been described with diabetes.
- Familial cases have been described.
- Distinct SNP polymorphisms in a candidate gene associated with ossification of the posterior longitudinal ligament (OPLL), collagen 6A1 (Col6A1), have been found in Japanese patients with DISH. Findings have not been reproduced in other populations.
- The pathophysiology is not well understood.

Clinical features
DISH may be asymptomatic, or present with variable degrees of pain and disability.
- If large, the anterior cervical syndesmophytes can cause dysphagia, lead to difficult intubations, cause stridor, dysphonia, and contribute to ventilatory difficulties. See Figure. 12.6.
- Spinal pain associated with DISH is thought to be due to mechanical damage at segments of the spine where there is compensatory excessive movement, as segments affected by DISH stiffen.
- Myelopathy has been reported rarely; neck trauma in the context of DISH may have greater potential adverse consequences.
- Examination is characterized by restricted spinal mobility, which may be regional or global.
- Enthesophytes and bony spurs can form in the peripheral skeleton (e.g. plantar calcaneal spur).
- There is a recognized association with DM and possibly metabolic syndrome.
- Long-term, the spine can stiffen and cause similar postural problems as those in ankylosing spondylitis (AS).

Investigations
Plain lateral radiographs of the spine are usually sufficient to confirm the diagnosis.
In difficult cases it may be necessary to request:
- ESR, CRP.
- HLA-B27 (a negative test might suggest against AS).
- AP pelvis or coned SIJ radiographs; if unclear, further imaging of the sacroiliac joint may be requested to confirm they are spared (e.g. MR though CT scan shows SIJ erosions. Bone scintigraphy can be informative.
- The main differential is from AS, where marginal syndesmophytes are seen, together with sacroiliitis.

Treatment
There are no RCTs of analgesics or disease modifying therapy for DISH. Management is focused on pain control, exercises to maintain range of movement, and addressing rare complications related to compression of surrounding structures.

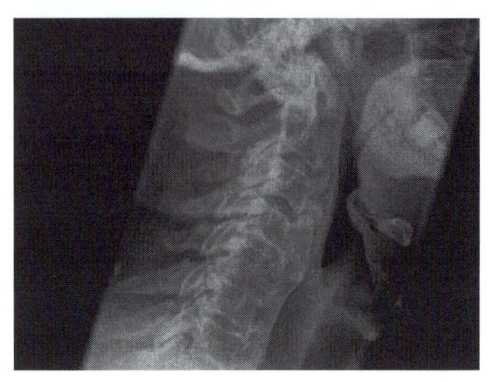

Figure 12.6 Radiographic appearance of DISH.

Neuropathic arthropathy
Neuropathic arthropathy or 'Charcot's joint' is a condition where peripheral (or central) neuropathy leads to secondary, painless, joint destruction.
- Prevalence is about 15% in DM, 20% in tabes dorsalis, 25% in syringomyelia.
- The dominant hypothesis is that loss of propio- and nociceptive input prevents protection the joint from excessive repetitive loading, leading to trauma, and progressive damage.
- The commonest clinical scenario in Europe and N America is involvement of hindfoot joints in DM.
- Plain radiographs show destruction of involved peripheral joints, without features of osteomyelitis. Early changes can mimic OA radiographically.
- Consideration should be given to potential metabolic, drug, toxic, mitotic, and vasculitic causes (of neuropathy), and MR imaging if central neurological disease suspected (e.g. multiple sclerosis, syringomyelia, spina bifida, etc.) Other useful tests might include:
  - FBC, U&E, LFT, γGT, ESR, CRP;
  - serum and urine protein electrophoresis; CXR;
  - B12, blood sugar and HbA1c;
  - complement, Igs RF, ANA, ENA, ANCA;
  - tests for localizing lesions if paraneoplastic syndrome suspected, e.g. colonoscopy for change of bowel habit.

Treatment
Is of the underlying neuropathy where treatable. For example, optimizing diabetic control to minimize progression. Patients find orthotics and joint protection helpful. Immobilization of the foot in plaster cast can be tried. There are case reports of the success of intravenous bisphosphonates, although controlled trial data is lacking for this and other therapies. In cases of hindfoot disease in DM failing to improve with conservative therapy, arthrodesis may be considered.

Major causes of neuropathic arthritis

- Trauma.
- Paraneoplastic sensory neuropathy – induced.
- Endocrine and metabolic causes:
  - diabetes;
  - pernicious anaemia;
  - Cushing's;
  - Alcohol;
  - Glucocorticoids.
- Leprosy.
- Neurological conditions:
  - Syphilis;
  - Syringomyelia;
  - spina bifida;
  - multiple sclerosis;
  - hereditary sensory-motor neuropathy;
  - cord compression.
- Inflammatory conditions:
  - Amyloid;
  - Scleroderma;
  - other autoimmune CTDs.

Osteonecrosis (ischaemic necrosis; see also p. 433)
This condition is also known as ischaemic/avascular or aseptic necrosis, although there are eponymous syndromes depending on the sites involved (e.g. Legg-Calvé-Perthes disease of femoral head in children). See Table on p. 433 for full list).

- The incidence has been estimated at 1 in 10 000–20 000 per year in the USA. Peak onset is from 20 to 50 years with an equal gender ratio.
- Osteonecrosis is usually idiopathic. The assumption is that vascular supply is compromised in bones prone to infarction – those without adequate collateral arterial supply. The commonest secondary causes are:
  - fracture mechanically compromising blood supply (e.g. femoral neck);
  - drugs – high dose glucocorticoids (e.g. post transplant), excessive alcohol, cyclophosphamide therapy, intravenous bisphosphonates (jaw);
  - diseases affecting blood flow – vasculitis, sickle cell disease, HIV, cancer;
  - low oxygen tension (Caisson's disease).

- Typically, osteonecrosis presents with refractory pain in the affected joint, although this is often not severe and the index of suspicion therefore needs to be high in appropriate patients.
- The affected bone may be tender if superficial (e.g. Kienbock's disease). Over time, range of movement and function can be progressively impaired if untreated.
- As collapse of the femoral head is quite common in end-stage hip disease, it can be impossible to discriminate whether the osteonecrosis is a primary or secondary process.
- If radiographs are uninformative (as is often the case in early disease) then bone scintigraphy, CT or, preferably, MRI should be performed. MR particularly can stage the lesion, monitor conservative management and can inform surgical approach.

Treatment
Conservative management includes analgesia, NSAIDs, resting, and passive stretching the affected joint. Surgical options include core decompression (for early hip disease), osteotomy, bone grafting, or arthroplasty. As with most other indications for surgery, controlled evidence of benefit is lacking.

Resources
Internet sites
http://www.osteonecrosis.org/nofbrochure/nonf-brochure.htm.

Khan NK. *Neuropathic arthopathy*. Available at: http://www.emedicine.com/radio/topic476.htm

Rothschild BM. *Diffuse idiopathic skeletal hyperostosis*. Available at: http://www.emedicine.com/orthoped/topic74.htm;

Centre for Osteonecrosis Research. http://www.osteonecrosis.org/pages/osteo.html.

See also
CPPD Depositor disease	p. 388
Gout	p. 384
Osteonecrosis	p. 433

Chapter 13

Crystal arthritis

Gout *384*
Calcium pyrophosphate dihydrate disease *388*
The basic calcium phosphate crystals *392*

Gout

Definition
The term gout is used to describe an inflammatory arthritis triggered by the crystallization of monosodium urate crystals in joints or soft tissue. The spectrum of disease is broad.

Classification and spectrum of disease
- Asymptomatic hyperuricaemia, which may not progress to acute gout.
- Acute gout due to monosodium urate deposition in joints or soft tissue.
- Recurrent attacks.
- Chronic tophaceous gout.
- Urolithiasis.
- Urate nephropathy (rare).

Diagnostic criteria
The presence of monosodium urate crystals in a joint, either during an attack or in asymptomatic joints, is the gold standard diagnostic test. Six or more criteria of the American College of Rheumatology guidelines make the diagnosis of gout highly likely.

Epidemiology
- In the UK, gout has an overall prevalence of 1.39% (male: female ratio of 3.6:1). Gout is rare in pre-menopausal women.
- The incidence is more difficult to determine. The incidence and prevalence of gout are both strongly age-related (prevalence >7% in men, and >4% in women, over the age of 75 years).

Aetiology and pathophysiology
- Hyperuricaemia is the most important risk factor for developing gout and, in most cases, results from impaired renal excretion rather than over-production.
- Not all people with hyperuricaemia or monosodium urate within a joint develop gout, although the 5-year cumulative risk is around one-third for those with a serum uric acid of greater than 0.6 mmol/l (10 mg/dl).
- Monosodium urate crystals cause inflammation and induce an attack of synovitis, but can also be found in asymptomatic joints.
- In younger patients (<25 years) underlying causes should be considered, such as myeloproliferative disease or rare inherited disorders, e.g. the Lesch–Nyhan syndrome or familial hyperuricaemia with renal failure.
- Tophi are formed from urate deposits in some patients in prolonged hyperuricaemia. They are usually subcutaneous and are seen in late disease. They contain amorphous urates, lipids, proteins, and calcific deposits.

Risk factors
A number of risk factors have been identified, including:
- Overall body weigh or central obesity.
- Very rapid weight loss through dieting may cause hyperuricaemia, and an acute attack.
- Hypertension.
- Loop and thiazide diuretics.
- Excessive alcohol intake.
- Occupations such as business executives or naval marine.

Causes of hyperuricaemia
Primary
Secondary
Causes of under excretion of urate
- Renal impairment.
- Hypertension.
- Hypothyroidism.
- Drugs, e.g. ethanol, aspirin, diuretics.
- Lead toxicity.

Causes of over production of urate
- Malignancy: lymphoproliferative diseases, tumour lysis syndrome.
- Severe exfoliative psoriasis.
- Excessive consumption.
- Drugs, e.g. ethanol, cytotoxics.
- Inborn errors of metabolism.

Clinical presentation
Key features in history
Acute gout
- First attacks of acute gout are usually monoarticular (up to 90% of patients) with the metatarsophalangeal joint of the great toe affected in more than 50%.
- Joints other than the 1st metatarsophalangeal joint (MTPJ) include weight bearing joints, the wrist, the elbow and small joints of the hand. Axial involvement is rare in early disease.
- Attacks are usually self-limiting after 5–7 days.
- Onset is often late at night or in the early morning.
- Low grade fever with malaise may occur.
- Precipitants of an attack include intercurrent illness, surgery and dehydration e.g. alcohol excess.

Chronic gout
- Polyarticular gout is often a feature of chronic disease.
- Repeated attacks get closer together and become more prolonged.
- Repeated attacks may result in deformity, reduced range of joint movement and chronic pain.
- Chronic gout is often associated with tophi.

Key features on examination
Acute gout
- A hot, swollen, exquisitely tender joint is typical.
- There may be involvement of the soft tissues, with cellulitis or tenosynovitis.
- Podagra is the term used to describe desquamation that occurs several days after the attack in the skin overlying the affected joint. It is not specific for gout.
- Bursitis may be present, most commonly affecting the olecranon bursa or prepatellar bursa.

Chronic gout
- Joints may become deformed by recurrent attacks, with consequential impaired function.
- Tophi are found subcutaneously, but can also occur in bone and end organs. Common sites for tophi are the bursa around elbows and knees, the pinna of the ear, the

Achilles tendon, and over MCPJs on the dorsum of the hand.
- Tophi are not associated with an inflammatory response.
- Tophi are usually painless, although a urate-rich, thick white/creamy discharge may occur from tophi if the skin is breached.

Natural history
- Recurrent acute attacks can be prolonged and may not resolve without treatment.
- Untreated, recurrent acute attacks of gout progress to chronic polyarthritis and/or tophus formation, with tophi reported in 12% of patients at 5 years.
- Tophi can develop after only one or two acute attacks of gout, usually in elderly women and at the site of Heberden's nodes.
- Chronic tophaceous gout is more likely in those with early disease onset, alcohol misuse, persistent hyperuricaemia, and poor drug compliance.
- The natural history of radiological progression and joint destruction in untreated recurrent gout has not been established in observational studies, but treatment may reduce disease progression.
- Gout is associated with a two-fold risk of renal calculi and is associated with high urinary urate excretion.

Co-morbidities
Compared with patients with osteoarthritis, patients with gout are more likely to have coronary artery disease, hypertension, diabetes, insulin resistance, the metabolic syndrome, and chronic renal failure. Serum urate may be an independent risk factor for both renal disease and coronary artery disease.

Investigations
Blood tests
- A mild to moderate leucocytosis is seen in acute gout, although not in chronic gout.
- An elevation of acute phase proteins is typical in acute attacks of gout
- Serum creatinine will establish baseline renal function prior to treatment.
- Serum urate is unreliable during an acute attack, as levels may fall, and may delay the diagnosis.
- Blood cultures will be negative but should be collected if septic arthritis is a possibility.

Synovial fluid
Joint aspiration with synovial fluid analysis is the most important diagnostic test. Synovial fluid should be cultured even if monosodium urate crystals are identified, as gout and sepsis can co-exist. Monosodium urate crystals are negatively birefringent and needle-shaped under polarized light. Crystals may deteriorate and if there is any delay in microscopy, the synovial fluid should be refrigerated.

Imaging
- Plain radiographs are unhelpful in early gout. Soft tissue swelling may be seen, but is a non-specific finding.
- The hallmarks of radiographic gout are the presence of tophi, which appear eccentric and nodular, sometimes with calcification, in the soft tissues near a joint.
- Erosions may occur if the tophus lies next to the cortex of the bone, with resulting new periosteal bone formation. The classical description is that of an erosion with an overhanging margin.
- If the tophus is found in a joint, the typical appearance of the erosion is of a punched out lesion with a sclerotic border.
- Erosions are commonly found on the head of the first metatarsal.
- In acute gout, ultrasound is useful to identify synovitis within the joint and can aid accuracy guiding the needle into the joint if blind aspiration has been unsuccessful. A granular or sparky appearance of the synovial fluid has been described in patients with gout, but does not replace the need for joint aspiration for diagnosis.

Histology
Gouty tophi can be surgically removed, although this is rarely necessary. The exudate from tophi contains monosodium urate, which can be identified on polarized light microscopy if the exudate is smeared onto a slide.

Differential diagnosis
Septic arthritis is the most important diagnosis to exclude, because of its associated mortality and morbidity. Other crystal arthropathies may result in similar clinical features, although the treatment modalities are less well defined in this group. Chronic gout may mimic nodal osteoarthritis, and polyarticular gout may mimic inflammatory arthritis. As both are self-limiting, each may be confused with palindromic rheumatoid arthritis.

General aims of treatment
- Asymptomatic hyperuricaemia does not require treatment.
- Septic arthritis should be considered in any patient with an acutely hot, swollen joint.
- Pain relief with NSAIDs and simple analgesia should be commenced.
- Terminate the attack as soon as possible.
- Assess patients for recognized co-morbidities.

Management of acute gout
- Acute gout is intensely painful, but is usually self-limiting, resolving spontaneously in 1–2 weeks.
- There is a wide spectrum of attacks of gout from mild monoarthritis to severe polyarticular flares.
- Ice therapy, NSAIDs, colchicine, and glucocorticoids are effective.
- The affected joint should be rested.

NSAIDs
- Indometacin has been the traditional NSAID of choice, although there is no evidence for the superiority of any one NSAID over another, in either efficacy or safety in an acute attack.
- Most have an effect within 4 h of administration.
- NSAIDs should be avoided in patients with heart failure, renal insufficiency, or a history of previous peptic disease

Colchicine
- Most patients respond to colchicine within 18 hours and joint inflammation subsides in 75–80% of patients.
- NSAIDs may work more quickly, but colchicine does have a role in patients in whom NSAIDs are absolutely contraindicated.
- BSR guidelines recommend doses of 500µg 2–4 times daily, which are less likely to induce diarrhoea than those doses recommended in the BNF but may be associated with a slower clinical response.

Glucocorticoids
- Glucocorticoids are useful in patients who cannot tolerate or are not improving with NSAIDs or colchicine.
- Intra-articular injections are effective in monoarthritis or oligoarthritis.
- Oral, intramuscular or, more rarely, intravenous glucocorticoids are more appropriate in patients with polyarticular gout.
- No consensus exists for the dose of oral glucocorticoid, but prednisolone for 20–50 mg daily for 2 weeks is appropriate. Intramuscular depomedrone in a dose of 120 mg is the standard dose for intramuscular glucocorticoids.

Management of further attacks
In general, fewer subsequent attacks are seen in those with lower plasma uric acid levels. 40% of patients will not experience any further attacks within a year of their first attack. Within 3 years some 80% of patients will have had a further attack. Therefore, current guidance recommends patients with a first attack of gout should not be treated with serum urate lowering drugs unless they have a second attack within a year. However, there are specific groups where treatment is recommended following a first attack of acute gout:
- Patients with visible gouty tophi.
- Patients with renal insufficiency (raised plasma creatinine, Ccreat or GFR <80 ml/min).
- Patients with uric acid stones and gout.
- Patients who need require diuretics.

Treatment should be continuous and long-term. Allopurinol maintains low serum urate levels for at least 20 years, with no increase in side-effects. The main choice for specific uric acid-lowering drugs lies between agents inhibiting urate production (uricostatic agents) and those promoting urate excretion (uricosuric agents).

Uricostatic agents
Inhibitors of the enzyme xanthine oxidase inhibit production of urate from hypoxanthine and xanthine.

Allopurinol: allopurinol is the drug of choice in long term treatment of gout.
- Allopurinol should not be commenced during an acute attack, but should be introduced 1–2 weeks later. However, if allopurinol results in a flare, it should be continued during the acute attack and prophylactic cover added.
- The current recommendation is to introduce low dose colchicine (500 µg bd) for up to 6 months following introduction of allopurinol to avoid attacks of gout, or NSAIDs for 4–6 weeks in patients who are intolerant of colchicine.
- The dose of allopurinol should be increased by 50–100 mg, in response to changes in serum urate levels, and aiming for a serum urate half the upper limit of the normal range (less than 300 µmol/l).
- Most patients will achieve a reduction in serum urate levels within 7 days and certainly within 4 weeks, allowing for adjustment of the allopurinol dosage at short intervals. This may take longer in patients with tophi who have a higher total urate burden.
- A dose of up to 900 mg/day of allopurinol may be required to suppress serum urate levels adequately in a few resistant cases.
- Side-effects: possible side-effects include transient rashes (2%), however a reduction in dose, usually results in resolution. A life-threatening allergic reaction may occur in 1:300, resulting in fever, exfoliative dermatitis, mucositis, vasculitis, hepatitis and renal damage.
- Drug interactions: warfarin and azathioprine.

Other uricostatic agents: a new xanthine oxidase inhibitor, febuxostat, is currently undergoing clinical trials. In those patients with allopurinol hypersensitivity, and who have also failed uricosuric therapy, oxipurinol, and thiopurinol are other options, although severe hypersensitivity to allopurinol may also predict a severe reaction to these agents.

Uricosuric agents
Uricosuric agents are not widely prescribed in the UK, but are available for second line use in patients who are intolerant of or resistant to allopurinol. They carry a risk of increased uric acid stone formation.
- **Suphinpyrazone (Anturan, Novartis)**: 200–800 mg/day is only useful in patients with normal renal function. Side-effects: gastrointestinal (10–15%), inhibition of platelet function causing gastrointestinal haemorrhage, marrow failure.
- **Probenecid:** 0.5–2.0 g/day can be obtained on a named patient basis, but is only effective in patients with a serum creatinine <200 mol/l. Side-effects: dyspepsia and reflux oesophagitis (10%).
- **Benzbromarone** 50–200 mg/day in patients with mild or moderate renal insufficiency (creatinine clearance 30–60 ml/min). Benzbromarone is unlicensed in the UK, but can be obtained on a named patient basis. It is the most potent of the uricosuric agents. *Side-effects:* diarrhoea (10%), rare hepatotoxicity, and fatal hepatic necrosis. It is useful in patients with renal impairment.

Uricolytic agents
Two forms of urate oxidase [uricozyme and rasburicase, (Fasturec)], are available for treatment of chronic gout and are administered intravenously. Their use is limited by the formation of antibodies, which result in infusion reactions, but these drugs may be of use in patients who cannot tolerate allopurinol.

Other agents
Low dosage (500 µg od/tds) colchicine has a role in long-term prophylactic treatment and is effective in over 80%, but use can be restricted because of the risk of diarrhoea with high doses. Losartan, fenofibrate, and to a lesser extent atorvastatin have a weak uricosuric effect, making these drugs useful in the treatment of gout in patients with other co-morbidities.

Combination therapy
Combination therapy with benzbromarone and allopurinol together is more effective at reducing plasma urate concentrations than either drug alone and is therefore useful in patients who cannot tolerate high doses of allopurinol.

Physical therapies
- Ice packs help with symptomatic relief.
- Rest should be advised in acute attacks with mobilization encouraged as the attack is settling.
- Following an attack, moderate physical exercise aids gradual weight reduction, and reduces serum urate. However, intense exercise and joint trauma may precipitate a further acute attack.

Follow-up
- Review at 4–6 weeks following the first acute attack of gout is recommended to assess lifestyle factors, blood pressure, serum urate, renal function, and blood glucose.
- In patients with recurrent attacks, 3-monthly serum urate and creatinine levels are indicated for the first year, followed by annual assessment.

Subgroups requiring precautions
- Patients with renal insufficiency. GFR, rather than serum creatinine should guide treatment. Allopurinol causes more rashes and other adverse events in patients with renal insufficiency. Probenecid and sulfinpyrazone are ineffective in renal failure, and colchicine and NSAIDs should be avoided in this patient group. Benzbromarone can be used in patients with a plasma creatinine up to 500 mol/l.
- Elderly patients may need lower doses of allopurinol, and colchicine, and NSAIDs should be prescribed cautiously.

Table 13.1 Modification of allopurinol dosage with reduced renal function

GFR	Usual dose of allopurinol
>80 ml/min	200–300 mg daily
60–80 ml/min	100–200 mg daily
30–60 ml/min	50–100 mg daily
15–30 ml/min	50–100 mg alternate days
On dialysis	50–100 mg weekly

Patient advice
- **Dietary advice:** avoid foods with very high purine content such as shellfish, offal, and sardines, and moderating intake of other foods with relatively high purine content, such as meat and game. Even though some vegetables are high in urate, vegetarian diets are less associated with gout suggesting different metabolic pathways. Restricting protein intake to 70 g/day may also be beneficial.
- **Fluid intake:** patients with nephrolithiasis should drink at least 2 l/day to reduce the risk of stone formation. Water, fruit juice, skimmed or semi-skimmed milk, sugar-free squashes, cordials, tea, and coffee are all suitable. High intake of dietary fructose, which is found in sugar sweetened soft drinks, has recently been associated with an increased risk of gout in men.
- **Alcohol** can raise the serum urate both by enhancing urate production and by reducing renal clearance. Advice about alcohol consumption therefore should include:
  - restricting alcohol consumption to less than 21 units per week (men) and 14 units/week (women);
  - avoid beer, stout, port and similar fortified wines;
  - have at least 3 alcohol-free days per week.

Resources
Guidelines
BSR.
Prodigy Guidance on Gout 1999, updated 2004.
EULAR Standing Committee for International Clinical Studies including Therapeutics (ESCISIT).

Patient organizations
UK Gout Society

Internet sites
www.ukgoutsociety.org

http://www.prodigy.nhs.uk/gout/management/quick_answers/scenario_acute_gout

http://www.prodigy.nhs.uk/gout/management/quick_answers/scenario_preventing_gout

http://rheumatology.oxfordjournals.org/cgi/content/full/kem056av1

Controversies
The NICE technology appraisal for Febuxostat is due in September 2008.

ICD-10 codes
M10.0	Idiopathic gout
M10.1	Lead-induced gout
M10.2	Drug-induced gout
M10.3	Gout due to impairment of renal function
M10.4	Other secondary gout
M10.9	Gout, unspecified

References
Wallace SL, Robinson H, Masi AT, Decker JL, McCarty DJ, Yu T-F. Preliminary criteria for the classification of the acute arthritis of primary gout. *Arthritis Rheum* 1977; **20**: 895–900.

Zhang W, Doherty M, Bardin T, Pascual T, Barskova V, Conaghan P, et al. EULAR evidence based recommendations for gout. Part I: diagnosis. *Ann Rheum Dis* 2006; **65**: 1301–11.

Calcium pyrophosphate dihydrate disease

Definition
Calcium pyrophosphate disease (CPPDD) deposition in joints results in both an acute and chronic arthropathy. The term pseudogout is used to describe the acute arthritis caused by CPPDD crystals. Chondrocalcinosis is the name used to describe the radiological appearances of crystal deposition within cartilage, but is not specific for CPPDD crystals and can occur with deposition of other minerals.

History
CPPDD crystals were first identified in 1962, but the pathophysiology of crystal formation and disease progression is poorly understood. Treatment is therefore symptomatic.

Diagnostic criteria
Demonstration of the presence of CPPDD crystals on polarized light microscopy is the gold standard diagnostic test.

Classification
Rosenthal and Ryan proposed diagnostic criteria for CPPDD disease in 2001 and, although useful, does not allow classification of all patients. A different classification is based on defining sporadic, familial and secondary causes.

Table 13.2 Rosethal and Ryan diagnostic criteria for CPPDD disease

Type A	Pseudogout/acute inflammatory monoarthritis
Type B	Pseudorheumatoid/polyarthritis with synovitis
Type C &D	Pseudo-osteoarthritis/joint degeneration with (type C) or without (type D) acute synovitic attacks
Type E	Asymptomatic (incidence unknown)
Type F	Pseudoneurotrophic/severe joint destruction with or without neuropathy
Others	Tophaceous CPPDD deposits, spinal CPPDD deposits, crowned dens syndrome, spinal stenosis

Epidemiology
- Prevalence and incidence have been difficult to determine in view of the broad spectrum of presentation, but an estimation of prevalence suggests CPPDD to be between half that or equivalent to gout.
- CPPDD is more prevalent in women, with an average age at presentation of 72.
- Both incidence and prevalence increase with age, with presentation unusual below the age of 50 years. The presence of CPPDD in patients less than this age should prompt investigation of underlying metabolic causes.
- Radiographic prevalence is estimated to be 8.1%, rising to 27.1% in those over 85.
- Familial CPPDD appears to be a heterogenous group of diseases mostly inherited by an autosomal dominant inheritance and associated with severe, premature CPPDD disease.

Aetiology and pathophysiology
It remains unclear why patients develop CPPDD crystals, although abnormalities in pyrophosphate metabolism seem to be central. Crystal deposition in cartilage appears to result, with deposition in both hyaline and fibrocartilage. Histologically, large chondrocytes can be identified, which are not found in osteoarthritis, although the role of these is unclear. How crystals reach a joint, cause inflammation, and how resolution of an acute attack occurs are also poorly understood. As with gout, a number of precipitants of an acute attack are recognized, which include intercurrent illness, stroke, trauma, surgery, and some drugs.

Clinical presentation
Key features in history and examination
Acute pseudogout (Type A)
- This is the commonest presentation of pseudogout.
- The term pseudogout reflects the clinical similarities between an acute attack of CPPDD and gout.
- A monoarticular presentation is typical.
- Pain is acute in onset with pain, swelling, and erythema.
- The knee, wrist, shoulder, and elbow are the commonest joints affected.
- Attacks are usually self-limiting, but tend to be more prolonged than gout.
- Fever with malaise may occur.
- Precipitants of an attack include intercurrent illness preceding the onset of an attack, trauma, and surgery.
- Elderly patients can present with systemic malaise, with hypotension and confusion, mimicking systemic sepsis or other conditions.

Pseudorheumatoid presentation (type B)
- Large joint symptoms are common, with history of generalized stiffness.
- Small joint involvement is rare.
- Early morning stiffness may be marked.
- Differentiation from rheumatoid arthritis may be difficult, but CPPDD is not associated with rheumatoid factor, CPPDD crystals are isolated from the joints and flares of CPPDD typically affect one joint at a time, whereas in rheumatoid arthritis flares are more generalized.

Pseudo-osteoarthritis (Types C and D)
- Pain and stiffness is the commonest presentation of the pseudo-osteoarthritis types.
- Examination reveals a restricted range of movement.
- The pattern of joint involvement may be useful as upper limb involvement may occur, a pattern less commonly seen in patients with osteoarthritis.
- Type C has acute flares of pseudogout on the background of pseudo-osteoarthritis.
- Treatment of type D is as for osteoarthritis.

Asymptomatic (Type E)
- These patients are picked up incidentally on plain radiographs.
- This may reflect the largest group of patients with CPPDD disease.

Neuropathic CPPDD disease (Type F)
This is rare, but describes those cases where CPPDD disease has been described in the presence of neuropathy in association with tertiary syphilis.

Other forms of CPPDD disease
Tophaceous deposits of CPPDD, similar to those seen in tophaceous gout are rare. They are described in tendons, bursae, and bone.

CHAPTER 13 **Crystal arthritis**

Spinal deposits occur in the ligametum flavum, resulting in clinical symptoms of cord compression, in either the cervical or lumbar spine.

The crowned dens syndrome describes acute attacks of neck pain due to CPPDD deposition around the atlanto-axial joint, and may be associated with fever and malaise.

Natural history
Unlike gout, there is no established progression from one type of CPPDD disease to another, although type D would be reclassified as type C following an acute episode of pseudogout.

Co-morbidities
There are a number of conditions which are thought to be associated with CPPDD. Screening for these is important if CPPDD disease is diagnosed in anyone under the age of 50.
- Haemochromatosis.
- Hypothyroidism.
- Wilson's disease.
- Hyperparathroidism.
- Hypomagnesaemia.
- Hypophosphataemia.

Other looser associations include gout, sustained hypercalcaemia, and diabetes mellitus.

Investigations in acute pseudogout
Blood tests
- A mild to moderate leucocytosis is seen in acute attacks.
- The inflammatory response is reflected in elevation of acute phase proteins including CRP and ESR.
- Serum creatinine to establish baseline renal function prior to treatment should be established.
- Blood cultures will be negative, but should be collected if septic arthritis is a possibility.
- Blood tests are unhelpful in chronic CPPDD disease.
- Screening of younger patients for underlying metabolic associations should include calcium, magnesium, and ferritin.

Joint aspiration and synovial fluid analysis
- Joint aspiration and synovial fluid analysis is the most important diagnostic test.
- Synovial fluid is frequently heavily blood stained.
- Synovial fluid should be cultured even if CPPDD crystals are identified as crystal arthropathy and sepsis can co-exist.
- CPPDD crystals are weakly positively birefringent rhomboid-shaped crystals under polarized light and are more difficult to identify than monosodium urate crystals.
- Crystals may deteriorate in synovial fluid so refrigeration should be considered if analysis is delayed.
- Crystals may be difficult to identify, and microscopy can therefore be negative. Crystals can be intra- or extracellular, making identification in synovial fluid more difficult.
- There is no correlation between the severity of an acute attack and the number of crystals found in the synovial fluid.

Imaging
- Plain radiographs may be normal and, therefore, unhelpful in acute pseudogout, although the presence of chondrocalcinosis does make the diagnosis more likely.
- Soft tissue swelling may be seen, but is a non-specific finding.
- Chondrocalcinosis reflects CPPDD/mineral deposition within both hyaline and fibrocartilage
- The commonest areas to find chondrocalcinosis include the medial and lateral menisci of the knee, the triangular fibrocartilage of the wrist, and the symphysis pubis.
- Eburnation, joint space narrowing and subchondral cysts, but with a relative paucity of osteophytes are typical.
- A destructive arthropathy in joints rarely affected by osteoarthritis may raise the possibility of CPPDD disease.
- Spinal disease, such as disc calcification and subchondral cysts occur in the facet joints.

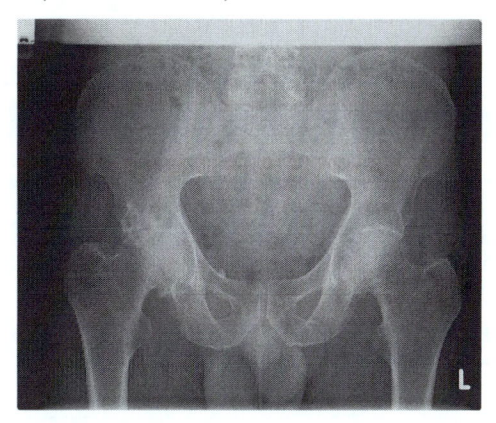

Figure 13.1 This plain radiograph was requested as the patient complained of hip pain, but incidental symphyseal chondrocalcinosis was evident.

Differential diagnosis
Septic arthritis is the most important diagnosis to exclude, because of its associated mortality and morbidity. Other crystal arthropathies may result in similar clinical features.

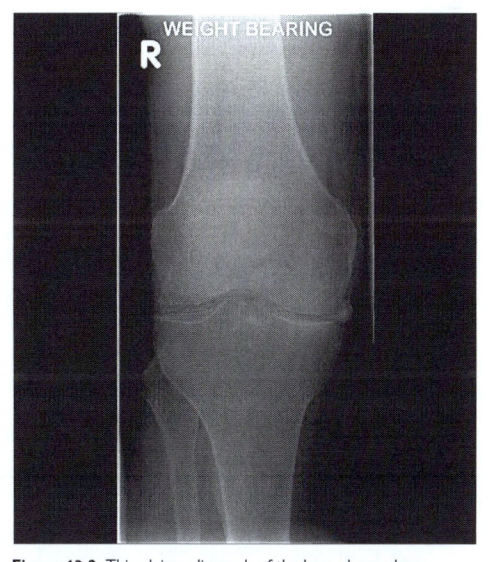

Figure 13.2 This plain radiograph of the knee shows dense tricompartmental chondrocalcinosis with early osteoarthritis. Chondrocalcinosis was detected within the symphysis pubis on a plain radiograph in this patient with osteoarthritis of the hip.

Treatment

Aim of treatment during the acute episode
- Exclude septic arthritis.
- Pain relief with NSAIDs and simple analgesia.
- Intra-articular injection of glucocorticoid has been shown to reduce the duration of attacks of acute pseudogout, although no randomized controlled trials exist.
- Treat any underlying precipitating cause.
- Rest the joint.

Aim of treatment during recurrent attacks/chronic CPPDD
- Low dose colchicine (1 mg/day) may reduce the frequency of attacks.
- Low dose oral prednisolone is sometimes used in patients with frequent attacks, but there is no evidence base to support this.
- Patients with pseudorheumatoid CPPDD may respond to DMARD therapy, and success has been reported with gold and hydroxychloroquine.
- Joint replacement surgery may be necessary for those joints in which there is extensive cartilage loss.

Prognosis
The natural history remains unclear in long-term disease.

Patient advice
- No lifestyle changes have been shown to alter the frequency of attacks.
- The joint should be rested in the event of an acute attack.
- Patients should be advised to seek medical attention in the event of a new attack in order to exclude other causes of hot swollen joint and to speed the administration of intra-articular glucocorticoid therapy to terminate an acute attack quickly.

Resources

Guidelines
There are no accepted guidelines for the management and treatment of CPPDD disease.

Internet sites
http://www.library.nhs.uk/musculoskeletal/ViewResource.aspx?resID=77860

www.patient.co.uk/showdoc/40001166/

Controversies
There are no targeted therapies in CPPDD disease because current understanding of the pathophysiology remains to be established.

There is no evidence base for the role of oral glucocorticoid therapy in patients with recurrent attacks of pseudogout.

In patients with severe destructive arthropathy, there are no randomized controlled data to demonstrate a disease modifying effect of any therapeutic agent.

ICD-10 codes
M11	Other crystal arthropathies
M11.1	Familial chondrocalcinosis
M11.2	Other chondrocalcinosis

References

Bouvet J, et al. Acute neck pain due to calcifications surrounding the odontoid process: the crowned dens syndrome. *Arthritis Rheum* 1985; **22**: 928–32.

Doherty M, Dieppe PA, Watt I. Pyrophosphate arthropathy: a propsepctive study. *Br J Rheumatol* 1993; **32**: 189–96

Kohn NN, Hughes RE, McCarty DJ, et al. The significance of calcium pyrophosphate crystals in the synovial fluid of arthritis patients: The 'pseudogout syndrome'. II. Identification of crystals. *Ann Intern Med* 1962; **56**: 738–45.

Reginato AJ, Tamesis E, Netter P. Familial and clinical aspects of calcium pyrophosphate deposition disease. *Curr Rheumatol Rep* 1999; **1**: 112–20.

Rosenthal AK. Pathogenesis of calcium pyrophosphate crystal deposition disease. *Curr Rheumatol Rep* 2001; **3**: 17–23.

Rosenthal AK, Ryan LM. Calcium pyrophosphate crystal deposition disease; pseudogout; articular chondrocalcinosis. In: Koopman WJ (eds) *Arthritis and Allied Conditions*, 14th edn. Philadelphia: Lea and Febiger, 2348–71.

The basic calcium phosphate crystals

Definition
The deposition of calcium containing crystals in joints or soft tissue surrounding joints causes localized pain, swelling and tenderness in the majority of patients. The crystals implicated in this process include those formed from calcium pyrophosphate dihydrate and basic calcium phosphate (BCP) crystals, which include carbonated-substituted hydroxyapatite, tricalcium phosphate, and octacalcium phosphate. BCP will be discussed here.

Classification and spectrum of disease
There are no classification criteria, but a number of clinical conditions are recognized and include:
- Calcific tendinitis/acute periarthritis of the joint capsule.
- Crystal associated osteoarthritis.
- Acute synovitis of small joints.
- Destructive arthropathy, e.g. Milwaukee shoulder syndrome.

Monoarticular presentation is the commonest presentation, although occasionally polyarticular disease may occur. The shoulder is the commonest joint involved and may occur bilaterally. Other less common sites include the elbow, wrist, hand, knee, ankle, foot, and spine.

Diagnostic criteria
- The identification of calcium containing crystals within the affected joint is diagnostic, although the crystals are small and not detected on routine microscopy with polarized light.
- Definitive diagnosis requires electron microscopy although alizarin red S stain and polarized light microscopy has been used as a basic screening test.
- No accepted diagnostic criteria have been developed, but the presence of typical clinical features and the presence of calcification on radiological investigations make the diagnosis probable.

Epidemiology
- Most cases occur in patients aged between 30 and 50, although BCP has been described in children.
- Men and women are equally affected.
- Calcium containing crystals are reported in up to 60% of patients undergoing knee arthroplasty due to the association with osteoarthritis.

Aetiology and pathophysiology
- The mechanism remains poorly understood.
- Extra-articular inorganic pyrophosphate is recognized as an important factor in the control of calcium crystal formation with high production by chondrocytes implicated in BCP crystal formation.
- Age and genetic factors are thought to increase extra-articular inorganic pyrophosphate

Risk factors
A number of predisposing factors, such as family history, trauma, and degenerative factors have been postulated, but remain tenuous.

Clinical features
Key features
- Pain usually arises from the periarticular tissues with patients describing acute onset of pain, and examination confirms swelling and tenderness of the affected area.
- Calcification can be asymptomatic and picked up on incidental radiological investigations.
- The site of involvement may be unusual, for example, toes, wrists, elbows, and ankles.
- Joint involvement results in a destructive arthropathy, for example, the Milwaukee shoulder.
- Symptoms are usually self-limiting.

Presentation of commonly involved joints
Milwaukee shoulder
- The classical presentation is in elderly women with rapidly accumulating shoulder effusions.
- Symptoms and disease are unresponsive to glucocorticoid injections or other treatment modalities.
- Joint disease results in underlying joint destruction and is often associated with a large rotator cuff tear.

Elbow
Calcification can occur in the tendons, bursae, and the joint capsule.

Hand and wrist
The commonest site of tendon involvement in the hand and wrist is in the flexor carpi ulnaris tendon.

Hip and pelvis
Tendinous calcification can occur in gluteus medius and minimus (around the greater and lesser trochanters of the hip).

Knee
The quadriceps and patellar tendons may be affected as may the bursae and the joint capsule.

Ankle and foot
The Achilles tendon may be affected along with a number of other different tendons and ligaments.

Spine
Paraspinal ligaments may develop calcification, with the longus coli tendon the most commonly affected.

Natural history
Acute calcific tendinitis is usually self-limiting, but destructive arthropathy in joints can be resistant to treatment and tends to be progressive.

Investigations
Blood tests
In the majority of cases, normal inflammatory markers and a normal white cell count are found. However, an acute inflammatory response may be seen in patients with acute calcific deposits.

Imaging
- The typical appearance on plain imaging is of calcific deposits, which may vary in size. These deposits may be unfragmented when found in asymptomatic joints but typically become fragmented in patients with acutely painful joints and an active inflammatory component.
- Radiographic appearances are of resolution of calcific material if radiographs are repeated.
- Erosion or breaching of the cortex of the bone may occur and CT is useful in excluding malignant causes of bone erosion.

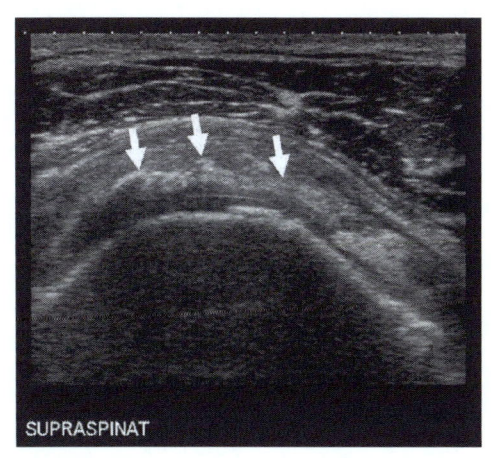

Figure 13.3 On US, calcium deposition can be visualized within the supraspinatus tendon, shown here by the arrows.

- Imaging of affected joints reveals osteoporosis, joint destruction and periarticular calcification.

Histology
Macroscopically, a cheesy calcified material is found in the periarticular soft tissues.

Differential diagnosis
The differential diagnosis includes those causes of acute localized pain:
- Septic arthritis
- Other acute crystal arthropathy
- AVN
- Acute tendon tears/tendinopathy
- Trauma
- Inflammatory arthritis, e.g. RA
- Other causes of extra-articular calcification, e.g. metabolic disease, or collagen vascular disease

Aims of treatment
- The management of crystal associated osteoarthritis is the same as that for uncomplicated osteoarthritis as no specific treatment options are available.

- Acute calcific tendinitis is treated symptomatically with NSAIDS, local glucocorticoid injections and physical therapies such as heat/cold compresses, and exercise.
- More specific therapies include needling the calcific deposits under ultrasound control, shock wave therapy and surgical removal, although the evidence base for these procedures remains primarily anecdotal.
- Arthroplasty is occasionally required in severe joint destruction.

Patient advice
- There is no specific advice to avoid flares of disease.
- Advice should include resting the inflamed joint and seeking medical advice to exclude other causes of acute joint pain.
- Treatment is limited in its success in treating destructive arthropathy.
- There are no recognized triggers for acute attacks.
- Calcific tendinitis may recur in different locations, but is usually self-limiting.

Resources
Guidelines
There are no guidelines for the treatment of basic calcium phosphate crystal disease.

ICD-10 codes
M11.0   Hydroxyapatite deposition disease

References
Bonavita JA, Dalinka MK, Schumacher HR Jr. Hydroxyapatite deposition disease. *Radiology* 1980; **134**: 621–5.

Dieppe PA, Huskisson EC, Crocker P, et al. Apatite deposition disease. A new arthropathy. *Lancet* 1976; **1**: 266–8.

Garcia GM, McCord GC, Kumar R. Hydroxyapatite crystal deposition disease. *Semin Musculoskel Radiol* 2003; **7**: 187–93.

Halverson PB, McCarty DJ, Cheung HS, et al. Milwaukee shoulder syndrome: eleven additional cases with involvement of the knee in seven (basic calcium phosphate crystal deposition disease. *Semin Arthritis Rheum* 1984; **14**: 36–44.

Paul H, Reginato AJ, Schumacher HR. Alizarin red S staining as a screening test to detect calcium compounds in synovial fluid. *Arthritis Rheum* 1983; **26**: 191–200.

Chapter 14

Bone diseases

Post-menopausal osteoporosis *396*
Therapeutics of post-menopausal osteoporosis *402*
Osteoporosis in men *406*
Glucocorticoid induced osteoporosis (GIO) *408*
Osteoporosis in children *412*
Primary hyperparathyroidism *414*
Paget's disease of bone (osteodystrophia deformans) *418*
Osteomalacia and rickets *422*
Renal bone disease *426*
Osteogenesis imperfecta *428*
Miscellaneous bone diseases 1 *432*
Miscellaneous bone diseases 2 *434*

Post-menopausal osteoporosis

Definition
Osteoporosis is a disease characterized by low bone mass and/or poor bone quality, leading to enhanced bone fragility and a consequent increase in fracture risk. Low bone mass as measured by bone mineral density (BMD) is one of the most important predisposing factors for osteoporotic fracture; however, osteoporosis is more than low BMD. It is a disease of compromised bone strength. The determinants of bone strength are: mass, geometry, and microstructure, material properties, and bone turnover.

Definition utilizing a measure of BMD
BMD changes with age, increasing to a peak in the third decade then changing little over a period of consolidation. BMD then decreases slowly with a usual accelerated phase of bone loss shortly after the menopause.

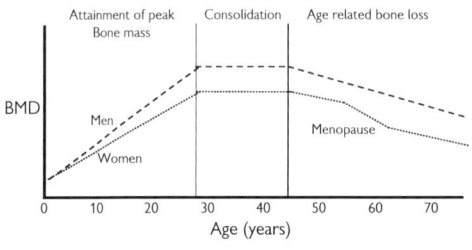

Figure 14.1 Changes in bone mass over time.

Post-menopausal osteoporosis (PMO) has been defined by the World Health Organization (WHO) as a low BMD (see below), ideally measured by hip or lumbar spine dual X-ray absorptiometry (DXA). See Table 14.1. This is an accepted definition. However, this is somewhat arbitrary and based on a surrogate, not true, measure of bone density. Currently, direct measures of the other parameters of bone strength are not incorporated either into an accepted definition of PMO or its diagnosis; however, some determinants of 'strength' would be encompassed by a definition of PMO, which includes bone fragility. Thus, a more comprehensive definition of PMO might be

> fracture sustained with low or no trauma (fragility) in association with osteoporotic range BMD (as defined by The WHO criteria).

Epidemiology
There is an increased incidence of osteoporotic fractures in women with advancing age reflecting deteriorating bone quality and mass, and an increasing tendency to fall. See Figure 14.2.

Table 14.1 The WHO definition of PMO

T-score	Interpretation
T ≤ −2.5	'Osteoporosis' – the BMD is at least 2.5 SDs below the peak mean BMD
T > −2.5, but ≤ −1.0	'Osteopaenia' – the BMD is 1–2.5 SDs below the peak mean BMD
T > −1.0	'Normal' – the BMD is less than 1 SD below the peak mean BMD

WHO definition of PMO based on multiples of the SD of the range of women's peak BMD ('about age 25–35 years).

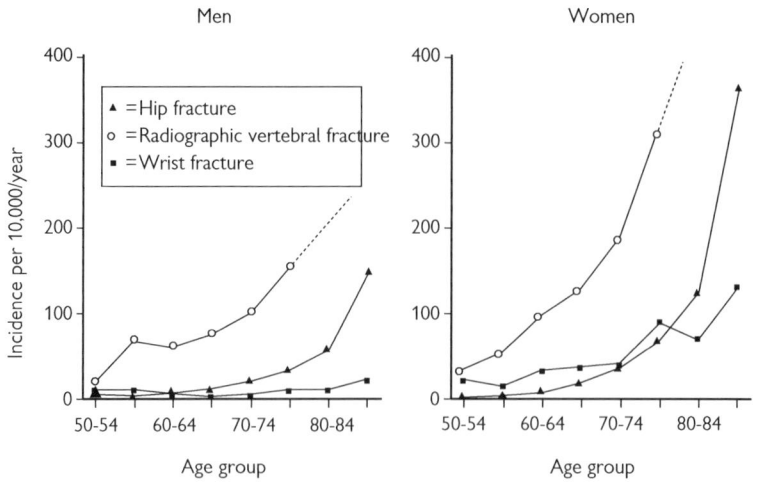

Figure 14.2 Incidence of fractures.

- Racial variation in fracture incidence exists with lower rates in Afro-Caribbean compared with Caucasian and Asian populations.
- Environmental factors such as dietary protein intake, vitamin D (25-OHD) status, and genetic factors (see below) are all likely to influence the gradient of fracture risk within any given population.
- The commonest sites of fracture associated with bone fragility are: spine, hip, distal forearm, proximal humerus, and pelvis.

Hip fractures
- Hip fractures are associated with 10–20% mortality in the first year after fracture and substantial morbidity particularly decreasing independence in the elderly.
- Worldwide it was estimated there were 1.2 m hip fractures in women in 1990. Rates of hip fracture worldwide increase with increasing latitude.
- In Western countries, above 50 years old there is a female:male ratio of hip fracture of 2:1.
- A lower rate of hip fracture incidence in some developing countries reflects the lower life expectancy.

Vertebral fracture
- The recent development of morphometric and semi-quantitative measures of vertebral fracture has facilitated some recent reliable studies of vertebral fracture.
- Only one-third of spinal fractures come to medical attention; only 25% follow a fall.
- Prevalence varies between 12 and 25% in post-menopausal women. Rates can vary owing to the difficulty in discriminating vertebral deformities from fracture – often difficult where fracture may lead to very minor changes in vertebral height. Prevalence increases with age and the gradient is steeper in women compared with men.
- Recent data from the EPIDOS study suggests fracture prevalence of 19% aged 75–79 years, 21% aged 80–84 years, and 41% in women aged 85 years and older.
- In Rochester, Minnesota the incidence was estimated as 18% per 1000 women over the age of 50 years.

Distal forearm fracture
- The incidence of wrist and distal forearm fractures increases after the menopause, although the gradient of increase with age is less steep notably after the age of 75 years compared with hip and vertebral fractures.
- Distal forearm fracture may be less frequently a consequence of a fall with advanced age given fall mechanics. Owing neuromuscular deterioration in the very elderly, a fall forwards onto an outstretched hand is less frequent compared with at a younger age. Falls tend to be more sideways or backwards with age, often causing trauma to the pelvis and posterior femur area.
- Fracture incidence rises from a premenopausal rate of 10 per 10 000 population/year to 120 per 10 000 population/year after the age of 85 years.
- There is a winter peak in presentation. Overall, there is a 4:1 ratio in favour of women compared with men.

Fracture is a risk for fracture
- Generally, the presence of one fragility fracture increases the risk of further fractures if no anti-osteoporosis treatment is given.
- Predictive power of further fracture is probably greatest for vertebral and hip fracture. Distal forearm fracture predicts an excess risk of fracture after 70 years old.

Consequences of fracture
- There are about 35 m women estimated to have/have had an osteoporotic fracture worldwide. Disability quantified as Disability Adjusted Life Years (DALYs), which incorporates mortality, was recently estimated to be greater for osteoporosis overall compared with cancer with the exception of lung cancer.
- 50% of those ambulatory prior to hip fracture are unable to walk independently after.
- One consequence of having a hip fracture is the need for permanent nursing home care <15% of women 50–55 years old, but >50% of women >90 years old.
- Given the projected increases in life expectancy it has been estimated that fractures in both women and men will increase from around 1.7m in 1990 to 6.3 m in 2050.
- Based on the above and other trends in hip fracture incidence, hip fracture is expected to rise from 46 000 in 1985 to 117 000 in 2016.

Aetiology and pathophysiology

Genetics
There is a significant heritable component to BMD, particularly peak BMD, bone turnover markers, and bone geometric parameters, each of which has been linked to fracture risk. It is estimated that 60–80% of the variation in peak BMD may be due to genetic factors.

- Fractures have an heritable component, shown in 3 large studies from the USA, Sweden, and an International Study (data from Europe, Canada, and Australia).
- Polymorphic markers in the vitamin-D receptor gene, in the promotor region of the collagen Iα1 (COL1A1) gene (Sp1) and in BMP2 (chromosome 20p12) have been linked to fracture risk in certain populations.
- Polymorphisms in the low-density lipoprotein receptor-related protein 5 (LRP5) have been linked to significant variations in BMD.
- As yet, studies have not consistently linked single gene polymorphisms to fracture and fracture risk in different populations.

Environment
Both exercise and nutritional factors have a role in determining peak bone density (a strong determinant of future PMO) and fracture risk.

- Weight-bearing exercise increases bone mass by 1–2%/year in adolescence. Exercise may also optimize skeletal growth and shape, structural aspects of skeletal growth, which may ultimately influence bone fragility.
- The type and extent of weight-bearing exercise necessary to optimize maintenance of bone mass and/or prevent increased bone turnover in post-menopausal women is unknown. Some is better than none!

Nutrition: calcium
Adequate calcium intake is important for optimal skeletal growth and gain in bone mass in children and adolescents, and maintenance of bone mass and reduction of abnormally increased bone turnover in the elderly.

- Calcium intakes are positively correlated with bone mass at all stages of life.
- Western diets typically high in protein and salt, and low in potassium can increase urinary calcium loss.
- Recommended daily intakes of calcium vary with age and skeletal development, and in the context of the country's/region's typical dietary constituents (Table 14.2).

- Calcium deficiency is most accurately determined by an elevation in PTH assuming there are no other reasons for PTH elevation. Calcium deficiency is usually a consequence of vitamin D deficiency, the two co-exist invariably to varying degrees.

Table 14.2 Recommended calcium intakes

Age group or person	Calcium intakes recommended by different authorities	
	US National Institute of Health	UK Dept., of Health*
Infants and children	From 270 mg at 7–12 months to 1300 mg age 12 years	350–550 mg
Teenagers	1300 mg	800–1000 mg
Women	1000 mg (1200 mg in women >51 years)	700 mg
Breast feeding women	No advice	1250 mg

For average calcium content in typical foods see: http://ods.od.nih.gov/factsheets/calcium.asp

*The UK NOS and others have questioned whether, for people with osteoporosis and the elderly, these amounts are sufficient.

Nutrition: vitamin D

Vitamin D facilitates calcium absorption. Over 90% of the body's vitamin D is derived (synthesized) in a UV-dependent mechanism in skin. An age-related decline in solar exposure and metabolic efficiency underscores the reason for widespread vitamin D deficiency in the elderly.
- The best current estimate for the lower limit of normal levels of vitamin D (by measurement of 25-OHD) is 30 µg/l (75 nmol/l).
- Oral intakes of vitamin D are generally low, although if UV-triggered skin generation of vitamin D is adequate, an oral intake of vitamin D is not necessary.
- In the USA and Canada, milk is fortified with vitamin D. Margarine and cereals are often carry small amounts of vitamin D. Generally, the best food source of vitamin D generally is oily fish, e.g. mackerel, salmon or sardines.
- Higher serum 25-OHD has been associated with higher BMD (NHANES III), improved lower limb neuromuscular function and fewer falls in elderly women.

Hormones

Oestrogen deficiency is a major risk for PMO.
- Oestrogen loss increases bone turnover activation frequency and contributes to remodelling imbalances though de-repressed effects on osteoblast generated IGF-1, osteoprotegerin, and TGFβ, for example, and bone marrow cytokines, such as Il-1, Il-6, and TNFα.
- The hypo-oestrogenic effects on fracture risk depend on its duration and severity, but also age-related BMD and skeletal integrity. Thus, the short-term fracture risk from hypo-oestrogenaemia in young women taking (certain) contraceptives is different to that in 51-year-old women just going through the menopause.

Other determinants of bone strength

Factors such as bone geometry and trabecular connectivity are undoubtedly important determinants of bone strength and fracture risk (see Plate 31).
- It is likely that variations in skeletal geometry achieved during skeletal growth are influenced by a complex integral of genetic and environmental factors.
- The rate of age-dependent skeletal deterioration (e.g. loss of trabecular connectivity) is more likely a function of environmental compared with genetic influences.

Risk factors

Risk factors can be considered to be intrinsic or environmental, mostly a consequence of lifestyle. Two major risks for PMO, low BMD, and falls, are influenced in turn by a combination of both intrinsic and environmental components.

Table 14.3 PMO: main risks for fracture

Intrinsic	Environmental/lifestyle
Age	Low body weight
Caucasian/Asian race	Cigarette smoking
Previous fragility fracture	Excessive alcohol
Oestrogen deficiency	Prolonged immobilization
Family history of fragility fracture	Low dietary calcium
Co-morbidities (e.g. RA)	Vitamin D deficiency

Intrinsic risk factors
- As the skeleton ages, BMD, and skeletal integrity diminishes. Age is an important determinant of fracture risk.
- Probably through an effect on having larger bones and BMD, an Afro-Caribbean skeleton is protected from the age-related effects in skeletal mass and bone quality compared with Caucasian and Asian origin skeletons.
- Oestrogen has important protective effects on the skeleton. Rapid bone loss follows oestrogen deficiency in early post-menopausal women. Also, lower levels of oestrogen measured in established post-menopausal women have been related to rates of bone loss.
- Studies are not conclusive on what family history of fracture constitutes an increased risk. The most relevant risk factor is a maternal hip fracture at a young age, say <70 years. Lesser degrees of fracture risk are possibly associated with a history of a fragility fracture in a first degree female relative and father.
- A number of conditions and medications are associated with an increased risk of PMO.

Lifestyle risk factors
- Leanness [body mass index (BMI) <20 kg/m^2] is a strong risk factor for fracture. It is dependent on BMD. Incremental changes in BMI above 20 kg/m^2 are not protective. Both mechanical effects of body mass on bone and greater circulating oestrogens after the menopause have been proposed as reasons for a protective effect of obesity.
- A lack of mechanical stimuli increases bone resorption. Hence, prolonged immobility causes a net loss of bone.
- Higher fracture risk in women who smoke is partly, although not wholly explained by lower BMD. Probable contributory factors to risk include lower body weight, earlier menopause and enhanced degradation of circulating oestrogen in smokers.
- Excessive alcohol has a number of effects: reducing gonadal hormone production, interfering with calcium absorption and vitamin D metabolism, affecting protein metabolism, causing sarcopaenia and increased falls risk. Alcoholics often also have poor nutritional intake.

- Very low calcium intake is a risk factor for PMO. Such severe calcium deficiency is usually a consequence, in part, of vitamin D deficiency. There is some controversy over whether mild or moderate calcium deficiency is an independent risk for fracture.
- High salt and caffeine intake may be risks for fracture. Increased calcium excretion may explain the risk.
- The list of conditions, which are associated with low BMD and increased bone turnover, is long. Many, but not all of these conditions, have been shown to increase the risk of fracture risk in women.
- A condition or long-term treatment associated with osteoporosis is an indication to measure BMD.

Some conditions and medications which increase the risk of osteoporosis

- *Endocrine diseases*: hyperparathyroidism, Type 1 diabetes, hyperthyroidism, Cushing's, hyperprolactinaemia.
- *Chronic inflammatory diseases*: rheumatoid arthritis, ankylosing spondylitis, Crohn's disease, coeliac disease.
- *Neuromuscular diseases*: paraplegia, multiple sclerosis.
- *Cancer*: breast cancer, multiple myeloma.
- *Transplantation*.
- *Pregnancy-induced osteoporosis*.
- *Anorexia nervosa*.
- *Rare conditions* (e.g. osteogenesis imperfecta, mastocytosis, homocystinuria).
- *Medications*:
  - glucocorticoids;
  - aromatase inhibitors;
  - long-term low molecular weight heparin;
  - anticonvulsants.

BMD (bone mass) as a risk factor for osteoporosis
- Prospective studies show the risk of osteoporotic fracture increases continuously as BMD declines. There is a 1.5–3-fold increase in risk of fracture for each standard deviation (SD) fall in BMD.
- A greater accuracy of fracture risk can be obtained by a site-specific BMD assessment.
- The highest gradient of risk is at the hip (2.6). BMD at different sites can be used to predict the future risk of fracture at the same or other sites.
- Currently BMD assessment is integral to overall osteoporosis/fracture risk assessment.

Falls (see Table 14.4)
- A fall is a prerequisite for a distal forearm and hip fracture in the majority of people. Falls increase with age particularly in post-menopausal women.
- Though just 1% of falls in the elderly leads to a fracture, a fall in the year preceding a wrist or hip fracture in the elderly is very common.
- There are numerous risk factors for falls, which in turn should be considered risks for osteoporotic fracture in elderly post-menopausal women.

Clinical features

PMO, though conventionally diagnosed on the basis of BMD (see below) is characterized clinically by fragility fracture. PMO can predate any clinical symptoms or signs.

Key features in the history
- Relevant points in the history are derived from a review of clinical risk factors (see above).
- Broadly, the history should explore age of menopause, co-morbidities, and use of medications associated with osteoporosis, nutrition, family history of fracture, previous fractures, and falls history (and causes thereof).

Table 14.4

Falls risk factors	Example causes
Previous falls	
Gait, balance, mobility, and muscle weakness	Sarcopaenia
Perceived functional ability and fear of falling	Low confidence; walking unaided
Visual deficiency	Poor eyesight; use of bifocals when walking
Cognitive impairment	Dementia
Incontinence	Diuretics; bladder pathology; neurological disease.
Home hazards	Trip hazard; poor lighting
Cardiac pathology or medications	Hypotension secondary to bradycardia or medications
Some specific medications and polypharmacy	Salt loss from diuretics (hypotension); dizziness from benzodiazepines

Key features on examination
A review of appendicular skeletal and pelvic fracture features is beyond the scope of this text. Please refer to orthopaedic texts.

Vertebral fractures (VFs)
- VFs are not always associated with pain.
- Multiple VFs in the thoracic spine can cause kyphosis. Kyphosis is not always due to VFs (e.g. multiple level intervertebral disc disease and biomechanical causes).
- Christmas tree pattern folds of skin falling down on the back can indicate multiple VFs (although is not specific).
- The lower rib cage can approximate to the iliac rim when the patient is standing if multiple VFs have caused substantial height loss.

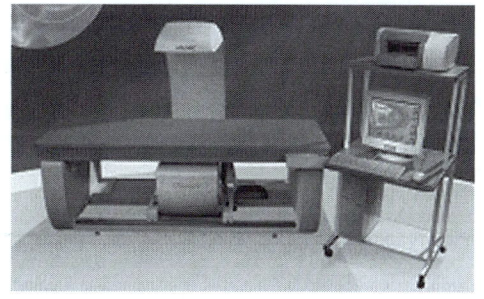

Figure 14.3 DXA scanner.

Investigations

DXA scanning

- Since 1994, a consensus report from The World Health Organization (WHO) has resulted in widespread adoption of a definition of PMO based on measurement of BMD from hip, spine, or forearm expressed in BMD standard deviation units (*T-scores*).
- DXA technique using appropriate software can estimate BMD at sites in the femoral neck, lumbar spine, forearm, and the whole skeleton.
- The T-score definition of osteoporosis has been adopted for men, but should not be used for children, adolescents, and premenopausal women.
- Greatest accuracy of specific fracture prediction derives from its site-specific BMD measurement. Hip and spine BMD are the best overall predictors of *any* fracture.
- Peripheral DXA scanners allow forearm bone BMD to be measured. Although forearm bone osteoporosis can be diagnosed, generalized PMO is not predicted well by low forearm BMD.
- As there are a number of technical issues regarding scan acquisition and interpretation there are a number of constraints on the use of DXA.

$$\text{T-Score} = \frac{\text{Measured BMD - young adult mean BMD}}{\text{Young adult BMD standard deviation (SD)}}$$

T-Scores were originally intended to be used only to interpret BMD results in post-menopausal women

Table 14.5 World Health Organization (WHO) definitions of osteoporosis and T-score classification of BMD in women

T-score	Interpretation
T ≤ −2.5	Osteoporosis – the BMD result is equal to, or more than, 2.5SDs below the young adult mean BMD
T ≤ −1, but is > −2.5	Osteopaenia – the BMD result is between 1 and 2.5 SDs below the young adult mean BMD
T > −1	Normal – the BMD result is less than 1 SD below the young adult mean BMD

See p. 401 for use of BMD in FRAX.

Spinal imaging

- Obvious vertebral fracture is shown on using DXA-based vertebral fracture analysis (VFA) or conventional lateral spinal radiographs (see Plate 29).
- Detecting mild vertebral fracture, where little change in shape of the vertebral body has occurred, is difficult using radiographs or VFA.
- There is a recognized pattern of appearance of vertebral body osteoporosis with MR, which can be useful to rule out malignancy-associated causes of fracture.
- Semiquantitative scales of vertebral morphology (e.g. after Genant or Jiang/Eastell) applied to conventional lateral spinal radiographs are useful for grading vertebral deformity and fracture for the purposes of studies. Knowledge of the scales and their derivation is useful for bone physicians, rheumatologists and radiologists.

Table 14.6 Interpretative aspects of DXA

DXA: technical or interpretative issue	Possible consequence
BMD estimated from mineralized content of bone scanned	BMD measure may reflect any condition, which affects bone mineralization in scanned area
BMD is estimated from an area (not volume) of bone	May falsely elevate vertebral body BMD from a spine where there is degenerative disease at any depth under scanned area
Gross obesity, ascites, or skeletal soft-tissue calcification in scanned area	Affects scanning acquisition – accuracy and precision.
High BMD may not always denote bone strength	Interpret scans cautiously if a condition is present that causes sclerotic, but fragile bones (e.g. renal osteodystrophy)
General assumptions from single site BMD measurement	May have low BMD in one place, but not the skeleton generally (e.g. low forearm BMD from selective effects of hyperparathyroidism)

Quantitative (heel) ultrasound (QUS)

- Though no definition of PMO using quantitative ultrasound exists and it cannot be used to *diagnose* osteoporosis, QUS may have a role in indicating and managing osteoporotic fracture risk.
- QUS machines are configured to measure broadband ultrasound attenuation (BUA) or speed of sound (SOS) through the os calcis.
- QUS scanners are portable and cheap. Both BUA and SOS predict hip fracture in post-menopausal women partly independently of DXA-derived BMD.

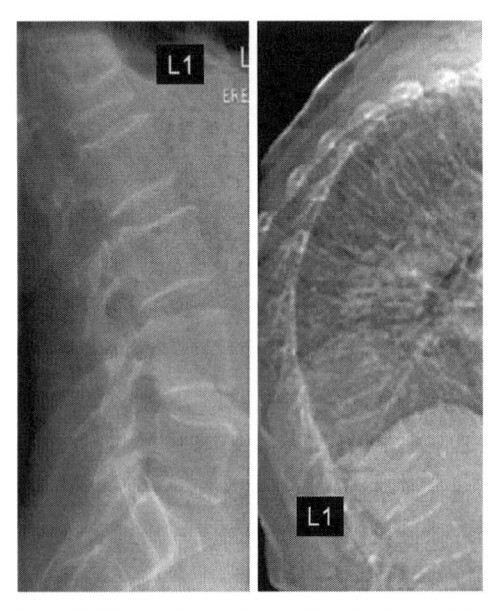

Figure 14.4 Lumbar fracture shown on lateral radiographs (left) and using DXA (Vertebral Assessment Mode). Reproduced from Osteoporosis (Oxford Rheumatology Library), Clunie & Keen, 2008, with permission from Oxford University Press.

- QUS may be useful to identify people at higher risk of low BMD measured by DXA and thus be used to reassure people that a DXA scan is not needed.
- All major therapeutic osteoporosis studies, which have proved fracture prevention, have done so in people who've had a fracture, and/or low hip and/or spine BMD measured by DXA. Fracture prevention using bisphosphonates or strontium ranelate has not been shown on patients defined at risk on the basis of QUS.
- The attributes of QUS suggest it may play a role in helping physicians manage osteoporosis risk. As no measure of bone mineral content or BMD is made, it cannot be used to diagnose osteoporosis.

Other imaging
- Conventional CT and bone scintigraphy can be helpful in some cases in characterizing fracture (e.g. pelvic), but are not routinely used to diagnose osteoporosis.
- Quantitative computed tomography (QCT) has been used in research to determine the true three-dimensional volumetric BMD of trabecular-rich bone.
- Using digital X-ray radiogrammetry (DXR), BMD of the metacarpals can be inferred from digitized radiographs of the hand. DXR has been shown to predict regional osteoporosis in certain condition, such as rheumatoid arthritis.

Laboratory investigations
- PMO typically occurs, existing without any abnormal laboratory test abnormalities.
- Frequently clinical, DXA, and other imaging investigations cannot discriminate PMO from secondary causes of osteoporosis. Laboratory tests are then indicated.
- Frequently conditions causing secondary osteoporosis can be clinically silent or difficult to detect clinically (e.g. subclinical hyperthyroidism, primary hyperparathyroidism, early osteomalacia, or myeloma). A high index of clinical suspicion is needed, although it would be
- prudent to consider a screen of laboratory tests regardless of clinical assessment where DXA scan has shown osteoporosis on T-score WHO criteria.

Laboratory tests useful in identifying causes of osteoporosis in post-menopausal women or conditions contributing to increased fracture risk in PMO
- Serum calcium, phosphate, ALP, albumen.
- 25-hydroxyvitamin D, PTH.
- TFTs, LFTs, creatinine (and estimated GFR).
- Serum and urine protein electrophoresis.
- Coeliac antibodies (e.g. tTG).

- Given that fragility, osteoporotic fracture can occur in elderly post-menopausal women at 'osteopaenic' levels of BMD above the T-score threshold ($-2.5 < T \leq -1$), it is wise to consider laboratory tests in some women who have had fragility fractures and osteopaenia, say at a certain age such as ≥65 years old.

Bone histopathology
This is the gold-standard method for diagnosing osteoporosis. A transiliac undecalcified bone biopsy is required.
- In practice obtaining a bone biopsy for routine diagnosis of osteoporosis is inappropriately invasive, costly, and unfeasible, but also, if obtained on iliac bone, might be viewed as from an inappropriate skeletal site.
- Biopsy is best reserved to clarify bone disease where multiple aetiologies may exist (e.g. associated with long-term anticonvulsants or in renal bone disease).
- In PMO findings are: cortical and trabecular bone deficit with trabeculation of endocortical bone and poor trabecular connectivity. Dynamic indices (e.g. activation frequency – the probability that a remodelling cycle will begin at any point) vary considerably.

FRAX® (WHO fracture risk assessment tool)
The FRAX tool evaluates fracture risk for patients. It is based on individual patient models integrating risks associated with clinical risk factors and femoral neck BMD. See www.shef.ac.uk/FRAX
- FRAX is based on data from large population cohorts (men and women).
- FRAX provides a 10y probability of fracture.
- FRAX can be applied for individuals in different countries.
- In the UK, FRAX on-line links directly to an online resource detailing guidance for therapy (NOGG).

References
Blake GM, Wahner HW, Fogelman I. Technical principles of X-ray absorptiometry. In: Blake GM, Wahner HW, Fogelman I, eds, *The Evaluation of Osteoporosis*. London: Martin Dunitz, 1999: 55.

Chang K, Center J, Nguyen ND, et al. Incidence of hip and other osteoporotic fractures in elderly men and women: Dubbo Osteoporosis Epidemiology Study. *J Bone Miner Res* 2004; **19**: 532–6.

Clunie G. The diagnosis of osteoporosis. In: Clunie G, Keen R, eds, *Osteoporosis*. 2007:17–32.

Grados F, Marcelli C, Dargent-Molina P, et al. Prevalence of vertebral fractures in French women older than 75 years from the EPIDOS study. *Bone* 2004; **34**: 362–7.

ISCD. The writing group for the ISCD position development conference. Exec. Summary. *J Clin Densitom* 2004; **7**: 7–12.

Jiang G, Eastell R, Barrington NA, Ferrar L. Comparison of methods for the visual identification of prevalent vertebral fracture in osteoporosis. *Osteoporos Int* 2004; **15**(11): 887–96.

Johnell O, Kanis JA. An estimate of the worldwide prevalence and disability associated with osteoporotic fractures. *Osteoporos Int* 2006; **17**: 1726–33.

Kanis JA, Johnell O, Oden A, De Laet C, Jonsson B. Ten year probabilities of osteoporotic fractures according to BMD and diagnostic thresholds. *Osteoporos Int* 2001; **12**: 989–95.

O'Neill TW, Felsenberg D, Varlow J, et al. The prevalence of vertebral deformity in European men and women: the EVOS. *J Bone Miner Res* 1996; **11**: 1010–7.

Thompson PW, Taylor J, Dawson A. The annual incidence and seasonal variation of fractures of the distal radius in men and women over 25 years in Dorset, UK. *Injury* 2004; **35**: 462–6.

WHO Scientific group on the assessment of osteoporosis at primary health care level., 2004. Available at: www.who.int/chp/topics/osteoporosis.pdf;

Therapeutics of post-menopausal osteoporosis

Acute fracture management
The orthopaedic management of acute fracture is beyond the scope of this text though Rheumatologists may be required to manage medical problems in such patients, advising on pain control and investigating underlying causes of fracture. All post-menopausal women who have had a fracture should be investigated for osteoporosis.

Pain control
Fracture units typically work to protocols for acute pain relief from fracture.
- There is some evidence that calcitonin injection 100–200 iu subcutaneously bd has analgesic properties. Its effect on fracture healing is not precisely known. Intolerance owing to effects of vasodilation is common.
- There is some debate over whether IV bisphosphonate given at the time of vertebral fracture is appropriate. Reducing bone turnover with bisphosphonate may impair fracture healing. Only anecdotal reports suggest efficacy at reducing pain.

Vertebroplasty
Vertebroplasty is the percutaneous injection of bone cement into painful fractured vertebrae.
- Vertebroplasty has been shown to reduce pain from both acute and chronic fractures in >85% patients. The effect is most notable with acute fractures.
- Pretreatment MR is important to identify symptomatic level, define posterior cortical margin, ensure pedicles are intact, characterizes the appearance of the fractured vertebra, and can point to other pathology, which might be contributing to the pain.
- Polymethylmethacrylate cement is used. The main complication is extravasation of cement into soft-tissues and epidural space.
- The most serious complication, although rare, is cement leakage into para-vertebral veins and consequent pulmonary emboli.
- Other complications include spinal cord compression and acute radiculopathy, pain, and fever, and slight increase in risk of fracture of adjacent vertebral body.

Kyphoplasty
Kyphoplasty describes the injection of cement into a balloon, which has been inflated within a collapsed vertebra. It aims to restore vertebral anatomy and spinal deformity, and is more technically demanding than vertebroplasty.
- Achieving restoration of vertebral height in the acute setting is a more realistic aim than where vertebral fractures are chronic.
- The procedure is safer than vertebroplasty given the containment of injected cement within the balloon.

Fracture prevention

Objectives of treatment
The over-arching importance of managing PMO is to prevent fractures. Thus, PMO management includes:
- Choice of, and supervising adherence to, long-term drug therapy.
- Avoiding lifestyle habits and general 'ill-health' factors that can increase fracture risk and surveillance for.
- Addressing, any conditions evolving over time that can contribute to bone fragility.

General bone health measures
There are some simple measures, which are logically and intuitively appropriate to recommend to post-menopausal women, regardless of any BMD measurement and specific fracture risk assessment to maximize the chance of maintaining good skeletal health in the long-term:
- Stop smoking.
- Reduce alcohol.
- Remain mobile and weight bearing.
- Remain vitamin D replete (>75 nmol/l or >25 µg/l).
- Avoid suboptimal dietary calcium intake specifically avoiding secondary hyperparathyroidism.

Added to this list and for the elderly, we might reasonably add the identification and addressing of factors, which would lead to an increased falls risk.

It is important also to address the above for women who are recommended to take specific treatment (see below).

When to recommend specific drug treatment
Most guidelines recommend treatment on the basis of high relative risk of fracture expressed by low hip or lumbar spine BMD, specifically a T-score of –2.5 or less. This approach, however, leads to some young post-menopausal women with a low T-score, but low risk of fracture being treated and some elderly women with T-scores higher than –2.5 not being treated despite a high risk of fracture primarily because of their age.

Current and future practice determining which women will 'benefit' from treatment is based on an integration of 4 aspects of fracture risk assessment (e.g. FRAX).
- **Age:** an important risk factor for fracture, chiefly independently of BMD.
- **BMD:** for each SD decrease in BMD, the relative risk of fracture increases by about 2.5.
- **Previous fragility fracture:** which roughly doubles any risk estimate of future fracture.
- **Clinical risk factors:** based currently on some evidence, but mostly assumption, that the more risk factors there are, the higher the fracture risk, again partly independent of BMD.

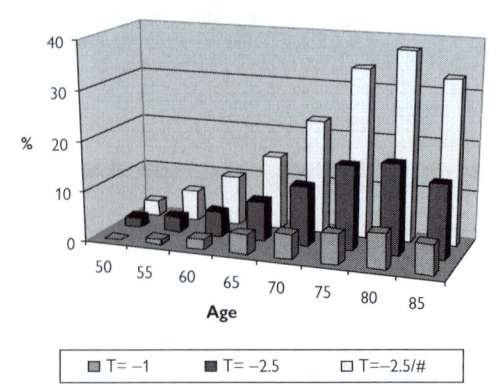

Figure 14.5 The 10-year risk of hip fracture (%) in post-menopausal women. Integrating age, BMD T-score, and previous fracture (#) into a risk assessment (graph from data derived chiefly from Kanis et al., 2001, and adapted).

- Thus, as shown in Figure 14.5, even if a 55-year-old woman has a T-score of −2.5 and has had a fracture, her 10-year risk of having a hip fracture is <5%; in fact lower than a 70-year-old woman who might have a higher T-score (of −1) and has not had a fracture.
- The integration of risk from individual fracture risk factors (with BMD) —see FRAX (www.shef.ac.uk/FRAX) —has been widely adapted in guiding decisions about therapy.

Pharmacological treatment (See Table 17.4)
Efficacy of drugs in PMO is measured in terms of fracture prevention. The 3 main ways drugs can work to reduce fracture incidence are by increasing bone mass, reducing bone turnover, and improving (or maintaining) the structural integrity of bone.

Hormone replacement therapy (HRT)
- In randomized-controlled trials (RCTs), HRT protects against loss of BMD, either as combined oestrogen-gestagen preparations or as unopposed oestrogen therapy in hysterectomized women. Oral, transdermal, and percutaneous delivery all show efficacy.
- Conflicting data for anti-fracture efficacy of HRT can be summarized from:
  - Wells' meta-analysis, which concludes that HRT is associated with a non-significant reduction in risk of vertebral (RR 0.66; 95%CI 0.41–1.07) and non-vertebral (RR 0.87; 95%CI 0.71–1.08) fracture, respectively;
  - the Women's Health Initiative (WHI) studies, which showed unopposed oestrogen in 10 739 post-menopausal hysterectomized women was associated with a hazard ratio for hip fracture of 0.61 (0.41–0.91) and in 16 608 women with an intact uterus (given oestrogen + gestagen) was 0.66 (0.45–0.98)
- In recommending HRT for osteoporosis, it's benefits (including the relief of climacteric symptoms) needs to be balanced against the adverse effects:
  - an increased risk of breast cancer and coronary heart disease in women with an intact uterus receiving combined oestrogen + gestagen therapy;
  - an increased risk of stroke and venous thromboembolism (VTE) in women receiving both oestrogen only and oestrogen + gestagen therapy.
- HRT thus would arguably be best considered in women with premature menopause where it might have a relatively low risk of side-effects (i.e. where the background rate of breast cancer, coronary and cerebral vascular disease, and VTE is relatively low).

Selective oestrogen receptor modulators (SERMs)
- SERMs are non-steroidal partial oestrogen agonists in bone, but act as antagonists in reproductive tissues.
- Raloxifene is the only SERM currently licensed for the treatment and prevention of PMO.
- Raloxifene suppresses bone turnover and prevents bone loss though effects are less potent than with oestrogen, in-keeping with partial agonist activity.
- In the MORE trial (7705 post-menopausal women), the risk of vertebral fracture risk was significantly reduced with raloxifene 60 mg daily (RR 0.7; 95%CI 0.5–0.8).
- Although Raloxifene exerts a similar effect on risk of vertebral fracture compared with HRT, no benefit was found in terms of risk of hip fracture.

Table 14.7 Choices for treating PMO

Treatment for PMO	Fracture prevention: a crude synthesis of strength of evidence data and size of prevention effect	
	Vertebral	Non-vertebral
HRT	++	+/-
Raloxifene	++	-
Etidronate	++	+
Alendronate	+++	++
Risedronate	+++	++
Ibandronate (oral)	+++	+
Zoledronate (IV)	++++	++
Strontium ranelate	+++	++
rhPTH	++++	+

Bisphosphonates: oral
Bisphosphonates localize to bone mineral surfaces exposed by osteoclasts then inhibit osteoclast activity. Bone turnover is reduced; trabecular bone tends to retain its connectivity and bone mass increases.
- Daily oral Alendronate, Risedronate, and Ibandronate and intermittent Etidronate (400 mg daily for 14 days continuous once in every 13-week cycle) have all been shown to reduce the risk of vertebral fracture.
- The entry criteria for index studies of the above have differed slightly (e.g. based on age, baseline BMD, fracture history, etc.), but basically, each therapy is associated with a 35–60% relative risk reduction in vertebral fracture rates over placebo – in (probably generally) vitamin D replete women (except Etidronate) without substantial secondary hyperparathyroidism.
- Further studies have shown intermittent dosing (weekly for Alendronate 70 mg and Risedronate 35 mg and monthly for Ibandronate 150 mg) results in similar changes in lumbar spine BMD occur over 1–2 years as daily dosing of the same drug. Such 'bridging' studies use BMD as a surrogate marker of anti-fracture efficacy.
- The same degree of trial rigour is not evident for studies where non-vertebral fracture has been the end-point. Studies suggest anti-hip (and other non-vertebral) fracture efficacy for daily Alendronate and Risedronate essentially, but only where baseline osteoporosis risk indices were most marked (e.g. very low BMD and or multiple fractures). Similar, but fewer data exist for Ibandronate.
- Larger improvements in lumbar spine BMD with bisphosphonates are associated with larger decreases in vertebral fracture risk.
- Non-adherence with bisphosphonates long-term is significant and associated with reduction in fracture prevention effect. Management strategies that increase patient contact and supervision while on treatment have been shown to improve compliance.
- Oral bisphosphonates can cause upper GI side effects, diarrhoea, arthralgia, and occasionally rashes.
- Oral bisphosphonates are absorbed poorly and need to be taken fasting (with water) then (ideally) patients need to wait 60 min before taking food, drink, or other medications.

- Oral bisphosphonate anti-fracture efficacy has been determined only in studies where attempts have been made to keep patients replete in vitamin D and calcium. It is convention to provide daily vitamin D3 and calcium supplements with bisphosphonate therapy.

Bisphosphonates: intravenous

Owing to intolerance of oral medications, small bowel disease/malabsorption, poor adherence, or inefficacy, it may be necessary to consider intravenous therapy. Historically Pamidronate has been used (e.g. 30–60 mg every 3–4 months), although no robust study data are available showing anti-fracture efficacy. Currently, 2 bisphosphonates – Ibandronate and Zoledronate – are licensed for use to treat PMO.

- Ibandronate 3 mg (bolus injection) given once every 3 months shows changes in BMD and bone turnover markers equivalent to changes seen with oral Ibandronate doses associated with vertebral fracture reduction. It is tolerated well.
- Zoledronate 5 mg given as yearly infusions reduces vertebral fractures by 70%, hip fractures by 41% and all non-vertebral fractures by 25% over 3 years in PMO. Adherence to treatment (return for serial yearly infusions) was very high in the study.
- Common side effects with all IV bisphosphonates appear to be mild fever, myoarthralgia and transient acute phase response (flu-like illness in 25–40%). These side effects may be reduced by continuous calcium supplementation through the treatment period.
- Acute uveitis and osteonecrosis of the jaw (ONJ) are rare, but recognized side effects from IV bisphosphonates. Most ONJ cases have been in cancer patients treated with recurrent infusions many of whom had had cranial radiotherapy and/or poor dentition.
- Acute nephritis and renal failure have been reported with Zoledronate. Atrial fibrillation may be a rare side effect of Zoledronate infusion.

Strontium ranelate (SR)

Strontium is incorporated into bone where it has a long half-life. Its mechanisms of action are unclear, but may be multifactorial.

- SR inhibits osteoclast recruitment, and activity at resorption sites and potentiates osteoblast proliferation and differentiation. As a result, endosteal bone forms and trabecular volume increases (shown in rats and from transiliac bone biopsies in some patients).
- Strontium appears to directly trigger calcium-sensing receptors on bone cells.
- Two major placebo-controlled RCTs have shown efficacy and tolerability of SR 2 g daily in PMO.
- A RCT of 1649 women with at least one vertebral fracture and low lumbar spine BMD showed after 3 years there was a relative risk reduction of 41% in vertebral fractures with SR compared with placebo (95%CI 0.48–0.73; $p < 0.001$).
- A RCT of 5000 women showed a relative risk reduction in non-vertebral (including hip) fractures of 16% with SR compared with placebo (95%CI 0.71–1.00, $p = 0.05$) after 3 years.
- Additional daily calcium and vitamin D3 supplements are advisable with SR therapy.
- SR is formulated as granules, which are dissolved in water therefore SR is drunk.
- Ideally, SR needs to be taken at least 2 h after food and drink, and at least 2 h before.
- The main side-effect with SR appears to be gut intolerance (diarrhoea). Increased risk of VTE and Drug Reaction with Eosinophilia and Systemic Symptoms (DRESS) syndrome have been reported, with the former listed as a relative contraindication to use.

Recombinant human parathyroid hormone (rhPTH)

Intermittent parathyroid hormone (PTH) has a stimulatory effect on bone turnover, which preferentially affects bone formation over resorption (as opposed to continuous bone exposure to PTH which overall results in bone loss through excessive resorption). Therapeutic PTH has been manufactured as recombinant human PTH (amino acids 1–34 or 1–84).

- Accretion of BMD occurs over 30 months or more with daily PTH injections. Changes also include cortical thickening and increased trabecular connectivity.
- Teriparatide (rhPTH 1-34) is licensed to treat PMO. It is given as a 20 µg SC injection daily for 18 months. It is supplied in a pre-filled syringe, which lasts for 28 days and must be stored at 2–8°C.
- A RCT of 1600 women showed a 65% relative risk reduction of vertebral fractures with rhPTH 1–34 over placebo (RR 0.35; CI 0.22–0.55). The study was not powered to detect a change in hip fractures though a significant reduction in non-vertebral fractures overall was observed (RR 0.47; CI 0.25–0.88).
- Follow-up of patients after 18 months showed an anti-fracture effect of rhPTH 1–34 extending for 18 months for vertebral and 30 months for non-vertebral sites.
- Preotact™/Preos© (rhPTH 1–84) is licensed to treat patients at high risk of fracture at a dose of 100 µg daily by SC injection for a maximum 24 months.
- Preotact™/Preos© rhPTH (1–84) is supplied in cartridges, which are placed in an injection pen device every 2 weeks and can be stored at room temperature for up to 1 week out of 2.
- A RCT in 2532 post-menopausal women, mean age 64 years 19% of whom only had had a previous vertebral fracture, showed that rhPTH 1–84 was associated with a significant 58% reduction in vertebral fracture risk. There were no data on non-vertebral fractures.
- Regarding patient selection: in many countries PTH treatment is targeted at patients at high risk of osteoporosis and/or where other treatments have failed.
- Mild hypercalcaemia and hypercalciuria are common, but clinically relatively insignificant effects. An effect of rhPTH on reducing spinal pain is also noted though it is not clear whether this is due to reduction of vertebral fractures or a independent mechanism.
- Because of the (theoretical) risk of osteosarcoma it is advisable that patients already at risk of this tumour are not treated with PTH (Paget's disease of bone, osteomalacia, bone metastases and patients who've had previous skeletal radiotherapy).

Denosumab

Denosumab is a human monoclonal antibody (IgG$_2$) that targets the receptor activator of nuclear factor kappa B ligand (RANKL), a key mediator of the resorptive phase of bone remodelling. RANKL, produced by osteoblasts, is preventing from binding its ligand RANK. Thus, Denosumab mimics the action of endogenous osteoprotegerin – the decoy receptor for RANKL. Initial studies in postmenopausal women with low BMD suggest twice yearly treatments by SC injection increases BMD and decreases biochemical markers of bone resorption significantly, and equivalent to changes seen with Alendronate. Fracture end-point studies are currently in progress.

Current controversies

- The nature of fracture risk assessment to guide treatment intervention thresholds is currently the focus of research (e.g. FRAX). Using such fracture risk algorithms incorporating BMD data, age, fracture prevalence, and risk factors, rather than relying on relative risk from BMD alone, has many theoretical advantages (see Tucker et al., 2007).
- What are the long-term effects of bisphosphonates? How long should treatment be continued?
- What is the optimum (if any) method of monitoring treatment? BMD alone? BMD and bone markers or markers alone?
- The cost-effectiveness of new (expensive) treatments is an important unresolved issue. What level of fracture risk justifies introduction of each preventive treatment? This question raises country (healthcare system)-specific issues about when to intervene with a preventive therapy. It is somewhat a socio-political question too, particularly if there is healthcare rationing within a fixed budget (see Ström et al., 2007).
- In the UK it remains to be seen whether NICE will incorporate absolute risk algorithms into their recommendations for osteoporosis management. At present, not!

Resources

Assessment tools

For algorithm to determine individuals' absolute risk of fracture with and without incorporating measurements of BMD see link at www.shef.ac.uk/FRAX/

Guidelines

NICE technology appraisals on the use of medicines for primary and secondary osteoporosis. Available at: www.nice.org.uk

Guidelines for professionals. Available at www.nof.org/. This is for US professionals with guidelines based on The US healthcare system.

Osteoporosis: clinical guidelines for prevention and treatment. RCP, London ISBN 9781860161391. Available at: www.rcplondon.ac.uk/pubs

European guidance for the diagnosis and management of osteoporosis in post-menopausal women (Kanis et al. 2008).

Patient support groups

National Osteoporosis Foundation (USA). Available at: www.nof.org

National Osteoporosis Society (UK). Available at: www.nos.org.uk

Other Internet sites

For average calcium content in typical foods, see http://ods.od.nih.gov/factsheets/calcium.asp

International Bone Mineral Society. Available at: www.ibmsonline.org. An organization for bone physicians facilitating generation and dissemination of knowledge about bone and mineral metabolism.

Interpreting DXA and BMD measurements. See listings at: www.noah-health.org/en/bjm/osteoporosis/diagnosis/testing.html.

ICD-10 codes

M80.0–9	Osteoporosis with pathological fracture
M81.0–9	Osteoporosis without pathological fracture
M82*	Osteoporosis in diseases classified elsewhere (e.g. myeloma M82.0*)

References

Adami S. Bisphosphonate anti-fracture efficacy. *Bone* 2007; **41**: S8–15.

Black DM, Greenspan SL, Ensrud KE, et al. The effects of parathyroid hormone and Alendronate alone or in combination in post-menopausal osteoporosis. *N Engl J Med* 2003; **349**: 1207–15.

Black DM, Delmas PD, Eastell R, et al. Once yearly zoledronic acid for treatment of postmenopausal osteoporosis. *N Engl J Med* 2007; **356**(18): 1809–22.

Ettinger B, Black DM, Mitlak BH, et al. Reduction of vertebral fracture risk in postmenopausal women with osteoporosis treated with raloxifene. *J Am Med Ass* 1999; **282**: 637–45.

Greenspan SL, Bone HG, Ettinger MP, et al. Effect of recombinant human parathyroid hormone (1–84) on vertebral fracture and bone mineral density in postmenopausal women with osteoporosis: a randomized trial. *Ann Intern Med* 2007; **146**(5): 326–39.

Kanis JA, Adams J, Bergstrom F, et al. The cost-effectiveness of Alendronate in the management of osteoporosis. *Bone* 2008; **42**: 4–15.

Layton KF, Thielen KR, Koch CA, et al. Vertebroplasty, first 1000 cases of a single centre: Evaluation of the outcomes and complications. *Am J Neuroradiol* 2007; **28**: 683–9.

Ledlie J, Renfro M. Balloon kyphoplasty: one year outcomes in height restoration, chronic pain and activity outcomes. *J Neurosurgery* 2006; **98**: 36–42.

Meunier PJ, Roux C, Seeman E, et al. The effects of strontium ranelate on risk of vertebral fracture in women with postmenopausal osteoporosis. *N Engl J Med* 2004; **350**: 459–68.

Tucker G, Metcalfe A, Pearce C, et al. The importance of calculating absolute rather than relative fracture risk. *Bone* 2007; **41**: 937–41.

Rossouw JE, Anderson GL, Prentice RL, et al. Risks and benefits of estrogen plus progestin in healthy postmenopausal women: principal results from the Women's Health Initiative randomized controlled trial. *J Am Med Ass* 2002; **288**: 321–33.

Russell RG, Xia Z, Dunford JE, et al. Bisphosphonates: an update on mechanisms of action and how these relate to clinical efficacy. *Ann NY Acad Sci* 2007; **1117**: 209–57.

Ström O, Bergström F, Sen SS, et al. Cost-effectiveness of Alendronate in the treatment of postmenopausal women in 9 European countries – an economic evaluation based on the fracture intervention trial. *Osteoporos Int* 2007; **18**: 1047–61.

Wells G, Tugwell P, Shea B, et al. Meta-analysis of the efficacy of hormone replacement therapy in treating and preventing osteoporosis in postmenopausal women. *Endocr Rev* 2002; **23**: 529–39.

Osteoporosis in men

Osteoporosis in men is under diagnosed and therefore under treated. For example in >1000 men diagnosed with osteoporotic fractures, <10% had received medication for osteoporosis and only 1% had had bone mineral density (BMD) measurement (Feldstein et al., 2005).

Epidemiology
The incidence of fractures in men is about half that in women for the same age. The known excess mortality risk a major fracture confers is greater in men compared with women.
- Men who have distal forearm fractures: have lower BMD than controls; have a 40% likelihood of having osteoporosis; have a 3 and 11 times the risk of having hip and vertebral fractures, respectively.
- About 50% of men with low trauma vertebral fractures have been shown to have BMD evidence of osteoporosis at the lumbar spine or femoral neck.
- There is great disability after hip fracture in men, with only 21% living independently in the community a year later, 26% require home care, and 53% needing institutional care.

Aetiology and pathogenesis of fracture
Genetic
BMD varies inversely with the incidence of vertebral and hip fractures in men. There is likely to be a strong genetic determinant of peak BMD contributing to primary osteoporosis in men.
- Genetic factors account for up to 80% of the variance in peak BMD – a variation in collagen type IA1, the vitamin D receptor, vitamin D binding protein, the oestrogen receptor, and insulin-like growth factor 1 (IGF-1) genes may all account for some variance in peak BMD.
- The genetic contribution to age-related bone loss caused by declining testosterone aromatization is unknown. Genetic, secondary pathological, and environmental factors may all be relevant (see below).

Environment
Men have larger bones thus a 12% greater peak BMD than women. Non-genetic determinants of peak BMD include calcium intake, exercise, delayed puberty, and intra-uterine development.
- Age-related bone loss after the age of 40 years contributes to osteoporosis in men. It is chiefly non-genetic in its aetiology, but data is sparse. It can be influenced by influenced by declining sex steroid concentrations, low body mass index, smoking, physical inactivity, impaired vitamin D production, and metabolism and secondary hyperparathyroidism (SHPT).
- Age-related decrease in circulating free testosterone, adrenal androgens, growth hormone and IGF-1 occur in men. Each hormone has been linked to decreased bone formation. Up to 20% of men with symptomatic vertebral fractures and 50% of men with hip fractures are hypogonadal. Testosterone actions on the skeleton are at least in part mediated by its aromatization to oestradiol and the effect of the latter on the skeleton. BMD and fracture risk in men associate with serum oestradiol levels more closely than with testosterone.

- Osteoporosis is often caused by underlying secondary causes of bone loss such as hypogonadism, oral glucocorticoids (GCs), and long-term excessive alcohol intake. These are found in over 50% of men presenting with symptomatic vertebral fractures.

Table 14.8 Causes of secondary osteoporosis in men

Major causes	Alcoholism; glucocorticoids (GCs); hypogonadism; transplantation
Metabolic and endocrine disease	Hyperparathyroidism; thyrotoxicosis; idiopathic hypercalciuria; Cushing's disease
GI disease	Chronic liver disease; IBD; coeliac disease; gastric surgery
Iatrogenic	Chemotherapy; androgen deprivation therapy (through rendering men completely hypogonadal); phenobarbitone, and phenytoin; warfarin; LMWt heparin
Other	Malignancy (e.g. myeloma); renal bone disease

Clinical features
Key features in history
- Previous fracture with minimal trauma particularly in proximal humerus, spine, pelvis, forearm, or hip.
- A history of features of one or more of the secondary causes of osteoporosis (e.g. alcohol consumption, GC and other drug use, low libido or erectile dysfunction, chronic bowel symptoms, enteric intolerance to gluten containing foods).
- Family history of fragility fracture in first-degree relative particularly parent.

Key features on examination
- Genuine loss of height, TSp kyphosis, approximation of lower ribs to iliac rim – all can be signs of osteoporosis though are not specific.
- Cutaneous and other stigmata of chronic liver disease.
- Signs of hypogonadism: passive demeanour, low/sparse body hair, centripetal obesity, small testicular size.
- Signs of Cushing's: centripetal obesity, skin striae

Co-morbidities
Secondary causes of osteoporosis are common in men compared with women.

Diagnosis and investigations
The diagnosis of osteoporosis in an elderly man with fragility fracture(s) can be straightforward though in men <80 years. It is appropriate to substantiate the diagnosis with a BMD scan. All men with fracture (or 'fragility' or low trauma fracture) after the age of 50 or 60 years, for example, might reasonably be referred for a dual X-ray absorptiometry (DXA) scan. Key issues are:
- Diagnosing spinal fractures.
- The interpretation of DXA results.
- The investigations to rule out secondary osteoporosis.

Diagnosing spinal fractures
There is well recognized under-reporting of spinal fractures in men and women.

- Owing to vertebral end-plate irregularities, non-osteoporotic vertebral deformities are commonly seen on radiographs of ageing men in the TSp. The deformities are often slightly wedge-shaped.
- BMD by DXA is often not low in men with wedge deformities of the TSp.
- The key appearance in a wedge shaped vertebra, which distinguishes the bone as fractured may be specific central end-plate depression (scalloped appearance), rather than a linear decline in height (posterior to anterior).
- Studies are being done to quantify vertebral size and continuous changes in vertebral height in association with indices of osteoporosis (e.g. low BMD).

Interpretation of DXA results
- In both sexes, the same inverse relationship between absolute BMD and incidence of fractures might indicate that the same absolute BMD threshold could be used for the diagnosis of osteoporosis in men and women. Then a T-score of −2.5 in women would be equivalent to a T-score of −2.8.
- The prevalence of osteoporosis using a T-score definition of −2.8 would be too low, but a T-score definition of −2.5 after the age of 50 years approximates to lifetime risk of fracture for men.
- There is a broad international agreement to use a DXA-derived hip or spine BMD T-score definition of −2.5 as the diagnostic threshold for osteoporosis in men.

Investigations to rule out secondary causes
The occurrence of a fragility fracture in a man >50 years or finding of a BMD T-score of hip or spine is −2.5 might reasonably be taken as an indication to screen for secondary causes of bone fragility whether or not history or examination (see above) is suggestive.

Treatment
All men with osteoporosis should be counselled about the need to optimize weight [BMI < 19 is associated with generalized osteoporosis, but obesity (BMI > 30) associated with hypovitaminosis-D and SHPT], stop any smoking, reduce alcohol if excessive and consider regular weight-bearing exercise.
- Secondary causes of osteoporosis need to be identified and addressed.
- Calcium and vitamin D supplements should be advised to maintain repletion in vitamin D (e.g. 25-hydroxyvitamin D >75 nmol/l) and to avoid SHPT.
- The most robust evidence for drug therapy comes from studies of Alendronate and teriparatide (rhPTH).
- The use of the on-line fracture risk tool (www.shef.ac.uk/FRAX) can apply for men, as well as for women. In the UK an online link to a site providing guidelines for treatment (NOGG).

Bisphosphonates
Oral (daily) Alendronate reduces vertebral fractures in eugonadal and hypogonadal men and is licensed to treat osteoporosis in men. It would be unlikely that weekly Alendronate would not be efficacious
Weekly Risedronate is a licensed option to Alendronate for which fracture prevention data exists.

Table 14.9 Investigation of causes of bone fragility in men

Initial investigations	Conditions
Full blood count; tissue transglutaminase (tTg) antibodies; ESR; CRP	Malignancy; coeliac disease
9 a.m. Testosterone and LH (±SHBG)	Hypogonadism
Prolactin, FSH, thyroid function tests	Pituitary disease and hyperthyroidism
Parathyroid hormone; bone biochemistry and 25-OHD	$1^e/2^e$ PHPT; hypovitaminosis-D or osteomalacia
Liver function tests	Liver disease; alcoholism
Urea, electrolytes, creatinine and GFR	Renal bone disease
24-h urinary calcium	Idiopathic hypercalciuria
24-h urinary cortisol	Cushing's disease
Serum and urine protein electrophoresis; PSA	Myeloma; prostate carcinoma

Teriparatide
Teriparatide is a recombinant human PTH molecule (1-34), which reduces vertebral fractures in men with osteoporosis (Orwoll et al., 2003). It is given by SC injection daily over an 18-month period.

Other treatments
- Strontium ranelate 2 g daily shows anti-fracture efficacy in women, but there are no data for men. It would be likely to work and offers an alternative if Alendronate fails and teriparatide is unavailable.
- Testosterone replacement may reduce fractures and increase BMD in hypogonadal men. Its role in eugonadal men is not yet known.

Resources
See under Post-menopausal osteoporosis

References
Feldstein AC, Nichols G, Orwoll E, et al. The near absence of osteoporosis treatment in older men with fractures. *Osteoporos Int* 2005; **16**: 953–62.
Orwoll ES, Ettinger M, Weiss S, et al. Alendronate treatment of osteoporosis in men. *N Engl J Med* 2000; **343**: 604–10.
Orwoll ES, Scheele WH, Paul S, et al. The effect of teriparatide therapy on bone density in men with osteoporosis. *J Bone Miner Res* 2003; **18**: 9–17.
Ringe JD, Faber H, Farahmand P, Dorst A. Efficacy of Risedronate in men with primary and secondary osteoporosis: results of a 1 year study. *Rheumatol Int* 2006; **26**: 427–3.

Glucocorticoid induced osteoporosis (GIO)

Glucocorticoids (GCs) are the commonest cause of secondary osteoporosis. About 1:200 of the population may be taking GCs in a course lasting 3 months or more. About 30% of individuals taking GCs for more than 3 years will have evidence of osteoporotic fractures.

Epidemiology
- The relative risk of fracture for those taking GCs is about 2.6 for vertebral and 1.6 for hip fractures.
- Fracture risk relates to GC dose and duration, low BMD, increasing age and the underlying condition.

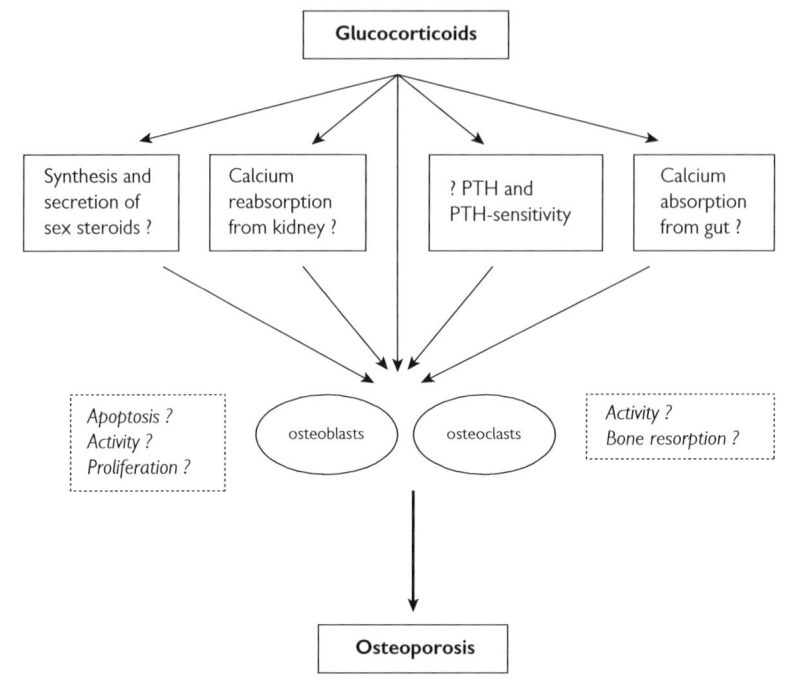

Figure 14.6 The likely major mechanisms of glucocorticoid-induced osteoporosis (GIO).

- Fractures can occur at a higher bone mineral density (BMD) compared with non-GC-treated populations.
- GCs have been identified as the commonest cause of osteoporotic fracture in the young.
- The prevalence of vertebral fractures in patients taking GCs is about 25–30%. The incidence of vertebral fractures is about 13–22% (data from control arms of randomized trials of therapy for GIO).
- GIO can occur even at low doses in some patients (<5 mg/day).

Aetiology and pathophysiology

GCs cause osteoporosis through direct effects on bone formation and resorption, by affecting bone mineral metabolism, and gonadal hormones. Fracture risk is enhanced through an increased falls tendency through GC-induced reduced muscle strength.

- GCs reduce osteoblast proliferation and function through an effect on IGF-1, IGF-2, and TGFβ1.
- GCs cause osteocytes apoptosis. This mechanism may be important in causing osteonecrosis.
- GCs may cause negative calcium balance by a combination of reducing calcium absorption by the gut and reabsorption in the kidney ultimately resulting in SHPT. A consensus for a direct molecular effect of GCs on vitamin-D metabolism is lacking, as data from animal and human studies are conflicting.
- GCs may reduce gonadal hormone production, which in turn may increase bone resorption.
- There is type II muscle fibre atrophy and decrease in Type I fibres in GC-treated patients.

Clinical features
Key features in history
- A thorough assessment of GIO requires an assessment of all osteoporosis risk factors (see 'Post-menopausal osteoporosis').
- Reviewing the diagnosis of the condition being treated with GC (e.g. is it really PMR?), when GCs are being taken (i.e. in the morning to reduce the risk of long-term GC dependence) and considering whether GC-sparing immunosuppressants can be introduced (e.g. can azathioprine be started – perhaps not if patient on allopurinol or TPMT activity status low) may provide information which may help to minimize the adverse effects of GCs.

Key features on examination
A TSp kyphosis may denote underlying spinal fractures owing to GCs, but features are not specific.

Investigations
DXA
- The earliest signs of GIO are seen in the lumbar spine.
- Some studies suggest that vertebral fractures caused by GCs occur at a higher BMD than fractures seen in other types of osteoporosis.
- Bone loss secondary to GCs, documented by BMD, is greatest in the first 12–18 months.
- Over time BMD loss can be 5–10% per year. For patients not treated with anti-osteoporosis therapy, while on GCs, yearly BMD assessments are appropriate.

Laboratory investigations
Tests to rule out conditions associated with osteoporosis are prudent when assessing patients for GIO. Undisclosed pathology relevant to bone 'ill-health', such as myeloma, hyperthyroidism, alcoholism, and chronic kidney disease (CKD) 3–5 and hyperparathyroidism are, when considered together, not infrequently encountered, particularly in the elderly. See Post-menopausal osteoporosis.

Differential diagnosis
Given the frequency of conditions, post-menopausal and other secondary causes of osteoporosis can contribute to low BMD, and fracture risk in patients taking GCs. Low BMD can also be due to osteomalacia/SHPT.

Treatment
Objectives of treatment
Some patients may be treated with GCs long-term. There are general principles for reducing GIO risk. Sadly, numerous studies show that despite guidelines from various organizations pertinent to different diseases and patient groups, the extent and appropriateness of management of osteoporosis risk in patients is disappointing.

Calcium and vitamin D
- Dietary increases in calcium or calcium supplements alone are insufficient to prevent GC-induced bone loss.
- Combination calcium and vitamin D therapy is universally advised for patient taking GCs.
- It is inconclusive whether combination treatment with vitamin D is more effective at reducing bone loss from GCs using 25-OHD, or either calcitriol or 1α-calcidol.
- Most GIO guidelines don't specify whether or how to assess calcium and vitamin-D status, although state it is important. Specific testing of vitamin-D and PTH at the outset of a long course of GCs might be prudent. If patients are replete in vitamin-D and have no SHPT, or abnormalities are slight, then advise daily calcium 0.5–1 g and vitamin-D3 400–800 iu, while GCs are being taken.

Bisphosphonates
- Numerous studies have examined the effects of a variety of bisphosphonates in reducing GC-induced bone loss with positive results.

Table 14.10 Assessment and managing GIO: overview

Assessment	Action
Prior to starting GCs	Exclude secondary[e] causes of osteoporosis; obtain fracture baseline (include lateral TSp + LSp radiographs).
When starting GCs	Treat osteoporosis according to risk of fracture (e.g. use guidelines)
While on GCs	Minimize GC dose; ensure adherence with GCs, calcium and vitamin D and specific anti-fracture therapy; monitor BMD; consider introducing GC-sparing immunosuppressants; consider treatment failure if incident fractures occur or BMD drops significantly on therapy

- Reliable vertebral and non-vertebral fracture prevention data in all relevant diseases at risk of osteoporosis, where GCs are used, have not been obtained.
- In The UK (2007–2008) the only drugs licensed to treat/prevent GIO are alendronic acid (Alendronate) and fosamax, although randomized controlled trial data suggests that Risedronate (Actonel) and cyclical Etidronate are all effective at preventing and treating GIO.
- Ibandronate, given as an intravenous bolus, prevents GC-induced bone loss and appears to prevent fractures though studies were not powered to assess fracture prevention. Clodronate also reduces bone loss associated with GCs and may prevent fractures.
- The effects of intravenous bisphosphonates (Pamidronate, Ibandronate and Zoledronate) on reducing fractures and bone loss in GIO are untested in large robust RCTs. Anecdotal evidence suggests bone turnover and BMD loss though can be reduced significantly.

Gonadal hormone replacement
- HRT reduces GC-induced bone loss in post-menopausal women. Fracture prevention has not been shown.
- Testosterone replacement should be considered in hypogonadal men on long-term GCs. Patient preferences often dictate the use of testosterone. When counselled about its benefits and risks, including prostate cancer, some men may choose not to be treated.
- If GIO risk is high, testosterone alone may not be sufficient to prevent GIO in hypogonadal men.

Other drugs
No RCT has yet shown a fracture prevention effect of strontium Ranelate or rhPTH in GIO; however, it would be a surprise if both do not given their effects on bone biomarkers and BMD in GIO patients.

When to introduce therapy
A number of guidelines exist (see below). All highlight the need to replenish calcium and vitamin D deficiency, use vitamin D and calcium combination supplements, and introduce specific anti-fracture therapy at a higher BMD threshold than would happen normally.
- The case for early (primary) prevention is greatest in post-menopausal women and people with low BMD.
- As bone loss occurs within the first year, fracture risk should be assessed and decisions made about therapy for GIO when GCs are started, not at a later date.

Resources

Guidelines
American College of Rheumatology. Recommendations for the prevention and treatment of GC-induced osteoporosis, update 2001 (ACR 2001; www.rheumatology.org/research/guidelines).

Chronic GC therapy-induced osteoporosis in patients with obstructive lung disease (Goldstein et al., 1999, Available at: www.chestjournal.org/cgi/content/full/116/6/1733).

GC-induced osteoporosis. RCP (UK) 2002. Available at: www.rcplondon.ac.uk/pubs/books/glucocorticoid

British Society of Gastroenterology. Guidelines for osteoporosis in coeliac disease and inflammatory bowel disease, 2000. Available at: www.bsg.org.uk/.

ICD-10 codes
M81.4   Drug-induced osteoporosis
Y42.0   Glucocorticoids and synthetic analogues

References

ACR ad hoc Committee on Glucocorticoid-induced Osteoporosis. Arthritis Rheum 2001; **44**: 1496–503.

Goldstein MF, Fallon JJ, Harning R. Chronic glucocorticoid therapy-induced osteoporosis in patients with obstructive lung disease. Chest 1999; **116**: 1733–49.

Patscan D, Loddenkemper K, Buttgereit F. Molecular mechanisms of glucocorticoid-induced osteoporosis. Bone 2001; **29**(6): 498–505.

Reid I. Glucocorticoid osteoporosis – mechanisms and management. Eur J Endocrinol 1997; **137**(3): 209–17.

Saag KG, Emkey R, Schnitzer TJ, et al. Alendronate for the prevention and treatment of glucocorticoid-induced osteoporosis. Glucocorticoid-Induced Osteoporosis Intervention Study Group. N Engl J Med 1998; **339**(5): 292–9.

Van Staa TP. The pathogenesis, epidemiology and management of glucocorticoid-induced osteoporosis. Calcif Tissue Int 2006; **79**: 129–37.

Bone diseases

Osteoporosis in children

There is no universally accepted or robust definition of osteoporosis in children. An emerging consensus exists that for a diagnosis of osteoporosis to be made there should be recurrent low trauma fractures together with low bone mass or vertebral fractures. Osteoporosis cannot be defined on the basis of low bone mineral density (BMD) alone. There are 3 main clinical situations:
- **Recurrent fractures:** low bone mass, but no obvious underlying condition.
- **Secondary osteoporosis:** secondary to systemic conditions or their treatment
- **Primary osteoporosis:** IJO – a self-limiting pre-pubertal condition with generalized osteoporosis – or osteoporosis associated with an hereditary disease of connective tissue.

The other differential diagnosis of osteoporosis in children is osteogenesis imperfecta (OI); see p. 428.

Epidemiology
- Fractures are common in healthy children: 25-40% of girls and 40–50% of boys sustain at least one fracture during growth (peak 11–15 years). 25% fracture repeatedly.
- There is some epidemiological data to suggest childhood osteoporosis is more prevalent in regions where calcium intake is low and in children with low BMD.
- An increased risk of osteoporotic fracture is recognized for a number of systemic conditions.
- Some conditions confer a potent fracture risk. The odds ratio (OR) for hip fracture associated with anorexia nervosa (AN) is >7.
- According to reviews of the topic, IJO is very rare, at least in the form originally described by Dent.
- IJO occurs in both sexes with a mean age of onset of 7 years (range 1–13 years)

Aetiology and pathophysiology
Low bone mass and fractures
- In healthy children there may be interactions between the factors determining growth and susceptibility to fracture. These effects may be most relevant when growth velocity is greatest.
- In these healthy children an integration of further factors such as activities and trauma risk, calcium and/or vitamin D status and genetic influences [e.g. allelic variation in the lipoprotein receptor-related protein 5 (LRP5)] might be important in conferring a deficit in load-adaptational skeletal integrity.

Secondary osteoporosis
- Immobilization is a contributory cause to bone loss associated with many chronic diseases particularly neurological diseases. The presumed mechanism is lack of bone formation as a result of suboptimal mechanical stimulation of bone.
- Chronic inflammation underscores bone loss or poor formation in Crohn's disease, juvenile idiopathic arthritis (JIA) and cystic fibrosis (CF), identifiable before any GC therapy is started. Ulcerative colitis probably isn't associated with secondary osteoporosis.
- Osteoporosis risk is greatest where multiple risk factors exist. For example, systemic inflammation, liver disease and relative immobility will all likely contribute to bone loss in CF; low body and muscle mass, poor oestrogen and nutritional status are all likely to contribute to low bone mass in anorexia nervosa (AN).
- Like the adult skeleton, the growing skeleton is sensitive to the effects of various hormonal abnormalities including thyroxine and endogenous GC production.

Secondary osteoporosis in children: the main causes

Endocrine disorders/treatment
- Cushing syndrome.
- Growth hormone deficiency.
- Thyrotoxicosis.

Gastrointestinal disorders
- Malabsorption (e.g. coeliac disease).
- Crohn's disease.
- Biliary atresia.
- Chronic hepatitis.
- Glycogen storage disease type 1.

Therapies
- Glucocorticoids
- Cyclosporin
- Methotrexate
- Anticonvulsants

Other
- Anorexia nervosa.
- Juvenile idiopathic arthritides.
- Cancer – notably leukaemia.
- Immobilization owing to neurological disease.
- Thalassaemia.
- Cystic fibrosis.
- Gaucher disease.
- Organ transplant.

IJO
- Pathophysiology is unknown.
- Bone biopsies from IJO children show reduced activation frequency, and low remodelling activity and osteoblast function. No increased bone resorption has been detected. The poor bone formation may be selective being confined to bone surfaces exposed to bone marrow. Intracortical and periosteal surfaces are less affected than trabecular-rich bone areas.
- No underlying genetic abnormality has been consistently reported.

Other forms of primary osteoporosis
- Though a condition caused by defective bone collagen formation, OI is considered to mimic childhood osteoporosis. It is almost universally associated with childhood bone fragility (see p. 428).
- The heritable conditions of connective tissue Ehlers–Danlos syndrome, Bruck syndrome, Marfan syndrome, homcystinuria and osteoporosis pseudoglioma syndrome are all rare causes of primary osteoporosis.

Clinical features
- Children and adolescents with osteoporosis are likely to present either with fractures alone, or secondary to systemic disease, or with typical features of IJO.

- Any assessment should include the appraisal of underlying diseases, which is beyond the scope of this chapter.
- Calcium intake is difficult to assess formally, but a cursory review of dietary habits might throw light on poor nutritional status.
- IJO classically presents with an insidious onset of pain in the back, hips, and feet with difficulty walking. Pain can involve extremities. Muscles may be weak.
- Fractures in IJO typically occur at bone metaphyses. Some recommend IJO be diagnosed only when there are vertebral compression fractures present.

Investigations
Laboratory tests
- Tests are aimed at characterizing the presence and activity of the condition causing the osteoporosis.
- Measuring vitamin D (25-OHD), parathyroid hormone (PTH), and routine bone biochemistry may be prudent whatever the likely cause of osteoporosis as calcium and vitamin-D deficiency can complicate any other cause of poor bone health, and would be easily correctable with supplements in most cases.

Radiographs and dual X-ray absorptiometry (DXA)
- Major fractures of the spine are simply detected by lateral spinal radiographs. Subtle vertebral fractures are not easily detected though algorithms for detecting relative vertebral height loss are being investigated.
- Careful radiological assessment of long bone appearances may be necessary where the differential diagnosis lies between OI and IJO. In IJO small radiolucent bands at sites of newly-formed metaphyseal bone are typical.
- DXA measurements are strongly influenced by changes in bone and body size related to age and pubertal development. BMD estimated from a measure of bone mineral content in a 2D area of growing bone is difficult to normalize for given the variety in growth rates for age in healthy children, but notably where growth deviates excessively from the mean – a situation more frequently encountered in association with pathology.
- The factors above are amplified for the hip and forearm compared with the spine.
- The comparison of a BMD measure with its reference range should be interpreted carefully. Different BMD correction algorithms have been proposed. One of the simplest divides bone mineral content (BMC) by the 3D volume of the bone calculated from the measured vertebral area and assuming the vertebra is a cube. This is called the bone mineral apparent density (BMAD).

Key points regarding diagnosis of osteoporosis in children
- The diagnosis should not be made on DXA results alone.
- DXA should be done only in specialist centres.
- Z-scores, ideally of the LSp, should be quoted, not T-scores, and compared with the best available reference interval data. The value of BMD to predict fractures has not yet been determined
- Age-related Z-scores are unreliable in children who are small for their age
- A variety of algorithms may help correct for bone size, growth variation and pubertal development. There is no consensus on which method to use
- Whole body BMC and quantitative Computerized Tomography (QCT) may offer advantages over hip and LSp BMD. Corrections may still need to be made for BMC and radiation doses are relatively high for QCT

Differential diagnosis
- The distinction of recurrent fractures with low bone mass in healthy children compared with secondary osteoporosis requires exclusion of systemic disease.
- IJO may need distinction from OI in certain children, notably those presenting with fractures <10 years old.
- Multiple fractures in infancy may be due to non-accidental injury/child abuse.

Table 14.11 The differential diagnosis of IJO and OI

	IJO	OI
Familial	No	Often
Onset	Late prepubertal	Birth or soon after
Fractures	Metaphyseal; incl. vertebral	Long bone diaphyseal
Growth rate	Normal	Normal or low
Connective tissues	No involvement	Hypermobility, blue sclerae,
Bone biopsy	↓Bone turnover	↑Bone turnover; hyperosteocytosis
Genetics	LRP5 mutations in some	Collagen type 1 in most patients

Treatment
- Where there is no secondary osteoporosis, and both IJO and OI have been excluded, then advice regarding trauma risk should be given, but patients and their families reassured.
- Although calcium supplementation has led to convincing increases in BMD in healthy children in the short-term, the long-term advantages are unproved.
- Studies of weight-bearing activity have been generally positive in terms of improving BMD. Adherence in the long-term, however, has proved a problem
- In all forms of osteoporosis, bisphosphonates are the treatment of choice, and should be given with additional calcium and vitamin D supplements.
- In secondary osteoporosis, robust long-term fracture end-point studies are lacking, but bisphosphonates are tolerated well for up to 3 years.
- Calcium supplements, usually with vitamin D should be considered in children with osteoporosis and chronic liver disease, those with fractures and low dietary calcium intakes, and those on anticonvulsants.

Resources
See under Post-menopausal osteoporosis

References
Adams J, Shaw N, on behalf of the Bone Density Forum. *A Practical Guide to Bone Densitometry in Children*. Bath: National Osteoporosis Society 2004. Available at: ww.nos.org.uk

Bianchi ML. Osteoporosis in children and adolescents. *Bone* 2007; **41**: 486–95.

Manias K, McCabe D, Bishop N. Fractures and recurrent fractures in children: varying effects of environmental factors as well as bone size and mass. *Bone* 2006; **39**: 652–7.

Ward L, Tricco A, Phuong P, et al. Bisphosphonate therapy for children and adolescents with secondary osteoporosis. *Cochrane Database Syst Rev* 2007; **17**(4): CD005324.

Writing Group for the ISCD Position Development Conference. Position statement: executive summary. *J Clin Densitom* 2004; **7**: 7–12.

Primary hyperparathyroidism

Primary hyperparathyroidism (PHPT) and malignancy account for >90% of all hypercalcaemic patients. PHPT is a hypercalcaemic state resulting from excessive secretion of PTH from one or more parathyroid glands. Although historically patients may have presented with marked neuromyopathic, or cardiac features, or even pancreatitis, PHPT is usually detected early in its course now and rarely presents with such severe clinical manifestations.

Epidemiology
- Benign PHPT is relatively common with an incidence of between 1:500 to 1:1000.
- A 4–5× increase in PHPT incidence was noted in the early 1970s because of the widespread use of the laboratory auto-analyser and the disclosure of hypercalcaemia in patients being tested for other problems.
- Women are affected more than men 3:1.
- PHPT can rarely be part of familial multiple endocrine neoplasia (MEN 1 or 2a).
- MEN1 has an estimated prevalence of 2–3/100 000 and typically PHPT associated with MEN1 presents by the age of 50 years. MEN2a is rarer.

Aetiology and pathophysiology
- PHPT is caused by a single benign solitary adenoma in 80% of cases. Four-gland hyperplasia is seen in 15–20%. MEN1 may account for around 2% of PHPT cases.
- PHPT due to carcinoma is rare (<0.5% of PHPT cases).
- There is loss of normal feedback control of PTH by extracellular calcium. Why precisely the control is lost at a molecular level is unknown.
- There is no change in calcium sensitivity of individual parathyroid cells ('set point') in PHPT due to adenomas. Excess PTH relates to parathyroid cell number.
- Underlying genetic causes postulated to be relevant in some cases of PHPT include: gene rearrangements leading to altered growth potential of parathyroid cells; over-expression of cyclin D1 a cell cycle regulator, loss of a copy of a MEN1 tumour suppressor gene.
- Both MEN1 and MEN2a are autosomal dominant conditions affecting men and women equally.
- MEN1 occurs secondary to a mutation of the MEN1 tumour suppressor gene (11q13). The gene encodes the protein 'menin' whose gene regulatory functions have not been fully elucidated. Tumour growth depends on (somatic) acquired mutations occurring in the normal gene copy in one cell. Thus, a critical check in clonal proliferation is removed for that cell
- MEN2a is due to a mutation in the RET proto-oncogene (chromosome 10) seen in >95% of MEN2a families. RET is a receptor tyrosine kinase.

Clinical features
- Patients are often asymptomatic or present non-specific symptoms, such as fatigue, a sense of weakness, intellectual weariness.
- A family history of hypercalcaemia or endocrine tumours raises the possibility of MEN1 and MEN2a.
- Although theoretically possible, symptoms from hypercalcaemia and hypercalciuria – excessive thirst, urinary frequency, nocturia, muscular and bone aches, and abdominal symptoms – are not always volunteered.
- Peptic ulcer disease is unlikely to be related to PHPT unless as part of a MEN syndrome. Severe pancreatitis is thought to be unusual nowadays.
- The association of PHPT with hypertension (and thus cardiac and renal disease) is debated. It may be that vascular calcification accounts for an increased risk of such disease in the long-term.
- Bone pain due to PHPT bone disease (osteitis fibrosa cystica) is likely to be rare nowadays. Radiographic representation of it (regardless of symptoms) may be seen in <5% of PHPT cases in the USA for example.

Table 14.12 Familial hyperparathyroid syndromes

	Heritable predisposition to tumours
MEN1	Parathyroid adenomas (PHPT), anterior pituitary and adrenocortical adenomas, pancreatic islet tumours, duodenal gastrinomas, bronchial or thymic carcinoids, lipomas, facial angiofibromas, truncal collagenomas.
MEN2a	Medullary thyroid cancer, phaeochromocytomas, multiglandular PHPT.

Co-morbidities
Renal disease
Patients with PHPT should be screened for hypercalciuria (see below) and renal calcification. Renal disease should be an important factor in deciding timing for parathyroidectomy and should be monitored for closely in conservatively managed PHPT patients.

Arthritis
Pseudogout is well recognized as a complication of PHPT. Pseudogout is just one form of CPPDD disease, however. The prevalence and impact of CPPDD disease in PHPT has been poorly evaluated. Caution in ascribing arthritis in PHPT patients to osteoarthritis alone is unwise until a skeletal survey reviewed by a musculoskeletal radiologist has shown an absence of erosive CPPDD disease/arthritis.

MEN1
- PHPT is the commonest and (typically) earliest manifestation of MEN1.
- Gastric hyperacidity symptoms in PHPT should raise awareness of the co-existence of a gastrinoma.
- Familial PHPT without a familial history of any other tumour does not rule out MEN1. Long-term surveillance of family members is not unreasonable.

MEN2a
PHPT is of low penetrance in MEN2a (20% cases). Overall, the commonest tumour is medullary thyroid cancer (calcitonin producing), which occurs in >90%.

Investigations
Laboratory
- The combination of hypercalcaemia and raised PTH are diagnostic. Phosphate tends to be low or low-normal.
- PHPT can be associated with normocalcaemia
- Urinary calcium excretion is elevated in 35–40%.
- 1,25-dihydroxyvitamin D levels are high in about 25% cases (PTH stimulates 1α-hydroxylase). 25-OHD is often in the insufficiency range.
- It is important to assess renal function, estimating GFR.

CHAPTER 14 **Bone diseases**

Imaging
- The majority of patients lack radiological manifestations. *Osteitis Fibrosa* (OF) can occur rarely in advanced PHPT and is manifest by sub-periosteal resorption of distal phalanges, tapering of distal clavicles, patchy ('salt and pepper pot') lucencies in of the skull, bone cysts and brown tumours of long bones.
- Dual X-ray absorptiometry (DXA) can show how PHPT causes a selective resorption of cortical compared with trabecular bone. Disproportionately low forearm bone mineral density (BMD) compared with LSp may indicate a selective cortical bone-erosive process of PTH. The changes also occur in SHPT.
- In patients with OF, bone scintigraphy can show the extent of the bone disease.
- Imaging to show any nephrocalcinosis/nephrolithiasis is important. The results influence management decisions.
- After a decision has been made to consider surgery then imaging to locate any parathyroid gland adenomata is done. Though there is controversy over whether imaging is necessary in patients who have not previously had neck surgery, many would advocate both neck ultrasound and ^{99m}Tc-sestimibi scintigraphy. The combination of scan results increases the accuracy of abnormal gland location over a single scan.

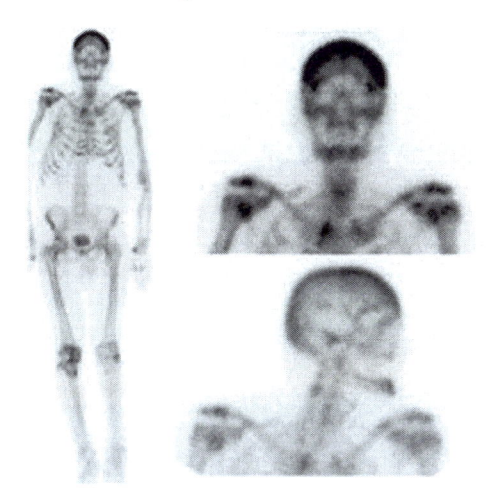

Figure 14.7 ^{99m}Tc-MDP scintigraphy in PHPT bone disease (OF): increased tracer/bone turnover in cranial bones and both humeral and femoral bone metaphyses

Treatment
Surgical
- Surgical removal of the adenoma or hyperplastic parathyroid gland(s) cures PHPT.
- The main factors determining a decision to operate are: the presence of significant bone or renal disease, if the patient is young or has marked hypercalcaemia.
- There is, despite guidelines, still considerable controversy when to operate in asymptomatic individuals. Some evidence suggests surgery improves quality of life and BMD measures compared with conservative management for asymptomatic PHPT.

- The NIH guidelines (1990) for managing PHPT have been widely criticized and a consensus has addressed outdated aspects of the guidelines (Bilezikian 2002).
- Surgery requires exceptional skill and experience. Options include a minimally invasive approach under local or general anaesthetic, useful in removing a single adenoma identified on pre-operative scans or neck exploration under general anaesthetic.
- In multiglandular disease, all parathyroid gland tissue is removed except for a remnant, which is left *in situ* or transplanted in the non-dominant forearm.
- Post-operative complications include prolonged ('hungry bone syndrome') or permanent (total gland removal) hypocalcaemia and recurrent laryngeal nerve palsy.
- In MEN1 it is especially important to consider when to operate as adenomas can re-occur and multiple operations may be needed in the future. A total neck exploration is necessary as multiple adenomas can be present and all glands need to be visualized
- In MEN2a, because undiagnosed phaeochromocytoma can cause death or substantial morbidity at operation, it is important to screen for phaeochromocytoma before undertaking parathyroid surgery.

Medical
- Asymptomatic PHPT patients can do well managed conservatively. Laboratory measures of biochemistry and BMD can remain stable for many years.
- However there are a number of caveats to the above:
  - 25% of patients will have progression of hypercalcaemia or a decline in BMD over 10 years;
  - the increase in fracture risk, and determinants of it, in medically-managed PHPT are not well known;
  - patients <50 years have high risk of progressive PHPT;
  - the effect of CPPDD disease on quality of life, disability and joint pain/failure in monitored compared with surgically treated PHPT is unknown.
  - specialist clinical, laboratory, and BMD monitoring long-term is required.
- PHPT patients should avoid thiazides, may benefit from a regular bisphosphonate avoid calcium supplements and should adopt a low calcium intake diet.
- Monitoring of renal function is required. To reduce effects of hypercalcaemia and hypercalciuria, patients should be advised to avoid prolonged immobility and ensure adequate hydration.
- Calcimimetics play a role in medical management by altering the 'setpoint' of the calcium sensing receptor. A biological effect has been demonstrated in the short term (normalizing serum calcium for up to 3 years).

Resources
Internet sites
www.endocrine.niddk.nih.gov/pubs/hyper/hyper.htm

www.ncbi.nlm.nih.gov/bookshelf/br.fcgi?book=endocrin&part=A742; (Review of PTH and vitamin-D biology/pathol.)

ICD-10 codes
E21.0   Primary hyperparathyroidsim

References

Arnold A. Familial hyperparathyroid syndromes. In: *Primer on the Metabolic Bone Diseases and Disorders of Mineral Metabolism*, 6th edn. Washington: ASBMR, 2006; 185-8.

Arnold A, Shattuck TM, et al. Molecular pathogenesis of PHPT. *J Bone Miner Res* 2002; **17**: N30–6.

Bilezikian JP, Potts JT, et al. Summary statement from a workshop on asymptomatic PHPT: a perspective for the 21st century. *J Bone Miner Res* 2002; **17** S2: N2–11.

Silverberg SJ, Shane E, Jacobs TP, Siris E, Bilezikian JP. The natural history of treated and untreated asymptomatic primary hyperparathyroidism: a ten year prospective study. *N Engl J Med* 1999; **41**: 1249–55.

Silverberg SJ, Bilezikan JP. The diagnosis and management of asymptomatic primary hyperparathyroidism. *Nat Clin Pract Endocrinol Metab* 2006; **2**(9): 494–503.

Paget's disease of bone (osteodystrophia deformans)

Described originally (but inaccurately) as an 'osteitis' (osteitis deformans) in 1877 by Sir James Paget (1814–99), this condition, named after him, is most accurately, but perhaps not most 'catchily', referred to as *osteodystrophia deformans*. Paget's Disease of bone (PDB) is a localized disease of bone remodelling. Structural changes in bone, notably expansion, occur as a result of increases in disordered osteoclast function. The site and severity of skeletal involvement varies considerably and many patients are asymptomatic. PDB has a variety of long-term consequences on joint and nerve function primarily as a result of local expansion of affected bone. PDB can be classified as symptomatic (bone pain) or asymptomatic and described by its local effect (e.g. deforming, secondary arthritis) and also its extent:

- **Monostotic:** one bone or portion of bone affected.
- **Polyostotic:** 2 or more bones affected.

Epidemiology
- Occurs in both men and women and is commonly diagnosed in the elderly. It is rare to make the diagnosis in adults <25 years and thought to occur primarily after 40 years.
- Ethnic and geographical clustering occurs. PDB is common in Europe, N America, Australia, and NZ.
- PDB has been described in East European, and Sub-Saharan African and Arabic populations, but the prevalence rates are very low. In both North and South America, rates are higher in people of European descent compared with indigenous groups and those with Afro-Caribbean origin.
- Prevalence in Europe is 0.5–4.5% and 3–4% in Australia and NZ. Rates decrease from north to south in Europe.
- In Lancashire, UK 6–8% people >55 years have PDB.
- Recent studies point to a decline in PDB prevalence – cause unknown.

Aetiology and pathophysiology
Genetic
- PDB commonly occurs in families: there is an AD pattern of inheritance, 1st degree relatives of an affected person are 7× more likely to get PDB.
- Several genetic loci have been linked to familial PDB:
  - Predisposition loci have been detected on chromosome 18 and 6. No specific genes identified.
  - A mutation in a gene (5q35) encoding an ubiquitin binding protein, sequestosome-1 (SQSTM14/p62^{ZIP}), has been detected in 11/24 French-Canadian families with PDB.
- There is current focus on a number of genes, which affect NF-kB signalling (e.g. data from PDB families and studies, which link PDB extent/severity to severity of mutation).
- SQSTM1 is a 'scaffold protein' important in the NF-κB activation pathway. SQSTM1 mutations probably relevant to PDB cluster at its C-terminus (ubiquitin-binding domain). However, direct evidence for a functional effect of SQSTM1 mutations *in vivo* is thin.
- If relevant to PDB pathophysiology, the SQSTM1-NF-κB signalling pathway may be abnormally complicated by factors, which affect the correct assembly and function of the multi-protein signalling complex (Apkc-SQSTM1-traf6). Thus, other genetic influences affecting this pathway may clearly be relevant in determining the heterogeneity of PDB.
- However, genetic influences alone are unlikely to account for PDB given the focal (not complete skeletal) nature of the condition.

Environment
- For >30 years studies have suggested PDB may be caused by a paramyxoviral infection.
- Originally, nuclear and cytoplasmic inclusions were described in PBD bone, which were thought to resemble paramyxoviral nucleocapsids.
- Subsequently, measles, canine distemper, and respiratory syncytial virus have been linked with PDB from a variety of studies using immunocytochemistry staining of PDB sections for nucleocapsid proteins and *in situ* hybridization of viral nucleocapsid transcripts in affected bone.
- Theories linking paramyxoviral infection with PDB have been weakened by the failure of some researchers to reproduce the results published by others.
- Some cogent arguments weaken the case for a viral aetiology alone. For example, if viruses are ubiquitous and found globally, why is PDB not found globally? Also, how do viruses persist for decades in immunocompetent people assuming most are contracted in childhood but PDB occurs in the elderly?

Pathology
- The hallmark is increase in bone resorption from multinucleate osteoclasts and increased osteoblasts.
- Increased bone turnover is shown by increases in serum and urinary resorption markers (e.g. deoxypyridinolene, type 1 collagen N- and C- telopeptides).
- Coupled osteoblast activity increases and is reflected in increases in ALP.
- In early PDB increased osteoclast activity predominates with lytic lesions ('blade of grass' lesion in long bones).
- New bone formation is coupled but accelerated and collagen fibres are laid down haphazardly. Ultimately, there is a mosaic pattern of woven bone.
- Bone marrow is infiltrated by excessive fibrous connective tissue and blood vessels. Bone matrix is normally mineralized

Clinical features
Key features in history
- The main symptom is bone pain. It often remains at rest and is deep seated. The commonest bones affected are pelvis, femurs, vertebrae, skull, and tibiae.
- Typical features in the history (though non-specific) from skull involvement include: deafness (skull PDB affecting VIIIth cranial nerve neural canal or inner ear bone function); change in shape of head/increase in hat size; neck/occipital pain or intrinsic headache; dental/gum problems (mandible involvement); change in timbre of voice (from changes in nasal bone shape and narrowing of the airway).
- Groin/anterior thigh pain might suggest hip OA secondary to pelvic or femur PDB.
- Symptoms of spinal claudication might suggest lumbar vertebral PDB (see also Plate 24).

Key features on examination
- Look for skeletal deformity (e.g. bowing of femur or tibia, enlarged head for body size/square head, widening of gap between teeth, kyphosis).

- Heat felt over suspected involved bones might represent hypervascularity of Pagetoid bone.
- Examination needs to be comprehensive and aimed at evaluating possible effects of expanded Pagetoid bone. Referral on to other specialties may be needed.
- Bowing of legs is associated with leg length discrepancy and mechanically-induced lower back and leg symptoms.

Table 14.13 Examination of a patient with PDB

Complication of PDB	Examination
Platybasia	Neurological: rule out myelopathy
Spinal canal encroachment	Neurological: to rule out spinal canal or radicular nerve exit foramen stenosis
Osteoarthritis	Rheumatological: to assess hip, knee, and shoulder (typically)
Hearing loss	Detailed ENT examination
Mandibular involvement	Maxillofacial examination and oral health assessment
Long bone deformities	Rheumatological/biomechanical to assess deformity, mobility and assess need for orthoses/mobility aids
Hyper-vascularity	Cardiac examination to assess any high output cardiac failure

Co-morbidities
- Hypercalcaemia and hypercalciuria associated with prolonged immobility.
- Secondary hyperparathyroidism typically seen in those patients with very high ALP levels. Mechanism unknown, but thought to be secondary to low serum calcium in patients requiring high calcium flux into active pagetoid bone. One possible result is associated (mainly peripheral bone fragility/osteoporosis).
- Sarcoma is a recognized but very rare complication of PDB. Intense and worsening pain in known PDB site needs investigation for sarcomatous change.
- Hyperuricaemia and gout. May be a consequence of increased cellular turnover in bone.
- Other co-morbidities occur primarily as a consequence of expansion of bone – see above.

Investigations

Laboratory
- Raised ALP. Raised resorption markers (e.g. urinary NTX or serum CTX).
- Always check blood calcium and phosphate and 25-hydroxyvitamin-D and PTH (see above).

Imaging
Radiographs.
- Appearances are pathognomonic.
- Bones are typically expanded, show cortical thickening, coarsened trabeculae, and a mixture of lytic and sclerotic areas.

Scintigraphy.
$99m$Tc-MDP isotope bone scans are the most sensitive way of detecting involved skeletal sites in PDB.

- Typical patterns of abnormality are well recognized. Polyostotic PDB is easily defined.
- Abnormalities point to foci of involvement for further clinical and radiographic assessment if necessary.

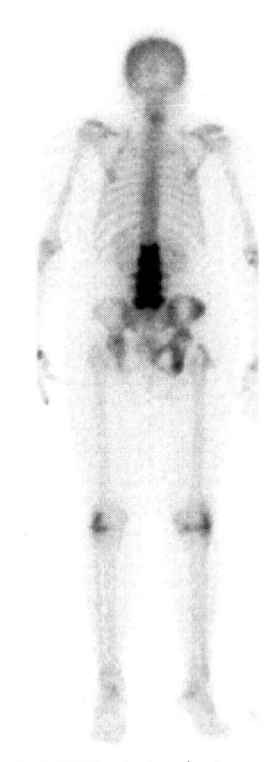

Figure 14.8 99mTc-MDP scintigraphy (posterior whole body view) showing PDB in contiguous lumbar spine vertebrae, right hemipelvis, and skull. Scan also shows osteoarthritic knees

CT and MR
CT is the imaging of choice where a fracture is not reliably disclosed on plain radiographs (e.g. fissure fracture of femur). MRI may be considered for:
- Characterizing radicular nerve root compression or spinal canal stenosis.
- Evaluating any myelopathy at axial (e.g. associated with platybasia) or subaxial spinal levels.
- Characterizing the range of lesions at joints affected by adjacent bone PDB.
- To assess any sarcomatous change or investigate potential bone metastases within pagetoid bone.

Histology/histomorphometry.
Bone biopsy is rarely required for a diagnosis of PDB.
- Cortical and trabecular bone area/volume is greatly increased. Within bone there is a mosaic appearance of packets of both woven and lamellar bone.
- Wide irregular trabeculae and poorly defined junction between trabecular and cortical bone.

- Osteoclast number may be 10× normal with the cells >100 μm wide containing 20–100 nuclei. These multinucleate osteoclasts are unique to PDB.
- Osteoblasts are numerous, plump and cuboidal.
- Osteoid area is moderately excessive and mineral apposition rate accelerated.
- Peritrabecular and marrow fibrosis is prevalent near osteoclasts and marrow blood vessels prominent. Haemorrhage may be noted.

Differential diagnosis
Malignancy, severe osteomalacia and fibrogenesis imperfecta ossium (FIO) are the main alternatives.
- FIO is often associated with a paraprotein and has distinct radiographic appearances without bone expansion or cortical thickening, and characteristically disordered bone collagen appearances on bone biopsy.
- In some cases, the discrimination of PDB and malignancy will require MR characterization of bone and associated soft-tissue lesions though
- Distinctive patterns of abnormal ^{99m}Tc-MDP scintigraphy, carefully interpreted, discriminates pathology.

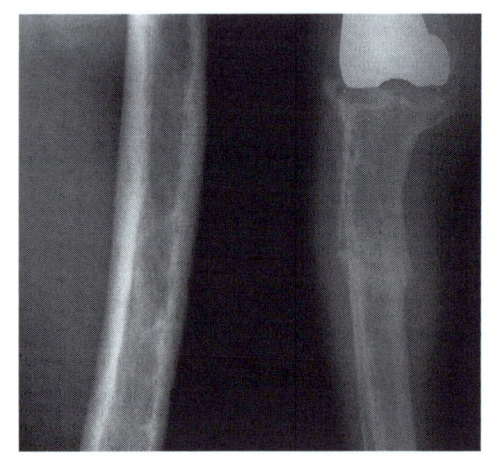

Figure 14.9 PDB femur (left) showing a number of transverse cortical fissure fractures. PDB tibia (right) with complete mid-shaft fracture.

Treatment
Between the mid-1970s and early 1990s the only therapies for PDB available were Etidronate and calcitonin.
- The more potent bisphosphonates – Alendronate, Risedronate, Clodronate, Ibandronate, neridronate, tiludronate, olpadronate, pamidronate and Zoledronate – have all now shown efficacy in PDB.
- The main indication for bisphosphonate treatment is bone pain. Improvement in pain correlates with drop in ALP and other bone turnover markers.
- Bisphosphonates vary in their ability to produce 'remission' from pain and duration of normalized ALP.
- Pain may not necessarily be from pagetoid bone, but from osteoarthritis in joints adjacent to pagetoid bone or radicular lesions (e.g. expansion of vertebrae).

- Though there are many long-term effects from untreated PDB (e.g. deafness, platybasia, cord compression, joint disease, fissure fractures, sarcoma, spinal stenosis), no studies convincingly show that bisphosphonates or other therapy, prevents these effects.
- All bisphosphonate regimes can cause hypocalcaemia, thus correction of vitamin D deficiency and regular calcium supplementation in PDB patients undergoing treatment courses is important.
- Various regimes for giving pamidronate have proved effective. The most commonly used regimes use 60–90 mg (in 500 ml 0.9% saline or 5% dextrose) 2–3 doses given 1–2 weeks apart.
- Normalizing ALP with pamidronate in PDB patients prior to orthopaedic operations reduces the amount of blood loss at the operation site.
- Calcitonin – well established though modestly effective therapy given by SC injection 100 units/day. Therapy over 3–6 months associated with reduction in bone pain in a majority and ALP in 50%. Remaining in biochemical remission after cessation of therapy is unusual and in some indefinite treatment might be needed. Escape from therapy (calcitonin receptor down-regulation or antibodies to the drug) is recognized. Flushing, nausea, and headaches are common and can be severe.

Prognosis and natural history
PDB is considered by many to be a benign condition and not needing treatment. In some however severe disease can cause deafness, fracture, aggressive arthritis, and neural spinal compromise. It remains controversial whether prophylactic therapy at an early stage can abrogate or prevent some of these complications.

Resources
Guidelines
See Selby et al.

Support groups
National Association for the relief of Paget's Disease: www.paget.org.uk;

ICD-10 codes
M88   Paget's disease of bone
M88.0   Paget's disease of skull
M88.8/9   Paget's disease of other bones/unspecified

References
Langston AL, Ralston SH. Management *of Paget's disease of* bone. *Rheumatology* 2004; **43**: 955–9.

Paget J. On a form *of* chronic inflammation *of* bones (osteitis deformans). *Trans Med-Chir Soc* 1877; **60**: 255–36.

Rebel A, Malkani K, Basle M, Bregeon C. Is Paget's Disease of bone a viral infection? *Calcif Tiss Res* 1997; **22**(Suppl): 283–6.

Scarsbrook a, Brown M, Wilson D. UK guidelines on management of Paget's disease of bone. *Rheumatology* 2004; **43**: 399–400.

Selby PL. Guidelines for the diagnosis and management of Paget's disease: a UK perspective. *J Bone Miner Res* 2006; **S2**: 92–3.

Siris ES, Roodman GD. Paget's disease of bone. In: Favus MJ (ed.) *Primer on the metabolic bone diseases and disorders of bone mineral metabolism*, 6th edn. Washington DC: ASBMR, 2006; 320–30.

Osteomalacia and rickets

Osteomalacia (in adults) and rickets (in children) is the consequence of low vitamin-D, calcium, or phosphorus. The manifestations of the severe condition are bone pain, fractures, myopathy, and calcium deficiency. In some forms of osteomalacia, phosphate depletion occurs as part of the primary defect. Mild hypovitaminosis-D is very common, can be associated with muscle and bone aches (rather than frank myopathy), and results in poor bone mineralization (osteoporosis) through SHPT.

Types of osteomalacia and rickets
- Nutritional deficiency.
- Drug induced.
- Pseudovitamin D deficiency rickets.
- Hereditary vitamin-D resistance rickets.
- Hypophosphataemic vitamin D resistant rickets.
- Tumour-induced osteomalacia.

Vitamin D biology
Vitamin D is formed from the effect of UV-B sunlight on 7-dehydrocholesterol in skin cells. Two forms (D2/ergocalciferol and D3/cholecalciferol) are formed. D2 is about 30% as effective as D3 at maintaining vitamin-D status. Both forms bind to vitamin-D binding protein in the blood and are hydroxylated in the liver (to 25-OHD). The production of this (still) inert form of vitamin-D is not tightly regulated and 25-OHD is the most reliable measure of total body vitamin-D status. The active vitamin-D form, 1,25-dihydroxyvitamin D, is generated in the kidney from hydroxylation of 25-OHD. 1,25-dihydroxyvitamin D has a variety of biological actions in tissues, but its known actions are primarily on gut and skeleton.

Biological functions of 1,25-dihydoxyvitamin-D
- Facilitates and enhances calcium (duodenal) and phosphate (entire small intestine) absorption from the gut.
- Triggers osteoblast RANKL which, through RANK interaction, activates osteoclasts to resorb bone releasing calcium into the circulation.
- Triggers osteoblast production of a number of mediators important for laying down bone osteoid.
- Decreases PTH synthesis and secretion.
- Non-calcaemic actions through genomic vitamin-D response elements (vitamin-D receptors):
  - effects on many different tissues;
  - broadly anti-proliferative and pro-differentiative;
  - *in vivo* consequences not well understood.

Nutritional deficiency
Epidemiology
- Hypovitaminosis-D is prevalent in extreme latitudes, in people who do not expose their skin to sun and is increasingly prevalent with age.
- Babies excessively breast-fed by mothers with dark skin and infants fed only non-dairy milk substitutes are at risk of rickets.
- Calcium deficiency may reflect chronically poor dietary intake, gut disease (poor absorption), or excessive calcium excretion.
- Vitamin D deficiency is common. Studies in places such as Boston, Finland, and Northern Europe show that substantial rates of deficiency occur in different ages and populations. Secondary hyperparathyroidism (SHPT) in these studies is not unusual.
- Isolated calcium deficiency rickets or osteomalacia is unusual. Low calcium intake in the infant's weaning period, diets high in phytate and oxalate. Some traditional African diets particularly can lead to calcium deficiency rickets age 4–8 years. Muscle weakness may be less common than in vitamin D deficiency states.

Aetiology and pathophysiology
Osteomalacia and nutritional deficiency rickets can be caused by either vitamin-D or calcium deficiency or (usually) both. Nutritional phosphate depletion causing osteomalacia/rickets is unusual given the ubiquitous presence of phosphate in foodstuffs. There are rare hereditary causes of rickets (see below).
- Low vitamin D leads to poor (vitamin-D dependent) calcium absorption from the small bowel and SHPT.
- Low 1,25-dihydroxyvitamin D can aggravate SHPT (reduction of suppression of PTH production). SHPT causes osteopaenia, renal tubular calcium retention, and urinary phosphate loss, which worsens the osseous lesion. Bone and growth plates become 'mineral-poor'.
- Vitamin D insufficiency is defined by consensus as the level below which it leads to an elevation of SHPT [essentially around 75 nmol/l (25 μg/l)].
- In disease due to calcium deficiency, 25-OHD is in the reference interval, but PTH and 1,25-dihydroxyvitamin D are elevated. The latter can lead to early degradation of 25-OHD and lead to vitamin D deficiency.

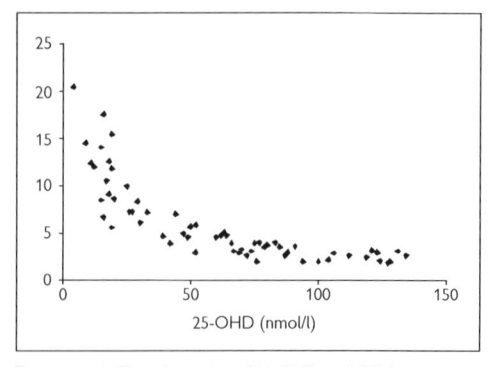

Figure 14.10 The relationship of 25-OHD with PTH in any given Caucasian population: the concept of vitamin D insufficiency.

As 25-OHD falls below 70–80 nmol/l, PTH (Y-axis shown in pmol/l) begins to rise. Thus at or below this level 25-OHD might be considered 'insufficient' to prevent compensatory secondary hyperparathyroidism (SHPT). The clinical consequences of 'insufficiency' are debated.

CHAPTER 14 **Bone diseases**

Clinical features
Key points in history
- Can exist without many symptoms. Bone and muscle pains, however, are common, often non-specific, chronic, and widespread.
- Patients have often been previously misdiagnosed with fibromyalgia, chronic fatigue, and depression.
- Bone pain is often unremitting. Myalgias and weakness in hip and proximal leg musculature is typical.

People/populations at risk of osteomalacia
- Institutionalized elderly.
- Elderly with little or no sun exposure.
- Excessive sunscreen use or sun avoidance (e.g. people with pale, sensitive skin, SLE).
- All people, particularly dark-skinned people, living at extreme latitudes.
- Where ethnicity/religion implies all skin is covered.
- Chronic liver disease.
- Previous gastro-duodenal surgery/duodenal pathology.
- Long-term anticonvulsant use.

Key points on examination
- Full examination is necessary to consider causes of widespread pain including: conditions characterized by axial and peripheral enthesitis and osteitis, particularly psoriatic arthritis/enthesitis, and chronic sarcoidosis, myositis/myopathies and other chronic arthritides.
- Check gait for myopathic features (waddling, leaning back, slow, slightly wide based, using walking aids).
- Examine for muscle weakness in quads, pelvic stabilizers (Trendelenberg), and shoulder girdle muscles.
- Tenderness of muscles, bony prominence points, tendons and ligaments is usually non-specific. Patients may satisfy ACR criteria for fibromyalgia – caution!

Investigations
Laboratory
- Bone biochemistry: calcium is usually normal, phosphate may be normal or low, ALP may be normal or raised. Urinary calcium excretion usually low.
- 25-OHD is usually <25 nmol/l (10 µg/l) and PTH raised >5 pmol/l, but often much higher.
- Renal function needs testing because low GFR is associated with phosphate retention and high PTH, and this complicates interpretation of tests.
- Liver function, folate, iron studies, celiac autoantibodies, autoimmune serology may all be useful in selected patients to rule out associated conditions or conditions causing non-specific pains mimicking symptomology.
- Bone biopsy. Rarely needed for uncomplicated clinical scenario but can be useful if >1 bone disease likely to exist (e.g. osteomalacia and osteoporosis). Main feature: excess unmineralized osteoid (see Plate 30)

Imaging
- Features of rickets can develop quickly. Defects occur at growth plates: initially blurring of the growth plate appearance then widening of physes with splaying of the long bone metaphyses.
- Pseudofractures – small radiolucent lines through bone cortices – typically in femoral neck, pelvis and ribs – are shown by radiographs and isotope bone scintigraphy and are present where osteomalacia is severe

- The commonest finding in osteomalacia is osteopaenia, demonstrated on radiographs or on DXA scans – often confused with osteoporosis.

Treatment
Vitamin D deficiency
There are a number of alternatives for achieving Vitamin D repletion. Increasing UV skin exposure and oily fish consumption can be recommended if there is insufficiency alone without bone and muscle disease or underlying pathological association, in the non-elderly.
- In infants and young children Vitamin D drops 5000–15 000 iu (125–375 µg) daily for 2 months usually corrects deficiency. Normalizing ALP and (rickets) radiographic features takes a few months longer.
- Adolescents and adults can be given daily (10 000 iu/250 µg) or weekly (50 000 iu/1.25 mg) ergocalciferol (D2) for several months.
- If adherence with prescribed oral therapy is likely to be an issue, intramuscular ergocalciferol 300,000iu every 6 weeks is an alternative.
- Initial replacement with 1,25-dihydroxyvitamin D is not usually necessary in simple nutritional deficiency but may be sensible if there is small bowel or liver disease.
- Calcium correction (and resolution of SHPT) can follow 25-OHD correction automatically unless there is malabsorption or marked calcium dietary restriction.
- Initially calcium replacement can be used (e.g. 25-50mg/kg/day) especially if dietary intake is poor.

Calcium deficiency
- 1g daily calcium supplements for 6 months is usually sufficient to correct deficiency unless there is malabsorption or co-existent vitamin D deficiency.

Prevention of Hypovitaminosis D and calcium deficiency (and osteomalacia/rickets)
- There is controversy over the recommended daily intake (RDI) of oral vitamin D and calcium in infants, adolescents and adults required to prevent calcium and vitamin D insufficiency and – in the long-term given dietary and lifestyle habits – deficiencies.
- RDI of calcium varies between 700 and 1500 mg for adults with the highest levels recommended for the elderly and breast-feeding mothers.

Calcium-containing food	Amount	Calcium (mg)
Cheese	100 g (≈3½ oz)	600–1000
Semi-skimmed milk	1 l (≈1¾ pints)	1285
Yoghurt	125 g (≈4½ oz)	225
Spinach	100 g (≈3½ oz)	130
Canned sardines in oil	100 g (≈3½ oz)	550

- RDI for vitamin D varies given the reference population. In The USA it is 200 iu (5 µg) per day for children and adults <50 years and 600 iu daily for those >70 years.
- In the absence of sunlight the RDIs for dietary vitamin D, however, are likely to be inadequate to maintain vitamin-D repletion.

Drug-induced osteomalacia
- Cholestyramine can reduce vitamin D gut absorption when used in the long-term for binding bile salts in post-iliectomy diarrhoea.
- Aluminium containing antacids can reduce phosphate absorption causing hypophosphataemic osteomalacia.
- Renal reabsorption of phosphate can be caused by cadmium and ifosfamide.
- The main causes of drug-induced osteomalacia however are anticonvulsants. The effect is greatest with (?exclusive to) hepatic enzyme inducing agents:
  - the most frequently implicated drugs are phenytoin and phenobarbitone;
  - phenytoin, and possibly phenobarbitone, may have direct toxic effects on bone thus contributing to bone fragility through causing osteoporosis as well as osteomalacia;
  - anticonvulsant induced osteomalacia risk is greatest in the institutionalized and in those who avoid sunlight or have poor calcium dietary intake (often the more socially disadvantaged);
  - biochemical abnormalities are typical though ALP can be raised owing to hepatic enzyme induction from the anti-epilepsy drug alone;
  - studies comparing the success of treatment with ergocalciferol (as above), compared with therapeutic 1,25-dihydroxyvitamin D (calcitriol) have not been done;
  - issues with adherence to oral therapy and a continual need to take anticonvulsants would suggest long-term monitoring for drug-induced osteomalacia in epilepsy patients is prudent.

Pseudovitamin D deficiency rickets
- Autosomal recessive condition caused by mutations in 25-hydroxyvitamin D 1α-hydroxylase gene.
- Presents in the first year of life with rickets, hypocalcaemic seizures, SHPT, hypophosphataemia and very low or undetectable levels of 1,25-dihydoxyvitamin D; however, there is normal circulating 25-OHD.
- The condition is cured with calcitriol and calcium supplements, which need to be continued life-long.

Hereditary vitamin D resistant rickets
- Autosomal recessive condition caused by mutations in vitamin D receptor (VDR). In affected patients mutations in all VDR functional domains have been demonstrated (DNA, ligand, and co-modulator binding).
- Often a history of parental consanguinity – parents typically functionally normal heterozygotes.
- Presents in infancy with rickets and hypocalcaemia symptoms – tetany/seizures, SHPT, hypophosphataemia, tooth enamel hypoplasia, and alopecia totalis.
- Distinguished biochemically from pseudovitamin D deficiency by high 1,25-dihydroxyvitamin D and by a poor/lack of response to calcitriol.
- In 50% patients there is some VDR function thus therapeutic response to calcitriol and calcium supplements can be seen. In total VDR function lack therapy with IV calcium can ameliorate the rickets lesions.
- Sporadic remission can occur after skeletal growth though is not usual. Management of condition through pregnancy and serious intercurrent illness is difficult.

Hypophosphataemic vitamin D resistant rickets/X-linked hypophosphataemia (XLH)
- Named as hypophosphataemia vitamin D resistant rickets by Albright in 1937, the most common form of this condition is also known as X-linked hypophosphataemia (XLH) – a dominant trait.
- Condition is due to mutations in *PHEX* gene, which encodes a Phosphate regulating gene with homologies to endopeptidases on the X chromosome (Xp22.1-22.2). More than 180 *PHEX* mutations have been identified (www.phexdb.mcgill.ca).
- PHEX protein primarily regulates fibroblast growth factor 23 (FGF-23) levels. It is presumed that mutations in PHEX can impair enzymatic cleavage (and deactivation) of FGF-23 (and probably other similar proteins termed 'phosphatonins').
- FGF-23 has a key role in regulating normal phosphate homeostasis in a number of tissues. Its levels vary inversely with the expression of Na-P co-transporters at cellular membranes in a variety of tissues.
- Abnormalities in FGF-23 and phosphate homeostasis are gradually being investigated in a number of conditions, particularly those involving renal pathology.
- Some but not all XLH patients do have high FGF-23 levels. High FGF-23 may simply be a consequence of a *PHEX* gene mutation. To date, no FGF-23 gene mutations have been found in XLH.
- Presentation is unusual before the child starts to walk though the condition can often be suspected from a positive family history.
- An affected child develops rickets, lower limb deformities, and is slow to walk. Skeletal growth is slow and dental abnormalities can be severe.
- Biochemically, there is hypophosphataemia, phosphaturia, and functionally low 1,25-dihydroxyvitamin D for the (low) level of serum phosphate. Serum calcium, PTH, and 25-OHD levels are normal.
- Treatment is with frequent daily dosing of phosphate initially 40 mg/kg/day increasing to 100 mg/kg/day, but not to exceed 3 g daily.
- Raising serum phosphate will cause functional hypocalcaemia and SHPT which will worsen phosphaturia so additional therapeutic (bd) calcitriol is given to suppress PTH (25–75 ng/kg/day).
- If growth is still poor growth hormone can be considered and some successes are noted.
- Continuing treatment in adults is somewhat debated. Symptomatic patients can derive benefit from continuing therapy. Whether to continue to use calcitriol alone or with phosphate supplements is also debated.
- The commonest long-term complications of treatment are nephrocalcinosis and hyperparathyroidism. Thiazides may slow the development of the former. Untreated SHPT can result in tertiary hyperparathyroidism for which parathyroidectomy is the only option.

Autosomal dominant hypophosphataemic rickets (ADHR).
- As in XLH there is a variable age in onset. Like XLH, however, presentation is generally in childhood or in young adults. A family history may be obtained.
- Clinically ADHR is very similar to XLH when it presents in infants (see above).

- ADHR is biochemically indistinguishable from XLH and TIO (see below). Serum FGF-23 levels are elevated.
- The defect in ADHR appears to be in the FGF-23 gene. Mutations probably render FGF-23 resistant to (deactivating) cleavage, thus lead to excessive levels. As a result there is a decrease in transmembrane phosphate transport and generation of 1,25-dihydroxyvitamin D.
- Treatment is as for XLH.

Tumour-induced osteomalacia/oncogenic hypophosphataemic osteomalacia

A rare acquired condition. Osteomalacia bone and muscle disease occurs because of severe hypophosphataemia caused by 'phosphatonins' produced by tumours.

Clinical and biochemical characteristics
- Presents usually in adults age 40–60 years with progressive, sometimes long-standing, myopathy, and bone pain. Often many different diagnoses have been made. Fragility fractures are common in established disease.
- Underlying tumours producing the phosphatonin (commonly FGF-23) are often small, benign and difficult to detect – often overlooked by patient or other doctors.
- Hypophosphataemia is often profound. There is renal phosphate wasting and inappropriately low 1,25-dihydroxyvitamin D for the level of serum phosphate. Serum calcium, 25-OHD and PTH are usually normal though ALP is invariably raised.
- Bone histomorphometry shows profound osteomalacia.
- FGF-23 and other phosphatonins (Secreted Frizzled Related Protein 4 [sFRP4], Matrix Extracellular Phosphoglycoprotein [MEPE] and Fibroblast Growth Factor 7 ([FGF-7]) cause urine phosphate loss owing to reduced proximal renal tubule phosphate reabsorption.

Pathophysiology
- Excessive FGF-23 is produced by a tumour. Excessive FGF-23 inhibits renal tubular phosphate reabsorption and down-regulates 25-hydroxyvitamin D 1α-hydroxylase enzyme activity in the kidney leading to low 1,25-dihydroxyvitamin D. Gross phosphate wasting occurs and leads to osteomalacia.
- Tumours are usually mesenchymal cell rich, often small, benign, slow-growing and located in discrete places. FGF-23 RNA is abundantly expressed in these tumours.
- TIO has been associated with a variety of carcinomas, neurofibromatosis and fibrous dysplasia of bone also.
- Gene expression profiles of tumours associated with TIO have suggested some other 'phosphatonin' candidates including sFRP4, MEPE, and FGF-7.

Differential diagnosis
- TIO patients often get diagnosed with fibromyalgia or chronic fatigue syndrome. As myopathy and bone lesions develop (and become positive on bone scintigraphy) then TIO can be mistaken for skeletal malignancy.
- In many reported cases, where correct diagnosis has been delayed, there is often a situation where persistent hypophosphataemia has been overlooked.
- TIO presenting in infants, children and young adults can appear similar to XLH and ADHR clinically and identical biochemically. Generally, TIO presents much later in adulthood than XLH or ADHR.

Finding the tumours
- Imaging with somatostatin receptor and bone scintigraphy can be useful in identifying tumour location and the extent of osteomalacia lesions respectively. Bone scintigraphy can disclose lesions of fibrous dysplasia, which can hide phosphatonin-producing tumours or activity.
- Positive [18]FDG PET can identify small tumours.
- Given the frequent disclosure of tumours in the facial bones/sinuses CT scanning of the sinuses has been suggested as a useful 'blind' investigation to arrange.
- In a high proportion of cases, imaging fails to initially identify tumours. In such patients treatment (see below) will help, but repeated investigations, sometimes years into the future, can ultimately reveal tumours.

Treatment
- Resection of tumours cures the condition. Frequently, tumours can't be found or resection is unfeasible.
- TIO is treated with calcitriol 1–3 µg/day and phosphorus (2 g/day in divided doses). Doses should be tailored to improve symptoms, maintain fasting phosphorus in the reference interval, normalize ALP, and control SHPT without causing hypercalcaemia or hypercalciuria.
- With optimal calcitriol and phosphorus usage the myopathy and osteomalacia regresses.
- Monitoring for nephrocalcinosis and renal dysfunction long-term is necessary (?hypercalciuria from calcitriol).

Resources

ICD-10 codes
M83	Adult osteomalacia
M83.0–9	Various classifications of osteomalacia (e.g. M83.2 adult osteomalacia due to malabsorption; M83.5 Other drug-induced osteomalacia in adults)
E55	Rickets
E55.9	Vitamin D deficiency, unspecified
E83.3	Disorders of phosphorus metabolism (includes vitamin-D-resistant osteomalacia/rickets)

References

Bischoff-Ferrari HA, Dietrich T, Orav EJ, Zhang Y, Karlson EW, and Dawson-Hughes B. Higher 25-hydoxyvitamin D levels are associated with better lower extremity function in active and inactive adults 60+ years of age. *Am J Clin Nutr* 2004; **80**: 752–8.

Dawson-Hughes B, Heaney RP, Holick MF, Lips P, Meunier PJ, Vieth R. Estimates of optimal vitamin D status. *Osteoporos Int* 2005; **16**: 713–16.

Holick MF. Evaluation and treatment of disorders of calcium, phosphorus and magnesium. In: Noble J (ed.) *Textbook of Primary Care Medicine*, 3rd edn. St Louis: Mosby, 2000; 886–98.

Holick MF, Garabedian M. Vitamin D: photobiology, metabolism, mechanism of action and clinical applications. In: Favus MJ (ed.) *Primer on the Metabolic Bone Diseases and Disorders of Mineral Metabolism*, 6th edn. Washington DC: ASBMR, 2006; 106–14.

Jan de Beur SM. Tumour-induced osteomalacia. *J Am Med Ass* 2005; **294**: 1260–7.

Veith R. Vitamin D supplementation, 25hydroxyvitamin D concentrations and safety. *Am J Clin Nutr* 1999; **69**: 842–56.

Renal bone disease

Chronic kidney disease (CKD) is associated with increased bone fragility and abnormalities of bone turnover traditionally referred to as renal osteodystrophy (ROD).

Definitions

The US National Kidney Foundation (NKF 2002) classifies CKD on estimated GFR calculated by the Modification of Diet in Renal Disease (MDRD) formula (NKF K/DOQI).

Table 14.14 Stages of CKD

CKD stage	GFR (ml/min/1.73 m^2)	
1	>90	Evidence of chronic kidney damage
2	60–89	Evidence of chronic kidney damage
3	30–59	
4	15–29	
5	<15	End-stage renal disease

The abnormalities of the skeleton in CKD are collectively known as renal osteodystrophy (ROD). ROD has recently been defined as an alteration of bone morphology in patients with CKD. ROD is associated with a 3–4× increase in fractures and is a complex disorder of compromised bone strength consisting of a spectrum of skeletal abnormalities.

Skeletal abnormalities in renal osteodystrophy (ROD)

Bone and bone mineral abnormalities
- Osteitis fibrosa and mild hyperparathyroidism.
- Osteomalacia.
- Vitamin D related.
- Non vitamin D related: Chronic metabolic acidosis; aluminium accumulation.
- Phosphate depletion.
- Adynamic bone disease (low bone turnover).
- Mixed uraemic osteodystrophy.
- Amyloid bone disease.
- Osteoporosis.

Epidemiology

The prevalence of ROD in end-stage renal disease (ESRD) can vary with dialysis modality. The frequencies of the main forms of ROD defined histologically in patients undergoing peritoneal dialysis (PD) are:
- Osteitis fibrosa (OF) <10%.
- Adynamic bone disease (ADB) 60%.
- Mixed (OF+ADB) <10%.
- Osteomalacia.

In those having haemodialysis, OF is about 4× more prevalent, but ADB about half as frequent as in PD.

ROD may complicate osteoporosis: 50–70% of elderly women presenting with hip fractures (mean age 84 years) have a GFR <35 ml/min.

Aetiology and pathophysiology

As GFR declines there is impaired excretion of phosphate and reabsorption of calcium and decreased renal 1α-hydroxylation of 25-OHD to calcitriol, despite initial appropriate PTH responses (secondary hyperparathyroidism [SHPT]). When the kidneys can no longer eliminate more phosphate in response to PTH, phosphate levels rise. Through the effects of hyperphosphataemia on PTH production and further suppression of 1α-hydroxylation – mediated probably through a variety of mechanisms (see Martin et al., 2006) – calcitriol is lowered, potentially further aggravating hypocalcaemia.

- Chronic PTH gland stimulation can eventually cause:
  - parathyroid gland nodular hyperplasia;
  - excessive PTH secretion even if hypocalcaemia is corrected (often leading to tertiary hyperparathyroidism);
  - calcium and phosphate to be released from bone exacerbating hyperphosphataemia and occasionally leading to hypercalcaemia.
- Hyperphosphataemia-induced fibroblast growth factor 23 (FGF-23) may additionally suppress 1α-hydroxylation of 25-OHD.

Clinical features

ROD is asymptomatic in the early stage. In advanced disease, bone pain is prominent particularly in OF. Focal skeletal pain may be due to microfractures. The assessment can be complicated by the presence of other musculoskeletal lesions associated with CKD.

Co-morbidities

SHPT and vascular disease
- High PTH >600 pg/ml (63 pmol/l), calcium >2.37 mmol/l and phosphorus (>1.6 mmol/l) are associated with an elevated risk of death and cardiovascular events.
- Arterial calcification either occurs in the intimal layer within atherosclerotic plaques or affects the tunica media causing medial wall calcification.
- The latter increases vascular stiffness, reduces vascular compliance, elevates systolic blood pressure, widens pulse pressure, and causes left ventricular hypertrophy.

CKD and osteoporosis.
WHO grades of BMD are not ideally used to diagnose osteoporosis or indicate fracture risk in CKD4/5 patients with GFR <30 ml/min or on dialysis because:
- WHO BMD grades only apply to healthy Caucasian post-menopausal women.
- All forms of ROD may be associated with low BMD.
- How ROD subtypes relate to T-scores and fracture risk is unknown.
- Aortic calcification may lead to misleading elevation of measured BMD of the spine on the AP projection.

Patients with end-stage renal disease have other risk factors for bone fragility: heparin and glucocorticoid (GC) use, hypogonadism, poor nutrition, 25-hydroxyvitamin D (25-OHD) deficiency and metabolic acidosis.

CKD and musculoskeletal conditions
Gout, calcium pyrophosphate dihydrate disease, and other arthropathies due to calcium and phosphate containing crystals can occur in advanced CKD patients. Secondary tendonopathies and mechanical joint failure can ensue. The incidence of osteonecrosis and septic arthritis is elevated in CKD compared with controls.

Investigations

Laboratory
Measurable PTH correlates with the predominant histological abnormality in bone. High iPTH levels suggest osteitis fibrosa and low iPTH reflects low bone turnover ROD. But overlap is common.

Secondary causes of osteoporosis may need excluding (e.g. 9 a.m. testosterone and LH in men)

Imaging
Radiographs, DXA, and other techniques measuring BMD cannot predict ROD subtype with accuracy.
- BMD data may not be a useful clinical tool in predicting fracture. Studies are lacking.
- Bone scintigraphy can highlight the distribution of OF. Patterns correlating to ADB are not well recognized.

Histology: bone biopsy
The diagnosis of ROD essentially requires a bone biopsy.
- Bone biopsies are reported using three histological descriptions – bone turnover, mineralization, and volume.
- Bone biopsies are used rarely in many centres perhaps owing to the number of pathologists skilled in the detailed analysis of bone tissue.

ROD features on undecalcified bone biopsy

ROD subtype	Histomorphometry/features
Osteitis fibrosa	High bone turnover
	Markedly increased remodelling activity
Adynamic bone disease	Low bone turnover
	Decreased remodelling activity and osteoid surfaces
Osteomalacia	Low bone turnover
	Decreased remodelling activity
	Increased osteoid surfaces
Mixed	Patchy areas of osteitis fibrosa
	Increased osteoid

Treatment
Osteoporosis risk in patients with CKD 1 or 2 and early CKD 3 should be managed routinely.

Management of metabolic abnormalities in CKD3
- When GFR is <60 ml/min iPTH should be measured and if elevated 25-OHD checked (NKF, 2002).
- 25-OHD deficiency is common and is a risk for severe hyperparathyroidism in CKD.
- If 25-OHD is insufficient (<75 nmol/l), supplemental vitamin-D3 and calcium can be given with advice to increase skin exposure to the sun.
- 25-OHD deficiency (<25 nmol/l) is often associated with osteomalacia bone and muscle lesions, and high dose 25-OHD repletion then may be needed.

Management of SHPT in ROD
In CKD 4 and 5 key components of management are to:
- Reduce phosphate retention by restricting dietary phosphate, using frequent dialysis and phosphate binders (e.g. sevalamer).
- Optimize PTH levels by judicious use of active vitamin-D analogues (e.g. 1α-calcidol, calcitriol or paricalcitol). Consider calcimimetics (e.g. Cinacalcet), which increase the sensitivity of the PTH gland calcium-sensing receptor thereby reducing PTH release.

Management of osteoporosis in ROD
- Oral bisphosphonates and strontium ranelate are probably safe in CKD 3, but cautioned in CKD 4 and 5.
- There are no fracture end-point studies for any therapy in CKD 4 and 5 patients.

Management of ROD post-transplant
Fracture risk post-transplant is 4× that of the normal population and chiefly relates to glucocorticoid use and is managed best in light of renal function.
- Tertiary PTH+, present pretransplant and can resolve spontaneously, but take years to do so.
- Replace 25-OHD insufficiency/deficiency.
- Consider calcimimetics or parathyroidectomy if:
  - PTH-induced hypercalcaemia persists;
  - hyperparathyroidism is severe;
  - there is severe bone fragility (fractures);
  - there is severe joint disease (e.g. CPPDD)
- Rule out hypogonadism in men.
- Stop smoking, reduce alcohol, increase weight-bearing exercise, and minimize doses of GCs.
- In those with fractures and high PTH oral bisphosphonate therapy would seem a logical choice, but no fracture outcome studies have been done.

Acknowledgements
With thanks to Dr Brian Camilleri, Consultant Nephrologist, for his important contribution on the text.

Resources

Guidelines
For physicians, guidelines on managing renal bone disease and other aspects of CKD are at www.renal.org.

ICD-10 codes
N25.0 Renal osteodystrophy
N25.8 SHPT of renal origin

References
Cunningham J, Sprague S. Osteoporosis in chronic kidney disease. *Am J Kidney Dis* 2004; **43**: 566–71.

EBPG Expert Group on Renal Transplantation. European best practice guidelines for renal transplantation. Section IV: long-term management of the transplant recipient. Bone disease. *Nephrol Dial Transplant* 2002; **17**(Suppl 4): 43–8.

Elder G. Pathophysiology and recent advances in renal osteodystrophy. *J Bone Min Res* 2002; **17**: 2094–15

Martin KJ, Ziyad Al-A, Gonzalez EA. Renal osteodystrophy. In: Favus MJ (ed.) *Primer on the Metabolic Bone Diseases and Disorders of Mineral Metabolism*, 6th edn. Washington DC: ASBMR, 2006:359–66.

Moe S, Dreuke T, Cunningham J, et al. Definition, evaluation, and classification of renal osteodystrophy: a position statement from kidney disease: improving global outcomes (KDIGO). *Kidney Int* 2006; **69**: 1945–53.

NKF. National Kidney Foundation K/DOQI clinical practice guidelines for chronic kidney disease: evaluation, classification, and stratification. *Am J Kidney Dis* 2002; **39**(Suppl 2): S1–246.

Ramsey-Goldman R, Dunn JE, Dunlop DD, et al. Increased risk of fracture in patients receiving solid organ transplants. *J Bone Miner Res* 1999; **14**: 456–63.

Osteogenesis imperfecta

Osteogenesis imperfecta (OI) is a rare autosomal dominant inherited disorder of connective tissue characterized by bone fragility and fracture. Forms are chiefly due to abnormalities in Type 1 collagen and clinically varied – from a lethal phenotype and mild forms that may only manifest as osteoporosis in adults.

Classification of OI by type

OI type	Clinical features	Inheritance
I	Normal stature. Little or no deformity. Blue sclerae. Hearing loss in 50%	AD
II	Lethal in the perinatal period	AD
III	Progressive deformity. Short stature. Sclerae vary. DI common. Hearing loss common	AD/AR (rare)
IV	Mild to moderate bone deformity. Variable short stature. DI common. Occasional hearing loss. Sclerae vary.	AD
V	Phenotypically the same as IV but also triad of hypertrophic callus formation, dense metaphyseal bands, interosseous membrane ossification. Normal Type 1 collagen	AD, gene unknown
VI	Phenotypically the same as IV. ↑ALP. Fish scale appearance of bone under microscope	Unknown
VII	Phenotypically the same as IV. Found only in small Quebecois community. Blue sclerae. Rhizomelia. Moderate to severe bone disease.	AR, gene at 3p22-24.1

AD=autosomal dominant; AR=autosomal recessive; DI=dentinogenesis imperfecta.

Classification
Broadly in keeping with general features associated with recognized phenotypes there are varying degrees of growth deficiency, dentinogenesis imperfecta, hearing loss, macrocephaly, blue sclerae, scoliosis, barrel chest, and hypermobility. OI is conventionally described according to Sillence.
- Sillence described 4 types according to clinical features. Three further types have been added though these have been described on the basis of additional non-clinical parameters.
- Types IV–VI appear to have normal type 1 collagen.

Epidemiology
OI is rare. Reliable figures of prevalence and incidence don't exist. Both males and females are affected. Cases, families, and disease clusters in small ethnically restricted groups have been described from across the world.

Aetiology and pathophysiology
- >90% of OI patients have abnormalities in type 1 collagen. Types V–VI do not have type 1 collagen mutations.
- Type 1 OI is due to reduced synthesis of structurally normal type 1 collagen and have an increase in type 3: type 1 collagen ratio.
- In types II–IV a mixture of normal and abnormal collagen is synthesized. With rare exceptions the structural defects are either glycine substitutions or an in-frame deletion from alternate exon splicing.
- Defects in collagen chains impair helix folding and expose chains to enzymes for longer thus chains become excessively modified.
- Recessive forms of OI are probably caused by parenteral mosaicism for a dominantly inherited mutation.

Clinical features
OI can present at different ages thus its differential diagnosis varies dependently (see below). A positive family history is absent because mutations occur *de novo*.

Some features are common to all OI types: flat mid-face, bluish sclerae, yellow or opalescent teeth, relative macrocephaly, barrel chest and pectus excavatum, joint laxity.

Type I OI
- Mildest form of OI. Fractures occur postnatally often when child starts to mobilize, but incidence of fracture decrease after puberty. Occasionally, presents in early middle age as 'early osteoporosis'.
- Hearing loss can occur – often late in childhood or early adulthood.
- Growth deficiency, long bone deformity, and dentinogenesis imperfecta are unusual.

Type II OI
- Generally lethal in the peri-natal period. Birth often premature and are small for gestational age.
- There are major skeletal deformities and demise usually follows respiratory insufficiency.

Type III OI
- Severe type with progressive deformity. Fractures occur very commonly. Bones deform from normal muscle tension.
- Extreme growth deficiency and scoliosis common.
- Type III is compatible with full life span, although respiratory insufficiency and cor pulmonale can occur in middle age.
- Respiratory problems frequently complicate and compromise long-term health.

Type IV OI
- Moderately severe. Diagnosis can be at birth although often not until becomes mobile or even starts school.
- Typically several fractures a year occur though decrease after puberty.
- Final stature is small and children may be responsive to growth hormone. Compatible with normal life-span.
- Radiographically, there is osteoporosis and many develop scoliosis and vertebral fractures.

CHAPTER 14 Bone diseases

OI/EDS subtype

A discrete subtype of OI may exist, where there are features suggestive also of Ehlers–Danlos syndrome (EDS). Joint laxity/hypermobility is prominent.

Type V–VII

Recent subtypes of OI indistinguishable from Type IV OI have been proposed on the basis of having distinguishing radiology and/or bone histology.

Investigations

Serum biochemistry is normal though sometime ALP is elevated after a fracture.

Imaging
- In all types of OI: generalized osteopaenia. Long bones have thin cortices and a gracile appearance. Long bones of the arm are less affected than those of the leg.
- In severe OI, long bones are bowed, have modelling deformities, metaphyseal flaring, and a popcorn appearance at metaphyses.
- Vertebral fractures are common and affect thoracolumbar segments first.
- Skull radiographs can show platybasia in types III and IV. In this situation surveillance for brain stem features and myelopathy is prudent, and imaging with MRI sometimes necessary.

Bone densitometry

DXA evaluation shows low BMD for age. Notably DXA can aid diagnosis in milder OI forms in adults. Generally, OI severity correlates inversely with Z-score.

Bone histomorphometry
- Usually defects in modelling are obvious. There is thickening of trabeculae.
- Cancellous bone volume and cortical width are always decreased – under polarized light the lamellae are thinner and less smooth than in controls.
- Mineral apposition rates are normal.

Differential diagnosis

Depends on the time of presentation.
- Prenatally: severe type II or III may be difficult to distinguish from achondrogenesis type 1.
- In neonates: infantile hypophosphatasia – low ALP in the latter usually distinguishes.
- In toddlers and older children non-accidental injury is often considered the cause of recurrent fractures.
- In the pre-pubertal child age 9–11 years idiopathic juvenile osteoporosis (IJO; see 'Osteoporosis in children')
- In adults: causes of osteoporosis.

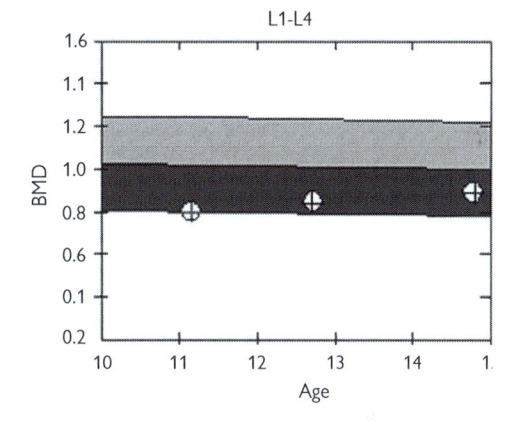

Figure 14.12 Changes in BMD (+12% from baseline) in a woman with mild OI and fragility fractures (at age <40y) with serial pamidronate injections (30mg once every 4 months)

Treatment

Physical therapy and rehabilitation are key interventions. Physiotherapy should begin in infancy and be undertaken by specialist physiotherapists cognisant with the aims and objectives of managing OI, and it's complications.

Orthopaedic care
- Involved orthopaedic surgeons should be experienced in managing OI. Preventive surgery is often necessary.
- Fractures should not be allowed to heal without reduction as function may be lost if deformity occurs.
- Long bones require fixation with an intramedullary rod with the smallest diameter to avoid cortical atrophy.

Surveillance for associated features
- Abnormal pulmonary function, particularly poor thoracic excursion, respiratory infections, and cor pulmonale are should be monitored for and managed early.
- Hearing loss and cord compression at the skull base can occur and can be monitored for. A radiograph showing platybasia at an early stage might denote those at risk of high cervical cord lesions.
- Recombinant human GH

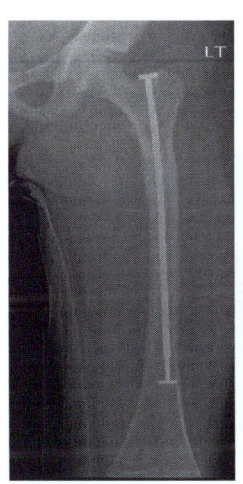

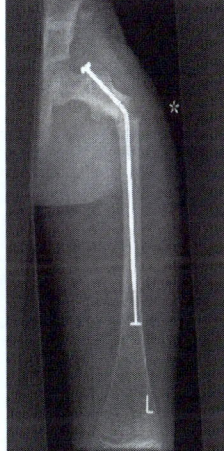

Figure 14.11 OI, girl aged 12 years. Left: despite an intramedullary (Sheffield) rod inserted as prevention against fracture, a shaft fracture has occurred. Right: the fracture has worsened and rod bends (radiograph on day of surgery). Note extendable lower part of rod has not fully extended with growth as intended and distal femur striations corresponding to cycles of intravenous pamidronate.

- Severe growth deficiency associated with OI can be treated with rhGH.
- Most type I OI and 50% type IV OI respond to rhGH. Type I OI children can respond to reach normal height.

Bisphosphonates
- RCTs in children with moderately severe OI suggest that IV bisphosphonates have therapeutic potential (ses also Plate 26)
- Bisphosphonate therapy increases BMD, iliac trabecular bone volume, and cortical width in the short-term, but effects on cortical bone may not be as obvious as on trabecular bone. Fracture prevention data in the long-term are not conclusive.
- The optimum duration of treatment with IV bisphosphonates in children and adults is unknown.
- Both oral and IV bisphosphonates have been used successfully to increase BMD in milder forms of OI particularly in adults. Long-term fracture prevention studies have not yet been completed.

Resources

Patient and physician resources
The OI Foundation is a repository of advice and information for patients, physicians and therapists: www.oif.org. A similar UK-based organization is www.brittlebone.org.

See excellent and comprehensive (open access) article by Steiner RD, Pepin MG and Byers PH. Available at: www.ncbi.nlm.nih.gov/books/bv.fcgi?rid=gene.chapter.oi.

ICD-10 codes
Q78.0   Osteogenesis imperfecta

References
Glorieux FH, Rauch F, Plotkin H, Ward L, Travers R. Type V osteogenesis imperfecta: a new form of brittle bone disease. *J Bone Miner Res* 2000; **15**: 1650–8.

Glorieux FH, Ward LM, Rauch F, Lalic L, Roughley PJ, Travers R. Osteogenesis imperfecta type VI: a form of brittle bone disease with a mineralization defect. *J Bone Miner Res* 2000; **17**: 12–18.

Kuivaniemi H, Tromp G, Prockop DJ. Mutations in fibrillar collagens and network forming collagen cause a spectrum of diseases of bone, cartilage and blood vessels. *Human Mutat* 1997; **9**: 300–15.

Marini JC. Osteogenesis Imperfecta. In: Favus MJ (ed.) *Primer on the Metabolic Bone Diseases and Disorders of Mineral Metabolism* 6th edn. Washington DC: ASBMR, 2006: 418–21.

Rauch F, Travers R, Plotkin H, Glorieux FH. The effects of intravenous pamidronate on the bone tissue of children and adolescents with osteogenesis imperfecta. *J Clin Invest* 2002; **110**: 1293–9

Sakkers R, Kok D, Engelbert R, et al. Skeletal effects and functional outcome with olpadronate in children with osteogenesis imperfecta. A 2y randomised placebo-controlled study. *Lancet* 2004; **363**: 1427–31.

Sillence DO, Senn A, Danks DM. Genetic heterogeneity in osteogenesis imperfecta. *J Med Genet* 1979; **16**: 101–16.

Ward LM, Rauch F, Travers R, et al. Osteogenesis imperfecta type VII: an autosomal recessive form of brittle bone disease. *Bone* 2002; **31**: 12–18.

Miscellaneous bone diseases 1

Fibrous dysplasia (FD)
A congenital non-inherited disorder usually diagnosed in childhood. Normal bone and bone marrow are replaced by highly vascular fibrous tissue and pre-osteoblastic cells.
- Aetiology – somatic mutations in the cAMP regulating protein Gsα, which is coded for by the GNAS gene.
- Children present with skeletal pain. FD can vary from a single lesion (monostotic) or involve multiple sites (polyostotic). FD can affect skull, spine, and long bones.
- FD frequently is associated with hyperpigmentation (café-au-lait spots) and hyperfunctioning endocrinopathies (e.g. growth hormone excess, hyperthyroidism, Cushing's). FD in combination with these features is termed McCune-Albright syndrome.
- FD can be associated with fractures, limb length discrepancy, and long bone deformity.
- FD lesions are characteristic on radiographs and bone scintigraphy is useful for staging disease, and in determining response to bisphosphonates.
- Hypophosphataemia and excess FGF-23 are associated features. Markers of bone turnover are increased.
- Pain can persist into adulthood and, generally, pain is often poorly addressed. Patients benefit from NSAIDs.
- Intravenous bisphosphonates have shown consistent efficacy in reducing pain, although there is some debate whether lesions change radiographically and long-term skeletal complications can be prevented.

Hypertrophic osteoarthropathy (HOA)
Primary HOA (pachydermal periostitis)
Autosomal dominant condition of unclear aetiology causing clubbing, hyperhydrosis, skin thickening (especially of the head termed cutis vertices gyrata), arthralgias, and periostitis affecting mainly distal limb bones.
- Affects men > women and blacks > whites. Onset typically in adolescence.
- Peripheries can enlarge and appear 'acromegalic'.
- Radiographs: periosteal thickening and ragged whiskering of proliferative bone. Distinguished from secondary HOA (smooth undulating periosteal thickening).
- Joint contractures and neurovascular compression from osteosclerotic lesions can require surgical intervention.

Secondary HO (90% of all HOA cases)

Secondary causes of HPOA are pulmonary (HPOA), pleural, cardiac, abdominal, and miscellaneous. Pleural causes include pleural fibroma and mesothelioma.
- Cyanotic heart disease with a right-to-left shunt is the only cardiac cause described.
- Pulmonary causes: bronchogenic carcinoma; tuberculosis; pulmonary abscesses; blastomycosis; bronchiectasis; emphysema; and *Pneumocystis carinii* infection in AIDS, Hodgkin disease, metastases, or cystic fibrosis.
- Abdominal causes: liver cirrhosis, IBD, amoebic and bacillary dysentery, polyposis, gastrointestinal tract neoplasms, lymphoma, Whipple's and biliary atresia.
- Digital clubbing is common. Initially, fibro-elastic tissue in the nailbed thickens. Then fluctuation, striations, shininess and increased curvature of the nail follows.
- Articular features occur in 30–40% of patients and are often the presenting features.
- Current theories of aetiopathogenesis focus on the possibility of enhanced exposure of peripheral tissues to vascular endothelial growth factor (VEGF) or COX2-derived PGE_2.
- Bone scintigraphy shows bone lesions but patterns are not specific. CT chest can determine cause of HPOA.
- A role for bisphosphonates in HOA management has been suggested, and clinical responses to pamidronate have been reported in both primary and secondary HOA. Beneficial effects of octreotide have been reported in two cases of refractory secondary HOA.

Fibrogenesis imperfecta ossium (FIO)
Rare bone disease of unknown aetiology characterized by diffuse coarse trabeculation – mixed sclerosis and lysis, which needs to be discriminated from Paget's Disease of Bone (see p. 418) and axial osteomalacia.
- Sporadic condition with no known genetic factors.
- Presents during middle age or later with bone pain usually in proximal distribution. Fractures occur.
- Many cases exhibit rapid deterioration and progressive disability. Patients have marked bony tenderness.
- In early disease, radiographs show osteopaenia, but later show abnormal trabeculation (dense fish-net) with blurring between trabecular and cortical bone.
- FIO is distinguished from PDB by a lack of bone expansion and cortical bone appearances. In FIO cortices are thin and often not visible. Cortex in PDB is usually highly visible and often thickened.
- ALP is increased, but calcium, phosphate, and PTH normal unless there is coincident hypovitaminosis-D.
- Histopathology: aberrant collagen structure lacking birefringence on polarized light microscopy. Electron microscopy shows collagen fibrils are thin and 'tangled'; abnormal mineralization; thick osteoid seams.
- In some, but not all reported cases there may be an association with paraproteinaemia.
- No proven effective treatment in all reported cases. Pulse melphalan (e.g. 4–6 mg bd daily) and prednisolone 0.25 mg/day for 5 days/month and continuous calcitriol 0.25–0.5 μg/day has facilitated long-term survival in one case and been reported 'successful' in another.

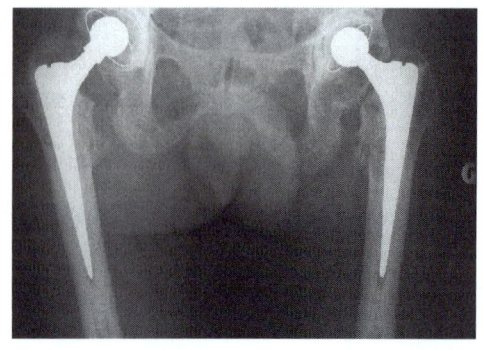

Figure 14.13 FIO. Coarse 'fishnet' trabecular pattern. Note: no bone expansion and absence of cortical features in pelvis

Osteonecrosis (ischaemic necrosis)
Regional vascular changes can cause bone ischaemia that, if sufficiently severe will cause bone cell death. Consequently, if resorption of dead tissue is compromised during skeletal repair then fracture can occur owing to focal bone weakness. See also pp. 168–171.

Major causes of osteonecrosis
- Endocrine/metabolic:
  - alcohol abuse, pancreatitis;
  - glucocorticoid therapy;
  - Cushing's syndrome, phaeochromocytoma;
  - Gout;
  - Osteomalacia.
- Storage diseases (e.g. Gaucher's disease).
- Haemoglobinopathies.
- Trauma, dysbaria.
- HIV infection.
- Radiotherapy.
- Idiopathic.

Legg–Calvé–Perthes disease (LCPD)
Idiopathic osteonecrosis of capital femoral epiphysis in children. It is common, complex, and controversial.
- Typically affects ages 2–12 years, mean age 7 years. Mainly boys.
- Aetiology is unknown. Interruption of blood flow at this site may be caused by raised intracapsular pressure, synovitis, venous thrombosis, or increased blood viscosity. Extensive femoral head involvement is invariable.
- The growth plate becomes ischaemic. Cartilage survives however. Reparative processes can succeed though if fracture occurs there is pain. Leg growth can be affected and the growth plate can fuse prematurely.
- Children with LCPD typically limp with pain, have reduced hip motion, and can develop permanent contractures if not addressed.
- Radiographs: should request AP and 'frogs legs' views. MR: often helpful to stage lesion.
- Prognosis depends on the degree to which the femoral head deforms and extent of epiphyseal involvement.
- Treatment usually conservative: analgesia, physiotherapy, monitoring for femoral head displacement.
- Surgical intervention is required for correction of femoral head deformity.

Skeletal sites prone to osteonecrosis
LCPD illustrates how subchondral bone is especially prone to osteonecrosis. The pathogenesis of interrupted blood flow is poorly understood though. Process has been linked to numbers of adipocytes within medullary space compressing sinusoids.

Osteochondroses
Refers to atraumatic ischaemic necrosis that typically affects an ossification (growth) centre. The extent and severity of lesions is variable. See also chapters on anatomy and regional musculoskeletal lesions.

Osteonecrosis of the jaw
Recently described in patients receiving intravenous bisphosphonates, notably Zoledronate and pamidronate.

Common sites of osteonecrosis and osteochondritis
Adult skeleton
- Osteochondritis dissecans (König).
- Osteochondritis of lunate (Kienböck).
- Proximal carpal scaphoid.
- Femoral or humeral head and fractured talus.

Growing skeleton
- LCPD femoral head.
- Slipped femoral epiphysis.
- Osgood Schlatter (tibial tuberosity osteochondrosis).
- Navicular osteochondrosis (Köhler).
- Medial tibial condyle osteochondrosis (Blount).
- Os calcis osteochrondrosis (Sever).
- Second metatarsal head osteochondrosis (Freiberg).
- Primary vertebral ossification centre osteochondrosis (Calvé).
- Secondary vertebral ossification centre (Scheuermann's).
- Humeral capitellum osteochondrosis (Pinner).

- Mostly reported in patients receiving bisphosphonates for bone cancer, typically in those who have had radiotherapy of head and/or neck.
- Incidence may also relate to the presence of poor oral health and may be triggered by dental work.
- The lesions can be persistent, often slow and sometimes impossible to heal, and can lead to recurrent infections.
- It is prudent to avoid intravenous bisphosphonates in those with poor oral health or delay treatment until after necessary dental work has been completed.

Resources
See explanation of the disease for patients at www.mayoclinic.com/health/fibrous-dysplasia/. See also, the Fibrous Dysplasia Foundation: www.fibrousdysplasia.org.

References
Chapurlat R, Delmas PD, Liens D. Long-term effects of intravenous pamidronate in fibrous dysplasia of bone. *J Bone Miner Res* 2002; **10**: 1746–52.

Kelly MH, Brillante B, Collins MT. Pain in fibrous dysplasia of bone: age-related changes and the anatomical distribution of skeletal lesions. *Osteoporos Int* 2008; **19**: 57–63.

Kozal KR, Milne GL, Morrow JD, Cuiffo BP. Hypertrophic osteoarthropathy pathogenesis: a case highlighting the potential role for cyclo-oxygenase-2-derived prostaglandin E_2. *Nature Clin Practice Rheumatol* 2006; **2**(8): 452–6.

Matucci-Cerinic M, Lott T, Jajic IVO, Pignone A, Bussani C, Cagnoni M. The clinical spectrum of pachydermoperiostitis (primary hypertrophic osteoarthropathy). *Medicine* 1991; **79**: 208–14.

Pazianas M, Miller P, Blumentals WA, Bernal M, Kothawala P. A review of the literature on osteonecrosis of the jaw in patients with osteoporosis treated with oral bisphosphonates: prevalence, risk factors, and clinical characteristics. *Clin Ther* 2007; **29**: 1548–58.

Swan CH, Shah K, Brewer DB, Cooke WT. Fibrogenesis imperfecta ossium. *Q J Med* 1976; **45**: 233–53.

Ralphs JR, Stamp TCB, Dopping-Hepenstal PJC, Ali SY. Ultrastructural features of the osteoid of patients with fibrogenesis imperfecta ossium. *Bone* 1989; **10**: 243–9.

Miscellaneous bone diseases 2

Sclerosing bone disorders
Many conditions cause either localized or general sclerosis of bone. The major ones are listed below.

Disorders characterized by bone sclerosis
- **Dysostoses:** osteopetrosis, melorheostosis, progressive diaphyseal dysplasia, endosteal hyperostosis, pycnodysostosis, osteopathia striata, osteopoikilosis.
- **Metabolic:** carbonic anhydrase II deficiency, hepatitis C associated sclerosis, fluorosis, LRP5 activation (high bone mass phenotype), renal osteodystrophy (see p. 426), X-linked hypophosphataemia (see p. 424).
- **Other:** axial osteomalacia, FIO (see p. 432), Erdheim Chester disease, hypertrophic osteoarthropathy (p. 432), Paget's (see p. 418), sarcoid (see p. 510), mastocytosis, leukaemia, lymphoma, myeloma, osteonecrosis (see p. 433), sickle cell disease, bone metastases (e.g. prostate), previous radiotherapy.

Osteopetrosis
Autosomal dominant (AD) form relatively benign and the recessive (AR) form invariably lethal in infants (not discussed here). There is diversity in clinical features and some heterogeneity in genotypes.
- All forms develop through a specific defect in osteoclast mediated bone resorption.
- There are 2 main adult forms: Type 1 AD osteopetrosis (ADO) is high bone mass phenotype with LRP5 activation. Type 2 ADO is Albers–Schonberg disease which has been associated with mutations in CLCN7 (a chloride channel gene).
- In adult disease radiographic changes have begun in childhood: symmetrical increase in bone mass; skull base sclerosis and vertebral end-plate thickening; 'bone-in-bone' appearance to vertebrae; alternating sclerotic/lucent bands in iliac/long bones. Fractures.
- Features: facial palsies; hearing deficit; slipped capital epiphysis; carpal tunnel syndrome.
- Bone biochemistry normal. Elevation in acid phosphatase. Histopathology diagnostic.
- In adults treatment is supportive (in children bone marrow transplant has improved some patients).

Progressive diaphyseal dysplasia (PDD)
AD condition (mutations in TGFβ1 gene). Also known as Camurati–Engelman disease.
- Presents in children with limping or waddling gait, leg pain, muscle wasting, and reduced extremity fat. If severe can cause enlarged head, proptosis, thin limbs.
- Features: cranial nerve palsies, skeletal tenderness, enlarged liver/spleen. Although progressive, severity is variable and clinical course unpredictable. Remission of symptoms can occur.
- Radiographs typically show smooth symmetrical hyperostosis of long bone diaphyses. Lesions show on bone scintigraphy.
- Bone biochemistry is normal. ALP sometimes elevated.
- Low dose GCs can reduce symptoms but bisphosphonates can increase pain. There is some interest in the therapeutic potential of losartan, which may have in vivo anti-TGFβ effects.

Pycnodysostosis
About 100 cases from 50 families described. AR inheritance. May have affected Henri Toulouse-Lautrec.
- Impaired collagen degradation a consistent feature. Recent studies point to deactivating mutation in cathepsin K gene.
- Low GH and IGF-1 levels have been described.
- Global prevalence though rare; particularly well reported in Japan.
- Presents with short stature, dysmorphic features.
- Shares many radiographic features with ADO. No consistent abnormal laboratory abnormalities.
- There is no known specific treatment.

Endosteal hyperostosis (EH)
Originally Van Buchem described a condition termed 'hyperostosis corticalis generalisata' in 1955. There are now two main types of EH recognized:

Van Buchem disease
Rare AR condition described in adults and children caused by 52 kb deletion downstream enhancer of *SOST*, which encodes for sclerostin – a peptide, which promotes osteoblast apoptosis, binds to LRP5/6 and antagonizes canonical Wnt signalling.
- Features: progressive asymmetrical jaw enlargement, cranial neural foraminae narrowing (facial nerve palsy, optic atrophy, deafness etc); tender long bones; ↑ALP.
- Endosteal cortical thickening is dense and homogenous; sclerotic skull, mandible, pelvis, and ribs.
- No known treatment. Surgery to relieve cranial nerve entrapment can be considered.

Sclerosteosis
Cortical hyperostosis with syndactyly. AR condition occurring primarily in Afrikaners or others of Dutch ancestry. Patients have a shortened life expectancy.
- Enhanced osteoblast activity owing to deactivating lesions in *SOST* gene.
- Features: patients generally tall ('gigantism'); cranial nerve palsies; square mandible; raised intracranial pressure; headache; syndactyly; finger nail dysplasia.
- Normal radiographs in early childhood. Radiographic features similar to Van Buchem disease otherwise.
- No specific treatment available.

Melorheostosis
Sporadic condition probably due to segmentary embryonic defect. Unknown aetiology.
- Presents in childhood often with bone pain and stiffness or soft-tissue abnormalities (fibromas, fibrolipomas, linear melorheostotic scleroderma, hypertrichosis, capillary haemangiomas, lymphangiectasias). Lesions appear typically in sclero/myotomes.
- Bone lesions: dense irregular, eccentric hyperostoses often in lower > upper limbs. Lesions are vascular, show intensely on bone scans, progress in childhood, but change is variable in adults.

- Bone pain can persist due to subperiosteal new bone. Marrow fibrosis can occur.
- Radiologically, lesions have been likened to hardened wax dripping down a candle.
- No specific treatment. Affected joints can deform requiring surgical correction of contractures.

Disorders of hyperostosis/heterotopic bone
Abnormal bone can arise from the skeleton (e.g. HME) or can form as a result of signals, which trigger mesenchymal tissue to form bone in periskeletal soft tissue.

Hereditary multiple hyperostosis (HME)
Also termed 'diaphyseal aclasia', this is an AD condition caused by various mutations in exostosin genes 1 or 2.
- Characterized by the development of bony protuberances mainly located on the long bones.
- Three HME loci have been mapped to chromosomes 8q24 (EXT1), 11p11-13 (EXT2), and 19p (EXT3).
- The EXT1 and EXT2 genes encode glycosyltransferases involved in synthesis of heparan sulphate proteoglycans.
- Exostoses can impair growth if near the growth plate, cause limb deformities, increase the risk of osteoarthritis in adjacent joints and interfere with nerve function.
- The most severe forms of the disease and malignant transformation of exostoses to chondrosarcomas were associated with EXT1 mutations.
- Surgery to excise hyperostoses can be helpful. Surveillance for malignant change is important.

Heterotopic ossification
Heterotopic ossification (HO) is the abnormal formation of true bone within extraskeletal soft tissues and is the more rational term for a group of conditions previously referred to as myositis ossificans. See Figure 14.14.
- HO can be, though is not always, triggered by trauma, can occur after panniculitis or associated with certain pastimes (e.g. Rider's bones – HO in hip adductors; Shooter's bones – HO in the deltoid muscle).
- There is a strong association between spinal cord injury and HO (twice as likely in male patients).
- HO is rare in children <10 years, occurs in all races and at any site; often starts as a painful mass and may require differentiation from malignancy.
- Although HO can, in theory, complicate trauma and neural injury in many, there may be a propensity in rare cases to develop spontaneous lesions (myositis ossificans nontraumatica).
- HO originates from osteoprogenitor cells lying in soft-tissue – possible muscle septae or fascia. The process, which starts with spindle cell proliferation takes about 6 weeks to develop established bone. Lesions evolve medially, so although they start in soft-tissue, they eventually lesions merge with the skeleton. The condition is discriminated from the very rare AD fibrodysplasia ossificans progressiva (FOP) where bone is relentlessly and extensively formed in soft-tissues through adolescence into adulthood. In FOP families there is linkage to 2q23–24, where there is a mutation in the activin A receptor type 1A (ACVR1) gene - a BMP type 1 receptor. ACVR1 is a critical regulator of BMP signalling in endochondral bone formation during embryogenesis.

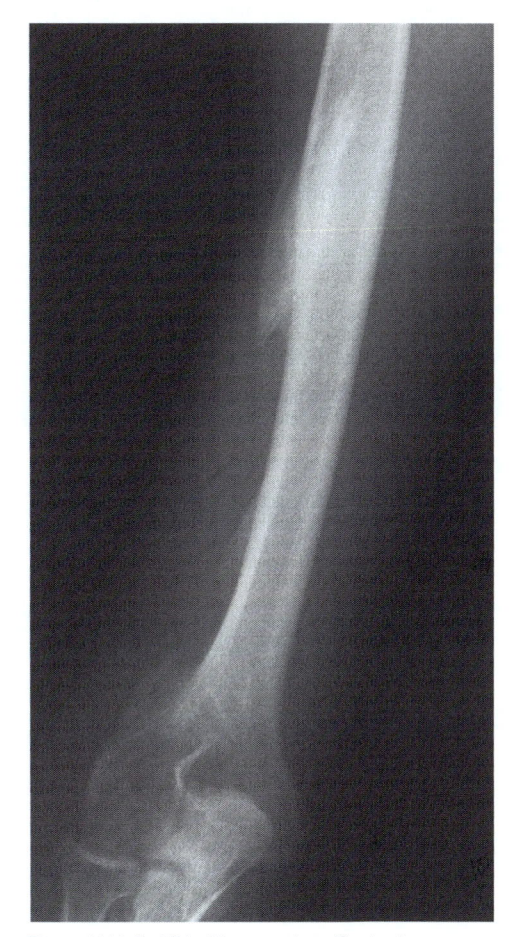

Figure 14.14 Established heterotopic ossification in upper arm: contiguous with diaphysis (two lesions) and one just above lateral epicondyle (patient with myositis ossificans nontraumatic.

Resources
Osteopetrosis web site: a self-funded voluntary 'sign post' site. Available at: http://www.osteopetrosis.org/. Also see UK based organization: http://www.osteopetrosis.co.uk

See comprehensive open access article by Beighton PH, Hamersma H, Brunkow ME. Available at: www.ncbi.nlm.nih.gov/books/bv.fcgi?rid=gene.chapter.sost

MHE coalition: www.familyvillage.wisc.edu/lib_mhe.htm – a site for patients and their families. Also, a useful site listing current research and medical/scientific information. Available at: www.mheresearchfoundation.org/homepage.html. See also the excellent, comprehensive article by Schmale GA. Available at: www.ncbi.nlm.nih.gov/books/bv.fcgi?rid=gene.chapter.ext.

Patient resources
The Melorheostosis Society: www.melorheostosis.com/
Melorheostosis UK: www.melo.eu.com

References

Azouz EM, Greenspan A. *Melorheostosis.* Orphanet encyclopedia 2005. Available at: www.orpha.net/data/patho/GB/uk-Melorheostosis.pdf.

Shore EM, Xu M, Feldman GJ, et al. A recurrent mutation in the BMP type I receptor ACVR1 causes inherited and sporadic fibrodysplasia ossificans progressiva. *Nat Genet* 2006; **38**: 525–7.

Wallace SE, Wilcox WR. *Camurati–Engelmann Disease.* Available at: http://www.genetests.org/profiles/ced/index.html

Whyte MP. Sclerosing bone disorders. In: Favus MJ (ed.) *Primer on the metabolic bone diseases and disorders of mineral metabolism*, 6th edn. Washington DC: ASBMR, 2006:398–414.

Chapter 15

Hereditary diseases of connective tissue

Marfan syndrome *438*
Ehlers–Danlos syndrome *440*
Joint hypermobility syndrome *442*

Marfan syndrome

Definition
An inherited disorder of connective tissue initially described by Marfan in 1896 and recently shown to be due to defects in the fibrillin gene (*FBN-1*).

Classification criteria
Criteria for the diagnosis of Marfan syndrome have been proposed – the Ghent nosology (De Paepe et al., 1996).

Epidemiology

Table 15.1 The Ghent nosology for Marfan syndrome

Skeletal system (≥ 4 required to be present)
• Pectus carinatum.
• Pectus excavatum.
• Span to height ratio >1.05.
• Wrist and thumb signs.
• Scoliosis > 20°.
• Elbow extension <170°.
• Pes planus.
• Protrusio acetabulae.
Dura
Lumbosacral ectasia demonstrated on CT or MRI.
Ocular
Ectopia lentis.
Cardiovascular
• Dilatation of ascending aorta involving at least the sinuses of valsalva.
• Dissection of ascending aorta.
Pedigree
• First degree relative with Marfan syndrome.
• Presence of *FBN-1* mutation.

For index case: diagnosis requires major criteria in at least two different organ systems and involvement of a third organ system.
For relative of an index case: major criterion in one system and involvement of a second organ system.

- The incidence of Marfan syndrome is 1 in 20 000 and it is one of the more common inherited disorders of connective tissues.
- There is no known gender, racial, or geographical influence on incidence.
- Inheritance is autosomal dominant.
- 25% of cases arise as a result of new mutations.

Aetiology
Marfan syndrome is due to a mutation in the fibrillin-1 gene on chromosome 15q21.1. Fibrillin-1 has a high degree of homology with the latent TGF-β binding proteins. The TGF-β family of cytokines are secreted as large latent complexes which are sequestered in the extracellular matrix, which may then play a role in regulation of TGF-β activity. Mutations in the gene coding for the type II TGF-β receptor replicate the classical Marfan phenotype. The current notion is that the features of Marfan syndrome are acquired postnatally as a result of failed regulation of TGF-β by the extracellular matrix. Increased activity of TGF-β has been demonstrated in the cardiac valve disease of fibrillin deficient mice.

The fibrillin-2 gene on chromosome 5 has 80% homology with fibrillin-1 and mutations are associated with cases of congenital contractural arachnodactyly.

Clinical features
Key features on history
- Presentation is often with tall stature (>95th centile), in combination with disproportionately long limbs and arachnodactylyl.
- There may be a family history of tall stature, arachnodactylyl, severe myopia, and sudden cardiac death.
- Myopia is common and may be severe due to increased axial length of the ocular globe.

Key features on examination
Skeletal
- Typical skeletal features include scoliosis, pectus excavatum or carinatum, high arched palate, ligamentous laxity, and flat feet.
- Bone mineral density on DXA is reduced.

Ocular
Slit lamp examination is required to detect the typical upward subluxation of the lens, which is present in about 60% of cases. This occurs bilaterally.

Cardiovascular
The most common cardiovascular features are mitral valve prolapse and dilatation of the ascending aorta, with development of mitral or aortic regurgitation. Dilatation of the aorta starts at the sinus of valsalva and is symmetrical. Aortic rupture or dissection may occur.

General investigations
- Routine haematological, biochemical and serological tests are all normal.
- Echocardiographic assessment of aortic root and arch dilatation is necessary.
- Mutation screening of all 65 exons of the *FBN-1* gene is available using genomic DNA extracted from leucocytes and can detect the majority of mutations.

Imaging
Plain radiographs of limbs, skull, spine, and chest.

Differential diagnosis
The Marfanoid habitus is no longer considered pathognomic for Marfan syndrome and can be found in a number of other conditions (see Tables 15.2, 3).
- Homocystinuria has similar musculoskeletal and ocular manifestations, but the lens dislocates downwards. Homocystine may be detected in the urine.
- Congenital contractural arachnodactyly has similar skeletal features, but there are no ocular or cardiovascular abnormalities. The contractures improve with age.
- Marfanoid hypermobility syndrome has no ocular or cardiovascular abnormalities, but the skin and joints are more hyperextensible than in Marfan syndrome.
- In EDS types I, II, and III valvular defects may be present, but joint laxity is more severe and skeletal proportions are normal.

CHAPTER 15 Hereditary diseases of connective tissue

Table 15.2 Features of the Marfanoid habitus

- Arachnodactyly.
- Span to height ≥1.05.
- Crown/pubis:pubis/floor ratio <0.89.
- Hand:height ratio >11%.
- Foot:height ratio >15%.
- Scoliosis.
- Pectus carinatum.
- Pectus excavatum.

Table 15.3 Conditions in which the Marfanoid habitus is found

- Congenital contractural arachnodactyly.
- Familial thoracic aortic aneurysm (Loeys-Dietz).
- Familial aortic dissection.
- Familial ectopia lentis.
- Familial Marfan-like habitus.
- Mass phenotype.
- Familial mitral valve prolapse.
- Stickler syndrome.
- Shprintzen–Goldberg syndrome.
- Homocystinuria.
- EDS, kyphoscoliotic Type (EDS type VI).
- Benign joint hypermobility syndrome.

Prognosis

- Life expectancy was previously reduced by 30–40% due to sudden cardiac death, but programs of regular echocardiography to assess aortic root diameter has improved life expectancy to around 50–70 years.
- Post-cardiac surgery prognosis is 88% at 5 years.

Patient advice

- Inherited condition of connective tissue with autosomal dominant pattern of inheritance.
- Multisystem involving joints, eyes, and heart.
- Risk of aortic dissection and aortic regurgitation. Neccessity for regular echocardiography and electrocardiography to monitor aortic root size. Possible need for cardiac surgery.
- Risk of pregnancy. Cardiac status.

Treatment

- Tight control of blood pressure reduces the risk of aortic dilatation.
- Surgical repair of both the aortic arch and aortic root should be performed electively when the aortic root diameter reaches about 50 mm.
- Pregnancy is high risk in patients with moderate aortic dilatation.
- Orthopaedic surgery to correct or prevent further progression of scoliosis should be considered when the angle >45°.

Follow-up

- Patients should be managed in centres with appropriate cardiological, ophthalmology, and orthopaedic expertise.
- Annual echocardiography and electrocardiography should be performed to monitor aortic dilatation and consideration of surgery should begin at 45 mm with more frequent echocardiography.
- Annual ophthalmology assessment,
- 6-monthly orthopaedic assessment of these at risk of scoliosis and intervention when the scoliosis exceeds 45°.

Resources

Patient organizations
National Marfan Foundation. www.marfan.org

Others
OMIM 154700: www.ncbi.nlm.nih.gov/omim/

ICD-10 coding
Q87.4   Marfan syndrome

References

Bird HA. Lessons from Marfan's syndrome. *Rheumatology* 2007; **46**: 902–3.

DePaepe A, Devereux RB, Dietz HC, et al. Revised criteria for the Marfan syndrome. *Am J Med Genet* 1996; **62**: 417–26.

Mizuguchi T, Collod-Beroud G, Akiyama T, et al. Heterozygous TGFBR2 mutations in the Marfan syndrome. *Nat Genet* 2005; **37**: 275–81.

Ng CM, Cheng A, Myers LA, et al. TGF-B dependent pathogenesis of mitral valve prolapse in a mouse model of Marfan syndrome. *J Clin Invest* 2004; **114**: 1586–92.

Pereiria L, DAlession M, Ramirez F, et al. Genomic organization of eh sequence coding for fibrillin, the defective gene product in Marfan syndrome. *Hum Mol Genet* 1999; **10**: 99–117.

Sakai LY, Keene DR, Engvall E. Fibrillin, a new 350-kD glycoprotein, is a component of extracellular microfibrils. *J Cell Biol* 1986; **103**: 2499–509.

See also

Joint hypermobility syndrome	p. 442
Ehlers–Danlos syndrome	p. 440
Osteogenesis imperfecta	p. 398

Ehlers–Danlos syndrome

Definition
The Ehlers–Danlos Syndrome (EDS) is a group of inherited defects in collagen types I, III, and V. They are clinically heterogeneous, but characterized by skin fragility, ligamentous laxity, spinal deformity, vascular fragility, and rarely retinal detachment

Classification criteria
The Villefranche classification scheme recognizes subtypes based on clinical features, and underlying biochemical and genetic defect (Table 15.4).

Table 15.4 Classification of Ehlers-Danlos syndrome

Name	Type	OMIM	Inheritance
Classical gravis	I	130 000	AD
Classical mitis	II	130 010	AD
Hypermobility	III	130 020	AD
Vascular	IV	130 050	AD
X-linked	V	305 200	XL
Kyphoscoliosis	VI	225 400	AR
Arthrochalasia	VIIA	130 060	AD
	VIIB	130 060	AD
Dermatospraxis	VIIC	225 410	AR
Periodontitis	VIII	130 080	AD
Fibronectin deficient	X	225 310	AR.

OMIM = On-line Mendelian inheritance in man (www.ncbi.nlm.nih.gov/omim/).
AD = autosomal dominant; AR=autosomal recessive.
XL = X-linked.

Epidemiology
The incidence varies depending on type, the most severe vascular type IV EDS occurs in less than 1:100 000 births. The classic EDS type I is estimated to occur 1:20 000 people.

Aetiology
- Type III collagen is a homotrimer encoded on chromosome 2q31. The constituent $\alpha 1$ (III) chains share with type I collagen the same arrangement of exons and Gly-X-Y repeats.
- The classic type of EDS (subtypes I and II) are usually caused by mutations in genes encoding collagen type V (*COL5A1* and *COL5A2*). These mutations interfere with fibrillogenesis and result in disrupted fibrils, which can be seen on electron microscopy. This only accounts for 30% of cases of classical EDS.
- Type IV EDS results from defects in structure or synthesis of type III collagen.
- Type VI is due to defects in lysyl hydroxylase.
- Type VII EDS has defects of the processing of N-terminal peptide of type I collagen, which results in abnormal fibril formation. The mutations cause skipping of exon 6 which contains the N-proteinase cleavage site or the N-terminal proteinase itself.
- Type X is due to defects in fibronectin.
- Tenascin-X is an extracellular matrix protein, mutations in gene for which result in a clinical phenotype similar to classic EDS.

Clinical features
Key features on history
Articular/periarticular
Joint laxity: this may be pronounced. When presenting in adult life, there is often a history joint laxity at school, and being relatively good at gymnastics or acrobatics. History of recurrent joint dislocations.

Cutaneous
- History of soft, thin, hyperextensible skin.
- Scar healing.
- Bruising.

Familial history
Joint laxity, poor wound healing or bruising.

Key features on examination
Skeletal
Joint hypermobility as assessed using the Beighton scale.

Cutaneous
- Hyperextensible skin.
- Poor wound healing with thin atrophic scars.

Key features of the types of EDS
- Type I EDS (previously the gravis form) is characterized by velvety and hyperextensible skin, marked joint laxity, thin atrophic scars and easy bruising.
- Type II EDS (previously mitis form) is a less severe form of Type I, but early osteoarthritis may develop.
- Type III EDS is associated with recurrent joint dislocation and osteoarthritis. Scars heal normally. This type overlaps with the joint hyper mobility syndrome.
- Type IV EDS is the severest form and has a poor prognosis. Complications include arterial rupture, colon or uterine rupture. The facies are characteristic with large eyes, thin nose and lips. There is marked bruising, the skin appears aged and there is joint hyperextensibility.
- Type V has similar features to Type II, but has X-linked inheritance.
- Type VI is characterized by scoliosis, ocular fragility, soft extensible skin and hypermobility.
- Type VII presents with recurrent joint dislocation, joint laxity, short stature, and skin bruising.
- Type VIII is characterized by generalized periodontitis, with soft extensible skin, easy bruising, and hypermobility.
- Type X presents with mild joint hypermobility, easy bruising, and abnormal platelet aggregation.

Diagnosis
Biochemical studies of collagens types I, III, V using fibroblasts are required to establish the diagnosis. Molecular analysis of *COL1A1*, *COL1A2*, *COL3A1*, *COL5A1*, *COL5A2*, genes are required to confirm the diagnosis.

Differential diagnosis
- The features of EDS overlap with other collagen disorders Marfan syndrome, osteogenesis imperfecta, and benign joint hypermobility syndrome. The first two are rare, but the third is common.
- Establishment of the precise type of EDS may be difficult solely on clinical grounds, but it is important to exclude type IV because of its serious manifestations.

CHAPTER 15 **Hereditary diseases of connective tissue**

- Retinal detachment and premature osteoarthritis should lead to consideration of Stickler's syndrome as an abnormality of collagen I.

Prognosis
- This depends on type.
- Type IV has the poorest prognosis because of arterial, bowel, or uterine rupture. The milder forms are associated with a normal life expectancy.

Patient advice
- EDS is due to an inherited defect of collagen. Most types are inherited in a autosomal dominant manner, with 50% of children being affected.
- Sports that hyperextend or otherwise stress joints should be avoided.
- Patients especially those with type IV need to be educated to inform all physicians of their condition.
- Skin is often fragile and care should be given to surgical procedures.
- Patients are often relatively resistant to local anaesthetics for reasons, which are unclear; this leads to anxiety on the part of the patient and a label of sensitive' patient being given.

Treatment
There are no randomized controlled trials of treatment in EDS.
- Treatment of presenting soft tissue or articular lesions using conventional approaches, such as rest, ice, elevation, physiotherapy, local steroid injections, and surgery. Corticosteroid injection with a depot preparation should be avoided where possible because they inhibit fibroblast collagen synthesis, thereby further weakening tendons and other collagen containing tissues. Surgical sutures may tear through weak skin leading to dehiscence.
- Conventional analgesics and NSAIDs may be helpful in the short term, but less so in the long term.
- Self-help is important and patients need to recognize that the precise cause of widespread pain may be difficult to establish.
- Physiotherapy with joint stabilization exercise can reduce pain and reduce excessive movement.

Resources
Patient organizations
Ehlers-Danlos National Foundation (www.ednf.org/)

Others
OMIM www.ncbi.nlm.nih.gov/sites/entrez, see Table 15.1.

ICD-10 coding
Q79.6 Ehlers–Danlos syndrome

References
Beighton P, De Paepe A, Steinmann B, Tsipouras P, Wenstrup RJ. Ehlers-Danlos syndromes: revised nosology, Villefranche, 1997. Ehlers-Danlos National Foundation (USA) and Ehlers-Danlos Support Group (UK). *Am J Med Genet* 1998; **77**: 31–7.

Malfait F, Hakim A, de Paepe A, Grahame R. The genetic basis of the joint hypermobility syndromes. *Rheumatology* 2006; **45**: 502–7.

See also
Marfan syndrome	p. 438
Joint hypermobility syndrome	p. 442
Osteogenesis imperfect	p. 444

Joint hypermobility syndrome

Definition
Joint hypermobility syndrome (JHS) is the occurrence of musculoskeletal symptoms in hypermobile subjects in the absence of demonstrable systemic rheumatological disease.

Classification criteria
Joint hypermobility is assessed using the nine point Beighton hypermobility scale (Table 15.5). However, this ignores other joints that may be hypermobile.

Table 15.5 Nine-point Beighton scoring system for joint hypermobility

Scoring 1 point each side
- Passive dorsiflexion of the fifth MCP joint to 90°.
- Apposition of the thumb to the flexor aspect of the forearm.
- Hyperextension of the elbow beyond 0°.
- Hyperextension of the knee beyond 0°.

Scoring 1 point
- Forward flexion of the trunk placing hands flat on the floor with knees extended
- Maximum score = 9

Adapted from Beighton et al. (1973).
Criteria for the diagnosis of the hypermobility syndrome have been proposed.

Table 15.6 1998 Brighton revised diagnostic criteria for the benign joint hypermobility syndrome

Major criteria
- A Beighton score >4/9 (either currently or historical).
- Arthralgia for > 3 months in 4 or more joint.

Minor criteria
- A Beighton score of 1, 2, or 3/9 (0, 1, 2, 3, if aged >50 years).
- Arthralgia (>3 months) in 1– 3 joints or back pain (>3 months), spondylosis, spondylolysis/spondylolisthesis.
- Dislocation/subluxation in more than one joint or in one joint on more than one occasion.
- Soft tissue rheumatism - ≥3 lesions (e.g. epicondylitis, tenosynovitis, bursitis).
- Marfanoid habitus: (tall, slim, span > height, upper segment: lower segment <0.89 and arachnodactyly).
- Abnormal skin: striae, hyperextensibility, thin skin, papyraceous scarring.
- Eye signs: drooping eyelids or myopia or antimongoloid slant.
- Varicose veins, hernia, uterine, or rectal prolapse.

Joint hypermobility syndrome is diagnosed in the presence of:
- 2 major criteria OR
- 1 major and 2 minor criteria OR
- 4 minor criteria

Two minor criteria will suffice in the presence of an unequivocally affected first degree relative.
JHS is excluded by the presence of Marfan's syndrome or EDS (other than type III – hypermobility type). NB Major criteria 1 and minor 1 are mutually exclusive as are major 2 and minor 2.
Adapted from Grahame et al. (2000).

Epidemiology
- Generalized ligamentous laxity occurs in up to 10% of the general population.
- The majority of people are asymptomatic.
- Hypermobility generally decreases throughout life.
- Women are more flexible than men.
- There is a greater range of joint mobility in Asians than sub-Saharan Africans who are also more mobile than white Caucasians.
- There is an occupational association with ballet dancers, musicians, gymnasts, and acrobats due to the requirement for great flexibility.

Aetiology
The genetic basis of JHS is unknown. Genes encoding collagens and collagen-modifying enzymes are considered to be good candidate genes. Mutations in the non-collagenous tenascin-X gene have been found in small number of patients with JHS. Complete absence of tenascin-X results in a phenotype reminiscent of the classic type of EDS. The heterozygotes have reduced levels of tenascin-X and about half have generalized joint hypermobility. This suggest that haploinsufficiency of tenascin-X may account for a small proportion (5–10%) of patients with JHS.

Mutations in genes encoding *COL1A1* and *COL1A2* also have a role in the development of hypermobility, although typically they are responsible for osteogenesis imperfecta.

Clinical features
Key features in history
Articular/periarticular
- Presentation is with traction injuries at enthesis, synovitis, tenosynovitis, bursitis, chondromalacia patellae, rotator cuff lesions.
- Joint instability with recurrent dislocation or subluxation especially shoulder, patella, MCP, and TMJ joints.
- Chronic low grade inflammatory synovitis with a traumatic background.

Cutaneous
- History of soft, thin, hyperextensible skin.
- Striae may develop at puberty, and are significant if not the result of pregnancy or obesity.

Skeletal
A history of stress fractures of metatarsals, fibula, pars interarticularis in the lumbar spine and vertebral bodies is common

Key features on examination
Skeletal
- Joint hypermobility that should be assessed using the Beighton hypermobility scale. Other joints may be hypermobile, which are not assessed in the scale.
- Joint instability may result in medial arch collapse in the foot.
- Absence of evidence of progressive inflammatory arthritis.
- Myofascial trigger spots may be present.

Cutaneous
- Soft, thin, hyperextensible skin.
- Striae.

CHAPTER 15 Hereditary diseases of connective tissue

Neurophysiological
- Impairment of joint proprioception.
- Relative lack of efficacy of topical local anaesthetics.
- Dysautonomia.

General investigations
- The acute phase response (ESR and CRP), and autoantibody profile are both normal or negative unless there is coincidental disease.
- DXA scanning reveals generalized osteopaenia.

Differential diagnosis
- JHS must be distinguished from more severe disorders of connective tissue such as Marfan syndrome, Ehlers Danlos syndrome type IV and osteogenesis imperfecta. There are a number of overlapping clinical features.
- EDS IV has a readily recognisable clinical phenotype, but the other types of EDS may be difficult to distinguish.
- The presence of skin hyperextensibility and bruising is suggestive of classic EDS (Types I and II); a history of congenital hip dislocation is suggestive of the arthrochalasis subtype of EDS.
- A history of bone fragility, short stature, and blue sclerae is suggestive of osteogenesis imperfecta.
- The presence of the Marfanoid habitus together with cardiovascular or ocular involvement suggests Marfan syndrome.

Prognosis
JHS is benign as life-threatening complications are not a feature.

Pathology
Skin biopsies from hypermobile subjects show abnormalities of in the structure of collagen bundles.

Patient advice
- Reassure patients that they do not have a more serious rheumatic disease (e.g. inflammatory arthritis) and that they do have a recognized condition.
- Advice about appropriate levels of exercise.

Treatment
- Devise and individual treatment plan.
- Treat soft tissue conditions in conventional style with rest, physiotherapy, local steroid injections, and surgery as needed.
- Depot injection should be avoided as these preparations can further weaken soft tissues.
- Care should be taken with surgery, especially in those with fragile skin because of the risks of wound dehiscence.
- Physiotherapy employing a variety of techniques – passive mobilization, exercises, traction, joint stabilization, and proprioceptive enhancement.
- Analgesia using NSAIDs or analgesics may useful in the short term.

Resources
Patient organizations
Joint Hypermobility syndrome association:
www.hypermobility.org

ICD-10 coding
M35.7   Hypermobility syndrome

References
Beighton PH, Solomon L, Soskolne C. Articular mobility in African populations. *Ann Rheum Dis* 1973; **32**: 413–17.

Grahame R, Bird HA, Child A, *et al.* British Society for Rheumatology Special Interest Group on Heritable Disorders of Connective Tissue Disease. The revised (Brighton 1998) criteria for the diagnosis of BJHS. *J Rheumatol* 2000; **27**: 1777–9.

Kirk JH, Ansell B, Bywaters EGH. The hypermobility syndrome. *Ann Rheum Dis* 1967; **26**: 425.

Malfait F, Hakim AJ, De Paepe A, Grahame R. The genetic basis of the joint hypermobility syndromes. *Rheumatology* 2006; **45**: 502–7.

See also
Marfan syndrome	p. 438
Ehlers–Danlos syndrome	p. 440
Osteogenesis imperfect	p. 428

Chapter 16

Musculoskeletal infection

Practical approach to a hot swollen joint 446
Septic arthritis 448
Gonococcal arthritis 452
Osteomyelitis 454
Soft tissue infection 458
Rheumatic fever 462
Brucellosis 464
Lyme disease 466
Viral arthritis 468
Mycobacterial infection 472
Fungal infection 476

Practical approach to a hot swollen joint

Definition
A patient presenting with a hot swollen joint requires emergency assessment and treatment, as the major cause of avoidable morbidity is untreated sepsis.

Epidemiology
Risk Factors for septic joint
- Pre-existing joint disease.
- Prosthetic joints.
- Low socioeconomic status.
- IV drug abuse.
- Alcohol abuse.
- Diabetes mellitus.
- Recent intra-articular steroid injections.
- Ulcerated skin.

Clinical features
Key features on history
- A septic joint usual presents with <2 weeks duration of symptoms.
- Any joint may be affected; hip and knee are probably the most common.
- In up to 22% of cases more than one joint may be affected.
- The presence or absence of fever is not a reliable indicator of infection.
- Risk factors for sepsis.
- Previous history of gout or pseudogout.
- History of trauma.

Key features on examination
- The joint is hot, swollen, and tender with a reduced range of movement.
- Overlying erythema without a joint effusion is suggestive of cellulitis. Evidence of swelling in either the supra- or infra patellar region is suggestive of bursitis.
- Look for portals of infection.
- A gouty joint is exquisitely tender and red.
- A tophus may be present overlying the joint. Tophi may be present elsewhere, e.g. ears, elbows, toes, and fingers.

Differential diagnosis
The hot swollen joint must always be considered septic in the absence of a definite alternative diagnosis.
- Sepsis.
- Inflammatory arthritis.
- Crystal arthritis (due to both gout and CPPDD).
- Haemarthrosis.
- Trauma.
- Bursitis/cellulitis.

General investigations
Synovial fluid examination
Synovial fluid should be aspirated, sent for Gram stain and cultured prior to starting antibiotics. Anticoagulation is not a contraindication to joint aspiration.
A prosthetic joint with suspected infection should always be referred to an orthopaedic surgeon.
Polarizing light microscopy should always be performed to look for crystals.

Other investigations
Blood cultures
These should always be taken in cases of suspected sepsis.

Full blood count
An FBC with differential white count should always be performed. The absence of raised neutrophil count does not exclude sepsis, especially if previous antibiotics have been given.

Acute phase response
Absence of a raised ESR or CRP does not exclude sepsis. The CRP and ESR may be a guide to response to treatment.

Biochemistry
- Serum uric acid is of no diagnostic value in the diagnosis of acute gout or sepsis.
- Renal and liver function should be measured, as evidence of renal or hepatic dysfunction is indicative of a worse prognosis.

Clotting
INR if the patient is anticoagulated, although anticoagulation is not a contraindication for joint aspiration. If INR is elevated above 3.5, then consideration should be given to correcting the INR before joint aspiration.

Imaging
Plain radiographs
Plain X-rays of the infected are of no value in the diagnosis of acute infection. They may, however, show chondrocalcinosis suggestive of pyrophosphate arthropathy. They are useful as a baseline against which future films can be evaluated.

Bone scintigraphy
This will show an infected joint as a hot joint, but is unable to distinguish this from other inflammatory process.

MRI
This is most useful in late untreated cases where there is a possibility of underlying bone damage or osteomyelitis.

Treatment
Antibiotic treatment for joint sepsis
This should be in accordance with local guidelines following advice from a local microbiologist. There is little high quality evidence as to the choice and length of treatment. Treatment should be initiated empirically and then modified when results are available.
Likely organisms are *Staph. aureus* or streptococci; therefore, initial antibiotic choice should reflect this, especially if there are no risk factors for atypical organisms.
In the elderly or immunocompromised patient, Gram-negative organisms are more likely.
MRSA should be considered in high risk patients.
Conventionally, IV antibiotics are given for 2 weeks and then orally for 4 weeks.

Joint drainage
Pus should be removed from an infected joint either by needle aspiration or arthroscopically. Repeated joint lavage may be required.

Other conditions

Crystal arthritis
- Aspirate joint and consider injection of intra-articular corticosteroids.
- Use NSAIDs or colchicine as appropriate.

Inflammatory arthritis
Aspirate joint and consider intra-articular corticosteroids. Use NSAIDs and oral/intramuscular steroids as necessary. Treat underlying inflammatory arthritis.

Haemarthrosis
Aspirate joint arthroscopically to dryness. Investigate for causes of bleeding if no history of trauma.

Resources

Guidelines

BSR, BHPR, BOA, RCGP and BSAC. *Guidelines for the Management of the Hot Swollen Joint in Adults.*

BSR and BHPR. *Guidelines for the Management of Gout.*

References

Jordan KM, Cameron JS, Snaith M, Zhang W, Doherty M, Seckl J, Hingorani A, Jaques R, Nuki G on behalf of the British Society for Rheumatology and British Health Professionals in Rheumatology Standards, Guidelines and Audit Working Group (SGAWG). British Society for Rheumatology and British Health Professionals in Rheumatology Guideline for the Management of Gout. *Rheumatology*, 2007; **46**: 1372–4.

Mathews C, Field M, Jones A, et al. BSR, BHPR, BOA, RCGP and BSAC guidelines for the management of the hot swollen joint in adults. *Rheumatology* 2006; **45**: 1039–41.

See also
Synovial fluid analysis
Bacterial infections
Crystal arthritis

Septic arthritis

Definition
Septic arthritis is a pyogenic infection within a joint, and is a medical emergency with an associated mortality and morbidity. Prompt diagnosis and appropriate treatment are imperative to limit cartilage destruction, and to preserve a good functional outcome.

Classification
Classification is usually on the basis of the causative organism. *Staphylococcus aureus* is the commonest organism isolated in septic arthritis.

Epidemiology
Incidence
- Septic arthritis is relatively rare and is estimated at 6 per 100 000 per year in developed countries, with those under 15 and over 55 representing the highest risk groups.
- Septic arthritis is more likely to occur in individuals with pre-existing joint disease, e.g. prosthetic joints or inflammatory arthritis. In patients with rheumatoid arthritis, the incidence is estimated to be around 70 per 100 000 per annum.

Common causative organisms
Gram positive septic arthritis
- Gram positive cocci cause 50–70% of bacterial septic arthritis with *Staph. aureus, S. epidermidis*, and streptococci (pyogenes, group B and G) the most commonly isolated organisms.
- In contrast, Group C Streptococci, pneumococci, and Gram positive bacilli are more rarely implicated.

Gram negative septic arthritis
- Gram negative infection is most commonly caused by *Neisseria* species, with *N. gonorrheoa* and *N. meningitides* the most common agents.
- *Haemophilus influenzae*, previously a commonly implicated pathogen in paediatric infection, is less frequently seen since the introduction of the HIB (*Haemophilus influenzae* type b) vaccine.
- Gram negative rods cause less than 20% of septic arthritis, with *E. coli, Proteus mirabilis, Klebsiella*, and enterobacter the most commonly implicated organisms in this group.
- *Pseudomonas aeruginosa* infection is rare and usually found in the elderly.
- Less than 1% of septic arthritis is caused by anaerobic bacteria.

Risk factors for septic arthritis
- **Age:** the extremes of ages are more susceptible.
- **Gender:** similar incidence is seen in men and women
- **Distal infection:** septic arthritis most usually arises from haematogenous spread from a distal focus.
- **Instrumentation:** sepsis following joint aspiration or arthroscopy is rare and is estimated at 1 in 15 000 to 1 in 50 000.
- **Immunosuppression:** for example, with glucocorticoids.
- **Alcoholism.**
- **Intravenous drug abuse:** the puncture site is the portal of entry for organisms, and is most commonly contaminated with *Staph. aureus*. Underlying concomitant Human Immunodeficiency virus (HIV) infection should be considered in intravenous drug abusers.
- **Pre-existing joint disease:** the risk of haematogenous spread is increased due to increased blood flow into abnormal joints.
- **Co-morbidities:** diabetes, malignancy, chronic organ failure, e.g. established renal or liver disease, skin disease.
- **Prosthetic joints.**

Staphylococcus aureus *immunopathology*
- *Staph. aureus* septic arthritis causes the most severe joint destruction because of the range of extracellular toxins and degradative enzymes produced by this particular organism.
- Some strains are encapsulated, which aids the virulence of the organism.
- Staphylococcal adhesions, expressed on the bacterial surface, enable the organism to adhere to and invade host tissue, and facilitate penetration of joints. Soft tissue infection is much more likely to be caused by staphylococcal strains without the ability to express adhesin.
- Some toxins, named superantigens, are responsible for the release of cytokines, such as tumour necrosis factor and interferon gamma, which result in fever, hypotension, and the features of severe systemic sepsis.
- The immune response of the host is also central to the severity of presentation of infection. T cell action, which occurs in the adaptive immune response, aggravates the damage caused by joint sepsis, and elimination of T cell activity reduces mortality and joint damage. B cell depletion appears to have no effect on outcome following septic arthritis. The innate immune system protects against infection by staphylococci, and the severity of infection is more marked in hosts in which there are complement deficiencies.

Clinical features
High clinical suspicion allows early diagnosis.

Key features in the history
- There is usually sudden onset of severe pain and swelling, with functional disability.
- Patients usually, but not always, feel systemically unwell.
- There may be a history of recent/continuing distant infection.
- Rigors occur in patients with fever, but may also be a feature of crystal arthritis.
- The age of the patient is relevant as extremities of age make septic arthritis more likely.
- There may be a history of pre-existing joint disease.
- Recent instrumentation, e.g. arthroscopy or joint aspiration and injection should be established.
- Immunosuppressive therapies, such as glucocorticoid therapy, are important risk factors.
- Anticoagulation is not a risk factor for infection, but it is important to check clotting prior to joint aspiration in those patients who are anticoagulated.
- Recent antibiotic treatment should be established as isolation of the causative organism is more difficult in this setting.
- Polyarticular infection occurs in up to 22% of cases.

Some patients have no fever and a subacute onset, making diagnosis more challenging. Polyarticular sepsis is rare and is usually found in patients with predisposing factors.

Key features on examination
- Fever is a non-specific feature, and may also occur in crystal arthritis. The absence of fever does not exclude septic arthritis.
- Tachycardia is uncommon in the elderly but is often present in younger patients.
- Hypotension occurs in patients with septicaemia.
- The joint is tender and the patient is reluctant to move it actively or to allow passive movement.
- Erythema of the overlying skin is common and there may be an associated cellulitis or bursitis.
- Effusion is usually present.
- Distant infection, e.g. skin, nasopharyngx, chest, urine, endocarditits should be sought.

Investigations
Laboratory
- A neutrophilia is typical, but not universally found.
- An inflammatory response is usual with CRP responding more quickly than ESR.
- Renal impairment may reflect systemic sepsis.
- Liver function tests may be deranged in sepsis.
- Autoantibodies are not helpful in diagnosing sepsis.
- Blood cultures are positive in around 33% of septic arthritis and should be collected in all patients.

Imaging
- Plain radiographs are unhelpful diagnostically in early septic arthritis, but establish pre-existing joint disease and non-specific soft tissue swelling.
- The earliest plain radiographs changes are seen after 2 weeks in patients with untreated infection.
- Ultrasound may be useful in determining synovitis and effusion, and aid accuracy of diagnostic aspiration.
- Nuclear medicine scans detect non-specific inflammatory joint disease.
- MR scans are helpful if soft tissue infection or osteomyelitis are suspected, but are unhelpful in early infection.

Synovial fluid aspiration
- Joint aspiration, with microscopy and culture of the synovial fluid, is the single most important diagnostic test.
- Frank pus may be aspirated, making the diagnosis more likely.
- The sample should be sent to the laboratory immediately it has been taken and not left for routine transport.
- Organisms are cultured in 50–70% of septic arthritis.
- Crystal arthritis and sepsis can co-exist.
- High neutrophil count, high lactate, and low glucose are the typical characteristics in septic synovial fluid.
- PCR on synovial fluid is often non-specific and 20% of RA cases have detectable bacterial DNA, rendering this an unhelpful test in septic arthritis.
- Hip aspiration should be undertaken under ultrasound/image intensifier control, and should be considered for other joints if blind aspiration is unyieldy.

Other tests
Cultures/swabs should be collected if distant site of infection is likely, e.g. genitourinary, respiratory.

Useful tips
- Cellulitis may co-exist, and iatrogenic septic arthritis may occur as a result of inserting a needle through infected skin. In this situation, the diagnosis of septic arthritis may need to be made pragmatically on the basis of clinical findings.
- If fluid cannot be aspirated from a potentially septic joint, consider asking another experienced doctor, or requesting an ultrasound-guided aspiration.
- If a patient is anticoagulated with warfarin, an urgent INR should be checked, and anticoagulation reversal considered if the INR is greater than 3.5. An icepack will induce vasoconstriction and may reduce the risk of haemarthrosis.

Differential diagnosis
- Crystal arthritis.
- Infection in the overlying soft tissues, e.g. bursitis, cellulitis.
- Monoarthritic presentation of inflammatory arthritis.
- Trauma.
- Haemarthrosis.

Objectives of management
Treat infection
- If clinical suspicion is high, but initial microscopy of synovial fluid negative, treatment with antibiotics should be commenced.
- Consult local policy for antibiotic choice in septic arthritis.
- Antibiotic choice should cover *Staph. aureus*, the commonest pathogen, unless clinical features suggest a different organism, whilst awaiting culture and sensitivities.
- Antibiotics must only be started after aspiration of synovial fluid and collection of blood for culture.
- Intravenous flucloxacillin (2 g qds) and benzyl penicillin (1.2 g qds) cover the majority of staphylococcal and streptococcal species. In penicillin allergic patients, clindamycin 450–600 mg qds IV or 2nd or 3rd generation cephalosporin IV is appropriate.
- If *methacillin resistant staphylococcus aureus* (MRSA) is a possibility, intravenous vancomycin is the antibiotic of choice.
- If there is a high risk of Gram negative sepsis, antibiotic choice should be 2nd or 3rd generation cephalosporin.
- Close liaison with microbiology colleagues is advised.
- The evidence base for the duration of antibiotic therapy is not established but current practice is to treat for a total of 6 week, with 2 week of intravenous therapy followed by 4 weeks of oral therapy.
- Markers of infections, such as inflammatory markers and white cell count should be monitored, and would be expected to fall over the first 7-14 days.
- All patients with possible septic arthritis of a prosthetic joint should be referred urgently to the on call orthopaedic team for aspiration and further management.

Remove pus
- Pus contains toxins and enzymes released by the organism, which are damaging to cartilage. Pus should therefore be removed as a matter of urgency.
- There are no studies comparing arthroscopic lavage with repeated joint lavage, but close liaison with orthopaedic colleagues is advised.
- The joint should be aspirated to dryness either by closed needle or arthroscopically, and may need to be repeated.

Pain relief
NSAIDs and analgesia should be given to all patients with no contraindication to these therapies. Short-term opioid analgesia should be considered in those patients with inadequate pain control.

Rehabilitation
- It is unclear at which point rehabilitation of the joint should occur.
- Early mobilization of the joint is a balance between reducing damage during infection and preventing muscle wasting/contractures.
- One approach is to start rehabilitation as the indicators of infection on blood tests are falling, and the patient is feeling more comfortable.

Management of immunosuppressive agents
- Patients on DMARD therapies for RA are at risk of infection due to their rheumatoid arthritis and the immunosuppressive effect of the DMARDs. There is no evidence to suggest stopping DMARD therapy in patients with septic arthritis.
- In patients treated with anti-TNFα agents, current BSR recommendation is to withhold anti-TNFα therapy for 12 months following infection. No studies have explored the possibility of introducing anti-TNFα earlier than this.
- In patients prescribed regular long term glucocorticoid therapy, additional glucocorticoid should be considered to prevent Addisonian crises.

Prosthetic joint infection
The possibility of prosthetic joint infection should be referred to the on call orthopaedic team who will be aspirate the joint under sterile conditions, usually in theatre, a technique which should not be undertaken by teams other than the orthopaedic surgeons except in exception circumstances because of the potential risk of introducing infection into a non-infected prosthetic joint.

Predisposing factors for prosthetic infection.
- Poor nutritional status.
- Underlying joint disease, e.g. rheumatoid arthritis.
- Obesity.
- Diabetes mellitus.
- Malignancy.
- Remote infection.
- Skin disease.
- Revision surgery (the risk of infection in revision surgery is estimated at 4% compared with 0.5% in first replacements).

Clinical features
- Early infection occurs within 3 months of surgery. Patients present with pain and systemic symptoms. On examination, the patient is pyrexial and has a tachycardia. Examination of the wound and joint reveal erythema, tenderness, and sometimes a hot, gaping wound. Early infection is usually due to *Staph. aureus* or Gram negative bacilli.
- Delayed infection occurs between 3 and 24 months after surgery, and is associated with subtle signs. Persistent pain arises as a result of inflammation and early loosening.
- Late infection occurs after an uncomplicated 2-year period following surgery and is always due to haematogenous spread. The main sources of infection are skin, respiratory, urinary, and dental sources.

Investigations
In early infection, inflammatory markers and neutrophil count will be elevated, although they are less reliable in delayed and late infection. Conventional radiographs are often unhelpful, but may show loosening and rarefaction of the bone surrounding the prosthesis. Imaging with US, CT and MR will be more helpful, and should be undertaken following discussion with radiological colleagues. Prosthetic joints should be aspirated by orthopaedic surgeons, usually in theatre under sterile conditions, and only if the risk of prosthetic infection is greater than the risk of introducing infection into a non-infected prosthetic joint.

Management of prosthetic infection
Management depends of the age of the patient and the length of time there has been infection present in the joint. Each case is assessed individually. Options include:
- Irrigation of the joint.
- Single stage procedure to replace the prosthesis.
- Two-stage procedure, with treatment with antibiotics between removal of the first prosthesis and the replacement with a second.
- Long-term antibiotics and leaving the prosthesis in place.
- Removal and arthrodesis.
- Amputation of the affected limb.

Close liaison with microbiology colleagues is essential. In those patients who undergo a revision, antibiotics can be mixed into the cement, and can make up to 20% of the cement mixture, although the addition of antibiotics may compromise the cement resulting in weakness.

Unusual sites for septic arthritis
- Septic arthritis of the symphysis pubis is rare and often follows uro-gynaecological surgery. The differential diagnosis includes osteitis pubis, a non-infectious inflammatory condition seen in athletes.
- Septic arthritis of the sacroiliac joint is uncommon and usually occurs as a result of *Staph. aureus* infection. Intravenous drug abusers are particularly at risk. Endocarditis should be excluded. *Brucella* infection can result in unilateral sacroiliitis.

Advice to patients with septic arthritis
- Bed rest during the acute episode is recommended.
- Pain management aids early rehabilitation.
- Soft tissue swelling may occur and doesn't necessarily indicate worsening of infection.
- Completing the course of antibiotics and good compliance is vital to the eradication of infection and preventing antibiotic resistance.
- Exercise should be undertaken within the limits of pain and as the signs and symptoms of infection improve.
- Modification of risk factors for risk factors, for example, high blood sugars in diabetic patients should be addressed.
- The risk of permanent deformity/loss of function may be should be discussed, especially in patients with a delayed diagnosis.

Prognosis and natural history
- Mortality is reported in up to 11%, but in elderly patients with rheumatoid arthritis and poylarticular sepsis, mortality may be as high as 50%.
- Functional impairment is as high as 70%.

Monitoring infection

A settling neutrophil count, inflammatory markers and fever are reassuring. If these indicators of infection are not settling, consider:
- Reculturing of blood and synovial fluid.
- Establishing patient compliance with antibiotics.
- Dose/route of delivery of antibiotics.
- Reviewing antibiotic sensitivities.
- Searching for distal or other deep seated infection, e.g. disciitis.

Follow-up

Follow-up is recommended at the end of antibiotic therapy and once more following cessation of antibiotic therapy. For those patients with permanent functional disability, joint replacement is an option. However, eradication of infection must be undertaken before surgery is contemplated.

Current controversies

- It remains unclear if glucocorticoid therapy or bisphosphonates may modify the inflammatory response during infection, and therefore reduce the potential structural and functional damage in a joint. It is unlikely there will ever be trials of intra-articular glucocorticoid or bisphosphonates in patients with septic arthritis. However, there is some limited data in children to suggest a beneficial effect on functional outcome at 1–2 years following sepsis in those who received a short course of oral prednisolone.
- There are no studies comparing joint lavage with arthroscopic washout, although removing pus from the joint, by either technique, is appropriate.
- There are no studies comparing the different durations of antibiotic therapy, and the proposed 6 weeks of antibiotic therapy has been adopted as standard practice on the basis of clinical experience.
- The potential for a vaccine to protect against *Staph. aureus*, remains a theoretical development for the future, although efforts to date have been unsuccessful.

Resources

Guidelines

C. Mathews, M. Field, A. Jones, et al on behalf of the British Society for Rheumatology Standards, Guidelines and Audit Working Group Rheumatology. *BSR & BHPR, BOA, RCGP, and BSAC. Guidelines for the Management of the Hot Swollen Joint in Adults* 2006; **45**: 1039–41.

Internet sites for patient group

www.patient.co.uk/showdoc/27000235

ICD-10 codes

M00–M03	Infectious arthropathies.
M00.0	Staphylococcal arthritis and polyarthritis
M00.1	Pneumococcal arthritis and polyarthritis
M00.2	Other streptococcal arthritis and polyarthritis
M00.8	Arthritis and polyarthritis due to other specified bacterial agents
M00.9	pyogenic arthritis, unspecified.

References

Kaandorp CJ, Dinant HJ, van der Laar M, et al. Incidence and sources of native and prosthetic joint infection: a community based prospective survey. *Annl Rheumat Dis* 1997; **56**: 470–5.

Odio CM, Ramirez T, Pharmd GA, et al. Double blind, randomized, placebo-controlled study of dexamethasone therapy for hematogenous septic arthritis in children. *Pediat Infect Dis J* 2003; **22**: 883–8.

Patti JM, Bremell T, Krajewska-Pietrasik D, et al. The *Staphylococcus aureus* collagen adhesin is a virulence determinant in experimental septic arthritis. *Infect Immun* 1994; **62**: 152–61.

Shirtliff ME, Mader JY. Acute septic arthritis. *Clin Microbiol Rev* 2002; **15**: 527–44.

Tarkowski A. Infectious arthritis. *Best Pract Res Clin Rheumatol* 2006; **20**: 1029–44.

Verdrengh M. Carlsten H. Ohlsson C. Tarkowski A. Addition of bisphosphonate to antibiotic and anti-inflammatory treatment reduces bone resorption in experimental Staphylococcus *aureus*-induced arthritis. *J Orthopaed Res* 2007; **25**: 304–10.

Gonococcal arthritis

Neisseria gonorrhoeae is the second commonest cause of all sexually transmitted infection in the UK. Transmission is via the mucosa, of the urethra, endocervix, pharynx, rectum, and the conjunctiva of the newborn. Occasionally, infection may involve the fallopian tubes, or can result in bacteraemia, involvement of the skin and/or arthritis. *N. gonorrhoeae* is an obligate human pathogen and a fastidious organism, and therefore requires a nutritious medium and supplements such as glucose and iron for growth.

Epidemiology and risk factors

- Young people are most commonly infected, with current rates highest in males aged 20–24 years and females aged 16–19 years.
- The highest rates are found in London and predominantly urban areas.
- Gonococcal infection tends to be concentrated in core prevention groups. In the UK these include homo- and bisexual men, and black ethnic minority populations.
- Multiple sexual partners leads to higher risk of exposure, and other co-existing sexually transmitted infections.
- In 2006, there were 19 007 cases diagnosed in sexual health clinics in the United Kingdom. The true number of cases is estimated to be considerably greater.
- Mucosal infection progresses to disseminated infection in 0.5–3% of patients.
- The associated arthritis is seen in sexually active young adults, with a ratio of men to women of 1:3. One explanation for this difference is that women may present later and, therefore, with more widely disseminated infection.
- Only 25%, mostly men, report genital infection.
- The incidence of gonococcal infection is falling in both the USA and Europe as a result of education programmes, and is currently lower in Europe than in the USA.
- The host factors that aid dissemination include pregnancy, menstruation, and immunosuppressed states such as lupus, HIV, and hypocomplementaemia.
- The Health Protection Agency has a role in monitoring the rates of gonococcal infection and antibiotic resistance in the UK.

Clinical features

- The polyarthralgia of gonococcal infection is asymmetrical, may be severe, and be associated with a fever.
- The pattern of joint involvement is typically migratory and may resolve spontaneously.
- The skin rash is typically discrete, with papular, pustular or vesicular lesions and is not itchy. The rash appears on the limb and trunk, but there is sparing of the face and scalp.
- Arthritis occurs in less than half of cases although tenosynovitis occurs in two-thirds, and can be difficult to differentiate from arthritis.
- Monoarticular joint involvement is more common than polyarticular disease, with knees, wrists, ankles, and finger joints being the most commonly affected.
- In cases where diagnosis is delayed, endocarditis, myocarditis, pericarditis, and conduction abnormalities indicate cardiac involvement.
- Other musculoskeletal manifestations include pyomyositis and osteomyelitis. Hepatitis and meningeal involvement are other life-threatening complications.

Investigations

- Leucocytosis and high inflammatory markers are typically found.
- Synovial fluid microscopy and culture is likely to reveal Gram negative diplococci in around 50% of cases, with a similar yield from blood cultures.
- Both intra- and extracellular organisms may be seen on Gram stain.
- Isolation of the organisms is difficult and transfer of synovial fluid to culture media should be undertaken as soon as possible and if practical, at the bedside.
- Cultures from the mucosa of the genital tract have a yield of around 80%. A detailed sexual history is imperative to identify which mucosal surfaces should be swabbed and in order to arrange contact tracing. Involvement of colleagues in the sexual health team is advised.
- Co-existing chlamydial infection should be excluded, along with other sexually transmitted diseases.
- PCR has a role in diagnosis, although is less useful than routine culture as antibiotic resistance and sensitivity are not possible with this technique. Specificity of PCR is high at 97% and sensitivity is between 78 and 80%.
- Nucleic acid amplification is a technique that enables earlier detection of gonococcal infection.

Management

- Antibiotic resistance has resulted in increased need to obtain microbiological confirmation prior to treatment.
- Antibiotic resistance has increased since the late 1980s, and has limited the use of penicillin in patients with gonococcal infection.
- In England and Wales, ciprofloxacin was the recommended first-line therapy until resistance reached 5% in 2002.
- Since then guidelines have been revised to recommend the use of the third generation cephalosporins, cefixime (oral) or ceftriaxone (intramuscular).
- Azithromycin is not a recommended first-line therapy for gonorrhoea, but should be used at a 2-g dose, rather than the 1-g dose used for *Chlamydia* infections.
- Parenteral antibiotics are recommended for the first 24–48 h, and this should be followed by a further 7 days of oral antibiotics.
- Repeat cultures should then be considered to ensure eradication.
- In gonococcal arthritis, the joints should be washed out/repeatedly aspirated to remove purulent fluid.
- Patients should be screened for other sexually transmitted infections
- Partners should be contacted for appropriate investigation and treatment, and contact screening.

Resistance mechanisms

Resistance to penicillin can result from the acquisition of a plasmid, which inactivates penicillin, (penicillinase-producing *N. gonorrhoeae*) or from multiple mutations, which reduce the permeability of the membrane (chromosomally-mediated resistant *N. gonorrhoeae*). Resistance to ciprofloxacin arises as a result of mutations in the DNA gyrase gene, and the topoisomerase gene IV, which are responsible for supercoiling of DNA within the bacterial cell. Resistance is usually high-level and affects all the quinolones.

Differential diagnosis
The differential diagnosis includes all causes of hot swollen joint, including septic arthritis due to all causes, monoarthritis due to inflammatory arthritis, trauma, etc.

Advice
- Limiting the number of sexual partners, and consistent and correct use of condoms helps to reduce the incidence of gonorrhoea and other sexually-acquired infections.
- Compliance with the full prescribed course of antibiotics ensures both eradication of infection and reduces the risk of antibiotic resistance.
- Contact tracing is vital to prevent transmission of gonococcal infection to other sexual partners, and to prevent morbidity due to unrecognized or silent infection.

Prognosis
- Untreated gonorrhoea may result in pelvic inflammatory disease in women, the consequences of which include chronic pain and dysparunia, infertility, and an increased risk of ectopic pregnancy.
- Infection in the mother can be transmitted to the baby during delivery, resulting in neonatal conjunctivitis, which is responsive to antibiotic treatment.
- Chronic infection may result in joint damage, but early treatment is associated with a favourable outcome with no long-term sequelae.

Current controversies
The development of a protective vaccine against *Neisseria gonorrhoea* is an area of ongoing research.

Resources
ICD-10 codes
A54.4 Gonococcal infection of unsculosketel system
M01.3 Arthritis
M73.0 Bursitis
M90.2b Osteomyeitis
M68.0 Synoritis
M68.0 Tenosynovitis

Websites
www.bashh.org

http://www.hpa.org.uk/infections/topics_az/hiv_and_sti/Stats/STIs/gonorrhoea/default.htm

References
Ghosn SH, Kibbi AG. Cutaneous gonococcal infections. *Clin Dermatol* 2004; **22**: 476–80.

Gray-Swain MR, Peipert JF. Pelvic inflammatory disease in adolescents. Curr Opin *Obstet Gynecol* 2006; **18**: 503–10.

Olshen E, Shrier LA. Diagnostic tests for chlamydia and gonorrhoeal infection. *Semin Paediat Infect Dis* 2005; **16**: 192–8.

Rice PA. Gonococcal arthritis (disseminated gonococcal infection). *Infect Dis Clin N Am* 2005; **19**: 853–61.

Tapsall JW. Antibiotic resistance in Neisseria gonorhoeae. *Clin Infect Dis* 2005; **41**(Suppl 4): S263–8.

Osteomyelitis

Osteomyelitis is one of the most difficult infectious diseases to treat. Progressive bony destruction and the formation of sequestra are hallmarks of this infectious process. It can arise as a result of:
- Haematogenous seedling.
- Contiguous spread of infection.
- Direct inoculation into intact bone.

Classification
There are two main systems of classification.
- The Waldvogel classification uses the duration of disease, the mechanism of infection, and the presence of vascular insufficiency within the bone.
- Cierny–Mader classification is based on portion of bone involved, the physiological status of the host, and other risk factors including pre-existing co-morbidities, such as malignancy, vascular disease, and diabetes.

Long bone osteomyelitis
Long bone osteomyelitis may arise either from haematogenous or contiguous spread of infection with the most commonly implicated organism being *Staph. aureus*. However, coagulase-negative staphylococcus, aerobic Gram negative bacteria (such as enterococci, *Pseudomonas*, *Proteus* and *E. coli*) and *Peptostreptococcus* species are also fairly commonly isolated from cultures in osteomyelitis. Less commonly, infection may be due to mycobacterial infection, *Mycoplasma*, *Salmonella*, *Brucella*, or fungal agents.

Clinical features
The presenting symptoms in subacute infection are vague and usually non-specific, for example, low grade fever and poorly localized pain of insidious onset. Examination may reveal fever, with local swelling and tenderness over the affected site. In those with co-existing soft tissue infection, the tissues may be tender and erythematous, and with a discharging sinus. Rarely patients may be acutely systemically unwell, with signs of sepsis. Signs of distant infection, such as endocarditis should be sought in all cases. A high index of suspicion is necessary in all cases.

Investigations
- Although there may be a neutrophilia in acute cases, a normal total white cell count may be found in chronic cases.
- Inflammatory markers, such as ESR and CRP are usually elevated, and may be used to monitor response to treatment.
- Imaging of bone using plain radiographs may indicate bone destruction and destruction of the cortex of the bone after 14 days following the onset of infection. MR and CT, however, provide greater resolution of bone and soft tissue. Figure 16.1 is an example of the MR appearance of osteomyelitis. Metal, such as that in prosthetic joints, interferes with image quality and therefore significantly reduces the ability of these techniques to provide detail in adjacent bone. Isotope bone scans are non-specific. Radiolabelled white cell scans may help localize infection.
- Microbiological investigations include blood cultures, bone biopsy, and culture either following needle biopsy or surgical exploration.
- Diagnosis is usually made of the combination of clinical, radiological, and culture of bone specimens.

Management
It is vital to obtain samples for microbiology prior to commencing antibiotic therapy. Bone sampling, blood culture, and surgical sampling, are all possible methods of isolating the causative organism. Culture of bone reveals the organism in 94% of cases. Wound swabs, however, in patients with sinus formation, are susceptible to normal skin flora colonization, and are therefore less sensitive and give rise to false positive cultures.

Treatment
A combination of surgical exploration, debridement, and adequate doses and duration of the appropriate antibiotic to eradicate infection is required. The aims of surgery are to drain infected tissue, debride necrotic tissue, and remove infected metal ware. Dead space is eliminated, and stabilization of bone with either bone grafts or using external fixation devices may be necessary, depending on the extent of the infection. There is no evidence base guiding the length of treatment of antibiotic therapy, but standard practice determines a course of 4–6 weeks of an antibiotic which is able to penetrate bone well.

Open fracture osteomyelitis
Between 2 and 25% of open fractures are complicated by infection, and the type of fracture, the degree of soft tissue damage and contamination of the wound at the time of injury influence the likelihood of the development of infection. A delay in surgical reduction and debridement of more than 5 h has been shown to be associated with a higher risk of infection. The tibia is the commonest site of osteomyelitis following an open fracture, usually in young men between 20 and 30 years of age. Infection results in non-union, chronic infection, and eventually, if untreated or refractory to treatment, amputation may be required.

Clinical features
Infection usually becomes clinically obvious a few months after the injury, with symptoms of bone pain and fever, and erythema and localized pain on examination.

Investigations
The need for microbiological cultures and the surgical management of open fracture osteomyelitis is identical to that of long bone osteomyelitis. Often more than one organism may be isolated as skin flora are more likely to be implicated in infection following open fracture than in osteomyelitis due to haematogenous spread of an organism.

Management of infection risk in open fractures
Parenteral antibiotic therapy should be administered within 6 h of injury and for a period of 7–10 days. More prolonged prophylactic antibiotic therapy is not indicated as there is no evidence this reduces the risk of chronic infection and bacterial resistance may result.

Vertebral osteomyelitis and disciitis
Vertebral osteomyelitis and disciitis usually arise from haematogenous spread from a distant focus of infection in the skin, the gastrointestinal, the genitourinary, or the respiratory tracts. The origin of infection may remain obscure. Gram negative aerobic bacilli and *Candida* are seen in patients who abuse intravenous drugs. The segmental arterial

circulation of the vertebrae is the most likely route of haematogenous spread to the spine. Lumbar vertebral infection is the most common site of infection and may result in epidural extension. If the abscess becomes more extensive, involvement of the subdural space may occur with paravertebral, mediastinal, retroperitoneal, and psoas muscle infection arising as a complication. Disc space infection may also arise.

Clinical features
The symptoms comprise insidious pain and spinal tenderness. 15% have symptoms and signs of nerve root compression at presentation. Fever is present in less than half of patients.

Investigations
- Inflammatory markers are normally elevated as is the neutrophil count.
- The organism may be isolated on blood cultures.
- MR is the imaging technique of choice and details the abscess clearly.

CT-guided biopsy may be undertaken of the abscess, but will only reveal an organism in around 50% of cases. *Staph. aureus* and coagulase negative staphylococci are the commonest organisms.

Management
- Management is normally conservative.
- Surgical debridement should be reserved for those patients with neurological compromise who are not responding to conservative treatment with antibiotics, or those who have significant bone destruction.
- Antibiotics should be continued for 4–6 weeks and repeat imaging with MR will confirm resolution of the infection.
- Inflammatory markers can be used to monitor the response to treatment in combination with the patient's clinical state.
- Neurological examination should be performed daily or if new symptoms develop to ensure early detection of spinal or nerve root involvement. These new symptoms should be investigated with further urgent imaging and may require surgery.
- Bony fusion occurs after 1–2 years of infection.

Osteomyelitis in diabetics
- 15% of patients with diabetic foot ulcers will develop osteomyelitis and, of these, 16% will require amputation to eliminate infection.
- 36% of patients develop recurrent infections. It can be difficult to differentiate between superficial foot ulcers and osteomyelitis, but in general, the larger the ulcer (>2 cm) and the greater the depth (>3 mm) and the more bone that is visible, the higher the risk of osteomyelitis.
- Surgical resection or amputation is often necessary, and the duration of antibiotic therapy should last for at least 4 weeks and be guided by clinical response.

Osteomyelitis in patients with rheumatoid arthritis
Patients with rheumatoid arthritis have a higher risk of osteomyelitis due to *Staph. aureus*, mycobacterial, and fungal infection than in the general population. Presentation, especially if there are multiple foci of infection, may present as a generalized rheumatoid flare.

Other forms of osteomyelitis
Osteomyelitis of the clavicle
This condition is rare and represents less than 3% of all cases of osteomyelitis, and may be associated with subclavian venous catheterization. *Staph. aureus* is the commonest implicated organism.

Frequency of follow-up
There are no clear guidelines recommending the frequency of follow-up in patients with osteomyelitis. However, persistently raised inflammatory markers indicating evidence of ongoing sepsis are an indication for close supervision. Persistent soft tissue changes on MR, especially in the spine, indicate an unfavourable prognosis.

Prognosis
Osteomyelitis remains a difficult management problem and the rate of relapse is as high as in 1 in 5.

Multidisciplinary team
Close liaison between orthopaedic surgeon, microbiologist, and spinal or neurosurgeons in patients with spinal infection is vital. Physiotherapy is important in the rehabilitation of the patient with osteomyelitis, and exercise aims to improve muscle tone and strength. Occupational therapists should be involved in all patients with functional impairment.

Patient advice
- Compliance with antibiotic therapy is vital for eradication/control of infection.
- The management plan is formed in each case depending on the individual clinical situation of the individual patient.

Resources
Websites
http://www.patient.co.uk/showdoc/40001112/
http://cks.library.nhs.uk/patient_information_leaflet/Osteomyelitis

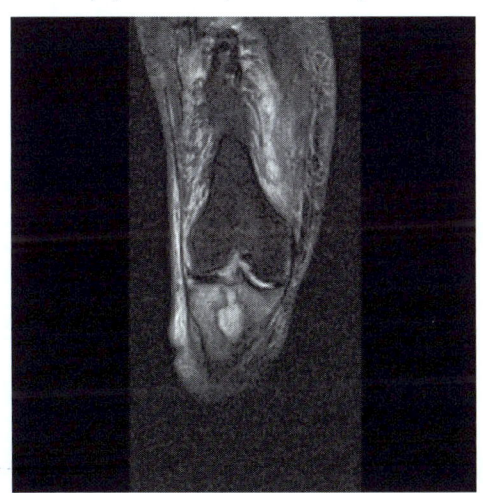

Figure 16.1 This is a coronal T2 fat saturated image showing a well circumscribed fluid collection within the proximal tibial metaphysis. It is surrounded by a bone enhancing wall and ill-defined enhancement in the adjacent bone. A tract I seen extending proximally to the articular surface of the lateral tibial plateau.

ICD-10 codes

M86.0　Acute haematogenous osteomyelitis
M86.1　Other acute osteomyelitis
M86.2　Subacute osteomyelitis
M86.3　Chronic multifocal osteomyelitis
M86.4　Chronic osteomyelitis with draining sinus
M86.5　Other chronic haematogenous osteomyelitis
M86.6　Other chronic osteomyelitis
M86.8　Other osteomyelitis
M86.9　Osteomyelitis, unspecified

References

Cierny 3d G, Mader JT, Penninck JJ. A clinical staging system for adult osteomyelitis. *Clin Orthopaed Related Res* 2003; **414**: 7–24.

Gold RH, Hawkins RA, Katz RD. Bacterial osteomyelitis: findings on plain radiography, CT, MR and scintigraphy. *Am J Roentol* 1991; **157**: 365–70.

Reihaus W, Waldbaur H, Seeling W. Spinal epidural abscess: a meta-analysis of 915 patients. *Neurosurg Rev* 2000; **23**: 175–204.

Sia IG, Berbari EF. Osteomyelitis. *Best Pract Res Clin Rheumatol* 2006; **20**: 1065–81.

Waldvogel FA, Medoff G, Swartz MN. Oteomyelitis: a review of the clinical features: therapeutic considerations and unusual aspects. *N Engl J Med* 1970; **282**: 198–206.

Soft tissue infection

Cellulitis

Definition
Cellulitis is an infection of the dermis and subcutis that produces a warm, red, tender area of skin. Erysipelas is the term used to describe superficial cellulitis, which often involves the face, but also involves the local lymphatic drainage, resulting in raised shiny plaques.

Clinical features
- Patients may be systemically unwell with malaise and fever.
- Locally, the skin appears warm with erythema and may be tender to touch. It is often poorly demarcated, and severe infection may result in oedema, vesicles, bullae, and necrosis.
- The lower limb is most commonly affected.
- Skin trauma and animal bites act as portals of entry for skin infection.
- Recurrent episodes of cellulitis in the same location often reflect local anatomical abnormalities, e.g. in the lymphatic system, which occur as a result of previous infection.

Pathogenesis
- The commonest causative organisms are *Staph. aureus* and *Strep. pyogenes*.
- The commonest site of cellulitis is the lower limb.
- Multi-organism cellulitis usually arises from infection with anaerobes and Gram negative aerobes, and is often implicated in patients with chronic ulcers.
- Necrotizing infection, where there is crepitus associated with the cellulitis and a thin discharge, may evolve into myonecrosis and is usually caused by *Clostridium perfringens*. *Bacteroides*, Peptostreptococci, Peptococci and *Prevotella* may also cause myonecrosis.
- Unusual or opportunistic infections are commoner in patients who are immunocompromised or immunosuppressed.

Investigations
- There may be no significant elevation of inflammatory markers or a neurophilia.
- Blood cultures are often negative.
- Skin biopsy may be useful in patients with resistant infection, especially when non-infectious causes are included in the differential diagnosis. Skin biopsies should undergo special stains for fungi and mycobacteria, and for culture.
- Bullae and ulcers should be swabbed, and the swab sent for culture.

Imaging
Imaging with MR or ultrasound is indicated if there is a possibility of deep soft tissue infection or a local collection, and MR is the imaging technique of choice where associated osteomyelitis is suspected.

Treatment of routine cellulitis
The majority of cases can be managed in an outpatient setting with oral antibiotics, the choice of which should cover both *Staph. aureus* and *Strep. pyogenes*. Patients who require admission to hospital include:
- Those who are systemically unwell.
- Those with systemic features of sepsis.
- Those with immunocompromise.
- Those patients with cellulitis that is resistant to oral antibiotic therapy.

It is important to consider cellulitis due to MRSA in those patients who are not responding to standard therapy. If multi-organism infection is likely, broad spectrum antibiotic therapy is necessary. Occasionally, prolonged antibiotic therapy lasting 6 weeks is necessary for complete resolution of infection.

> **Differential diagnosis**
>
> *Infection*
> - Bacterial.
> - Viral, e.g. herpes simplex virus.
> - Fungal, e.g. *Candida*.
> - Parasitic, e.g. Mycobacterium.
>
> *Non-infectious causes*
> - Panniculitis, e.g. erythema nodosum, lupus panniculitis.
> - Neutrophilic disease, e.g. Sweet's syndrome.
> - Connective tissue disease, e.g. acute phase of systemic sclerosis, calcinosis cutis on dermatomyositis, relapsing polychondritis.
> - Others, e.g. sarcoidosis, erythromelalgia, compartment syndrome.
> - Neoplastic.
> - Metastatic.
> - Vascular.
> - Metabolic, e.g. gout.
> - Iatrogenic, e.g. drug eruption, radiotherapy, foreign body.

Bursitis

Bursae may be classified as deep (beneath fibrous fascia) or superficial, and are closed sacs lined with synovium that in normal circumstances produce a small amount of lubricating fluid. There are around 150 bursae, and these act as buffers against friction and facilitate movement of adjacent tissues over one another. While some bursae are present from birth, others are acquired in response to recurrent pressure. Bursitis may arise as part of a localized or systemic inflammatory process, or secondary to infection.

Non-septic bursitis
- Non-septic bursitis due to recurrent trauma or pressure is associated with specific activities or occupations. Recurrent pressure over specific bursae resulting in non-septic inflammation has been linked with specific occupations. For example, housemaid's knee is used to describe a prepatellar bursitis and clergyman's knee is used to describe infrapatellar bursitis.
- Non-septic bursitis is common in gout and rheumatoid arthritis

Septic bursitis
- Infection is more likely in superficial, rather than deep bursae because of the increased risk of trauma in superficial tissues.
- The bursae that most commonly become infected are the olecranon, prepatellar, and superficial infrapatellar.

- The route of infection is thought to be due to direct inoculation from local trauma, which may be chronic or acute. Infection due to haematogenous spread is rare.
- Predisposing features include diabetes mellitus, alcohol abuse, and previous non-septic bursitis.

Causative organisms
- 80% of cases are caused by *Staph. aureus*.
- The remainder are caused by β haemolytic streptococci, coagulase negative staphylococci, enterococci, and occasionally Gram negative organisms.
- *Brucella*, tuberculosis, and *Candida* have all been isolated in refractory cases of bursitis.

Clinical features
- The typical presentation is of pain and erythema over the affected bursa.
- There may be a history of trauma.
- There may be a previous history of bursitis.
- Patients may be systemically unwell with a fever.
- Joint mobility is preserved in uncomplicated bursitis.

Investigations
- The total white cell count is normally elevated, typically with a neutrophilia.
- There may be an elevation of inflammatory markers.
- Imaging may reveal bursal fluid, bursal synovitis, and associated abscesses.
- Aspiration of the affected bursae may reveal purulent fluid, which should be sent for gram stain, culture, and microscopy under polarized light.
- Fluid should be examined for acid fast bacilli in resistant cases.

Treatment
- Uncomplicated superficial bursitis responds well to antibiotics.
- Gram stain and cultures should guide antibiotic choice.
- If cultures are negative, antibiotics should cover *Staph. aureus* and streptococci.
- Standard therapy starts with intravenous antibiotics until the infection starts to settle, followed by oral antibiotics.
- Total duration of antibiotics is usually up to 4 weeks, although some cases settle within this time allowing discontinuation of therapy.
- Broad spectrum antibiotics may be required in patients with resistant bursitis.
- Surgical incision and drainage may be required in cases where resolution is slow.

Prognosis
The prognosis of bursitis is good, although infection due to tuberculosis or *Brucella* may require prolonged therapy, and may relapse on cessation of treatment.

Infectious tenosynovitis

Definition
Infectious or suppurative tenosynovitis occurs when infection occurs in a closed synovial tendon sheath.

Causative organisms
The organisms implicated in infectious tenosynovitis depend on the exposure and trauma.
- Streptococci, *Staph. aureus*, and *S. epidermidis* are mostly implicated, with Gram negative organisms and enterococci implicated less commonly.
- Bite wounds are associated with mulitorganism infection, and include *Eikenella corrodens*, *Haemophilus* sp., and anaerobes such as *Veillonella*.
- *N. gonorrhoeae* is the commonest cause of infection due to haematogenous spread.
- Mycobacterial tenosynovitis is associated with fresh and salt water exposure, when *M. marinum* is often isolated.

Clinical features
- Those tendons most commonly involved are the flexor tendons of the hand, although infectious tenosynovitis can occur in any tendon sheath.
- There is usually a history of trauma in which introduction of the causative organism, such as via an animal bite or scratch, occurs.
- Haematogenous spread is, however, recognized and in particular with *N gonorrhoeae*.
- In the hand, communication may exist between the tendon sheath and adjacent bursae, allowing spread of infection into adjacent tissues. In the thumb or little finger a communicating bursa allows infection on both the dorsum and palm of the hand in the shape of a horseshoe, with the collection termed a horseshoe abscess.
- The typical findings include tenderness, symmetrical enlargement of the affected finger, a flexed finger at rest, and exquisite pain on passive extension.
- Gonococcal infection most commonly affects the extensor tendons, unlike other infections.
- Mycobacterial infection presents with a chronic, insidious onset. Atypical infection presents 2–4 weeks after inoculation, and a nodular cellulitic process, called a fish tank granuloma, develops.
- There may be an obvious puncture wound that may reveal evidence of infection.
- Necrosis of the tendon may occur if infection is untreated.
- Host immunity is important in determining response to infection, and immunocompromised or immunosuppressed patients may have more extensive infection than those with normal immunity.

Investigations
- There may be an elevated total white cell count, but this is not a universal finding.
- Plain radiographs are unhelpful.
- Ultrasound may reveal inflammation within the tendon sheath.
- MR is useful in to determine the extent of infection.

Diagnosis
Diagnosis is made on the basis of Gram stain and culture, either by needle aspiration or at the time of surgical exploration.

Treatment
- Prophylactic antibiotics should be administered to all patients with animal bites.
- If infectious tenosynovitis is suspected, empirical antibiotics should be started following needle aspiration of the tendon sheath.
- Antibiotic choice should be guided by the history and likeliest organism
- Surgical treatment is advised due to the high rate of tendon necrosis, and should be undertaken in all but the earliest cases of infection, and in these cases too if infection is not improving with antibiotics in the first 24 h.

- Repeat debridement and extensive tenosynovectomy may be necessary in cases where infection is resistant to antibiotic therapy.

Myositis

Infectious myositis may be caused by viruses, bacterial infection, fungi, and parasites. The pattern may be focal or diffuse depending on the cause, but in general, bacteria and fungi cause focal myositis whereas viral and parasitic myositis is more diffuse.

Viral myositis

A large number of viral infections may result in myalgia or myositis and include adenovirus, Coxsackie B, Echovirus, Epstein-Barr, Hepatitis B, HIV, HTLV-1, mumps, Parvovirus, *Rubella* virus, *Varicella zoster* and West Nile virus. Influenza virus, especially influenza B virus may result in myositis, with a preponderance for the muscle in the calf. Coxsackie B infection causes chest wall myalgias, and is known as Bornholm disease or pleurodynia syndrome.

Bacterial myositis

Bacterial myositis is classified as:
- Staphylococcal.
- Streptococcal.
- Gram negative organisms, e.g. Enterobacteria, *Pseudomonas, Aeromonas*, etc.
- Anaerobes, e.g. clostridium, bacteroides, Fusobacterium, Peptostreptococcus, etc.

Systemic infection, such as endocarditis, may also result in myalgias, with small abscess formation the cause.

Pyomyositis

Pyogenic myositis is classified as:
- Clostridial myonecrosis (gas gangrene).
- Group A streptococcus necrotizing myositis.
- Non-clostridial myositis, e.g. anaerobic streptococcal myonecrosis.

Pyomyositis is commoner in the developing world than in the west, and results from trauma, poor nutrition, and concomitant infection. Immunocompromised patients, such as those with HIV infection, patients prescribed glucocorticoids, or those with co-morbidities such as diabetes mellitus or malignancy are at increased risk. Infection is thought to arise from bacteraemia and seedlings of infection within a focal area of muscle. Three stages occur of pyomyositis occur:
- Bacteria are deposited within the muscle.
- Suppurative stage, with abscess formation.
- Systemic infection with septicaemia.

Clinical features

Pain and swelling of the affected muscle, with systemic upset is typical, although often there is little to find clinically as the infection is deep. As the abscess grows, the cardinal features of inflammation become more apparent. The most commonly areas affected are the large muscle groups of the lower limb, and is multifocal in around 20% of cases. Diagnosis may be challenging. For example, an iliopsoas abscess may resemble appendicitis and an obturator internus abscess may mimic septic arthritis of the hip.

Investigations

Imaging with MR or CT are the preferred methods of imaging in pyomyositis. There is normally an acute phase response seen on routine blood tests and a leucocytosis is usual except in patients who are immunocompromised. Creatinine kinase is usually within the normal range, and blood cultures are positive in up to 30% of cases. *Staph. aureus* is the commonest organism, implicated in 70% of cases in the developed world. Fungi and microsporidia are rarely seen in patients who are not immunocompromised.

Treatment

A combination of surgical drainage and broad spectrum antibiotics is usually required, pending microbiological culture. Culture of the pus obtained at the time of drainage is mandatory to isolate the underlying organism. Antibiotic cover should cover *Staph. aureus*. If MRSA is suspected, vancomycin should be introduced as part of the broad spectrum cover. Close liaison with microbiological colleagues is necessary pending culture sensitivities. Treatment results in an excellent prognosis in those patients who do not have septicaemia, and should be continued intravenous for 3–4 weeks.

Psoas abscess

Psoas infection often arises from nearby sources, such as the gastrointestinal tract, e.g. in patients with Crohn's disease, diverticular disease, or malignancy. Other sources of infection include gynaecological infection or rarely haematogenous spread. *Staph. aureus* or mycobacterium tuberculosis may arise from vertebral osteomyelitis.

Clinical features

Patients present with back or lower abdominal pain, fever, and pain on weight bearing, with an antalgic gait. The psoas sign (passive extension of the hip) may be positive.

Investigations

CT or MR are the investigation of choice.

Treatment

Treatment consists of surgical drainage and antibiotic therapy tailored to the organism. Gram negative cover should be considered, especially if a gastrointestinal origin is implicated.

Gas gangrene

This is a rapidly progressive infection with necrosis of muscle tissue and severe systemic upset. The infectious agent is almost always clostridium perfringes and the commonest presentation is following trauma, where the wound has been contaminated with soil or dirt, although infection may arise in wounds following gastrointestinal surgery, infection sites, or in ischaemic tissue. *Clostridium septicum* may result in gas gangrene, but in the absence of an entry wound. Bacteraemia is usually associated with gastrointestinal pathology, such as colitis or malignancy. *C. novyi*, and other clostridia species account for a small number of cases of gas gangrene.

History

Rapid tissue necrosis presents with swelling, lack of bleeding and loss of elasticity. The pathological process occurs as a result of a toxin – alpha toxin, which splits lecithin and inhibits leukocytes. The history varies from 6 h to 21 days following injury, and is associated with severe pain. The wound is often offensive smelling and inflamed. Gas bubbles may appear in the adjacent skin, resulting in crepitus and gas may be emitted from the wound. Patients are normally systemically unwell with hypotension and shock.

Investigations

The total WBC is normally elevated. Haemolysis may result. Blood cultures are positive in 15% and a Gram stain on the biopsied tissue may confirm Gram positive bacilli.

Treatment
Urgent surgical exploration and debridement, with fasciotomies or amputation is required. Antibiotic regimes include high dose intravenous penicillin and clindamycin.

Outcome
Even with aggressive treatment, mortality is high, and in the region of 25%.

Group A streptococcal necrotising myositis
This is a common cause of cellulitis and soft tissue infection. Occasionally, this organism results in myositis, for which the terms are group A streptococcal necrotizing myositis, streptococcal myonecrosis, or gangrenous myositis. It usually arises in patients under 50 and with no other co-morbidities or history of trauma, but often arises in conjunction with a systemic, toxic shock-like syndrome.

Presentation
- **Stage 1:** prodromal illness, often with sore throat and myaligia/arthralgia lasting 3–7 days.
- **Stage 2:** rapid onset and worsening of pain, usually in the leg, with skin involvement including discolouration and bullae formation.
- **Stage 3:** overwhelming sepsis with multi-organ failure.

Investigations
Microbiological culture of tissue removed at surgical exploration and debridement is mandatory. Leucocytosis and high inflammatory markers may not be present in the early stages. Creatine kinase may be elevated.

Treatment
Urgent surgical debridement, and high dose penicillin and clindamycin are necessary, but mortality may be as high as 85%.

Anaerobic streptococcal myonecrosis
This is very similar to gas gangrene and may be caused by streptococcal infection, both anaerobic and group A, or *Staph. aureus*. Treatment is with surgical debridement and antibiotics.

Other bacterial causes of myonecrosis
Other causative agents include *Bacillus* and *Aeromonas*.

Parasitic infection

Trichinosis
This parasitic infection occurs after eating under-cooked infected meat, normally pork. Incubation is 1–2 weeks following ingestion. The larvae penetrate the intestinal wall of the host and are then spread by haematogenous carriage.

Symptoms
Mild gastrointestinal symptoms may occur, then muscle pain and tenderness develop. Involved muscles often include those in the head and neck, such as the masseter, peri-orbital, and tongue muscles. The diaphragm may also be involved. Neurological and cardiac complications also occur.

Investigations
An eosinphilia is usually found, but may be the only abnormality on blood tests. Significant infection is required to cause a rise in CK. 3 weeks following infection, serological tests will become positive and diagnosis is normally made on this basis, rather than on muscle biopsy; this may show larvae, but identifying which species they belong to may be difficult.

Treatment
Albendazole or mebendazole are effective, but mostly in the gastrointestinal phase of the infection. Muscle larvae are very difficult to treat. In life-threatening complications, there is a role for high dose glucocorticoid therapy. Disease prevention includes careful food preparation and cooking.

Cysticercosis
This parasitic infection arises from the ingestion of undercooked pork infected with *Taenia solium* eggs. Infected water is also implicated as a source of infection. The eggs enter the body via the gastrointestinal tract and reach the muscles via the bloodstream. They may be deposited in the central nervous system, heart, and eye, in addition to muscle. Incubation takes from weeks to years.

Symptoms
Myalgias, fever and eosinophilia may occur, although the neurological manifestations include seizures, headaches, or psychiatric manifestations.

Investigations
Serological tests are the main method of diagnosis. Plain radiographs may reveal calcified casts within the muscles. This appearance is described as puffed rice in appearance.

Treatment
Treatment is with praziquantel or albendazole with concomitant glucocorticoid therapy as antifungal agents may cause swelling of the infected lesions, which is of particular clinical relevance in neurological infection.

Other parasitic infections
Other parasitic infections include acute schistosomiasis, Chaga's disease, and toxocariasis.

Resources

ICD-10 codes

L03	Cellulitis
M71.0	Bursitis
M71.2	Bursitis
M73.0	Bursitis
M73.1	Bursitis
M65.0	Infectious tenosynovitis
M65.1	Infectious tenosynovitis
M60.0	Myositis

References

Kroshinsky D, Grossman ME, Fox LP. Approach to the patient with presumed cellulitis. *Semin Cutan Med Surg* 2007; **26**: 168–78.

Small LN, Ross JJ. Suppurative tenosynovitis and septic bursitis. *Infect Dis Clin N Am* 2005; 991–1005.

Wadia NH, Katrak SM. Muscle infection: viral, parasitic, bacterial, and spirochaetal. In Schapira AHV, Griggs RC (eds) *Muscle Diseases*. Boston: Butterworth Heinemann, 1999: 339–62.

Rheumatic fever

Definition
Rheumatic fever is a delayed, multisystem disease that occurs following group A streptococcal infection of the pharynx.

Spectrum of disease
Rheumatic heart disease is a major cause of morbidity and mortality in low and middle income countries, and among underprivileged communities in high income countries. Primary prevention of acute rheumatic fever is possible with adequate antibiotic treatment of streptococcal throat infections.

Diagnostic criteria
- The modified Jones criteria are commonly used to diagnose the initial attack of acute rheumatic fever.
- The probability of acute rheumatic fever is high when there is evidence of recent streptococcal infection (increase in the antistreptolysin O titre) with either two major, or one major and two minor manifestations.
- Permanent damage to heart valves may result from recurrent attacks of rheumatic fever.
- The other major manifestations are transient and do not lead to permanent damage but are important in the diagnosis.

> **Modified Jones criteria for diagnosis of acute rheumatic fever, 1992**
>
> *Major criteria*
> - Carditis
> - Polyarthritis
> - Erythema marginatum
> - Subcutaneous nodules
> - Chorea
>
> *Minor criteria*
> - Prolonged P–R interval on electrocardiogram
> - Arthralgia
> - Fever
> - Acute phase reactants
>
> Plus supporting evidence of a preceding streptococcal infection for both major and minor criteria

Epidemiology
- Acute rheumatic fever is prevalent in developing countries, where there is overcrowding and poor access to health care.
- The highest reported incidence of acute rheumatic fever is in indigenous populations of Australia and New Zealand, although incidence is yet to be established in many developing countries.
- The estimated annual number of cases in those populations with a high incidence is 374 per 100 000 population in the 5–14 years age group with 60% estimated to develop rheumatic heart disease.
- In the west, the incidence has dropped to fewer than 1 per 100 000 population.

Aetiology and pathophysiology
- It is well established that group A beta haemolytic streptococcus causes acute rheumatic fever, but not by a direct toxic effect.
- The pathogenesis and immune mechanisms are still not completely understood.
- The host's humoral and cell-mediated immune response to the bacterium's antigens determine the severity of the individual clinical response, although the virulence of the streptococcal species is also important.
- The strains of group A streptococcus associated with acute rheumatic fever may express an M protein or antiphagocytic component in their cell wall.
- A decreasing incidence of acute rheumatic fever in the United States over the past 50 years is correlated with the falling incidence of streptococcal pharyngitis in children. This may be due to changing strains of group A streptococcal infection.

Clinical presentation of acute rheumatic fever
Key features in history and examination
- There is normally a history of sore throat, which precedes other symptoms by an average of 3 weeks (range 1–5 weeks).
- The modified Jones criteria for the diagnosis of acute rheumatic fever are necessary as the presentation is variable. A high index of clinical suspicion is necessary.

Arthritis
- A migratory pattern of joint involvement is seen, with several joints being affected at any one time, with synovitis persisting for around a week before settling.
- However, despite the use of NSAIDs, the pain is often more severe than the clinical findings.
- Those joints involved normally include the large weight bearing joints, with a very small minority presenting with only small joint involvement.

Carditis
- Cardiac symptoms are variable, and include non-specific chest discomfort or symptoms of heart failure.
- New or changing murmurs may be found on examination. The commonest is a mitral regurgitant murmur, although aortic regurgitation is also a feature.
- If extensive valvular disease occurs, signs of congestive cardiac failure may be detected, needing urgent and aggressive therapy.
- Varying degrees of heart block are recognized. First degree heart block is asymptomatic and other symptomatic forms may require pacing.

Chorea
- An abrupt, non-rhythmic, involuntary movement disorder is characteristic of Sydenham's chorea or St Vitus' dance. Classically, these movements disappear during sleep but recur on waking and are present at rest.
- Facial muscles may also be involved and involuntary grimacing and smiling may occur.
- Muscle weakness can be detected in the milking sign when the patient is asked to squeeze the fingers of the examiners hand. The patients grip contracts and releases continuously as if the patient were milking.
- Inappropriate behaviour is a manifestation of neurological involvement

Skin involvement
- Subcutaneous nodules lasting less than a month are painless and firm. They vary in size, but may be as large as 2 cm, when they may mimic rheumatoid nodules.

- Erythema marginatum is a pink or red rash generally found on the trunk and limbs, but with sparing of the face. The term marginatum describes the resolution of the rash from the centre giving a ring like appearance. The lesions may come and go, and are normally associated with carditis.

Minor manifestations
- Fever, up to 40°C, normally settles after 1–3 weeks.
- Abdominal pain is non-specific and usually begins at the start of the illness.
- Acute phase reactants are a non-specific finding.

Investigations
- Throat cultures should be performed but are usually negative by the time rheumatic fever presents.
- Antistreptolysin O and anti-DNAse in paired sera at baseline and 2 weeks later may indicate recent streptococcal infection if there is an elevation in titres.
- ECG and echocardiography are useful to diagnose and monitor cardiac involvement, and will detect mild cases of carditis in patients who are asymptomatic. ECG is necessary to pick up elongated P–R intervals. Typical valvular lesions such as valve leaflet and chordal thickening, leaflet shortening, mitral annular dilation, leaflet prolapse, and chordal elongation are easily identified.
- Synovial fluid is sterile.
- Joint involvement may be picked up on plain radiographs as non-specific soft tissue swelling.

Natural history
- Mortality occurs in 5%.
- 60% develop rheumatic heart disease within 10 years of infection.

Differential diagnosis
The differential diagnosis of acute rheumatic fever includes septic arthritis, connective tissue diseases, Lyme disease, sickle cell anaemia, infective endocarditis, leukaemia, and lymphoma.

Treatment
Drug therapy
- A Cochrane review identified no cardiac benefit in treating rheumatic fever with glucocorticoids, aspirin, or intravenous immunoglobulin.
- There is no evidence to support the use of glucocorticoids in acute decompensating cardiac disease.
- Penicillin during the acute attack has been inadequately studied.

Primary prevention
- A recent systematic review concluded that giving antibiotics to patients with sore throats and symptoms suggestive of a streptococcal infection (pharyngeal exudates and enlarged tender cervical lymph nodes) reduced the risk of rheumatic fever by 70%.
- Eradicating poverty and overcrowding, and improving access to medical care in the developing world is also vital.

Secondary prevention
- Prevention of recurrent attacks of rheumatic fever is the most cost effective way of preventing rheumatic heart disease.
- Penicillin remains the antibiotic of choice.

- Intramuscular penicillin is preferred as it is more effective than oral penicillin and ensures better compliance.

Surgery
Urgent valve replacement may be life saving in a patient with decompensating cardiac failure, and is a more common cause of heart failure than myocardial disease in rheumatic fever. If possible, repair of a damaged valve is preferred to prosthetic replacement.

Physical therapies
Current practice is that physical activity should be restricted until the acute episode has settled, and then should be built up slowly. There is no evidence-base for this advice.

Follow-up
Regular follow-up is necessary and optimizes timing of valvular heart disease surgery.

Patient advice
- Good compliance with antibiotics is imperative to ensure lower risk of rheumatic heart disease.
- Patients should be encouraged to seek medical attention for future sore throats.

Resources
Guidelines
WHO guidelines. Report of a WHO Expert Consultation. World Health Organization. ISBN-13 9789241209236

Internet sites
http://cks.library.nhs.uk/patient_information_leaflet/Rheumatic_fever

http://www.patient.co.uk/showdoc/40000571/

www.who.int/cardiovascular_diseases/resources/trs923/en/

http://www.worldheart.org/

http://kidshealth.org.nz/index.php/ps-pagename/centralpage/pi-id/58

ICD-10 codes
Acute rheumatic fever (I00–I02)

I00	Rheumatic fever without mention of heart involvement (arthritis, rheumatic, acute or subacute)
I01	Rheumatic fever with heart involvement Excludes: chronic diseases of rheumatic origin (I05–I09) unless rheumatic fever is also present or there is evidence of recrudescence or activity of the rheumatic process
I01.0	Acute rheumatic pericarditis
I01.1	Acute rheumatic endocarditis
I01.2	Acute rheumatic myocarditis
I01.8	Other acute rheumatic heart disease
I01.9	Acute rheumatic heart disease, unspecified
I02	Rheumatic chorea
I02.0	Rheumatic chorea with heart involvement
I02.9	Rheumatic chorea without heart involvement
I05–I09	Chronic rheumatic heart diseases

References
Del Mar CB, Glasziou PP, Spinks AB. Antibiotics for sore throat. *Cochrane Database Syst Rev* 2004; **2**: CD000023

Manyemba J, Mayosi MB. Penicillin for secondary prevention of rheumatic fever. *Cochrane Database Syst Rev* 2002; **3**: CD002227.

World Health Organization. Rheumatic Fever and Rheumatic Heart Disease: Report of a WHO Expert Consultation. Geneva: WHO, 2001.

Brucellosis

Brucellosis is a chronic granulomatous infection caused by intracellular bacteria, and is the commonest zoonotic infection worldwide.

Epidemiology

Brucella infection is widespread in the developing world, but is also recognized in the developed world. A high rate of infection has been reported in countries such as Turkey, Peru, Mexico, and Syria, although the reported cases are likely to be a significant under-estimate of the true incidence. There is a relationship between the disease and socio-economic status, with lower social classes reflecting the greater likelihood of ingestion of unpasteurized dairy products.

Aetiology

- *Brucella* belongs to the proteobacteria species, and there are six classic pathogens, of which four are recognized human zoonoses. The four species are *B. melitensis*, *B. abortus*, *B suis*, and *B canis*. *B. ovis* is common is sheep, but has not been identified in humans. *B. maris* affects mammalian sea life, but not land-based animals.
- *Brucella* are small, Gram negative bacteria, unusual as classic virulence factors, such as exotoxins or endotoxins, are not produced, but infection occurs as a result of host invasion and persistence in that host through inhibition of programmed cell death.
- The presence of rough or smooth lipopolysaccharide correlates with the virulence of the disease in humans.
- *Brucella* invades the mucosa, after which phagocytes ingest the organisms.
- The majority of brucellae are rapidly eliminated by phagolysosome fusion.
- 15–30% of bacteria survive in gradually evolving brucellae-containing compartments that limit antibiotic action.
- Replication of the bacterium takes place in the endoplasmic reticulum without affecting host-cell integrity.
- After replication, brucellae are released with the help of haemolysins and induced cell necrosis.

Risk factors for infection

- Infection in humans occurs primarily through the consumption of infected, unpasteurized animal-milk products, but can also occur through direct contact with infected animal parts (such as the placenta), and through the inhalation of infected aerosolized particles.
- Brucellosis is an occupational disease in shepherds, abattoir workers, veterinarians, dairy-industry professionals, and personnel in microbiological laboratories.
- One important epidemiologic step in containing brucellosis in the community is the screening of household members of infected persons.
- Airborne transmission of brucellosis has created interest in *Brucella* as a potential biological weapon.

Clinical features

- Fever is invariable, and can be spiking and accompanied by rigors if bacteraemia is present, but may be relapsing, mild, and protracted.
- Malodorous perspiration is almost pathognomonic.
- Constitutional symptoms are generally present with non-specific malaise.
- Examination is often unremarkable, though lymphadenopathy, hepatomegaly, or splenomegaly may be present.

Musculoskeletal manifestations

Musculoskeletal involvement is the most common complication of brucellosis, affecting up to one-third of patients.
- Three distinct forms exist – peripheral arthritis, sacroiliitis, and spondylitis.
- Osteoarticular complications are sometimes linked to a genetic predisposition, with recent data suggesting an association with HLA-B39.
- Sacroiliac involvement and spondylosis may occur especially in adults, while children are more likely to develop a peripheral arthritis, osteomyelitis or soft tissue infection, e.g. bursitis.

Peripheral arthritis
- Peripheral arthritis is the most common musculoskeletal manifestation and is non-erosive.
- Monoarthritis is the commonest presentation, although oligoarthritis is also relatively common.
- A symmetrical small joint polyarthritis may reflect a reactive mechanism, rather than true polyarticular sepsis.
- Prosthetic joints can also be affected in peripheral arthritis.
- Children are particularly likely to present with peripheral arthritis. Although any joint may be affected, the large weight bearing joints are most commonly involved.

Sacroiliitis
- Sacroiliitis in *Brucella* infection is almost always unilateral. Typically, a young male adult presents with severe gluteal pain.
- There is an inflammatory response on routine blood testing but plain radiographs are unhelpful.
- MR demonstrates bone oedema and is the investigation of choice.

Spondylitis
- Spondylitis, is difficult to treat in this context and often results in residual damage.
- It is commoner in older patients who have chronic disease.
- Patients complain of subacute/acute back pain.
- The lumbar spine is the usual site of involvement and the cervical spine the least frequently involved.
- Spondylitis is usually diagnosed with plain radiography, in which the characteristic Pons sign (a step-like erosion of the anterosuperior vertebral margin) can be identified, or with scintigraphy and magnetic resonance imaging. MR also has the benefit of imaging nerve root involvement.
- Infection is aggressive causing extensive bone destruction, often requiring a combination of antibiotic therapy and surgical debridement with stabilization.

Multisystem disease

- The reproductive system is the second most common site of focal brucellosis. Brucellosis can present as epididymoorchitis in men and can be difficult to diagnose. Whether or not testicular infection results in subsequent infertility remains to be established. In women, brucellosis in pregnancy poses a risk of spontaneous abortion.
- Hepatitis is common, usually presenting as a mild rise in transaminases. Liver abscess and jaundice are rare complications. Granulomas can be present in liver-biopsy specimens in cases of both *B. melitensis* and *B. abortus*. Ascites is not uncommon.

- The central nervous system is involved in 5 to 7 percent of cases and may present with meningitis, encephalitis, meningoencephalitis, meningovascular disease, brain abscesses, or demyelinating syndromes. The prognosis is often poor in these situations.
- Endocarditis remains the principal cause of mortality in infection due to brucellosis. It usually involves the aortic valve and urgent surgical valve replacement is often necessary. Early recognition, adequate antibiotic treatment, and the absence of signs of heart failure are all features which allow conservative management in the first instance although clinical deterioration indicates the need for surgical intervention.
- Respiratory complications of brucellosis are rare. Respiratory complications include lobar pneumonia and pleural effusions but are found in only around 16% of all cases of brucellosis.

Investigations
- Blood tests reveal a non-specific inflammatory response.
- There may be a mild lymphocytosis, but with an overall leuopaenia.
- Anaemia may be present, but is mild.
- There may be a thrombocytopenia.
- Rarely, there may be a pancytopenia, thought to arise as a result of bone marrow involvement and hypersplenism.
- Cytopenias, either in combination or in isolation, may arise as a result of diffuse intravascular coagulation, haemophagocytosis, or immunologically mediated cellular destruction.
- Synovial fluid microscopy and culture is negative.
- Synovial biopsies reveal non-specific histological changes.
- Aspirates from the olecranon or prepatellar bursae are negative for microscopy and culture.

Diagnosis
The absolute diagnosis of brucellosis requires isolation of the bacterium from blood or tissue samples. The sensitivity of blood culture varies, from 15 to 70%. Bone marrow cultures are considered the gold standard for the diagnosis of brucellosis, since the relatively high concentration of *Brucella* in the reticuloendothelial system makes it easier to detect the organism. Bacterial elimination from the bone marrow equates to a full and adequate response to antibiotic therapy, although repeated bone marrow examination is both invasive and uncomfortable, and therefore not routinely repeated. Cure is based on clinical grounds, and by the absence of symptoms. A residual bacterial load is found in a significant number of patients who are clinically well, even 3 years after 'successful' treatment.

Serology
- The serum agglutination test remains the most popular diagnostic tool for brucellosis. Titres above 1:160 are considered diagnostic with a relevant clinical presentation.
- Seroconversion can also be used in diagnosis.
- Drawbacks of this include the inability to diagnose *B. canis* infections; cross-reactions with a number of other organisms including *E. coli*, *Salmonella urbana*, *Yersinia enterocolitica*, and *Vibrio cholerae*, and the percentage of cases in which seroconversion does not occur.
- Serum agglutination tests have a major drawback in that they are not suitable for patient follow-up, since titres can remain high for a prolonged period.
- Indirect enzyme-linked immunosorbent assays (ELISAs) typically use cytoplasmic proteins as antigens. ELISA measures class M, G, and A immunoglobulins, which allows for a better interpretation of the clinical situation. A comparison with the serum agglutination test yields higher sensitivity and specificity.
- The development of a specific polymerase chain reaction (PCR) is a recent advance. PCR is fast, can be performed on any body tissue, and can yield positive results as soon as 10 days after infection.

Treatment
- Combination therapy is necessary as all monotherapies have an unacceptably high relapse rate.
- The optimal treatment regime remains a matter of debate.
- In 1986, the World Health Organization issued guidelines for the treatment of human brucellosis with both regimes including doxycycline for a period of 6 weeks, in combination with either streptomycin for 2–3 weeks or rifampin for 6 weeks. More recently, triple therapy with doxycycline, aminoglycoside, and rifampicin has been advocated.
- Most complications of brucellosis can be adequately treated with standard regimens.
- A prolonged triple regimen is used for neurobrucellosis.
- In spondylitis a duration of treatment of at least 3 months is standard.
- Rifampin is the mainstay of treatment in cases of brucellosis during pregnancy, in various combinations.
- Brucellosis in children is treated with combinations that are based on rifampin and trimethoprim–sulfamethoxazole, and with aminoglycosides.

Future developments
A worldwide database is in development to record all cases of brucellosis and to facilitate large randomized controlled trial of therapy.

Patient advice
Advice includes avoiding ingestion of unpasteurized dairy products, and careful hygiene in those who work closely with animals. Good compliance with antibiotic regimes must be stressed, as rates of relapse are higher in those with poor compliance.

Resources
ICD-10 codes
A23   Brucellosis

References
Al Dahouk S, Tomaso H, Nockler K, Neubauer H, Frangoulidis D. Laboratory-based diagnosis of brucellosis – a review of the literature. Part I: techniques for direct detection and identification of *Brucella* spp. *Clin Lab* 2003; **49**: 487–505.

Ariza J, Bosilkovski M, Cascio A, et al. Perspectives for the treatment of brucellosis in the 21st century: the Ioannina recommendations. *PloS Med* 2007; **4**: e317.

Ariza J, Pujol M, Valverde J, et al. Brucellar sacroiliitis: findings in 63 episodes and current relevance. *Clin Infect Dis* 1993; **16**: 761–5.

Pappas G, Akritidis N, Bosilkovski M, Tsianos E. Brucellosis. *N Engl J Med* 2005; **352**: 2325–36.

Reguera JM, Alarcon A, Miralles F, Pachon J, Juarez C, Colmenero JD. Brucella endocarditis: clinical, diagnostic, and therapeutic approach. *Eur J Clin Microbiol Infect Dis* 2003; **22**: 647–50.

Shaalan MA, Memish ZA, Mahmoud SA, et al. Brucellosis in children: clinical observations in 115 cases. *Int J Infect Dis* 2002; **6**: 182–6.

Young EJ. Serologic diagnosis of human brucellosis: analysis of 214 cases by agglutination tests and review of the literature. *Rev Infect Dis* 1991; **13**: 359–72.

Lyme disease

Lyme disease, named after Old Lyme, Connecticut, where it was first described, is the most common tick borne infection. The clinical features were originally described in 1977 and *Borrelia burgdoferi* was isolated in 1982.

Epidemiology
In the UK, the incidence is estimated at 0.3/100 000, and is up to 155/100 000 in Slovakia, where the highest incidence is reported. Incidence is also high in Austria, Germany, and Sweden. In the USA, incidence is estimated at 8.2/100 000. In the UK, more than half the cases are acquired in south west England, with the majority of cases reported in the summer months. Lyme disease is not a notifiable disease. Global warming is expected to increase the incidence of vector-borne diseases as milder weather increases tick activity for a longer proportion of the year. An increase in tick numbers of 10-fold is believed to have occurred since 1986.

Aetiology
Borrelia burgdorferi is a Gram negative, highly motile, corkscrew-shaped bacterium. There are 3 species, *B. burgdoferi* sensu *strictu*, *B. garinii*, and *B. afzelli*. The first is the only species found in USA, whereas all 3 are found in Europe. All 3 species cause arthritis, but *B. garinii* may cause neuroborreliosis and *B. afzellii* is the species most likely to cause chronic skin involvement.

Pathogenesis
Around 80 ticks are implicated in the transmission of infection to humans. *Ixodes ricinus* is the hard tick which carries *B. burgdorferi*. It is has a lifecycle of 3 years, and feeds on hosts such as deer, which may be infected with *B. burgdorferi*. Once infected, the adult tick then feeds on other uninfected mammals such as deer, small rodents and humans, and therefore transmits infection. It is estimated 25% of ticks are infected with *B. burgdorferi*. Ticks are almost invisible on human skin. However, they grow up to 10 mm and are visible as black specks having ingested the blood of the host. They feed primarily in the spring and summer and feeding can take up to 6 days to complete. Ticks are able to move about on the host and therefore can be found on unexposed skin.
- Infection of the host occurs via the tick bite. The reaction site contains lymphocytes, macrophages, and plasma cells, which release pro-inflammatory cytokines.
- The spirochaete then disseminates widely over the next weeks to blood, heart, brain, muscle, bone, spleen, liver, brain, and eye, although some hosts are asymptomatic.
- Most patients recover with treatment, although 10% of patients develop a chronic arthritis. Whether this is due to resistant infection or an autoimmune-medicated inflammatory response remains unclear.

Clinical features
Erythema migrans, lymphadenosis cutis benigna, meningopolyneuritis (Bannwarth syndrome) and acrodermatitis chronica atrophicans are pathognomonic features of Lyme disease. These are discussed below.

Natural history
Early Lyme disease
- Erythema migrans is the most common clinical manifestation (75%). The incubation period varies from 3 to 32 days, and the macule expands to a red-purple well demarcated rash, near or around the site of the tick bite. This may remain uniform or become ring like. The area of erythema varies from 2 to 60 cm in diameter. The area of erthyema grows by 1cm per day, and usually last between 3–4 weeks before settling spontaneously.
- Other symptoms include fever, malaise, headache, arthralgia/myalgia, and lymphadenopathy.
- Lymphadenosis cutis benigna is a rare manifestation, which is a purple nodule that forms on the skin of the face or on the nipple.
- Acute neuroborreliosis develops in around 15% of patients within months of infection. Symptoms of neuroborreliosis include meningitis, cranial neuropathies (particularly of the facial nerve), and radiculopathy. The radiculopathy usually combines motor and sensory components and is associated with severe pain.
- Carditis occurs in less 5% of patients, and presents as atrioventricular heart block, or left or right bundle branch block.
- Eye involvement presents as conjunctivitis or uveitis.
- Joint pain is often migratory although synovitis is rare.

Late Lyme disease
- Borrellia infection may persist for years.
- Acrodermatitis chronica atrophicans is a chronic skin condition that is oedematous and violacious in colour. It is not normally seen until 12 months after infection. It may progress over years to a paper like skin atrophy. Rare complications include squamous cell carcinoma and B cell lymphoma.
- Chronic neuroborelliosis is rare, but may present with chronic encephalitis, encephalomyelitis, peripheral neuropathy, and cerebral vasculitits.

Lyme arthritis
In the USA, 60% of patients with untreated borelliosis develop joint manifestations, although this is less common in Europe reflecting the spectrum of clinical features caused by the different *Borellia* species. Joint disease typically occurs in late disease and is usually intermittent with acute flares followed by ever-shortening remissions. The distribution is usually mono- or oligoarticular, involving knees, elbows, and ankles, although other joints may be affected. Large joint effusions are common. Tenosynovitis and bursitis are rare.

Investigations
A low grade inflammatory response may be seen, although bloods may also be normal. RF and ANA are usually normal, although chronic infection may result in a low grade seropositivity. Synovial aspirates reveal leucocytosis, but cultures are negative.

Prognosis
Erosions are rare even in chronic arthritis. 90% of patients are asymptomatic following treatment. Oral antibiotics are useful even in chronic disease. A minority of patients do not respond to antibiotics, suggesting an autoimmune response from the host against infection. Long-term antibiotic therapy to eradicate chronic disease remains controversial.

Post-Lyme syndrome
A small number of patients who are treated for Lyme disease continue to complain of fatigue, myalgias, and memory disturbance, which are usually mild.

Diagnosis
IgM and IgG antibodies specific for Borrelia burgdoferi should be performed, with a rise in IgM detectable from 2 to 4 weeks following infection and the peak in IgM at 6–8 weeks. After that a rise in IgG antibodies is detected. For screening, a sensitive ELISA is appropriate, followed by an immunoblot, with a higher sensitivity for confirmation. Culture of erythema migrans biopsies has a yield of 50%, similar to that of plasma during the early stages of infection. CSF culture has a yield of 10% in neuroborelliosis.

PCR
PCR is not routinely available, although DNA can be isolated in a number of different tissues, e.g. skin, CSF, synovial fluid, blood, and urine. A negative PCR does not exclude Lyme disease.

Treatment
Antibiotics should be prescribed on the basis of clinical symptoms. Asymptomatic patients with positive serology should not be treated on the basis of serology alone. Oral therapy is usually with doxycycline, with amoxicillin reserved for children or in pregnancy. Intravenous therapy is usually with ceftriaxone or cefotaxime. Jarisch–Herxheimer reaction is reported in the first few days of therapy and glucocorticoid cover is necessary in symptomatic patients. NSAIDs and simple analgesia have a role. The risks of oral, parenteral, and intra-articular glucocorticoid therapy remain controversial because of the potential risk of reactivation of infection.

Erythema migrans
Antibiotics should be initiated as soon as erythema migrans is diagnosed. The antibiotic of choice is doxycycline 200 mg daily for 14–21 days.

Arthritis and acrodermatitis
Most patients will respond to oral antibiotics, although some will require antibiotics intravenously for up to 3 months to abolish joint symptoms. The benefit of doxycycline is that it also has a mild anti-inflammatory effect, although this should be borne in mind when planning antibiotic duration as it may mask ongoing joint symptoms. Acrodermatitis responds well to oral antibiotics. Neurological involvement requires intravenous antibiotic therapy.

Neuroborelliosis
3 weeks of therapy is probably sufficient in patients with neurological involvement. Oral therapy is adequate in facial palsy alone, although parenteral therapy is more appropriate in a patient with extensive disease.

Treatment resistant disease
This needs to be distinguished from post-Lyme syndrome and continuing infection should be established by PCR or culture. Eradication is usually undertaken using parenteral antibiotic therapy.

Post-Lyme syndromes
This does not appear to be improved by antibiotic therapy.

Other treatment options
NSAIDs, simple analgesia, and physiotherapy have important roles. DMARDs have a role in patients with treatment resistant disease who have not settled with eradication therapy.

Controversies
The role of long-term antibiotics in patients with chronic symptoms remains an area of great debate, especially in the USA. Current medical opinion does not support the use of long-term antibiotic therapy, despite a vocal patient body. There are calls for Lyme disease to become a notifiable disease, especially since the incidence of infection is increasing.

Patient advice
Education should cover those who enjoy woodland or forest walks or cycling, with awareness of where ticks are found, the time of year when ticks are more common, their appearance on the skin, and the importance of seeking medical advice if a skin rash should develop. Clothing should cover arms and legs. Removal of ticks from the skin should be encouraged using tweezers, but care should be taken to remove all the tick's body.

Resources
Support groups
www.lymediseaseaction.org.uk

Internet support
Health protection agency centre for infection control. Holborn, London. Available at:

http://www.hpa.org.uk/infections/about/surveillance/surveillance_menu.htm. and

www.cdc.gov/mmwR/review/mmwrhtml/mm5317a4.htm

ICD-10 codes
M01.2   Arthritis in Lyme disease

References
Blackwood T. The ubiquitous tick. *Br Trav Health Ass J* 2007; **10**: 34.

Luger SW, Paparone P, Wormser GP, et al. Comparison of cefuroxime axetil and doxycycline in treatment of patients with early Lyme disease associated with erythema migrans. *Antimicrob Agents Chemother* 1995; **39**: 661–7.

Mullegger RR. Dermatological manifestations of manifestations of Lyme borreliosis. *Eur J Dermatol* 2004; **14**: 296–309.

Schnarr S, Franz J, Krause A, Zeidler H. Lyme borreliosis. *Best Pract Res Clin Rheumatol* 2006; **20**: 1099–118.

Tonks, A. Lyme Wars. *Br Med J* 2007; **335**: 910–12.

Viral arthritis

Arthralgia associated with viral infection is common and usually self-limiting over a period of weeks, although occasionally follows a more chronic course. Viral arthropathy is also reported following vaccination. The pattern of joint involvement is usually a symmetrical polyarthropathy, with women more commonly affected than men or children. Permanent joint damage is rare. Some viral infections are commonly associated with arthralgia, such as mumps or rubella, although it is less common in others, such as varicella or adenovirus. Virus is seldom isolated from synovial fluid.

Pathogenesis
The pro-inflammatory consequences of viral infection are complex and involve a number of different pathways. Different viruses modify or influence particular cellular responses. The main effects of viral infection include:
- Target the cells of innate immunity, by infecting monocytes promoting pro-inflammatory cytokine secretion.
- Impairment of antigen presenting cell function, e.g. HIV, CMV, and EBV infection result in impaired B cell function.
- Induction of autoantibody production, e.g. EBV induced IgG production with cross-reactivity against lupus associated autoantigens, and parvovirus B19 may induce antibodies against other cellular antigens.
- Induction of T cell immunity by depletion of thymic T cells, or modification of autoreactive T cell function, a mechanism also implicated in the pathogenesis of autoimmune diseases such as rheumatoid arthritis.
- Directly damage synovial cells, e.g. EBV, HTLV-1, rubella, and Ross River virus may directly infect synovial cells, and with an increased expression of double stranded RNA which is arthritogenic. Parvovirus B19, an extracellular virus, results in immune complex formation and deposition within the joint resulting in an inflammatory response and antibody formation.

Human parvovirus B19
Human parvovirus B19 is one of the Erythrovirus genus and is a small DNA virus. Transmission is usually via inhalation, but can occur via blood products or vertically from mother to foetus. Infection is often seen in early spring.

Clinical features
- The majority of infections are subclinical.
- Most present 2 weeks after infection with fever and erythema infectiosum or a 'slapped cheek' appearance.
- 50% of adults and 10% of children are reported to have a symmetrical small joint and knee arthralgia.
- Joint symptoms are commoner in women than men.
- Resolution of arthralgia within 3 weeks is usual, although 1 in 5 women have more prolonged symptoms.
- An erosive arthropathy is reported, but is rare.
- New presentations and flares of lupus have been linked with infection due to parvovirus B19.
- Non-rheumatological manifestations include hydrops foetalis and foetal death. Haematological, neurological, and cardiac sequelae of infection have been reported.

The association of human parvovirus B19 and rheumatoid arthritis
- Although an association between parvovirus B19 and rheumatoid arthritis has been postulated, the link remains tenuous.
- IgG antibodies against B19 are within the range expected for age, and B19 DNA has been found within the tissues of patients with normal joints.
- Patients with acute parvovirus B19 infection can meet the criteria for rheumatoid arthritis, and may transiently become seropositive. B19 DNA has been isolated from synovial fluid and tissue from patients with rheumatoid arthritis, and those patients who express HLA-DR4 are more likely to develop chronic arthritis following parvovirus infection.

Investigations
- Acute parvovirus B19 causes the presence of IgM antibodies and, later, IgG antibodies are detectable.
- PCR is useful in patients who are immunocompromised and unable to mount an antiviral antibody response, but may be positive for over 12 months following infection making interpretation difficult.

Treatment
Symptom relief is the mainstay of therapy, with either simple analgesics or non-steroidal anti-inflammatory drugs. There is no vaccine currently available.

Alphaviral infections
There are 26 viruses in the genus Alphavirus. These are spherical viruses that contain an RNA-containing nucleocapsid surrounded by a lipid layer. Transmission is cyclical and occurs between arthropods (normally mosquitos) and mammalian hosts, such as humans. Infection rates rise when mosquitos are prevalent, usually in the monsoon season. Recognizing a history of travel in patients with alphavirus infection is paramount to making the diagnosis. Ross River virus causes more than 8000 cases per annum in Australia and the West Pacific. Barmah Forest virus is less prevalent in Australia and causes myalgias, and occasionally arthritis. Ockelbo and Pogosta are prevalent in Scandanavia. Chikungunya is found mostly in Africa and Asia.

Clinical features
- The most common symptoms include rash, fever, arthralgia and systemic upset after an incubation period of up to 10 days.
- Subclinical infections are thought to be common and children are often spared joint involvement.
- The joint involvement ranges from a mild migratory polyarthralgia to a systemic synovitis involving the small joints primarily.
- Myalgia may be prominent.

Diagnosis
- The history of travel is particularly important in patients with rash, fever, and arthralgia/myalgia who have travelled to endemic areas.
- Paired sera are needed, as IgM specific for alphavirus may persist for years, and should be collected around 10 days apart. A 4-fold increase in the titre is usually characteristic.

Treatment of alphavirus
Treatment is mainly supportive and consists of simple analgesia, non-steroidal anti-inflammatory drugs, and mobilization as joint symptoms settle.

Mumps
Mumps is more likely to affect men, with an incidence of 0.44%.

Clinical features
- The joint pain may start just before the onset of parotitis, but may be delayed for up to 15 days.
- Both large and small joints are affected.
- Arthralgia is the commonest presentation, although synovitis can occur.

Treatment
Symptoms are usually self-limiting after a fortnight, but can persist for up to 3 months.

Hepatitis B
- Up to 20% of patients infected with hepatitis B report symptoms of arthritis, often with urticaria, between 2 days and 6 weeks before the onset of jaundice.
- The symptoms usually settle spontaneously before or coinciding with the onset of jaundice.
- The small joints are most commonly affected, although knee and ankles involvement is recognized.
- Effusions are a rare finding.

Hepatitis C
Infection with this agent is only rarely associated with joint symptoms, unless associated with a cryoglobulinaemia.

Human T-lymphotropic virus type 1
A proliferative synovitis may occur in people infected with human T-lymphotropic virus type 1, which usually results in a chronic oligoarthritis. Large joints are predominantly affected, and atypical lymphocytes are often found in the synovial fluid.

Rubella arthritis
Rubella is a genus of the Togaviridae family of viruses. It has a single-stranded RNA and is a member of the Rubivirus subfamily. Transmission is by the airborne route, but vertical transmission from mother to foetus is also possible.

Clinical features
- The incubation period is 1–2 weeks, and presents with lymphadenoapathy, followed by a rash 6 days later.
- Complications of rubella infection include encephalopathy, Guillain–Barre syndrome, and rarely haematological abnormalities, such as thrombocytopenia and haemolytic anaemia.
- 50% of adult women report joint symptoms, but this is less common in girls or males, and usually follow the appearance of the rash. Joint symptoms are typically a symmetrical small joint polyarthritis, which may progress to larger weight bearing joints.
- The natural history is of a self-limiting illness, which resolves within a month. However, a more chronic course has been reported in some and following vaccination.
- Rubella infection in the foetus is particularly significant in the first trimester of pregnancy resulting in congenital rubella syndrome, characterized by congenital malformation of the nervous system, cardiac abnormalities, and ocular and auditory involvement.

Diagnosis
The most reliable way of confirming infection is the detection of IgM antibodies to rubella. A rise in the IgM titre in paired sera collected 2 weeks apart is also indicative of recent infection.

Treatment
Vaccination programmes are well established in the UK, and are now being introduced in a number of developing countries with a significant reduction in rubella infections and congenital rubella syndrome. However, one disadvantage of the vaccination programme is the frequency of self-limiting arthralgia, particularly in women. This is normally short lived and responds well to non-steroidal anti-inflammatory drugs.

Human immunodeficiency virus
Human Immunodeficiency Virus (HIV) was first isolated in 1983, but has since caused a pandemic and has had particularly devastating consequences in developing countries, such as Africa. It is now estimated that over 40 million people are infected worldwide and more than 3 million have died of AIDS. In the UK, at the end of 2006, 73 000 people were estimated to infected with HIV, and one-third were estimated to be unaware of their infection. In 2007, 6393 new cases were reported. Effective antiviral treatments, called HAART (highly active antiretroviral treatment) have prolonged life, but have also resulted in a spectrum of rheumatological and autoimmune manifestations of HIV infection.

Transmission
- Sexual contact is the commonest route of transmission and rectal intercourse, the presence of very early or advanced infection, concurrent genital ulcers or the presence of other sexually transmitted disease make transmission more likely.
- Blood or blood product infusion is now a much less likely source of infection, since heat treatment and HIV testing is routine.
- Intravenous drug abuse and shared needles carries significant risks of HIV transmission.
- Rising HIV transmission rates were originally through homosexual intercourse and via blood products, although since 1999 heterosexual transmission has taken over as the main cause of rising HIV prevalence.
- Vertical transmission is the commonest route of infection in children worldwide, although in the UK the introduction of HIV testing in pregnant women has diminished this route of transmission.

Pathogenesis
- HIV is a lentivirus from the family of retroviruses.
- The virus attaches to host cells by the membrane protein CD4 receptor on helper T lymphocytes, macrophages and other antigen presenting cells.
- As viral replication occurs, significant destruction of CD4 lymphocytes occurs.
- Quantitative PCR is the most commonly available technique for quantifying viral load, which is usually higher during seroconversion, early on in infection, and also in late disease.
- Some 4–6 months after infection, control of viral replication occurs and the viral load plateaus. The level of this plateau varies from individual to individual and is called the 'set point'. Those individuals with a lower set level are more likely to progress slowly towards AIDS defining illness than those with a higher set point.
- The set point rises slowly as infection progresses and during intercurrent illnesses.

Clinical features
- A severe decline in the number of CD4+ helper T lymphocytes occurs during HIV infection and, as a result, cell-mediated immunity becomes significantly impaired and results in opportunistic infection and malignancy.
- Hypergammaglobulinaemia occurs and is associated with the development of a number of different autoantibodies with clinical consequences, idiopathic cytopenias and severe drug allergies.

Natural history
Following infection there is an asymptomatic period of 2–4 weeks, which is then followed by a seroconversion illness, consisting of a 1–2-week self-limiting illness comprising mild glandular fever-like symptoms, with a sore throat, fever, lymphadenopahy, and a non-itchy maculopapular rash. A period of latency then ensues and is of varying length, but is prolonged with the introduction of HAART. Finally, there is progression to AIDS, and opportunistic and life-threatening infection.

Rheumatological manifestations
Arthralgia
Arthralgia is reported in 5% of patients with HIV and can be disabling. Most do not progress to significant arthritis. Treatment is with simple analgesia.

Painful articular syndrome
This is reported when HIV was first recognized, but is much less common now. Presentation is with self-limiting bone pain, but with no abnormalities on examination. Treatment is with analgesia.

HIV associated arthritis
- Arthritis associated with HIV infection is usually self-limiting (within 6 weeks) and presents with an oligoarticular arthritis, often involving weight-bearing joints, and with no long-term sequelae.
- A more chronic course is also recognized, resembling a seronegative polyarthritis, often with entheitis and with progressive joint space narrowing on plain radiographs.
- Mucocutaneous involvement include keratoderma blenorrhagicum and circinate balanitis (see Plate 10). Urethritis is also a feature.
- Axial involvement and uveitis are much less common.
- Over 80% of patient with HIV and this pattern of involvement are HLA B27 positive.
- Treatment success is reported with sulphasalazine and hydroxychloroquine in more severe cases. Caution should be used with methotrexate and there is emerging evidence for success with anti-TNFα therapy.

Psoriasis and psoriatic arthritis
Psorasis in HIV is often gutate in appearance and may be very extensive. The psoriatic rash in HIV infection often coincides with the point in disease progression where opportunistic infection starts to emerge. Success in treating the skin disease is reported with HAART, as well as with ciclosporin, methotrexate, and etanercept, although close monitoring of all these agents is advised.

Undifferentiated spondyloarthritis
Enthesopathy without joint involvement is common, and therapeutic success is reported with NSAIDs and sulphasalazine. Success is also reported with HAART.

HIV-associated muscle disease
Myalgia, fibromyalgia, asymptomatic elevation in CK, polymyositis, and inclusion body myositis are recognized. Glucocorticoids normally result in a rapid lowering of CK and an improvement in symptoms in HIV associated polymyositis. Immunsuppression with methotrexte and azathioprine has been successful. Prognosis of HIV polymyositis is in general good. Pyomyositis is usually due to Staph. aureus and is rarely seen in the UK

Diffuse infiltrative lymphocytosis syndrome (DILS)
This is characterized by salivary gland involvement, with or without sicca symptoms and an associated lymphocytosis. DILS is estimated to occur in 3–8% of HIV positive patients in the period before HAART was developed. Biopsies reveal a focal sialadenitis similar to that seen in Sjogren's syndrome, although there is less destruction in HIV associated disease. Other manifestations of DILS include lymphocytic interstitial pneumonitis, VII cranial nerve palsy, peripheral neuropathy and lymphoma. It is reported that those patients that develop DILS as a manifestation of their HIV infection have a better survival and prognosis than other patients with HIV.

Treatment
Symptomatic treatment includes artificial tears and saliva. HAART is effective at reducing the salivary gland swelling, and some of the extra-glandular features of DILS, such as peripheral neuropathy. However, there maybe a role for prednisolone in a dose of 30–40 mg daily in those cases which are resistant.

Vasculitis associated with HIV
A wide range of vasculitides have been reported in patients with HIV, including polyarteritis nodosa, Henoch–Schonlein purpura, Behcet's disease, and hypersensitivity vasculitis. Treatment of HIV vasculitis is normally responsive to high dose glucocorticoids, although cytotoxics have a role in resistant disease.

Autoantibody formation in HIV
Rheumatoid factor and antinuclear antibodies are found in up to 17% of patients with HIV. IgG anticardiolipin antibodies are found in 95% of patients with AIDS and 20–30 of patients with HIV overall. They are probably of little clinical significance. Cryoglobulins (usually in association with Hepatitis C) and ANCA have also been reported.

Effects of HAART on musculoskeletal system
Symptoms include:
- Zydovudine myopathy.
- Zydovudine rhabdomyloysis.
- Adhesive capsulitis.
- Duprytrens contracture.
- Tenosynovitis.
- Avascular necrosis (hyperlipdaemia, high dose glucocorticoids, APLS).

Resources
Support groups
www.hiv-aids-carers.org.uk
www.dhiverse.org.uk/localsupport.htm

ICD-10 codes
B20–B24

References
Chantler JK, Ford DK, Tingle AJ. Persistent rubella infection and rubella-associated arthritis. *Lancet* 1982; **1**: 1323–5.
Dalakis MC, Pereshkpour GH, Gravell M, Sever JL. Polymyositis associated with the AIDS retrovirus. *J Am Med Ass* 1986; **256**: 2381–3.

Poole BD, Scofield RH, Harley JB, James JA. Epstein–Barr virus and molecular mimicry in systemic lupus erythematosis. *Autoimmunity* 2006; **39**: 63–70.

Schattner A. Consequences or coincidence? The occurrence, pathogenesis and significance of autoimmune manifestations after viral vaccines. *Vaccine* 2005; **23**: 3876–86.

Speyer I, Breedveld FC, Dijkmans BAC. Human parvovirus B19 infection is not followed by inflammatory joint disease during long term follow up. A retrospective study of 54 patients. *Clin Exp Rheumatol* 1998; **16**: 576–8.

White DG, Mortimer PP, Blake DR, et al. Human parvovirus arthropathy. *Lancet* 1985; **1**: 419–21.

Winchester R, Bernstein DH, Fischer HD, et al. The co-occurrence of Reiter's syndrome and acquired immunodeficiency. *Annl Intern Med* 1987; **106**: 19–26.

Mycobacterial infection

Tuberculosis

Prevalence
Approximately 80% of new cases of mycobacterium tuberculosis (MTB) occur in developing regions, such as sub-Saharan Africa and Asia. This may, in part, be related to the rising prevalence of HIV infection. In the UK, 44% of all cases are in London, with the highest rates around 40 per 100 000 of the population, similar to those in some developing countries. Emerging multi-drug resistant MTB is an increasing concern and is a worldwide issue. Extra-pulmonary MTB is also increasing, partly in patients with HIV, but also in patients who are immunosuppressed.

Classification
Musculoskeletal MTB is classified as
- Spinal.
- Arthritis with synovial disease.
- Osteomyelitis.
- Soft tissue disease.

Aetiology
- Mycobacterium tuberculosis is almost always the causative agent in tuberculous infection. Atypical mycobacterial infection is rare.
- Primary MTB infection is transmitted via inhalation of droplet nuclei released by the infected host on coughing, sneezing, or speaking. Lungs are therefore usually the site of primary infection with other sites more rarely involved.
- The endogenous host immunity influences the risk of infection. Mycobacteria that reach the lungs are phagocytosed by macrophages within the alveolar tissue, resulting in release of a number of different interferons and cytokines, which up-regulate the innate immune system. Intracellular growth of those bacteria that survive phagocytosis results in rupture of the macrophage with release into the blood and haematogenous spread to distant tissues. Granuloma formation occurs as a result of macrophage recruitment, which forms a Ghon focus, an important step in the development of immunity.
- It is estimated that 10% of infected individuals will develop active MTB eventually.
- The term primary MTB is used to describe clinical infection directly following exposure to MTB. Secondary MTB is the term used to describe infection within 2 years of that original exposure due to reactivation on a tuberculous focus.
- In joint and bone MTB, the infection is almost always secondary to haematogenous spread although rarely spread from an osteomyelitic focus may occur.

Pathology
The synovitis resulting from infection causes joint swelling, granulation tissue formation, and pannus, which in turn causes destruction of bone by eroding cartilage and subchondral bone. Necrosis, cold abscess formation, and fistulae may then result. This follows a much more indolent course than pyogenic infection.

Tuberculous arthritis
85% of MTB arthritis presents with chronic monoarthritis, usually involving the hip or knee. However, unilateral sacroiliac, shoulder, elbow, ankle, carpal, and tarsal involvement are reported. Oligo- or polyarticular presentations are rare. A high index of suspicion is necessary to make the diagnosis.

Tuberculous osteomyelitis
Osteomyelitis due to mycobacterium accounts for 2–3% of musculoskeletal infection. The short bones, such as metacarpal, metatarsals, and phalanges are common involved. Onset is insidious with involvement of the diaphysis, which causes a fusiform, tender swelling. There may be abscess formation. The radiological appearances eventually confirm enlargement of the shaft of the bone due to new subperiosteal bone formation. Prognosis is good as infection responds well to anti-tuberculous therapy.

Pott's disease of the spine
Tuberculous spondylitis was originally described by Percival Pott, a London surgeon in the 18th century. Infection may affect any part of the spine, but most commonly involves the thoracic spine, and may involve both vertebrae and intervertebral disc (as demonstrated in Figure 16.2). Presenting symptoms include back pain, with systemic symptoms of fever, weight loss, and anorexia. Vertebral collapse causes deformity and kyphosis. Neurological involvement may present with sensory or motor symptoms, or paraplegia due to spinal cord compression by the spinal abscess or vertebral collapse. Treatment with antituberculous drugs is central, and surgical options include debridement and drainage of the abscess and spinal stabilization.

Reactive arthritis (Poncet's disease)
Poncet's disease is defined as an aseptic polyarthritis associated with extrapulmonary disease. The typical picture is of a large joint arthritis primarily affecting children and young adults, associated with systemic features, often with effusion in the joints.

Panniculitis associated with MTB
The commonest manifestation of this is erythema nodosum. Erythema induratum is a form of lobular panniculitis associated with vasculitis. Response to anti-tuberculous therapy is good.

Atypical mycobacterium
Infection due to atypical mycobacteria is rare and is more likely to cause soft tissue than bone infection. M. kansaii infection is the commonest, although infection due to M. xenopi, M. marinum, M. avium intracellulare, M. chelonei, and M. fortuitum is reported.

Investigation of mycobacterium tuberculosis
Typically, an acute phase response in seen, although this is a non-specific test. Synovial microscopy (20–40% yield), and culture (yield of 80%) should be undertaken, and if necessary, synovial biopsy (yield of 90%). The tuberculin skin test is useful in patients who have not had previous exposure to MTB or had a previous BCG (Bacille Calmette–Guerin) vaccination. Immunocompromise, however, results in a high rate of false negative tests. A new commercial enzyme-linked immunospot assay (T spot MTB) detects gamma interferon-producing T cells and is sensitive (sensitivity of 97.2%) in detecting patients with active or latent MTB.

Imaging
Juxta-articular osteoporosis, peripheral erosions, and gradual joint space loss are the typical appearances seen on plain radiographs, and are termed Phemister's triad.

CHAPTER 16 **Musculoskeletal infection** 473

for multi-drug resistance. Monitoring of liver function tests is important as transaminases may rise, and a level 5–6 times baseline is an indication for withdrawal of therapy and then gradual reintroduction when the liver function test have returned to normal.
- Avoidance of alcohol and other hepatotoxic drugs is recommended. Active liver disease precludes use of isoniazid and rifampicin. Pyrazinamide may precipitate attacks of gout. Rifampicin can cause orange discolouration of urine and tears, so patients should be warned about this.
- A high success rate is achieved in treating osteoarticular MTB with multi-drug regimens.

The role of surgery
Surgery may be required in specific circumstances:
- Synovial tissue biopsy to aid diagnosis.
- Joint lavage if there is thick purulent effusion.
- Drainage of cold abscesses.
- Surgical correction of deformity.

Prognosis
There is usually resolution of symptoms in those patients with musculoskeletal infection who have good compliance with antituberculous therapy.

Leprosy
Mycobacterium leprae causes a spectrum of disease, possibly influenced by host immunity, with the extremes of the clinical spectrum defined as:
- **Tuberculous disease:** characterized by hypopigmented, desensitized skin.
- **Lepromatous disease:** characterized by severe, and often painful damage to nerves and other organs.

In tuberculous leprosy, characteristic granulomas are found at involved sites, with only a few bacilli demonstrated on biopsy. In lepromatous disease, infection results in cartilage destruction in the nose, ears, and larynx with large numbers of bacilli seen histologically. The term borderline leprosy is reserved for the majority of patients who lie between these two extremes.

Musculoskeletal manifestations of leprosy
- Neuropathic joints.
- Bacterial sepsis.
- Acute polyarthritis (associated with lepra reactions).
- Chronic/subacute symmetrical polyarthritis, either as a result of direct infection or an autoimmune reaction. Erosions have been reported as has treatment success with sulphasalazine and hydroxychloroquine. Sacroiliitis and tenosynovitis are also reported.

Treatment
Treatment of leprosy involves combination therapy including dapsone, rifampicin, and clofazimine. Lepra reactions (response to treatment) involve pain and swelling at the site of infection, especially in skin, nerves, eyes, and ears. Neuropathic deterioration is often very marked. Leprosy is characterized by the response to treatment which can be divided into two patterns of lepra reaction.

Type 1
There is either a downgrading to tuberculous disease or up grading to lepromatous disease in those patients with borderline leprosy, in both clinical and immunological terms.

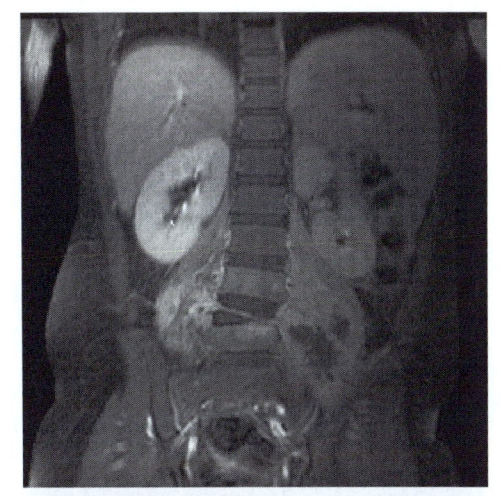

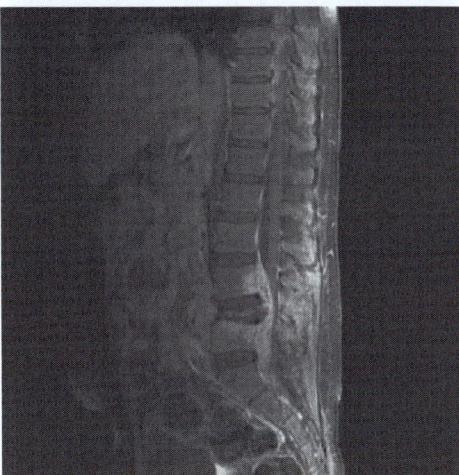

Figure 16.2 This is a post-contrast coronal T1 fat saturated MR showing bilateral psoas collections and the collapsed L4 vertebra. The lateral view demonstrates the extension of the abscess posteriorly into the epidural space.

Treatment
- Early diagnosis and full assessment of the patient improves the prognosis.
- Multidrug regimens are mandatory, partly because of drug resistance and secondly because of the different growth patterns of the bacilli. For example, some multiply rapidly and are vulnerable to particular anti-tuberculous therapy, and other are much slower and therefore respond to different agents. There may be an increase in efficacy using different agents together, so that treatment regimes can be shortened to 6–9 months from the original 12–24-month treatment regimes. Combinations of antituberculous therapy include 3 or 4 agents from isoniazide, rifampicin, pyrazinamide, ethambutol, and streptomycin.
- Monitoring for compliance and side effects is central to treatment. Poor compliance may in part be responsible

Type 2
An immune complex syndrome, erythema nodosum leprosum, develops in patients with lepromatous or borderline lepromatous disease.

Resources

Internet support

www.dh.gov.uk/en/Publicationsandstatistics/Publications/PublicationsPolicyandGuidance/DH_075621

ICD-10 codes
M01.1, M49.0

References

Meier T, Eulenbruch HP, Wrighton-Smith P, et al. Sensitivity of a new commercial enzyme-linked immunospot assay (T spot TB) for diagnosis of tuberculosis in clinical practice. Eur J Clin Microbiol Infect Dis 2005; **24**: 529–36.

CHAPTER 16 Musculoskeletal infection

Fungal infection

Musculoskeletal infection due to fungal infection is rare and difficult to diagnose. The majority occur mainly in the tropics and are rare in Europe. The course tends to be slow and prolonged, with skin and lung involvement.

Histoplasmosis

- Histoplasmosis capsulatum is endemic in Ohio and Mississippi in the USA, and is also found in Central and West Africa. The African species has larger spores than that found in the USA.
- Infection is caught by the inhalation of spores, which are found in soil.
- Those individuals particularly at risk of developing pulmonary histoplasmosis are those with underlying lung disease and those who are immunocompromised. Lung involvement, and lymphoreticular and bone marrow involvement then occurs.
- Presentation is often a flitting polyarthralgia or polyarthritis with erythema nodosum.
- Osteomyelitis and joint infection are rare in the USA, but reported in 50% of African infections.
- Vertebral involvement may lead to spinal cord compression and paraplegia. The differential diagnosis includes tuberculosis or, if widespread, sickle-cell osteomyelitis.
- Diagnosis is made on histology, which confirms giant cell granulomas containing yeast cells.
- Treatment is with amphotericin B and fluconazole, or itraconozole.

Cryptococcosis

- Cryptococcus neoformans causes initial infection in the lung.
- Dissemination is rare and usually only in patients with immunocompromise. In this situation, presentation is often with meningitis.
- Vertebral osteomyelitis is rare.
- The differential diagnosis includes tuberculosis.
- Arthritis due to cryptococcal infection is rare.
- Diagnosis is made histologically.
- Treatment is with amphotericin B or fluconazole and 5-fluorocytosine. Surgical debridement is often necessary.

Paracoccidioidomycosis

- Paracoccidioides brasiliensis is the fungus which causes paracoccidioidomycosis, also called 'South American blastomycosis' as it is found in central and southern America.
- The primary infection involves the lungs and is often asymptomatic.
- Dissemination occurs to both skin and lymphoreticular tissue.
- Presentation may be with chronic skeletal manifestations involving scapula, acromium, clavicle, rib, humerus, radius, or phalanges. Symptoms include slowly progressive bone pain and signs of inflammatory arthritis if infection spreads to a joint.
- Differential diagnosis includes tuberculosis, histoplasmosis, sarcoidosis, and malignancy.
- Diagnosis is made histologically.
- Treatment is with amphotericin or trimethoprim for musculoskeletal disease and may be required for up to 4 years.

Sporotrichosis

- Sporothrix schenkii, the dimorphic fungus implicated in infection, is found in soil and decaying vegetation.
- This is the most common subcutaneous infection in South Africa and Mexico.
- A monoarthritis occurs if infection involves lymph nodes.
- Disseminated infection occurs in the immunocompromised patient.
- Diagnosis is made histologically.
- Treatment is with amphotericin B combined with ketaconazole.

Blastomycosis

- Blastomycosis dermatitidis is found in North and South America and Africa.
- Infection occurs following inhalation.
- Dissemination results in skin involvement in 80% and osteolytic lesions in 60%.
- Differential diagnosis in the spine includes tuberculosis.
- Monoarthritis is rare, resulting from spread from local bone involvement.
- Histology from synovial tissue or bone may be diagnostic, although Blastomycosis dermatitidis can also be seen in synovial fluid.
- Treatment is with surgical debridement, drainage and amphotericin B.

Penicilliosis

- Penicillium marneffei is endemic in Thailand and Southern China.
- Presentation is usually with a chronic mono or oligoarthritis. Osteomyelitis and subcutaneous abscesses can also occur.
- The diagnosis is confirmed when encapsulated yeast is seen on microscopy of smears, stained with Wrights stain.
- The differential diagnosis includes histoplasma capsulatum.

Mycetoma

This term encapsulates a group of chronic infections of subcutaneous tissue, bones and joints.

Actinomycetes.
These are aerobic bacteria that resemble fungi. They cause chronic suppuration with sinus formation.

Fungi
Madurella mycetomatis is one example and causes maduromycetoma. These infections are generally treatment resistant.

Parastic infection

An oligo/polyarthritis may result as an immune phenomenon following infection with helminths, filariasis, or Bancroftian filiariasis.

Chylous arthritis

Chyle within a joint is caused by lymphatic obstruction due to Wuchereria bancrofti, a nematode worm. The effusion is normally sterile, but can look creamy and may resemble pus. Treatment is with diethylcarbamazine.

Loiasis
- This is caused by the worm Loa-Loa and is found in the African rainforests and in South America.
- The microfilaria migrate under the skin, appearing as Calabar swellings.
- Arthritis results from microfilaria within the joint and mimics septic arthritis.
- Treatment is with diethylcarbamazine.

Onchocerciasis
- Infection with the nematode *Onchocerca volvulus* from black fly results in dermatitis with nodules, river blindness, and a monoarthritis.
- The joint involvement may worsen with diethylcarbamazine.

Guinea worm
- An eosinophilic synovitis occurs following ingestion of the worm *Dracunculus medinensis*, which is found in drinking water. The worm invades the joint, resulting in synovitis.
- Ulceration and sinus formation with superimposed bacterial sepsis may result.
- Treatment is difficult and surgical removal of the worm is necessary.

Gnathosostomiasis
The nematode *Gnathostoma spinigerum* causes abscess formation in muscle.

Schistosomiasis
Two species of nematode fluke are describe: *S. mansoni* and *S. haemotobium*, which can cause a reactive arthritis with enthesitis.

Strongyloides
This may result in a reactive arthritis or vasculitis.

Echinococcus (hydatid disease)
Cysts may form in bone and muscle and inflammatory arthritis may also occur.

Trichinosis
Trichinella spiralis results in an eosinophilic myositis. Myositis is associated with cystericercosis.

Protozoa
Both arthritis and myositis are described.

Resources
Internet support
Health protection agency centre for infection control, Holborn, London. Available at:

http://www.hpa.org.uk/infections/about/surveillance/surveillance_menu.htm.

ICD-10 codes
M01.6, M01.8

Reference
Blackwood T. The ubiquitous tick. *Br Trav Health Ass J* 2007; **10**: 34

Chapter 17

Chronic pain

Chronic pain *480*
Fibromyalgia syndrome *484*
Complex regional pain syndrome type I *488*

Chronic pain

Background
Pain of more than 3 months is defined as chronic even though the features that characterize chronic pain can occur much more quickly. It is the commonest reason for a patient to seek consultation with a rheumatologist. Perhaps more than any other medical condition, it epitomizes the biopsychosocial model of healthcare.

The characteristics and management of arthritis or inflammatory pain; cancer pain; pain associated with nerve lesions; and acute pain are specifically not discussed for the purposes of this chapter.

The International Association for the Study of Pain defines any pain as all of the following:
- An unpleasant sensory experience.
- An unpleasant emotional experience.
- An experience associated with actual or potential tissue damage, or described in terms of such damage.
- Always subjective.

Many people with chronic pain report pain in the absence of tissue damage or any likely pathophysiological cause.
As a general approach:
- It is important to identify cases where there are specific treatments.
- Pain needs to be distinguished from 'distress' (i.e. the emotional response).
- Sleep and mood disturbances are common. It can be helpful to address these.
- Pain interrupts attention and causes cognitive dysfunction, such as memory loss. It can be helpful to recognize this.
- The consequences of pain may be more problematic than pain itself. It can be helpful to focus on this.

Epidemiology
Pain that lasted more than 3 months was estimated to affect about 14% of the population 'significantly' and 6% 'severely' in a community survey in the Grampian region. This survey described all forms of chronic pain and did not differentiate between regional and widespread. People were more likely to indicate significant chronic pain if they were:
- Unable to work (odds ratio 11.1).
- Older than 75 years (4.4).
- Achieved no educational qualifications (2.9).
- Lived in rented council housing (2.2).
- Female (1.3).

Pathophysiology
Peripheral pain fibres
These are slowly conducting C and Aδ fibres that release glutamate, substance P, and calcitonin gene-related peptide (CGRP). Patients with fibromyalgia have 3 times the spinal level of substance P in their CSF obtained from lumbar puncture when compared with healthy volunteers.

Spinal cord
The spinal gate is controlled by local spinal mechanisms [glutamate, glycine and γ-aminobutyric acid (GABA)] and descending pathways releasing serotonin and noradrenaline). Opioids are effective at blocking spinal transmission. Patients with chronic pain demonstrate 'wind-up' and central sensitization of the spinal cord.

Brain stem
The peripheral pain 'message' divides into two and is carried primarily through contralateral, anterolateral, and dorsolateral pathways. One pathway, the 'somatic' experience of pain, is modulated through the brainstem, where it activates the reticular formation before going on to the thalamus and somatosensory cortex. This pathway is needed to localize pain. The other pathway, the 'emotional' component of pain also passes through the thalamus before going into the anterior cingulate and frontal cortex.

Descending pathways
Interconnections between the ascending pathways at the level of the medulla and midbrain activate the peri-aqueductal grey, raphe nucleus, and the rostroventral medulla to excite descending pathways that release noradrenaline and serotonin. Diffuse noxious inhibitory control (DNIC) is another descending spinal pathway probably opioid-mediated.

Brain
The primary and secondary somatosensory cortex, insular, anterior cingulated, and prefrontal cortex invariably activate following an acutely painful stimulus in functional brain imaging using MRI or PET scanning. Bilateral brain activation can also be seen, as well as activity in the amygdale, hippocampus, basal ganglia, and posterior parietal lobe depending upon patient and protocol. Patients with chronic pain demonstrate disrupted neural network dynamics when compared with controls. The integrative properties of the brain allows the 'perceptual categorization' resulting from this neuromatrix activity to interact with pre-existing 'value-category memory' to generate a conscious awareness or qualia.

Treatment options
Pharmacological therapies
No single strategy will 'cure' the problem. It is necessary to have a number of different treatment options and to empower the patient to think laterally. Rotating treatments; concentrating on function, rather than pain; goal setting; and keeping a diary, as an objective reflection may be helpful.

Conventional analgesics
A pain ladder approach is appropriate, although this has no evidence-base in chronic non-malignant pain.

Paracetamol/NSAIDs
- Paracetamol is preferred by a minority of patients with rheumatoid arthritis, osteoarthritis, and fibromyalgia for its effectiveness and side effect profile.
- In one study 14% rated paracetamol more effective than non-steroidal anti-inflammatory drugs (NSAIDs), 26% the same and 60% less effective. This is a poorly researched area.
- NSAIDs are useful for chronic arthritis and there is no evidence to distinguish any benefit or harm in head-to-head trials conducted between them.
- Anecdotally, if one NSAID doesn't work, another NSAID may be helpful.
- Long-term use needs to be weighed against the serious risks to a patient, in particular gastrointestinal (GI) bleeds, renal, and cardiovascular disease.

- A proton pump inhibitor or higher dose histamine (H2) antagonist should be prescribed if one or more of the following risk factors for gastrointestinal bleeding is present:
  - age over 65 years;
  - previous history of GI bleed;
  - serious co-morbidity;
  - prolonged use of high NSAID doses;
  - aspirin or anticoagulants.
- Cyclo-oxygenase-II (COX-II) inhibitors are associated with a reduced incidence of upper GI adverse events, but have significant cardiovascular risk profiles. It is unclear whether this applies to all NSAIDs or is a specific feature of COX-II inhibitors.
- NSAID use is a complex area and the patient needs to be consulted in how to manage their chronic pain. Two-thirds of patients with osteoarthritis were willing to accept increased risk of heart attack, stroke, or stomach bleeding for a 2/10 point reduction in pain. Half would accept risk at the level of 1 in 50. Pain is the area of health that almost 70% of rheumatoid arthritis patients would most like improved.

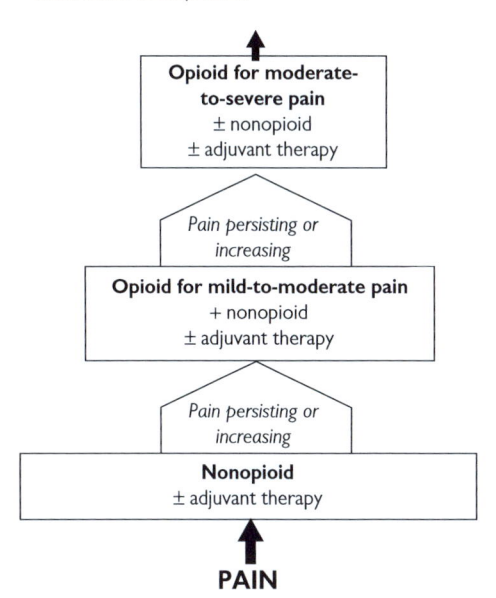

Figure 17.1 The WHO Pain Ladder. Reproduced with permission from WHO.

The WHO Pain Ladder
Opioids
Codeine is a pro-drug that is metabolized by the liver (cytochrome P450 enzyme CYP2D6) to morphine.
- About 6–10% of Caucasians do not have this enzyme and codeine will not be effective for them yet they will still get side effects.
- Randomized, controlled studies of various opioids given to adults with arthritis and other causes of chronic pain have demonstrated their efficacy and safety.

- The problems with administering strong opioids in patients with chronic pain are:
  - opioids are not as effective for chronic pain as they are for acute pain, especially where pain is secondary to a damaged nervous system;
  - opioids also may not be given in adequate doses due to the fears of addiction.
- Opioid-like drugs [Tramadol and (dextro) propoxyphene] combine opioid actions with serotonergic actions and this dual effect allows them theoretical benefit over traditional opioids.
- Slow-release strong opioids, including the use of patches, can be used in the treatment of chronic pain.

Adjunct medications
The following drugs have been demonstrated to improve pain relief, although were not developed primarily for analgesia. Such drugs include anti-depressants and anti-convulsants.
- Antidepressants, such as amitriptylline, nortriptylline and imipramine, selective serotonin re-uptake inhibitors (SSRIs), and serotonin-norepinephrine re-uptake inhibitors (SNRIs), such as fluoxetine, duloxetine, and venlafaxine. For neuropathic pains, the number needed to treat (NNT) is about 3 for a 50% reduction in pain. 4% have to stop treatment, however, due to adverse reactions.
- Anticonvulsants, such as gabapentin, pregabalin, carbamezepine, valproate, lamotrigine, clonazepam, and phenytoin may have a role to play.
- A systematic review of the efficacy of tetrahydrocannabinol in the management of pain suggests it is roughly equivalent to codeine 50 mg, but with a higher incidence of psychotropic adverse effects.

Topical rubs
Topical NSAIDs provide effective pain relief with a NNT figure of 3.1 (2.7–3.8) for at least 50% pain relief at 2 weeks after beginning treatment.
- Topical application of NSAIDs is not associated with serious side effects.
- Topically applied capsaicin is useful in alleviating the pain associated with diabetic neuropathy, osteoarthritis and psoriasis with NNT figures of 4.2 (2.9 to 7.5), 3.3 (2.6–4.8) and 3.9 (2.7–7.4), respectively.
- Lidocaine patches may also have a role for local chronic pain syndromes.

Non-pharmacological therapies
Transcutaneous electrical nerve stimulation (TENS)
TENS may be useful, but there is no conclusive evidence that TENS is effective for chronic pain.
- There are 19 randomized trials of TENS, including one of a parallel cross-over design involving 658 patients and using Sham-TENS and other controls looking at a variety of outcomes.
- Most of the TENS trials were small and difficult to blind as active TENS gives a tingling feeling. 10/15 studies using inactive controls gave a positive treatment effect.

Relaxation
Relaxation does not appear to be effective in relieving chronic non-malignant pain. Although some trials report benefit with relaxation, it is unclear whether this is clinically meaningful. There appear to be no demonstrable long-term benefits of relaxation. It may be useful as part of combined therapies programme.

Psychological-based treatments
Cognitive behavioural therapy, behavioural therapy, and biofeedback. are effective in reducing the pain experience, and improving positive behaviour expression, appraisal, and coping in individuals with chronic pain.

Complementary therapies
There are a host of complementary therapies, the commonest in the UK being acupuncture, homeopathy, herbal medicines, and topical devices (magnets, bracelets, crystals). There is no good evidence for the efficacy of any complementary therapy. Some points need to be made:
- There is known harm for some complementary therapies (herbal remedy drug interactions, acupuncture needle infections).
- There is a definite cost.
- The placebo effect is linked to patient expectation.
- Some people find complementary therapies helpful.

Clinical tips
- Patients value the time to give their history and appreciate a thorough examination.
- The following clinician characteristics have been demonstrated to help patients with unexplained medical symptoms (irritable bowel):
  - questions concerning symptoms, relationships, lifestyle;
  - how the patient understands the 'cause' and 'meaning' of the symptoms;
  - warm, friendly manner, active listening, empathy, and positive expectation.
- Understanding and describing pain as a functional nervous disturbance can lead to a change in the 'number needed to offend' (NNO) from 2 to 10 when compared with other strategies for explaining to patients the cause of their symptoms.
- Aiming for control, rather than a cure can be helpful. Changes in both pharmacological and non-pharmacological interventions may lead to improvements.
- Be aware of common causes of distress and attempt to address these with either onward referral via primary or secondary care or empowering the patient to self-refer to direct-access services.
- Honesty is the best policy. Western medicine does not have the solution to every patient's symptoms. Complementary therapies, providing they do no harm, can be helpful.
- Pain pathways can be divided into two broad areas – somatic localizing acute pain and ill-defined emotional distress. A single peripheral insult activates both of these. Reflecting this to the patient in a non-judgemental fashion can be helpful.

Resources

Assessment tools
Brief Pain Inventory. Available at: http://www.mdanderson.org/pdf/bpilong.pdf

SF-36. Available at: http://www.sf-36.org/tools/SF36.shtml

British Pain Society's Good practice guide to assessing pain in older people> Available at: http://www.britishpainsociety.org/book_pain_older_people.pdf

Guidelines
Guidelines on Pain Management, National Library for Health. http://www.library.nhs.uk/guidelinesfinder/

Evidence-based medicine for pain management. Bandolier. http://www.jr2.ox.ac.uk/bandolier/

British Pain Society's 2007 Guidelines on Pain Management Programmes for Adults. http://www.britishpainsociety.org/book_pmp_main.pdf

Patient organizations
Action on Pain, Tel: (Helpline) 0845 603 1593. Available at: www.action-on-pain.co.uk/

Arthritis Care HelpLine, Tel: 0808 8004050. Available at: www.arthritiscare.org.uk

NHS patient support. Available at: www.patient.co.uk

Pain Concern, Tel: 01620 822572. Available at: www.painconcern.org.uk

Pain Association Scotland, Tel (enquiries only): 0800 783 6059. Available at: www.chronicpaininfo.org

NHS expert patients. Available at: www.expertpatients.nhs.uk

Talking Life, Tel (enquiries): 0151 632 1206. Available at: www.talkinglife.co.uk

CRUSE Bereavement Helpline 0844 477 9400. Available at: www.crusebereavementcare.org.uk

Unwind Helpline is 0191 384 2056

Politically active groups include www.paincoalition.org.uk

Internet sites
Pain Web for Health Professionals. Available at: www.thepainweb.com

International Association of Pain. Available at: www.iasp-pain.org

British Pain Society. Available at: www.britishpainsociety.org

Royal National Hospital for Rheumatic Disease, Bath. Available at: www.bath.ac.uk/pain-management/

INPUT, Guy's and St Thomas' Hospitals, London. Available at: www.gstt.nhs.uk/services/acutepatient/perioperative/pain/input.aspx

ICD-10 codes
R52.2; R52.9

References
Baliki MN, Geha PY, et al. Beyond feeling: chronic pain hurts the brain, disrupting the default-mode network. *J Neurosci* 2008; **28**: 1398–403.

Caldwell J, Hale ME, et al. Treatment of osteoarthritis pain with controlled release oxycodone or fixed combination oxycodone plus acetaminophen added to nonsteroidal antiinflammatory drugs: a double blind, randomized, multicenter, placebo controlled trial. *J Rheumatol* 1999; **26**: 862–9.

Campbell FA, Tramèr MA, et al. Are cannabinoids an effective and safe treatment option in the management of pain? A qualitative systematic review. *BMJ* 2001; **323**: 13–16.

Carroll, D, Moore RA, et al. Transcutaneous electrical nerve stimulation (TENS) for chronic pain (Cochrane Review), in: *The Cochrane Library* 2002; Issue 2, Update software, Oxford.

Dickenson AH. Gate control theory of pain stands test of time. *BJA* 2001; **88**: 755–7.

Eckardt K, Li S, Ammon S, et al. Same incidence of adverse drug events after codeine administration irrespective of the genetically determined differences in morphine formation. *Pain* 1998; **76**: 27–33.

Edelman GM. Naturalizing consciousness: a theoretical framework. *PNAS* 2003; **100**: 5520–4.

Furlan AD, Sandoval JA, et al. Opioids for chronic noncancer pain: a meta-analysis of effectiveness and side effects. *CMAJ* 2006; **174**: 1589–94.

Heiberg T, Kvien KV. Preferences for improved health examined in 1024 patients with rheumatoid arthritis: pain has highest priority. *Arthritis Rheum* 2002; **47**: 391–7.

Jadad AR, CarrolD, et al. Morphine responsiveness of chronic pain: double-blind crossover study with patient controlled analgesia. *Lancet*. 1992; **339**: 1367–71.

Kaptchuk TJ, Kelley JM, et al. Components of placebo effect: randomised controlled trial in patients with irritable bowel syndrome. *BMJ* 2008; **336**: 999–1003.

McQuay H, Carroll D. Anticonvulsant drugs for management of pain: a systematic review. *BMJ* 1995; **311**: 1047–52.

Moore RA, Carroll D. A systematic review of topically-applied non-steroidal anti-inflammatory drugs. *BMJ* 1998; **316**: 333–8.

Morley S, Eccleston C. systematic review and meta-analysis of randomised controlled trials of cognitive behaviour therapy and behaviour therapy for chronic pain in adults, excluding headache. *Pain* 1999; **80**: 1–13.

Richardson CG, Chalmers A, et al. Pain relief in osteoarthritis: patients' willingness to risk medication-induced gastrointestinal, cardiovascular, and cerebrovascular complications. *J Rheumatology* 2007; **34**: 1579–85.

Smith BH, Elliott AM, et al. The impact of chronic pain in the community. *Fam Pract* 2001; **18**: 292–9.

Stone J, Wojcik W, et al. What should we say to patients with symptoms unexplained by disease? The 'number needed to offend'. *BMJ* 2002; **325**: 1449–50.

Wolfe F, Zhao S. Preference for nonsteroidal antiinflammatory drugs over acetaminophen by rheumatic disease patients. *Arthritis & Rheum*. 2000; **43**: 378–85.

Zhang WY, Li Wan Po A. The effectiveness of topically applied capsaicin. A meta-analysis. *Eur J Clin Pharmacol* 1994; **46**: 517–22.

Fibromyalgia syndrome

Definition
Fibromyalgia syndrome (FMS) is defined as chronic widespread (bilateral, axial, and above and below waist) unexplained pain associated with at least 11 of 18 specified tender points. Characteristic features include: fatigue, sleep disturbances, subjective memory loss, swelling (e.g. lymph nodes), paraesthesiae, stiffness.

History
Froriep described 'rheumatic' patients with hard tender muscles

- **1904** Gowers used term 'fibrositis' to describe patients with sleep disturbances, fatigue, and sensitivity to touch.
- **1930s** Lewis and Kellgren injected saline into deep muscles of healthy volunteers who described non-dermatomal, but consistent patterns of pain
- **1970s** Smith and Moldofsky described tender points in patients with stage 4 sleep disturbances. They then showed the onset of symptoms and muscle tenderness similar to that seen in patients with fibromyalgia by sleep-depriving healthy volunteers. Several investigators corroborated these findings in the 1980s.
- **1990** American College of Rheumatology criteria for the classification of fibromyalgia. 293 patients with FMS, and 265 age- and sex-matched controls with a rheumatic disorder were evaluated by blinded assessors using the definition provided above. This gave a sensitivity of 88% and specificity of 81%.

Epidemiology
The reporting of chronic widespread pain appears higher now than in 1950s. The point prevalence of chronic widespread pain in a community-based questionnaire survey in Manchester, UK, was about 5% with associations with:
- Fatigue (Risk ratio 3.8).
- Mental disorder (anxiety, panic disorder) (3.2).
- Psychological disturbance (2.2).
- Low levels of self-care (2.2).
- Reporting of other somatic symptoms (2.0).
- Reporting multiple symptoms aged 7 (1.5).

Ethnic minorities have also reported higher prevalence of chronic pain and this may reflect social, cultural and psychological differences. Around Manchester these include:
- Indian.
- Pakistani.
- Bangladeshi.
- African (not specified).
- Caribbean.

A higher tender point count (>4) is associated with low levels of self-care with the following risk factors:
- Abuse (Odds ratio 6.9).
- Adverse childhood experiences (2.1).

Aetiology and pathophysiology
Central pain pathways are sensitized in patients with FMS. The brain's pain neuromatrix is active in patients with FMS in a different way to healthy controls. Furthermore, Substance P, a key neuropeptide in pain transmission pathways, is three times elevated in the cerebrospinal fluid (CSF) of patients with FMS compared with healthy age- and sex-matched controls.

- Disturbed sleep clearly has an interesting relationship with unexplained pain both in clinical anecdotes and in the laboratory. Large, well-controlled studies are required.
- Hormonal profiling is consistent with a chronic stress reaction with evidence of low urinary free cortisol levels, decreased cortisol response to cortisol-releasing hormone, low neuropeptide Y plasma levels, and low growth hormone levels. Growth hormone, insulin growth factor-1 (IGF-1) and prolactin levels may also be different in FMS patients.
- Although major depressive illness occurs more commonly in patients with FMS and, more commonly, in their family members, there is no evidence for a specific personality type predisposed to developing FMS and evidence that pain contributes to the development and maintenance of the depression.
- Muscle abnormalities have been described in patients with FMS including type II fibre atrophy, changes in glycogen and lipids and mitochondrial abnormalities. However, these are likely to be secondary to inactivity and pain.

Clinical features
Key points in the history
The presence of co-morbidities related to FMS should alert the physician and increase the pre-test probability for FMS.

Co-morbidities
- Chronic fatigue.
- Chronic spinal pain.
- Chronic regional pain syndromes.
- Irritable bowel.
- Irritable bladder.
- Restless legs.
- Endometriosis.
- Anxiety.
- Depression.
- Joint hypermobility syndrome.
  Although classically described as a diagnosis of exclusion, features of the syndrome usually include the following:
- Low mood (pain that causes tearfulness).
- Subjective memory loss.
- Disturbed or unrefreshed sleep.

There are several other useful questions that might include feeling.

Key points on examination
Examination focuses around identifying secondary causes (e.g. hypothyroidism) and the tender points.
All locations are bilateral:
- **Occipit:** suboccipital muscle insertions.
- **Low cervical:** anterior aspects of intertransverse spaces at C5–7.
- **Trapezius:** midpoint of upper border.
- **Supraspinatus:** above scapula spine near medial border at origins.
- **Second rib:** second costochondral junction.
- **Lateral epicondyle:** 2 cm distal to epicondyles.
- **Gluteal:** upper outer quadrant in anterior fold of muscle.
- **Greater trochanter:** posterior to trochanteric prominence.
- **Knee:** medial fat pad proximal to the joint line.

Investigations
Laboratory
To rule out secondary fibromyalgia, the following blood tests should be taken:
- FBC.
- Urea and electrolytes.
- Creatinine.
- LFTs.
- ESR.
- TSH.

Other blood tests to consider include: vitamin D, PTH, serum ACE, CRP, ANA, RF, 9am cortisol, synacthen, fasting glucose.

Imaging
No imaging modality rules in or out the diagnosis of FMS and, therefore, imaging is not helpful unless another diagnosis is being investigated.

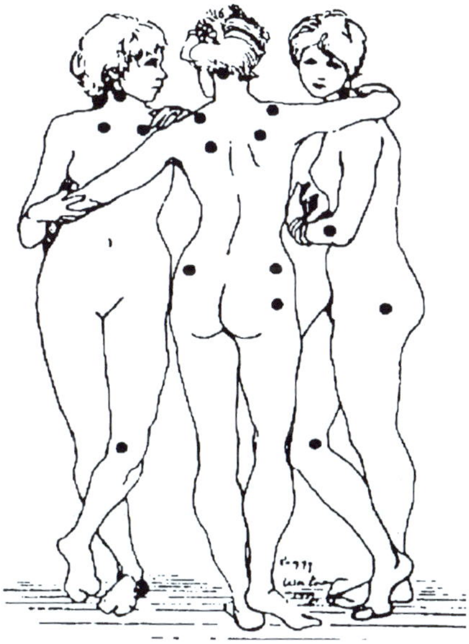

Figure 17.2 FMS: The tender points

Differential diagnosis
- Endocrine disease (e.g. hypothyroidism, vitamin D insufficiency/deficiency).
- Autoimmune disease (e.g. SLE, RA).
- Anaemia, renal disease or hepatic disease.

Treatment
Objectives of management
- Functioning.
- Mood.
- Pain experience.
- Coping skills.

Physical therapies
Aerobic exercise may be helpful for both pain and functioning, and certainly has beneficial effects on other systems, chiefly cardiovascular. It is likely that greater success will be afforded if the programme is tailored to the individual needs of the patient and paced.

Heated pool therapy is effective in improving pain and functioning for patients with FMS.

Pharmacological therapies
Simple analgesics and NSAIDs can be helpful.
- Tramadol may be of value, and been has demonstrated improved pain and functioning in patients with FMS.
- Careful consideration of the risk-benefit ratio for NSAIDs and COX-II inhibitors should be used. Further consideration is important if prescribing strong opioids.

Antidepressants
These are useful and valid studies have been published mainly using amitriptylline and fluoxetine. Both appear to improve pain and functioning within 6–12 weeks.
- Duloxetine (NNT 6 to reduce pain by more than 50%) and milnacipran, both dual selective serotonin-noradrenaline reuptake inhibitors may be helpful.
- Moclobemide and pirlindole, reversible inhibitors of monoamine oxidase A, also reduce pain. Function was not assessed, but side effects were low and non-serious.

Anticonvulsants
Gabapentin may be useful. There was a NNT of 5 to achieve 30% reduction in pain, and also help sleep and functioning. Tender points were not affected and it was generally well tolerated. Pregabalin also reduces pain (NNT 6 for more than 50% pain reduction), but functioning was not assessed and this could be used if there are side effects with gabapentin.

Pramipexole and tropisetron
Pramipexole is a non-ergoline dopamine agonist shown to improve pain scores. Tropisetron, a 5-HT3 antagonist, also reduces pain scores with no effect on functioning.

Glucocorticoids (GCs)
GCs may help in the short-term, but can not be justified given the long-term potential side effects.

Intravenous lignocaine
Intravenous lignocaine may be effective in FMS, but no long-term studies have been done and there are significant side effects, including some cardiovascular.

Psychological treatments

Cognitive-behavioural therapy (CBT)

CBT is likely to be of benefit, although there is an absence of good quality evidence. Multi-method CBT may be more effective than targeted approaches. Multi-disciplinary pain management programmes in either primary or secondary care are perhaps most effective.

Relaxation

Relaxation and education programmes are less likely to induce improvement in pain, functioning, and mood unless combined with other modalities.

Complementary therapies

There is no good evidence to support any of the complementary therapies in patients with FMS. Nevertheless, some patients find complementary therapies helpful for their symptoms. Sadly, most patients who attend such therapies are not informed of potential side effects, the industry remains unregulated and there is uncertainty as to the long-term impact of their interventions.

Prognosis and natural history

Only 15% of patients who reported chronic widespread pain in a postal survey reported no pain when the survey was repeated after 7 years. Poorer prognosis was associated with being >50 years old, reporting dry eyes or mouth, and daytime tiredness.

Current controversies

The genetics of pain suggests that many hundreds of genes, if not thousands are involved suggesting that mechanisms are even more complex than outlined here. Mechanistic-based approaches for helping patients with chronic pain appear some way off.

Serotonergic descending pathways from the brainstem and midbrain that are thought to be 'raising' the spinal gate to prevent spinal cord sensitization may, in fact, be 'lowering' it and cause such central sensitization.

Patients with chronic pain have a higher incidence of mortality although this may be accounted for by adjusting for smoking and obesity confounders.

Resources

Guidelines

Carville SF, Arendt-Nielsen A, et al. EULAR evidence based recommendations for the management of FMS. *Ann Rheum Dis* 2007. E-pub Oct 3.

Jain AK, Carruthers BM, et al. Fibromyalgia syndrome: Canadian clinical working case definition, diagnostic and treatment protocols – a consensus document. *J Musculoskel Pain* 2003;**11**: 3–107.

US-based National Guideline Clearing House, 2005. Available at: http://www.guideline.gov/summary/summary.aspx?doc_id=7352

Patient organizations

Fibromyalgia Association UK Helpline 0845 345 2322. Available at: www.fibromyalgia-associationuk.org

Arthritis Research Campaign. Available at: www.arc.org.uk

See also www.ukfibromyalgia.com; www.myopain.org

ICD-10 codes

M79.0; M79.7

References

Jones GT, Silman AJ, et al. Are common symptoms in childhood associated with chronic widespread body pain in adulthood? Results from the 1958 British Birth Cohort Study. *Arth Rheum* 2007; **56**: 1669-1675.

Allison TR, Symmons DPM, et al. Musculoskeletal pain is more generalised among people from ethnic minorities than among white people in Greater Manchester. *Ann Rheum Dis* 2002; **61**: 151–6.

Arnold LM, Goldenberg DL, et al. Gabapentin in the treatment of fibromyalgia: a randomized, double-blind, placebo-controlled, multicenter trial. *Arthritis Rheum.*2007; **56**: 1336–44.

Arnold LM, Keck PE. Antidepressant treatment of fibromyalgia: a meta-analysis and review. *Psychosomatics* 2000; **41**: 104–13.

Arnold LM, Lu Y, et al. A double-blind, multicenter trial comparing duloxetine with placebo in the treatment of fibromyalgia patients with or without major depressive disorder. *Arthritis Rheum* 2004; **50**: 2974–84.

Arnold LM, Rosen A, et al. A randomized, double-blind, placebo-controlled trial of duloxetine in the treatment of women with fibromyalgia with or without major depressive disorder. *Pain* 2005; **119**: 5–15.

Benjamin S, Morris S. The association between chronic widespread pain and mental disorder. A population-based study. *Arth Rheum* 2000; **53**: 561–7.

Carroll D, Seers K. Relaxation for the relief of chronic pain: a systematic review. *J Adv Nurs* 1998; **27**: 476–87.

Cowan D, Wilson-Barnet J, et al. A randomized, double-blind, placebo-controlled, cross-over pilot study to assess the effects of long-term opioid drug consumption and subsequent abstinence in chronic non-cancer pain patients receiving controlled-release morphine. *Pain Med* 2005; **6**: 113–21.

Crofford LJ, Pillemer SR, et al. Hypothalamic-pituitary-adrenal axis perturbations in patients with fibromyalgia. *Arthritis Rheum* 1994; **37**: 1583–92.

Crofford LJ, Rowbotham MC, et al. Pregabalin for the treatment of fibromyalgia syndrome. *Arthritis Rheum* 2005; **52**: 1264–73.

Goldenberg DL. Fibromyalgia and related syndromes. In: Klippel JH, Dieppe PA (eds) *Rheumatology*, 2nd edn. New York: Mosby, Section 4.15, 1–12.

Gøtzsche PC. Reporting of outcomes in arthritis trials measured on ordinal and interval scales is inadequate in relation to meta-analysis. *Ann Rheum Dis.* 2001; **60**: 349–52.

Gracely R, Petzke F, et al. Functional magnetic resonance imaging evidence of augmented pain processing in fibromyalgia. *Arthritis Rheum.* 2002; **46**: 1333–43.

Hunt IM, Silman AJ, et al. The prevalence and associated features of chronic widespread pain in the community using the ,Manchester definition of chronic widespread pain. *Rheumatology* 1999; **38**: 275–9.

Kalso E, Tramèr MR, et al. Systemic local anaesthetic type drugs in chronic pain: a systematic review. *Eur J Pain* 1998; **2**: 3–14.

Main CJ, Waddell G. Behavioural responses to examination. A reappraisal of the interpretation of 'nonorganic signs'. *Spine* 1998; **23**: 2367–71.

McBeth J, MacFarlan GJ, et al. The association between tender points, psychological distress, and adverse childhood experiences. A community-based study. *Arthritis Rheum* 1999; **42**: 1397–404.

Papgeorgiou AC, Silman AJ, Macfarlance GJ. Chronic Widespread pain in the population: a seven year follow-up study. *Ann Rheum Dis*; 2002; **61**: 1071–4.

Russell IJ, Orr MD, et al. Elevated cerebrospinal fluid levels of substance P in patients with the fibromyalgia syndrome. *Arthritis Rheum* 1994; **37**: 1593–1601.

Tofferi JK, Jackson JL. Treatment of fibromyalgia with cyclobenzaprine: a meta-analysis. *Arthritis Rheum* 2004; **51**: 9–13.

Wolfe F, Smythe Ha, et al. The ACR 1990 criteria for the classification of fibromyalgia. Report of the Multicentre Criteria Committee. *Arthritis Rheum* 1990; **33**: 160–72.

Complex regional pain syndrome type I

Background
As common as rheumatoid arthritis this condition affects peripheral and central nervous systems, and all of the tissues in the affected limb. The result is intractable pain, deformity, loss of function, and even amputation.

History
1864 Silas Weir Mitchell described causalgia in wounded soldiers of the US Civil War.
1900 Sudek described localized osteoporosis in the condition.
1947 Evans coined the term 'reflex sympathetic dystrophy'.
1959 Curtiss and Kincaid described 3 cases of transient osteoporosis.
1994 International Association for the Study of Pain (IASP) recommended the terms Complex regional pain syndrome (CRPS) type I (no nerve damage) and CRPS type II (nerve damage).

Definition
CRPS-1 is formerly known as reflex sympathetic dystrophy (RSD) or osteodystrophy. The new definition requires:
- An initiating noxious event/immobilization.
- Spontaneous pain (allodynia/hyperalgesia), disproportionate to the initiating event and non-dermatomal.
- Evidence of vascular instability, local changes in growth or function of connective tissues (skin, nails, hair, etc.).
- CRPS-1 to be a diagnosis of exclusion.

Epidemiology
2 population-based studies have been performed.
- De Mos estimated an incidence of 26 per 100 000 in the Netherlands.
- Sandroni et al estimated an incidence of 5 per 100 000 in Minnesota with a period prevalence of 21 per 100 000. as 75% underwent spontaneous resolution.

The following characteristics were apparent from these two studies:
- 7th decade gave the highest presentation.
- Upper extremity more commonly affected than lower.
- Female:Male ratio 3–4:1.
- Antecedent event (fracture commonest cause – 45%).

Aetiology and pathophysiology
Central nervous system changes can be seen and intriguingly reorganize into a more normal pattern when the disease gets better. Thalamic and somatosensory changes are the most obvious.
- Nociceptive loop, whereby noradrenaline release from the sympathetic nervous system activate nociceptors may propagate peripheral pain.
- The sympathetic nervous system, autonomic nervous system, spinal cord, peripheral fibres are all seen to demonstrate abnormalities.
- Peripheral mechanisms for the syndrome, including ischaemia, neurogenic inflammation, and immobilization have been put forward.
- Psychological factors do not appear to be any different than other patients who exhibit chronic pain.

Clinical features
Key features in the history
- Rule out other causes of syndromes similar to CRPS.
- Assess for risk factors such as co-morbidities.

A large sample of patients meeting IASP criteria for CRPS report:
- Colour and temperature asymmetry (87%).
- Spontaneous burning or stinging pain (81%).
- Hyperaesthesia (61%).
- Sweating asymmetry (53%).
- Altered skin (24%).
- Altered nail growth (21%).
- Hair growth (18%).

Other features related to cortical plasticity may be reported by the patient. These might include a change in the perception of their body schema:
- Feeling that their affected limb does not belong to them (depersonalization).
- Lack of awareness of their affected limb.
- Feeling of swelling.
- Desire to get rid of their limb (autotomy-wish).
- Neglect-like syndrome.

Key features on examination
Features related to IASP criteria:
- Mechanical and thermal allodynia (71%).
- Decreased range of movement (70%).
- Colour asymmetry (66%).
- Temperature asymmetry (56%).
- Abnormal sweating (24%).
- Dystonia (14%).
- Tremor (9%).
- Hair or nail changes (9%).
- Skin changes (20%).

Features related to cortical plasticity:
- Altered body schema (described with eyes closed).
- Digit misperception (eyes closed, which finger touched).
- Parietal lobe dysfunction (neuropsychological tests).
- Referred sensations (hand-face commonest).

Co-morbidities
Depression, anxiety and panic disorders, disorders of body image (obesity, eating disorders).

Differential diagnosis
- Fracture.
- Nerve injury.
- Infection.
- Vascular insufficiency (arterial or venous).
- CNS lesion.

Investigations
As a diagnosis of exclusion, investigations should be tailored to rule out infection, inflammation, crystal arthritis, trauma (stress fracture), and osteonecrosis or other diagnoses on the differential dependent upon clinical findings.
- Venous or lymphatic obstruction or arterial ischaemia can also be confused with CRPS-1.
- Routine blood tests and local radiographs can therefore be helpful.

- Specialized tests, such as thermography, triple phase radionuclide bone scans and MRI can give characteristic appearances, but are neither sensitive nor specific enough to confirm or refute the diagnosis.

Treatment
Objectives of management
The overriding aim of management is the functional restoration of the affected limb.

Physical therapies
Desensitization and gentle mobilization using occupational therapists and physiotherapists form the mainstay of treatment, and should be supported by nerve blocks, medications, and cognitive-behavioural therapy. A multidisciplinary team is therefore essential.

Pharmacological therapies
- Randomized controlled trials with intravenous clodronate and alendronate have demonstrated that these treatments, as well as intranasal calcitonin, are beneficial for improving pain, movement and function.
- Gabapentin is perhaps the best-studied adjunct treatment and appears to help patients, although can cause weight gain, light-headedness, and poor concentration.
- Tricyclic antidepressants may also be useful in CRPS-1, but have more side effects than SSRIs. Good trial data for CRPS-1 is lacking.
- A controlled trial of GCs in a small number of patients demonstrated improved outcome over placebo.
- Intravenous phentolamine and other sympatholytic agents, including reserpine, phenoxybenzamine, and clonidine have not demonstrated efficacy in small trials, but anecdotally help some patients.
- Thalidomide and anti-TNFα agents are being actively studied after case report evidence.
- Topical capsaicin might be useful, but is painful and difficult to apply.
- Topical lidocaine patch may be useful.
- Topical DMSO, a free radical scavenger, may also be efficacious. High dose oral vitamin C may work for similar reasons.

Interventional therapies
- There is no evidence from existing trials that guanethidine used in intravenous regional sympathetic blockade reduces the pain associated with CRPS-1 above that of placebo.
- Based on a small number of patients, there is weak evidence that ketanserin and bretylium may provide some relief. Blocks anecdotally may be helpful for patients with mechanical allodynia, and burning pains accompanied with changes in temperature and colour, or to help rehabilitation that has stalled.
- There is limited evidence of long-term benefit of *spinal cord stimulators* from a single randomized trial and a number of case series, and as technology improves this may change.
- Less data exists for spinal cord pumps with morphine, baclofen, clonidine, or ziconotide, a conotoxin-derived agent.
- Chemical or surgical sympathectomy also has little good published evidence, and the true risk-benefit balance is difficult to establish for this intervention.
- Deep brain stimulation has been tried, but is not widely available or recommended.

Psychological treatments
Hypnotherapy, imagery, progressive muscle relaxation, autogenic training, and EMG, or thermal biofeedback all have been used in treating 'learned disuse'. Cognitive approaches may also be helpful. There are no good studies to date.

Prognosis and natural history
It's likely that the majority of patients with CRPS will spontaneously resolve. What propagates the condition in some people is an area for active research. Some people will have many years of intractable pain and disrupted functioning.

Current controversies
Patients with CRPS are seen to have brain changes in the somatosensory cortex and changes in the body schema able to be detected clinically. Mechanisms involved in neuroplasticity are related to the pathophysiology of CRPS and may be therapeutic targets of the future.

Using neuropsychological techniques to study differences in patients with chronic pain, and healthy volunteers may be a productive method for studying differences in their cognitive and emotional responses that can be used for therapies and outcome measures.

There may be an autoimmune component as well as an endocrine component to CRPS that may allow treatment modalities, such as IVIg.

Resources
Assessment tools
Pain assessments (e.g. Brief pain inventory, Short form McGill); Functional assessments (e.g. upper extremity functional index; lower extremity functional index); Health quality (e.g. SF-36); Emotional assessments (e.g. HAD, BDI)

Patient organizations
UK Patient-led information and links. Available at: www.rsd-crps.co.uk

USA websites: www.rsdfoundation.org; www.rsds.org

Guidelines
American guidelines. Available at: http://www.guidelines.gov/summary

Internet sites
RNHRD, Bath inpatient programmes. Available at: www.rnhrd.nhs.uk/departments/rheumatology/complex_regional_pain_syndrome.htm

ICD-10 codes
M89.0 Algoneurodystrophy, shoulder-hand syndrome, Sudeck's atrophy, sympathetic reflex dystrophy.
G56.4 Causalgia

References
Bruehl S, Chung OY. Psychological and behavioural aspects of complex regional pain syndrome. *Clin J Pain* 2006; **22**: 430–7.

De Mos M, De Bruijn AG, et al. The incidence of complex regional pain syndrome: a population-based study. *Pain* 2007; **129**: 12–20.

Forouzanfar T, Koke AJ, et al. (2002). Treatment of complex regional pain syndrome type I. *Eur J Pain* 2002; **6**: 105–22.

Harden RN, Swan M, et al. Treatment of complex regional pain syndrome. *Clin J Pain* 2006; **22**: 420–4.

Jadad, A. R, Carroll, D, et al. Intravenous regional sympathetic blockade for pain relief in reflex sympathetic dystrophy: a systematic review and a randomized, double-blind crossover study. *J Pain Symptom Manage* 1995; **10**: 13–20.

Kingery WS. A critical review of controlled clinical trials for peripheral neuropathic pain and complex regional pain syndromes. *Pain* 1997; **73**: 123–39.

Lewis JS, Kersten P, et al. Body perception disturbance: a contribution to pain in complex regional pain syndrome. *Pain* 2007; **133**: 111–19.

McQuay HJ, Tramer M, et al. A systematic review of antidepressants in neuropathic pain. *Pain*.1996; **68**: 217–27.

Mellick GA, Mellick LB. Reflex sympathetic dystrophy treated with gabapentin. *Arch Phys Med Rehabil* 1997; **78**: 98–105.

Nelson DV, Stacey BR. Interventional therapies in the management of complex regional pain syndrome. *Clin J Pain* 2006; **22**: 438–42.

Rowbotham MC. Pharmacologic management of CRPS. *Clin J Pain* 2006; **22**: 425–9.

Sandroni P, Benrud-Larson LM, McClelland RL, Low PA. Complex Regional Pain Syndrome type I: incidence and prevalence in Olmsted county. A population-based study. Pain, 2003; **103**: 199-207.

Severens JL, Oerlemans HM, et al. Cost-effectiveness analysis of adjuvant physical or occupational therapy for patients with reflex sympathetic dystrophy. *Arch Phys Med Rehabil*. 1999; **80**: 1038–43.

Shenker NG, Cohen HC, et al. Developing concepts in allodynic pain. *Clin Med* 2008; **8**: 79–82.

Silber T. Eating disorders and reflex sympathetic dystrophy syndrome: is there a common pathway. *Med Hypotheses*, 1997; **48**: 197–200.

Taylor RS. Van Buyet JP. Spinal cord stimulation for complex regional pain syndrome: a systematic review of the clinical and cost-effectiveness literature and assessment of prognostic factors. *Eur J Pain* 2006; **10**: 91–101.

van Hilten BJ, van de Beek W-JT, et al. Intrathecal baclofen for the treatment of dystonia in patients with reflex sympathetic dystrophy. *N Engl J Med* 2000; **343**: 625–30.

Chapter 18

Miscellaneous diseases

Acromegaly *492*
Diabetes mellitus *494*
Adult onset Still's disease *496*
Amyloidosis *498*
Autoinflammatory syndromes *500*
Hyperimmunoglobulinaemia D with periodic fever syndrome *502*
TNF-receptor-associated periodic syndrome *503*
Cryopyrin-associated periodic syndrome *504*
Haemochromatosis *506*
Haemoglobinopathies *508*
Haemophilia *510*
Sarcoidosis *512*
Panniculitis *514*
Alkaptonuria *516*
Gaucher's disease *518*
Eosinophilia-myalgia syndrome and toxic oil syndrome *520*
Metabolic myopathies *522*
Synovial osteochondromatosis *526*
Pigmented villonodular synovitis *527*
Bone tumours *528*

Acromegaly

Acromegaly is caused by over secretion of growth hormone usually by a pituitary tumour.

Definition
Acromegaly is caused by over secretion of growth hormone usually by a pituitary tumour, resulting in soft tissue over-growth in adults and gigantism in children.

Aetiology
- Acromegaly is usually caused by a benign pituitary tumour (acidophilic tumour), resulting in over-production of growth hormone (GH).
- Growth hormone stimulates the growth of all tissue, with an increase in protein synthesis. Epiphyseal chondrocytes proliferate and in adults there is reactivation of chondral proliferation. Excess GH accelerates the aging process and increases the occurrence and severity of OA.

Clinical features
Acromegaly progresses slowly with enlargement of the head, face, hands, and feet.

Key features on history
Musculoskeletal
- Back pain occurs in 50%, predominately in the lumbar spine.
- 70–90% of patients develop arthralgia.

Neuropathy
Parasthesiae and pain in the hand suggestive of carpal tunnel syndrome is common, due to compression and hypertrophy of the median nerve. Carpal tunnel syndrome occurs in 50% of patients.

Myopathy
Proximal muscle weakness occurs in 50%.

Key features on examination
Soft tissue over-growth
- Characteristic facies – prominent supraorbital ridge, large nose, prognathism, thickened lips and tongue.
- Coarse thickened skin. Increased thickness of the heal pad.

Musculoskeletal
- 'Spade-like' hands due to soft tissue over-growth.
- Thoracic kyphosis and rib enlargement leading to barrel chest.
- Signs of OA: crepitus, loss range of movement, and deformity of large joints, knees, hips, and shoulders. The first MCP is typically involved.
- Palpable bursae may be thickened.

Neuropathy
- Signs of carpal tunnel syndrome: median motor and sensory impairment, positive Phalen's and Tinel's sign.
- Ulnar and popliteal nerves may be enlarged and palpable.
- Spinal cord compression and cauda equina syndrome are rare.

Muscle disease
Proximal weakness out of proportion to the increased muscle mass. Decreased exercise tolerance.

General investigations
Radiological investigations
- Cartilage hypertrophy. Widening of the joint space occurs combined with soft tissue and synovial hypertrophy. Most frequently seen in the knees, MCP, and interphalangeal (IP) joints.
- Cartilaginous and osseous degeneration. Thickened cartilage is prone to premature degeneration. The earliest sign is the vacuum sign in the knee joints. Small osteophytes and increased joint space are very suggestive of acromegaly.
- In the terminal phalanges a typical feature is the enlargement of the tuft and base of the distal phalange.

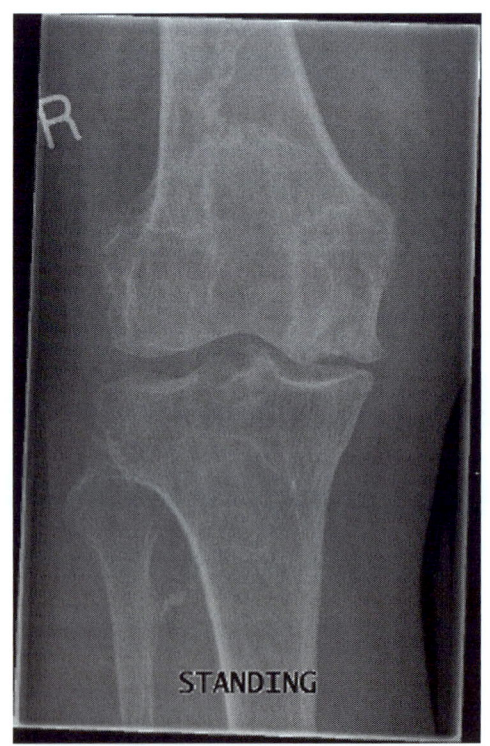

Figure 18.1 Standing plain radiograph of knee, showing early osteoarthritic changes and an increase in joint space.

Differential diagnosis

The combination of clinical and radiological features should make the diagnosis straightforward. In acromegaly, non-weight bearing joints, such as elbows and shoulders are involved unlike primary OA. Hyperostosis may resemble DISH.

Treatment

- Treatment is of the primary pituitary tumour. Soft tissue over-growth manifestations are often improved by reduction in GH levels.
- Degenerative hyperostotic manifestations do not improve after reduction of GH levels.

References

Liote F, Orcel P. Osteoarticular disorders of endocrine origin. *Baillieres Best Pract Res Clin Rheumatol* 2000; **14**: 251–76.

Forgacs S. Acromegaly. In: Hochberg M, Silman A, Smolen J, Weinblatt M, Weisman M (eds) *Rheumatology*, 3rd edn. Ottawa: Mosby 2003

Diabetes mellitus

Diabetes mellitus is characterized by chronic hyperglycaemia this leads to metabolic dysfunction and protein disorders. A variety of musculoskeletal disorders occur in long duration diabetics.

Diabetic osteoarthropathy

This is a late complication of diabetes mellitus, occurring in up to 1.4% of diabetics predominately in the over 50 years of age group.

It affects predominately the foot joints, with the MTPJs most commonly involved.

Clinical features

Key features on history
The pain is much less severe than expected because neuropathy is always also present.
- **Musculoskeletal:** swelling of the foot joints that is relatively painless.
- **Neurological:** parasthesiae and numbness.
- **Cutaneous:** ulcer formation.

Key features on examination
- **Musculoskeletal:** increased joint mobility due laxity of the joint capsule.
- **Soft tissue swelling:** metatarsal joint destruction with foot shortening, collapse of the medial arch led to development of the 'rocker bottom foot'.
- **Neurological:** sensory neuropathy, loss of vibration sense and decreased reflexes.
- **Cutaneous:** neuropathic plantar ulcers occur in association with bone destruction.

Radiological investigation
Plain radiology is the best means of making the diagnosis. Three stages can be identified on plain radiographs
- Porosis, cortical defects, and subluxation.
- Osteolysis, fragmentation, fractures, periosteal reaction.
- Cortical defect filing, deforming arthritis, ankylosis.

MRI is useful for distinguishing diabetic osteoarthropathy from osteomyelitis.

Differential diagnosis
Diabetic osteoarthropathy must be distinguished from infection, osteoarthritis, other neuropathic arthropathies, tumours, and inflammatory arthritis.

Pathogenesis
- Neuropathy is the major cause of osteoarthropathy and the osteolysis is due to neurogenic factors and not inflammation.
- Infection and microangiopathy play a less significant role.

Prognosis
Osteolysis may stop spontaneously with healing.

Treatment
- Conservative management is key with good care of ulcers; a combined approach with a diabetic foot care team is essential. Surgery should be avoided if possible.
- Good control of diabetes is essential both to treat established disease, and also to prevent developvment of late complications of diabetes such as neuropathy and osteoarthropathy.

Diabetic cheiroarthropathy

Most commonly occurs in long-standing type I diabetics.

Clinical features

Key features on history
- Parasthesiae and pain are the earliest features, which progresses very slowly.
- Loss of hand function.

Key features on examination
- Thick, tight waxy skin.
- Joint restriction and sclerosis of tendon sheaths.
- Typical prayer sign with the patient unable to press the hands together.

Pathogenesis
Diabetic microangiopathy is thought to be the main factor.

Treatment
There is no specific treatment apart from good diabetic control, analgesia and symptomatic management.

Diabetic femoral amyotrophy

- Diabetic femoral amyotrophy is characterized by severe unilateral anterior thigh pain followed by wasting and weakness of quadriceps muscles and loss knee reflex. It is bilateral in 50% of patients.
- Recovery begins at 3 months and is usually complete by 18 months.

Muscle infarction

- Muscle infarction is a rare cause of severe pain in diabetics. There is acute severe pain and swelling of muscle, typically the thigh.
- Muscle biopsy shows necrosis and oedema.
- Resolution occurs over a few weeks, but recurrence is common.

References

Liote F, Orcel P. Osteoarticular disorders of endocrine origin. *Baillieres Best Pract Res Clin Rheumatol* 2000; **14**: 251–76.

CHAPTER 18 Miscellaneous diseases

Adult onset Still's disease

Definition
Adult onset Still's disease (AOSD) is a rare condition characterized by recurrent episodes of inflammation.

Diagnostic criteria
There are several sets of diagnostic criteria of which the Yamaguchi are the most sensitive (93.5%).

> **Yamaguchi criteria for Adult onset Still's disease**
>
> *Major criteria*
> - Arthritis.
> - Swelling or limitation of motion, warmth, pain, stiffness.
> - Duration of 6 weeks.
> - Exclusion other reasons for arthropathy.
> - Fever (>39.0°C) persisting, intermittent.
> - Typical rash: persistent eruption is NOT characteristic of the disease.
> - Elevated WBC > 10 000.
>
> *Minor criteria*
> - Sore throat.
> - Lymphadenopathy or splenomegaly.
> - Abnormal LFTs – not attributable to drug toxicity or allergy.
> - Negative ANA or RF.
>
> *Exclusion criteria*
> Infection, malignancy, vasculitis.
>
> To establish a diagnosis of AOSD, patients require five criteria including two major criteria. From Yamaguchi et al. (1992).

Epidemiology
- The incidence is 1–2/million/year.
- Sex distribution is equal.
- The peak age of onset is 16–35 years.

Aetiology
- The aetiology is unknown, but the clinical presentation with fever, rash, sore throat, and lymphadenopathy suggests an infectious cause. A viral aetiology has most often been suggested, but no agent has yet been identified.
- There is no clear association with HLA or other genetic markers. No clear environmental factors have been found.
- Pro-inflammatory cytokines, such as IL-1, Il-6, IL-18, interferon gamma, TNF, and macrophage colony stimulating factor are raised, and thought to have role in the pathogenesis.

Clinical features
AOSD affects many organs. The full spectrum of clinical features may not be present at onset and only may develop over a few weeks.

Key features on history
Systemic
- Fever is almost universal with virtually all patients exhibiting a fever > 39°C, spiking usually during the evening or night.
- Sore throat occurs in up to 92% of cases.
- Weight loss of > 10% occurs in 75%.
- Lymphadenopathy occurs in 65%. Hepatosplenomegaly occurs in 50%.

Musculoskeletal
- Joint pain is a common feature and is greatest during febrile episodes.. It becomes worse during the course of illness and may be very mild at presentation.
- Myalgia (75%) can be severe and also increases during febrile episodes.
- Abdominal pain is usually mild and infrequently severe enough to warrant laparotomy.
- Pleurisy and pericarditis occur in 30–40% of patients.

Key features on examination
Musculoskeletal
- Initially the synovitis is migratory and additive, but becomes more persistent. This can involve both large and small joints (both PIPJ and DIPJ of the hands), with the knee being most commonly involved (84%).
- The axial skeleton is infrequently involved.

Skin
- The rash is characteristically salmon pink, macular, or maculopapular.
- It is evanescent and occurs during febrile attacks lasting for several hours.
- Lymphadenopathy (65%) most commonly occurs in the cervical region, the nodes are mobile and tender.

General investigations
The diagnosis is often delayed due to the non-specific nature of the illness.
- FBC anaemia of chronic disease, leucocytosis (WBC>15 $\times 10^9$/l in 80%), thrombocytosis.
- Acute phase response (ESR and CRP) is raised in all patients.
- Liver function abnormal in 75%.
- Ferritin: hyperferritinaemia with extreme elevation is common. It is unrelated to iron metabolism and is due to cytokine-induced increased synthesis by the reticuloendothelial system.

Serological investigations
- ANCA, ANA, RF, anticardiolipin antibodies. These are usually negative.
- Complement levels are normal.
- Cryoglobulins.

Synovial fluid
Synovial fluid is inflammatory with raised white cell count.

Biopsy
Lymph node and skin biopsy are not needed for the diagnosis, but is often performed to exclude malignancy or vasculitis.

Differential diagnosis
- The differential diagnosis is broad and the diagnosis is essentially that of exclusion. Granulomatous disorders, vasculitis, infection, malignancy, and connective tissue disease all need to be ruled out.

- Schnitzler syndrome is rare, but shares many features with AOSD, including high fever, lymphadenopathy, hepatosplenomegaly, raised acute phase response, and leucocytosis. However, there is urticaria and a monoclonal IgM gammopathy and less marked elevation in ferritin.

Prognosis
- The course is monophasic in 61.5% of cases and relapsing in 38.5%. The median duration of treatment is 10 years.
- Chronic articular involvement occurs in one-third.
- Presence of polyarthritis especially shoulder or hip joint early in the disease course is predictive of a chronic course.
- Death is uncommon, but is due to infection, hepatic failure, and disseminated intravascular coagulation.

Pathology
- Lymph node histology shows infiltrates of plasma cells, and polymorphonuclear leucocytes and reactive hyperplasia.
- Skin biopsy shows a mild perivascular inflammation of the superficial dermis with few lymphocytes or neutrophils.
- Liver biopsy mononuclear sinusoidal and portal tract infiltrates with mild Kupffer cell hyperplasia. Focal hepatitis is less common.

Patient advice
- Diagnosis of exclusion.
- Requires long-term therapy, but in general the prognosis is good.

Treatment
- There are no randomized controlled trials in AOSD.
- Often, in the first instance, around 20–25% of patients respond well. Aspirin is often still used in relatively high doses.
- Oral corticosteroids usually give quick symptom relief. 0.5–1.0 mg/kg may be required initially. Pulse intravenous corticosteroids are not usually needed. Depending on response the dose may be tapered quite quickly
- Chronic polyarthritis is managed with low dose oral corticosteroids. Immunosuppressive agents, such as methotrexate, may have a place in reducing steroid exposure and preventing long-term joint damage. Other immunosuppressive drugs that have been utilized include azathioprine, leflunomide, ciclosporin, and cyclophosphamide.
- Other agents used experimentally include intravenous gamma globulin, inhibitors of TNF-alpha, IL-1, and Il-6.

Follow-up
Every 3–6 months as patients condition dictates. AOSD is a relapsing condition and lifelong follow-up is required.

Resources
Guidelines
There are no guidelines specifically for AOSD, but reference should be made to local guidance on steroid induced osteoporosis, use and monitoring of immunosuppressive therapy and vaccination.

Patient organizations
International Still's Disease Foundation.
www.stillsdisease.org

ICD-10 coding
M06.1   Adult-oset Still's disease.

References
Efthimiou P, Kontzias A, Ward CM, Ogden N. Adult-onset Still's disease: can recent advances in our understanding of its pathogenesis lead to targeted therapy. *Nat Clin Pract Rheumatol* 2007; **3**: 328–35.

Esdaile JM. Adult Still's disease. In: Hochberg M, Silman A, Smolen J, Weinblatt M, Weisman M (eds) *Rheumatology*, 3rd edn. Ottawa: Mosby, 2003: 793–80.

Kadar J, Petrovicz E. Adult-onset Still's disease. *Best Prac Res Clin Rheumatol* 2004; **18**: 663–74.

Yamaguchi M, Ohta A, Tsunematsu T, *et al.* Preliminary criteria for classification of adult-Still's disease. *J Rheumatol* 1992; **19**: 424–30.

Amyloidosis

Definition
The amyloidoses are a group of disorders characterized by deposition of extracellular amyloid fibrils.

Epidemiology
AA type
The most common type of systemic amyloidosis worldwide is AA type. The most common associations in Western countries are chronic inflammatory conditions, whilst in regions where infection is common it is associated with tuberculosis and leprosy (Table 18.1). The reported frequency of AA amyloidosis in inflammatory disease varies widely across the world is probably dependent on the means of diagnosis.

AL type
In the USA, AL type is most common, the incidence in Olmsted County was estimated to be 1/100 000 between 1950 and 1989. In Holland, the prevalence is 1/75 000. 20% of people with multiple myeloma develop AL amyloidosis.

Aβ2-microglobulin
Aβ2-microglobulin amyloidosis occurs in chronic haemodialysis.

Aetiology
- Amyloid deposition reflects a conformational change in the structure of the precursor protein and is the final common endpoint of several different processes.
- There are at least 23 amyloid precursors. A common feature is a β-pleated sheet either in the native protein or after conformational change, which is deposited, and disrupts the organization and function of tissues and organs.
- In the AA type the fibrils are derived from the acute phase protein serum amyloid A (SAA) through a process of cleavage, misfolding and aggregation into a highly ordered abnormal β-sheet conformation. SAA is an apolipoprotein constituent of high-density lipoprotein, which is synthesized by hepatocytes stimulated by pro-inflammatory cytokines. Prolonged over synthesis of SAA is a requirement for development of AA amyloidosis, but why only a small proportion of patients with chronic inflammation develop amyloidosis is unknown.
- In the AL type, the precursor is Ig light chain (κ or λ), λ light chains are more amyloidogenic. Structural changes in the light chain may be responsible for amyloidogenesis, either deletions resulting in small chains or glycosylation.
- In Aβ2-microglobulin amyloidosis, the precursor protein is β2-microglobulin. Improved haemodialysis techniques have reduced the frequency of this complication.

Clinical features
Key features on history
General
Symptoms suggestive of amyloidosis include proteinuria especially developing in the context of chronic inflammatory disease or infection. In a recent series of AA amyloid the mean duration of symptomatic inflammatory disease before development of amyloidosis was 17 years (Lachmann et al, 2007). The clinical features of AA amyloid are the same irrespective of the underlying inflammatory disease.

Musculoskeletal
- In AL type amyloidosis joint involvement is infrequent. Joint stiffness occurs more than pain. Involves both large and small joints either in a symmetrical or asymmetrical manner.
- Aβ2-microglobulin amyloidosis occurs in the setting of chronic dialysis. Always involves the joints and skeleton. There is infiltration of the carpal ligament leading to symptoms of carpal tunnel syndrome, which in this setting should prompt investigation for amyloidosis. Neck pain is due to a destructive spondyloarthropathy.
- Musculoskeletal involvement is not a feature of familial transthyretin amyloidoses, but neuropathic joints can develop due to the severe neuropathy.

Renal disease
Renal disease is the typical presentation of AA (97% at presentation) and AL amyloidosis. Development of proteinuria in a patient with longstanding active inflammatory disease should prompt investigation for AA amyloidosis.

Neuropathy
A sensorimotor proximal or distal polyneuropathy is the presenting feature in 10–20% of AL amyloidosis. Occurs in the familial TTR amyloidoses

Cardiac
Cardiac involvement occurs in 20% of AL patients, but is much rarer (<10%) in AA amyloidosis, and results in a cardiomyopathy and arrhythmias.

Key features on examination
Musculoskeletal
- In AL amyloidosis there is stiffness of joints with little swelling. Infiltration of the skin may produce palpable pads e.g. over the shoulders.
- Aβ₂-microglobulin. Stiff painful peripheral joints with a destructive arthropathy, most common sites are wrist, shoulders, hips, knees, and spine.

Table 18.1 Associations of AA amyloidosis

Inflammatory arthritis (60%)
• Rheumatoid arthritis (most common worldwide (33%))
• Juvenile idiopathic arthritis (17%)
• Others including ankylosing spondylitis (10%)
Chronic Infection (15%)
• Bronchiectasis (5%)
• Injection drug abuse (4%)
• Complication paraplegia (ulcers etc) (2%)
• Osteomyelitis (1%)
• Tuberculosis (1%)
Periodic fever syndromes (9%)
• Familial Mediterranean fever (5%)
• TNF-receptor-associated periodic fever syndrome (2%)
Inflammatory Bowel Disease (5%)
Malignancy (1%)

Percentages from a series of 374 patients (Lachmann et al., 2007).

Neuropathy
- Proximal and distal sensorimotor neuropathy. Autonomic neuropathy may occur with postural hypotension, and incontinence. Neuropathy is not seen in AA amyloidosis.
- Signs of carpal tunnel syndrome especially in $A\beta_2$-microglobulin amyloidosis.

General investigations
There are no specific serological or urine markers of amyloidosis. CRP, SSA, and other acute phase reactants are not specific markers, as they are raised in chronic inflammation and most patients with chronic inflammation do not develop amyloidosis.
- Assessment of renal function with quantification of proteinuria (nephrotic range > 3 g/24 h). Hypoproteinaemia supports a diagnosis of nephrotic syndrome.
- Serum and urine immunofixation, serum-free light chains. The presence of monoclonal Ig or free light chains suggests AL amyloidosis.
- Bone marrow aspiration may be required to demonstrate monoclonal plasma cell proliferation and production of free light chains.
- Investigations for hereditary forms of amyloidosis – mutations in genes encoding for transthyretin, fibrinogen A -chain, apolipoprotein A-I, apolipoprotein A-II, and lysozyme.

Biopsy
Rectal biopsy or subcutaneous fat aspiration are the techniques of choice for obtaining tissue for diagnosis.

Imaging
X-ray
Plain radiographic features of amyloidosis include osteoporosis, lytic lesions, pathological fractures, osteonecrosis, subchondral cysts and erosions.

Ultrasound
US may show thickening of soft tissues around joints and especially in the wrist.

MRI
- MRI may show thickened synovium and soft tissue infiltration.
- MRI is the method of choice for investigating possible amyloid deposits, especially in $A\beta_2$-microglobulin amyloidosis.

Nuclear medicine
Serum amyloid P (SaP) scanning uses iodinated SaP that binds to amyloid fibrils. It is useful in demonstrating the extent of amyloid deposition and can be used to measure response to treatment.

Synovial fluid
The synovial fluid is characteristically non-inflammatory and may contain amyloid fibrils.

Differential diagnosis
This is from other causes of nephrotic syndrome or neuropathy. Drugs particularly gold and penicillin may cause proteinuria.

Pathology
Samples for assessment of possible amyloidosis should be stained using Congo red and examined under polarizing light microscopy. Amyloid fibrils will have apple green birefringence.

Treatment
- **AA amyloidosis:** the treatment is to control the underlying inflammatory condition or chronic infection. With treatment regression of amyloid deposits can be observed using serial SaP scanning.
- **AL amyloidosis:** the aim is to reduce production of amyloid forming monoclonal light chain by treatment of the underlying plasma cell dyscrasia.

Prognosis
- The median survival in AA amyloidosis is 133 months.
- Factors associated with a poor prognosis are age at presentation and end-stage renal failure.

Resources
Patient organizations
Amyloidosis support network. www.amyloidosis.org.

ICD-10 coding
E.85   Amyloidosis

References
Buxbaum J. Amyloidosis. In: Hochberg MC, Silman A, Smolen JS, Weinblatt M, Weisman MH (eds) *Rheumatology*. Ottawa: Mosby, 2004: 2015–25.

Comenzo RL. Current and emerging views and treatments of systemic immunoglobulin light-chain (Al) amyloidosis. *Contrib Nephrol* 2007; **153**: 195–210.

Kiss E, Keusch G, Zanetti M, et al. Dialysis-related amyloidosis revisited. *Am J Res* 2005; **185**: 1460–7.

Lachmann HJ, Goodman HJ, Gibertson JA, et al. Natural history and outcome in systemic AA amyloidosis. *N Engl J Med* 2007; **356**: 2361–71.

See also
Rheumatoid arthritis
Autoinflammatory syndromes.

Autoinflammatory syndromes

The autoinflammatory syndromes are a group of inherited conditions characterized by inflammation, arthralgias, and a propensity for development of secondary AA amyloidosis.

The conditions include: familial Mediterranean fever (FMF), hyperimmunoglobulin D with periodic fever syndrome (HIDS), tumour-necrosis factor (TNF)-receptor-associated periodic syndrome (TRAPS), cryopyrin associated periodic syndrome (CAPS). They are distinguished from systemic onset JIA in the child because children are usually well between attacks. The conditions are all very rare and are best investigated at specialized centres.

Familial Mediterranean fever

Classification criteria
The Tel Hashomer criteria are widely used to clinically define FMF.

Tel Hashomer criteria for FMF

Major criteria
- Recurrent febrile episodes accompanied by peritonitis, synovitis or pleuritis
- Amyloidosis of the AA-type without predisposing disease
- Favourable response to colchicine treatment

Minor criteria
- Recurrent febrile episodes
- Erysipelas like erythema
- FMF in a first degree relative

Definitive diagnosis: 2 major or 1 major and 2 minor. Probable diagnosis: 1 major and 1 minor.
The specificity in a Jewish population is > 95%.

Epidemiology
- Autosomal recessive condition
- Most frequent in individuals of non-Ashkenazi Jewish, Armenian, Arab, or Turkish ethnic origin.
- Relatively common amongst non-Ashkenazi (Eastern European) Jews and Italians.
- Carrier frequencies of 1:3 and 1:5 have been reported in some populations.

Aetiology
Molecular genetics
The FMF gene, MEFV, is located on the short arm of chromosome 16p13.3 and is a 10-exon gene encoding pyrin a 781 amino acid protein.

There are 4 common missense mutations – substitution of isoleucine for methionine at codon 680 (M680I); valine for methionine at 694 (M694V); of isoleucine for methionine at codon 694 (M694I); alanine for valine at 726 (V726A), but over 100 variants have been described.

The MEFV gene produces a pyrin and is expressed in myeloid cells. Pyrin is believed to regulate inflammation by via apoptosis. Mutated variants of pyrin are unable to regulate inflammation especially pathways involving IL-1B and NFkB.

Clinical features
Key features on history
- The acute attacks of FMF are characterized by fever, serositis, rash, and arthralgia. The duration of attacks is 24–72 h, but joint pain can last for 1 week.
- Attacks are not truly periodic, but can occur at widely varying intervals and, thus, are episodic.
- There is often no obvious precipitant, but emotion, exercise, and menstruation have all been associated.
- Between attacks patients are asymptomatic.

Systemic
The height of the fever varies between patients, but is higher in children.

Cutaneous
Tender red plaques on the legs.

Serosal
- Abdominal pain is the second most common feature and occurs in >90%.
- Pleurisy is common and often occurs with abdominal pain. Sharp, stabbing chest pain, worse on inspiration, coughing. Pain may be referred to the shoulder from the diaphragm.
- Pericardial chest pain is uncommon.

Musculoskeletal
- Arthralgias with or without joint swelling present initially in childhood. Most frequently, monarticular, typically involving the knee or ankle. Polyarticular or oligoarticular presentations are less common.
- Prolonged episodes of myalgia can develop in association with fever (protracted febrile myalgia); and are thought to be due to vasculitis.

Key features on examination
Cutaneous
The most characteristic lesion is a tender erythematous plaque on the dorsum of the foot, ankle, or calf.

Musculoskeletal
- Inflammatory synovitis most commonly affecting the lower limb joints, in a monarticular pattern. The effusion may be quite large.
- Destructive arthritis rarely occurs.

Serosal
- Diffuse abdominal tenderness, which may be sufficiently severe to mimic an acute abdomen.
- Signs of a pleural effusion may be present.
- Pericarditis is uncommon.

General investigations
Investigation is directed at establishing the diagnosis.
- FBC anaemia (only if severe GI or renal haemorrhage), leucocytosis.
- Acute phase response. The ESR, CRP, serum amyloid A (SAA), fibrinogen, and haptoglobin are all raised.

Serological investigations
- ANA, ANCA, RF should all be negative. A positive ANA or ANCA suggests the presence of a connective tissue disease or other vasculitis.
- Complement levels are normal.

Genetic screening
Patients with typical clinical features should be screened for the common mutations (see above)

Differential diagnosis
The diagnosis is based on clinical manifestations. Patients with typical clinical features may not have demonstrable mutations. Since the advent of genetic screening patients with milder features are being discovered who do not fulfil recognized criteria.

Prognosis
- Overall prognosis is determined by the risk of development of AA amyloidosis.
- The risk of amyloidosis varies between mutations with the risk apparently highest for patients with the M694V mutation. A family history of amyloidosis also increases the risk suggesting that other genes are important including the SAA1 a/a genotype.

Patient advice
- Recessively inherited condition. Recurrent attacks of abdominal pain, fever, and joint pain.
- Amyloidosis is the most serious complication.

Treatment
- Colchicine (1–2 mg/day) is the basis of treatment. The dose is limited by gastrointestinal side effects – diarrhoea, cramping, and bloating.
- Colchicine prevents acute inflammatory attacks and also the long-term development of amyloidosis.
- Glucocorticoids appear to be ineffective.
- Anecdotal reports describe successful use of TNF-alpha blockade and Anakinra in colchicine resistant cases.

Follow-up
Long-term follow-up is required with regular urinalysis is necessary to detect development of amyloidosis.

Resources
Internet resources
OMIM 249100 www.ncbi.nlm.nih.gov/entrez/

ICD-10 code
E85.0 Non-neuropathic heredofamilial amyloidosis. Familial Mediterranean fever

References
Livneh A, Langevitz P, Zemer D, et al. Criteria for the diagnosis of familial Mediterranean fever. *Arthritis Rheum* 1997; **40**: 1879–85.

Ozel AM, Demitürk L, Yazgan Y, Avsar K, Günay A, Gürbüz AK et al. Familial Mediterranean fever: a review of the disease and clinical and laboratory findings in 105 patients. *Dig Liver Dis* 2000; **32**: 504–9.

Yao Q, Furst D. Autoinflammatory diseases: an update of clinical and genetic aspects. *Rheumatology* 2008; **47**: 946–51

Hyperimmunoglobulinaemia D with periodic fever syndrome

HIDS is characterized by recurrent attacks similar to FMF, but with the presence of raised levels of IgD in serum.

Epidemiology
A rare condition, most pedigrees are clustered in northern Europe.

Aetiology
Molecular genetics
HIDS is a recessively inherited condition defined by mutations in the mevalonate kinase gene (*MVK*) located at 12q24, which catalyses the conversion of mevalonic acid to 5-phosphomevalonic acid, a key stage in the biosynthesis of cholesterol and isoprenoid. The most common mutation is a substitution of isoleucine for valine at codon 377 (V377I). The exact mechanism is uncertain, defective apoptosis of lymphocytes may be important, and the role of raised IgD is unknown. IgD can increase TNF-α and IL-1 levels.

Clinical features
Key features on history
- The median age of onset is <6 months.
- Vaccinations may trigger attacks, as well as infections, emotion, trauma, and surgery.
- The usual length of attacks of high fever is 3–7 days. The interval between attacks is variable, but typically 4–6 weeks.

Serosal
The majority of patients have attacks of abdominal pain, which may be severe enough to require laparotomy. Diarrhoea is seen more frequently than in FMF.

Musculoskeletal
- 70% of patients experience arthralgias, with knees and ankles most commonly involved.
- Attacks may be polyarticular in contrast to FMF.

Key features on examination
Lymphadenopathy
Widespread, tender lymphadenopathy is more common in HIDS than the other autoinflammatory syndromes. Swelling varies with attacks.

Musculoskeletal
Large joint arthritis varying with severity of the febrile episode and with abdominal pain.

Mucocutaneous
- Crops of erythematous red macules 0.5–2.0 cm in diameter are the most common feature.
- Painful aphthous orogenital ulcers are sometimes found.
- Hepatosplenomegaly is seen.

General investigations
- FBC leucocytosis with left shift.
- Acute phase response. The ESR, CRP, serum amyloid A (SAA), fibrinogen and haptoglobin are all raised.
- Serum IgD elevation > 14.1mg/dl on two occasions at least 1 month apart.
- Urine mevalonic acid levels are raised during attacks.
- Genetic screening
- Mutational analysis initially looking for the most common mutations V377I or I268T mutations. If this is negative a more comprehensive genome screen can be conducted.

Differential diagnosis
This is from the other autoinflammatory conditions. Some patients have MVK mutation, but normal IgD levels and are termed variant HIDS.

Prognosis
Unlike the other autoinflammatory syndromes amyloidosis has not been reported in HIDS. The frequency and severity of attacks tend to diminish with age.

Treatment
There is no proven treatment. NSAIDs may control fever and joint pain. Corticosteroids may help some patients. Colchicine is ineffective.

Resources
Internet resources
OMIM 260920
www.ncbi.nlm.nih.gov/entrvez/

References
Drenth JP, Haagsma CJ, van der Meer JM. Hypergammaglobulinae-miaD and periodic fever syndrome. *Medicine (Baltimore)* 1994; 73: 133–44.

Yao Q, Furst D. Autoinflammatory diseases: an update of clinical and genetic aspects. *Rheumatology* 2008; **47**: 946–51.

TNF-receptor-associated periodic syndrome

TRAPs comprise a group of dominantly inherited fever syndromes, which were previously known under a variety of terms including, e.g. familial Hibernian fever. The discovery of the genetic basis led to the syndromes being linked, being due to mutations in the 55 Kd receptor for TNF-α.

Epidemiology
The original pedigrees were described in Hibernian families, but a broad ethnic distribution has since been described.
The condition is inherited as an autosomal dominant.

Aetiology
Molecular genetics
TNF-α has two receptors a 55kDa molecule (p55) and a 75kDa molecule (p75). The p55 receptor is encoded by *TNFRSF1A* on chromosome 12p13.2, whilst the p75 receptor is encoded by *TNFRSF1B* on chromosome 1p36.3-p36.2. The p55 receptor is expressed on a wide variety of cell types, whilst the p75 is restricted to leucocytes and endothelial cells. TRAPs is caused by mutations in *TNFRSF1A*.

The most frequent mutation is R92Q. Levels of TNFRSF1A protein is low in plasma and the aberrant form of TNFR1 is present on cell surface. Neutralization of TNF-α is impeded and TNF-α driven inflammation is uncontrolled. However, the precise pathogenesis of the clinical features is not completely understood.

Clinical features
- The median age of onset is 3 years.
- The duration of attacks is longer than for the other syndromes lasting longer than 1 week.

Serosal
- Abdominal pain and serositis may be severe.
- Pleurisy with chest pain occurs.
- Scrotal pain due to inflammation of the tunica vaginalis occurs but uncommonly.

Musculoskeletal
- Arthralgia is more frequent than arthritis occurring in two-thirds of patients. Usually non-erosive, and monarticular or oligoarticular.
- Myalgia occurs frequently, unlike FMF. There is a region of muscle pain, which is warm and tender. There is an overlying area of erythema which blanches with pressure. Biopsy shows a panniculitis, fasciitis and perivascular inflammation, but no myositis.

Ocular
8% of patients experience conjunctivitis, periorbital oedema, and or periorbital pain. Iritis and uveitis are less common.

General investigations
- FBC leucocytosis with left shift. Anaemia of chronic disease.
- Acute phase response. The ESR, CRP, serum amyloid A (SAA), fibrinogen and haptoglobin are all raised.
- Polyclonal increase in gamma globulins.
- Mevalonic aciduria.

Serological investigations
- ANA, ANCA, RF should all be negative. A positive ANA or ANCA suggests the presence of a connective tissue disease or other vasculitis.
- Complement levels are normal.

Genetic screening
Mutational analysis initially looking for the most common mutations.

Differential diagnosis
This is from the other autoinflammatory conditions. The diagnosis is made by establishing a mutation in *TNFRSF1A* in a patient with an unexplained fever syndrome.

Prognosis
14% of patients develop AA amyloidosis.

Treatment
- Colchicine is ineffective in preventing the febrile attacks and also it does not prevent amyloidosis.
- Glucocorticoids can be used to treat acute attacks.
- Etanercept has been used with mixed results, but is considered useful as a steroid sparing agent.

Resources
Internet resources
OMIM 142680 www.ncbi.nlm.nih.gov/omim

References
Dodé C, André M, Bienvenu T, Hausfater, Pêcheux C, Bienvenu J, et al. The enlarging clinical, genetic, and population spectrum of tumour necrosis factor receptor-associated periodic syndrome. *Arthritis Rheum* 2002; **46**: 2181–8.

Yao Q, Furst D. Autoinflammatory diseases: an update of clinical and genetic aspects. *Rheumatology* 2008; **47**: 946–51.

Cryopyrin-associated periodic syndrome

The cryopyrin associated periodic syndrome (CAPS) is a group conditions previously considered to be separate entities, but recently shown to be due to mutations in the CIAS1 gene. The group includes Muckle Well syndrome (MWS), familial cold inflammatory condition (FCAS), and neonatal onset multi-system inflammatory disease (NOMID)/chronic infantile neurological cutaneous and articular syndrome (CINCA).

MWS is characterized by attacks of fever, malaise, arthralgias, and urticaria.

Epidemiology
- A rare condition, the initial cases were all described in Europe.
- The inheritance is autosomal dominant.

Aetiology
Molecular genetics
CAPS is caused by mutations in the CIAS1 gene located on chromosome 1q44. The encoded protein is cryopyrin and >40 mutations are known. The CIAS1 gene product cryopyrin (also known as PYPAF1 or NALP3) is part of the inflammasome and is essential for activation of caspase 1 and processing of IL-1 and IL-18. Thus, the effects of mutations may be mediated by their effects on IL-1, IL-18, and NFkB.

Clinical features
Key features on history and examination
- The age of onset is variable from infancy to adolescence.
- Attacks last 12–48 h.
- FCAS is the mildest syndrome. CINCA/NOMID is the most severe.

Musculoskeletal
Arthralgias are more common and affect predominantly large joints. The pattern is typically oligoarticular.

Cutaneous
The rash is erythematosus geographical plaque, reminiscent of urticaria, but they do not itch. They 'ache'.

Sensorineural hearing loss
- 70% of cases with MWS develop progressive sensori neural hearing loss.
- Deafness also occurs in CINCA/NOMID.

General investigations
- FBC leucocytosis with left shift.
- Acute phase response. The ESR, CRP, serum amyloid A (SAA), fibrinogen, and haptoglobin are all raised.

Genetic screening
Mutational analysis initially looking for the most common mutations.

Differential diagnosis
This is from the other autoinflammatory conditions.

Prognosis
25% of patients develop AA amyloidosis.

Treatment
- There is no proven treatment. NSAIDs may control fever and joint pain. Corticosteroids may help some patients.
- Therapy targeting the IL-1B pathway with IL-!ra (anakinra) have been effective in a small number of patients.

Table 18.2 Major discriminating features of the auotinflammatory condition

	FMF	TRAPS	HIDS	CAPS
Age of onset	<20 years	<20 years	Median 6 months	<6 months
Fever duration	1–3 days	> 7 days	3–7 days	1–2 days
Serositis	±±	±±	±	±
Musculoskeletal	Monarthritis	Monarthritis, myalgia	Polyarthritis	Deforming arthritis
Cutaneous	Erysipeloid	Erysipeloid	Macules, papules, urticaria	Urticaria
Adenopathy	Rare	Rare	Yes	Rare
Deafness	No	No	No	Yes
Amyoidosis	±±±	±±	±	±
Inheritance	Recessive	Dominant	Recessive	Dominant
Gene mutation	MEFV	TNFRSF1A	MVK	CIAS1
Gene product	Pyrin/marenostrin	TNFR1A	Mevalonate kinase	Cryopyrin
Therapy				
Colchicine	±±	–	–	–
Glucocorticoids	–	±	–	–
TNF-α blockers	±	±	±	–
IL-1 antagonists	–	±	±	±±

Adapted from Yao & Furst (2008).

Resources

Internet resources
OMIM 191100
www.ncbi.nlm.nih.gov/omim

References

Aksentijevich I, Putnam C, Remmer EF, Mueller JL, Le J, Kolodner RD, et al. The clinical continuum of cryopyrinopathies: novel CIAS1 mutations in North American patients and a new cryopyrin model. *Arthritis Rheum* 2007; **56**: 1273–85.

Yao Q, Furst D. Autoinflammatory diseases: an update of clinical and genetic aspects. *Rheumatology* 2008; **47**: 946–51.

Haemochromatosis

Haemochromatosis is an inherited condition of iron storage, which results in a characteristic arthropathy, first described in 1964.

Epidemiology
- Haemochromatosis is most common in Northern European populations – the highest prevalence being Ireland, UK, Brittany and Scandinavia.
- The annual incidence is 2–4/100 000 with a prevalence of 20–80/100 000.
- In the USA 1 in 227 white Caucasians are homozygous for the *HFE* C282Y mutation. In Ireland the rate is 1 in 83.
- Males and females are affected equally. Males present typically between ages 25–70 and females after the menopause.
- There is an association with HLA-A3-B14 (relative risk 23).

Aetiology
- Iron is poorly excreted in man and in haemochromatosis there is increased absorption from the diet leading to iron overload.
- Hepcidin controls extracellular iron concentration by binding to and inducing the degradation of the cellular iron exporter ferroportin. Iron absorption is related to hepcidin, which has a key position in the pathological changes in haemochromatosis. Deficiency of hepcidin is seen in many iron overload states with increased iron absorption. The precise mechanism by which the HFE C282Y protein, ferroportin and hepcidin interact is unclear.

Genetics
Haemochromatosis is an autosomal recessive condition, due to mutation in the HFE gene located on the short arm of chromosome 6p21.3. The most common mutation is C282Y reflecting mutation of cys to tyr at locus 282. A number of other mutations have been described, e.g. H63D (his to asp at locus 63). In Northern Europe 90% patients are homozygous for C282Y and 5% heterozygous C282Y/H63D. The compound heterozygotes are less severely affected. However, 25% of C282Y homozygotes do not develop iron overload.

Clinical features
Key features on history
- Onset of iron overload is uncommon before 30 years of age.
- Presentation is with gradual stiffness, pain on use and enlargement of the MCP joints. There is evolution into a polyarticular arthropathy.
- There may be episodes of acute pseudogout, which may involve the knee, wrist, intervertebral disk and symphysis pubis.
- Fatigue is a common feature.
- Non-specific abdominal pain and discomfort may be the presentation of liver disease.

Key features on examination
Arthropathy
Patients develop a characteristic pattern of OA, with involvement of the 2nd and 3rd MCP joints. The tenderness is mild and the joint is not warm. There is an absence of soft tissue swelling.

Cardiac
Cardiac involvement is uncommon, but an arrhythmia may be an early feature.

Liver
Cirrhosis is a late feature.

Endocrine
Diabetes is late manifestation and occurs when cirrhosis is established. Hypogonadism is also a late feature.

Cutaneous
Skin pigmentation is not diagnostic and is a slate grey colour, rather than brown. It is caused by melanin and not iron.

General investigations
- Investigation is directed at establishing the diagnosis and assessing the extent and severity of organ involvement.
- Initial screening for the diagnosis is measurement of serum iron, transferrin, and ferritin. A transferrin saturation of >62% makes haemochromatosis very likely. Serum ferritin alone may be misleading as it is elevated in inflammatory states.
- A liver biopsy is only needed for prognostic purposes in patients with severe iron overload (ferritin >1000 μg/l) and abnormal liver function.
- The acute phase response is normal and the rheumatoid factor negative.

Genetic screening
HFE genotyping should be performed when screening iron studies are abnormal. Homozygosity for the C282Y mutation or for the compound heterozygous C282Y/H63D confirms the diagnosis.

Imaging
- There are typical changes of OA with joint space narrowing, subchondral sclerosis, and cysts. Prominent hook-like osteophytes are present especially at the MCP joints.
- The pattern of joint involvement is not typical for OA, with involvement of the MCP, midcarpal, radiocarpal, elbows and glenohumeral joints. The 2nd and 3rd MCPs are typically involved.
- 30% of patients have radiological evidence of chondrocalcinosis.

Differential diagnosis
- This is from other types of osteoarthritis and inflammatory arthritis.
- Secondary iron overload is excluded by an absence of a history of blood transfusions, parenteral iron administration and anaemia (b-thalassaemia, sideroblastic anaemia).
- Porphyria cutanea tarda may present with raised transferrin saturation and ferritin concentration with abnormalities of liver function. The skin is more fragile with blisters and the pigmentation is deeper. The diagnosis is made on the demonstration of the presence of uroporphyrins.
- Alcoholic liver disease may be associated with increased ferritin and transferrin saturation.

Prognosis

- The rate of progression of the arthropathy is extremely variable, but regular venesection does not improve the arthropathy. The damage to synovial membrane and cartilage is irreversible.
- The overall prognosis is excellent if venesection is started early in the disease. Patients with cirrhosis have 200-fold risk of hepatocellular carcinoma.

Pathology

Synovial biopsies characteristically show haemosiderin deposition in type B synovial lining cells.

Synovial fluid

Synovial fluid is mildly inflammatory and calcium pyrophosphate crystals may be present.

Patient advice

- Family members should be screened as early initiation of regular phlebotomy can prevent development of systemic disease.
- Alcohol and excess vitamin C should be avoided as this can increase iron absorption.

Treatment

- Therapy is directed to removing excess iron by venesection. Initially this is weekly until transferrin saturation is normal with a ferritin 20–50 g/l. Maintenance phlebotomy is thereafter required to maintain normal transferrin saturation.
- Venesection does not appear to have a significant impact on progression of the arthropathy. Treatment is otherwise symptomatic with analgesics, NSAIDs, and exercises.
- Liver function improves with venesection, as does the cardiomyopathy.

Resources

Patient organization
The haemochromatosis society UK.
www.haemochromatosis.org.uk

Other
OMIM:
www.ncbi.nlm.nih.gov/entrez/
OMIM 235200

ICD-10
E83.1 Disorders of iron metabolism

References

Adams PC, Barton JC. Haemochromatosis. *Lancet* 2007; **370**: 1855–60.

Bacon BR, Olynk JK, Brunt EM et al. HFE genotype in patients with haemochromatosis and other liver disease. *Ann Intern Med* 1999; **130**: 953–62.

Puechal X. Genetic haemochromatosis: why is discovery of the HLA-H gene of such interest to rheumatologists. *Rev Rhumatisme* 1997; **64**: 527–9. [in English.]

Schumacher HR. Haemochromatosis and arthritis. *Arthritis Rheum* 1994; **7**: 41–50.

See also

Osteoarthritis
Calcium pyrophosphate deposition disease

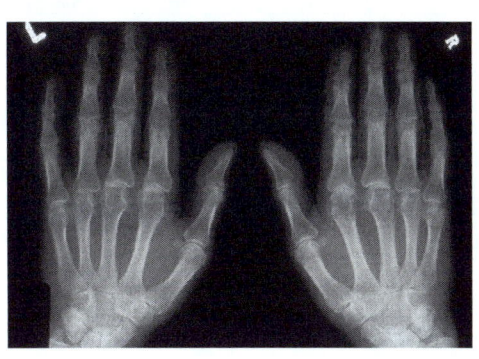

Figure 18.2 Haemochromatosis, showing osteoarthritis MCPs joints.

Haemoglobinopathies

Haemoglobinopathies result from inherited defects in the structure and function of haemoglobin. Sickle cell disease is the most common haemoglobinopathy causing an arthropathy.

Epidemiology
- Sickle cell disease occurs in people from Africa, Southern Italy, Northern Greece, Southern Turkey, Saudi Arabia, and Central and Southern India.
- Painful crisis are more common men than women. In men they occur most frequently between ages 15 and 25 years, in women the frequency is constant between ages 15 and 40 years.

Aetiology
Sickle cell haemoglobin (HbS) occurs when there is a single nucleotide substitution in the β-globin gene, at position B6, valine is substituted for glutamic acid. The β-globin gene is located at 11p15.5. In hypoxic conditions HbS forms liquid crystals that deform the erythrocytes into rigid sickle shaped cells. This leads to vaso-occlusion. This also occurs in the other sickle syndromes.

Genetics
Sickle cell disease is an autosomal recessive condition, due to inheritance of the HbS gene from both parents (i.e. homozygous). The heterozygous state sickle cell trait is not associated with rheumatic disease. Other sickle cell syndromes occur when HbS is combined with other abnormal Hb genes, e.g. sickle cell HbC disease (HbS from one parent and HbC from the other), or HbS with β-thalassaemia (S- $β^+$-thalassaemia.)

Clinical features
Key features on history
Painful crisis
- A history of sickle cell disease is usually available but should be sort in a patient presenting with painful veno-occlusive disease, dactylitis, or osteonecrosis from an appropriate ethnic background.
- Painful crisis is the typical feature of sickle cell disease. One or more joints may become inflamed. The may spread either in an additive manner or be migratory.
- Pain occurs most frequently in the juxta-articular regions of long bones, but also occurs the back, ribs, and rarely the abdomen. Acute back pain may be the only feature.
- Duration of the crisis is from a few minutes to several weeks, but persistence beyond 2 weeks is unusual in uncomplicated crisis.

There are four distinct phases to the crisis:
- **Prodromal:** the patient is restless and vaguely unwell.
- **Initial:** jaundice and increasing pain.
- **Established:** pain reaches it maximum.
- **Resolution:** pain gradually decreases and resolves over 2 weeks.

Precipitating factors include:
- Cold
- Pregnancy
- Emotional stress
- High altitude travelling

Dactylitis
- In children aged 6 months to 2 years vaso-occlusive crisis occur in bones of hand and feet leading to dactylitis.
- Symptoms improve over 1 week but may recur.

Osteonecrosis
- Occurs in up to 20% of patients at the femoral head. Initially may be indistinguishable from an acute crisis, but the pain does not settle after 2 weeks. Pain gets worse on walking and at night.
- Osteonecrosis can occur at other joints particularly the shoulder, where there is pain and loss of range of movement.

Osteomyelitis
- Usually follows an episode of painful crisis and should be considered if the crisis lasts more than 2 weeks.
- Multiple sites may be involved, which can be symmetrical.

Septic arthritis
- Uncommon in sickle cell disease, occurs in the presence of acute osteomyelitis, but more often as a result of haematogenous spread.
- Acute increase in pain in patients with known osteonecrosis of the hip should be assessed for septic arthritis.

Key features on examination
Painful crisis
- There may be marked localized joint swelling.
- Patients develop jaundice.

Dactylitis
- Acute painful non-pitting swelling of hands and feet.
- Shortening of digits due to necrosis of the epiphysis is a consequence of previous dactylitis.

Osteonecrosis
- Osteonecrosis is a late feature.
- Pain and marked loss of range of movement, especially at the hip and shoulder.

Osteomyelitis and septic arthritis
- Soft tissue swelling and persistent pyrexia.

General investigations
- Initial screening for the diagnosis is a sickle cell test, which should be performed in unexplained bone pain or osteonecrosis. If positive it should be followed with haemoglobin electrophoresis.
- In each painful crisis haemoglobin and reticulocyte count should be determined to exclude an aplastic crisis.
- A raised ESR and leucocytosis suggest infection. In uncomplicated SS, the ESR is normal, but rises during the resolving phase of the crisis and to a much higher level in infection. The CRP is a more sensitive measure of the inflammatory response.
- Hyperuricaemia is common (40%), but acute gout is rare.
- Blood cultures and joint aspiration should be performed when sepsis is suspected. Sickle cell patients are particularly prone to infections with *Haemophilus influenzae*, *Streptococcus pneumoniae* and *Salmonella*.

CHAPTER 18 Miscellaneous diseases

Imaging

Plain radiographs
- Plain radiographs are not useful in the early stages of osteomyelitis.
- Osteonecrosis can be assessed using the Steinberg classification system, but early in the process the X-ray is normal and MRI is more useful.

MRI
- MRI shows abnormalities due to osteonecrosis much earlier than X-ray and should be used. The overall sensitivity is reported to be 91%.
- Gadolinium-enhanced MRI demonstrates osteomyelitis with irregular marrow enhancement. Acute infarcts appear as thin linear enhancement.

Ultrasound
A finding of >4 mm of subperiosteal fluid is suggestive of osteomyelitis.

Differential diagnosis
- Infection of bone or joint should always be considered. Rarely a chronic destructive synovitis occurs, which needs to be differentiated from rheumatoid disease.
- Rheumatic fever is common in the same regions as sickle cell disease and the migratory arthritis of rheumatic fever must be differentiated.
- The ANA is often positive, but SLE occurs no more frequently in these patient.

Pathology
- The occlusion of small blood vessels in the bone marrow leads to many of the complication of sickle disease, such as painful crisis, dactylitis, and osteonecrosis. Polymerization of HbS in a deoxygenated state leads to increased rigidity of red cells and vaso occlusion. This leads to hypoxia and tissue damage.
- *Salmonella* infection especially osteomyelitis is common in sickle cell disease. The reason is unclear, but may relate to reticuloendothelial failure, iron overload, and defects in the alternate complement pathway.

Synovial fluid
Synovial fluid is non-inflammatory, straw coloured and sterile in uncomplicated arthritis.

Patient advice
- Family members should be screened for the presence of abnormal haemoglobins.
- Advice about avoidance of sickle crisis.

Treatment
- Appropriate analgesia including is necessary. In severe crisis opiates may be needed.
- Rehydration is essential and may be intravenous.
- Intravenous antibiotics should be started if infection is suspected.

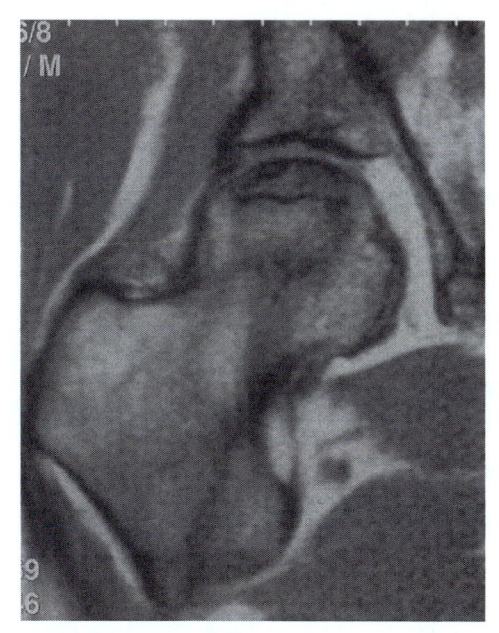

Figure 18.3 Avascular necrosis of the hip in a patient with sickle cell disease.

- Osteonecrosis of the femoral head should be treated with rest and avoidance of weight bearing. Decompression should be considered in early osteonecrosis.

Resources
Patient organizations
Sickle Cell Association of America. Available at: www.sicklecelldisease.org

Others
OMIM: www.ncbi.nlm.nih.gov/entrez/
OMIM 603903 (sickle cell disease)

ICD-10 coding
D57 Sickle cell disease

References
Cordner S, De Ceular K. Musculoskeletal manifestations of haemoglobinopathies. *Curr Opin Rheumatol* 2003;

See also
Osteoarthritis
Calcium pyrophosphate deposition disease
Osteonecrosis
Osteomyelitis
Septic arthritis

Haemophilia

Definition
Deficiency of factor VIII (Haemophilia A) or factor IX (Haemophilia B or Christmas disease) is due to X-linked inherited defects in the blood coagulation cascade resulting in recurrent musculoskeletal haemorrhage.

Epidemiology
- Factor VIII deficiency has an incidence of 1:5000 male births and Factor IX deficiency an incidence of 1:30 000 male births.
- There are no ethnic or geographical variations, and no HLA associations.

Aetiology
- Haemophilia is inherited as a sex-linked recessive trait. Thus, males only are affected and females are carriers.
- The factor VIII gene is located on the long arm of the X chromosome at Xq28. It is 168kb long and has 26 exons. Factor VIII is a plasma glycoprotein which circulates in a non-covalent association with von Willebrand factor. A variety of mutations have been described, the most common of which is a translocation in intron 22 which causes 40–50% of cases.
- The factor IX gene is located on the long arm of the X chromosome at Xq27. It is 34kb long and has eight exons. Missense and nonsense mutations account for 80% of mutations. There is no common mutation.
- Deficiencies of other clotting factors are very rare, as is the acquired form of factor VIII deficiency.
- The severity of the bleeding disorder depends on the levels of plasma coagulation factors that, in turn, reflect the precise mutation.
- Iron deposition appears to be important in the development of synovitis. Ferritin-induced production of superoxide anions and OH radicals causes damage to both cartilage and synovium, which leads to fibrosis of the joint.

Clinical features
Key features on history
General
Try to establish the nature and severity of the bleeding disorder. Does the patient receive factor VIII injections and which haemophilia centre does the patient attend.

Acute haemarthrosis
The diagnosis of haemophilia is usually well established before the first musculoskeletal bleeding episode.
- Age of onset depends on the severity of the bleeding disorder.
- Weight-bearing joints on the dominant side are most commonly affected and the child's ability to walk is affected. Knee, elbow, and ankle are the most commonly affected joints.
- Intra-articular bleeding can occur spontaneously in severe disease and after minor trauma in moderate disease.
- Intra-articular haemorrhage presents with initial joint stiffness followed by acute pain, warmth, and swelling. Rising intra-articular pressure eventual stops the bleeding.
- Milder bleeding episodes are less dramatic, and may be restricted to the subsynovium or be unrecognized by the patient.
- Muscle haemorrhage is acutely painful and may be crippling.

Subacute arthropathy
Follows recurrent haemorrhage into one or more joints, there is pain without evidence of acute haemorrhage.

Key features on examination
Acute haemarthrosis
- The joint is swollen, hot, and very tender.
- Bruising appears as the swelling subsides.

Subacute arthropathy
- Examination reveals a 'boggy synovitis', with synovial thickening and chronic effusion.
- Peri-articular muscles are weak and the joint ligaments lax.

Chronic arthropathy
- The affected joint is disorganized. There is bony thickening, deformity, loss of range of movement, and crepitus.
- Joint contractures are present due to fibrosis or ankylosis.
- Soft tissue swelling and effusions are uncommon at this stage.

Haemophiliac pseudotumour
Destructive lesion occurring in bones associated with fracture, local infection and ulceration. Due to recurrent haemorrhage into the subperiosteal region, which then becomes encapsulated and subsequently enlarges.

General investigations
- Coagulation screen including bleeding time, platelet count, prothrombin time, partial thromboplastin time, factor VIII and factor XI levels will confirm the diagnosis.
- The acute phase response is normal. RF and ANA are negative.
- The joint should be aspirated and the synovial fluid cultured, if there is doubt about the diagnosis.

Imaging
X-rays
Plain radiographic appearances depend on the stage of disease.

Early disease
- Periarticular soft tissue swelling.
- Periarticular demineralization.
- Increased radiodensity of synovium.

Intermediate
- Growth arrest lines (Harris lines).
- Widening or premature fusion of the epiphysis.
- Widening of the femoral or humeral intercondylar notches.
- Squaring of the inferior border of the patella.
- Proximal radial head enlargement.
- Increased talotibial slant and flattening of talus.

Late
- Irregularity of cartilage with narrowing.
- Central and marginal erosions.
- Subarticular sclerosis, bone cysts, osteophyte formation.
- Joint disorganization.
- Bony ankylosis.

Ultrasound
- Useful to demonstrate degree of synovial hypertrophy.
- Assess soft lesions, such as muscle haematoma.

MRI
- Demonstrates blood in the joint cavity and subsynovium.
- Detect changes in hyaline cartilage before changes become apparent using plain radiography.
- Assess degree synovial hypertrophy.

Synovial fluid
The synovial fluid is characteristically bloody, the first sample being heavily blood stained.

Differential diagnosis
- Acute arthropathy is usually readily recognized in previously diagnosed patients. The main differential diagnosis of the single hot joint is infection, which should be excluded by synovial fluid culture.
- Rarely musculoskeletal haemorrhage is the presenting event. The differential of haemarthrosis then includes trauma (intra-articular fracture), bleeding disorder (platelet deficiency, anti-coagulant therapy, acquired factor VIII deficiency), blood dyscrasia, villonodular synovitis, joint neoplasms
- Von Willebrand disease (deficiency or dysfunction of the adhesive glycoprotein von Willebrand factor), although more common does not present with acute haemarthrosis.

Pathology
Haemophiliac synovitis is characterized by synovial hypertrophy, monocyte infiltration, deposition of haemosiderin in the synovium, and subsynovium, and new vessel formation.

Patient advice
- Genetic counselling. X-linked recessive condition, which runs true in families. 80% of mothers of an isolated patient are expected to be haemophilia carriers.
- Rare condition resulting in bleeding disorder and arthropathy.
- Avoidance of trauma both accidental and surgical.
- Avoidance aspirin and other drugs affecting platelet function.
- Avoidance of intramuscular injection.

Treatment
Management is best performed in specialist haemophilia centre with an appropriate multi disciplinary team.

Acute arthropathy
- Immediate factor replacement is required and may already been started by the patient at home.
- Prompt treatment of haemarthrosis is essential, aspiration is only needed when the diagnosis is unclear, the joint very distended or where infection needs to be excluded.
- The joint should be iced, elevated, rested, and appropriate analgesics used. Graduated physiotherapy, local ultrasound, isometric exercises are required to mobilize the patient.

Subacute arthropathy
- The development of the characteristic boggy synovitis indicates potential destructive disease.
- Acute rapid treatment of bleeding is required. The use of early prophylactic therapy with factor replacement before joint damage occurs successfully prevents development of subacute arthropathy.
- Physiotherapy to maintain muscle strength and prevent contracture development is necessary.
- Intra-articular or oral corticosteroids only produce a short-term benefit.

Chronic arthropathy
May not be completely preventable even with modern treatment and prophylactic regimen. Joint arthroplasty (elbow, knee) should be considered, but is technically difficult. Ankle arthroplasty is less successful and consideration is still given to arthrodesis.

Resources
Patient organizations
Haemophila Society (UK): www.haemophilia.org.uk

Others
OMIM: www.ncbi.nlm.nih.gov/entrez/
OMIM: haemophilia A 306700
OMIM: haemophilia B 306900

ICD-10 coding
D66 Hereditary factor VIII deficiency
D67 Hereditary factor IX deficiency

References
Bolton-Maggs PHB, Pasi KJ. Haemophilias A and B. *Lancet* 2003; **361**: 1801–9.
Resnick D. Bleeding disorders. In: Resnick D. *Diagnosis of Bone and Joint Disorders*, 4th edn. Saunders, 2002; 2346–73.

Sarcoidosis

Sarcoidosis is a multisystem granulomatous disease of unknown cause.

Definition
Sarcoidosis is a multisystem disease of unknown aetiology characterized by the formation of non-caseating granulomata in affected organs.

Epidemiology
- In the USA the incidence is 10.9/100 000 in Caucasians and 35.5/100 000 in Afro-Americans. The incidence in Scandinavia is 15–20/100 000.
- Females are affected more frequently.
- Onset is typically aged <40 years.
- There is seasonal clustering of acute sarcoidosis in the spring.

Aetiology
- The aetiology is unknown. However, three factors seem to be important. Exposure to a triggering antigen, acquired cellular immunity to the antigen, and development of effector cells that promote a non-specific inflammatory response.
- Inflammatory alveolitis precedes granuloma formation and is composed of CD4+ T-cells and mononuclear phagocytes. Accumulation and activation antigen-specific Th1 lymphocytes is critical to granuloma formation. The mechanisms of granuloma resolution are not well understood.
- Acute sarcoidosis in is associated with HLA B8, DR3. HLA-DR3. No consistent non-HLA associations have been established.

Clinical features
Acute sarcoidosis occurs typically as Löfgren's syndrome: a triad of constitutional illness, polyarthritis and erythema nodosum

Key features on history
Systemic
Fever and malaise are common.

Musculoskeletal
Typically begins in the ankles and may spread to knees, wrists, elbows, PIPs, and MCPs. Occurs in 70%. Monarthritis is uncommon. The axial skeleton and sacroiliac joints are spared.

Cutaneous
Erythema nodosum occurs in up to two-thirds of patients with acute sarcoidosis.

Key features on examination
Musculoskeletal
The ankle joints are typically warm, red, and very tender.

Cutaneous
Raised warm tender nodules (erythema nodosum) are typically present over the calves, but may occur on the forearms.

Chronic sarcoidosis
This is uncommon and most cases occur in Afro-Carribean patients.

Key features on history
Musculoskeletal
- Chronic oligo- or polyarticular arthropathy occurs late in the disease, and is associated with interstitial lung disease and other organ involvement.
- Dactylitis: diffuse swelling of a digit that may be tender.

Key features on examination
Musculoskeletal
- Oligo or poly articular involvement knees, ankles, wrists, and small joints of the hands and feet. Joint destruction is rare.
- Dactylitis with soft tissue swelling over digits, and tenderness and stiffness of neighbouring joints is common.

Muscle disease
- Asymptomatic skeletal muscle involvement is common and a random muscle biopsy may confirm the diagnosis.
- Acute sarcoid myopathy is rare and indistinguishable from acute polymyositis, with development of acute proximal myopathy, raised CK, and myopathic changes on EMG.
- Chronic sarcoid myopathy presents with bilateral symmetrical proximal muscle wasting and weakness. The CK is usually normal.

Osseous sarcoidosis
Bone lesions occur in up to 5% of patients, usually in those with chronic cutaneous or internal organ involvement.

Pulmonary
Pulmonary fibrosis is present in 25%.

Cutaneous
- Skin involvement is common (25–35%). Macules, papules, and plaques may arise as single or isolated lesions.
- Lupus pernio: violaceous lesions on nose, cheeks, lips and ears.

General investigations
Investigation is directed at establishing the diagnosis, and assessing the extent and severity of organ involvement.
- FBC: anaemia of chronic disease.
- Acute phase response (ESR and CRP).
- Liver function: ALP may be raised in one-third of patients.
- Bone biochemistry: activated in macrophages in the granulomata increase hydroxylation of 25-hydroxyvitamin D to 3 to 1,25 hydroxyvitamin D3 and this leads to hypercalcaemia in 10% and hypercalciuria in 40%. Plasma 1,25 hydroxyvitamin D3 levels are raised.
- ACE: angiotensin-converting enzyme (ACE) is produced by epithelioid cells of the granulomata and activated alveolar macrophages. Elevated ACE levels are seen in 40–90% of cases. Elevated ACE levels are seen in other granulomatous diseases and in some non-granulomatous diseases such as Gaucher's disease, thyrotoxicosis, liver cirrhosis and diabetes mellitus.

Radiological investigations
- Chest X-ray: this is abnormal in 95% of cases. In acute disease this may show bilateral hilar lymphadenopathy. There may evidence of interstitial lung disease, which will need assessment with high resolution CT.

- Osseous sarcoidosis cysts, lytic lesions with periosteal reaction, reticular lace-like changes, sclerosis, and destructive changes.

Nuclear medicine
- Gallium-67 citrate scintigraphy reveals increased uptake by sarcoid granulomata typically in the parotid and lachrymal glands (Panda sign). Uptake is non-specific and occurs in lymphoma, TB, and fungal infection.
- ^{18}F-FDG-PET may be useful in assessing extent organ involvement and identifying potential biopsy sites.

Bronchoscopy and bronchiolar alveolar lavage
- The lavaged fluid typically shows a 30–50% lymphocytosis with a CD4/CD8 T-cell ratio >3.5.
- Pulmonary function testing. This shows restrictive pattern with reduction in vital capacity, residual volume, and total lung capacity. 65% of patients have airflow limitation at presentation.

Biopsy of an affected organ should be obtained where possible to confirm diagnosis and, in particular, to exclude infection or malignant disease.

Kveim test: the reagent is no longer available.

Differential diagnosis
- This is from other types of acute inflammatory arthritis, including reactive arthritis, rheumatoid disease, and occasionally gout.
- Chronic sarcoid arthritis may resemble RA, but is generally milder. Monarticular disease must be differentiated from infection.
- Upper airways disease needs to be distinguished from Wegener's granulomatosis, keratoconjunctivitis, and parotid involvement from Sjögren's syndrome. The uveitis needs to be distinguished from spondyloarthropathy and Behçet's syndrome
- Erythema nodosum has many causes. Other granulomatous diseases, such as Mycobacterial infection, fungal infection, berylliosis, and local reactions to tumours or lymphoma. Appropriate serological investigations, biopsies and cultures may be required in regions where Mycobacterial/fungal diseases are common.

Disease assessment
- Severity of involvement of target organs should be carefully assessed
- Slit lamp examination is required to assess asymptomatic eye involvement.

Prognosis
- Acute sarcoidosis (including Löfgren's syndrome) has an excellent prognosis with a 90% remission rate. The arthritis lasts from 2 weeks to 4 months. In a Spanish series 8% had active disease at 2 years and 6% relapsed (Mana et al., 1999).
- Overall, 60% of cases remit spontaneously with 10-20% responding to corticosteroids. In 10–30% there is a chronic course, of these 50% have progressive pulmonary disease.

Pathology
The sarcoid granuloma is well circumscribed; round or oval, non-caseating, and made up of compact radially arranged epithelioid cells. The giant cells are Langerhans type. The centre of the granuloma is composed of CD4+ Th1 T cells and macrophage derived cells.

Patient advice
- **Acute disease:** self-limiting process most likely to be a reaction to infection and typically no treatment is required.
- **Chronic disease:** life-long condition requiring treatment with corticosteroids.

Treatment
- *Acute sarcoid arthritis:* most patients respond well to NSAIDs. Occasional patients with severe arthropathy require a short course of corticosteroids (prednisolone 15–40 mg/day).
- *Chronic sarcoid arthritis:* many patients simply require NSAIDs. Those with major organ involvement need corticosteroids.
- *Cutaneous sarcoidosis* may respond to hydroxychloroquin. Low dose once weekly oral methotrexate may permit reduction in prednisolone dosage.
- The role of other immunosuppressive agents and TNF-alpha blockade is unknown, although positive isolated case reports support their use.

Resources
Patient organizations
American lung association: www.lungusa.org

Foundation for sarcoidosis research: www.stopsarcoidosis.org

ICD-10 coding
D86   Sarcoidosis

References
ManaJ, Gomez-Vaquero C, Montero A et al. Löfgren's syndrome revisited: a study of 186 patients. Am J Med 1999; 107: 240-5.

Iannuzzi MC, Rybicki BA, Teirstein AS. Sarcoidosis. N Engl J Med 2007;357:2153-65.

Panniculitis

Panniculitis is inflammation of adipose tissue most typically within subcutaneous fat. Erythema nodosum (EN) is the most common variety.

Classification

Panniculitis can be divided into four categories based on the histopathological appearance.

Table 18.3 Classification of the panniculitides

Septal panniculitis	Erythema nodosum
	Vilanova's disease
Lobular panniculitis	Weber-Christian disease
	Rothmann–Makai syndrome
	Subcutaneous fat necrosis of the newborn
	Post-steroid
	Calcifying
	Enzymatic
	Pancreatic
	Alpha1-antitrypsin deficiency
	Physical or factitious
	Histiocytic cytophagic syndromes
	Lipodystrophy syndromes
	Connective tissue associated
	Lipodermalosclerosis
Mixed panniculitis	Lupus profundus
	Behçet's erythema nodosum
Panniculitis/vasculitis	Leucocytoclastic vasculitis
	Polyarteritis nodosa
	Erythema induratum

From Callen (2004)

Epidemiology

- The panniculitides can occur at any age, but most typically in young adults.
- They occur more commonly in women.
- EN has an annual incidence of 2–3/100 000; other types of panniculitis are much rarer.
- EN is associated with HLA-B8.

Erythema nodosum

Key features on history

EN is usually acute and self-limited, and heals without scar formation.
- Acute development of one or more tender red nodules on the anterior shins.
- Prodromal fever, malaise, arthralgias.

Key features on examination

- Tender red palpable nodules over the anterior shins.
- Older lesions appear bruised, ulceration is rare.

Aetiopathogenesis of EN

- Up to 50% of cases of EN have an underlying cause, with sarcoidosis and infection being the most common.
- Löfgren's syndrome is a triad of EN, acute arthropathy, and bilateral hilar lymphadenopathy.

Table 18.4 Causes of erythema nodosum

Systemic	Sarcoidosis
	Pregnancy
	Inflammatory bowel disease
	Connective tissue diseases
	Malignancy
	Sweet's syndrome
	Behçet's disease
Infections	Streptococcal pharyngitis
	Mycobacterial
	Coccidioidomycosis
	Blastomycosis
	Histoplasmosis
	Psittacosis
	Yersinosis
	Salmonellosis
	Cat scratch fever
	Leprosy
Drugs	Antibiotics – penicillin, sulphonamides
	Oral contraceptive pill

Weber–Christian disease

Key features on history

Fever

- Recurrent tender nodules that can occur anywhere.
- Arthralgias, myalgias.
- Abdominal pain due to mesenteric panniculitis.

Key features on examination

Recurrent multiple subcutaneous nodules, these result in fat destruction and scar formation.

Investigation

Biopsy reveals lobular panniculitis with fat degeneration, foamy histiocytes, and giant cell formation.

Pancreatic panniculitis

Patients with a wide variety of pancreatic conditions may develop a lobular panniculitis.

Key features on examination

- Subcutaneous fat necrosis.
- There may be an accompanying polyarthritis with osseous intramedullary fat necrosis.

Lupus profundus

Key features on history

- Panniculitis is a rare complication of SLE occurring in 1–3% of patients with SLE.
- Activity of panniculitis appears not to mirror activity of SLE.

Key features on examination
- The lesions are tender red-blue subcutaneous nodules, which may ulcerate.
- Typically they occur on face, upper arms thighs, and buttocks.

Alpha-1 antitrypsin deficiency
Alpha-1 antitrypsin is associated with panniculitis. Histologically, the appearances are a lobular, septal, or a mixed panniculitis.

Post-steroid panniculitis
Panniculitis may follow steroid therapy especially in children. It may recur with reuse of corticosteroids. The pathogenesis is not known.

Histiocytic cytophagic panniculitis
This is a chronic histiocytic disease of subcutaneous fat, accompanied with panniculitis, fever, serositis, and lymph adenopathy. The haemophagocytic syndrome may occur. Prednisolone and immunosuppression may be useful.

Lipoatrophic panniculitis
Rothmann–Makai syndrome (lipogranulomatosis subcutanea) is a form of subcutaneous lipoatrophy that occurs after an inflammatory disease in children. There are multiple erythematous lesions on the extremities which heal with subcutaneous atrophy. Fever may be present. Treatment is uncertain.

Investigation
Histologically, there is evidence of both septal and lobular panniculitis.

General investigations
- Infection screen, especially looking for evidence of upper respiratory tract infection, throat swab, and ASO titre.
- Chest radiograph looking for infection (especially Mycobacterial) or bilateral hilar lymphadenopathy suggestive of acute sarcoidosis.
- Appropriate serological investigations, biopsy, and cultures may be required in areas where Mycobacterial and fungal infections are common.
- Investigation for inflammatory bowel disease is unnecessary in asymptomatic patients, as this usually symptomatic when accompanied by panniculitis.
- Autoantibody serology if there is evidence of a connective tissue disorder
- Amylase and lipase should be measured in patients possibly with pancreatic disease.
- Biopsy if the diagnosis is in doubt. A deep wedge biopsy including subcutaneous fat is necessary

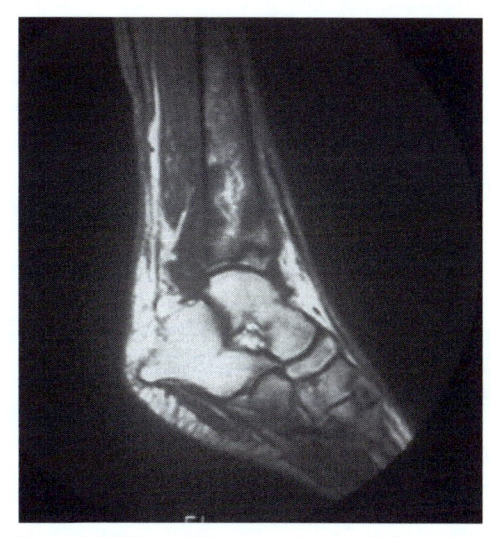

Figure 18.4 MRI Sagittal T1-weighted showing multiple low signal areas indicating osteonecrosis and marrow oedema. In a patients with metastatic pancreatic fat necrosis.

Differential diagnosis
The differential diagnosis of EN includes other forms of panniculitis, insect bites (history and evidence of a puncture wound), thrombophlebitis, and cellulitis.

Treatment
- EN is usually self-limiting, NSAIDs may be needed for arthralgias/myalgias.
- Chronic relapsing forms of panniculitis may respond to corticosteroids or other immunosuppressive drugs.

References
Callen JP. Panniculitis. In: Isenberg DA, Maddison PJ, Woo P, Glass D, Breedveld FC (eds) *Oxford Textbook of Rheumatology*, 3rd edn. Oxford: 2004: 1031–35.

See also
Sarcoidosis
SLE

Alkaptonuria

Definition
A rare autosomal recessive condition resulting from lack of homogentisic acid oxidase, and the accumulation of homogentisic acid causing ochronosis and ochronotic arthropathy. Ochronosis is the characteristic black pigmentation seen in alkpatonuric patients.

Alkaptonuria was the first human condition in which the pattern of Mendelian inheritance was recognized by Garrod in 1902. Garrod in 1908 hypothesized that a specific enzyme was lacking.

Epidemiology
- The highest frequency occurs in Slovakia (1/19 000).
- The overall frequency is 1/250 000 – 1/million live births.

Aetiology
- Alkaptonuria is due to lack of the enzyme homogentisic acid oxidase (HGO). The gene for this enzyme is located on 3q21–23. A variety of different mutations have been described including nonsense, missense and frame shift mutations. There does not appear to be any correlation between the HGO mutation and severity of disease. Homogentisic acid oxidase catalyses the oxidative cleavage of the ring of homogentisic acid into maleylacetoacetic acid. Homogentisic acid then accumulates slowly in the tissues, resulting in the characterstic black pigmentation. The renal clearance of homogentisic acid is high suggesting active renal tubular excretion.
- Inheritance as an autosomal recessive condition.
- The exact mechanism by which pigment deposition results in arthropathy is not known.

Clinical features
Key features on history
- In infancy, the first feature may be the mother noticing a dark discolouration of the nappies.
- In adults there is often a history of dark urine (in half of patients this is the presenting feature) or urine that darkens on standing.

Musculoskeletal
- Joint pain often starts before the age of 30 years. Initially, this is spinal and then a peripheral arthritis develops.
- Episodic joint inflammation occurs later.

Cutaneous
- Pigmentation of the sclera and ear is rarely seen before 20–30 years of age.
- Adult alkpatonuric patients may have dark urine or urine that darkens on standing.

Key features on examination
Musculoskeletal
- Marked spinal stiffness at all levels with kyphosis.
- Large joint osteoarthritis is common, particularly knee, hip, and shoulder.
- Small joint involvement is unusual.
- They may be a joint effusion.

Cutaneous
- Ochronotic pigmentation in the eye is visible at the insertion of the rectus muscles, and may spread to the conjunctiva and sclerae.
- Pigmentation of the auricular cartilage appears as a slate-blue or grey colour in the concha, antihelix, and tragus.

General investigations
- The acute phase response is normal. RF and ANA are negative. HLA-B27 is generally negative.
- A sample of urine should be left to stand. It will darken if it contains excessive amounts of homogentisic acid.
- Homogentisic acid levels in plasma and urine may be determined by high-performance liquid chromatography.

Imaging
X-rays
On plain radiography of the lumbar spine the characteristic findings are:
- Wafer like calcification of intervertebral discs.
- Narrowing of disc spaces.
- Ossification of the of the ligaments.

In peripheral joints the appearances of osteoarthritis develop about 10 years after the spinal changes. Multiple intra-articular radio-opaque loose bodies may be seen in the knees.

Synovial fluid
Effusions occur in around 50% of patients. The synovial fluid is characteristically non-inflammatory, containing mainly mononuclear cells (100–700 cells/mm^3). Pyrophosphate and apatite crystals have been found in alkaptonuric patients.

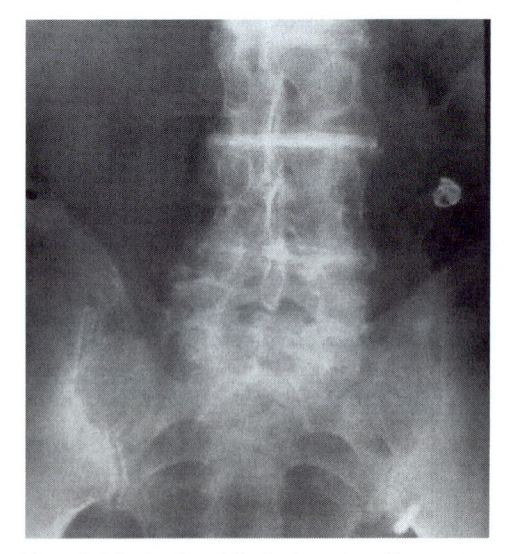

Figure 18.5 Lumbar disc calcification in a patient with longstanding ochronosis.

Differential diagnosis
- The main differential diagnosis is from osteoarthritis, ankylosing spondylitis, and calcium pyrophosphate deposition disease.
- Ankylosing spondylitis can be distinguished from ochronosis by the presence of syndesmophytes, erosion, and fusion of the sacroiliac joints.

- Osteophytosis on X-ray is not present in ochronosis, but is a typical feature of osteoarthritis. Ochronosis affects shoulders and sacroiliac joint, which are less frequently involved in osteoarthritis.

Pathology
Biopsies show ochronotic pigment in the cartilage. This is located within collagen bundles causing loss of striation, swelling, and fracture.

Patient advice
- Genetic counselling about mode of inheritance. Screening of first degree relatives.
- Rare inherited condition resulting in arthropathy.

Treatment
- There is no treatment for the underlying enzymatic defect. Vitamin C has been used, but is not effective. Nitisinone has been used on an experimental basis and reduces urinary HGA levels. The long-term effect on joint function is unknown.
- Analgesics, NSAIDs, physiotherapy as required.
- Joint replacement may be required in severe cases.
- Lumbar spinal stenosis may require surgical decompression.

Resources
Patient organizations
The Alkaptonuria society. www.alkaptonuria.info

Others
OMIM: www.ncbi.nlm.nih.gov/entrez/
OMIM 203500

ICD-10 coding
E70.2 Disorders of tyrosine metabolism

References
Phornphutkul C, Introne W, Perry M, et al. Natural history of alkaptonuria. *N Engl J Med* 2002; **347**: 2111–21.

Suwannarat P, O'Brien K, Perry MB, et al. Use of nitisinone in alkaptonuria. *Metabolism* 2005; **7**: 719–28.

See also
Osteoarthritis
Spondyloarthropathy

Gaucher's disease

Definition
Gaucher's disease results from accumulation of glucosylceramide in organs in the storage Gaucher cells.
Three types of Gaucher's disease are recognized.

> **Types of Gaucher's disease**
> *Type 1 (non-neuronopathic)*
> - Organomegaly.
> - Hypersplenism leading to haematological abnormalities.
> - Bone lesions due to medullary infiltration by Gaucher cells.
> - No CNS involvement.
>
> *Type 2 (acute neuronopathic)*
> - Early CNS involvement.
> - Fatal by age 2 years.
>
> *Type 3 (subacute neuronopathic)*
> - Organ involvement.
> - Medullary lesions.
> - CNS involvement, but less severe than in type 2.

Epidemiology
Gaucher's disease is an autosomal recessive condition
Type 1 is the most common and occurs most frequently in Ashkenazi Jew (prevalence 15–40/100 000), but occurs in all ethnic groups (1/100 000). Can occur at any age, but the median age is 30 years.
Type 2 and 3 are much rarer and predominately occur in non-Jewish patients. Type 2 presents age <6months and type 3 age <20 years.

Aetiology
Biochemistry
Gaucher's disease arises from a defect in the gene for glucocerebrosidase, which results in decreased activity. Glucocerebrosidase is 65 kDa membrane associated monomeric protein, which hydrolyses β-glucosidic ester bonds. Decreased activity of the enzyme results in accumulation of glucosylceramide linked by a β-glucosidic bond. Glucosylceramide is the end product of glycosphingolipid catabolism and is normally degraded into ceramide and glucose by glucocerebrosidase.

Molecular genetics
The gene for β-glucocerebrosidase is located at 1q21. The most common mutations are N370S. and L444P. A wide phenotypic difference is seen with some mutations leading to a mild phenotype (e.g. R496H), whilst some lead to loss of catalytic activity and enzyme stability (e.g. L444P).

Clinical features
Type 1
Key features on history
There is a broad spectrum of severity, with onset at any age. Mental development is normal.

Musculoskeletal
- Episodic arthralgias. Most frequently involving the spine, hips, legs, and shoulders.
- Fractures may occur to bone fragility.
- Acute pain, tenderness possibly with fever may occur in osteonecrosis.

Key features on examination
Haematological
Hepatosplenomegaly.

Musculoskeletal
- Pain and limitation of movement occur in osteonecrosis.
- Growth retardation.

Type 2
Key features on history
- Early onset of oculomotor abnormalities.

Key features on examination
Haematological
- Hepatosplenomegaly

Neurological
- Bilateral fixed strabismus and oculomotor apraxia are early signs.
- Hypertonia neck muscles and opisthotonus.

Type 3
Intermediate between types 1 and 3. The neurological features are similar to type 2.

General investigations
- Investigation is directed at establishing the diagnosis.
- FBC anaemia, leucopaenia, thrombocytopaenia due to hypersplenism.
- Cholestatic enzymes may be increased but liver failure is uncommon.
- Serum ACE, tartrate resistant acid phosphatase is raised.
- Leucocyte glucocerebrosidase is elevated.

Genetic screening
Patients with typical clinical features should be screened for the common mutations.

Imaging
- Plain radiographs show typical appearances.
- Failure of skeletal remodelling leads to development of the 'Erlenmeyer flask' deformity with expansion of the contours of long bones, there is cortical thinning and loss of the normal concavity. Vertebral bodies show depression of the superior and inferior endplates 'H-vertebra'.
- Bone marrow infiltration results in osteolytic lesions.
- Osteonecrosis results in joint damage with appearances identical to idiopathic osteonecrosis.
- MR is the most sensitive method of assessing for assessing bone marrow infiltration by Gaucher cells and can be used to assess response to treatment.

Bone marrow biopsy
The diagnosis is made on the demonstration of Gaucher cells in bone marrow biopsy. The cells are large mono- or multinucleated cells with a typical 'wrinkled tissue paper' appearance of the cytoplasm.

Differential diagnosis
The diagnosis is based on clinical manifestations and the radiological appearances. The plain radiographic appearances

are not specific for Gaucher's disease. The diagnosis should be considered in a patient with hepatosplenomegaly, osteopaenia, focal osteosclerosis, osteonecrosis, and Erlenmeyer flask deformities.

Prognosis
- The prognosis is variable dependent on the precise mutation as there is a very broad clinical heterogeneity.
- The more severe forms have a worse prognosis with progressive hypersplenism, bone pain, skeletal deformity, and fracture. However, enzyme replacement therapy reverses hypersplenism and bone pain, and reduces fractures.
- Type 2 is fatal before age 2 years.

Patient advice
- Gaucher's disease is a recessively inherited condition.
- The prognosis is dependent on the exact gene mutation and is quite good with enzyme replacement therapy.

Treatment
Enzyme replacement with macrophage targeted glucocerebrosidase reverses haematological and hepatosplenomegaly within a few weeks, but the osseous complications take longer to reverse. The optimum treatment regimens for milder type 1 disease is still uncertain.

Resources
Patient organizations
www.gaucher.org.uk
Others
OMIM www.ncbi.nlm.nih.gov/entrez/
Gaucher's disease type 1 OMIM 230800
Gaucher's disease type 2 OMIM 230900
Gaucher's disease type 3 OMIM 231000

ICD-10 code
E55.2   Other sphingolipidosis

References
Vom Dahl S, Poll L, Di Rococco M, Ciana G, Denes C, Mariani G, Mass M. Evidence-based recommendations for monitoring bone disease and the response to enzyme replacement therapy in Gaucher patients. *Curr Med Res Opin* 2006; **22**: 1045–64.

Eosinophilia-myalgia syndrome and toxic oil syndrome

Definition
Eosinophilia-myalgia syndrome (EMS), toxic oil syndrome and eosinophilic fasciitis are united by the clinical features of eosinophilia and fasciitis. They should however be considered separate illnesses as toxins have been implicated in the development of EMS and Toxic Oil Syndrome but not eosinophilic fasciitis. The latter condition will be dealt with separately.

First defined in 1989 EMS was an epidemic associated with the ingestion of L-tryptophan preparations from a single Japanese manufacturer (Showa Denko). L-tryptophan, an essential amino acid, has been available over the counter since the 1970s and has been used to treat insomnia, depression and premenstrual symptoms.

Diagnostic criteria
The US Centres for Disease Control and Prevention (CDC) defined the syndrome according to 3 criteria:
- Eosinophil count greater than 1000/mm^3.
- Incapacitating myalgia.
- Exclusion of other infectious or neoplastic illness that could account for the other two findings.

Epidemiology
EMS was initially described in 3 patients in New Mexico in October 1989. In excess of 1500 cases were subsequently reported within the US over the following two years.

The syndrome occurred most commonly in Caucasian females over 35 years of age. The daily dose ranged from 10–15 000 mg (median 1500 mg) with the development of symptoms occurring at a median of 127 days after first ingestion of the formulation. It is worth noting, however, that up to 14% of cases of EMS were not related to L-tryptophan. Nevertheless, since the epidemic only a few incident cases have been described.

Toxic oil syndrome was another epidemic occurring in Spain in 1981 which followed the ingestion of adulterated rapeseed cooking oil. The oil had been denatured with 2 percent aniline for industrial use, refined, then sold illegally as pure olive oil.

Aetiology and pathophysiology
Due to the epidemic nature of EMS and its association with a single source of L-tryptophan, a contaminant was highly likely to be the culprit. This was subsequently found to be ethylidene bis[tryptophan] (EBT). Experiments revealed that mice administered L-tryptophan from the batch in question developed myofascial thickening. Further analysis found a second contaminant (phenylamino)alanine to be associated with the condition. This was found to be chemically similar to an aniline derivative implicated in toxic oil syndrome.

Abnormal tryptophan metabolism in patients with both syndromes has been found however this may simply be a consequence of an inflammatory response. Up-regulation of pro-inflammatory cytokines is a feature. In addition, excessive amounts of tryptophan inhibit histamine degradation which leads to eosinophilia and myalgia. The exact pathogenesis of the conditions however remains unknown.

Clinical features
EMS most commonly presented with a flu-like illness with marked myalgia and arthralgia as well as profound weakness and fatigue. By definition all patients suffered from myalgia and eosinophilia.

Toxic oil syndrome usually manifest as an atypical pneumonia with non-productive cough, pleuritic chest pain, headache, fever and pulmonary infiltrates on CXR.

Clinical features common to both conditions were protean and included:

Symptoms and signs
- Myalgia.
- Arthralgia.
- Rash.
- Peripheral oedema.
- Cough.
- Dyspnoea.
- Fever.
- Alopecia.
- Neuropathy (sensory or sensorimotor involvement in a glove and stocking distribution).
- Hepatomegaly.

Investigations
- Leucocytosis.
- Eosinophilia (>500 mm^3).
- Elevated ESR.
- Elevated aldolase.
- Abnormal CXR.
- Abnormal LFTs.

Scleroderma-like skin change was unique to eosinophilia-myalgia syndrome.

General investigations
Relevant investigations to exclude differential diagnoses should be performed (see individual chapters).

Salient investigation for the syndromes include:
- Eosinophilia (mandatory for EMS, although may be missed if present in early disease only).
- Leukocytosis.
- Raised IgE levels (toxic oil syndrome only).
- ANAs especially in EMS.
- Normal CK levels in almost all patients.
- Elevated aldolase.
- Abnormal LFTs common (transaminitis).

Imaging
- CXR: normal to acute infiltrates, pleural effusion.
- Other helpful imaging modalities include: MR brain, PFTs, EMG/NCS.

Histology
Histological analysis of affected tissue reveals:
- Capillary endothelial cell hyperplasia with swelling and necrosis.
- Inflammatory cell infiltrate in connective tissue, nerve, and muscle.
- Fibrosis particularly in the fascia.

Differential diagnosis
- Churg–Strauss syndrome.
- Eosinophilic pneumonia.
- Hypereosinophilic syndrome.
- Systemic sclerosis.

- Polymyalgia rheumatica.
- Trichinosis.
- Hypothyroidism.
- Occult malignancy.

Treatment
Avoidance of the offending toxins was critical. Symptomatic relief of the myriad clinical features was required as no drug was found to alter the natural history of the conditions. NSAIDs and corticosteroids were frequently used, especially in early disease. Chronic symptoms have been found to be extremely resistant to treatment.

Physiotherapy and occupational therapy was necessary for musculoskeletal manifestations and functional impairment.

Prognosis
When L-tryptophan was recalled from the market in November 1989, the incidence of EMS plummeted. The mortality rate for the first year was 2.7% for EMS and 1.5–3.6 % for toxic oil syndrome. Death resulted from progressive polyneuropathy and myopathy in the majority of patients with EMS. Both conditions were associated with long-term morbidity most commonly patients complaining of myalgia, muscle cramps, and neuropathy. Only 10% of patients surveyed 4 years after disease onset were symptom free.

Resources
Assessment tools
Not applicable

Guidelines
Not applicable

Patient organizations
The National Eosinophilia-Myalgia Syndrome Network: http://www.nemsn.org/

ICD-10 codes
M35.8   Other specified systemic involvement of CTD

References
Kilbourne EM, Philen RM, Kamb ML, Falk H. Tryptophan produced by Showa Denko and epidemic eosinophilia-myalgia syndrome. *J Rheumatol Suppl.* 1996; **46**: 81–91.

Posada de la Paz M, Philen RM, Borda AI. Toxic oil syndrome: the perspective after 20 years. *Epidemiol Rev* 2001; **23**: 231–47.

Sullivan EA, Staehling N, Philen RN. Eosinophiliamyalgia syndrome among the non-L-tryptophan users and pre-epidemic cases. *J Rheumatol* 1996; **23**: 1784–7.

Tabuenca JM. Toxic-allergic syndrome caused by ingestion of rape-seed oil denatured with aniline. *Lancet* 1981; **2**: 567–8

Varga J, Kähäri VM. Eosinophilia-myalgia syndrome, eosinophilic fasciitis, and related fibrosing disorders. *Curr Opin Rheumatol* 1997; **9**: 562–70.

Metabolic myopathies

Definition
The metabolic myopathies are a diverse group of disorders characterized by abnormalities of skeletal muscle energy production. They arise as a consequence of inherited defects in glycogen, lipid, purine, or mitochondrial metabolism. The term 'secondary metabolic myopathy' has been used to describe muscle damage from miscellaneous insults, such as drugs, toxins, and endocrinopathy.

Metabolic myopathies are traditionally managed within a neurology setting; however, it is imperative that rheumatologists are aware of these diseases as they often mimic other conditions, particularly inflammatory myositis. Furthermore, they can be life threatening and are potentially treatable.

Epidemiology
The metabolic myopathies are rare diseases and epidemiological data are limited. McArdle's disease is one of the more common with a prevalence of approximately one per 100 000. Symptoms may develop at any age, but usually appear in childhood or early adult life.

General clinical features
Metabolic myopathies classically present with episodes of reversible muscle dysfunction induced by exercise.
- Symptoms include muscle cramps, pain, weakness, stiffness, and myoglobinuria.
- Less commonly, they manifest as persistent, progressive muscle weakness.
- In rare cases, there may be a mixture of dynamic and permanent muscle symptoms.
- Children typically present with severe multisystem manifestations, whereas adult-onset disease primarily affects muscles.

Aetiology and pathophysiology
The specific genetic and biochemical abnormalities responsible for many of the metabolic myopathies have been identified. The majority are enzyme defects that lead to a block in muscle adenosine triphosphate (ATP) production. A basic understanding of muscle energy metabolism is fundamental to understanding the pathogenesis of these conditions.

Overview of muscle energy metabolism
Glycogen, glucose and free fatty acids (FFAs) are the main substrates for muscle ATP production.
- Glycogen is metabolized in the cytoplasm to pyruvate, which then diffuses into mitochondria.
- Short and medium chain fatty acids cross freely into the mitochondria.
- Long-chain fatty acids require binding to carnitine for transport across the mitochondrial membrane. This process is mediated by the carnitine palmitoyltransferases I and II.
- Within the mitochondria, oxidative decarboxylation of pyruvate and B-oxidation of FFAs results in acetyl-co-enzyme A formation, ultimately driving ATP production.
- Additional sources of ATP include anaerobic glycolysis (pyruvate is converted to lactate) and the purine nucleotide cycle.

The potential for dysfunction
Episodic muscle dysfunction may be the end result of defects anywhere along the pathway. However, the pattern of symptoms may allow prediction of the likely site of the abnormality.
- FFAs are the principal muscle energy substrate at rest and during prolonged low intensity exertion, e.g. walking. Lipid oxidation defects therefore tend to produce symptoms several hours into moderate exercise or on fasting.
- Utilization of glycogen is necessary for more strenuous exertion, such as running, or on intense, isometric exercise, e.g. lifting weights. Disorders of glycogen metabolism typically cause symptoms within a few minutes of commencing vigorous exercise.
- In mitochondrial myopathies, muscle pain and fatigue may be precipitated by normal daily activities.

The mechanisms by which these defects may lead to rhabdomyolysis are not well understood. In addition, the pathological processes underlying progressive muscle weakness are unclear. These patients tend to have more extensive glycogen or lipid deposition within muscle, which could potentially interfere with contraction; however, this is not universally seen.

Disorders of glycogen metabolism
These conditions are commonly termed the 'glycogen storage disorders' or 'glycogenoses'. They result from a variety of enzyme defects leading to derangements in glycogen synthesis, glycogenolysis, or glycolysis.
- Inheritance is autosomal recessive, with the exception of type VIII (hepatic form) and type IX, which are X-linked recessive traits.
- The clinical manifestations of these conditions are extremely diverse, ranging from severe multisystem disease in infancy to isolated progressive muscle weakness in the elderly.
- Amongst the more common of these, myophosphorylase (McArdle's disease) or phosphofructokinase (PFK) deficiencies typically cause episodic muscle symptoms, whereas acid maltase or debranching enzyme deficiencies are more likely to present with a progressive myopathy.

Myophosphorylase deficiency (McArdle's disease)
- Symptoms often develop in childhood but may not become clinically significant until adolescence
- Muscle fatigue, weakness and aching pain characteristically emerge during the first few minutes of strenuous exertion
- Brief rest or intake of carbohydrate when symptoms appear may subsequently improve exercise tolerance, termed the 'second wind' phenomenon.
- Acute, painful muscle contractures are seen. These differ from ordinary cramps in that they solely occur on exercise, may last for hours, pain is exacerbated by stretching the muscle and electrical activity is absent on EMG.
- Symptoms may culminate in muscle necrosis, myoglobinuria (cola coloured urine) and rarely renal failure.
- Muscle function usually returns to normal between episodes, although mild permanent weakness may develop in long-standing disease.

Phosphofructokinase deficiency (Tarui's disease)
- Clinical presentation may be indistinguishable from McArdle's disease.
- Symptoms are exacerbated, rather than improved by carbohydrate intake.

CHAPTER 18 Miscellaneous diseases

Table 18.5 Glycogenoses

Type	Enzyme defect	Clinical features
II	Acid maltase (α-glucosidase)	Adult form: proximal myopathy with respiratory involvement
III	Debrancher	Hepatomegaly, hypoglycaemia, progressive myopathy
IV	Brancher	Hepatosplenomegaly, cirrhosis, cardiomyopathy, myopathy
V	Myo-phosphorylase	Exercise intolerance, myoglobinuria
VII	Muscle PFK	Exercise intolerance, myoglobinuria, haemolytic anaemia
VIII	Phosphorylase b kinase	Various types affecting liver, heart Muscle form: exercise intolerance, myoglobinuria
IX	PGA kinase	Seizures, mental impairment Exercise intolerance, myoglobinuria
X	Muscle PGA mutase	Exercise intolerance, myoglobinuria
XI	Muscle LDH	Exercise intolerance, myoglobinuria
XII	Aldolase A	Haemolytic anaemia, exercise intolerance, myopathy
XIII	ββ-Enolase	Exercise intolerance
*	AMP-activated protein kinase	Cardiomyopathy, Proximal myopathy

PFK, phosphofructokinase; PGA phosphoglycerate; LDH, lactate dehydrogenase; *not yet classified

- May be a mild haemolytic anaemia (phosphofructokinase is also found in red blood cells).
- Rarely manifests as progressive myopathy in older adults.

Acid maltase deficiency (Pompe's disease)
- Deficiency of lysosomal acid α-glucosidase.
- Classic infantile form is rapidly fatal.
- Late onset variant manifests at any age from early childhood onwards; onset as late as 68 has been reported. Prognosis improves with older age onset.
- Slowly progressive proximal muscle weakness is almost universal and is the presenting symptom in 80%.
- Propensity for respiratory muscle involvement. About 70% patients die from respiratory failure.
- May be increased risk of cerebral aneurysm.

Debranching enzyme deficiency
- May cause progressive myopathy in the 2nd to 3rd decade.
- Weakness and wasting is often predominantly distal.
- Respiratory muscles are occasionally involved.
- A mild sensory axonal polyneuropathy is frequently seen.

Disorders of lipid metabolism
These include:
- Carnitine deficiency syndromes: muscle or systemic.
- Fatty acid transport defects: carnitine palmitoyltransferase II deficiency is the most common.
- Defects of β oxidation enzyme.

Clinical features
Reversible muscle symptoms are classically precipitated by prolonged moderate exertion, e.g. walking, but may also be induced by fasting, cold exposure, infection, or general anaesthesia. Muscle pain is a frequent symptom but cramps are less common than in the glycogenoses and acute, painful contractures, and 'second wind' phenomena are not seen.

- Episodes of hypoketotic hypoglycaemia and coma may result from depletion of glycogen stores on fasting in conjunction with failure of hepatic conversion of fatty acids to ketoacids.
- Lipid deposition may lead to progressive myopathy, cardiomyopathy and fatty infiltration of the liver.
- Abnormal tissue and serum carnitine levels.

Carnitine deficiency syndromes
- Primary muscle carnitine deficiency causes a lipid storage myopathy. It usually presents in early life with progressive, proximal muscle weakness.
- Systemic carnitine deficiency often presents in infancy. Features include recurrent episodes of hypoketotic hypoglycaemia, encephalopathy, and cardiomyopathy.
- Muscle carnitine deficiency may also be seen in mitochondrial disorders or may be acquired, notably secondary to haemodialysis or drugs, e.g. valproate.

Fatty acid transport defects [carnitine palmitoyltransferase (CPT) II deficiency]
- Commonest cause of recurrent rhabdomyolysis and myoglobinuria. The associated risk of acute tubular necrosis is higher than in the glycogenoses.
- Clinical manifestations are usually evident by the age of 20, but may appear as late as the fifth decade.
- The Ser113Leu mutation is found in 65% of patients.
- Episodic muscle pain and stiffness on sustained low intensity exercise or fasting is characteristic.
- Attacks of rhabdomyolysis may be life threatening due to respiratory failure, renal failure, or cardiac arrhythmias.
- Muscle function is usually normal between attacks.

Defects of oxidation enzymes
These affect a variety of mitochondrial enzymes, including the short, medium, long, and very long-chain acyl-CoA dehydrogenases (VLCAD), and produce a wide spectrum of clinical phenotypes. VLCAD deficiency presents similarly to CPT II deficiency and may be clinically indistinguishable.

Disorders of purine metabolism
Adenosine monophosphate (myoadenylate) deaminase (AMPD) deficiency
About 1.2–3.7% of the general population are homozygous for AMPD mutations and deficiency of AMPD has been reported in up to 3% of muscle biopsies. However, the clinical significance of this is debatable. It has been suggested that AMPD deficiency may result in exercise intolerance and myalgia in a subset of affected individuals. Conversely, the prevalence of AMPD deficiency does not appear to be increased in patients with muscle symptoms compared with the general population.

Mitochondrial myopathies
These are a diverse group of multisystem diseases resulting from abnormalities of the respiratory chain. Inheritance is either maternal or Mendelian according to whether genetic defects affect mitochondrial or nuclear DNA.

- Muscle involvement is common but the predominant symptoms are usually extra-muscular, e.g. blindness, deafness, encephalopathy, ophthalmoplegia, and seizures.
- There are numerous recognized syndromes, such as MERRF (myoclonic epilepsy with ragged red fibres), MELAS (mitochondrial encephalomyopathy with lactic acidosis and stroke-like episodes), and PEO (progressive external ophthalmoplegia).
- A subset of patients may present with progressive muscle weakness in the absence of overt systemic manifestations, and a detailed family history and thorough evaluation for potential associated features is therefore required.

Investigation of metabolic myopathies
Investigation beyond basic blood and urine tests is generally undertaken in a specialist setting.

Laboratory
General
- FBC: haemolytic anaemia can occur in some glycogenoses.
- LFTs, renal profile, bone profile, LDH, urate.
- Rhabdomyolysis may lead to elevated creatinine, potassium, urate, phosphate, and reduced calcium.
- Serum myoglobin may be detectable in acute rhabdomyolysis, but is cleared rapidly (within 1–6 h).

Creatine kinase (CK)
- CK should be tested at rest and during acute attacks of muscle symptoms.
- Glycogenoses tend to cause a persistently raised CK. Elevation is usually mild to moderate, although CK may be very high in acid maltase deficiency.
- In lipid oxidation defects, CK is usually normal between episodes of rhabdomyolysis.

Urine myoglobin
- Dark urine, positive for blood on dipstick, but with no red cells/casts on microscopy may indicate myoglobinuria.
- Semi-quantitative assay for haem pigments have approximately 80% sensitivity for myoglobin.
- Crucially, lack of detectable urine myoglobin does not exclude rhabdomyolysis.

Imaging
MR and CT scanning have been utilized in glycogen storage disorders to characterize muscle pathology and are useful to guide muscle biopsy. Nuclear MR spectroscopy provides an assessment of muscle metabolism, and may be useful in detecting glycolytic and mitochondrial defects.

Histology
Muscle biopsy
Diagnosis often rests on specific biochemical testing of muscle tissue for enzyme activity. However, given the large number of potential defects, this should be targeted according to initial clinical evaluation. Microscopy may reveal lipid or glycogen storage vacuoles but equally may be normal. Ragged red fibres suggest mitochondrial myopathy, but are not pathognomonic.

Other
Forearm ischaemic lactate test
- Involves exercising the forearm with an inflated blood pressure cuff *in situ* to create anaerobic conditions, and serial blood tests for lactate, pyruvate, CK, and ammonia.
- This test carries a risk of rhabdomyolysis and a non-ischaemic version has been advocated.
- Glycogenoses cause absence or blunting of the normal rise in lactate (with the exception of acid maltase, brancher and phosphorylase b kinase deficiencies).
- Results are normal in disorders of lipid metabolism.
- Lactate and pyruvate may be elevated in mitochondrial myopathies.

Electromyography (EMG)
- May show myopathic features in glycogenoses, especially in patients with progressive weakness. Marked insertional irritability may be evident in acid maltase deficiency.
- Often normal in mitochondrial disorders and between symptomatic episodes in CPT II deficiency.

Further tests
These should be directed by the clinical presentation.
- Carnitine levels may be abnormal in disorders of lipid metabolism. Serum and urine analysis for fatty acid metabolites is often informative.
- Enzyme testing in white blood cells or skin fibroblasts may be useful in acid maltase deficiency.
- Identification of the responsible genetic defect is now possible in many of the metabolic myopathies.

Differential diagnosis of myopathy
Muscle pain, fatigue, and cramps are ubiquitous complaints, and it may be difficult to determine whether an underlying pathological process is likely. However, severe, aching pain on exertion, prolonged cramps, and myoglobinuria are suggestive of metabolic muscle disease. A thorough family history and evaluation for extramuscular features are mandatory. The numerous alternative causes for muscle cramps should also be considered, including:
- Electrolyte abnormalities: low calcium, magnesium.
- Peripheral vascular disease.
- Hypothyroidism, hyperparathyroidism.
- Drugs/toxins, e.g. diuretics, statins, alcohol.
- Motor neurone disease: leg cramps are common.
- Peripheral neuropathy and radiculopathy.

In patients presenting with progressive muscle weakness, the differential is wide and includes the idiopathic inflammatory myopathies, muscular dystrophies, endocrinopathies, and drugs.

Treatment
General management strategies include:
- Avoidance of activities that precipitate symptoms.
- Dietary modification: A high protein diet and pyridoxine supplements have been advocated for McArdle's disease; however, a recent Cochrane Review concluded there was insufficient evidence to recommend any specific intervention. A low fat, high carbohydrate diet with supplementary intake before exercise appears useful in CPT II deficiency.
- Carnitine, riboflavin, and medium chain triglycerides have been trialled in disorders of lipid metabolism with some success.
- Low dose creatine supplements have been shown to be beneficial in McArdle's disease, although higher doses appeared to be detrimental.
- Moderate intensity exercise programme have been shown to improve symptoms in mitochondrial disorders and glycogenoses and are likely to be helpful in other metabolic myopathies.

Novel therapeutic strategies include enzyme replacement and gene therapies. Intravenous recombinant acid α-glucosidase has been shown to have beneficial effects in acid maltase deficiency. Progress towards gene therapy has been made using animal models, although it remains to be seen whether this is transferable to humans.

Resources

ICD-10 codes
E74.0   Glycogen storage disease
E75.6   Lipid storage disorder unspecified
G71.3   Mitichondrial myopathy

References

Bonnefont JP, Djouadi F, Prip-Buus C, Gobin S, Munnich A, Bastin J. Carnitine palmitoyltransferases 1 and 2: biochemical, molecular and medical aspects. *Mol Aspects Med* 2004; **25**: 495–520.

Darras BT, Friedman NR. Metabolic myopathies: a clinical approach; part I. *Pediatr Neurol* 2000; **22**(2): 87–97.

Dimauro S, Lamperti C. Muscle glycogenoses. *Muscle Nerve* 2001; **24**: 984–99.

DiMauro S. Muscle glycogenoses: an overview. *Acta Myol* 2007; **XXVI**: 35–41.

Haller RG. Treatment of McArdle disease. *Arch Neurol* 2002; **57**: 923–4.

Hanisch F, Joshi P, Zierz S. AMP deaminase deficiency in skeletal muscle is unlikely to be of clinical relevance *J Neurol* 2008;255: 318–22.

Kishnani PS, Corzo D, Nicolino M, et al. Recombinant human acid [alpha]-glucosidase: major clinical benefits in infantile-onset Pompe disease. *Neurology*. 2007; **68**: 99–109.

Niranjanan N, Holton J, Hanna M. Is it really myositis? A consideration of the differential diagnosis. *Curr Opin Rheumatol* 2004; **16**: 684–91

Pierelli PL, Amabile G, Valente G, et al. Muscular cramps: proposals for a new classification. *Acta Neurol Scand* 2003; **107**: 176–86.

Quinlivan R, Beynon RJ, Martinuzzi A. Pharmacological and nutritional treatment for McArdle disease (Glycogen Storage Disease type V). *Cochrane Database Syst Rev.* 2008; 2:CD003458.

Vorgerd M, Zange J, Kley R, et al. Effect of high-dose creatine therapy on symptoms of exercise intolerance in McArdle disease: double-blind, placebo-controlled crossover study. *Arch Neurol* 2002; **59**: 97–101.

Winkel LP, Van den Hout JM, Kamphoven JH, et al. Enzyme replacement therapy in late-onset Pompe's disease: a three-year follow-up. *Ann Neurol.* 2004; **55**: 495–502.

Wortmann RL. Metabolic and mitochondrial myopathies. *Curr Opin Rheumatol* 1999; **11**(6): 462–7.

See also
Polymyositis (p. 282)
Dermatomyositis (p. 290)

Synovial osteochondromatosis

Definition
Synovial osteochondromatosis is a rare condition of synovium causing multiple loose bodies with in a joint cavity.

Epidemiology
- Occurs equally in males and females.
- Onset is typically aged 30–50 years.

Aetiology
Results from metaplasia of synovial tissue into cartilage, which can subsequently calcify or ossify. The trigger for the condition is unknown.

Clinical features
Key features on history
- Usually occurs in a single joint and rarely polyarticular.
- Most commonly affects the knee (>50% cases) hip, shoulder, elbows, TMJ and hands.
- Presentation is with pain and swelling of the joint.
- Joint locking.

Key features on examination
- A firm mass may be palpable.
- There is often restriction of movement, with pain and swelling.

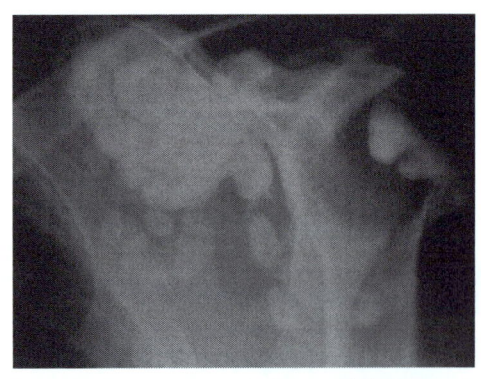

Figure 18.6 Shoulder arthrography showing multiple intra-articular loose bodies typical of synovial osteochondromatosis.

General investigations
Imaging
X-ray
- There is the characteristic appearance of popcorn in the joint if the loose bodies are calcified.
- Secondary OA may develop.

MRI
MRI can demonstrate the chondromata before calcification.

Differential diagnosis
Similar calcified loose bodies can be seen following joint trauma, osteochondritis dessicans, tumoural calcinosis, and severe OA.

Prognosis
Progression is generally slow with eventual development of secondary OA. The condition may be self-limiting with cessation of production of new chondromata. Synovial chondromata do not become malignant.

Pathology
The synovium is hyperplastic with numerous villi. There are cartilaginous nodules within the synovium and also within the joint space.

Synovial fluid
Non-specific inflammatory changes may be seen

Patient advice
- Rare condition, for which symptomatic treatment is usually adequate.
- Surgical removal of loose bodies may be necessary

Treatment
- NSAIDs for pain relief and reduction inflammation.
- Arthroscopy or open arthrotomy for removal of loose bodies and synovectomy. These may need to be repeated as the condition may recur.

References
Crotty JM, Monu JU, Pope TL. Synovial osteochondromatosis. *Radiol Clin N Am* 1996; 34: 327–42.

Pigmented villonodular synovitis

Definition
Pigmented villonodular synovitis (PVNS) is a group of benign proliferative conditions of the synovium and mesenchyme.

Epidemiology
- Occurs equally in males and females.
- The incidence is around 2/million/year.

Aetiology
The aetiology is clonal in nature and PVNS is now considered to be a benign neoplasm of synovium.

Clinical features
Key features on history
There are three modes of presentation
- *Isolated tenosynovitis:* this typically presents in the hand with a painless mass on a finger adherent to a tendon.
- *Diffuse form:* the diffuse form of PVNS usually affects the knee. Presentation is a gradual onset of pain, swelling, and stiffness, affecting a single joint. Less commonly the hip, ankle, hand, shoulder, or spine are involved.
- *Localized form:* this is the least common. Presentation is with joint swelling and locking due to a free floating pedunculated intra-articular mass.

Key features on examination
- *Isolated tenosynovitis:* a painless mass adherent to a tendon.
- *Diffuse form:* warm swollen joint with restricted range of movement.
- *Localized form:* swollen joint, which may lock..

Investigation
Imaging
X-rays
Plain radiographs do not show the lesion, but in joints with a tight capsule there may be scalloped lesions with sclerotic margins, due to local erosion or pressure from the mass.
CT
CT scanning shows high attenuation because of the presence of haemosiderin pigment.

MRI
MRI is the investigation of choice. The lesion appears dark on all sequences because of the ferromagnetic nature of haemosiderin causing shortening of the T1 and T2 relaxation time. The extent of the lesion can be delineated and used to plan surgery.

Joint aspiration
Aspirated synovial fluid is haemorrhagic or brown in colour, due to recurrent haemorrhage.

Differential diagnosis
The isolated form needs to be distinguished from other lesions such as ganglions and foreign body granulomata.
PVNS as a cause of haemarthrosis needs to be distinguished from other causes of bloody knee effusions, such as trauma, clotting disorders, neuropathic joints, sickle cell anaemia, and hypermobility. Recurrent haemorrhagic effusions should raise the possibility of PVNS.
Localized form needs to differentiated from other causes of joint locking, such as meniscal tears.

Prognosis
Progression is generally very slow; however, the diffuse form can cause significant disability.

Pathology
Exuberant proliferation of synovial lining cells. They are invasive and form finger-like extensions or villi, which fill the joint space with lobulated masses that invade into the subsynovial connective tissue leading to bone erosions and destruction. Histologically, there are multinucleated giant cells and haemosiderin laden macrophages, giving rise to the characteristic colour of the lesion.

Patient advice
- Benign lesion.
- Surgery is curative in the isolated and localized forms.
- Diffuse form requires extensive removal synovium and possible joint replacement, and may be disabling.

Treatment
- *Isolated tenosynovitis:* surgical treatment is aimed at removing the mass from the tendon sheath and is curative.
- *Diffuse form:* there are no randomized controlled trials in PVNS. Surgery is usually synovectomy, but it is usually difficult to achieve a curative resection. No medical treatment is successful. Radiation synovectomy has been used in combination with extensive surgical debridement. In the hip and knee total synovectomy followed by total arthroplasty has been successful with a low recurrence rate.
- *Localized form:* surgical excision of the free floating mass is curative.

Resources
ICD-10 coding
M12.2 villonodular synovitis (pigmented)

References
Tyler WK, Vidal AF, Williams RJ, Healey JH. Pigmented villonodular synovitis. *J Am Acad Orthop Surg* 2006; **14**: 376–85..

Bone tumours

Definition
Primary tumours of bone are generally rare and comprise a spectrum from benign lesions to aggressively malignant lesions.

Epidemiology
Generally rare conditions that can occur at any age group. Certain lesions, however, have very clearly defined age-specific occurrence.

Classification
The World Health Organization has developed a classification system for bone tumours based on histopathological criteria.

Classification of bone tumours

Bone-forming tumours
- **Benign:** osteoma, osteoid osteoma.
- **Intermediate:** malignant osteoblastoma.
- **Malignant:** osteosarcoma.

Cartilage-forming tumours
- **Benign:** chondroma, osteochondroma, chondroblastoma, chondroidmyxoid fibroma.
- **Malignant:** chondrosarcoma.

Giant cell tumour (osteoclastoma)

Marrow tumours (round cell tumours)
- Ewing sarcoma, neuroectodermal tumour, lymphoma, myeloma

Adapted from Dixon (2004).

Osteoma
Slowly growing benign lesion of well-differentiated mature bone tissue.

Key features on history
- Usually present in between ages 20 and 40 years.
- Often asymptomatic.
- Presents with a slow growing hard mass.

Key features on examination
Hard, firm swelling or mass.

General investigations
Imaging
- *X-ray:* dense radio-opaque well defined <3 cm in diameter.

Differential diagnosis
Multiple osteomata are part of Gardner's syndrome – colonic polyposis, osteomata, and soft tissue tumours.

Pathology
Thick trabeculae of mature bone.

Treatment
Excision for symptoms or cosmetic reasons.

Osteoid osteoma
Benign osteoblastic lesion, with a clearly demarcated outline.

Key features on history
- Present between age 5 and 30 and is more common in men.
- Pain is constant, worse at night, poorly localized, and not relieved by rest. Pain may be worsened by alcohol and relieved by aspirin.
- Most commonly located in the femur or tibia, but also occurs in short bones and the spinal column.

Key features on examination
Muscle atrophy, localized swelling, and tenderness.

General investigations
Imaging
- *X-ray:* small round area of osteolysis (nidus), surrounded by a halo of hyperostosis.
- *CT scan:* shows the nidus clearly and enables surgery to be planned.
- *Bone scintigraphy:* shows an area of increased uptake of radioisotope.

Differential diagnosis
This is from other bone tumours. When occurring close to a joint, may be mistaken for a monarthropathy.

Pathology
Cellular, highly vascular with immature bone and osteoid.

Treatment
- Surgical removal of the nidus.
- Incomplete resection may lead to recurrence.

Osteosarcoma
Malignant tumour of bone. Characterized by formation of bone or osteoid by tumour cells.

Key features on history
Pain arising from the tumour is often not very severe, and is increased by activity. In the later stages lump may be palpable. Pathological fracture may occur. The course is usually quite rapid.

Key features on examination
Localized tenderness with a palpable mass. Overlying skin may be warm due to marked vascularity of the tumour.

General investigations
Imaging

X-ray

The characteristic radiological features are:
- Periosteal reaction with formation of long spicules of bone radiating perpendicular to the bone giving a 'sunburst' appearance. This can also be seen in benign lesion such as haemangioma and other malignant lesions such as Ewing's sarcoma.
- Codman's triangle reflects elevation of the periosteum from the underlying cortex and can also occur in osteomyelitis or Ewing's sarcoma.

CT
- CT is useful to assess the local extent of bone.
- CT of the thorax should be performed at presentation because pulmonary metastasis is common.

MRI
MRI is the optimum method to assess extent of the lesion in bone.

Differential diagnosis
Osteosarcoma needs to be distinguished from other malignant bone tumours.

Pathology
There is a wide spectrum of pathological appearances, but the production of osteoid or bone is essential for the diagnosis.

Treatment
Pre- and post-operative chemotherapy and surgery.

Prognosis
The combination of chemotherapy and surgery has improved survival rates to 60–70% at 5 years.

Chondroma
Benign tumour characterized by formation of mature cartilage. Solitary lesions arising in the medulla (enchondroma)

Key features on history
- Often asymptomatic.
- When superficial may become palpable as lump.
- Pain occurs if there is a pathological fracture or malignant transformation.

Key features on examination
Palpable mass. Due to swelling of the bone.

General Investigations
Imaging
X-ray
- Small or moderate-sized osteolytic round or ovoid areas with well-defined margins, which expand and thin the cortex.
- Usually located in the metaphysis.

Differential diagnosis
- Radiologically from epidermal cysts in the terminal phalanges.
- Multiple enchondromata often unilateral occur in Ollier's disease. Maffucci syndrome is multiple enchondromata occurring in association with haemangiomata.

Pathology
The lesion is composed of mature cartilage.

Treatment
Surgical resection or curettage of small lesions.

Prognosis
Generally good, but there is a risk of malignant transformation, especially in multiple enchondromatosis.

Osteochondroma
Cartilage capped bony projection on the outside surface of bone.

Key features on history
- Osteochondromata are the most common bone tumour, comprising 40% of benign tumours and 20% of all bone tumours.
- Most common sites are metaphysis of long bones.
- Multiple osteochondromata are associated with disturbance of growth with shortness and deformity.
- Diagnosis is usually aged <20 years.
- Usually diagnosed as an incidental finding or presents as a painless mass.
- Pain is due fracture.

Key features on examination
Painless bony deformity.

General Investigations
Imaging
X-ray
Plain X-rays show a bony projection with a cartilage capped surface.

Treatment
Surgical resection only for symptomatic lesions.

Prognosis
The risk of malignant transformation to a chondrosarcoma is < 1%. The risk is much higher in cases of multiple osteochondromatosis.

Chondrosarcoma
Malignant tumour characterized by formation of cartilage.

Key features on history
- Pain is usually the first symptom, with a firm swelling.
- Variable duration of symptoms from weeks to years.

Key features on examination
Firm swelling.

General investigations
Imaging
X-rays
Intra-osseous osteolytic tumour. May show thickening and expansion of cortex. Extension into soft tissue suggests a high-grade malignancy.

MRI/CT
Best method of delineating extra-osseous extent.

Pathology
Cartilage forming tumour, with pleomorphic cells.

Treatment
Surgical resection is required. They are relatively radio-resistant and chemotherapeutic regimens are poorly developed.

Prognosis
- The 5-year survival is 50–50%.
- The most common site of metastasis is the lung.

References
Dixon. Bone Tumours. In: Hochberg M, Silman A, Smolen J, Weinblatt M, Weisman M (eds) *Rheumatology*, 3rd edn. Ottawa: Mosby 2004; 2185–99.

Schajowicz F. *Tumours and tumour like lesions of bone*, 2nd edn. Berlin: Springer Verlag, 1994.

Chapter 19

DMARDs and immunosuppressive drugs

Methotrexate *532*
Sulfasalazine *538*
Leflunomide *540*
Anti-malarials (hydroxychloroquine and chloroquine) *544*
Gold: intramuscular (sodium aurothimalate) and oral (auranofin) *546*
Penicillamine *550*
Azathioprine *552*
Mycophenolate mofetil *556*
Ciclosporin (previously cyclosporin A) *558*
Cyclophosphamide *562*
Biologics: anti-TNF (infliximab, etanercept, adalimumab), anti-CD20 (rituximab), anti-IL-1 (anakinra), CTLA4–Ig (abatacept), and anti-IL-6R (tocilizumab) *568*

Methotrexate

History
- **1940s**: aminopterin, a recently developed folic acid antagonist, being used in children with leukaemia, is found to be efficacious in the treatment of patients with rheumatoid arthritis.
- **1950s**: methotrexate (amethopterin; MTX; a less potent folic acid antagonist) is developed. Weekly pulses of methotrexate are anecdotally shown to have similar efficacy but less toxicity than aminopterin.
- **1960/70s**: anecdotal evidence accumulates for the use of MTX in rheumatoid arthritis and psoriatic arthritis.
- **1980s**: double-blind placebo controlled studies (DBPCS) confirm the efficacy of weekly pulsed MTX treatment in rheumatoid arthritis and psoriatic arthritis.
- **1990s**: folic acid supplementation is shown in DBPCS to reduce MTX toxicity and side effects but to have no effect on efficacy. MTX becomes the first choice disease modifying agent (DMARD) in rheumatoid arthritis. MTX combination treatments with other DMARDs is shown to be efficacious in patients not responding to MTX monotherapy. MTX combination treatment with other DMARDs is shown to be efficacious in early inflammatory arthritis. 'Inverting the pyramid' – early, rather than late treatment of rheumatoid arthritis with MTX is advocated
- **2000s**: MTX combination treatment with anti-TNF treatment is more efficacious than MTX monotherapy.

Possible mechanisms of action

Folate antagonist
MTX was developed as a folate antagonist, competitively inhibiting dihydrofolate reductase. Inhibition of dihydrofolate reductase results in reduced thymidine nucleotide synthesis and, therefore, reduced DNA synthesis and reduced lymphocyte proliferation. This is certainly its mode of action at the higher doses used in chemotherapy. Whether this is the mechanism of action in inflammatory arthritis is less clear. Methotrexate efficacy is not inhibited by folinic or folic acid co-treatment and regular folic acid supplementation is frequently given with methotrexate.

Adenosine release
Adenosine is an endogenous anti-inflammatory that is affected by MTX administration. Caffeine – an antagonist of adenosine – has been shown to have inhibitory effects on the efficacy of methotrexate, in keeping with the rationale for folate supplementation.

T cell adhesion molecule expression
In vitro studies show that MTX reduces the expression of adhesion molecules (e.g. VCAM-1, CLA and ICAM-1) on T cells. The effects on CLA (cutaneous lymphocyte-associated antigen) may be particularly important in psoriasis.

Evidence base: the clinical trials with MTX and what they showed

Summary
There is good evidence for MTX efficacy in rheumatoid arthritis and combination therapy should be considered early in the disease. MTX combines well with anti TNF treatments and most other DMARDS (except possibly sulfasalazine).

- MTX is useful in psoriatic arthritis, but may not be as good as sulfasalazine.
- MTX is useful as maintenance therapy, but not induction treatment, of ANCA associated vasculitis.
- MTX can be useful in SLE for the articular and cutaneous manifestations.
- There is no evidence to support MTX use in giant cell arteritis

Rheumatoid arthritis

MTX monotherapy
Weinblatt ME, Coblyn JS, Fox DA (1985) Efficacy of low-dose methotrexate in rheumatoid arthritis. *N Engl J Med* **312**(13): 818–22. A short study in a small group of patients (28) in a crossover placebo controlled study showed MTX to be superior to placebo.

William HJ, Willkens RF, Samuelson CO Jr, et al (1985) Comparison of low-dose oral pulse methotrexate and placebo in the treatment of rheumatoid arthritis. A controlled clinical trial. *Arthritis Rheum* **28**:721–30. The first large study (180 patients) showing clinical benefit of MTX over placebo.

Combination therapy methotrexate combines well with most other DMARDs

1. *MTX, hydroxychloroquine and sulfasalazine*
O'Dell JR, Leff R, Paulsen G, et al. (2002) Treatment of rheumatoid arthritis with methotrexate and hydroxychloroquine, methotrexate and sulfasalazine, or a combination of the three medications: results of a two-year, randomized, double-blind, placebo-controlled trial. *Arthritis Rheum* **46**:1164–70. The COBRA Study: triple combination treatment with MTX, hydroxychloroquine and sulfasalazine is better than MTX and sulfasalazine in combination. MTX and hydroxychloroquine is almost as good.

2. *MTX and leflunomide*
Kremer JM, Genovese MC, Cannon GW, et al. (2002) Concomitant leflunomide therapy in patients with active rheumatoid arthritis despite stable doses of methotrexate. A randomized, double-blind, placebo-controlled trial. *Ann Intern Med* **137**(9): 726–33. Good efficacy for the combination treatment, but problems with elevated liver transaminases

3. *MTX and ciclosporin*
Tugwell P, Pincus T, Yocum D, et al. (1995) Combination therapy with cyclosporine and methotrexate in severe rheumatoid arthritis. The Methotrexate-Cyclosporine Combination Study Group. *N Engl J Med* **333**(3): 137–41.

Ciclosporin with MTX is efficacious in MTX partial responders.

1. *MTX and gold*
Lehman AJ, Esdaile JM, Klinkhoff AV, et al. (2005) A 48-week, randomized, double-blind, double-observer, placebo-controlled multicenter trial of combination methotrexate and intramuscular gold therapy in rheumatoid arthritis: results of the METGO study. *Arthritis Rheum* **52**: 1360–70. Addition of IM Gold to MTX is advantageous in patients who have an inadequate response to MTX alone.

2. MTX and doxycycline
O'Dell JR, Elliott JR, Mallek JA, et al. (2006) Treatment of early seropositive rheumatoid arthritis: doxycycline plus methotrexate versus methotrexate alone. *Arthritis Rheum* **54**:621–7. Treatment with doxycycline (either 40 or 200 mg per day) and MTX in early seropositive inflammatory arthritis was superior to MTX alone.

3. MTX and anti-TNF
Maini R, St Clair EW, Breedveld F, et al. (1999) Infliximab (chimeric anti-tumour necrosis factor α monoclonal antibody) versus placebo in rheumatoid arthritis patients receiving concomitant methotrexate: a randomised phase III trial. ATTRACT Study Group. *Lancet.* **354**(9194): 1932–9.

Weinblatt ME, Kremer JM, Bankhurst AD, et al. (1999) A trial of etanercept, a recombinant tumor necrosis factor receptor:Fc fusion protein, in patients with rheumatoid arthritis receiving methotrexate. *N Engl J Med* **340**(4): 253–9.

The two initial anti-TNF studies (with etanercept and infliximab) showing that combination treatment with MTX and anti-TNF is efficacious in MTX non-responders

Goekoop-Ruiterman YP, de Vries-Bouwstra JK, Allaart CF, et al. (2005). Clinical and radiographic outcomes of four different treatment strategies in patients with early rheumatoid arthritis (the BeSt study): a randomised controlled trial. *Arthritis Rheum* **52**: 3381–90. The BeSt study showing that early combination treatment with methotrexate and anti-TNF, or methotrexate, sulfasalazine, and prednisolone, resulted in more rapid improvement clinically and joint damage suppression than sequential monotherapy or step-up combination therapy.

Psoriatic arthritis

MTX monotherapy
Willkens RF, Williams HJ, Ward JR, et al. (1984) Randomized, double-blind, placebo controlled trial of low-dose pulse methotrexate in psoriatic arthritis. *Arthritis Rheum* **27**: 376–81. Showed that MTX is more efficacious than placebo – in the Cochrane systematic review of 2000 it was concluded: 'The magnitude of the effect seen with ... oral low dose methotrexate suggests that it may be effective, but that further multicentre clinical trials are required to establish its efficacy'. Sulfasalazine and parenteral high dose MTX were seen to be more efficacious

MTX combination therapy
In psoriatic arthritis the only good evidence is for ciclosporin and MTX combination treatment:
Fraser AD, van Kuijk AW, Westhovens R, et al. (2005) A randomised, double blind, placebo controlled, multicentre trial of combination therapy with methotrexate plus ciclosporin in patients with active psoriatic arthritis. *Ann Rheum Dis* **64**: 859–64. Showed that patients responding inadequately to MTX alone benefited from additional DMARD treatment with ciclosporin.

Giant cell arteritis
There is no evidence for the use of methotrexate in GCA. Hoffman GS, Cid MC, Hellmann DB, et al. (2002) A multicenter, randomized, double-blind, placebo-controlled trial of adjuvant methotrexate treatment for giant cell arteritis. *Arthritis Rheum.* **46**: 1309–18. One of several good quality studies that have failed to show any benefit for MTX in giant cell arteritis.

ANCA associated vasculitis
De Groot K, Rasmussen N, Bacon PA, et al. (2005) Randomized trial of cyclophosphamide versus methotrexate for induction of remission in early systemic antineutrophil cytoplasmic antibody-associated vasculitis. *Arthritis Rheum* **52**: 2461–9. Methotrexate is effective, but less so than cyclophosphamide, and in patients with significant end organ involvement MTX should be used as maintenance treatment following remission induction with cyclophosphamide.

SLE
Carneiro JR, Sato EL (1999) Double blind, randomized, placebo controlled clinical trial of methotrexate in systemic lupus erythematosus. *J Rheumatol* **26**: 1275–9. This and one other controlled study in SLE show efficacy for MTX for articular and cutaneous manifestations of SLE

Prescribing considerations

What do I need to do before starting the treatment?
- Patient education with regard to dosing, side effects, monitoring, drug interactions, etc.
- Ensure your patient has a patient held monitoring booklet such as the one advised by the National Patient Safety Agency (http://www.npsa.nhs.uk/display?contentId=5085).

Record at baseline	
FBC	Allows monitoring of changes
LFTs	Allows monitoring of changes
ESR or CRP	Monitor disease activity
Renal function	Impaired renal function increases MTX levels
Varicella status	Either history or serology
CXR	Allows comparison in pulmonary toxicity

- An abnormal CXR is not a contraindication to treatment, but the patient should be monitored carefully, since there is an increased risk of MTX pneumonitis in patients with pre-existing lung disease.
- Some clinicians advocate pre-treatment pulmonary function to facilitate monitoring in the event of pneumonitis (see below under pneumonitis), but this is not universal
- Liaise with the patients GP represcribing and appropriate monitoring of the treatment

What dose should I prescribe?
- Oral methotrexate: 7.5–25 mg/**week**.
- Methotrexate should not be crushed or chewed.
- **Methotrexate is a weekly treatment,**
    e.g. **M** is for **M**ethotrexate on a **M**onday.

Various protocols are used for dosage escalation. Some use a more rapidly escalating regime than others.

> **Example regime:**
> - 10 mg/week starting dose increasing at 6 weeks (if blood test monitoring satisfactory) to 15 mg/week. Thereafter, 3 monthly increases of 2.5 mg/week (if blood test monitoring satisfactory) until dose of 25 mg/week or disease adequately controlled.
> - In vasculitis the usual starting dose in 15 mg/week.
>
> *Oral versus parenteral treatment*
> - Above 20 mg/week the bioavailability of oral methotrexate is variable and partial responders may benefit from a change to parenteral (usually subcutaneous) treatment
> - Overall dose should be adjusted on conversion due to improved bioavailability
> - 20 mg/week of oral MTX =~ 15 mg/week of SC. MTX

Folic acid prescription?
- Folic acid supplementation reduces side effects (mucocutaneous and hepatic) without affecting efficacy and is generally prescribed routinely. It should not be given the same day and is usually given weekly like MTX,

e.g. F for Folic Acid on a Friday

Important drug interactions
- Trimethoprim and Cotrimoxazole (Septrin) can cause acute pancytopenia and should be avoided.
- Phenytoin can increase the anti-folate effects of MTX.
- Probenecid decreases MTX excretion.
- NSAIDs do not significantly interfere with MTX at the doses used rheumatologically..

Monitoring
- **FBC & LFTs:** the British National Formulary advises weekly until therapy is stabilized and thereafter 2–3 monthly.
- **ESR:** useful for monitoring response to treatment

Side effects and what to discuss with your patients

Common
Nausea, abdominal discomfort, diarrhoea, anorexia, oral ulceration.

Haematological toxicity
Neutropenia, thrombocytopenia, pancytopenia. Warn patients to report infections/sore throat/bruising

Pulmonary toxicity
- Acute interstitial pneumonitis (an acute presentation).
- This is a hypersensitivity reaction to methotrexate.
- Note: MTX does not appear to cause pulmonary fibrosis Warn patients to report new: dry cough +/- dyspnoea.

Hepatic toxicity
- MTX can cause hepatic fibrosis and cirrhosis.
- More problematic in patients with psoriatic arthritis.
- Alcohol exacerbates this problem.
- Warn patients to avoid alcohol (psoriatic) and to minimize alcohol (rheumatoid).

FAQs
How long does it take to work?

A clinical response is usually seen after 3 months of treatment with methotrexate

What if I want to get pregnant?

Methotrexate is teratogenic, and should be avoided before and during pregnancy. It can have effects on both sperm and ova. It can also cause miscarriage. Methotrexate should be discontinued at least 3 months prior to planned conception by men and women

What about fertility?

Methotrexate may affect fertility in both and men and women although this has not been extensively studied.

What about injections?
- Live attenuated vaccines need to be avoided by patients taking methotrexate: yellow fever, MMR and rubella, BCG, oral polio, oral typhoid.
- Other vaccines will not be a problem.
- Patients should be advised to have an annual influenza immunization since they are at an increased risk of influenza.

What if I miss a dose?

Methotrexate can be taken at the normal dose up to 48 h after the usual time of the weekly dose. If later than 48 h the dose for that week should be omitted and the normal dose taken the following week.

Can I drink alcohol?

Patients with psoriatic arthritis should be advised to avoid alcohol. Patients with rheumatoid arthritis should be advised to minimize alcohol consumption

What to do if side effects occur

Common side effects
- Reduce the dose of MTX.
- Consider increasing folic acid dose.

CHAPTER 19 **DMARDs and immunosuppressive drugs** 535

ASYMPTOMATIC PATIENT

Persistent
Neutropenia (<1.5x10⁹/L) or
Thrombocytopenia (<150x10⁹/L)

↓

Stop MTX and monitor response

├── Resolved → Consider Retreatment at Lower dose
└── Persists → Assessment with Haematologist

SYMPTOMATIC PATIENT

Neutropenia (<1.5x10⁹/L) or
Thrombocytopenia (<150x10⁹/L)

↓

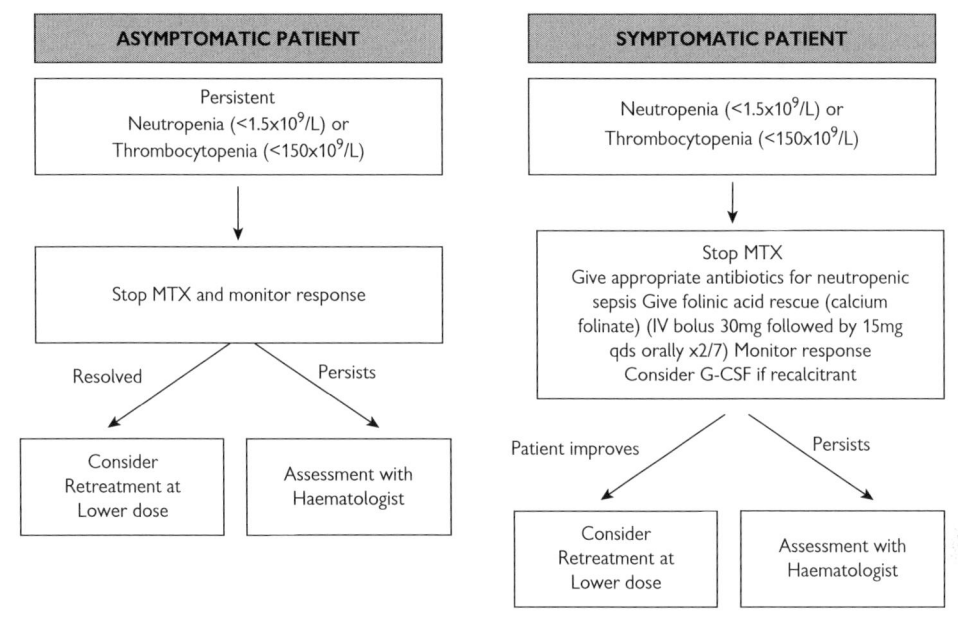

Stop MTX
Give appropriate antibiotics for neutropenic sepsis Give folinic acid rescue (calcium folinate) (IV bolus 30mg followed by 15mg qds orally x2/7) Monitor response
Consider G-CSF if recalcitrant

├── Patient improves → Consider Retreatment at Lower dose
└── Persists → Assessment with Haematologist

Figure 19.1 Haematological toxicity.

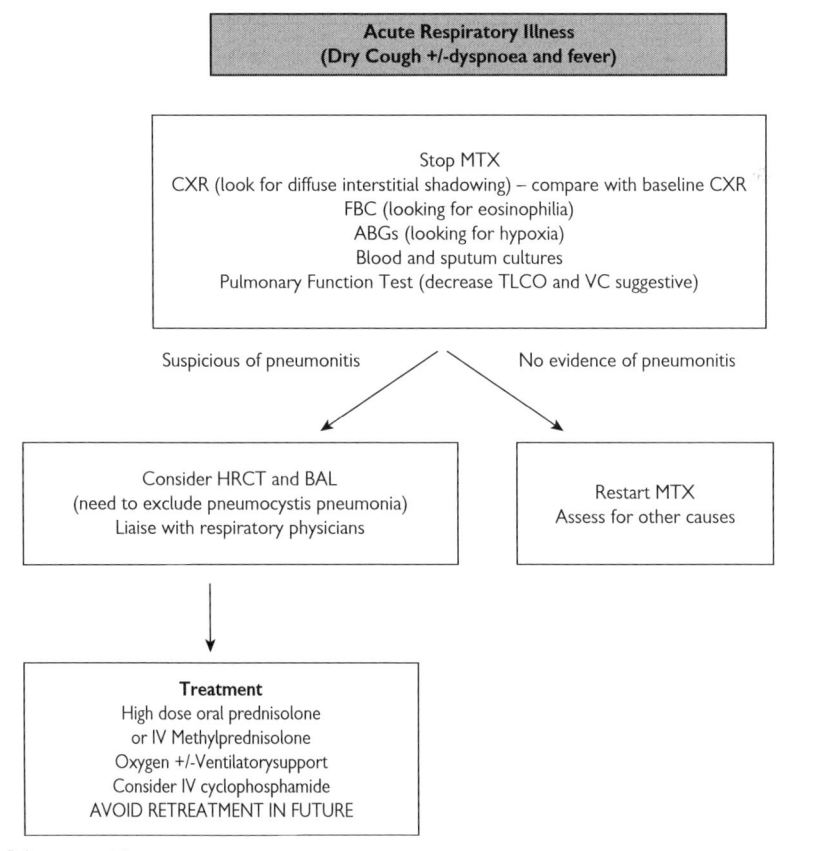

**Acute Respiratory Illness
(Dry Cough +/-dyspnoea and fever)**

↓

Stop MTX
CXR (look for diffuse interstitial shadowing) – compare with baseline CXR
FBC (looking for eosinophilia)
ABGs (looking for hypoxia)
Blood and sputum cultures
Pulmonary Function Test (decrease TLCO and VC suggestive)

├── Suspicious of pneumonitis → Consider HRCT and BAL (need to exclude pneumocystis pneumonia) Liaise with respiratory physicians
└── No evidence of pneumonitis → Restart MTX Assess for other causes

↓

Treatment
High dose oral prednisolone
or IV Methylprednisolone
Oxygen +/-Ventilatorysupport
Consider IV cyclophosphamide
AVOID RETREATMENT IN FUTURE

Figure 19.2 Pulmonary toxicity.

Figure 19.3 Hepatic toxicity.

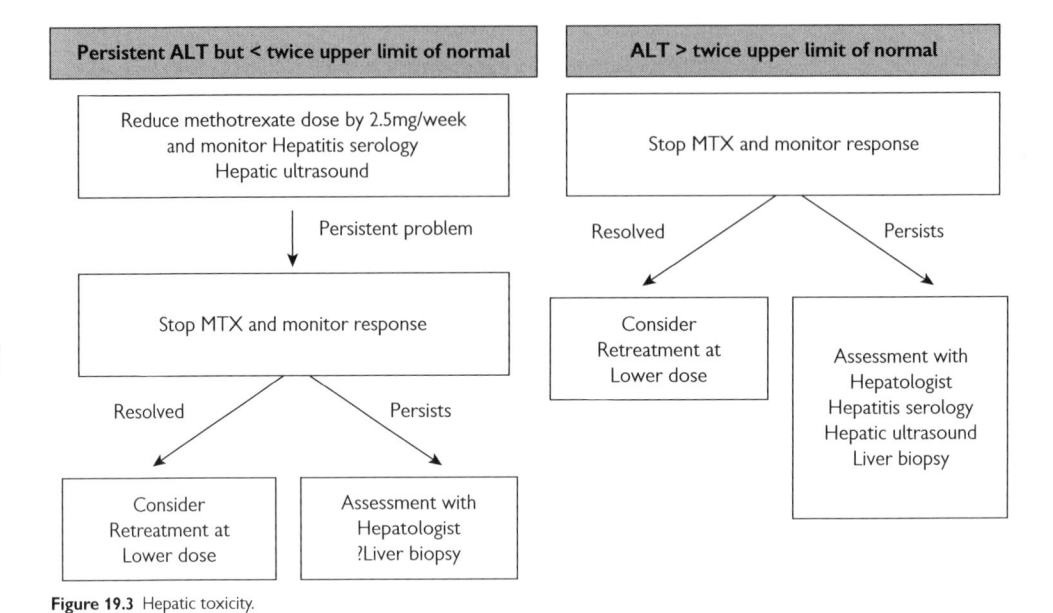

Surgical considerations
It is safe to continue MTX in the perioperative period and stopping the treatment may be associated with worse post-operative outcomes due to impaired rehabilitation.

Sulfasalazine

Trade name Salazopyrin

History
- **1942:** Dr Svartz synthesizes sulfasazaline – a combination of an anti-inflammatory (5-aminosalicylic acid) and an antibiotic (sulfapyridine).
- **1973**: sulfasalazine shown to have efficacy in ulcerative colitis.
- **1983**: sulfasalazine shown to have efficacy in rheumatoid arthritis.
- **1990**: sulfasalazine shown to have efficacy in psoriatic arthritis.

Possible mechanisms of action
Sulfasalazine (SSZ) is a combination of 5-amino salicylic acid and sulfapyridine. The anti-inflammatory, 5-aminosalicylic acid is produced following metabolism of SSZ in the intestine and is not well absorbed. It is this non-absorbed 5-aminosalicylic acid component that accounts for the efficacy of SSZ in inflammatory bowel disease. The sulfapyridine moiety is absorbed systemically and probably accounts for much (but not all) of the efficacy of SSZ in inflammatory arthritis.

Inhibition of NFkB activation
NFkB is important in T cell activation and can be induced by TNF-α. This mechanism of action may underline the efficacy of sulfasalazine in inflammatory arthritis. Sulfapyridine in isolation does not appear to have the same effect.

Induction of apoptosis of activated T cells
This effect may be linked to the NFkB inhibition, since NFkB inhibits the action of tumour necrosis factor (TNF)-related apoptosis-inducing ligand (TRAIL). Activity of this ligand results in apoptosis of T cells, which is enhanced following in vitro treatment with sulfasalazine.

Cytokine Inhibition (IL-1 and TNF α)
Sulfasalazine has been shown to inhibit TNF expression in monocytes in vitro and to reduce IL-1 and TNF α levels in vivo, which may clearly be an important mechanism of action in inflammatory arthritis.

Inhibition of folate uptake
Although probably not important as a mechanism of action, this action interferes with the uptake of MTX and predisposes patients on sulfasalazine to folate deficiency.

Evidence base: the main clinical trials with SSZ and what they showed
Summary
- SSZ is effective as monotherapy in psoriatic arthritis and appear more efficacious than methotrexate in this condition.
- SSZ is less effective in rheumatoid arthritis than methotrexate, but is nonetheless efficacious as monotherapy. It is more beneficial when combined with methotrexate, alongside hydroxychloroquine or prednisolone.

Psoriatic arthritis
Farr M, Kitas GD, Waterhouse L, et al. (1990) Sulphasalazine in psoriatic arthritis: a double-blind placebo-controlled study. Br J Rheumatol **29**: 46–9.

Dougados M, van der Linden S, Leirisalo-Repo M, et al. (1995) Sulfasalazine in the treatment of spondylarthropathy. A randomized, multicenter, double-blind, placebo-controlled study. Arthritis Rheum **38**: 618–27.

Gupta AK, Grober JS, Hamilton TA, et al. (1995) Sulfasalazine therapy for psoriatic arthritis: a double blind, placebo controlled trial. J Rheumatol **22**: 894–8.

Clegg DO, Reda DJ, Mejias E, et al. (1996) Comparison of sulfasalazine and placebo in the treatment of psoriatic arthritis. A Department of Veterans Affairs Cooperative Study. Arthritis Rheum **39**: 2013–20.

A selection of the placebo-controlled trials showing efficacy for SSZ in patients with psoriatic arthritis. A review of the evidence in favour of SSZ in psoriatic arthritis was published by the Cochrane Review Group in 2000.

Rheumatoid arthritis
SSZ monotherapy
Pullar T, Hunter JA, Capell HA (1983) Sulphasalazine in rheumatoid arthritis: a double blind comparison of sulphasalazine with placebo and sodium aurothiomalate. Br Med J (Clin Res Ed) **287**(6399): 1102–4. The first study showing the efficacy of SSZ in rheumatoid arthritis.

SSZ combination therapy
Sulfasalazine is efficacious in combination with MTX and steroid, particularly when hydroxychloroquine is used as well.

SSZ, hydroxychloroquine, and methotrexate
O'Dell JR, Leff R, Paulsen G, et al. (2002) Treatment of rheumatoid arthritis with methotrexate and hydroxychloroquine, methotrexate and sulfasalazine, or a combination of the three medications: results of a two-year, randomized, double-blind, placebo-controlled trial. Arthritis Rheum **46**: 1164–70.

Mottonen T, Hannonen P, Leirisalo-Repo M, et al. (1999) Comparison of combination therapy with single-drug therapy in early rheumatoid arthritis: a randomised trial. FIN-RACo trial group. Lancet. **353**(9164): 1568–73. Triple combination treatment with MTX, hydroxychloroquine, and sulfasalazine (the COBRA regime, or MTX and hydroxychloroquine) is better than MTX and sulfasalazine in combination.

SSZ, methotrexate, and prednisolone
Goekoop-Ruiterman YP, de Vries-Bouwstra JK, Allaart CF, et al. (2005) Clinical and radiographic outcomes of four different treatment strategies in patients with early rheumatoid arthritis (the BeSt study): a randomised controlled trial. Arthritis Rheum **52**: 3381–90. The BeSt study showed that early combination treatment with methotrexate and anti-TNF, or methotrexate, sulfasalazine, and prednisolone, resulted in more rapid improvement clinically and joint damage suppression than sequential monotherapy or step-up combination therapy.

Prescribing considerations
What do I need to do before starting the treatment?
- Patient education: dosing, side effects, monitoring.
- Ensure your patient has a monitoring booklet.

CHAPTER 19 DMARDs and immunosuppressive drugs

Record at baseline	
FBC	Allows monitoring of changes
LFTs	Allows monitoring of changes
ESR or CRP	Monitor disease activity
Renal function	Adjust dose if impaire

What dose should I prescribe?
The usual treatment dose in both rheumatoid arthritis and psoriatic arthritis in 1 g bd. The dosage is built up over the first 4 weeks of treatment:

Week 1 500 mg od.

Week 2 500 mg bd.

Week 3 1 g mane, 500 mg nocte.

Week 4 1 g bd.

The dose can be increased to 3 g if an inadequate response is achieved at the 1 g bd dose. In the author's experience this is more likely to be beneficial in patients with psoriatic arthritis.

Folic acid prescription?
Folic acid supplementation has not been shown to be beneficial in reducing the side effects of sulfasalazine (unlike methotrexate). However, sulfasalazine can cause elevation of homocysteine levels and a macrocytosis. In these instances, folic acid supplementation (as is used with methotrexate) can be considered.

Important drug interactions
Digoxin: sulfasalazine may reduce digoxin levels by interfering with absorption.

Monitoring of SSZ
FBC & LFTs

> **Example monitoring regime (local guidelines may vary)**
> - Fortnightly for the first 2 weeks.
> - Monthly, thereafter, for the first 3 months.
> - Thereafter, 3 monthly.

Renal function

6-monthly (the benefits of monitoring renal function with sulfasalazine are questionable).

ESR

Useful for monitoring response to treatment.

Side effects and what to discuss with your patients
Common

Nausea, abdominal discomfort, diarrhoea, skin rashes, malaise, headache, anorexia, oral ulceration, orange discolouration of body secretions.

Haematological toxicity
- Neutropenia, thrombocytopenia, pancytopenia.
- Warn patients to report infections/sore throat/bruising.
- These usually occur within the first 6 months of starting treatment with sulfasalazine.

Dermatological toxicity

As well as causing photosensitization, SSZ can rarely cause hypersensitivity reactions, including acute Stevens Johnson syndrome, and the treatment should be discontinued immediately if these reactions occur.

Orange body fluids

SSZ may cause body secretions to become an orange colour – urine, tears, sweat. This can cause staining of clothes and contact lenses, but is otherwise not clinically significant. Patients should be warned of this possibility.

Sperm counts

SSZ can cause a reversible oligospermia/azospermia. Male patients should be advised of decreased fertility. Sulfasalazine should be discontinued 3 months prior to planned conception in males.

FAQs
How long does it take to work?

A clinical response is usually seen after 3 months of treatment with sulfasalazine.

What do I do if I want to get pregnant?

No major teratogenic effects have been seen with sulfasalazine and it is generally considered reasonably safe in pregnancy. However, adequate folic acid supplementation prior to conception and during pregnancy should be assured given the anti-folate effects of sulfasalazine. As in all cases, the risk versus the benefits of continuing treatment should be discussed in an individual case

What about breastfeeding?

Sulfasalazine appears to be safe to use during lactation. However, the available data only relate to healthy non-kernicteric term infants. It is unclear whether this is applicable to premature infants or those with haemolysis.

Can I drink alcohol?
- There is no evidence that alcohol interferes with sulfasalazine.

What to do if side effects occur
Common side effects

These frequently resolve if the patient can continue with treatment for 2–3 weeks. If they fail to resolve and the patient cannot tolerate, reduce the dose of SSZ and try to increase a few weeks later.
- WBC <3.5 × 10^9/l: stop sulfasalazine and review.
- Platelets <150 × 10^9/l: stop sulfasalazine and review.
- ALT >twice upper limit: stop sulfasalazine and review.

Macrocytosis
Check B12 and folate and consider folic acid supplementation.

Leflunomide

Trade name Arava.

History
- **1992**: leflunomide (HWA 486 – 5-methyl-N-(4-trifluoromethylphenyl)-4-isoxazole carboximide), an immunosuppressant with an unknown mechanism of action, is demonstrated in-vivo to have benefit in a murine arthritis model.
- **1995:** leflunomide's mechanism of action *in vitro* is elucidated – inhibition of *de novo* pyrimidine synthesis by competitive inhibition of dihydro-orotate dehydrogenase resulting in inhibited uridine synthesis and reduced lymphocyte proliferation (particularly T cells).
- **1995**: leflunomide is shown in Phase II clinical studies to be efficacious in rheumatoid arthritis.
- **1999:** leflunomide is shown in 2 large Phase III clinical studies to have similar efficacy to methotrexate and sulfasalazine in rheumatoid arthritis.
- **2000**: leflunomide is licensed in the UK for patients with active rheumatoid arthritis.

Mechanism of action
Leflunomide is rapidly metabolized following absorption to an active substrate A77 1726. This active compound causes inhibition of dihydro-orotate dehydrogenase, resulting in inhibited uridine nucleotide synthesis and impairment of cellular progression through the cell cycle from G1 to S phase.
- **T cells:** there is good evidence that the uridine synthesis pathway is particularly important in T cell proliferation, and this may be the major mechanism of action in rheumatoid arthritis.
- **Dendritic cells**: A77 1726 also interferes with dendritic cell function, reducing the expression of co-stimulatory molecules on these key antigen presenting cells. This may be an additional important mechanism of action.

The active metabolite A77 1726 is cleared extremely slowly (due to high levels of protein binding) by renal and hepatobiliary clearance. Plasma levels therefore remain detectable for up to 2 years following discontinuation of treatment.

Evidence base: the clinical trials with leflunomide and what they showed

Summary
There is good evidence for efficacy of leflunomide monotherapy in rheumatoid arthritis and psoriatic arthritis.

Combination treatment with methotrexate is efficacious in rheumatoid arthritis, but there is a high prevalence of elevated liver transaminases.

There is no trial data to support leflunomide use in combination with other DMARDs or with biologics.

There is some limited evidence for leflunomide use in SLE and in remission maintenance in vasculitis (Wegener's granulomatosis).

All the trial studies in inflammatory arthritis use a 3-day 100 mg loading dose followed by 20 mg/day regular dosing.

Rheumatoid arthritis
Leflunomide monotherapy
Smolen JS, Scott DL, Rozman B, et al. (1999)Efficacy and safety of leflunomide compared with placebo and sulphasalazine in active rheumatoid arthritis: a double-blind, randomized, multicentre trial. European Leflunomide Study Group. *Lancet* **353**(9149): 259–66. MN301 study – (358 patients) leflunomide is significantly better than placebo and similar in efficacy to sulfasalazine (up to 2 g/day).

Strand V, Cohen S, Schiff M, et al. (1999) Treatment of active rheumatoid arthritis with leflunomide compared with placebo and methotrexate. Leflunomide Rheumatoid Arthritis Investigators Group. *Arch Intern Med* **159**: 2542–50. US301 study (482 patients) showing that leflunomide is significantly better than placebo and similar in efficacy to methotrexate (up to 15 mg/week).

Leflunomide combination therapy
Leflunomide and methotrexate
Kremer JM, Genovese MC, Cannon GW, et al. (2002) Concomitant leflunomide therapy in patients with active rheumatoid arthritis despite stable doses of methotrexate. A randomized, double-blind, placebo-controlled trial. *Ann Intern Med* **137**(9): 726–33. Good efficacy for the combination treatment, but problems with elevated liver transaminases

Leflunomide and sulfasalazine
Dougados M, Emery P, Lemmel EM, et al. (2005) When a DMARD fails, should patients switch to sulfasalazine or add sulfasalazine to continuing leflunomide? *Ann Rheum Dis* **64**: 44–51. No significant benefit in adding sulfasalazine to leflunomide (in leflunomide partial-responders) in this placebo controlled study (106 patients).

Psoriatic arthritis
Monotherapy
Kaltwasser JP, Nash P, Gladman D, et al. (2004) Efficacy and safety of leflunomide in the treatment of psoriatic arthritis and psoriasis: a multinational, double-blind, randomized, placebo-controlled clinical trial. *Arthritis Rheum* **50**: 1939–50. The TOPAS study – a placebo controlled study showing that in patients with psoriatic arthritis (with skin disease) leflunomide was significantly better than placebo for both the joints and the skin (190 patients).

Systemic lupus erythematosis
Tam LS, Li EK, Wong CK, et al. (2004) Double-blind, randomized, placebo-controlled pilot study of leflunomide in systemic lupus erythematosus. *Lupus*.**13**(8): 601–4. A small placebo controlled study showing efficacy in mild to moderate SLE.

Wegener's granulomatosis
Metzler C, Fink C, Lamprecht P, et al. (2004) Maintenance of remission with leflunomide in Wegener's granulomatosis. *Rheumatol (Oxf)* **43**: 315–20. A small open label study showing efficacy of 20–40 mg/day of leflunomide in maintenance of remission in Wegener's granulomatosis.

Prescribing considerations

What do I need to do before starting the treatment?
Counselling regarding conception is particularly important for leflunomide given the teratogenic risks and the long half-life of the active metabolite. This needs to be discussed before commencing treatment (in both men and women). Patients should be advised that contraception use is essential and conception should be avoided for 2 years post-treatment in women and 3 months post-treatment in men.
- Patient education re: dosing, side effects, monitoring, drug interactions, etc., is needed.
- Ensure your patient has a patient held monitoring booklet

Record at baseline	
FBC	Allows monitoring of changes.
LFTs	Allows monitoring of changes. Avoid if elevated baseline transaminases or significantly decreased serum protein levels
ESR or CRP	Monitor disease activity
Renal function	Impaired renal function increases leflunomide levels. Moderate/severe impairment is a relative contraindication.
Varicella status	Either history or serology
CXR	Allows comparison in pulmonary toxicity.
BP	Allows comparison for monitoring.

What dose should I prescribe and should I use a loading dose?
The clinical trials all use a 3-day loading regime of 100 mg/day followed by 20 mg/day.

Regular dosing at 20 mg/day (without the 3-day loading dose) is associated with less side effects (particularly gastrointestinal), but a delay in the onset of action.

Important drug interactions
- **Phenytoin:** increases plasma concentration.
- **Warfarin:** enhances effects of warfarin.
- **Tolbutamide:** enhances hypoglycaemic effect.

Monitoring
FBC & LFTs
The British National Formulary advises:
- Fortnightly for the first 6 months of treatment.
- Thereafter, 2 monthly.

ESR
Useful for monitoring response to treatment

BP
Should be checked every 3 months.

Side effects and what to discuss with your patients
Common
Nausea, abdominal discomfort, diarrhoea, mouth ulcers, weight loss, allergic reactions (including skin rashes and rarely anaphylaxis), taste disturbance, headache, and hair loss. The gastrointestinal side-effects are by far the commonest and are more frequent when the loading regime is used.

Teratogenic risk
Patients should be advised that contraception use is essential and conception should be avoided for 2 years post-treatment in women and 3 months post-treatment in men.

Haematological toxicity
- Neutropenia, thrombocytopenia, pancytopenia.
- Warn patients to report infections/sore throat/bruising.

Pulmonary toxicity
- Acute interstitial pneumonitis (as seen with methotrexate) has been reported with leflunomide.
- This is a hypersensitivity reaction to leflunomide.
- Counsel patients re: acute shortness of breath.

Hepatic toxicity
- Leflunomide can cause an acute (potentially life threatening) hepatitis (most commonly in the first few months of treatment), but there is no evidence to suggest it causes progressive cirrhosis.
- Warn patients minimize alcohol intake.

Hypertension
Leflunomide can cause hypertension and BP should be monitored regularly. It can usually be managed with a reduced dose +/– appropriate anti-hypertensive treatment.

If significant side effects occur or a patient conceives whilst on treatment a washout with colestyramine/activated charcoal or activated charcoal is required.

Colestyramine/activated charcoal/activated charcoal washout regime
Colestyramine 8 g 3 times a day for 11 days OR activated charcoal 50 g 4 times a day for 11 days.

FAQs

What if I want to get pregnant?
Leflunomide is teratogenic in women and should be avoided before and during pregnancy. Women should generally be advised to have a 2-year washout period prior to conception to allow full elimination of leflunomide. An alternative is a colestyramine/activated charcoal washout 3 months prior to conception. In either case, the serum concentration of the active metabolite should be measured prior to conception and should be less than 0.02 mg/l.

It is unclear whether leflunomide has effects on the sperm, but men should be advised to have a similar washout regime to women 3 months prior to conception.

Breast feeding on leflunomide is also contraindicated.

What about fertility?
There is no evidence that leflunomide effects fertility in either men or women

How long does it take to work?
With a loading dose clinical response is usually seen in 4–6 weeks. Without a loading dose clinical response usually takes longer (~12 weeks).

What about injections?
- Live attenuated vaccines need to be avoided by patients taking leflunomide: yellow fever, MMR and rubella, BCG, oral polio, oral typhoid.
- Other vaccines will not be a problem.
- Patients should be advised to have an annual influenza immunization since they are at an increased risk of influenza.

LEFLUNOMIDE

Can I drink alcohol?
Although there is no evidence for an interaction, it is advisable for patients to minimize alcohol consumption given the hepatotoxic potential of the treatment.

What if I miss a dose?
Take the missed dose as soon as the patient remembers. If it is close to the next due dose omit the missed dose and take the normal daily dose (do not double doses).

What to do if side effects occur

Common side effects
Reduce the dose of leflunomide (the lowest evidence based dose for treatment is 10mg/day)

Unplanned pregnancy
Immediate colestyramine/activated charcoal washout.

Surgical considerations
There is inadequate data on the safety of continuing leflunomide in the perioperative period. However, the long half-life of the active metabolite means that stopping the treatment would be impractical and may be associated with worse post-operative outcomes due to impaired rehabilitation.

ASYMPTOMATIC PATIENT

Persistent Neutropenia ($<1.5 \times 10^9$/L) or Thrombocytopenia ($<150 \times 10^9$/L)

↓

Stop leflunomide and monitor response

Resolved ↙ ↘

- Consider Retreatment at Lower dose
- Colestyramine or activated charcoal Washout regime

↓ Persists

Assessment with Haematologist

SYMPTOMATIC PATIENT

Neutropenia ($<1.5 \times 10^9$/L) or Thrombocytopenia ($<150 \times 10^9$/L)

↓

Stop leflunomide
Give appropriate antibiotics for neutropenic sepsis Give colestyramine or activated charcoal washout Monitor response
Consider G-CSF if recalcitrant

Patient improves ↙ ↘ Persists

- Consider Retreatment at Lower dose
- Assessment with Haematologist

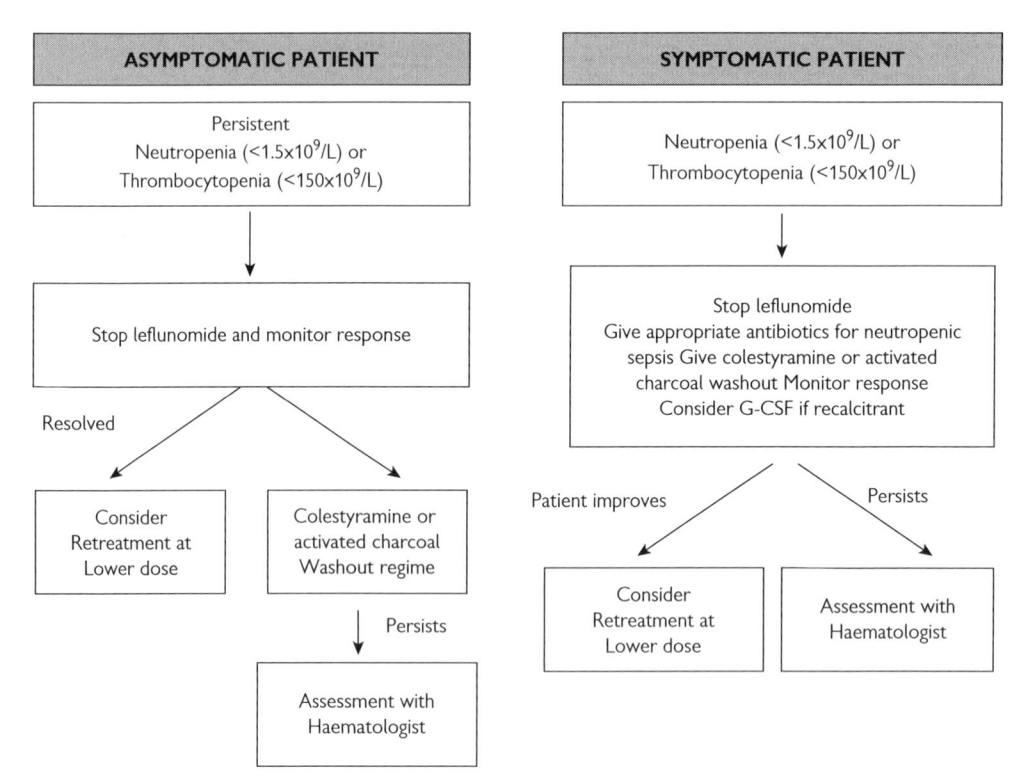

Figure 19.4 Haematological toxicity.

CHAPTER 19 **DMARDs and immunosuppressive drugs** 543

```
┌─────────────────────────────────────┐
│      Acute Respiratory Illness      │
│  (Dry Cough +/- dyspnoea and fever) │
└─────────────────────────────────────┘
                  │
┌─────────────────────────────────────────────────────────┐
│                    Stop leflunomide                      │
│ CXR (look for diffuse interstitial shadowing) – lesmpale with baseline CXR │
│              FBC (looking for eosinophilia)              │
│                 ABGs (looking for hypoxia)               │
│                 Blood and sputum cultures                │
│    Pulmonary Function Test (decrease TLCO and VC suggestive)    │
└─────────────────────────────────────────────────────────┘
```

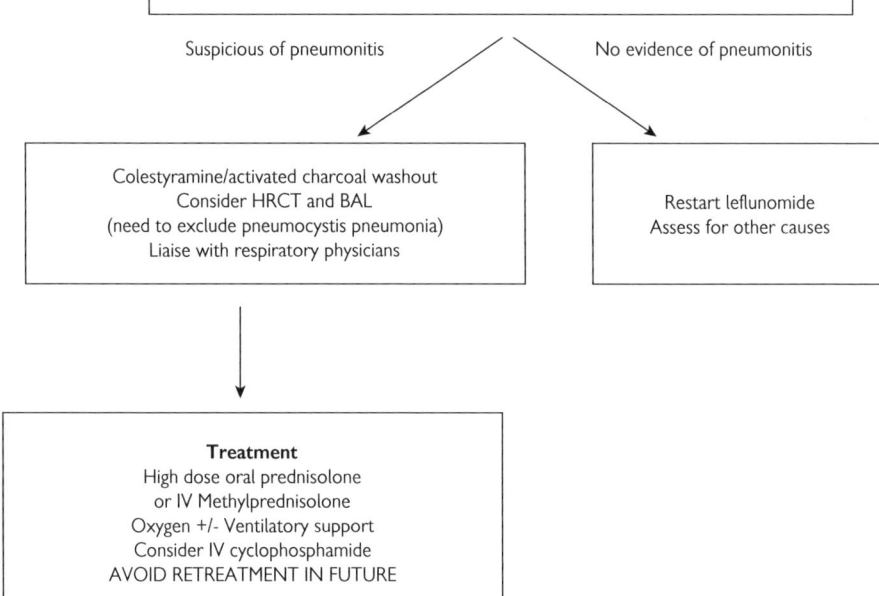

Suspicious of pneumonitis / No evidence of pneumonitis

- Colestyramine/activated charcoal washout
  Consider HRCT and BAL
  (need to exclude pneumocystis pneumonia)
  Liaise with respiratory physicians

- Restart leflunomide
  Assess for other causes

Treatment
High dose oral prednisolone
or IV Methylprednisolone
Oxygen +/- Ventilatory support
Consider IV cyclophosphamide
AVOID RETREATMENT IN FUTURE

Figure 19.5 Pulmonary toxicity.

Persistent ALT but < twice upper limit of normal

Reduce leflunomide dose and monitor

↓ Persistent problem

Stop leflunomide and monitor response
Hepatitis serology

Resolved / Persists

- Consider Retreatment at Lower dose
- Colestyramine or Activated charcoal Washout

ALT > twice upper limit of normal

Stop leflunomide and monitor response

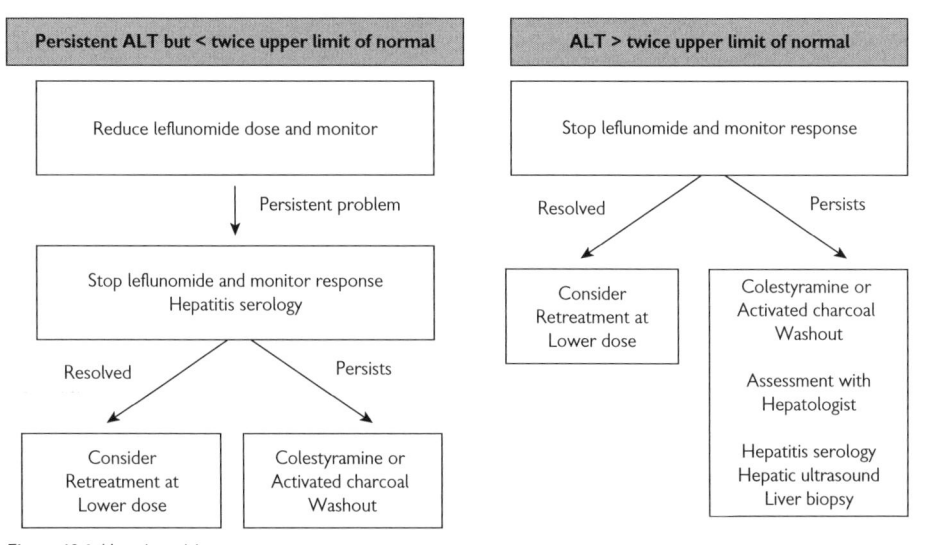

Resolved / Persists

- Consider Retreatment at Lower dose
- Colestyramine or Activated charcoal Washout

  Assessment with Hepatologist

  Hepatitis serology
  Hepatic ultrasound
  Liver biopsy

Figure 19.6 Hepatic toxicity.

Anti-malarials (hydroxychloroquine and chloroquine)

Trade name Hydroxychloroquine = Plaquenil.

History
- **Antiquity**: bark of the cinchona tree of South America (found in the Andes Mountains); recognized as having benefits in treating fever.
- **1600s**: Spanish Jesuits introduce the cinchona bark to Europe.
- **1670s**: powder of cinchona bark used to treat fever in King Charles II.
- **1820:** quinine (the active compound) isolated from cinchona bark.
- **1895:** Dr Thomas Payne (Physician, St Thomas' Hospital London), successfully uses quinine for patients with lupus erythematosus.
- **1931:** quinacrine (mepacrine), the first synthetic quinine derivative is synthesized (Bayer, Germany).
- **1934:** chloroquine; the first synthetic aminoquinolone is synthesized (Bayer, Germany). Hydroxychloroquine, another aminoquinolone, is synthesized soon after.
- **1951:** Page publishes evidence for mepacrine in SLE in *Lancet*
- **1957:** data published on the efficacy of chloroquine in SLE.
- **1959:** data published on the efficacy of hydroxychloroquine in SLE.
- **1960s:** retinal toxicity of the anti-malarials (particularly chloroquine) highlighted.
- **1970s:** hydroxychloroquine is found to be as efficacious as chloroquine, but associated with less retinal toxicity.
- **1980s:** monitoring protocols developed for hydroxychloroquine.

Possible mechanisms of action

Inhibition of antigen presentation
The aminoquinolones increases the pH within a number of cytoplasmic compartments. This is likely to interfere with the antigen presentation function of B cells and macrophages by affecting the assembly of MHC Class II molecules with peptide. This may be an important effect of antimalarials when used in combination treatments in rheumatoid arthritis.

Induction of apoptosis
Aminoquinolones have been shown to increase apoptosis in certain cell types. Given the proposed defect in apoptosis in SLE this may be an important mechanism in SLE.

Reduced levels of B-cell activating factor
BAFF is a serum factor (part of the TNF family) that appear to be important in autoantibody production in SLE. The quinolones appear to reduce the levels of BAFF.

Evidence base: the clinical trials with HCQ and what they showed

Summary
Despite widespread usage, there is a relative lack of good quality trial evidence to support the use of anti-malarials in SLE. There is some evidence to support HCQ treatment of the mucocutaneous manifestations of SLE and evidence that HCQ treatment reduces the frequency of flares in mild/moderate disease. There is a lack of good evidence for the articular manifestations.

Although there is some *in vitro* data to support an anti-thrombotic effect of HCQ in antiphospholipid antibody syndrome there is a lack of good quality trial data to support it's routine use.

There is good quality trial evidence for HCQ, particularly in combination with MTX (+/- Sulfasalazine) in rheumatoid arthritis

SLE
The Canadian Hydroxychloroquine Study Group (1991) A randomized study of the effect of withdrawing hydroxychloroquine sulfate in systemic lupus erythematosus. *N Engl J Med.* **324**(3): 150–4. Withdrawal of hydroxychloroquine is associated with an increased prevalence of lupus flares.

Drugs for discoid lupus erythematosus (2001) *Cochrane Database Syst Rev* 1:CD002954. A review of the trials in discoid lupus concluding that hydroxychloroquine is efficacious.

Williams HJ, Egger MJ, Singer JZ, et al. (1994) Comparison of hydroxychloroquine and placebo in the treatment of the arthropathy of mild systemic lupus erythematosus. *J Rheumatol* **21**: 1457–62. A small study (71 patients) that showed minimal benefits for hydroxychloroquine in treating the arthropathy of SLE.

Rheumatoid arthritis

HCQ monotherapy
The HERA Study (1995) A randomized trial of hydroxychloroquine in early rheumatoid arthritis: the HERA Study. *Am J Med.* **98**: 156–68. A DBPCS of 120 rheumatoid patients showing the efficacy of hydroxychloroquine as monotherapy in early rheumatoid arthritis (<2 years duration). A subsequent follow-up study showed that the treatment had long term benefit.

HCQ combination therapy
Hydroxychloroquine is efficacious in combination with MTX.

HCQ and methotrexate
O'Dell JR, Leff R, Paulsen G, et al. (2002) Treatment of rheumatoid arthritis with methotrexate and hydroxychloroquine, methotrexate and sulfasalazine, or a combination of the three medications: results of a two-year, randomized, double-blind, placebo-controlled trial. *Arthritis Rheum* **46**: 1164–70.

Mottonen T, Hannonen P, Leirsalo-Repo M, et al. (1999) Comparison of combination therapy with single-drug therapy in early rheumatoid arthritis: a randomised trial. FIN-RACo trial group. *Lancet* **353**(9164): 1568–73. Triple combination treatment with MTX, hydroxychloroquine and sulfasalazine (or MTX and hydroxychloroquine) is better than MTX and sulfasalazine in combination.

Prescribing considerations

What do I need to do before starting the treatment?
- Patient education re: dosing, side effects, monitoring, drug interactions, etc. It is particularly important to discuss visual considerations (see below).

CHAPTER 19 DMARDs and immunosuppressive drugs

Record at baseline

FBC	Allows monitoring of changes
LFTs	Adjust dose if impaired
ESR or CRP	Monitor disease activity
Renal function	Adjust dose if impaired

Baseline visual assessment, Royal College of Ophthalmologists 2004

- Ask about visual impairment.
- Record near visual acuity of each eye (with glasses where appropriate).

Hydroxychloroquine is consider safe in pregnancy, with no evidence of foetal toxicity at therapeutic doses. In SLE studies have shown that there is a significantly greater risk of flares, if the treatment is discontinued. In SLE it is therefore reasonable to continue treatment. See College of Opthalmologists website: http://www.rcophth.ac.uk/docs/publications/Oculartoxicity2004.pdf

- If no abnormality is detected with the above, treatment with HCQ can be commenced.
- If visual impairment is present an assessment, initially by an optometrist, is advised.
- If chloroquine is being prescribed ALL patients require regular ocular examinations by an ophthalmologist and liaison with the local ophthalmologists is required before commencing treatment

What dose should I prescribe?
- The maximum daily dose of hydroxychloroquine is 6.5 mg/kg/day.
- The usual treatment dose in both rheumatoid arthritis and SLE is 200 mg bd.
- This can be reduced to 200 mg od once a response has occurred or if side effects are problematic.
- The maximum daily dose of chloroquine is 2.5 mg/kg/day.
- The usual treatment dose in both rheumatoid arthritis and SLE is 150 mg od.

Important drug interactions
Amiodarone and moxifloxacin: there is a significant increased risk of ventricular arrhythmias when used with either of these drugs concomitantly.

Monitoring of HCQ
Blood tests
There is no requirement for regular blood test monitoring.

Visual monitoring
See Royal College of Ophthalmologists 2004.
Ask patient about visual symptoms and monitor visual acuity annually using the reading chart http://www.rcophth.ac.uk/docs/publications/Oculartoxicity2004.pdf. This can be undertaken by either a rheumatologist or an optometrist.
Refer to ophthalmologist if:
- Visual acuity changes: treatment should be stopped.
- Vision reported blurred.

Side effects and what to discuss with your patients
Common
Nausea, abdominal discomfort, headache, skin reactions.

Rare
Prolonged QT syndrome and predisposition to ventricular arrhythmias.

FAQs
How long does it take to work?
A clinical response is usually seen within 3 months with both hydroxychloroquine and chloroquine

What do I do if I want to get pregnant?
Rheumatoid improves in pregnancy, HCQ treatment is frequently discontinued and restarted post-delivery.

Do I have to take other anti-malarials if I am travelling?
Yes – hydroxychloroquine is not an effective monotherapy for malaria. Other anti-malarial quinolones should generally be avoided.

Gold: intramuscular (sodium aurothimalate) and oral (auranofin)

Trade names: Myocrisin, Intramuscular Gold, Ridaura, Oral Gold.

History
- **~2000 BC:** records suggest that the Egyptians and Chinese ingested solid gold for medicinal purposes.
- **1300s:** the Islamic alchemist Geber produces 'aqua regia' – soluble gold salts (using nitric and hydrochloric acid to dissolve gold).
- **1500s:** paracelsus uses soluble gold salts as a treatment for melancholy.
- **1700s:** gold salts included in Culpepper's pharmacopoeia for general malaise.
- **1800s:** gold salt use re-emerges as a treatment of syphilis.
- **1905:** Robert Koch awarded the Nobel Prize for Medicine for identification of *Mycobacterium tuberculosis* as the cause of tuberculosis. Koch also demonstrated that Gold cyanide inhibited the growth of *Mycobacterium in vitro*.
- **1920s:** gold salts used to treat pulmonary tuberculosis despite a lack of clinical evidence of efficacy, on the basis of Koch's *in vitro* findings.
- **1920s:** gold salts used to treat rheumatoid arthritis on the basis that the mycobacterium may be important in the aetiology.
- **1927:** a German study demonstrates the efficacy of gold treatment in rheumatoid arthritis.
- **1976:** oral gold (auranofin) introduced for treatment of rheumatoid arthritis.
- **1970s/1980s:** most commonly used DMARD in rheumatoid arthritis.

Possible mechanisms of action
Sodium aurothiomalate (intramuscular gold) is a water soluble gold thiolate salt. Auranofin is an orally bioavailable lipophilic gold salt (also a thiolate salt) developed in the 1980s. Serum gold levels with auranofin are lower than those with aurothiomalate (probably accounting for both the improved side effect profile and the reduced efficacy). Nevertheless, the presumed mechanisms of action of both gold salts are presumed to be similar. Gold thiolate salts appear to have potentially important actions at every stage of immune activation – potential effects at the different levels are indicated below. These effects appear to be predominantly mediated by interactions of the gold thiolate salts with thiols (compounds containing an –SH group) such as cysteine. These thiol-mediated effects are probably also important in the aetiology of the side effects of gold salt treatment.

Innate immune system
Toll-like receptor 4 (TLR4) is part of the recognition arm of the innate immune system. Gold salts have been shown to interfere with TLR4 activation, thereby interfering with NFkB activation in antigen presenting cells and reduced expression of COX-2.

Antigen presentation
Gold salts inhibit the differentiation of dendritic cells from their precursor cells thereby interfering with antigen presentation. This effect on maturation may be secondary to gold salts actions on Toll-like receptors or Class II MHC function.

T cell activation
Gold salts have been shown to interfere with peptide presentation by Class II MHC molecules and impair subsequent T cell activation.

Cytokine production (TNFα, IL-12, IL-1 and IL-10)
Gold salts inhibit TNFα and IL-12 secretion by activated monocytes. Gold salts also inhibit IL-1 converting enzyme activity thereby reducing IL-1 secretion. Furthermore, gold salts have been shown, *in vivo*, to increase serum levels of IL-10, an anti-inflammatory cytokine that reduces TNFα, IL-1 and IL-6 expression by monocytes.

Metalloproteinases
Gold salts can react with the thiol groups in metalloproteinases, such as collagenase, to inhibit their activity.

Evidence base: the main clinical trials with gold salts and what they showed

Summary
IM gold is more effective than PO gold. There is evidence of short-term benefit in rheumatoid arthritis, as monotherapy or in combination with methotrexate. Side effects limit it's utility.

Rheumatoid arthritis
Gold monotherapy
Clark P, Tugwell P, Bennett K, et al. (1989) Meta-analysis of injectable gold in rheumatoid arthritis. *J Rheumatol.* **16**: 442–7. A meta-analysis of trials with injectable gold as monotherapy showing a significant improvement in active synovitis, function and inflammatory markers. 11% of trial patients discontinued due to side effects.

Ward JR, Williams HJ, Egger MJ, et al. (1983) Comparison of auranofin, gold sodium thiomalate, and placebo in the treatment of rheumatoid arthritis. A controlled clinical trial. *Arthritis Rheum* **26**: 1303–15. A placebo controlled study (193 patients) showing that both oral and injectable gold salts are efficacious. The oral preparation (auranofin) was less efficacious, but better tolerated than the injectable preparation.

Gold combination therapy
1. *Gold and methotrexate*
Lehman AJ, Esdaile JM, Klinkhoff AV, et al. (2005) A 48-week, randomized, double-blind, double-observer, placebo-controlled multicenter trial of combination methotrexate and intramuscular gold therapy in rheumatoid arthritis: results of the METGO study. *Arthritis Rheum* **52**: 1360–70. The METGO study: IM gold is statistically better than placebo as step-up combination in MTX partial responders.

Prescribing considerations
What do I need to do before starting the treatment?
- Patient education re: dosing, side effects, and monitoring.
- Ensure your patient has a patient held monitoring booklet

For either oral or intramuscular gold:

Record at baseline	
FBC	Allows monitoring of changes
Urinalysis	Allows monitoring of changes
ESR or CRP	Monitor disease activity
Renal function	Avoid if significantly impaired
Liver function	Avoid if significantly impaired
Chest X-ray	Allows monitoring of changes

What dose should I prescribe?
Intramuscular gold (either deltoid or gluteal)
Initial treatment is weekly
- Week 1 – 10 mg: this is a test dose to ensure no immediate hypersensitivity reaction (ideally, this should be undertaken in hospital and patient observed for 1 h).
- Thereafter, 50 mg weekly until a total dose of 1000 mg (excluding the test dose).
- Then reduce dose to 50 mg every 2–4 weeks dependent on response (usually monthly).
- A response will usually take 12–15 weeks and should not be expected before at least 500 mg total dose has been achieved.
- If a patient fails to significantly respond after a total dose of 1 g the treatment should be discontinued.
- A maximum duration of 5 years of treatment with intramuscular gold is advised by some.

Oral gold
The normal starting dose is 3 mg od increasing to 3 mg bd after 1 month if tolerated. The dose should then be increased at 6 months to 9 mg (3 mg tds) if inadequate response. Discontinue after 9 months if no significant response.

Why do you give the test dose for intramuscular gold?
Approximately 5% of patients develop an acute vasomotor reaction to intramuscular gold, within the first hour of the first dose (a nitritoid reaction). This may include a rash, flushing, hypotension, and collapse. It should be managed as an anaphylactic reaction according to the clinical severity. The test dose should therefore be given where appropriate facilities for management./resuscitation are available – usually this is within hospital.

Important drug interactions
ACE inhibitors: there appears to be an increased risk of a first dose reactions in patients on ACE inhibitors.

Monitoring of gold
Intramuscular gold
Before every dose of intramuscular gold check:
- **Urinalysis:** look for developing proteinuria/haematuria.
- **FBC:** look for evidence of bone marrow suppression. Look for eosinophilia – it may precede a skin reaction.
- **Renal function:** look for worsening renal function.
- **LFTs:** look for developing hepatotoxicity.
- **Skin:** inspect for developing skin rash.

Approximately every 2–3 months:
ESR or CRP: useful for monitoring response to treatment.
An annual Chest X-ray is advised on gold treatment

Oral gold
Every 2 weeks for 2 months then monthly thereafter:
- **Urinalysis:** look for developing proteinuria/haematuria.
- **FBC:** look for evidence or bone marrow suppression. Look for eosinophilia – it may precede a skin reaction.
- **LFTs/CRP/ESR:** every 2–3 months.

Side effects and what to discuss with your patients
Approximately 1/3 of patients experience side effects with IM gold salts. Oral gold (auranofin) has a wider therapeutic index with less side effects, but lower efficacy. Although the side effects below are more common with intramuscular gold, they can still occur with the oral preparation.

Common
Nausea, abdominal discomfort, skin rashes, malaise, headache, anorexia, oral ulceration.

Haematological toxicity
- Neutropenia, thrombocytopenia, pancytopenia.
- Warn patients to report infections/sore throat/bruising.
- These usually occur within the first 6 months of starting treatment with sulfasalazine.

Dermatological toxicity
Can cause local pruritis to severe exfoliative dermatitis. In addition, long-term treatment with gold can cause a persistent blue-grey photosensitive skin pigmentation (chrysiasis). Patients should be advised to inform their doctor of any skin rashes developing on gold treatment.

Renal toxicity
In approximately 10% of patients, gold can cause proteinuria (usually reversible) and, rarely, haematuria, secondary to membranous glomerulonephritis. This can progress to nephrotic syndrome and renal impairment. Patients should be aware of the importance of urine dipstick monitoring

Hepatic toxicity
Gold can cause hepatotoxicity with cholestatic jaundice. Patients should be aware that liver function is monitored as part of the regular blood testing

Pulmonary toxicity
Gold can cause a progressive pulmonary fibrosis. This is monitored with an annual chest X-ray.

FAQs
How long does it take to work?
A clinical response is usually seen after 3 –4 months of treatment with gold

What do I do if I want to get pregnant?
There is evidence of transplacental transfer of gold to the foetus. Although there are no specific data on teratogenicity, it is advisable to discontinue gold treatment 3 month prior to a planned conception.

What about breastfeeding?
Weight adjusted serum gold levels in a breastfeeding child have been shown to be higher than those in the mother. Gold treatment should be avoided during breast feeding.

Can I drink alcohol?
There is no evidence that alcohol interferes with gold

What to do if side effects occur
Common side effects
- Mouth ulcers can be improved with a regular mouth wash.
- Abdominal pain can be improved with a high fibre diet.
- Mild skin rashes can improve with anti-histamines or 1% hydrocortisone.
- Mild side effects may improve with a reduction in the dose or frequency of gold treatment.

Haematological toxicity
- WBC <3.5 × 10^9/l.
- Platelets < 150 × 10^9/l Stop gold and review.
- Eosinophilia This may precede a skin rash. If it occurs reduce dose or frequency of gold and observe.

Dermatological toxicity
- Dependent on severity of skin reaction reduce dose or frequency or discontinue.
- Try with 1% hydrocortisone with or without antihistamines.
- Chrysiasis is generally irreversible, but gold should be discontinued if it develops.

Renal toxicity
Proteinuria
- \+ on dipstick on 1 occasion – continue treatment and monitor.
- ++ or greater on urine dipstick or + on more than 2 occasions.
- Check MSU to exclude infection.
- Arrange 24-h urine collection.
- If 24-h protein excretion >0.1, but <0.5 g/24 h – continue treatment and monitor.
- If 24-h protein excretion >0.5 g/24 h, stop treatment.

Haematuria
++ or greater on urine dipstick – stop treatment, check MSU, consider other causes.

Hepatic toxicity
- Acute jaundice or persistent elevation of ALT >twice upper limit of normal.
- Stop treatment,

Penicillamine

Trade name: Distamine®.

History
- **1943:** penicillamine is identified as a degradation product of penicillin.
- **1956:** Dr J Walshe identifies penicillamine as a heavy metal chelator and describes it's use as a copper chelator in the treatment of Wilson's disease.
- **1950s/60s:** D and L isoforms of penicillamine are studied – L-isoforms are identified as toxic in rats [due to greater pyridoxine (vitamin B6) antagonism], whilst D isoforms emerge as therapeutic agents. D-penicillamine is used to treat cystinuria, Wilson's disease, and primary biliary cirrhosis.
- **1963:** penicillamine is identified as being efficacious in rheumatoid arthritis when used as a possible chelator of rheumatoid factor.
- **1966:** penicillamine is identified as having potentially favourable effects on collagen in systemic sclerosis.

Possible mechanisms of action
Penicillamine is a cysteine analog that contains a free thiol group. Like the gold thiolate salts, penicillamine can therefore interact with compounds containing an –SH group, such as the amino acid cysteine.. These thiol mediated effects are likely to important in the mechanism of action and the side effects of penicillamine, as they are with gold. Like gold penicillamine may have effects on the immune system at multiple levels. There are relatively few studies of the mechanism of action of penicillamine, but there is evidence for cytokine effects (but not on TNF) and effects on metalloproteinases.

Cytokine production
Penicillamine has been shown *in vitro* and in animal models to produce a more Th2 type cytokine profile with increased IL-4 production and decreased interferon gamma production.

Metalloproteinases
Penicillamine has been shown *in vivo* to inhibit the activity of gelatinase B (MMP-9), a neutrophil and monocyte derived metalloproteinase that may be important in rheumatoid synovitis.

Rheumatoid factor
Penicillamine has been shown both *in vivo* and *in vitro* to reduce rheumatoid factor production.

Penicillamine inhibits collagen cross-linking *in vitro*, maintaining collagen in a more soluble form. This is probably through thiol mediated effects. This action was the reason penicillamine treatment was considered in patients with systemic sclerosis.

Penicillamine is also a heavy metal chelator and is used for copper chelation in Wilson's disease and treatment of arsenic poisoning. This does not seem to be important in it's mechanism of action in rheumatoid or systemic sclerosis

Evidence base: the main clinical trials with penicillamine and what they showed

Summary
Penicillamine is less effective than other DMARDs in rheumatoid arthritis and is associated with more toxicity. Trials have failed to demonstrate efficacy in systemic sclerosis.

Rheumatoid arthritis
Penicillamine monotherapy
Van Jaarsveld CH, Jacobs JW, van der Veen MJ, et al. (2000) Aggressive treatment in early rheumatoid arthritis: a randomised controlled trial. On behalf of the Rheumatic Research Foundation Utrecht, The Netherlands. *Ann Rheum Dis* **59**(6): 468–77. A randomized trial of several treatments showing that penicillamine was less efficacious and associated with more toxicity than other treatments including methotrexate, sulfasalazine and hydroxychloroquine.

Systemic sclerosis
Penicillamine monotherapy
Clements PJ, Furst DE, Wong WK, et al. (1999) High-dose versus low-dose D-penicillamine in early diffuse systemic sclerosis: analysis of a two-year, double-blind, randomized, controlled clinical trial. *Arthritis Rheum.* **42**: 1194–203. A 2-year trial of 134 patients with systemic sclerosis comparing high dose (750–1000 mg/day) with low dose (125 mg alt days) penicillamine. No significant difference was demonstrated. There was no placebo arm so it is possible that low dose penicillamine may be effective, but there is no trial data to support that assumption.

Prescribing considerations
What do I need to do before starting the treatment?
- Patient education re: dosing, side effects, and monitoring.
- Ensure your patient has a patient held monitoring booklet.

Record at baseline	
FBC	Allows monitoring of changes
Urinalysis	Allows monitoring of changes
ESR or CRP	Monitor disease activity
Renal function	Avoid if significantly impaired

What dose should I prescribe?
- **Month 1:** 125–250 mg (usually 250 mg) od.
- **Thereafter:** Increasing by 125–250 mg/month to usual maintenance of 750mg/day [maximum dose 1.5 g/day (1 g/day in the elderly)].

Important drug interactions
- **Antipsychotics:** increased risk of agranulocytosis with clozapine.
- **Iron and antacids:** reduce the absorption of penicillamine.

Monitoring of penicillamine
Every 2 weeks for first month and then monthly thereafter:
- **Urinalysis:** look for developing proteinuria/haematuria.
- **FBC:** look for low platelets or low white cell count.
- **ESR or CRP:** useful for monitoring response to treatment.

Side effects and what to discuss with your patients

Penicillamine treatment is associated with a wide spectrum of side effects. Approximately 2/3 of patients discontinue penicillamine in the first 2 years of treatment and the majority of these are due to side effects. It is estimated that 50% of patients experience side effects with penicillamine. The most important side effects are given below.

Common
Nausea, abdominal discomfort, skin rashes, taste disturbance, malaise, headache, anorexia

Haematological toxicity
- Occurs in approximately 5% of patients.
- Neutropenia, thrombocytopenia, pancytopenia all seen.
- Warn patients to report infections/sore throat/bruising.

Renal toxicity
Occurs in approximately 10% of patients. Penicillamine can cause proteinuria (usually reversible), and rarely haematuria, secondary to membranous glomerulonephritis (in approximately 90% of cases). Proteinuria most frequently develops after 4–6 months of treatment (75% of cases within 1 year). This can progress to nephrotic syndrome and renal impairment if treatment is continued. Patients should be aware of the importance of urine dipstick monitoring.

Systemic reactions
Rarely penicillamine can cause a febrile reaction, drug-induced lupus, and a myasthenia-like syndrome.

FAQs

How long does it take to work?
A clinical response is usually seen after 3–4 months of treatment with penicillamine.

What do I do if I want to get pregnant?
Penicillamine is contraindicated in pregnancy. In animal models it has adverse effects on lung development. Advise discontinuation 3 months prior to conception.

What about breastfeeding?
Penicillamine treatment should be avoided during breast feeding.

Can I drink alcohol?
There is no evidence that alcohol interferes with penicillamine

What to do if side effects occur

Common side effects
Mild side effects may improve with a reduction in the dose of penicillamine.

Haematological toxicity
- WBC <3.5 × 10^9/l.
- Platelets < 150 × 10^9/l. Stop penicillamine and review.

Renal toxicity
- Proteinuria.
- + on dipstick on 1 occasion – continue treatment and monitor.
- ++ or greater on urine dipstick or + on more than 2 occasions – check MSU to exclude infection. Arrange 24-h urine collection.
- If 24-h protein excretion >0.1, but <0.5 g/24 h – continue treatment and monitor.
- If 24-h protein excretion >0.5 g/24 h stop treatment.
- Spontaneous resolution of proteinuria may take >12 months.
- Consider corticosteroids treatment for more rapid resolution

Haematuria
++ or greater on urine dipstick – stop treatment, check MSU, consider other causes.

Azathioprine

Trade name: Imuran®

History
- **1951**: Elion and Hitchings (working at the Burroughs Wellcome Research Laboratories) develop 6-mercaptopurine (a thiopurine) as part of a programme to design purine analogues to interfere with nucleic acid synthesis (they are subsequently awarded the Nobel Prize for medicine in 1988 for their work).
- **1952**: 6-mercaptopurine is shown to be efficacious in childhood leukaemia.
- **1963**: azathioprine (a pro-drug of 6-mercaptopurine) is developed and found to be less toxic than 6-mercaptopurine, but similarly efficacious.
- **1960s**: Professor Sir Roy Calne uses 6-mercaptopurine and subsequently azathioprine as immunosuppressants to prevent transplant rejection. Reports of azathioprine having efficacy in a variety of rheumatic diseases accumulate.
- **1969**: DBPCS confirm the efficacy of azathioprine in rheumatoid arthritis and systemic lupus erythematosus.
- **1986**: DBPCS shows efficacy in PMR/GCA.
- **1990**: DBPCS shows efficacy in Behcet's.

Possible mechanisms of action

Azathioprine (AZA) is a pro-drug consisting of the thiopurine 6-mercaptopurine (6-MP) and a nitro-imadazole ring (6-thioinosinic acid). AZA is metabolized *in vivo* to 6-MP that is then further converted into several active metabolites by two main enzymes – TPMT (thio-purine methyltransferase) and IMPDH (inosine monophosphate dehydrogenase). TPMT also metabolizes 6-MP to an inactive metabolite (see below for the importance of this in toxicity). The anti-proliferative effects of AZA and 6-MP are mediated through the purine antagonist properties of 6-MP metabolites, inhibiting DNA replication. However, whether this wholly accounts for the immunosuppressive properties is unclear. Other possible mechanisms are outlined below:

Inhibition of CD28 co-stimulation
AZA (through 6-MP) interferes *in vitro* with T cell co-stimulation through CD28. This is analogous to the effects of CTLA4-Ig and may, in part, explain the immunosuppressant properties of azathioprine.

Antigen presentation
AZA has been shown to inhibit *in vitro* antigen presentation by antigen presenting cells, another possible immunomodulatory mechanism of action.

Inhibition of activated T cells
Genomic studies have shown that AZA and 6-MP have effects on the expression of a variety of potentially relevant genes in activated T cells (but not quiescent T cells), including a number of TNF receptor related genes.

Evidence base: the main clinical trials with AZA and what they showed

Summary
- AZA is effective as monotherapy in rheumatoid arthritis, systemic lupus erythematosus, and Behcet's.
- AZA is a weakly effective steroid sparing agent in GCA/PMR.
- AZA is effective in maintaining remission (but not inducing remission) in ANCA associated vasculitis and in lupus nephritis.

Rheumatoid arthritis

AZA monotherapy
Barnes CG, Currey HL, Dunne JF, et al. (1969) Azathioprine: a controlled double-blind trial in rheumatoid arthritis. *Ann Rheum Dis* **28**: 327–8. A double blind placebo controlled study with 49 patients over 1 year showing that azathioprine (2.5 mg/kg/day) facilitated a statistically significant reduction in steroid requirements.

Suarez-Almazor ME, Spooner C, Belseck E. (2000) Azathioprine for treating rheumatoid arthritis. *Cochrane Database Syst Rev* **2**: CD001461. A meta-analysis showing that azathioprine has short-term efficacy in patients with rheumatoid arthritis. Long-term efficacy could not be assessed due to a lack of data and azathioprine was associated with more toxicity than other DMARDs

AZA combination therapy
There is some data to suggest azathioprine is a safe alternative to use in combination with infliximab, but there is no evidence of efficacy in combination with other DMARDs

Anti-TNF and azathioprine
Perdriger A, Mariette X, Kuntz JL, et al. (2006) Safety of infliximab used in combination with leflunomide or azathioprine in daily clinical practice. *J Rheumatol* **33**: 865–9. One of several observational studies suggesting azathioprine combination therapy with anti-TNF is not associated with any less efficacy or any more adverse events than combination treatment with leflunomide or methotrexate.

PMR/GCA
De Silva M and Hazleman BL (1986) Azathioprine in giant cell arteritis/polymyalgia rheumatica: a double-blind study. *Ann Rheum Dis.* **45**: 136–8. A small double blind study (31 patients) showing that treatment with azathioprine (2.5 mg/kg/day) enabled a significantly greater reduction in steroid requirements at 1 year than placebo treatment.

Behçet's disease
Yazici H, Pazarli H, Barnes CG, et al. (1990) A controlled trial of azathioprine in Behçet's syndrome. *N Engl J Med.* **322**(5): 281–5. A double blind study (73 patients) showing that treatment with azathioprine (2.5 mg/kg/day) reduced the occurrence and recurrence of eye disease and reduced orogenital ulceration compared with placebo.

ANCA associated vasculitis (AAV)
Jayne D, Rasmussen N, Andrassy K, et al. (2003) A randomized trial of maintenance therapy for vasculitis associated with antineutrophil cytoplasmic autoantibodies. *N Engl J Med* **349**: 36–44. A controlled study of 144 patients who had achieved disease remission with cyclophosphamide. Patients were randomly assigned to treatment with either azathioprine (2 mg/kg/day) or continued cyclophosphamide. There was no significant difference in relapse rates in the two groups.

CHAPTER 19 DMARDs and immunosuppressive drugs

Systemic lupus erythematosus (SLE)

Although there is good trial evidence to support the use of azathioprine to maintain remission, post-cyclophosphamide, in patients with lupus nephritis, there is a lack of good trial data to support it's use in other patients with SLE.

Houssiau FA, Vasconcelos C, D'Cruz D, et al. (2002) Immunosuppressive therapy in lupus nephritis: the Euro-Lupus Nephritis Trial, a randomised trial of low dose versus high dose intravenous cyclophosphamide. *Arthritis Rheum* **46**: 2121–31. A controlled study of 90 patients showing that azathioprine maintenance treatment, following remission induction with cyclophosphamide, was not significantly different to continued cyclophosphamide treatment.

Prescribing considerations

What do I need to do before starting the treatment?
- Patient education re: dosing, side effects and monitoring.
- Ensure your patient has a patient held monitoring booklet

Record at baseline	
FBC	Allows monitoring of changes
LFTs	Allows monitoring of changes
ESR or CRP	Monitor disease activity
Renal function	Monitoring if renal disease activity (reduce dose if significantly impaired)
dsDNA in SLE	Allows monitoring of changes
ANCA in AAV	Allows monitoring of changes

What about checking TPMT status?

TPMT converts 6-MP to both active and inactive metabolites. The active metabolites produced by this route seem to correlate with hepatotoxicity. IMPDH metabolizes 6-MP to an active metabolite associated with more marrow toxicity. TPMT has significant genetic polymorphism. TPMT activity can be graded, with appropriate screening, as high, intermediate or low. Low levels of TPMT activity are associated with significantly more marrow toxicity because 6-MP becomes preferentially metabolized via the IMPDH route (see Figure 19.7).

Both the availability and the use of TPMT screening is variable and whether it alters clinical decision making is debated, since all patients treated with AZA are closely monitored for marrow toxicity. Furthermore, TPMT screening does not allow assessment of the risks of potential hepatic toxicity.

What dose should I prescribe?

Usual protocol for AZA prescription (local protocols may vary):
- **Week 1:** 50 mg od – then if tolerated
- **Week 2:** 2.5 mg/kg/day (usually 100–150 mg/day)

The dose can be increased to 3 or 3.5 mg/kg/day if necessary.

Important drug interactions
- **Allopurinol:** increased risk of all toxicity.
- **Captopril:** increased risk of marrow suppression.
- **Trimethoprim/cotrimoxazole:** increased risk of marrow suppression.
- **Phenytoin:** interferes with absorption of azathioprine.

Monitoring of AZA
- **FBC & LFTs:** example monitoring regime (local guidelines may vary). Fortnightly for the first 4 weeks. Monthly thereafter.
- **ESR:** useful for monitoring response to treatment

Side effects and what to discuss with your patients

Common
Nausea, abdominal discomfort, headache, anorexia.

Uncommon
Interstitial nephritis, pancreatitis, pneumonitis.

Haematological toxicity
- Neutropenia, thrombocytopenia, pancytopenia.
- Warn patients to report infections/sore throat/bruising.
- These usually occur within the first 6 months of starting treatment with azathioprine.

Sperm toxicity
- A small, but significant increased risk of congenital abnormalities and spontaneous abortion is seen in men taking thiopurines within 3 months of conception.
- Advise male patients to discontinue AZA for 3 months prior to conception

FAQs

How long does it take to work?
A clinical response is usually seen after 3 months of treatment with AZA

What do I do if I want to get pregnant?
AZA is generally considered reasonably safe in pregnancy, although some studies have shown a small, but significant increase in congenital abnormalities and pre-term birth. Given the risks to patients of activation of SLE and vasculitis during pregnancy, the risk benefit ratio is often in favour of continuing treatment in these patients.

What about breastfeeding?
Although listed as a contraindication in the BNF, AZA appears to be relatively safe to use during lactation. Studies have shown that the active metabolites are only detectable at significantly sub-therapeutic levels in the breast milk of mothers taking therapeutic doses of AZA. Furthermore,

azathioprine
↓
6-mercaptopurine
↙ ↘
IMPDH TPMT

Active metabolites with potential marrow toxicity | Active metabolites with potential hepatotoxicity | Inactive metabolites

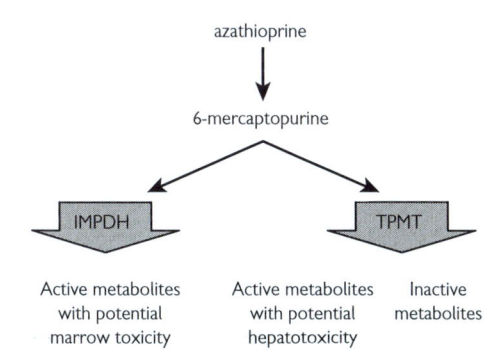

TPMT = thio-purine methyltransferase
IMPDH = inosine monophosphate dehydrogenase

Figure 19.7

neonatal blood levels are undetectable and the infants show no evidence of immunosuppression.

Does azathioprine cause cancer?
There is some data to suggest a small increased risk of lymphoma amongst patients taking azathioprine. However, there is also an increased risk associated with the autoimmune rheumatic diseases. Overall, the risk with azathioprine appears to be slightly greater, but the data is inconclusive.

Can I drink alcohol?
There is no evidence that alcohol interferes with azathioprine, although significant hepatic impairment would be a relative contraindication and dose adjustment would be required.

What about immunizations?
- Live vaccines should be avoided: live polio, rubella, varicella, and yellow fever.
- Influenza vaccination is recommended and is safe.

What to do if side effects occur

Common side effects
These frequently resolve if the patient can continue with treatment for 2–3 weeks. If they fail to resolve and patient cannot tolerate, reduce the dose of AZA, and try to increase a few weeks later.
WBC <3.5 × 10^9/l. Stop AZA and review.
Platelets <150 × 10^9/l. Stop AZA and review.
ALT > twice upper limit. Stop AZA and review.

Hypersensitivity reactions
- Dizziness, vomiting, diarrhoea, myalgia, rash, hypotension.
- Stop AZA and treat as appropriate.

Interstitial nephritis
Stop AZA and treat as appropriate.

Pancreatitis
Stop AZA and treat as appropriate.

Pneumonitis
Stop AZA and treat as appropriate.

Mycophenolate mofetil

Trade name: CellCept.

History
- **1800s**: mycophenolic acid is identified in *Penicillium* fungus.
- **1969**: mycophenolic acid is shown to inhibit inosine monophosphate dehydrogenase (IMPDH).
- **1980s**: mycophenolate mofetil (a pro-drug of mycophenolic acid) is developed and used in renal transplantation.
- **1990s**: placebo-controlled studies (PCS) confirm the efficacy of mycophenolate mofetil in renal transplantation.
- **1999**: open pilot study of mycophenolate shows efficacy in SLE nephritis.
- **2000s**: increasing evidence of efficacy in both renal and non-renal SLE.
- **2004**: evidence for mycophenolate in remission maintenance in vasculitis.

Possible mechanisms of action
Mycophenolate mofetil (MMF) is a pro-drug which is de-esterified to mycophenolic acid (MPA). MPA is an inhibitor of the inducible inosine monophosphate dehydrogenase (IMPDH -2), which is particularly important in T and B lymphocyte guanine nucleotide synthesis. It has less effect on the constitutively expressed isoform (IMPDH-1). Enteric-coated mycophenolate sodium is an alternative pro-drug that has been developed and used more recently in the field of transplantation. The enteric-coated sodium salt appears to have less gastrointestinal side effects (see below), but similar efficacy. However, there is, as yet, very little data on its use in rheumatology.

As well as inhibiting T and B cell proliferation MMF has a number of other potentially beneficial immunomodulatory effects.
- Induction of T cell apoptosis.
- Inhibition of dendritic cell maturation.
- Inhibition of adhesion molecule expression.

Evidence base: the main clinical trials with MMF and what they showed
Summary
Apart from in renal SLE there is a relative lack of good randomized controlled studies, but
- MMF is as effective as pulsed IV cyclophosphamide in remission induction in renal SLE.
- MMF appears effective in non-renal SLE.
- MMF appears effective in remission maintenance in ANCA associated vasculitis.
- MMF may be an alternative to cyclophosphamide in remission induction in certain patient with vasculitis.
- MMF may be effective in dermatomyositis.
- MMF is not effective in rheumatoid arthritis or Behcet's disease.

Systemic lupus erythematosus (SLE)
Ginzler EM, Dooley MA, Aranow C, et al. (2005) Mycophenolate mofetil or intravenous cyclophosphamide for lupus nephritis. *N Engl J Med* **353**: 2219–28. A large randomized open label study of 140 patients comparing oral MMF with IV pulsed cyclophosphamide in remission induction in renal SLE. The study showed that MMF is more effective and better tolerated than cyclophosphamide.

Karim MY, Alba P, Cuadrado MJ, et al. (2002) Mycophenolate mofetil for systemic lupus erythematosus refractory to other immunosuppressive agents. *Rheumatol (Oxf)* **41**: 876–82. An open label study of 21 patients with refractory disease showing benefit for MMF in both renal and non-renal disease

ANCA associated vasculitis (AAV)
Open label studies and anecdotal reports show efficacy in remission maintenance – less robust evidence for remission induction.

Langford CA, Talar-Williams C, Sneller MC (2004) Mycophenolate mofetil for remission maintenance in the treatment of Wegener's granulomatosis. *Arthritis Rheum* **51**: 278–83.

Stassen PM, Cohn Tervaert JW, Stegeman CA (2007) Induction of remission in active anti-neutrophil cytoplasmic antibody-associated vasculitis with mycophenolate mofetil in patients who cannot be treated with cyclophosphamide. *Ann Rheum Dis* **66**: 798–802.

Two small open label studies (14 and 32 patients, respectively) showing efficacy for mycophenolate in vasculitis [both remission maintenance and induction (in patients who could not be treated with cyclophosphamide)].

Dermatomyositis
Majithia V, Harisdangkul V. (2005) Mycophenolate mofetil (CellCept): an alternative therapy for autoimmune inflammatory myopathy. *Rheumatol (Oxf)* **44**: 386–9. One of several small open studies showing potentially beneficial results in patients with dermatomyositis.

Rheumatoid arthritis
Mycophenoloate monotherapy
Unpublished clinical trials have been undertaken with MMF, but have failed to show benefit

Behçet's disease
Adler YD, Mansmann U, Zouboulis CC (2001) Mycophenolate mofetil is ineffective in the treatment of mucocutaneous Adamantiades–Behçet's disease. *Dermatology* **203**(4): 322–4. A prospective open label study of 30 patients showing that treatment with MMF is ineffective in Behcet's.

Prescribing considerations
What do I need to do before starting the treatment?
- Patient education re: dosing, side effects and monitoring.
- Ensure your patient has a monitoring booklet

CHAPTER 19 **DMARDs and immunosuppressive drugs**

Record at baseline	
FBC	Allows monitoring of changes
LFTs	Allows monitoring of changes
ESR or CRP	Monitor disease activity
Renal function	Monitoring if renal disease activity (reduce dose if significantly impaired; MMF is 95% renally excreted so if in doubt measure creatinine clearance)
Lipid profile	Although recommended the rationale is unclear – some animal models actually suggest favourable effects of MMF on atherogenesis. It may reflect the post-transplant effects of other immunosuppressants
dsDNA in SLE	Allows monitoring of changes
ANCA in AAV	Allows monitoring of changes
BP	Mycophenolate can cause hypertensive changes

What dose should I prescribe?
Usual protocol for MMF prescription (local protocols may vary):
- **Week 1:** 500 mg od, then if tolerated
- **Week 2:** 500 mg bd
- **Week 3:** 1 g morning, 500 mg evening
- **From week 4:** 1 g bd. The dose can be increased to 1.5 g bd if necessary

Note: mycophenolate sodium: 720 mg is approximately equivalent to 1 g of MMF.

Important drug interactions
- **Antacids and colestyramine:** reduce the absorption of MMF by ~1/3.
- **Phenytoin:** absorption is reduced by MMF.
- **Aciclovir/ganciclovir:** increased plasma concentrations with MMF.

Monitoring of MMF
FBC, renal function, and LFTs and BP

Example monitoring regime
• Weekly for the first month.
• Fortnightly for the next 2 months.
• Monthly thereafter.

ESR or CRP
Useful for monitoring response to treatment (check monthly)

Side effects and what to discuss with your patients

Common
Nausea, abdominal discomfort, diarrhoea, headache, anorexia.

Uncommon
Rash (rarely Stevens–Johnson syndrome), pancreatitis.

Haematological toxicity
- Neutropenia, thrombocytopenia, pancytopenia.
- Warn patients to report infections/sore throat/bruising.

- These usually occur within the first 6 months of starting treatment with MMF.

Gastrointestinal toxicity
- The gastrointestinal side effects are the most troublesome with MMF, and can be reduced by slowly increasing the dose or by splitting the dose from bd to qds.
- The new enteric-coated mycophenolate sodium may be less problematic and similarly efficacious but has not yet been extensively studied in non-transplant use

Contraception
Mycophenolate is potentially toxic in pregnancy and appropriate contraception should be advised.

What to do if side effects occur
Common side effects
- The gastrointestinal effects are discussed above. Other minor side effects frequently resolve if the patient can continue with treatment for 2–3 weeks.
- If they fail to resolve and patient cannot tolerate, one can consider dose reduction or try a qds, rather than a bd regime.

Hypertension
- Consider dose reduction in first instance.
- If necessary treat with appropriate anti-hypertensive.

Haematological toxicity
- WBC <3.5 × 10^9/l: stop MMF and review.
- Platelets < 150 × 10^9/l: stop MMF and review.
- ALT > twice upper limit: stop MMF and review.

FAQs
How long does it take to work?
A clinical response is usually seen after 3 months of treatment with MMF.

What do I do if I want to get pregnant?
The transplant literature shows an increased prevalence of congenital abnormalities, premature birth and low birth weight amongst babies born of patients taking MMF. Ideally, MMF should therefore be discontinued at least 6 weeks prior to conception. However, this decision need to be balanced with the potential risk of stopping or changing treatment, and needs careful discussion with the patient.

What about breastfeeding?
There is a lack of good data with which to advise in this area, but the general guidance is to avoid the use of mycophenolate if breast feeding

Does MMF cause cancer?
There is conflicting data on whether MMF is associated with an increased risk of lymphoma and skin malignancy. Indeed, some studies suggest an anti-tumour effect. Patients should generally be advised to use high factor suntan cream and avoid excessive sunlight exposure.

Can I drink alcohol?
There is no evidence that alcohol interferes with MMF, although given the potentially hepatotoxic and pancreatitic effects of MMF moderation should be advised.

What about immunizations?
- Live vaccines should be avoided: live polio, rubella, varicella and yellow fever.
- Influenza vaccination is recommended and is safe

Ciclosporin (previously cyclosporin A)

History
- **1971:** ciclosporin is identified as an 11 amino acid peptide product of the soil fungus *Tolypocladium Inflatum*, itself identified as part of a programme at Sandoz (subsequently Novartis) to identify fungally derived antibiotics.
- **1972:** animal studies demonstrate immunosuppressive effects of ciclosporin, subsequently shown to be due to T cell mediated effects, as well as nephrotoxicity.
- **1979:** ciclosporin use, in preventing organ transplant rejection, is published by Prof Sir Roy Calne.
- **1983:** ciclosporin approved by the FDA for use in transplantation.
- **1984:** synthetic ciclosporin produced.
- **1991:** ciclosporin is identified (in an open label study) as being efficacious in rheumatoid arthritis, but with significant renal toxicity.
- **1995:** micro-emulsion synthetic ciclosporin developed with improved bio-availability (neoral).

Possible mechanisms of action
Ciclosporin inhibits the early activation of helper T cells (CD4+ T cells) by inhibition of IL-2 production. Ciclosporin binds to an intracellular protein (immunophilin) in CD4+ T cells. This complex in turns inhibits the action of calcineurin – a calcium dependent enzyme that is important in the regulation of interleukin 2 (IL-2) expression in T cells. IL-2 is critically important in early T cell activation and proliferation. CD4+ T cells are thought to have an important role in rheumatoid arthritis – they are key regulators of both the innate and the acquired immune response, they can be identified in the rheumatoid synovium, and there is the Class II MHC association with HLA-DRB0401.

Evidence base: the main clinical trials with ciclosporin and what they showed

Summary
Ciclosporin is efficacious in both rheumatoid arthritis and psoriatic arthritis. It is more effective as a combination treatment with both methotrexate and leflunomide than as monotherapy. There are no large randomized controlled studies, but a number of small studies show efficacy in both renal and non-renal SLE, as well as myositis. There is anecdotal data and small series showing efficacy in Behcet's syndrome.

Rheumatoid arthritis
Ciclosporin monotherapy
Ahern MJ, Harrison W, Hollingsworth P, et al. (1991) A randomised double-blind trial of cyclosporin and azathioprine in refractory rheumatoid arthritis. *Aust N Z J Med* **21**: 844–9. A randomized study showing that monotherapy with ciclosporin is similar to azathioprine in terms of efficacy

Ciclosporin combination therapy
1. Ciclosporin and Methotrexate
Tugwell P, Pincus T, Yocum D, et al. (1995) Combination therapy with cyclosporine and methotrexate in severe rheumatoid arthritis. The Methotrexate-Cyclosporine Combination Study Group. *N Engl J Med* **333**(3): 137–41. A double blind placebo-controlled study in 148 patients showing that step-up combination treatment with ciclosporin and methotrexate was more efficacious than methotrexate alone in patient inadequately responding to methotrexate.

Hetland ML, Stengaard-Pedersen K, Junker P, et al. (2006) Combination treatment with methotrexate, cyclosporine, and intraarticular betamethasone compared with methotrexate and intra-articular betamethasone in early active rheumatoid arthritis: an investigator-initiated, multicenter, randomized, double-blind, parallel-group, placebo-controlled study. *Arthritis Rheum.* **54**: 1401–9. The CIMESTRA Study: a randomized controlled trial in 160 patients showing benefit from the addition of ciclosporin to methotrexate and intraarticular steroids in patients with early rheumatoid.

2. Ciclosporin and leflunomide
Karanikolas G, Charnlambopoulos D, Andrianakos A, et al. (2006) Combination of cyclosporine and leflunomide versus single therapy in severe rheumatoid arthritis. *J Rheumatol* **33**: 486–9. A randomized controlled trial in 106 patients showing that the combination of leflunomide (20 mg) and ciclosporin (2.5–5 mg/kg/day) was better than either treatment as monotherapy in chronic rheumatoid arthritis

3. Ciclosporin and hydroxychloroquine
Miranda JM, Alvarez-Nemegvei J, Saavedra MA, et al. (2004) A randomized, double-blind, multicenter, controlled clinical trial of cyclosporine plus chloroquine vs. cyclosporine plus placebo in early-onset rheumatoid arthritis. *Arch Med Res* **35**: 36–42. A randomized controlled trial in 149 patients showing that the combination of antimalarials and ciclosporin (2.5–5 mg/kg/day) was no better than ciclosporin alone.

Psoriatic arthritis
Ciclosporin monotherapy
Spadaro A, Riccieri V, Sili-Scavalli A, et al. (1995) Comparison of cyclosporin A and methotrexate in the treatment of psoriatic arthritis: a one-year prospective study. *Clin Exp Rheumatol* **13**: 589–93. A small randomized study (35 patients) showing that ciclosporine monotherapy is similarly efficacious to methotrexate monotherapy in psoriatic arthritis.

Ciclosporin combination therapy
1. Ciclosporin and methotrexate
Fraser AD, van Kuijk AW, Westhovens R, et al. (2005) A randomised, double blind, placebo controlled, multicentre trial of combination therapy with methotrexate plus ciclosporin in patients with active psoriatic arthritis. *Ann Rheum Dis* **64**: 859–64. A randomized controlled study in 72 patients with psoriatic arthritis only partially responsive to MTX, showing significant, but limited efficacy of additional ciclosporin.

Systemic lupus erythematosis
Caccavo D, Lagana B, Mitterhofer AP, et al. (1997) Long-term treatment of systemic lupus erythematosus with cyclosporine A. *Arthritis Rheum* **40**: 27–35. An open label prospective study in 30 patients showing efficacy of ciclosporin in non-renal SLE.

Tam LS, Li EK, Leung CB, et al. (1998) Long-term treatment of lupus nephritis with cyclosporin A. *QJM.* **91**(8): 573–80. A small open label study (17 patients) showing efficacy of ciclosporin in renal SLE (WHO Type IV).

CHAPTER 19 **DMARDs and immunosuppressive drugs**

Dermatomyositis/polymyositis
Vencovsky J, Jarosova K, Machacek S, et al. (2000) Ciclosporine A versus methotrexate in the treatment of polymyositis and dermatomyositis. *Scand J Rheumatol* **29**: 95–102. A randomized study of 36 patients with inflammatory myositis showing similar efficacy for methotrexate and ciclosporin.

Prescribing considerations
What do I need to do before starting the treatment?
- Patient education re: dosing, side effects, and monitoring.
- Ensure your patient has a patient held monitoring booklet

Record at baseline	
FBC	Allows monitoring of changes
LFTs	Allows monitoring of changes
ESR or CRP	Monitor disease activity
Renal function	(Ciclosporin is nephrotoxic). Measure ×3 serum creatinine (record average baseline creatinine). Measure creatinine clearance
Urine	Allows monitoring of changes
BP	Treat hypertension before commencing

What dose should I prescribe?
Usual protocol for ciclosporin prescription (local protocols may vary):
- Starting dose 2.5 mg/kg/day (twice daily divided dose).
- After 6 weeks (if tolerated).
- Increase by 25 mg per day every 2–4 weeks
- Maximum dose 4 mg/kg/day (in rheumatoid arthritis/psoriatic arthritis).
- In other conditions doses up to 5 mg/kg/day may be used.
The brand of ciclosporin should be specified. Generally neoral (the micro-emulsion of ciclosporin) is the oral version of ciclosporin that is used. If changing from neural to sandimmun the bioavailability is less but generally a conversion of 1:1 is reasonable. If converting from sandimmun to neoral, an initial small dose reduction should be considered.

Important drug interactions
- There is an increased risk of nephrotoxicity and hyperkalaemia when ciclosporin is given with other nephrotoxic agents (NSAIDs, ACE inhibitors, aminoglycoside antibiotics, amphotericin, ciprofloxacin, melphalan, trimethoprim, colchicines, potassium sparing diuretics).
- St John's Wort also potentiates the action of ciclosporin.
- Statins: there is an increased risk of myopathy on statins [probably due to effects of ciclosporin on the hepatic transport of statins (+/– an effect on the cytochrome P450-mediated metabolism of the statins)].
- Grapefruit juice: grapefruit juice increases the plasma concentration of ciclosporin by interfering with gastrointestinal cytochrome P450 function.

Monitoring of ciclosporin
Monitor 2-weekly for the first 3 months:
- Serum creatinine.
- FBC.
- Blood pressure.
- Urinalysis.

Thereafter, monitor monthly.
ESR or CRP: useful for monitoring response to treatment (check monthly).

Side effects and what to discuss with your patients
Common
Nausea, abdominal discomfort, diarrhoea, headache, tremor, paraesthesia

Uncommon
Hirsutism and gum hyperplasia, seizures. Advise patients on oral hygiene to prevent gum disease and on cosmetic approaches to any hirsuitism.

Nephrotoxicity
- Rising serum creatinine and hyperkalaemia: discuss with patients what is being monitored and why.
- Warn patients about the interaction of ciclosporin with grapefruit juice, and the importance of monitoring of renal function and blood pressure

What to do if side effects occur
Common side effects
The common side effects will usually subside once treatment becomes established. If persistent consider dose reduction.

Hypertension on treatment
- Consider dose reduction in first instance.
- If necessary treat with an appropriate anti-hypertensive and continue treatment.
- Stop treatment if hypertension remains uncontrolled.

Nephrotoxicity
- Nephrotoxicity is monitored with reference to the baseline average creatinine.
- If there is a rise in serum creatinine >30% above baseline:
  - consider dose reduction;
  - if failure to improve after 1 month, discontinue.
- Rise in serum creatinine >50% above the average baseline creatinine should trigger discontinuation of treatment.

FAQs
How long does it take to work?
A clinical response is usually seen after 3 months of treatment with ciclosporin

What do I do if I want to get pregnant?
The transplant literature suggests an increased prevalence of low birth weight and prematurity amongst babies born of patients taking ciclosporin (possibly due to interference with foetal uptake of the amino acid taurine). Ideally, ciclosporin should therefore be discontinued at least 6 weeks prior to conception. However, the risk appears small and ciclosporin has certainly been used successfully in pregnancy. The serum concentration of ciclosporin falls during pregnancy so if dose escalation is required during pregnancy, the pre-pregnancy dose should be returned to postpartum to avoid nephrotoxicity.

What about breastfeeding?
Ciclosporin is excreted in the breast milk so in general it is advisable to avoid ciclosporin if breast feeding. However, anecdotal data from the transplantation experience suggests that the drug is not significantly absorbed by the infant since in one study serum levels in an infant breast feeding, whilst their mother was on ciclosporin were undetectable (despite detectable levels in breast milk).

Does ciclosporin cause cancer?
There is some data to suggest an increased risk of non-melanoma skin cancer. Patients should generally be advised to use high factor suntan cream and avoid excessive sunlight exposure.

There does not seem to be an increased risk of other malignancies.

Can I drink alcohol?
There is no evidence that alcohol interferes with ciclosporin.

What about immunizations?
- Live vaccines should be avoided: live polio, rubella, varicella, and yellow fever.
- Influenza vaccination is recommended and is safe

Cyclophosphamide

Trade name: Endoxana

History
- **1958:** Brock (working for ASTA Werke pharmaceutical company in Germany) publishes in *Nature* the development of a cyclic nitrogen mustard phosphamide ester (cyclophosphamide), which shows selective *in vivo* activation. This oxazaphosphorine was synthesized in a transport form which is enzymatically activated to the active nitrogen mustard.
- **1960s:** cyclophosphamide is shown to be efficacious in cancer treatment and in the late 1960s is shown to have immunosuppressive effects (in transplantation).
- **1960s:** urothelial toxicity of cyclophosphamide is recognized as problematic.
- **1968:** animal studies report the benefits of cyclophosphamide in lupus nephritis.
- **1971:** a placebo controlled study shows efficacy of oral cyclophosphamide treatment in lupus nephritis.
- **1978:** the protective effects of MESNA (sodium-2-mercaptoethane-sulfonate) in preventing urothelial toxicity are identified.
- **1980s/90s:** randomized controlled studies (the NIH studies) show the efficacy of IV pulsed cyclophosphamide (in combination with IV methylprednisolone) in lupus nephritis.
- **1990s:** randomized controlled studies with cyclosphosphamide show efficacy in ANCA associated vasculitides.

Mechanism of action
Cyclophosphamide is a pro-drug (an inactive cyclic phosphamide ester of phosphoramide mustard) that undergoes an *in vivo* activation process. It is initially hepatically metabolized via cytochrome P450 to an equilibrium mixture of 4-hydroxycyclophosphamide and aldophosphamide.

Aldophosphamide can be metabolized to phosphoramide mustard (the active guanidine alkylating agent responsible for the therapeutic effects) and acrolein (the agent responsible for bladder toxicity). Aldophosphamide can also be inactivated via aldehyde dehydrogenase (ALDH). The therapeutic effects of cyclophosphamide are therefore seen predominantly in cells with relatively low levels of ALDH.

The phosphoramide mustard moiety causes alkylation of guanidine nucleotides and inhibits DNA polymerization, thereby preventing cell replication in susceptible cell types. It is non-cell cycle phase specific. The most susceptible cell types are those which are most rapidly dividing, such as those of the immune system and the bone marrow.

The immunoregulatory effects of cyclophosphamide appear to be mediated, in part, through effects on T cell activity. There is some evidence that cyclophosphamide suppresses Th1-mediated immune responses whilst enhancing Th2-mediated responses. More recently there has been interest in a possible role of cyclophosphamide in modifying immune tolerance. There is evidence, from the transplantation literature, that cyclophosphamide reduces CD4+CD25+ regulatory T cells which could modulate immune tolerance and might, in part, account for it's efficacy in autoimmune diseases like SLE and AAV.

Evidence base: the clinical trials with cyclophosphamide

Summary
Overall, the data in SLE with renal involvement from controlled studies (such as the NIH (National Institute of Health) studies) support the use of IV pulsed cyclophosphamide (in combination with IV methylprednisolone) for remission induction in lupus nephritis. The NIH regime uses 0.5–1 g/m^2 cyclophosphamide monthly with IV methylprednisolone for induction. There is some evidence that lower dose regimens (500 mg IV fortnightly) may be as efficacious as these higher dose regimens. Maintenance treatment with cyclophosphamide also has proven efficacy in lupus nephritis, but for such longer-term treatment other immunosuppressive regimens (such as azathioprine, methotrexate or mycophenolate) may be as efficacious (and less toxic). There is less robust, but nonetheless significant, data to support the use of IV cyclophosphamide in other patients with severe non-renal neuropsychiatric SLE.

Cyclophosphamide (particularly intravenous pulsed therapy in combination with intravenous pulsed steroid) is also effective in both inducing and maintaining remission in ANCA associated vasculitis (AAV). The standard regimes in AAV use 10–15 mg/kg doses of cyclophosphamide given fortnightly for 6 weeks then 3-weekly for 9 weeks for remission induction. This regimen is also known as the CYCLOPS regimen, since it is the regime that has been studied in an ongoing large multicentre study of pulsed versus oral cyclophosphamide for remission induction

In both AAV and SLE intravenous pulsed treatment is associated with less toxicity than continuous oral treatment with similar efficacy.

Oral cyclophosphamide shows weak efficacy as monotherapy in rheumatoid arthritis, but toxicity and side effects are severe.

SLE
Steinberg AD, Kaltreider HB, Staples PJ, *et al.* (1971) Cyclophosphamide in lupus nephritis: a controlled trial. *Ann Intern Med* **75**: 165–71. The first randomized placebo controlled study of oral cyclophosphamide (3–4 mg/kg/day – a relatively high dose regime) in lupus nephritis. 13 patients treated over 10 weeks – significant benefit in cyclophosphamide treated group relative to placebo

Austin HA, Klippel JH, Balow JE, *et al.* (1986) Therapy of lupus nephritis. *N Engl J Med* **314**: 614–19. The first of the NIH studies, in 107 patients, using a variety of regimes. The study showed that IV pulsed cyclophosphamide (0.5–1 g/m2) was significantly better in proliferative lupus nephritis (reduced rate of end stage renal failure after 5 years) than oral steroids. The other regimes (oral cyclophosphamide and azathioprine) were not shown to be statistically different from IV pulsed cyclophosphamide, but neither were they shown to be significantly better than oral steroids.

Boumpas DT, Austin HA, Vaughan EM, et al. (1992) Controlled trial of pulse methylprednisolone versus two regimens of pulse cyclophosphamide in severe lupus nephritis. Lancet **340**: 741–5. The second NIH study, in 65 patients, showing that pulsed IV cyclophosphamide [either over 6 months (0.5–1 g/m^2 monthly) or 30 months (0.5–1 g/m^2 monthly ×6/12 then 3-monthly ×2 years) was better (as measured by increasing creatinine) than pulsed IV methylprednisolone. Relapses were more common in the 6-month study group than the 30-month group, but the 6-month group was not given any treatment to maintain remission.

Gourley MF, Austin HA, Scott D, et al. (1996) Methylprednisolone and cyclophosphamide, alone or in combination, in patients with lupus nephritis. Ann Intern Med **125**: 549–57. The third NIH study, in 82 patients, demonstrating the superior efficacy of combination treatment with pulsed IV cyclophosphamide (0.5–1 g/m^2 monthly ×6/12 then 3-monthly ×2 years) and IV methylprednisolone, compared with pulsed IV methylprednisolone alone. There was a trend to improved efficacy of combination treatment over pulsed IV cyclophosphamide alone, but this failed to reach statistical significance.

Flanc RS, Roberts MA, Strippoli, et al. (2004) Treatment for lupus nephritis. Cochrane Database Syst Rev **1**: CD002922. A meta-analysis of all cyclophosphamide studies concluding that cyclophosphamide treatment, in combination with steroids, is efficacious in proliferative lupus nephritis. A significant risk of gonadal failure (relative risk 2.18) was also noted.

Yee CS, Gordon C, Dostal C, et al. (2004) EULAR randomized controlled trial of pulse cyclophosphamide and methylprednisolone versus continuous cyclophosphamide and prednisolone followed by azathioprine and prednisolone in lupus nephritis. Ann Rheum Dis **63**: 525–9. A randomized controlled study in 32 patients showing no significant difference in efficacy between pulsed treatment (10 mg/kg IV initially than pulsed oral treatment thereafter) and continuous treatment with cyclophosphamide (2 mg/kg/day × 3 months) in remission induction and maintenance in renal SLE. However, the IV/pulsed regime was better tolerated.

Houssiau FA, Vasconcelos C, D'Cruz D, et al. (2002) Immunosuppressive therapy in lupus nephritis: the Euro-Lupus Nephritis Trial, a randomized trial of low dose versus high dose intravenous cyclophosphamide. Arthritis Rheum **46**: 2121–31. A controlled study of 90 patients showing that fortnightly pulsed low dose IV cyclophosphamide (500 mg/2 weeks) was as effective in remission induction as high dose treatment (0.5 g/m^2 increasing by 250 mg with each pulse to a maximum of 1500 mg/pulse), but with less infection risk.

Barile-Fabris L, Ariza-Andraca R, Olguin-Ortega L, et al. (2005) Controlled clinical trial of IV cyclophosphamide versus IV methylprednisolone in severe neurological manifestations in systemic lupus erythematosus. Ann Rheum Dis **64**: 620–5. A controlled study of 32 patients with severe neurological SLE. The study showed that, after an initial 3 g IV methylprednisolone treatment, pulsed IV cyclophosphamide (0.75 g/m^2 monthly for 1 year and then 3-monthly thereafter for another year) was significantly better (>20% neurological improvement) than pulsed IV methylprednisolone (1 g monthly ×4/12, 2-monthly ×6/12, 3-monthly × 1 year) alone.

ANCA associated vasculitis
Adu D, Pall A, Luqmani RA, et al. (1997) Controlled trial of pulse versus continuous prednisolone and cyclophosphamide in the treatment of systemic vasculitis. Q J Med **90**(6): 401–9. A randomized controlled study in 54 patients comparing (A) pulsed cyclophosphamide (15 mg/kg) and prednisolone (10 mg/kg, every 2 weeks for 6 weeks then every 3 weeks). (B) Continuous oral cyclophosphamide (2 mg/kg) for 3 months (followed by oral azathioprine) and prednisolone (0.85 mg/kg/day). The study showed that the continuous oral treatment regimen was associated with more toxicity and similar efficacy to the pulsed treatment regimen.

Guillevin L, Cordier JF, Lhote F, et al. (1997) A prospective, multicenter, randomised trial comparing steroid and pulsed cyclophosphamide versus steroids and oral cyclophosphamide in the treatment of generalised Wegener's granulomatosis. Arthritis Rheum **40**: 2187–98. A randomized controlled study of 50 patients. All patients prior to randomization received ×3 IV pulses of methylprednisolone, oral prednisolone (1 mg/kg) and a single IV pulse of cyclophosphamide (0.7 g/m^2). Thereafter, the study compared oral cyclophosphamide (2 mg/kg/day) with IV pulsed treatment (initially 0.7 g/m^2 every 3 weeks reducing to 6-weekly) over 1 year. The study again showed similar efficacy but fewer side effects with the IV pulsed cyclophosphamide regimen.

Haubitz M, Schellong S, Gobel U, et al. (1998) Intravenous pulse administration of cyclophosphamide versus daily oral treatment in patients with antineutrophil cytoplasmic antibody-associated vasculitis and renal involvement: a prospective, randomized study. Arthritis Rheum **41**: 1835–44. A randomized controlled study of 47 patients. All patients prior to randomization received ×3 IV pulses of methylprednisolone. Thereafter, the study compared IV pulsed cyclophosphamide (0.75 g/m^2 every month) with oral cyclophosphamide (2 mg/kg/day) over 1 year. The study again showed similar efficacy, but fewer side effects with the IV pulsed cyclophosphamide regime.

Rheumatoid arthritis
Suarez-Almazor ME, Belseck E. Shea B, et al. (2000) Cyclophosphamide for rheumatoid arthritis. Cochrane Database Syst Rev **4**: CD001157. A meta-analysis showing that oral cyclophosphamide is efficacious – benefit was shown for symptoms and signs of rheumatoid arthritis (similar to sulfasalazine, but less than methotrexate). However, it was associated with significant toxicity (haemorrhagic cystitis, GI side effects, bone marrow suppression, alopecia, amenorrhoea and herpes zoster).

Prescribing considerations
What do I need to do before starting the treatment?
Patient education re: dosing, side effects, monitoring, drug interactions, etc.

The risks of haemorrhagic cystitis, alopecia, bladder cancer, sepsis, teratogenicity, infertility, and future malignancy should all be explicitly discussed with patients as part of the informed consent process before treatment is initiated.

Neutropenic sepsis is a significant risk of cyclophosphamide treatment and patients should be cautioned to seek urgent medical advice if they become febrile or unwell during treatment.

Record at baseline	
FBC	Allows monitoring of changes
LFTs	Allows monitoring of changes
ESR or CRP	Monitor disease activity
Renal function	Dose adjustment in renal impairment
Urine dipstick	Monitor disease activity and evidence of urothelial toxicity
Varicella status	Either history or serology
Gonadal toxicity	Males are at a significant risk of oligospermia (particularly those requiring more than 3 months of treatment). Cryopreservation of sperm should be offered to all males before the first pulse of treatment. At least 50% of males will develop azoospermia as a result of cyclophosphamide treatment using standard SLE/AAV protocols

Females are at risk of premature ovarian failure although the threshold is thought to be higher than that for oligospermia in men. It is estimated that between 30–50% of women will experience permanent ovarian failure following 1 year of treatment with cyclophosphamide – older women (>30 years) are at the greatest risk. There is no routine ovarian cryopreservation programme for women, although some areas have experimental programmes (for preservation of both fertilized and unfertilized ova) and local policies should be investigated.

What dose should I prescribe?
Oral treatment
Pulsed IV cyclosphosphamide is generally preferred to continuous oral treatment since it has been associated with less toxicity in a number of trial studies. However, continuous oral treatment is still used occasionally.

Cyclophosphamide is available as 50–100 mg tablets
- Usual oral dose: 1.5–2 mg/kg/day rounded down to the nearest 50 mg.
- The maximum dose of oral cyclosphosphamide is usually 200 mg (although doses up to 4 mg/kg have been used in some studies).
- The dose should be reduced by 25% for patients >60 years and by 50% for patients >75 years.
- Usual practice is to induce remission with 2 mg/kg for ~3 months and to maintain remission with 1.5 mg/kg before changing to alternative maintenance therapy within 6 months.

Intravenous treatment
- Dosage is calculated either on the basis of mg/kg (in AAV) or body surface area (in SLE).
- Calculation for body surface area (BSA) in m^2 (Mosteller):
- BSA = square root {[weight (kg) × height (cm)]/3600}
- [usual adult BSA in men (~1.9m^2), in women (~1.6m^2)].

Examples of common dose regimens for remission induction
Note: induction regimes are generally given with IV Methylprednisolone (500 mg–1 g IV daily by intravenous infusion for 3 days) and concomitant oral steroid (usually a reducing regime) – see below for details.

A commonly used AAV regimen (based on BSR guidelines and the CYCLOPS study regimen)
- 15 mg/kg IV cyclophosphamide (maximum 1500 mg) (in 500 ml N. saline over 1 h (or longer if necessary)) every 2 weeks for 6 weeks then every 3 weeks for 3 months (reduce initial dose according to Table 1 for the elderly and those with a reduced creatinine clearance).
- Subsequent maintenance therapy may be with a reducing frequency of IV cyclophosphamide (e.g. 3 monthly) or with alternative immunosuppressive agents (e.g. azathioprine, mycophenolate, methotrexate)

Table 19.1 Pulsed cyclophosphamide dose reductions according to age and creatinine/creatinine clearance

Age	Creatinine <300 μmol/l (calculated creatinine clearance >30 ml/min)	Creatinine >300 μmol/l (calculated creatinine clearance <30 ml/min)
<60	15 mg/kg/pulse	12.5 mg/kg/pulse
60–70	12.5 mg/kg/pulse	10 mg/kg/pulse
>70	10 mg/kg/pulse	7.5 mg/kg/pulse

A commonly used SLE regimen
- 0.75–1 g/m^2 IV cyclophosphamide (maximum 1500 mg) (in 500 ml N saline over 1 h (or longer if necessary)) every month for 6 months (reduced to an initial dose of 0.5 g/m^2 for the elderly, those at risk of leucopenia or those with a creatinine clearance of <30 ml/min) – a commonly used regimen in lupus nephritis
- Subsequent maintenance therapy may be with a reducing frequency of IV cyclophosphamide (e.g. 3-monthly) or with alternative immunosuppressive agents (e.g. azathioprine, mycophenolate, methotrexate)

Other treatment considerations when prescribing IV pulsed cyclosphosphamide?
MESNA

MESNA reduces the urothelial toxicity of cyclophosphamide. One dose (either oral or IV) is given just prior to the infusion. Two further doses (usually oral) are then given 2 and 6 h post-infusion.
- **Dose 1:** IV 20% of cyclophosphamide dose in 500 ml of N saline over 1 h, given just prior to cyclophosphamide treatment; OR PO 40% of cyclophosphamide dose just pre treatment.
- **Dose 2:** PO 40% of cyclophosphamide dose 2 h post-infusion.
- **Dose 3:** PO 40% of cyclophosphamide dose 6 h post-infusion.

CHAPTER 19 **DMARDs and immunosuppressive drugs**

Antiemetic
Prophylactic antiemetic usage is advised for IV cyclophosphamide

> **Prophylactic antiemetic usage: an example regimen**
> - Ondansetron 8 mg IV just prior to cyclophosphamide infusion
> - Metoclopromide 10 mg po tds for 72 h post-infusion.
> - If vomiting is problematic, despite the above regime, change from metoclopromide to post-dose oral ondansetron and oral domperidone for subsequent infusions. If still problematic consider 1.5 mg haloperidol bd on day 1 and consider regular IV methylprednisolone with cyclophosphamide(see below)

IV glucocorticoids
The first dose of induction regimes of cyclophosphamide are frequently given with ×3 pulses of IV methylprednisolone 500 mg–1 g IV daily.

> Subsequent infusions can be given with progressive reduction regimes.
> **Subsequent infusions example**
> - 2nd pulse 500 mg IV methylprednisolone.
> - 3rd pulse 250 mg IV methylprednisolone.
> - IV steroid has both an anti-emetic effect and an immunosuppressive effect

Oral glucocorticoids
An example reducing oral steroid regime, for use in conjunction with IV pulsed cyclophosphamide regimes, is shown in Table 19.2. Doses may be reduced if IV methylprednisolone is used concomitantly.

Table 19.2 An example oral steroid reduction regime

Time from entry (weeks)	Dosage (max 80 mg)
0	1 mg/kg/day – 60 mg
1	0.75 mg/kg/day – 45 mg
2	0.5 mg/kg/day – 30 mg
3	0.4 mg/kg/day - 25 mg
4	0.33 mg/kg/day – 20 mg
5	0.3 mg/kg/day – 17.5 mg
6-12	0.25 mg/kg/day – 15 mg
Thereafter	Reduce by 2.5 mg/month according to clinical response

Hydration
- Adequate hydration reduces the risk of haemorrhagic cystitis. Consider 500 ml IV N. saline pre-treatment (particularly if not receiving IV MESNA).
- Advise patients to drink 3 l/day for 3 days post-infusion.

Infection
Cotrimoxazole 960 mg 30×/week (or 480 mg daily) should be given as prophylaxis against PCP during treatment with cyclophosphamide.

Monitoring
Monitoring of WBC after IV cyclophosphamide
Leucopenia/neutropenia and associated sepsis is a significant risk. The WCC should therefore be monitored on days 0, 7, 10, and 14 post-first infusion and with any subsequent infusions where there is a dose change. Thereafter, the WCC should be checked on the day of infusion or the previous day.

If the total WCC fails to drop below 5×10^9/l the dose of the subsequent infusion can be increased by 250 mg/m^2 to a maximum of 1 g/m^2 or 1500 mg.

If the total WCC drops to a nadir of $2-3\times10^9$/l or the neutrophils counts drops to $1-1.5 \times 10^9$/l the subsequent dose should be delayed until the neutrophil count rises about 2×10^9/l and the total WCC >4×10^9/l. Subsequent doses should be reduced by 20% and monitored using the same WCC monitoring regime.

If the total WCC drops to a nadir of $1-2 \times 10^9$/l or the neutrophils counts drops below 1×10^9/l the subsequent dose should be delayed until the neutrophil count rises about 2×10^9/l and the total WCC >4×10^9/l. Subsequent doses should be reduced by 40% and monitored using the same WCC monitoring regime.

It should always be ensured that the WCC is recovering before administration of the next dose of cyclophosphamide.

Urgent FBC in patients with infection/fever

Monitoring with oral cyclophosphamide
- FBC and urine.
- Leucopenia/neutropenia and associated sepsis are significant risks as is haemorrhagic cystitis.
- Monitor FBC and urine dipstick weekly for 4 weeks
- Monitor FBC and urine dipstick fortnightly for 2nd/3rd months.
- Monitor FBC and urine dipstick monthly thereafter.

Side effects and what to discuss with your patient
Common
- **Nausea and vomiting:** prophylactic antiemetic treatment should always be used in patients receiving cyclophosphamide.
- **Hair loss** (usually transient) can occur during treatment and patients should be forewarned of this.
- **Mouth ulcers** can also be problematic and patients should be advised of the importance of oral hygiene.
- **Skin rashes** can occur and patients should be aware of the increased risk of herpes zoster with cyclophosphamide/'steroid regimes.

Haemorrhagic cystitis
Patients should be advised of the importance of maintaining an adequate fluid intake when taking cyclophosphamide to reduce the chances of developing haemorrhagic cystitis (generally advise 8–10 glasses of water per day). They should also be advised to report any blood in the urine.

Infection and bone marrow toxicity
- As well as the risks of neutropenic sepsis highlighted above, there is an increased of all infections with cyclophosphamide treatments and the presentation of infections may be atypical.
- Patients should be advised to urgently contact a health care professional for any unexplained illness during treatment with cyclophosphamide and an urgent FBC obtained. Evidence of prior exposure to varicella (chicken pox) should, if possible, be confirmed before commencing treatment and if necessary VZV serology checked. If non-immune advise patients to avoid contact and consider immunization pre-treatment. All patients should receive PCP prophylaxis with cotrimoxazole.
- There is also a risk of thrombocytopenia with cyclophosphamide and patients should be advised to report unusual/easy bruising or other evidence of bleeding (e.g. tarry stools, etc.).

Infertility risk
Cyclophosphamide causes infertility (both reversibly during treatment and in a proportion of patients irreversibly (see above under gonadal toxicity) in both men and women. If possible, frozen storage of sperm or ova should be considered prior to commencing treatment. The risk of inducing irreversible infertility is significantly greater in older patients and patients having more prolonged treatment courses.

Malignancy
- Cyclophosphamide treatment has mutagenic/carcinogenic potential due to the alkylation of DNA.
- The incidence of all malignancies is increased in patients with SLE/AAV treated with cyclophosphamide (SIR approx. 2).
- The incidence of haematopoietic malignancy (most notably acute myeloid leukaemia) is significantly increased (SIR approx. 20) compared with the expected levels.
- Cyclophosphamide is also associated with an increased long-term risk of bladder cancer (SIR approx. 4) and non-melanoma skin cancer (SIR approx. 5).
- The risks of all malignancies are dose-dependent and malignancies can occur several decades after treatment so patients should be monitored long term.

Contraception
Cyclophosphamide is teratogenic due to the alkylating effects, and both male and females should use contraception during and for 3 months after cyclophosphamide treatment. Patients should be advised that even if the treatment stops a regular monthly menstrual cycle, it is still possible to conceive if appropriate contraception is not used.

Drug interactions
Possible drug interactions with cyclophosphamide include:
- **Allopurinol:** there have been conflicting reports concerning an increased risk of marrow toxicity in patients taking allopurinol alongside cyclophosphamide.
- **Phenytoin:** cyclophosphamide redutes the absorption of phenytoin.
- **Warfarin:** both increased and decreased effects have been reported with cyclophosphamide.
- **Thiazide diuretics:** prolonged leucopenia has been reported in patients treated with combination thiazide diuretics and cyclophosphamide, and thiazides should be used with caution in these patients

FAQs
How long does it take to work?
Advise patients that cyclophosphamide may take several weeks before the treatment takes effect.

What if I want to get pregnant?
Cyclophosphamide should not be used in pregnancy. Cyclophosphamide treatment should be discontinued at least 3 months prior to conception (in men and women). It is important for both men and women to take contraceptive precautions during cyclophosphamide treatment. Patients should be advised that even if the treatment stops a regular monthly menstrual cycle it is still possible to conceive if appropriate contraception is not used.

What about breast feeding?
Cyclophosphamide treatment should be avoided in patients who are breast feeding

What about immunizations?
- Live attenuated vaccines need to be avoided by patients on cyclophosphamide treatment: yellow fever, MMR and rubella, BCG, oral polio, oral typhoid.
- Other vaccines are not a problem.
- Patients should be advised to have an annual influenza immunization since they are at an increased risk of influenza.

Can I drink alcohol?
Alcohol does not interfere with cyclophosphamide

Biologics: anti-TNF (infliximab, etanercept, adalimumab), anti-CD20 (rituximab), anti-IL-1 (anakinra), CTLA4–Ig (abatacept), and anti-IL-6R (tocilizumab)

History

Infliximab, adalimumab and etanercept (Anti-TNF (antibodies and recombinant soluble receptor))

- **1890s:** Dr William Coley identifies that bacterial infections can trigger the immune system to produce anti-tumour effects.
- **1975:** tumour necrosis factor is identified as a monocyte derived cytotoxic factor by Dr Lloyd Old.
- **1986:** tumour necrosis factor is demonstrated to have detrimental effects on cartilage *in vitro*.
- **1988:** elevated levels of TNF are demonstrated in both synovial fluid and serum of patients with rheumatoid disease.
- **1992:** chimeric anti-TNF antibodies are shown to be efficacious in mouse models of inflammatory arthritis.
- **1993:** chimeric anti-TNF antibodies are shown to be efficacious in patients with rheumatoid arthritis.
- **1997:** recombinant human TNF receptor (etanercept) is shown to have efficacy in rheumatoid arthritis.
- **2002:** adalimumab (a non-chimeric anti-TNF antibody) is developed for treatment of rheumatoid arthritis. NICE TAG32 supports the use of anti-TNF in rheumatoid arthritis.

Rituximab (anti B cell (anti-CD20 antibody))

- **1992:** chimeric anti-CD20 antibodies are shown to deplete B cells in mouse models.
- **1997:** chimeric anti-CD20 antibody (Rituximab) is used successfully in the treatment of lymphoma.
- **2002:** Rituximab is shown to have efficacy, in different studies, in ANCA associated vasculitis, SLE, and rheumatoid arthritis.
- **2007:** NICE TAG126 supports the use of rituximab in rheumatoid arthritis patients who have failed anti-TNF.

Anakinra [anti IL-1 (IL-1 receptor antagonist)]

- **1982:** IL-1 is shown to be important in the pathogenesis of rheumatoid arthritis.
- **1984:** IL-1 receptor antagonist, a naturally occurring antagonist of IL-1, is identified.
- **1991:** recombinant IL-1 receptor antagonist is shown to be efficacious in a rabbit model of inflammatory arthritis.
- **1996:** preliminary data suggest some benefit for recombinant human IL-1 receptor antagonist (anakinra) in rheumatoid arthritis.
- **1996-2000:** several studies show limited efficacy with anakinra for symptoms but some reduction in radiographic progression in rheumatoid arthritis.
- **2003:** NICE TAG72 advises against the use of anakinra for rheumatoid arthritis.

Abatacept [anti-T cell (CTLA4-Ig fusion protein)]

- **1993:** CTLA4 (cytotoxic T lymphocyte antigen 4) is identified as a CD28-like molecule expressed on T cells, following activation, which inhibits T cell activation when it interacts with the CD80/86 ligand on antigen presenting cells. This is in contrast to the CD28/CD80/86 interaction which is stimulatory for T cells.
- **1994:** CTLA4-Ig fusion protein is shown to inhibit synovial T cell proliferation *in vitro* (by inhibiting CD28/CD80/86 interactions).
- **1995:** CTLA4-Ig is shown to inhibit inflammatory arthritis in a rat model.
- **2003:** CTLA4-Ig is shown to be efficacious in the treatment of rheumatoid arthritis.

Tocilizumab (Anti IL-6 (non-stimulatory anti-receptor antibody))

- **1988:** interleukin 6 levels are shown to be elevated in rheumatoid arthritis synovial fluid and serum. The Interleukin 6 receptor is isolated.
- **2000:** Tocilizumab (an anti-IL-6 receptor antibody) is shown to be efficacious in multicentric Castleman's disease (a condition characterized by high IL-6 levels).
- **2002:** Tocilizumab is shown to have efficacy in rheumatoid arthritis

Possible mechanisms of action

Conventional DMARDs are molecules that characteristically have a multiplicity of anti-inflammatory actions. By contrast, the biologics are variants of the endogenous proteins of the immune system (usually antibodies), which are bioengineered to specifically target individual components of the inflammatory response. Most commonly, these biologics target cytokines or co-stimulatory molecules, which have previously been demonstrated to be important in the inflammatory response. Antibodies may be chimeric (usually incorporating a murine binding region (Fab fragment), which gives the molecule it's specificity, and a human signalling component (Fc region) – see Figure 19.7. The mechanisms of action and the molecular structure of the common biologics used in rheumatology are shown in Table 19.3.

CHAPTER 19 DMARDs and immunosuppressive drugs

Table 19.3 A table of the biologics indicating their structure and their mechanism of action

Generic Name	Trade Name	Protein Structure	Mechanism Of Action
Infliximab	Remicade	Chimeric anti-TNF monoclonal antibody	Binds both membrane bound and circulating TNF preventing it's binding to the TNF receptor
Adalimumab	Humira	Humanized anti-TNF monoclonal antibody	Binds both membrane bound and circulating TNF preventing it's binding to the TNF receptor
Etanercept	Enbrel	Recombinant human TNF receptor	Binds circulating TNF preventing it's binding to the TNF receptor
Rituximab	Mabthera	Chimeric anti-CD20 monoclonal antibody	Binds CD20 on B cells resulting in B cell depletion through complement mediated cytotoxicity (interacting with the Fc component of the antibody)
Abatacept	Orencia	Recombinant Immunoglobulin/CTLA4 fusion protein	Binds with high affinity to CD80/86 on antigen presenting cells, preventing T cell activation through CD28 interactions with CD80/86
Anakinra	Kineret	Recombinant human IL-1 receptor antagonist	Binds to the IL-1 receptor and therefore prevents activation through IL-1 binding
Tocilizumab	Actemra	Recombinant human anti-IL-6 receptor antibody	Binds to but does not activate the IL-6 receptor. Prevents binding by constitutively secreted IL-6

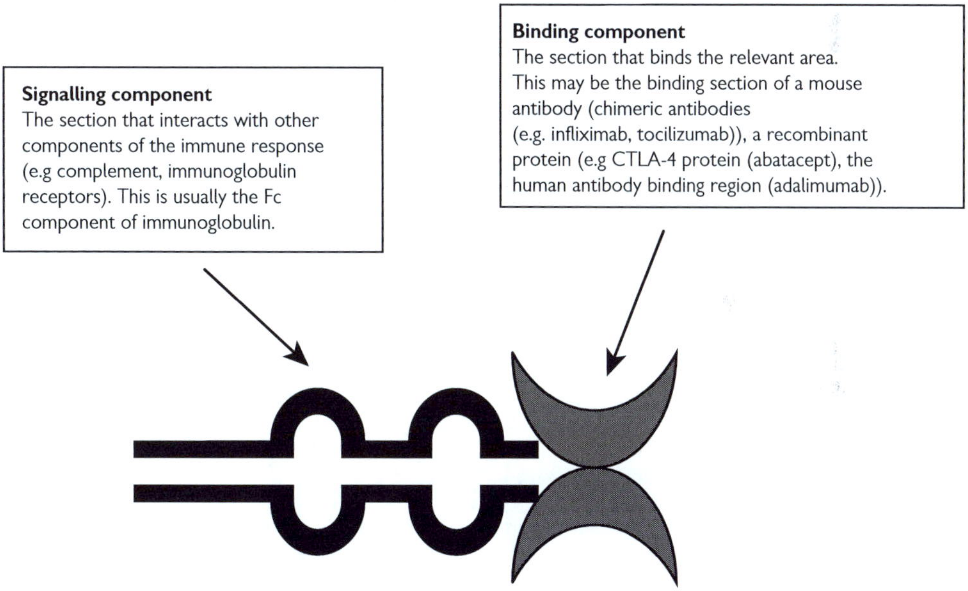

Signalling component
The section that interacts with other components of the immune response (e.g complement, immunoglobulin receptors). This is usually the Fc component of immunoglobulin.

Binding component
The section that binds the relevant area. This may be the binding section of a mouse antibody (chimeric antibodies (e.g. infliximab, tocilizumab)), a recombinant protein (e.g CTLA-4 protein (abatacept), the human antibody binding region (adalimumab)).

Figure 19.8 A figure showing the characteristic structure of the biologics with a binding component and a signalling component.

Evidence base: the clinical trials with biologics

Summary

Anti-TNF

There is good evidence for anti-TNF therapy, in rheumatoid arthritis in both symptom relief and prevention of radiographic progression/structural damage. Radiographic benefit may be seen even in the absence of symptomatic relief. All anti-TNF treatments are more effective if given as combination treatment with methotrexate. There appears to be similar efficacy for all three anti-TNF treatments although the infliximab has more robust evidence of efficacy in early disease, in inducing disease remission.

There also is good evidence for anti-TNF treatment of patients with psoriatic arthritis and ankylosing spondylitis.

Trial results in ANCA associated vasculitis are conflicting with some evidence in favour of infliximab but a large trial with etanercept showing no benefit.

There is limited data suggesting efficacy for infliximab in ocular Behçet's and in GCA, but further studies are needed in these areas.

Rituximab (anti-CD20 (B cell depletion)

There is good evidence for rituximab in rheumatoid arthritis, SLE and ANCA-associated vasculitis. In rheumatoid arthritis, where the evidence base is most robust, it is effective in combination with methotrexate and is effective in patients responding inadequately to anti-TNF.

Anakinra [IL-1 receptor antagonist (Anti-IL-1)]
Although studies have shown clinical efficacy, the symptomatic improvements seen are relatively small. The studies undertaken have shown efficacy in reducing radiographic progression.

Abatacept [CTLA4-Ig Fusion protein (Anti T cell)]
Studies have shown efficacy in patients partially responsive to conventional DMARDs, as well as those partially responsive to anti-TNF, in combination with conventional DMARDs (generally methotrexate)

Tocilizumab (Anti-IL6 receptor antibody)
Studies have shown efficacy for both symptom relief and radiographic progression in patients previously inadequately responsive to conventional DMARDs. Improved efficacy is seen when used in combination with methotrexate.

Anti-TNF (Infliximab, etanercept and adalimumab)
Rheumatoid arthritis
Elliott MJ, Maini RN, Feldmann M, et al. (1994) Randomized double-blind comparison of chimeric monoclonal antibody to tumour necrosis factor α (cA2) versus placebo in rheumatoid arthritis. *Lancet.* **344**(8930): 1105–10. The original DBPCS of anti-TNF treatment demonstrating the efficacy of infliximab as a single injection in rheumatoid arthritis

Lipsky P, van der Heijde, et al. (2000) Infliximab and methotrexate in the treatment of rheumatoid arthritis. Anti-Tumor Necrosis Factor Trial in Rheumatoid Arthritis with Concomitant Therapy Study Group. *N Engl J Med* **343**: 1594–602. The ATTRACT study – a DBPCRS of 428 patients showing the efficacy of infliximab in combination with methotrexate, in both symptom control and radiographic progression.

Smolen JS, Han C, Bala M, et al. (2005) Evidence of radiographic benefit of treatment with infliximab plus methotrexate in rheumatoid arthritis patients who had no clinical improvement: a detailed subanalysis of data from the anti-tumor necrosis factor trial in rheumatoid arthritis with concomitant therapy study. *Arthritis Rheum* **52**: 1020–30. A follow-up from the original ATTRACT study showing that even in patients who failed to respond clinically there was evidence of improved radiological outcome.

Quinn MA, Conaghan PG, O'Connor PJ, et al. (2005) Very early treatment with infliximab in addition to methotrexate in early, poor-prognosis rheumatoid arthritis reduces magnetic resonance imaging evidence of synovitis and damage, with sustained benefit after infliximab withdrawal: results from a twelve-month randomized, double-blind, placebo-controlled trial. *Arthritis Rheum* **52**: 27–35. A DBPCS showing that early treatment with infliximab (in patients with less than 12 months of symptoms) could induce a disease remission which was sustained despite stopping treatment.

Goekoop-Ruiterman YP, de Vries-Bouwstra JK, Allaart CF, et al. (2005) Clinical and radiographic outcomes of four different treatment strategies in patients with early rheumatoid arthritis (the BeSt study): a randomised controlled trial. *Arthritis Rheum* **52**: 3381–90. The BeSt study showing that early combination treatment, with methotrexate and infliximab, resulted in more rapid improvement clinically and joint damage suppression than sequential monotherapy or step-up combination therapy.

Smolen JS, Van Der Heijde DM, St Clair EW, et al. (2006) Predictors of joint damage in patients with early rheumatoid arthritis treated with high-dose methotrexate with or without concomitant infliximab: results from the ASPIRE trial. *Arthritis Rheum* **54**:702–10. The ASPIRE study – a double-blind controlled study showing that infliximab treatment (in combination with methotrexate) reduced radiographic progression of disease irrespective of the inflammatory response.

Weinblatt ME, Kremer JM, Bankhurst AD (1999) A trial of etanercept, a recombinant tumor necrosis factor receptor: Fc fusion protein, in patients with rheumatoid arthritis receiving methotrexate. *N Engl J Med* **340**(4): 253–9. The first DBPCS (89 patients) with etanercept which showed the efficacy of etanercept when used as combination treatment with methotrexate over 6 months of treatment

Keystone EC, Schiff MH, Kremer JM, et al. (2004) Once-weekly administration of 50 mg etanercept in patients with active rheumatoid arthritis: results of a multicenter, randomized, double-blind, placebo-controlled trial. *Arthritis Rheum* **50**: 353–63. A DBPCS in 420 patients showing that 50 mg weekly of etanercept was of equivalent efficacy to 25 mg twice weekly.

Weinblatt ME, Keystone EC, Furst DE (2003) Adalimumab, a fully human anti-tumor necrosis factor α monoclonal antibody, for the treatment of rheumatoid arthritis in patients taking concomitant methotrexate: the ARMADA trial. *Arthritis Rheum* **48**: 35–45. The ARMADA study - the initial DBPCS with adalimumab (271 patients) showing the efficacy of a number of different dosage regimes, every other week, in combination with methotrexate, over 6 months. Subsequent studies showed a reduction in radiographic progression of the disease, as well as symptom control.

Furst DE, Schiff MH, Fleischmann RM, et al. (2003) Adalimumab, a fully human anti tumor necrosis factor-α monoclonal antibody, and concomitant standard antirheumatic therapy for the treatment of rheumatoid arthritis: results of STAR (Safety Trial of Adalimumab in Rheumatoid Arthritis). *J Rheumatol* **30**: 2563–71. The STAR study – a DBPCS in 636 patients showing that 40 mg every other week of adalimumab was an effective and same treatment when added to conventional treatment in patients showing only partial responses to other treatment.

Psoriatic arthritis
Antoni CE, Kavanaugh A, Kirkham B, et al. (2005) Sustained benefits of infliximab therapy for dermatologic and articular manifestations of psoriatic arthritis: results from the infliximab multinational psoriatic arthritis controlled trial (IMPACT). *Arthritis Rheum* **52**: 1227–36. The IMPACT study – a double-blind placebo controlled cross-over treatment study (104 patients) showing that infliximab (5 mg/kg) is efficacious in patients with psoriatic arthritis and psoriasis

Mease PJ, Gotte BS, Metz J, et al. (2000) Etanercept in the treatment of psoriatic arthritis and psoriasis: a randomised trial. *Lancet* **356**(9227): 385–90. A DBPCS in 60 patients with psoriatic arthritis (and psoriasis) showing the efficacy of etanercept monotherapy over a 12-week treatment period.

Gladman DD, Mease PJ, Ritchlin CT, et al.(2007) Adalimumab for long-term treatment of psoriatic arthritis: forty-eight week data from the adalimumab effectiveness in psoriatic arthritis trial. *Arthritis Rheum* **56**: 476–88. The ADEPT study – a double blind placebo controlled trial (292 patients) with showing efficacy for adalimumab over a 6-month study period for both psoriatic arthritis and psoriasis.

Ankylosing spondylitis
Braun J, Brandt J, Listing J, et al. (2002) Treatment of active ankylosing spondylitis with infliximab: a randomised controlled multicentre trial. *Lancet* **359**(9313): 1187–93. A DBPCS in 70 patients with ankylosing spondylitis showing efficacy of infliximab over a 3-month treatment period.

Davis JC Jr, Van Der Heijde D, Braun J, et al. (2003) Recombinant human tumor necrosis factor receptor (etanercept) for treating ankylosing spondylitis: a randomized, controlled trial. *Arthritis Rheum* **48**: 3230–6. A DBPCS in 277 patients with ankylosing spondylitis showing the efficacy of etanercept monotherapy over a 6-month treatment period

ANCA associated vasculitis
Booth A, Harper L, Hammad T, et al. (2004) Prospective study of TNFα blockade with infliximab in anti-neutrophil cytoplasmic antibody-associated systemic vasculitis. *J Am Soc Nephrol* **15**: 717–21. An open label prospective study in 28 patients with ANCA associated vasculitis showing efficacy in disease remission with infliximab. A significant relapse rate was seen and further studies are required.

Wegener's Granulomatosis Etanercept Trial (WGET) Research Group (2005) Etanercept plus standard therapy for Wegener's granulomatosis. *N Engl J Med* **352**(4): 351–61. A randomized placebo-controlled study of 180 patients with Wegener's granulomatosis which failed to show any significant benefit for etanercept in the maintenance of remission.

Behçet's disease
Ohno S, Nakamura S, Hori S, et al. (2004) Efficacy, safety, and pharmacokinetics of multiple administration of infliximab in Behçet's disease with refractory uveoretinitis. *J Rheumatol* **31**: 1362–8. A small open label study showing efficacy for infliximab in Behcet's complicated by uveitis

RITUXIMAB (anti-CD20)
Rheumatoid arthritis
Edwards JC, Szczepanski L, Szechinski J, et al. (2004) Randomised efficacy of B-cell-targeted therapy with rituximab in patients with rheumatoid arthritis. *N Engl J Med* **350**:2572–81. The original randomized controlled study of rituximab treatment, of rheumatoid arthritis, (161 patients) demonstrating the efficacy of 2 infusions of rituximab either as monotherapy or in combination with cyclophosphamide or methotrexate.

Emery P, Fleischmann R, Filipowicz-Sosnowska, et al. (2006) The efficacy and safety of rituximab in patients with active rheumatoid arthritis despite methotrexate treatment: results of a phase IIB randomized, double-blind, placebo-controlled, dose-ranging trial. *Arthritis Rheum* **54**: 1390–400. The DANCER study – a DBPCS (465 patients over 6 months) showing that Rituximab 500mg on days 1 and 15 was as efficacious as 1000 mg on days 1 and 15. Treatment was given as combination treatment with methotrexate.

Cohen SB, Emery P, Greenwald MW, et al. (2006) Rituximab for rheumatoid arthritis refractory to anti-tumor necrosis factor therapy: Results of a multicenter, randomized, double-blind, placebo-controlled, phase III trial evaluating primary efficacy and safety at twenty-four weeks. *Arthritis Rheum* **54**: 2793–806. The REFLEX study – a DBPCS (519 patients) showing that rituximab was effective treatment (in combination with methotrexate over 6 months) in anti-TNF non responders.

SLE
Leandro MJ, Cambridge G, Edwards JC, et al. (2005) B-cell depletion in the treatment of patients with systemic lupus erythematosus: a longitudinal analysis of 24 patients. *Rheumatol (Oxf)* **44**: 1542–5. One of several open-label studies showing efficacy of rituximab in SLE. In this study 2 doses of rituximab (1 g) were given 2 weeks apart. Each rituximab dose was given with intravenous cyclophosphamide (750 mg) and methylprednisolone (250 mg). Responses were maintained over at least 6 months.

ANCA-associated vasculitis
Stasi R, Stipa E, Del Poeta G, et al. (2006) Long-term observation of patients with anti-neutrophil cytoplasmic antibody-associated vasculitis treated with rituximab. *Rheumatol (Oxf)* **45**: 1432–6. An open label prospective study, in 10 patients with relapsed ANCA associated vasculitis, showing efficacy for rituximab (375 mg/m^2 weekly for 4 weeks) in inducing remission.

Anakinra (IL-1 receptor antagonist)
Rheumatoid arthritis
Cohen SB, Moreland LW, Cush JJ, et al. (2004) A multicentre, double blind, randomised, placebo controlled trial of anakinra (Kineret), a recombinant interleukin 1 receptor antagonist, in patients with rheumatoid arthritis treated with background methotrexate. *Ann Rheum Dis* **63**: 1062–8. A DBPCT (506 patients) of 100 mg daily of anakinra as combination treatment with methotrexate. Although statistically significant clinical responses were seen at 24 weeks, compared with placebo, the magnitude of the difference was relatively small. Other studies have shown improved radiographic outcome.

Abatacept (CTLA4-Ig Fusion protein)
Rheumatoid arthritis
Kremer JM, Westhovens R, Leon M, et al. (2003) Treatment of rheumatoid arthritis by selective inhibition of T-cell activation with fusion protein CTLA4Ig. *N Engl J Med* **349**: 1907–15. The AIM study – a double blind placebo controlled, dose finding trial (339 patients), showing clinical efficacy of 10 mg/kg of abatacept (days 1, 15, 30, and thereafter monthly) in combination with methotrexate (in patients inadequately responsive to methotrexate).

Kremer JM, Dougados M, Emery P, et al. (2005) Treatment of rheumatoid arthritis with the selective costimulation modulator abatacept: twelve-month results of a phase iib, double-blind, randomized, placebo-controlled trial. *Arthritis Rheum* **52**: 2263–71. The ATTAIN trial – a DBPCS (258 patients), showing clinical efficacy of 10 mg/kg of abatacept (days 1, 15, 29, and thereafter monthly) over 6 months in combination with conventional DMARDs (75% of these were methotrexate) in patients previously inadequately responsive to anti-TNF treatment.

Tocilizumab (anti-IL-6 receptor antibody)
Rheumatoid arthritis
Maini RN, Taylor PC, Szechinski J, et al. (2006) Double-blind randomized controlled clinical trial of the interleukin-6 receptor antagonist, tocilizumab, in European patients with rheumatoid arthritis who had an incomplete response to methotrexate. *Arthritis Rheum* **54**: 2817–29. The CHARISMA Study – a randomized dose finding placebo controlled trial (359 patients) showing that 4–8 mg every 4 weeks of tocilizumab is symptomatically efficacious in patients who have inadequately responded to methotrexate. Improved responses were seen in combination with methotrexate than when tocilizumab was used as monotherapy.

Nishimoto N, Hashimoto J, Miyasaka N, et al. (2007) Study of active controlled monotherapy used for rheumatoid arthritis, an IL-6 inhibitor (SAMURAI): evidence of clinical and radiographic benefit from an × ray reader-blinded randomised controlled trial of tocilizumab. Ann Rheum Dis **66**: 1162–7. The SAMURAI study – a randomized controlled study (306 patients) showing improved radiographic outcome with tocilizumab monotherapy (8 mg/kg monthly) over 12 months compared with conventional DMARD treatment.

Prescribing considerations

What do I need to do before starting biologic treatment?
- Patient education re: dosing, side effects, monitoring, drug interactions, etc.
- Patients should be warned of the risks of infusion reactions with IV preparations, the potential risks of malignancy and the infection risks (see below).
- Ensure there is no history of SLE or multiple sclerosis before prescribing anti-TNF. Anti-TNF treatment should also be avoided in moderate – severe heart failure.
- Check weight (to calculate doses).

Subcutaneous injections
- Discuss with the patients the requirements for self injection and arrange appropriate delivery/support/cvollection at home.
- Ensure patient is happy and competent to self inject.
- Train/educate patient on: injection technique, sharps disposal, appropriate storage/disposal of treatment.
- Provide telephone helpline support for the patients.
- Warn patient,s at baseline that if they fail to respond adequately to the treatment it will need to be discontinued.

Record baseline disease activity

DAS28, BASDAI, SLEDAI, BILAG, BVAS (or other appropriate disease monitoring tools).

FBC	Consider monitoring neutrophils with Anakinra
Renal function	Monitoring disease activity (SLE, AAV)
ESR or CRP	Monitoring disease activity
Radiographs	Assessing disease progress
ANCA	If treating vasculitis
ANA/ENA	In patients for anti-TNF (due to the risk of developing ANA/SLE).

Infection risks
The major concern, with biologic treatments, is infection risk and serious life-threatening infections are a risk with all biologics. In comparison with the anti-TNF treatments, the risks seem to be less with rituximab, abatacept and tocilizumab but the data is more limited than that with anti-TNF. Do not start biologic treatments in patients with active infection or significant recurrent infections.

Patients receiving biologic treatments should be advised against eating un-pasteurized milk, mould ripened soft cheeses (e.g. camembert and brie), blue cheeses, pate and raw egg due to the risks of *Listeria* and *Salmonella* infection.

For anti-TNF treatment there is a particular risk of reactivation of latent TB. Furthermore, when TB occurs, there is an increased risk of extrapulmonary disease and disseminated infection.

Appropriate screening (see Figure 19.9) should be undertaken to exclude infection with TB before commencing treatment with anti-TNF.

If there is evidence of (or suspicion of) latent TB prophylactic treatment with isoniazid should be instituted (after consultation with a respiratory or infectious diseases physician)

Patients should be advised, when on treatment, to report any symptoms suggestive of TB (cough, weight loss or fever).

Monitoring and DMARDs
Ensure appropriate DMARD monitoring is in place.

Note: In addition to improved efficacy when methotrexate is used in combination with all biologics, the chimeric biologics (infliximab, rituximab and tocilizumab) are capable of inducing an antibody response [human anti-chimera antibodies (HACA)]. This response appears to be reduced by maintenance treatment with conventional DMARDs.

What dose should I prescribe?
Anti-TNF

1. *Rheumatoid arthritis*
- **Infliximab:** 3 mg/kg, 0, 2 and 6 weeks then 8 weekly by intravenous infusion.
- **Adalimumab:** 40 mg alternate weeks subcutaneously.
- **Etanercept:** 25 mg twice weekly subcutaneously or 50 mg weekly subcutaneously.

2. *Ankylosing spondylitis*
- **Infliximab:** 5 mg/kg 0,2 and 6 weeks then 8 weekly by intravenous infusion.
- **Adalimumab:** 40 mg alternate weeks subcutaneously.
- **Etanercept:** 25 mg twice weekly subcutaneously.

3. *Psoriatic arthritis*
- **Infliximab:** 5 mg/kg 0,2 and 6 weeks then 8 weekly by intravenous infusion.
- **Adalimumab:** 40 mg alternate weeks subcutaneously.
- **Etanercept:** 25 mg twice weekly subcutaneously.

Rituximab

1. *Rheumatoid arthritis*
- **Dose:** 1 g by intravenous infusion on days 0 and 14. Dose can then be repeated after >6 months if symptoms recur and B cell have reconstituted (ideally recheck B cell levels by measuring CD19 levels in PBMC).
- Rituximab should be given with 100 mg methylprednisolone IV and antihistamine/paracetamol PO to prevent infusion reaction.
- Rituximab should be given with regular methotrexate in rheumatoid arthritis

2. *SLE*

Dose: different studies have used different doses and there is no agreed regime. An evidence-based regime is:

Days 0 + 14   Rituximab 1 g IVI

                Cyclophosphamide 750 mg IVI

                With high dose oral prednisolone

Rituximab should be given with 100–250 mg methylprednisolone IV (higher doses of steroid have been used in

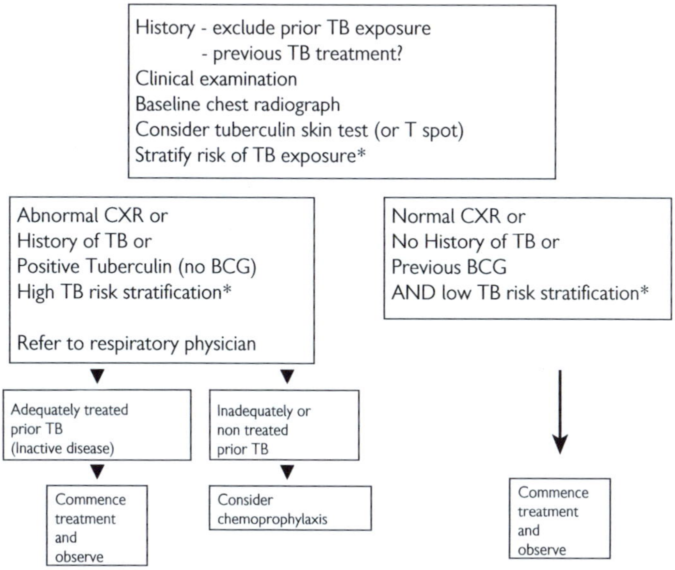

CHAPTER 19 **DMARDs and immunosuppressive drugs**

Figure 19.9 Screening Patients for TB (* see British Thoracic Guidelines 2004).

SLE studies) and antihistamine PO to prevent infusion reaction.

Anakinra

1. Rheumatoid arthritis

100 mg daily by subcutaneous injection.

Abatacept

1. Rheumatoid arthritis
- 10 mg/kg by intravenous infusion, 0, 2 and 4 weeks, thereafter every 4 weeks.
- Abatacept should be given as combination therapy with a DMARD (methotrexate is advised)

Tocilizumab

1. Rheumatoid arthritis
- 4–8 mg/kg every 4 weeks (8 mg/kg is the standard dose).
- Given by IV infusion.
- Tocilizumab should be given as combination therapy with a DMARD (methotrexate is advised).

Important drug interactions

There are currently no recognized drug interactions with the biologics. However the treatments are relatively new and any suspected drug interaction should be reported.

Monitoring

- Patients on biologics should be monitored initially at least every 3 months, for response to treatment. In the UK appropriate monitoring data should be submitted to the BSR Biologics Register http://www.medicine.manchester.ac.uk/arc/BSRBR/
- In patients on anti-TNF treatment a CXR should be undertaken after 3 months of treatment and thereafter annually. An ANA should be monitored annually.
- Patients should be assessed before all infusions to ensure there is no evidence of infection or developing side effects.

Side effects and what to discuss with your patients

Infection risk (see above)

- Advise patients of the increased infection risk (see above) and to seek medical advice early, in the event of unexplained illness.
- Advise patients to avoid eating un-pasteurized milk, mould ripened soft cheeses (e.g. camembert and brie), blue cheeses, pate and raw egg due to the risks of *Listeria* and *Salmonella* infection.

Infusion reactions

These characteristically occur during or shortly after the initial infusions of the intravenous biologics. They are characterized by high temperatures, nausea, shaking, headaches, skin rashes/itching. Occasionally, there may be hypotension, shortness of breath, and wheeze. Usually these can be controlled by stopping the infusion for a period of time then slowing the infusion rates and management with antihistamines, paracetamol and corticosteroids (see below).

Injection site reactions

A local skin reaction can occur at sites of subcutaneous injections (with adalimumab, etanercept and anakinra). These occur in 20–30% of patients. There is local redness, swelling, pain, and itching which can persist for up to 1 week after administration. The severity of these local reactions often reduces over time with treatment. The reactions can be reduced by frequently changing the area used for injections and by cooling the area (e.g. with a cold wet towel) post-injection.

Autoimmune reactions

The development of anti-nuclear antibodies and lupus-like syndromes have been reported in patients on anti-TNF treatment. The incidence of demyelinating disease is also possibly increased in patients on anti-TNF treatment. These reactions are thought to be due to altered cytokine balance and the development of symptoms suggestive of either SLE or demyelination should trigger discontinuation of the treatment. An ANA should be documented at baseline and during treatment in patients having anti-TNF treatment.

Congestive cardiac failure
Patients with moderate or severe congestive cardiac failure (NYHA Grade 3 or 4) should not be treated with anti-TNF due to the increased risk of CCF noted in trials with both infliximab and etanercept. If a patient develops CCF or experience worsening of mild symptoms, whilst being treated with anti-TNF the treatment should be discontinued. Patients should therefore be advised to report any worsening dyspnoea or oedema and should be monitored regularly.

FAQs

How long does it take to work?
This is dependent on the mechanism of action of the biologic in question. Anti-TNF treatments characteristically act quickly (the infusion treatments can work within a few days) and a response should certainly be evident within 12 weeks of treatment. By contrast the response to abatacept and rituximab can take longer. 3–6 months may be required before the benefits become apparent with these latter agents.

What if I miss a dose of a subcutaneous injection?
Inject the missed dose as soon as possible and then give the next dose as usual

What if I want to get pregnant?
Little is known about the toxicity/teratogenicity of the biologic treatments during pregnancy. There are reports of successful healthy deliveries but in general the treatments should be avoided during pregnancy. Women of child bearing age should therefore be advised on contraception. Furthermore, most biologics should be discontinued 3–6 months prior to conception, although rituximab should be discontinued 12 months before. It is important to also be aware of the risks of the concomitant DMARDs and advise accordingly.

What about breast feeding?
As for the pregnancy associated risks, the data is limited, but the advice should be to avoid biologic treatments whilst breast feeding.

What about immunization??
- Live attenuated vaccines need to be avoided by patients taking on biologic treatments (i.e. yellow fever, MMR and rubella, BCG, oral polio, oral typhoid).
- Other vaccines will not be a problem.
- Patients should be advised to have an annual influenza immunization, since they are at an increased risk of influenza. A pneumovax inoculation is also advisable, especially in the elderly.

Can I drink alcohol?
There is no known interaction of the biologics with alcohol, but patients should be advised accordingly for the DMARD treatments (particularly if taking methotrexate).

What to do if side effects occur

Infusion reactions
Mild infusion reaction (mild fever, shaking, itching)
Slow rate of infusion and give oral paracetamol 1 g and anti-histamine (e.g. chlorpheniramine (piriton) 4 mg)

Patient on anti-TNF treatment admitted with pyrexia

↓

1) Stop anti-TNF
2) Assess clinically for common infections
3) Arrange CXR
4) Send appropriate cultures (blood, urine, sputum etc)
5) Treat as indicated
6) Recommence anti-TNF 2-4 weeks post resolution of infection

↓

No obvious source identified but continued pyrexia

↓

INVESTIGATE FOR POSSIBLE TUBERCULOSIS

1) Arrange T-spot test if possible
2) Arrange tuberculin skin testing if T spot unavailable

1) Liaise with local microbiologists and respiratory physicians
2) Send EMUs x3 for TB culture (separate days)
3) Send sputum x3 for AFBs (separate days)
4) Lymph node aspirate if lymphadenopathy
5) Consider CT chest +/- bronchoalveolarlavage
6) Consider MRI brain +/- lumbar puncture

Figure 19.10

Moderate infusion reaction (fever, shaking, itching, chest pain, hypotension)
- Stop infusion.
- Consider hydrocortisone 100 mg IV and possibly IM adrenaline 1 ml 1:1000.
- Give paracetamol 1 g and anti-histamine (e.g. piriton 4 mg).
- Consider restarting infusion at a slower rate after 30–60 min.

Severe infusion reaction (anaphylactic hypotensive reaction – this is rare)
- Stop infusion and give IV fluids.
- Administer IM adrenaline 1 ml 1:1000.
- Consider IV adrenaline 1 ml 1:10 000.
- IV hydrocortisone 200 mg.
- IV chlorpheniramine 10 mg.
- Additional resuscitation as required.

Previous infusion reaction with treatment
Give prophylactic treatment with paracetamol 1 g and anti-histamine (e.g. piriton 4 mg) 30 min before treatment.
Patient admitted with a pyrexia.
Stop biologic drug and screen for common infections.

Surgical considerations

All biologics should be discontinued 2–4 weeks before and after surgery (due to the increased risk of infection). For infliximab surgery should ideally be scheduled for between infusions. The time to onset of action for rituximab is up to 6 months and routine surgery should ideally be scheduled 6 months after an infusion.

INDEX

A

abatacept 568–75
abdomen
  acute surgical 88
  examination 85–6
Abrams pleural biopsy 58
acalculous cholecystitis 83
accessory navicular bone 194
acetabular labral tears 169
acetabular rim syndrome 170
Achilles tendon and bursa injections 114
Achilles tendonopathy 192
acid maltase deficiency 523
acne fulminans 101
acrodermatitis chronica atrophicans 466, 467
acrodermatitis continua of Hallopeau 101
acromegaly 492
acromioclavicular joint 137
  injections 109
  osteoarthritis 142–3
actinomycetes 476
action potentials 44
active movement 9
acute cutaneous lupus erythematosus (ACLE) 98
acute renal failure 79–80
acute surgical abdomen 88
adalimumab 84, 568–75
adductor longus injury 171
adductor pollicis longus 147
adductor tendinitis injections 113
adenosine monophosphate (myoadenylate) deaminase (AMPD) deficiency 523
adjunct analgesics 481
adolescents, history taking 6–7
adult onset Still's disease (AOSD) 66, 496–7
airways 54, 55, 56, 58, 59, 62
alcohol 20
alkaptonuria 516–17
allergic conjunctivitis 50
allopurinol 84, 386, 387
alpha-1 antitrypsin deficiency 515
alphaviral infections 468
ALT/AST 86
amyloid 83, 88
amyloidosis 83, 498–9
anaerobic streptococcal myonecrosis 461
anakinra 568–75
analgesics 480–1
ANCA-associated vasculitis (AAV)
  general management 330–1
  kidney disease 74
  nervous system 94, 95
anconeus 147
ankle
  anatomy 184–5
  impingement syndrome 190–1
  injections 114–15
  regional musculoskeletal conditions 190–3
ankylosing spondylitis (AS) 214–19
  anti-TNFα therapy 217
  chest disease 54
  discriminating from DISH 216
  eye problems 48
  heart disease 66
  HLA B27 214
  measurement scale (BASFI) 4
  modified New York Criteria for diagnosis 214
  nervous system 92, 93
anserine bursa injections 113

anserine bursitis 179
antalgic gait 9
anterior cruciate ligament 174–5, 181
anterior lateral tract 121
anterior uveitis 49, 51
anti-C1q antibodies 39–40
anticardiolipin antibodies 39
anti-CD20 568–75
anticonvulsants
  inducing osteomalacia 424
  pain control 481
anti-cyclic citrullinated peptide (CCP) antibodies 40–1
anti-IL-1 568–75
anti-IL-6R 568–75
anti-malarials 544–5
anti-neutrophil cytoplasmic antibodies (ANCA) 41
antinuclear antibodies (ANA) 21, 38–9
antiphospholipid antibodies 39
antiphospholipid syndrome (APLS) 274–80
  definite 274
  eye problems 48
  heart disease 66, 67, 71, 276
  nervous system 93, 95
  pregnancy 274, 276, 279, 367
  skin disease 98
anti-synthetase syndrome 284
anti-TNF 71, 568–75
aortic insufficiency/regurgitation 69
aortitis 66, 67, 68, 70, 72
apatite-like clumps 42
appendicitis 83
arterial blood gases 59
ascending tracts 121
aseptic necrosis 381
aspiration
  joints 16, 106–7
  oesophageal dysmotility 82, 87
atlanto-axial instability 125
atrophoderma of Pasini and Pierini 99
auranofin 546–8
aurothiomalate 546–8
autoimmune connective tissue diseases 52, 239–311
autoimmune pancreatitis 84–5
autoimmune serology 38–41
autoinflammatory syndromes 500–5
autosomal dominant hypophosphataemic rickets (ADHR) 424
avascular necrosis 168–9, 381
axillary nerve injury 144
azathioprine 84, 552–4

B

back pain 130
bacterial meningitis 95
bacterial myositis 460
bacterial overgrowth 84, 88
Baker's (popliteal) cyst 181–2, 188
Bankart lesion 142
Barmah Forest virus 468
Barrett's metaplasia 82, 87
basic calcium phosphate crystals 392–3
basilar invagination 125
Bath Ankylosing Spondylitis Functional Index (BASFI) 4
behavioural therapy 482
Behçet's disease 15, 340–1
  chest disease 54

eye problems 48, 55, 340
gastrointestinal disease 82, 340
heart disease 66
nervous system 93, 95
pregnancy 368
skin disease 101
Beighton score 442
benign angiopathy of the CNS 93
benign joint hypermobility (BJH) 442–3
biceps 138, 146
bicipital tendinitis 143, 149
biofeedback 482
biologics 568–75
bisphosphonates 403–4
blastomycosis 476
blepharitis 49, 52
blind loop dermatosis-arthritis syndrome 101
blood gases 61
body habitus 9
bone
  diseases 395–436
  mineral density 396, 399
  pain 2, 19
  proliferation 25
  scanning 36–7
  sclerosis 434–5
  tumours 528–9
Borrelia burgdoferi 19, 466
Bouchard's nodes 374
brachialis 146
brachioradialis 146, 147
bronchiectasis 55, 56, 62
bronchiolitis 55, 56, 62
bronchoalveolar lavage (BAL) 60
bronchomalacia 55
brucellosis 15, 464–5
Buergher's disease 348–9
bullhorn sign 237
bullous lupus erythematosus 98
bupivacaine injections 107
bursa
  foot 187
  knee 175
  shoulder 139
  ultrasound 27
bursitis 458–9
  anserine 179
  crystal 149
  hip 168
  iliopsoas 168
  infrapatellar 179
  intermetatarsal 194
  ischiogluteal 168
  lateral pre-malleolar 191
  non-septic 458
  olecranon 149
  prepatellar 178–9
  retrocalcaneal 192
  septic 149, 458–9
  subcutaneous calcaneal 192
  traumatic 149
  trochanteric 112, 168
Buschke scleredema 99

C

calcific tendinitis, rotator cuff 141
calcium intake 397–8, 422, 423
calcium oxalate crystals 42
calcium pyrophosphate dihydrate (CPPD) crystals 42

calcium pyrophosphate dihydrate (CPPD) disease 14, 15, 388–90
Camurati–Engelman disease 434
cANCA 41
candidiasis 82, 87
capsaicin 481
cardiac amyloid 71
cardiac nodules 71
cardiovascular disease 20, 66–72
carnitine deficiency syndrome 523
carnitine palmitoyltransferase (CPT) II deficiency 523
carpal tunnel 152
carpal tunnel syndrome 160–1
 injections 112
 neurophysiology 45
carpometacarpal joint osteoarthritis 158
cataract 49
caudal epidural 115
cellulitis 458
cerebrospinal fluid 92
cervical spine 119, 122, 124–7
chest disease 31, 54–64
chest wall 54, 55–6, 57–8, 61, 128–9
Chikungunya virus 468
chilblain lupus erythematosus 98
Child Health Assessment Questionnaire (CHAQ) 4
children
 dermatomyositis (JDM) 298–300
 examination 10–11
 GALS examination 11
 growing pains 7
 history taking 3–4, 6–7
 osteoporosis 412–13
 pain 2, 6–7
 rickets 422–5
 torticollis 126–7
 see also juvenile idiopathic arthritis
chloroquine 544–5
cholecystitis 89
cholesterol crystals 42
chondrocalcinosis 388
chondroma 529
chondrosarcoma 529
Chopart joint 187
chorea 462
choroidal neovascular membrane 51
Christmas disease 510–11
chronic kidney disease (CKD) 80–1, 426
chronic pain 479–90
Churg–Strauss syndrome (CSS) 326–7
 gastrointestinal disease 82
 heart disease 66
 nervous system 93
 pregnancy 368
 treatment 330–1
chylous arthritis 476
ciclosporin 84, 558–60
CINCA/NOMID 504
clavicle 136
 osteomyelitis 455
clergyman's knee 179, 458
clinical assessment 1–23
clinical neurophysiology 44–5
'closed chain' 9
Clostridial myonecrosis 460–1
club foot 185
coccydynia 133
codeine 481
coeliac disease 83
Cogan's syndrome 338–9
cognitive behavioural therapy 482
colchicine 84
colitis 83, 88, 230
collagen disorders 437–43
collateral ligaments 174, 180–1
compartment syndromes 184, 188
complementary therapies 376–7, 482
complex regional pain syndrome type I (CRPS-I) 488–90
compound muscle action potential (CMAP) 44

computed tomography (CT) 30–2
conduction system disease 66–7, 68, 69, 70
conduction velocity (CV) 44
congenital contractural arachnodactyly 438
congenital heart block 67, 71
conjunctivitis 49
constipation 83, 88
co-prevalent conditions 3
coronary artery disease (CAD) 66, 67, 68, 70, 71
coronary ligament injections 113
costochondritis 55, 61
COX-II inhibitors 481
coxa valga 164
coxa vara 164
cranial setting 125
cricoarytenoiditis 55, 62
Crithidia luciliae assay 39
Crohn's disease 83, 230
cruciate ligaments 174–5, 181
cryoglobulinaemia 75, 82, 334–5
cryopyrin-associated periodic syndrome (CAPS) 504–5
cryptococcosis 476
crystal arthritis 15, 383–93
crystal bursitis 149
crystals, features 42
CT pulmonary angiogram (CTPA) 60
CTLA4-Ig 568–75
cubital tunnel syndrome 151, 161
cuneate tracts 121
cutaneous calcinosis 99
cutaneous lupus erythematosus 98, 244, 249
cutaneous vasculitis 100
cyclo-oxygenase-II (COX-II) inhibitors 481
cyclophosphamide 84, 562–6
cyclosporin A 558–60
cysticercosis 461
cytomegalovirus (CMV) 241

D

dactylitis 195
daytime somnolence 96
De Quervain's tenosynovitis 26, 159
 injections 111
debranching enzyme deficiency 523
deep morphea 99
delayed gastric emptying 83, 87
deltoid 137, 138
denervation 44–5
denosumab 405
depomedrone injections 107
dermatomes 120
dermatomyositis (DM) 290–6
 chest disease 54
 eye problems 48
 gastrointestinal disease 82
 heart disease 66
 juvenile 298–300
 nervous system 93, 95
 skin disease 98–9
descending tracts 121
diabetes mellitus 100, 494
diabetic cheiroarthropathy 162, 494
diabetic femoral amyotrophy 494
diabetic foot ulcers 455
diabetic osteoarthropathy 494
diabetic osteomyelitis 455
diaphyseal aclasia 435
diarrhoea 83, 88
diet
 gout 387
 post-menopausal osteoporosis 397–8
diffuse alveolar damage (DAD) 56
diffuse cutaneous systemic sclerosis 264, 271
diffuse idiopathic skeletal hyperostosis (DISH) 216, 380
diffuse infiltrative lymphocytosis syndrome (DILS) 470
diplopia 51
disability measurement 4

disc herniation 124–5, 131–2
discitis 126, 133, 454–5
discoid lupus erythematosus 98
disease modifying anti-rheumatic drugs (DMARDs) 531–75
distal interphalangeal joint (DIPJ) 152
distal motor latency (DML) 44
distal radio-ulna joint
 injections 111
 osteoarthritis 158
DNA antibodies 39
double vision 51
Dranunculus medinensis 477
driving 96
drug history 20
drug-induced problems
 gastrointestinal tract 84
 lupus 20, 241, 248–9
 myopathies 20, 292–3
 osteomalacia 424
 pneumonitis 56, 62
 side-effects of rheumatological drugs 49, 94
Dupuytren's disease 162
DXA scanning 400

E

echinococcus 477
echocardiography 60, 61, 69
Ehlers–Danlos syndrome (EDS) 82, 440–1
elbow
 anatomy 146–7
 differential diagnosis of pain 148
 injections 110
 nerve entrapment 150–1
 osteoarthritis 149–50
 regional musculoskeletal conditions 148–51
elderly, history taking 6
electrocardiogram (ECG) 61, 69
electroencephalogram (EEG) 92
electromyography (EMG) 22, 44–5, 92
ELISA 39
empyema 62
encephalitis 95
endocardial disease 66
endocrine disorders 285
endosteal hyperostosis (EH) 434
enteric arthritis 83, 226
enteric spondyloarthropathy 230
enteropathic spondyloarthropathy 230–1
enthesitis 14
 chest wall 61
 knee 178
 pelvis 171
enthesitis-related arthritis (ERA) 232–4, 352
eosinophilia-myalgia syndrome 520–1
eosinophilic fasciitis 310–11, 520
episcleritis 49, 52
Epstein-Barr virus (EBV) 241
equipment, examination 8
erosions 25
erosive osteoarthritis 375, 376
erythema migrans 466, 467
erythema nodosum 514
erythroderma 102
etanercept 84, 568–75
examination 8–12
exercise tests 61
exocrine pancreatic insufficiency 83, 88
extensor carpi radialis brevis 147
extensor carpi radialis longus 147
extensor carpi ulnaris 147
 tenosynovitis 159
extensor digiti minimi 147, 154
extensor digitorum communis 147, 154
extensor indicis proprius 147, 154
extensor pollicis brevis 147, 154
extensor pollicis longus 147, 154
extractable nuclear antigens (ENA) 39, 40
eye problems 15, 48–53

F

F wave 44
facial pain 90, 95
faecal incontinence 83
falls 399
familial cold inflammatory condition (FCAS) 504
familial Mediterranean fever (FMF) 15, 101, 500–1, 504
family history 15
fat pad impingement syndrome 178
fatty acid transport defects 523
feet, see foot
femoral head 164, 165
  avascular necrosis 168–9
femoroacetabular impingement (FAI) 169–70
FEV_1 58, 59
FEV_1/FVC 58, 59
fibre optic bronchoscopy 59
  with bronchoalveolar lavage (BAL) 60
fibrogenesis imperfecta ossium (FIO) 432
fibromyalgia 21
fibromyalgia syndrome (FMS) 484–6
fibroplastic rheumatism 100
fibrous dysplasia (FD) 432
fibular tunnel syndrome 189
first metatarsal phalangeal joint injections 114
fitness to fly 61
flat foot 185
flexor carpi radialis 147, 154
flexor carpi ulnaris 147, 154
flexor digiti minimi brevis 154
flexor digitorum profundus 154
flexor digitorum superficialis 147, 154
flexor pollicis brevis 154
flexor pollicis longus 154
flexural psoriasis 101
flow-volume loop 59
fluorescein angiography 51
follicular bronchiolitis 55, 56, 62
foot
  anatomy 185–7
  arches 185
  club foot 185
  flat foot 185
  foreign body granulomas 194
  injections 114–15
  regional musculoskeletal conditions 188–95
  ulcers 455
foot slap gait 9
forced expiratory volume in 1s (FEV_1) 58, 59
forced vital capacity (FVC) 58, 59
forearm fractures 397
foreign body granulomas 194
Forestier's disease 380
fractures
  CT 30–1
  osteomyelitis 454
  post-menopausal osteoporosis 397, 399, 402
  stress fractures 188, 194
Freiberg's infarction 194
frozen shoulder 141–2
functional assessment 9
fundoscopy 50
fungal infection 476–7
funny turns 90
FVC 58, 59

G

gait 9, 166
gallbladder 82, 83, 84, 85, 86, 88
GALS examination 9–10
  paediatric 11
ganglia 27, 162
gas gangrene 460–1
gas transfer factor 59
gastric antral vascular ectasia (GAVE) 83, 87
gastric emptying, delayed 83, 87
gastric masses 87
gastric ulcers 83, 87
gastritis 83, 87

gastroeosophageal reflux disease (GORD) 85
gastrointestinal problems 20, 82–9
Gaucher's disease 518–19
generalized morphea 99
generalized pustular psoriasis 102
giant cell arteritis (GCA) 48, 52, 66, 82, 93, 95, 318–19
giant diverticulae 83, 88
glaucoma 48
glenohumeral joint 136
  capsule 136
  injections 108–9
  osteoarthritis 143
glomerulonephritis 74–6
glucocorticoid crystals 42
glucocorticoid-induced osteoporosis (GIO) 408–10
glycogen storage disorders (glycogenoses) 522–3
gnathosostomiasis 477
gold 84, 546–8
golfer's elbow, see medial epicondylitis
gonococcal arthritis 14, 452–3
gout 14, 15, 384–7
  allopurinol 386, 387
  heart disease 66
  radiographs 16
  tophi 16, 384, 385
Gower's sign 10
gracile tracts 121
gram negative septic arthritis 448
gram positive septic arthritis 448
granulomas, foreign bodies 194
granulomatous dermatitis 98
groin
  anatomy 164–6
  regional musculoskeletal conditions 168–72
group A streptococcal necrotising myositis 461
growing pains 7
guinea worm 477
gut disease 82–9
guttate psoriasis 101
Guyon's canal 161

H

H reflex 44
HAART 469, 470
haemochromatosis 66, 83, 89, 506–7
haemoglobinopathies 508–9
haemolytic uraemic syndrome 278
haemophilia 510–11
hallux rigidus 194–5
hand
  anatomy 152–6
  injections 110–12
  main causes of pain 158
  osteoarthritis 158, 372, 374
  regional musculoskeletal conditions 158–62
  soft tissue injury 162
headaches 90, 95
Health Assessment Questionnaire (HAQ) 4
heart disease 66–72
heart valve disease 66, 67, 68, 70, 71
Heberden's nodes 374
HELLP 278
Henoch–Schönlein purpura (HSP) 74, 82, 342–3
HEp-2 cells 38
hepatic fibrosis 82
hepatitis 83, 88
hepatitis A 83
hepatitis B 19, 83, 469
hepatitis C 83, 241, 469
hepatobiliary disease 82–9
hepatosplenomegaly 83
hepcidin 506
hereditary multiple hyperostosis (HME) 435
hereditary periodic fever syndromes 101
hereditary vitamin D resistant rickets 424
heterotopic ossification 435
hidebound chest 55, 61
high resolution CT (HRCT) 31, 58, 59, 60

high-stepping gait 9
hip
  anatomy 164–6
  bursitis 168
  differential diagnosis of pain 168
  fractures 397
  injections 112–13
  osteoarthritis 372
  regional musculoskeletal conditions 168–72
  symmetry of movement 8–9
histiocytic cytophagic panniculitis 515
histoplasmosis 476
history taking 2–7
HIV 15, 469–70
HLA B27 214
Hoffa's disease 178
Hoffman (H) reflex 44
homocystinuria 438
hormone replacement therapy (HRT) 403
hot swollen joints 446–7
housemaid's knee 458
Hughes' syndrome 274
human immunodeficiency virus (HIV) 15, 469–70
human parvovirus B19 468
human T-lymphotrophic virus type 1 469
hydatid disease 477
hydrocortisone injections 107
hydroxyapatite crystals 42, 392
hydroxychloroquine 84, 544–5
  eye screening 52–3
hyperimmunoglobulinaemia D with periodic fever syndrome (HIDS) 101, 502, 504
hypermobile joints 442–3
hyperostosis
  endosteal (EH) 434
  hereditary multiple (HME) 435
hyperostosis corticalis generalisata 434
hyperparathyroidism 414–16
hypertrophic osteoarthropathy (HOA) 432
hyperuricaemia 384
hypophosphataemic vitamin D resistant rickets 424

I

ilioinguinal nerve entrapment 170
iliopsoas
  bursitis 168
  tendonitis 171
iliotibial band syndrome (ITBS) 179
ill patients, history taking 6
imipramine 481
immunization 241
immunosuppressive drugs 531–75
inclusion body myositis 93, 95, 285, 302–4
infection 445–77
  chest 63
  nervous system 91
  oligoarticular arthritis 15
  widespread pain 19
infectious tenosynovitis 459–60
inflammatory bowel disease (IBD) 48, 84, 230
infliximab 84, 568–75
infrapatellar bursa injections 113
infrapatellar bursitis 179
infraspinatus 138
inherited muscular dystrophies 285
injection therapy 105–16
intermetatarsal bursitis 194
interossei 154
interphalangeal joints 187
interpretative styles 5–6
intersection syndrome 159
interstitial lung disease (ILD) 55, 56, 62, 283–4
interventional procedures
  CT 31
  ultrasound 27–8
intervertebral discs 119
  discitis 126, 133, 454–5
  herniation 124–5, 131–2
intestinal bypass surgery 83
intoeing 10

intussusception 83, 88
investigations 23–45
iridocyclitis 49
iritis 49
ischaemic necrosis 168–9, 381, 433
ischaemic pain 19
ischiogluteal bursitis 168
Ixodes ricinus 466

J

Jaccoud's arthropathy 244
joint fluid 16
joint space 25
joints
  aspiration 16, 106–7
  hot swollen 446–7
  hypermobile 442–3
  malalignment 25
jumper's knee 178
juvenile dermatomyositis (JDM) 298–300
juvenile idiopathic arthritis (JIA) 351–7
  eye problems 48, 52, 53
  heart disease 66
  oligoarticular (oligo-JIA) 352, 358
  rheumatoid factor (RF) negative polyarticular 352, 359
  rheumatoid factor (RF) positive polyarticular 352, 360
  systemic onset 352, 362–3
juvenile idiopathic inflammatory myopathies (JIIMs) 298
juvenile psoriatic arthritis 352, 364
juvenile spondyloarthropathy 232–4

K

Kawasaki disease 66, 82, 344–5
keratoconjunctivitis sicca 52, 257
kidney disease 74–81
Kienböcks disease 159–60
knee
  alignment 175
  anatomy 174–6
  differential diagnosis of pain 180
  injections 113
  menisci 175, 180
  osteoarthritis 372
  regional musculoskeletal conditions 178–83
  symmetry of movement 8
Kussmaul's sign 68
kyphoplasty 402
kyphosis 62

L

L-tryptophan 520
laboratory investigations 17, 22
labral tears 169
Lachman's test 181
language barrier 6
large intestine 82, 83, 84, 85, 86, 88
large plaque psoriasis 101
laryngeal destruction 62
lateral collateral ligament 174, 180–1
lateral epicondylitis 110, 148–9
lateral femoral cutaneous nerve entrapment 170
lateral pre-malleolar bursitis 191
latissimus dorsi 137, 138
'Ledderhose' disease 194
leflunomide 84, 540–3
Legg–Calvé–Perthes disease (LCPD) 433
leprosy 473–4
levator scapulae 138
Libman–Sacks endocarditis 67, 276
lidocaine
  injections 107
  patches 481
limited cutaneous systemic sclerosis 264, 271
limited systemic sclerosis 264
limping 9
linear morphea 99

lipid liquid crystals 42
lipid metabolism disorders 523
lipoatrophic panniculitis 515
lipogranulomatosis subcutanea 515
lipomas 27
Lisfranc joint 187
Lister's tubercle 152
liver 82, 83, 84, 85, 86, 88
lobular panniculitis 515
local anaesthetic injections 106, 107
localized scleroderma 99–100
Löfgren's syndrome 512, 513, 514
loiasis 477
long bone osteomyelitis 454
long head of biceps, tendon rupture 143
longus capitus 120
longus colli 120
low back pain 130
lower leg
  anatomy 184
  pain 188
  regional musculoskeletal conditions 188–9
lucencies 25
Lulworth Cove erosions 16
lumbar spine 119, 122, 130–4
lumbricals 154
lung function tests 58, 59, 60
lung parenchyma 54, 55, 56, 58, 59, 62
lupus erythematosus tumidus 98
lupus nephritis 244, 249, 251
  pregnancy 366
lupus panniculitis 98
lupus pernio 100
lupus profundus 98, 514–15
Lyme disease 15, 19, 466–7
lymphadenopathy 57
lymphocytic interstitial pneumonia (LIP) 56
lymphoma 57, 63, 257–8

M

maculopathy 49, 50
maduromycetoma 476
magnetic resonance imaging (MRI) 16, 34–5
malabsorption 83, 87–8
malalignment 25
malignancy, investigations 22
manual muscle testing (MMT) 288
Marfanoid habitus 438–9
Marfanoid hypermobility syndrome 438
Marfan's syndrome 82, 438–9
McArdle's disease 522
McMurray's test 180
mechanical neck pain 124
medial collateral ligament 174, 180–1
  injections 113
medial epicondylitis 110, 149
median nerve 155
  entrapment 150–1, 160–1
megacolon 82, 83
megaesophagus 82, 87
MELAS 524
melorheostosis 434–5
meningitis, bacterial 95
menisci 175, 180
meralgia paraesthetica 170
MERRF 524
mesenteric arterial rupture 83
mesenteric ischaemia 88
metabolic myopathies 285, 524–5
metacarpophalangeal joint (MCPJ) 152
metatarsal stress fracture 194
metatarsophalangeal joints (MTPJ) 187
  synovitis 194
methotrexate 84, 532–6
methylprednisolone injections 107
microscopic polyangiitis (MPA) 93, 328–9, 330–1
midtarsal joint injections 114
Milwaukee shoulder 392
mitochondrial encephalomyopathy with lactic acidosis and stroke-like episodes (MELAS) 524
mitochondrial myopathies 522–3

mitral regurgitation 69
mixed connective tissue disease (MCTD) 307, 309
mixed panniculitis 515
monosodium urate (MSU) crystals 42, 384
morphea 99–100
Morton's neuroma 194
motor conduction velocity (MCV) 44
mouth 82, 83, 85, 86, 87
mouth ulcers 16, 83–4, 87
movement
  active/passive 9
  symmetrical 8–9
moya-moya 278
Muckle–Wells syndrome (MWS) 101, 504
mucocutaneous lymph node syndrome 344
mucosal telangectasiae 83, 88
mucosal ulceration 83, 87
mucous cyst 158
Mueller–Weiss syndrome 194
multiple musculoskeletal symptoms 3
mumps 469
muscle
  biopsy 22
  infarction 494
myalgia 19
mycetoma 476
mycobacterial infection 472–4
mycophenolate mofetil 84, 556–7
myelopathy 11–12
myocardial disease 66–7, 68, 69, 70
myocarditis 70, 71
myoclonic epilepsy with ragged red fibres (MERRF) 524
myopathies 19
  drug-induced 20, 292–3
  gait pattern 9
  neurophysiology 45
myophosphorylase deficiency 522
myositis 61, 460–1
myositis ossificans 435

N

nails 20
  psoriasis 101–2
navicular bone, accessory 194
neck, mechanical pain 124
needle electromyography (EMG) 44–5
Neisseria gonorrhoeae 452–3
neonatal cutaneous lupus 98
neonatal lupus 66, 67, 98
neonatal onset multi-system inflammatory disease (NOMID)/chronic infantile neurological cutaneous and articular syndrome (CINCA) 504
nephritic syndromes 74–6, 244
nephrogenic fibrosing dermopathy 100
nephrotic syndromes 76–8, 244
nerve conduction studies 44, 92
nerve entrapment 150–1, 160–1, 170–1, 189, 191
nerve roots 120, 121
nervous system 20, 90–7
neuroborreliosis 466, 467
neurogenic pain 12
neurological examination 11–12
neurological symptoms 20
neuropathic arthropathy 380–1
neuropathic CPPD disease 388
neuropathic pain 90–1, 96
neurophysiology 44–5
neurorehabilitation 96
neutrophilic dermatoses 101
non-septic bursitis 458
non-specific interstitial pneumonia (NSIP) 56
non-steroidal anti-inflammatory drugs (NSAIDs) 84, 87, 480–1
normality 8
nuclear medicine 36–7
nutrition
  osteomalacia and rickets 422, 423
  post-menopausal osteoporosis 397–8

O

obliterative bronchiolitis 55, 56, 62
observation 9
obstruction 83
ochronosis 516
Ockelbo virus 468
octacalcium phosphate crystals 392
ocular coherence tomography (OCT) 51
oedema 21
oesophageal candidiasis 82, 87
oesophageal dysmotility 82, 87
oesophageal perforation 82
oesophageal varices 82, 87
oesophagus 82, 84, 85, 86, 87
oestrogen, post-menopausal osteoporosis 398
olecranon bursa injections 110
olecranon bursitis 149
olecranon impingement syndrome 150
oligoarticular juvenile idiopathic arthritis (oligo-JIA) 352, 358
oligoarticular pains 14–17
onchocerciasis 477
oncogenic hypophosphataemic osteomalacia 425
open fracture osteomyelitis 454
opioids 481
optic disc 50
optic neuropathy 48
oral fissures 87
oral ulcers 16, 83–4, 87
organizing pneumonia (OP) 56
os trigonum 187
Osgood–Schlatter's syndrome (OSS) 180
osteitis fibrosa (OF) 415
osteitis pubis 170
osteoarthritis 14, 372–8
  elbow 149–50
  erosive 375, 376
  hand 158, 372, 374
  hip 372
  knee 372
  shoulder 142–3
osteoarthritis-related disorders 380–1
osteochondral lesion of talus (OLT) 191
osteochondritis 433
osteochondritis dissecans 150, 191
osteochondroma 529
osteochondroses 433
osteodystrophia deformans 418–20
osteodystrophy 488
osteogenesis imperfecta 428–30
osteoid osteoma 528
osteoma 528
osteomalacia 422–5
osteomyelitis 454–6, 472
osteonecrosis 168–9, 381, 433
osteopaenia 24
osteopetrosis 434
osteophytes 25
osteoporosis
  children 412–13
  glucocorticoid-induced (GIO) 408–10
  men 406–7
  post-menopausal 396–405
osteosarcoma 528–9
out toeing 10
overlap syndromes 291, 308, 309
oxidation enzyme defects 523

P

pachydermal periostitis 432
paediatrics, see children
Paget's disease of the bone 418–20
pain
  anterior knee 180
  bone 2, 19
  children 2, 6–7
  chronic 479–90
  descriptors 2
  elbow 148
  facial 90, 95
  hand 158
  hip 168
  history taking 2
  ischaemic 19
  ladder 481
  low back 130
  lower leg 188
  neck 124
  neurogenic 12
  neuropathic 90–1, 96
  oligoarticular 14–17
  referred 2, 9
  shoulder 140
  treatment 480–2
  widespread 18–22
  wrist 158
painful articular syndrome 470
palindromic rheumatism 199
palmaris longus 147, 154
palmoplantar pustulosis 102
pANCA 41
pancreas 82, 83, 84, 85, 86, 88
pancreatic arthritis syndrome 83
pancreatic panniculitis 514
pancreatitis 83, 84–5, 88
panniculitis 472, 514–15
panuveitis 49
papular mucinosis 99
papular sarcoid 101
paracetamol 480–1
paracoccidioidomycosis 476
parasites 461, 476
Parkinson's disease 11
parvovirus B19 19, 468
passive movement 9
patellar tendinosis 178
patellofemoral instability 178
patellofemoral joint 174
patterns
  of disease 14–17
  of symptoms 3, 6–7
pectoralis major 137, 138
pectoralis minor 138
pectus excavatum 55, 62
pelvis
  anatomy 164–6
  regional musculoskeletal conditions 168–72
penicillamine 550–1
penicilliosis 476
PEO 524
perforation 83
pericardial disease 66, 67, 68, 69, 70
perimetry 92
perineal ulcers 88
periosteal reaction 25
periostitis 189
peripheral limb pain 12
peripheral ulcerative keratitis 49
peroneal tendon injections 114
peroneal tendonitis 191
pharynx 82, 83
phosphofructokinase deficiency 522–3
piano key sign 199
pigmented villonodular synovitis (PVNS) 527
pinna inflammation 16
plain radiographs 24–5
plantar fascia 187
plantar fasciitis (PF) 115, 192–3
plantar fibromatosis 194
plantar plate disruption 194
plaque morphea 99
pleura 54, 55–6, 57–8, 61
pleural aspirate 58
pleural effusions 55–6, 61
pleuritis 55–6
plicae 179
pneumonia 55, 56
pneumonitis, drug-induced 56, 62
podagra 384
POEMS syndrome 100
Pogosta virus 468
polyarteritis nodosa (PAN) 48, 66, 82, 93, 332–3

polymyalgia rheumatica 320–1
polymyositis (PM) 282–9, 291
  chest disease 54, 283–4
  eye problems 48
  gastrointestinal disease 82
  heart disease 66
  HIV 470
  nervous system 93, 95
Pompe's disease 523
Poncet's disease 472
popliteal cyst 181–2, 188
porphyria cutanea tarda 100
portal hypertension 82
portal vein thrombosis 82
positron emission tomography (PET) 37
post-injection flare 106
post-Lyme syndrome 467
post-menopausal osteoporosis 396–405
post-steroid panniculitis 515
post-streptococcal arthritis 19, 226
posterior cruciate ligament 174–5, 181
posterior interosseous nerve 147
posterior tibial tendon dysfunction 191
posterior uveitis 49, 51
posture 9
Pott's disease of spine 472
pregnancy 365–9
  antiphospholipid syndrome 274, 276, 279, 367
  Behçet's disease 368
  Churg–Strauss syndrome 368
  drug treatment during 368–9
  rheumatoid arthritis 366
  Sjögren's syndrome 367
  spondyloarthropathy 367
  systemic lupus erythematosus 67, 250, 366–7
  systemic sclerosis 367
  Takayasu arteritis 3770
  vasculitides 367–8
  Wegener's granulomatosis 368
Preisser's disease 160
prepatellar bursitis 178–9
primary angiitis of the CNS (PACNS) 93
primary biliary cirrhosis 83, 84, 88
primary central nervous system vasculitis (PCNSV) 336–7
primary hyperparathyroidism 414–16
procaine injections 107
progressive diaphyseal dysplasia (PDD) 434
progressive external ophthalmoplegia (PEO) 524
pronator teres 147
pronator teres syndrome 150–1
prosthetic joint infection 450
protozoa 477
proximal interphalangeal joint (PIPJ) 152
pseudogout 388, 389
pseudo-obstruction 83, 88
pseudo-osteoarthritis 388
pseudovitamin D deficiency rickets 424
psoas abscess 460
psoas muscles 120
psoriasis vulgaris 101–3
psoriatic arthritis 220–5
  eye problems 48
  HIV 470
  juvenile 352, 364
psoriatic onycho pachydermo periostitis (POPP) 195
psychiatric problems 96
psychological therapies 96, 482
psychosocial history 20
pulmonary arterial aneurysm 63
pulmonary arterial hypertension (PAH) 55, 57, 63, 66, 69
pulmonary embolism 63
pulmonary haemorrhage 56, 62–3
pulmonary vasculature and lymphatics 54, 55, 57, 58, 60, 63
pulse oximetry 61
pulsus alternans 68
pulsus paradoxus 68
'pump bumps' 192

purine metabolism disorders 523
pus removal 449
pycnodysostosis 434
pyoderma gangrenosum 101
pyomyositis 460–1

Q

Q angle 175
quantitative ultrasound 400–1
questionnaires 4

R

racial background 18
radial nerve compression 161
radial tunnel syndrome 150
radiculopathy 45
radiocarpal joint 152
radiographs 16, 24–5
  chest 58, 60
radionuclide imaging 36–7
rashes 16, 20–1
Raynaud's phenomenon (RP) 99, 246, 266, 267, 271
reactive arthritis 15, 48, 66, 226–9, 472
recombinant human parathyroid hormone (rhPTH) 404
rectus abdominis injury 171
rectus femoris injury 171
referred pain 2, 9
reflex sympathetic dystrophy (RSD) 488
Reiter's syndrome 82, 226
relapsing polychondritis (RP) 48, 54, 66, 93, 95, 346–7
relaxation 481
renal bone disease (osteodystrophy) 426–7
renal disease 74–81
renal failure, acute 79–80
renal tubular acidosis 258
reporting styles 5
residual volume 59
respiratory muscle function tests 58
respiratory symptoms 20
restless legs syndrome 96
reticent patients 5
retina 48
retinaculae 184–5
retinal vasculitis 49, 52
retinitis 49
retinovascular disease 49, 50–1, 52
retrocalcaneal bursitis 192
rheumatic fever 19, 66, 67, 462–3
rheumatoid arthritis (disease) 14, 197–208
  chest disease 54, 62, 200
  eye problems 48, 200
  gastrointestinal disease 82
  heart disease 66, 67, 71, 200
  human parvovirus B19 468
  nervous system 92, 93, 95, 200
  osteomyelitis 455
  pregnancy 366
  rheumatoid nodules 56, 98, 199
  shoulder 143
  skin disease 98
  spine 125–6
  treatment 203–5
rheumatoid cutaneous vasculitis 98
rheumatoid factor 21, 40
rheumatoid factor (RF) negative polyarticular juvenile idiopathic arthritis 352, 359
rheumatoid factor (RF) positive polyarticular juvenile idiopathic arthritis 352, 360
rheumatoid nodules 56, 98, 199
rheumatology questionnaire tools 4
rhomboid minor/major 138
rhupus 308
rickets 422–5
right heart catheterization 60, 61
rituximab 84, 568–75
rocker bottom foot 494
Rodnan skin score 271
Roos manoeuvre 161

Ross River virus 468
rotator cuff 137
  disease 140–1
  injections 109
Rothmann–Makai syndrome 515
Rowell syndrome 98
RS3PE syndrome 21
rubella 19, 469

S

sacral epidural 115
sacroiliac joint 122
sacroiliac pain 133
SAPHO 16, 236–7
sarcoidosis 16, 512–13
  eye problems 48, 49
  heart disease 66
  lung sarcoid 54, 56–7, 62
  nervous system 93, 95
  skin disease 100–1
scalene muscles 120
scalp psoriasis 101
scaphoid non-union and advanced collapse (SNAC) 158
scapho-lunate advanced collapse (SLAC) 158
scapular 136
scar sarcoid 101
Schirmer's test 51, 257
schistosomiasis 477
Schnitzler syndrome 497
Schueurmann's disease 128
Schulman syndrome 310
scleritis 48, 49, 52
scleroderma, localized 99–100
sclerodermal renal crisis 267
sclerodermatomyositis 308
scleromyositis 308
scleromyxoedma 99
sclerosing bone disorders 434–5
sclerosis 25
sclerosteosis 434
scoliosis 55, 62, 133–4
seborrhoeic psoriasis 101
secondary gain 5
secondary metabolic myopathy 522
selective oestrogen receptor modulators (SERMs) 403
sensory action potentials (SAP) 44
septal panniculitis 514
septic arthritis 14, 15, 16, 448–51
septic bursitis 149, 458–9
septic joints 446–7
serial peak expiratory flow rate (PEFR) 59
serology 38–41
serratus anterior 138
sesamoiditis 194
sexual history 20
shoulder
  anatomy 136–9
  differential diagnosis of pain 140
  frozen 141–2
  instability 142
  Milwaukee 392
  nerve disorders 143–4
  osteoarthritis 142–3
  rheumatoid 143
  symmetry of movement 8
shoulder girdle 138, 140–4
  injections 108–9
'shrinking lung' syndrome 55, 61
sickle cell disease 508–9
sinus tachycardia 71
sinus tarsi syndrome 191
Sjögren's syndrome (SS) 254–62
  chest disease 54
  eye problems 48, 257
  gastrointestinal disease 82
  heart disease 66
  nervous system 93, 95
  pregnancy 367
  skin disease 100, 257
skin 16, 20–1, 85, 98–103

SLAC 158
sleep studies 61
slit lamp examination 51
small bowel ischaemia/infarction 83
small intestine 82, 83, 84, 85, 86, 87–8
SNAC 158
Sneddon's syndrome 276, 278
sniff test 58
social history 15
sodium aurothimalate 546–8
soft tissue infection 458–61
soft tissue swelling
  hand and wrist 162
  plain radiographs 24
  ultrasound 27
spinal accessory nerve injury 144
spinal cerebellar tracts 121
spinal cord 120–2
spinal stenosis 132–3
spinal tracts 120–1
spine 118–34
  anatomy 118–22
  cervical 119, 122, 124–7
  lumbar 119, 122, 130–4
  MRI 34, 35
  osteotomy 218
  rheumatoid arthritis 125–6
  thoracic 119, 122, 128–9
  see also intervertebral discs
spirometry 58, 59, 60
spondyloarthropathies (SpA) 14, 15, 209–37
  disease spectrum 210–13
  enteropathic 230–1
  juvenile 232–4
  pregnancy 367
spondylolisthesis 131
spondylolysis 131
spondylosis 372
  lumbar 130–1
  thoracic 128
sporotrichosis 476
sputum analysis 59
St Vitus' dance 462
Staphylococcus aureus 448
sternoclavicular joint 136
  injections 109
  osteoarthritis 142–3
steroid
  injections 106, 107
  post-steroid panniculitis 515
stiff skin syndrome 100
stiffness
  examination 11–12
  history taking 2
Still's disease, adult onset (AOSD) 66, 496–7
stoma, defunctioning 88
stomach 82, 83, 84, 85, 86, 87
stress fractures 188, 194
stroke 95
strongyloides 477
strontium ranelate (SR) 404
student's elbow 149
subacromial bursa 139
subacromial space injections 109
subacute cutaneous lupus erythematosus (SACLE) 98, 244
subaxial subluxation 125
subclavius 138
subcutaneous calcaneal bursitis 192
subscapularis 138
subtalar joint injections 114
sulfasalazine 84, 538–9
supinator 147
suppurative tenosynovitis 459–60
suprascapular nerve
  block 116
  injury 144
supraspinatus 138
Sweet's syndrome 101
Sydenham's chorea 462
symmetry 8–9

symptoms
  emphasis 5
  multiple 3
  non–musculoskeletal 4–5
  patterns 3, 6–7
synovial biopsy 17
synovial chondromatosis 16
synovial fluid analysis 42–3
synovial osteochondromatosis 526
synovial plica syndrome 179
synovitis 14
  MTPJ 194
  ultrasound 26
  villonodular 527
systemic lupus erythematosus (SLE) 240–52
  chest disease 54, 61, 62, 245
  drug-related 20, 241, 248–9
  eye problems 48, 49
  gastrointestinal disease 82, 245
  heart disease 66, 67, 71, 244, 245, 250, 251
  kidney disease 74, 244, 249, 251
  nervous system 92, 93, 95, 244–5, 249
  pregnancy 67, 250, 366–7
systemic onset juvenile idiopathic arthritis 352, 362–3
systemic sclerosis (SSc) 264–72
  chest disease 54, 57, 61, 62, 267
  eye problems 48
  astrointestinal disease 82, 266–7
  heart disease 66, 67, 267
  nervous system 93, 95
  pregnancy 367
  sclerodermal renal crisis 267
  sine scleroderma 264
  skin disease 99–100, 266

T

T-spot assay 58–9
Taenia solium 461
Takayasu arteritis 66, 93, 95, 322–3, 368
talus, osteochondral lesion 191
tarsal tunnel syndrome 191
Tarui's disease 522–3
technetium scan 36–7
temporal artery biopsy 318
temporomandibular joint (TMJ) arthritis 87
tendinitis
  bicipital 143, 149
  pelvis 171
  peroneal 191
  rotator cuff 141
  triceps 149
tendon tears 26
tennis elbow, *see* lateral epicondylitis
tenosynovitis
  hand and wrist 158–9
  infectious/suppurative 459–60
  ultrasound 26–7
TENS 481
teres major/minor 138
tetrahydrocannabinol 481
Thessaly test 180
thiopurine methyltransferase (TPMT)
  genotype 248

thoracic outlet syndrome 161–2
thoracic spine 119, 122, 128–9
thromboangiitis obliterans (TAO) 348–9
thromboembolic disease 57
thumb carpometacarpal joint 152
  injections 111
tibia
  periostitis 189
  stress fracture 188
tibiofemoral joint 174
tibiofibular joints 184
Tinnel's test 12
TNF-receptor-associated periodic syndrome (TRAPS) 101, 503, 504
tocilizumab 568–75
tonometry 51
tophi 16, 384, 385
topical rubs 481
torticollis 126–7
total lung capacity 58, 59
toxic myopathies 292–3
toxic oil syndrome 520–1
Toxoplasma gondii 19
tracheomalacia 55, 62
transbronchial biopsy 60
transcutaneous electrical nerve stimulation (TENS) 481
trapezius 138
TRAPS 101, 503, 504
traumatic bursitis 149
Trendelenberg gait 9
triamcinolone injections 107
triangular fibrocartilage (TFCC) 152
tricalcium phosphate crystals 392
triceps 146
trichinosis 461, 477
trigger finger 112, 159
trochanteric bursitis 112, 168
tryptophan 520
tuberculosis 472–3
tubulointerstitial nephritis (TIN) 78–9
tumours
  bone 528–9
  cervical spine 126
  osteomalacia induction 425

U

ulcerative colitis 83
ulnar nerve 147, 155–6
  compression 161
ultrasound 16, 26–8
undifferentiated arthritis 352
undifferentiated (autoimmune) connective tissue disease (UAICTD/UCTD) 306, 309
urogenital reactive arthritis 226
usual interstitial pneumonia (UIP) 56
uveitis 15, 48, 49, 51

V

valvular disease 66, 67, 68, 70, 71
Van Buchem disease 434
vascular malformations 27

vasculitis 313–49
  chest disease 54
  classification 314, 315
  clinical features 314–15
  cutaneous 100
  HIV 470
  liver 84
  pregnancy 367–8
  primary central nervous system (PCNSV) 336–7
  retinal 49, 52
  rheumatoid cutaneous 98
  small intestine 83, 88
ventilation-perfusion (V/Q) scan 36–7, 60
verbose patients 5
vertebra 118–19
  fractures 397, 399
  osteomyelitis 454–5
vertebroplasty 402
villonodular synovitis 527
viral arthritis 468–71
viral myocarditis 71
viral myositis 460
visual perimetry 92
vitamin D 398, 422, 423

W

Wadsworth test 161
walking 166
Weber–Christian disease 514
Wegener's granulomatosis (WG) 324–5
  eye problems 48
  gastrointestinal disease 82
  heart disease 66
  nervous system 93, 94
  pregnancy 368
  treatment 330–1
whiplash 125
Whipple's disease 82, 83, 84
WHO pain ladder 481
widespread pain 18–22
Wilson's disease 83, 89
WOMAC 4
wrist
  anatomy 152–6
  fractures 397
  ganglion 162
  injections 110–12
  main causes of pain 158
  regional musculoskeletal conditions 158–62
  soft tissue lesions 162
Wuchereria bancrofti 476

X

X-linked hypophosphataemia (XLH) 424
xerostomia 85, 87, 257

Printed and bound by CPI Group (UK) Ltd, Croydon, CR0 4YY